Contents in Brief

ESSENTIALS of Maternity, Newborn, AND Women's Health Nursing

FOURTH EDITION

ESSENTIALS of
Maternity, Newborn,
AND Women's
Health Nursing

FOURTH EDITION

Susan Scott Ricci, ARNP, MSN, M.Ed., CNE

Nursing Faculty
University of Central Florida
Orlando, Florida
Former Nursing Program Director and Faculty
Lake Sumter State College
Leesburg, Florida

. Wolters Kluwer

Philadelphia • Baltimore • New York • London
Buenos Aires • Hong Kong • Sydney • Tokyo

Acquisitions Editor: Natasha McIntyre
Product Development Editor: Annette Ferran
Editorial Assistant: Dan Reilly
Design Coordinator: Terry Mallon
Illustration Coordinator: Jennifer Clements
Production Project Manager: Priscilla Crater
Manufacturing Coordinator: Karin Duffield
Prepress Vendor: Aptara, Inc.

4th Edition

9 8 7 6 5 4 3

Printed in China

Library of Congress Cataloging-in-Publication Data

Names: Ricci, Susan Scott, author.
Title: Essentials of maternity, newborn & women's health nursing / Susan
   Scott Ricci.
Other titles: Essentials of maternity, newborn, and women's health nursing
Description: Fourth edition. | Philadelphia : Wolters Kluwer, [2017] |
   Includes bibliographical references and index.
Identifiers: LCCN 2016021183 | ISBN 9781451193992
Subjects: | MESH: Maternal-Child Nursing | Obstetric Nursing | Pregnancy
   Complications–nursing
Classification: LCC RG951 | NLM WY 157.3 | DDC 618.2/0231–dc23
LC record available at https://lccn.loc.gov/2016021183

LWW.com

CCS0418

This book is lovingly dedicated to my husband Glenn, for his unfailing patience, encouragement,—and whose support and sense of humor make anything possible. And also to my children, Brian and Jennifer, and my grandchildren—Alyssa, Leyton, Peyton, Wyatt, Michael, Rylan, and Brody—who continue to inspire me throughout my life. You make it all worthwhile.

Susan Scott Ricci

About the Author

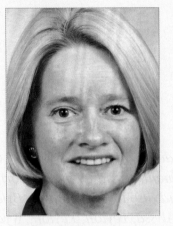

Susan Scott Ricci earned a diploma in nursing from the Washington Hospital Center School of Nursing, with a BSN and MSN, from Catholic University of America located in Washington, D.C., a M.Ed. in Counseling from the University of Southern Mississippi. She is licensed as a Women's Health Nurse Practitioner (ARNP) from the University of Florida. She recently acquired her national certification as a Certified Nurse Educator (CNE). She has worked in numerous women's health care settings including labor and birth, postpartum, prenatal, and family planning ambulatory care clinics. Susan is a women's health care nurse practitioner, who has spent 30+ years in practice and in nursing education teaching in LPN, ADN, and BSN programs. She is involved in several professional nursing organizations and holds memberships in Sigma Theta Tau International Honor Society of Nursing, National Association of OB/GYN Nurses, Who's Who in Professional Nursing, American Nurses Association, and the Florida Council of Maternal–Child Nurses.

With Susan Scott Ricci's wealth of practical and educational experience, it is essential to concentrate on evidence-based nursing practice and reduce the amount of "nice to know" information that is presented to students. As an educator, she recognized the tendency for nursing educators to want to "cover the world" when teaching, rather than focusing on the facts that students need to know to practice nursing safely. With this mission in mind, Susan has directed her energy to the *birth* of these essential facts in this textbook.

She recognizes that instructional time is shrinking as the world of health care is expanding exponentially. Therefore, with the valuable instructional time allotted, she has recognized the urgent need to present pertinent facts as concisely as possible to promote application of knowledge within nursing practice.

Reviewers

Vicki Aaberg, PhD, RN
Nursing Instructor
Seattle Pacific University
Seattle, Washington

Robin Adams-Weber, DNP, RN, WHNPBC
Associate Professor of Nursing
Women's Health Nurse Practitioner
Malone University
Canton, Ohio

Nancy Ahern, PhD, RN
Associate Professor of Nursing
California State University
Fullerton, California

Louise Aurilio, PhD, RN-BC, NE-BC
Associate Professor
Youngstown State University
Youngstown, Ohio

Kathleen Beebe, PhD, RN
Associate Professor
Dominican University of California
San Francisco, California

Tammy Bryant, MSN, RN
Program Director/Nursing Instructor
Southern Regional Technical College
Thomasville, Georgia

Stephanie Butkus
Associate Professor
Kettering College of Medical Arts
Dayton, Ohio

Amanda Campbell, PhD, RN
Associate Professor
Tyler Junior College
Tyler, Texas

Yasmin Cavenagh, MSN, MPH, RN
Instructor
Resurrection University
Chicago, Illinois

Tracy Colburn, MSN, BSN, RN, CEFM
Assistant Professor
Lewis and Clark Community College
Godfrey, Illinois

Denise Condra, MSN, RN, FNP-C
Associate Professor
Mount San Antonio College
Walnut, California

Patricia Davidson, MSN, RN
Clinical Associate Professor
University of Texas Health Science Center
San Antonio, Texas

Tamara Dennis, PhD, RNC
Associate Professor of Nursing
Abraham Baldwin Agricultural College
Tifton, Georgia

Barbara Derwinski-Robinson, MSN-RNC-WH-BC
Associate Professor
Montana State University
Billings, Montana

Susan Dougherty, DNO, MS, RNC, WHNP
Assistant Professor
Augusta University
Augusta, Georgia

Judith Drumm, RN, DNSc
Associate Professor
Palm Beach Atlantic University
West Palm Beach, Florida

Brooke Flinders, MSN, RN, CNM
Assistant Professor
Miami University Hamilton
Miami, Florida

Helen Gordon, MS, RN, CNM
Assistant Professor
Duke University
Durham, North Carolina

Susan Hall, MSN, RNC
Nursing Instructor
Winston-Salem State University
Winston-Salem, North Carolina

Elva Hammarstrand, RN, BScN, MN
Nursing Instructor
Red Deer College
Winnipeg, Manitoba, Canada

Marie Hanna, RN, MS, WHNP-C
Professor of Nursing
Suffolk County Community College
Selden, New York

Christina Harkins, MSN, RN
Assistant Professor
Lasalle University
Philadelphia, Pennsylvania

Sally Hartman, RNC, MSN, IBCLC, FACCE
Clinical Assistant Professor
Indiana Purdue University
Fort Wayne, Indiana

Mary Jane Hopkins, ARNP, BSN, MSN
Nursing Instructor
Indian River Community College
Fort Pierce, Florida

Carmen Kiraly, RN, MS, C-WHNP
Assistant Professor
Suffolk County Community College
Brentwood, New York

Joan Kuhnly, MS, RN, IBCLC
Nursing Instructor
University of Connecticut
Storrs, Connecticut

Christine Kuoni, MSN
Assistant Professor
San Antonio College
San Antonio, Texas

Diwana Lowe, MSN, RNC-OB
Associate Professor - Retired
Georgia Perimeter College
Georgia State University
Atlanta, Georgia

Maria Marconi, RN, MS
Assistant Professor
University of Rochester
Rochester, New York

Lucy Martinez-Schallmoser, PhD, RNC
Assistant Professor
Loyola University
Chicago, Illinois

Tammy McInerney, DNP, RN, NNPBC, CPNP
Assistant Professor
Delta College
University Center, Michigan

Anne Mitchell, PhD, RN, CNM
Assistant Professor
Oakland University
Rochester, Michigan

Anna Morris, MSN, RN
Assistant Professor
Northwestern State University
Natchitoches, Louisiana

Gretchen A. Nelson, BSN, MN, RNFA, FNP-c
Nursing Faculty
Fresno City College
Fresno, California

Valerie O'Dell, DNP, RN, CNE
Associate Professor/MSN Program Director
Youngstown State University
Youngstown, Ohio

Ann Marie Paraszczuk, EdD, MS, RNC
Professor
Molloy College
Rockville Center, New York

Cynthia Payne, BSN, MS, NP-BC, CNM
Assistant Professor
Georgia State at Perimeter College
Atlanta, Georgia

Audrey Perry, DNP, CNM, RN
Faculty Nurse Midwife
Reading Health School of Health Sciences
West Reading, Pennsylvania

Deborah A. Raines, PhD, EdS, RN, ANEF
Associate Professor
University at Buffalo: The State University of New York
Buffalo, New York

Anne Marie Rameika, MSN, FNP
Associate Professor
Community College of Rhode Island
Newport, Rhode Island

Frances Reynolds, MSN, RN
Assistant Professor of Nursing
Howard Community College
Columbia, Maryland

Margaret Riden, RN, MSN
Program Director
Blue Ridge Community and Technical College
Martinsburg, West Virginia

Aissa Yolanda Scott, MS, ARNP, CNM
Nurse Educator
Saint Petersburg College
Pinellas Park, Florida

Carol Siegmund, MSN, RN
Assistant Professor of Nursing
Leigh Carbon Community College
Schnecksville, Pennsylvania

Joyce Sizemore, MSN, RN
Professor of Nursing
Collin College
McKinney, Texas

Lauren Stehling, MSN/Ed, APRN, FNP-BC
Family Nurse Practitioner/Professional Nursing Faculty
Baptist Health System School of Health Professions
San Antonio, Texas

Barbara Stoner, RN, MSN
Nursing Faculty
Arapahoe Community College
Littleton, Colorado

Diane Thulier, PhD, RN
Assistant Professor
University of Rhode Island
Kingston, Rhode Island

Lois Tschetter, EdD, RN, IBCLC, CNE
Associate Professor
South Dakota State University
Brookings, South Dakota

Becky Weatherly, MSN, RN
Assistant Professor
Touro University
Henderson, Nevada

Deborah Whittaker, EdD, RN, RNC-MNN
Assistant Professor of Clinical Nursing
DeSales University
Center Valley, Pennsylvania

Angela Watkins, MSN, RN
Program Director
Calhoun Community College
Decatur, Alabama

Carol Wiggs, PhD, RN, CNM
Associate Professor
University of Texas Medical Branch
Galveston, Texas

Barbara Wilford, MSN, MBA, RN
Assistant Professor
Lorain County Community College
Elyria, Ohio

Barbara Wilson, PhD, RNC
Associate Professor
Arizona State University
Tempe, Arizona

Beth Youngblood, MSN, BSN
Associate Professor
Belmont University
Nashville, Tennessee

Preface

This textbook is designed as a practical approach to understanding the health of women in a maternity context and the health of their newborns. Women in our society are becoming empowered to make informed and responsible choices regarding their health and that of their newborns, but to do so they need the encouragement and support of nurses who care for them. This textbook focuses on the reproductive issues of women throughout the lifespan and arms the student or practicing nurse with essential information to care for women and their families and to assist them to make the right choices safely, intelligently, and with confidence.

Since the health care focus of women and their families has expanded well beyond our nation's borders, more cultural and global aspects of maternity and women's health care have been added to this fourth edition. The United States is part of the international community, and as such nurses must understand and respect diverse cultures and their customs to truly play an important role as a global partner. Nurses care for a variety of women from many continents, thus they have to be armed with appropriate tools to meet their client's diverse needs. Also, more evidence-based research findings have been included in this fourth edition for nurses to validate their practice and interventions.

ORGANIZATION

Each chapter of this textbook reviews an important dimension of a woman's general health throughout her life cycle and addresses risk factors, lifestyle choices that influence her well-being, appropriate interventions, and nursing education topics to preserve her health and that of her newborn.

The text is divided into eight units.

Unit 1: Introduction to Maternity, Newborn, and Women's Nursing

Unit 1 helps build a foundation for the student beginning with the study of maternal–newborn and women's health nursing by exploring contemporary issues and trends and community-based nursing.

Unit 2: Women's Health Throughout the Life Span

Unit 2 introduces the student to selected women's health topics, including the structure and function of the reproductive system, common reproductive concerns, sexually transmitted infections, problems of the breast, and benign disorders and cancers of the female reproductive tract. This unit encourages students to assist women in maintaining their quality of life, reducing their risk of disease, and becoming active partners in their own health promotion activities and with their health care professional.

Unit 3: Pregnancy

Unit 3 addresses topics related to normal pregnancy, including fetal development, genetics, and maternal adaptation to pregnancy. Nursing management during normal pregnancy is presented in a separate chapter encouraging application of basic knowledge to nursing practice. This nursing care chapter covers maternal and fetal assessment throughout pregnancy, interventions to promote self-care and minimize common discomforts, and client education.

Unit 4: Labor and Birth

Unit 4 begins with a chapter on the normal labor and birth process, including maternal and fetal adaptations. This is followed by a chapter discussing the nurse's role during normal labor and birth, which includes maternal and fetal assessment, pharmacologic and nonpharmacologic comfort measures and pain management, and specific nursing interventions during each stage of labor and birth.

Unit 5: Postpartum Period

Unit 5 focuses on maternal adaptation during the normal postpartum period. Both physiologic and psychological aspects are explored. Paternal adaptation is also considered. This unit also focuses on related nursing management, including assessment of physical and emotional status, promoting comfort, assisting with elimination, counseling about sexuality and contraception, promoting nutrition, promoting family adaptation, and discharge planning.

Unit 6: The Newborn

Unit 6 covers physiologic and behavioral adaptations of the normal newborn. It also delves into nursing management of the normal newborn, including immediate assessment and specific interventions as well as ongoing assessment, physical examination, and specific interventions during the early newborn period.

Unit 7: Childbearing at Risk

Unit 7 shifts the focus to at-risk pregnancy, childbirth, and postpartum care. Pre-existing conditions of the woman, pregnancy-related complications, at-risk labor, emergencies associated with labor and birth, and medical conditions and complications affecting the postpartum woman are covered. Treatment and nursing management are presented for each medical condition. This organization allows the student to build on a solid foundation of normal material when studying the at-risk content.

Unit 8: The Newborn at Risk

Unit 8 continues to focus on at-risk content. Issues of the newborn with birth weight variations, gestational age variations, congenital conditions, and acquired disorders are explored. Treatment and nursing management are presented for each medical condition. This organization helps cement the student's understanding of the material.

RECURRING FEATURES

To provide the instructor and student with an exciting and user-friendly text, a number of recurring features have been developed.

Key Terms

A list of terms that are considered essential to the chapter's understanding is presented at the beginning of each chapter. Each key term appears in boldface, with the definition included in the text. Key terms may also be accessed on thePoint.

Learning Objectives

Learning objectives included at the beginning of each chapter guide the student in understanding what is important and why, allowing him or her to prioritize information for learning. These valuable learning tools also provide opportunities for self-testing or instructor evaluation of student knowledge and ability.

WOW

Each chapter opens with inspiring Words of Wisdom, which offer helpful, timely, or interesting thoughts. These WOW statements set the stage for each chapter and give the student valuable insight into nursing care of women and newborns.

Case Studies

Real-life scenarios present relevant maternity, newborn, and women's health information that is intended to perfect the student's caregiving skills. Questions about the scenario provide an opportunity for the student to critically evaluate the appropriate course of action.

Evidence-Based Practice

The consistent promotion of evidence-based practice is a key feature of the text. Throughout the chapters, pivotal questions addressed by current research have been incorporated into Evidence-Based Practice boxes, which cite studies relevant to the chapter content.

Healthy People 2020

Throughout the textbook, relevant *Healthy People 2020* objectives are outlined in box format. The nursing implications or guidance provided in the box serves as a road map for improving the health of women, mothers, and newborns.

Teaching Guidelines

An important tool for achieving health promotion and disease prevention is health education. Throughout the textbook, Teaching Guidelines raise awareness, provide timely and accurate information, and are designed to ensure the student's preparation for educating women about various issues.

Drug Guides

Drug guide tables summarize information about commonly used medications. The actions, indications, and significant nursing implications presented assist the student in providing optimum care to women and their newborns.

Common Laboratory and Diagnostic Tests

Common Laboratory and Diagnostic Test tables in many of the chapters provide the student with a general understanding of how a broad range of disorders is diagnosed. Rather than reading the information repeatedly throughout the narrative, the student is then able to refer to the table as needed.

Common Medical Treatments

Common Medical Treatment tables in many of the nursing management chapters provide the student with a broad awareness of how a common group of disorders is treated either medically or surgically. The tables serve as a reference point for common medical treatments.

Nursing Care Plans

Nursing Care Plans provide concrete examples of each step of the nursing process and are provided in numerous chapters.[1] Found within the nursing process overview section of the chapter, the Nursing Care Plans summarize issue- or system-related content and outline a guide for delivering care.

Comparison Charts

These charts compare two or more disorders or other easily confused concepts. They serve to provide an explanation that clarifies the concepts for the student.

Nursing Procedures

Step-by-step Nursing Procedures are presented in a clear, concise format to facilitate competent performance of relevant procedures as well as to clarify any variations when appropriate.

Icons

Watch and Learn

A special icon throughout the book directs students to free video clips located on thePoint that highlight growth and development, communicating with children, and providing nursing care to the child in the hospital.

Concepts in Action Animations

These unique animations, also located on thePoint, bring physiologic and pathophysiologic concepts to life and enhance student comprehension.

Consider This!

In every chapter, the student is asked to *Consider This!* These first-person narratives engage the student in real-life scenarios experienced by their patients. The personal accounts evoke empathy and help the student to perfect caregiving skills. Each box ends with an opportunity for further contemplation, encouraging the student to think critically about the scenario.

Take Note!

The *Take Note!* feature draws the student's attention to points of critical emphasis throughout the chapter. This feature is often used to stress life-threatening or otherwise vitally important information.

Tables, Boxes, Illustrations, and Photographs

Abundant tables and boxes summarize key content throughout the book. Additionally, beautiful illustrations and photographs help the student to visualize the content. These features allow the student to quickly and easily access information.

Key Concepts

At the end of each chapter, Key Concepts provide a quick review of essential chapter elements. These bulleted lists help the student focus on the important aspects of the chapter.

References and Websites

References that were used in the development of the text are provided at the end of each chapter. The websites are located on thePoint. These listings enable the student to further explore topics of interest. Many online websites are provided as a means for the student to electronically explore relevant content material. These resources can be shared with women, children, and their families to enhance patient education and support.

Chapter Worksheets

Chapter worksheets at the end of each chapter assist the student in reviewing essential concepts. Chapter worksheets include:

- **Multiple-Choice Questions**—These review questions are written to test the student's ability to apply chapter material. Questions cover maternal–newborn and women's health content that the student might encounter on the national licensing exam (NCLEX).
- **Critical Thinking Exercises**—These exercises challenge the student to incorporate new knowledge with previously learned concepts and reach a satisfactory conclusion. They encourage the student to think critically, problem-solve, and consider his or her own perspective on given topics.
- **Study Activities**—These interactive activities promote student participation in the learning process. This section encourages increased interaction/learning via clinical, online, and community activities.

Teaching–Learning Package

Instructor's Resources

Tools to assist you with teaching your course are available upon adoption of this text on thePoint at http://thePoint. lww.com/Ricci3e.

- An **E-Book** on thePoint gives you access to the book's full text and images online.
- A **Test Generator** lets you put together exclusive new tests from a bank containing o**ver 800 questions** (twice as many as last edition) to help you in assessing your students' understanding of the material. Test questions link to chapter learning objectives.
- **PowerPoint presentations** with **Guided Lecture Notes** provide an easy way for you to integrate the textbook with your students' classroom experience, either via slide shows or handouts. Multiple-choice and true/false questions are integrated into the presentations to promote class participation.
- An **Image Bank** lets you use the photographs and illustrations from this textbook in your PowerPoint slides or as you see fit in your course.
- **Case Studies** with related questions (and suggested answers) give students an opportunity to apply their knowledge to a client case similar to one they might encounter in practice.
- **Pre-Lecture Quizzes** (and answers) are quick, knowledge-based assessments that allow you to check students' reading.
- **Discussion Topics** (and suggested answers) can be used as conversation starters or in online discussion boards.
- **Assignments** (and suggested answers) include group, written, clinical, and Web assignments.
- Sample **Syllabi** provide guidance for structuring your pediatric nursing courses and are provided for four different course lengths: 4, 6, 8, and 10 weeks.
- **Journal Articles**, updated for the new edition, offer access to current research available in Lippincott Williams & Wilkins journals.

Contact your sales representative or check out LWW.com/Nursing for more details and ordering information.

Student Resources

An exciting set of free resources is available to help students review material and become even more familiar with vital concepts. Students can access all these resources on thePoint using the codes printed in the front of their textbooks.

- **NCLEX-Style Review Questions** for each chapter help students review important concepts and practice for NCLEX. **Over 700 questions** are included, more than twice as many as last edition!
- **Multimedia Resources** appeal to a variety of learning styles. Icons in the text direct readers to relevant videos and animations:
  - **Watch and Learn Videos**
    A special icon throughout the book directs students to free video clips located on thePoint that highlight growth and development, communicating with children, and providing nursing care to the child in the hospital.

- **Concepts in Action Animations**
  These unique animations, also located on thePoint, bring physiologic and pathophysiologic concepts to life and enhance student comprehension.
- A **Spanish–English Audio Glossary** provides helpful terms and phrases for communicating with patients who speak Spanish.
- **Journal Articles** offer access to current research available in Lippincott Williams & Wilkins journals.
- **And more!**

Susan Scott Ricci

[1]Nursing Process Overview contains NANDA-I approved nursing diagnoses. Material related to nursing diagnoses is from Nursing Diagnoses—Definitions and Classification 2012-2014 © 2009, 2007, 2005, 2003, 2001, 1998, 1996, 1994 NANDA International. Used by arrangement with Wiley-Blackwell Publishing, a company of John Wiley & Sons, Inc. In order to make safe and effective judgments using NANDA-I nursing.

Contents

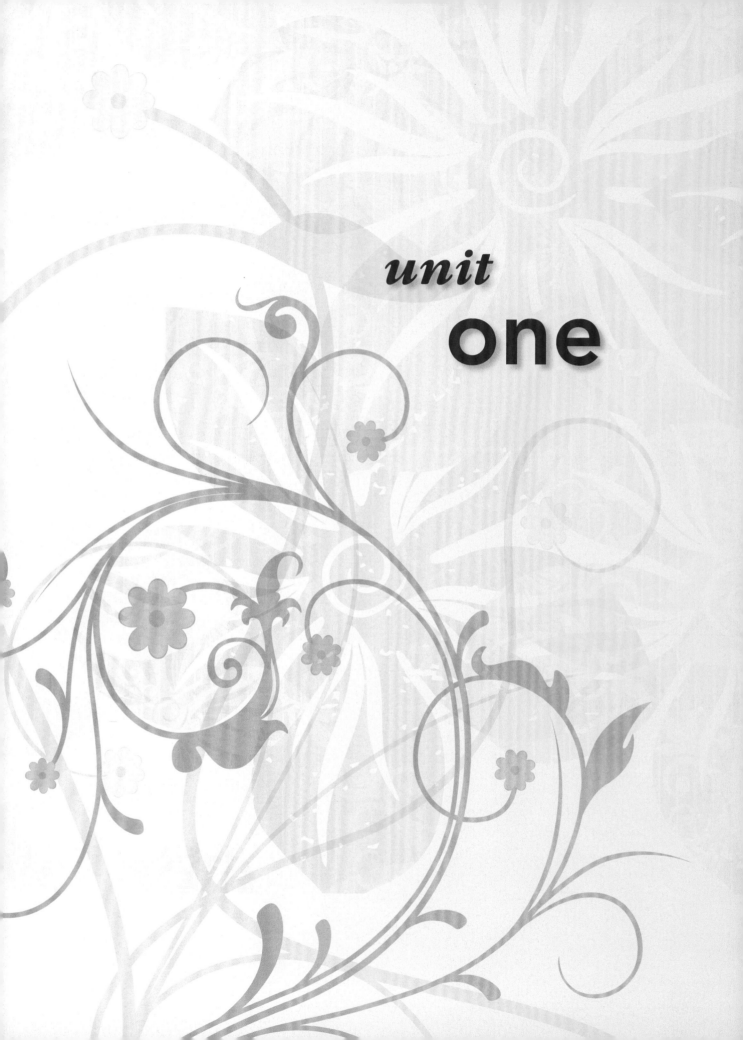

unit
one

Introduction to Maternity, Newborn, and Women's Nursing

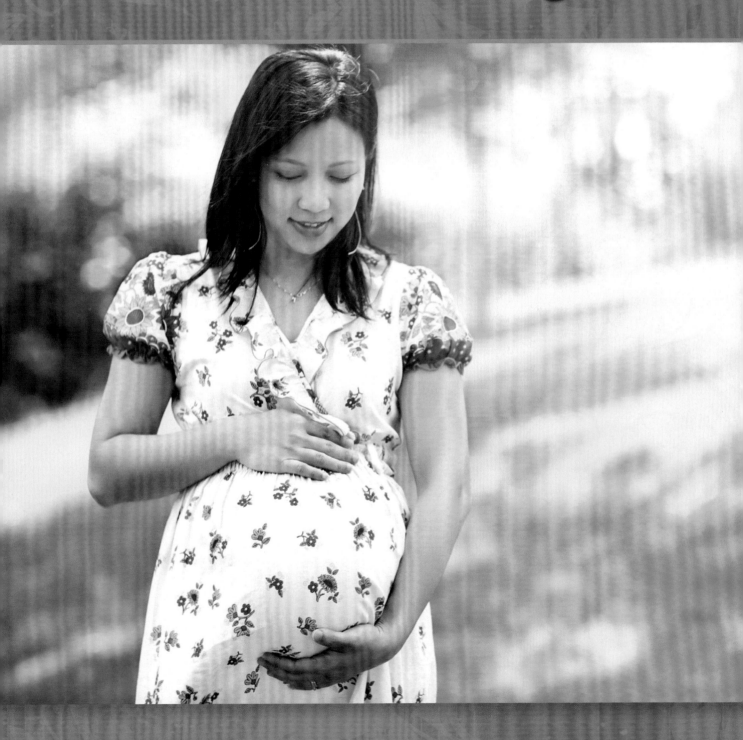

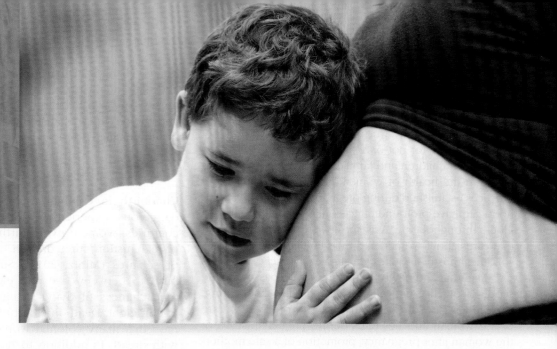

1

Perspectives on Maternal, Newborn, and Women's Health Care

Learning Objectives

Upon completion of the chapter, you will be able to:

1. Characterize the key milestones in the evolution of childbirth in America.

2. Outline the major components, concepts, and influences associated with the nursing management of women and their families.

3. Compare the past definitions of health and illness with the current definitions.

4. Examine the factors that affect maternal, newborn, and women's health.

5. Evaluate how society and culture can influence the health of women and their families.

6. Distinguish the health care barriers affecting women and their families.

7. Review the ethical and legal issues that may arise when caring for women and their families.

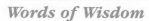

Sophia Nappo, a 38-year-old woman pregnant with her third child, comes to the prenatal clinic for a routine follow-up visit. Her mother, Betty, accompanies her because Sophia's husband is out of town. Sophia lives with her husband and two children, ages 4 and 9. She works part-time as a lunch aide in the local elementary school. What factors may play a role in influencing the health of Sophia and her family?

Words of Wisdom
Being pregnant and giving birth is like crossing a narrow bridge: people can accompany you to the bridge, and they can greet you on the other side, but you walk that bridge alone.

INTRODUCTION

A person's ability to lead a fulfilling life and to participate fully in society depends largely on his or her health status. This is especially true for women, who commonly are responsible for not only their own health but that of others: their children and families. Thus, it is important to focus on the health of women and families. Habits and practices established during pregnancy and in early childhood can have profound effects on a person's health and illness throughout life. As a society, creating a population that cares about women and their families and promotes solid health care and lifestyle choices is crucial.

Maternal and newborn nursing encompasses a wide scope of practice typically associated with childbearing. It includes care of the woman before pregnancy, care of the woman and her fetus during pregnancy, care of the woman after pregnancy, promotion of a safe motherhood, and care of the newborn, usually during the first 6 weeks after birth. The overall goal of maternal and newborn nursing is to promote and maintain optimal health for the woman and her family.

Nurses today have an unprecedented opportunity to improve the health and well-being of women and families. Events from birth to death, and every health care emergency in between, will likely involve the presence of a nurse. Involvement of a knowledgeable, supportive, comforting nurse often leads to a positive health care experience. Skilled nursing practice depends on a solid base of knowledge and clinical expertise delivered in a caring, holistic manner. Nurses, using their knowledge and passion, help meet the health care needs of their clients throughout the life span, whether the client is a pregnant woman, a fetus, a partner, or a woman with health-related problems. Nurses fill a variety of roles in helping clients to live healthier lives by providing direct care, emotional support, comfort, information, advice, advocacy, support, and counseling. Nurses are often "in the trenches" advocating for issues, drawing attention to the importance of health care for the client, and dealing with the lack of resources, the lack of access to health care, and the focus on acute care rather than education and prevention.

This chapter presents a general overview of the health care of women and their families and describes the major factors affecting maternal, newborn, and women's health. It also addresses health care information available to women and their families and improvements in diagnosis and treatments. Nurses need to be knowledgeable about these concepts and factors to ensure that they provide up-to-date professional care.

EVOLUTION OF MATERNAL AND NEWBORN NURSING

The health care of women has changed over the years due in part to changes in childbirth methods, social trends, changes in the health care system, and federal and state regulations. By reviewing historical events, nurses can gain a better understanding of the current and future status of maternal, newborn, and women's health nursing (Box 1.1).

Historical Perspective

Childbirth in colonial America was a difficult and dangerous experience. During the 17th and 18th centuries, women giving birth often died as a result of exhaustion, dehydration, infection, hemorrhage, or seizures (Mintz, 2013). Since most women gave birth to between five and eight children, their lifetime chances of dying in childbirth ran as high as one in eight. Death in childbirth was sufficiently common that many colonial women regarded pregnancy with dread. In addition to her anxieties about pregnancy, an expectant mother was filled with apprehension about the possible death of her newborn child. Approximately 50% of all children died before age 5 (King et al., 2015), compared with an infant mortality rate today of 6.17 infant deaths/1,000 live births (World Factbook, 2015).

Centuries ago, "granny midwives" handled the normal birthing process for most women. Midwifery skills have traditionally been passed from one woman to another within families, grandmothers to mothers to daughters, and also through apprenticeship with a more experienced midwife. Physicians usually were called only in extremely difficult cases, and all births took place at home (Simmons, Rothman, & Norman, 2013).

During the early 1900s, physicians attended about half the births in the United States. Midwives often cared for women who could not afford a doctor. Many women were attracted to hospitals because this showed affluence and hospitals provided pain management, which was not available in home births. In the 1950s, natural childbirth practices advocating birth without medication and focusing on relaxation techniques were introduced (Rabor, Taghipour, & Najmabadi, 2015). These techniques opened the door to childbirth education classes and helped bring the father back into the picture. Both partners could participate by taking an active role in pregnancy, childbirth, and parenting (Fig. 1.1).

Current Trends

In many ways, childbirth practices in the United States have come full circle, as we see the return of the nurse midwife and the *doula*. The concept of women helping other women during childbirth is not new; women who labored and gave birth at home were traditionally attended by relatives and midwives (Evidence-Based Practice 1.1). A **certified nurse midwife** (CNM) has

BOX 1.1

CHILDBIRTH IN AMERICA: A TIME LINE

1700s   Men did not attend births because it was considered indecent.
Women faced birth, not with joy and ecstasy, but with fear of death.
Female midwives attended the majority of all births at home.

1800s   There is a shift from using midwives to doctors among middle-class women.
The word *obstetrician* was formed from the Latin, meaning "to stand before."
Puerperal (childbed) fever was occurring in epidemic proportions.
Louis Pasteur demonstrated that streptococci were the major cause of puerperal fever that was killing mothers after delivery.
The first cesarean section was performed in Boston in 1894.
The x-ray was developed in 1895 and was used to assess pelvic size for birthing purposes.

1900s   Twilight sleep (a heavy dose of narcotics and amnesiacs) was used on women during childbirth in the United States.
The United States was 17th out of 20 nations in infant mortality rates.
Fifty to 75% of all women gave birth in hospitals by 1940.
Nurseries were started because moms could not care for their babies for several days after receiving chloroform gas.
In 1933, Dr. Grantley Dick-Reed wrote a book entitled *Childbirth Without Fear* that reduced the "fear–tension–pain" cycle women experienced during labor and birth.
In 1984, Dr. Fernand Lamaze wrote a book entitled *Painless Childbirth: The Lamaze Method* that advocated distraction and relaxation techniques to minimize the perception of pain.
Amniocentesis was first performed to assess fetal growth in 1966.
In the 1970s, the cesarean section rate was about 5%. By 2000 it rose to 34%, where it stands currently.
The 1970s and 1980s saw a growing trend to return birthing back to the basics—nonmedicated, nonintervening childbirth.
In the late 1900s, freestanding birthing centers—LDRPs—were designed, and the number of home births began to increase.

2000s   One in three women undergoes a surgical birth (cesarean).
Certified nurse midwives once again assist couples at home, in hospitals, or in freestanding facilities with natural childbirths. Research shows that midwives are the safest birth attendants for most women, with lower infant mortality and maternal rates, and fewer invasive interventions such as episiotomies and cesareans.
Childbirth classes of every flavor abound in most communities.
According to the latest available data, the United States ranks 50th in the world in maternal deaths.
The maternal mortality rate is approximately 11 in 100,000 live births.
According to the latest available data, the United States ranks 41st in the world in infant mortality rates.
The infant mortality rate is approximately 6 in 1,000 live births.

Adapted from Centers for Disease Control and Prevention [CDC]. (2015e). *Pregnancy-related deaths*. Retrieved from http://www.cdc.gov/reproductivehealth/MaternalInfantHealth/Pregnancy-relatedMortality.htm; King, T. L., Brucker, M. C., Kriebs, J. M., Fahey, J. O., Gegor, C. L., & Varney, H. (2015). *Varney's midwifery* (5th ed.). Burlington, MA: Jones & Bartlett Learning; and MacLean, M. (2015). *Midwives in 19th century America*. Retrieved from http://www.womenhistoryblog.com/2014/06/19th-century-midwives.html

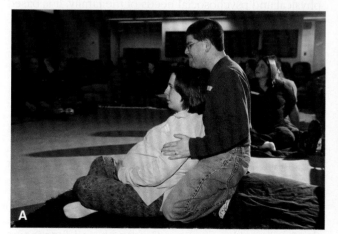
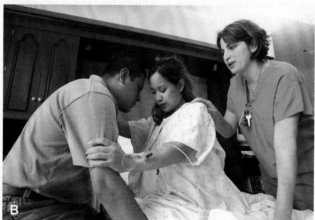

FIGURE 1.1 Today fathers and partners are welcome to take an active role in the pregnancy and childbirth experience. **A.** A couple can participate together in childbirth education classes. (Photo by Gus Freedman.) **B.** Fathers and partners can assist the woman throughout her labor and childbirth experience. (Photo by Joe Mitchell.)

EVIDENCE-BASED PRACTICE 1.1   **WOMEN'S RESPONSE TO CONTINUOUS LABOR SUPPORT**

Throughout history, women have been helping other women in labor by providing emotional support, comfort measures, information, and advocacy. However, in recent years, this practice has waned, and facilities frequently adhere to strict specific routines that may leave women feeling "dehumanized."

STUDY

A study was done to assess the effects on mothers and their newborns of continuous, one-to-one intrapartum care compared to usual care. The study also evaluated routine practices and policies in the birth environment that might affect a woman's autonomy, freedom of movement, and ability to cope with labor; who the caregiver was (a staff member of the facility or not); and when the support began (early or late in labor). All published and unpublished randomized clinical trials comparing continuous support during labor with usual care were examined. One author and one research assistant used standard methods for data collection and analysis and extracted the data independently. Clinical trial authors provided additional information. The researchers used relative risk for categorical data and weighted mean difference for continuous data. Twenty one studies from 15 countries involving 15,061 women were examined.

Findings

Women receiving continuous intrapartum support had a greater chance of a spontaneous vaginal birth, reduced

intrapartum analgesia, caused no harm; labors were shorter, and women were less likely to have a cesarean section or instrumental birth, regional analgesia, or a newborn with a low 5-minute Apgar score. These women also reported increased satisfaction with their labor and childbirth experience. Overall, the support, when provided by someone other than a facility staff member and initiated early in labor, proved to be more effective.

Nursing Implications

Based on this research, it is clear that women in labor benefit from one-to-one support during labor. Nurses can use the information gained from this study to educate women about the importance of having a support person during labor and birth. Nurses can also act as client advocates in facilities where they work to foster an environment that encourages the use of support persons during the intrapartum period. The focus of nursing needs to be individualized, supportive, and collaborative with the family during their childbearing experience. In short, nurses should place the needs of the mother and her family first in providing a continuum of care.

Although the study found that support is more effective when provided by someone other than a staff member, support from an individual is the key. Assigning the same nurse to provide care to the couple throughout the birthing experience also fosters a one-to-one relationship that helps meet the couple's needs and promotes feelings of security. By meeting the couple's needs, the nurse is enhancing their birthing experience.

Hodnett, E. D., Gates, S., Hofmeyr, G. J., Sakala, C., & Weston, J. (2013). Continuous support for women during childbirth. *Cochrane Database of Systematic Reviews*, 7(2), CD003766.

---

postgraduate training in the care of normal pregnancy and childbirth and is certified by the American College of Nurse Midwives. A **doula** is a birth assistant who provides emotional, physical, and educational support to the woman and family during childbirth and the postpartum period. Many nurses working in labor and birth areas today are credentialed in their specialty so that they can provide optimal care to the woman and her newborn. Childbirth choices are often based on what works best for the mother, child, and family.

CORE CONCEPTS OF MATERNAL, NEWBORN, AND WOMEN'S HEALTH NURSING

Maternal, newborn, and women's health nursing provides evidence-based care to the client within the context of the family unit. This care involves the implementation of an interdisciplinary plan in a collaborative manner to ensure continuity of care that is cost effective, quality oriented, and outcome focused. It involves family-centered, evidence-based, case-managed care.

Family-Centered Care

Family-centered care is the delivery of safe, satisfying, high-quality health care that focuses on and adapts to the physical and psychosocial needs of the family. It is based on mutual trust and collaboration between the woman, her family, and the health care provider. It is a partnership approach of families and their caregivers that recognizes the strength and integrity of the family. These are the basic principles of family-centered care:

- Childbirth is considered a normal, healthy event in the life of a family.
- Childbirth affects the entire family, and relationships will change.
- Families are capable of making decisions about their own care if given adequate information and professional support (Young, 2014).

The philosophy of family-centered care recognizes the family as the constant. The health and functioning of the family affect the health of the client and other members of the family. Family members support one another well beyond the health care provider's brief time with them, such as during the childbearing process or during a child's illness. Birth is viewed as a normal life event rather than a medical procedure.

Family-centered care requires the nurse to apply sensitivity to the client's and family's beliefs and those supporting their culture. This involves listening to the family's needs and shifting the nurse's authoritarian role to the family to empower them to make their own decisions within the context of a supportive environment. A true family perspective should be applied in maternity care and the new parents viewed as a family unit, not as a medical case. Nurses providing family-centered care means that they identify, respect, and care about client's differences, values, preferences, and expressed needs; relieve pain and suffering; coordinate continuous care; listen to, clearly inform, communicate with, and educate clients; share decision making and management; and continuously advocate for them (Denham et al., 2016).

With family-centered care, support and respect for the uniqueness and diversity of families are essential, along with encouragement and enhancement of the family's strengths and competencies. It is important to create opportunities for families to demonstrate their abilities and skills. Families can also acquire new abilities and skills to maintain a sense of control. Family-centered care promotes greater family self-determination, decision-making abilities, control, and self-efficacy, thereby enhancing the client's and family's sense of empowerment. When implementing family-centered care, nurses seek caregiver input; these suggestions and advice are incorporated into the client's plan of care as the nurse counsels and teaches the family appropriate health care interventions. Today, as nurses partner with various experts to provide high-quality and cost-effective care, one expert partnership that nurses can make is with the client's family. Nurses empower mothers with freedom of choice based on knowledge of alternatives. This means the mother's birth plan would be honored in an environment where the mother's choices are respected. Nurses must partner with women and their families for optimal care and quality outcomes (Beal, Dalton, & Maloney, 2015).

The impact of family-centered care can be seen in the models of care delivery for women. Families are kept together after childbirth, not separated as in past years. From the 1980s to the present, increased access to care for all women (regardless of their ability to pay) and hospital redesigns have focused on keeping families together during their childbirth experience (Clark, Beatty, & Reibel, 2015). Hospital redesigns include labor, delivery, and recovery rooms that incorporate all three activities in one room, and labor, delivery, recovery, and postpartum (LDRP) spaces that incorporate all four activities in one room, so that families don't have to move from place to place during the birth experience (Fig. 1.2).

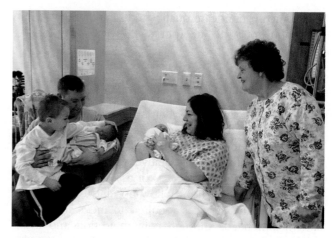

FIGURE 1.2 Providing an opportunity for the "big brother" to interact with his new siblings is an important component of family-centered nursing care.

Evidence-Based Care

Evidence-based practice (EBP) is a problem-solving approach to making nursing clinical decisions (Hanrahan et al., 2015). It involves the collection, interpretation, and integration of validated research-derived evidence from a variety of resources such as research findings, internal evidence from outcome management or process improvement processes, and patient preferences. Nurses need to find a way to integrate the best available evidence to translate into practice to achieve the best outcomes consistent with the aim of health care—to improve the experience of care, to improve the health of mothers and infants, and to reduce the costs of health care (Hain & Kear, 2015). **Evidence-based nursing practice** involves the use of research to establish a plan of care and to implement that care. This model of nursing practice includes the use of the best current evidence in making decisions about care. Widespread use of EBP may lead to a decrease in variation of care while at the same time increase in quality.

Scientific research findings help nurses not only stay current in their clinical specialties, but also in their choice of the most effective interventions. Many of the professional organizations—for example, the Association of Women's Health, Obstetric and Neonatal Nurses (AWHONN), the American Nurses Association (ANA), and the National League for Nursing (NLN)—have developed evidence-based clinical practice guidelines for the safest and most effective delivery of family-centered nursing care. Nurses should be diligent in seeking out these evidence-based guidelines to ensure excellence in their daily practice. When EBP is delivered in a context of caring and in a supportive organizational culture, the highest quality of care and best client outcomes can be achieved. The landmark report by the Health and Medicine Division (HMD) (2011), *The Future of Nursing: Leading Change, Advancing Health*, listed EBP as a competency required to enhance patient care quality and safety. Thus, it is no longer an option to incorporate EBP into our practice, but a necessity!

Case-Managed Care

Modern health care focuses on an interdisciplinary plan of care designed to meet a client's physical, developmental, educational, spiritual, and psychosocial needs. This interdisciplinary collaborative type of care is termed **case management**, a process of assessment, planning, application, coordination, follow-up, and evaluation of the options and services required to meet an individual's health needs through communication and available resources to promote quality cost-effective results. Operational excellence, quality of care, and sound financial performance are increasingly linked as key drivers of health care performance. Quality case management for all families contributes toward fewer complications, reductions in length of stay, and lowered costs. Case management is a continuous process that requires critical thinking about how care is delivered and its effect on the entire care progression of a client. It has, at its core, the values of care coordination, utilization management, and client advocacy across the continuum of care (Summers, 2016) and involves the following components:

- Advocacy, communication, and resource management
- Client-focused comprehensive care across a continuum
- Coordinated care with an interdisciplinary approach (Treadwell et al., 2015)

When the nurse effectively functions in the role of case manager, client and family satisfaction is increased, fragmentation of care is decreased, and outcome measurement for a homogenous group of clients is possible.

Think back to Sophia and her mother, Betty, who were described at the beginning of the chapter. Sophia and her husband are planning to use natural childbirth and to have their children present for the birth. While Sophia is waiting to be called for her appointment, Betty says, "Things have changed so much since I was pregnant. It's amazing what happens nowadays." Explain how things have changed in maternal and newborn health care, focusing on the concept of family-centered care.

HEALTH STATUS GOALS

At one time, health was defined simply as the absence of disease; health was measured by monitoring the mortality and morbidity of a group. During the past century, however, the focus on health has shifted to disease prevention, health promotion, and wellness. The World Health Organization (WHO, 2015a) defines health as "a state of complete physical, mental, and social well-being, and not merely the absence of disease or infirmity." The definition of health is complex; it is not merely the absence of disease or an analysis of mortality and morbidity statistics.

Healthy People 2020

In 1979, a surgeon general's report titled *Healthy People* presented a prevention agenda for the nation that identified the most significant preventable threats to the health of the United States. *Healthy People* is a set of goals and objectives with 10-year targets designed to guide national health promotion and disease prevention efforts to improve the health of all people in the United States. The current initiative is *Healthy People 2020*, which is the country's comprehensive, nationwide health promotion and disease prevention agenda that promotes the goal of improving the health and well-being of women, infants, children, and families (U.S. Department of Health & Human Services [USDHHS], 2015a). Ten specific health indicators serve as a way to evaluate progress made in the public health arena and to coordinate the national health improvement efforts. *Healthy People 2020* highlights the major health indicators of the 21st century that need to be addressed. This also outlines major goals intended to increase the quality and years of healthy life and to eliminate health disparities among ethnic groups by targeting the lifestyle choices and environmental conditions that contribute to over half of all premature deaths in the United States. *Healthy People 2020* identifies specific national health goals related to maternal, infant, and child health.

Improving the well-being of mothers, infants, and children is an important public health goal for the United States. Their well-being determines the health of the next generation and can help predict future public health challenges for families, communities, and the health care system. The objectives of the maternal, infant, and child

---

HEALTHY PEOPLE 2020 • 1.1

Major Health Concerns of the 21st Century

- Physical activity
- Overweight and obesity
- Tobacco use
- Substance abuse
- Responsible sexual behavior
- Mental health
- Injury and violence
- Environmental quality
- Immunizations
- Access to health care

Healthy People objectives based on data from http://www.healthypeople.gov.

National Health Goals—Maternal, Infant, and Child Health

- Reduce the rate of fetal and infant deaths.
- Reduce the rate of maternal mortality.
- Reduce the 1-year mortality rate for infants with Down syndrome.
- Reduce maternal illness and complications due to pregnancy.
- Reduce cesarean births among low-risk (full-term, singleton, vertex presentation) women.
- Reduce low-birth-weight (LBW) and very-low-birth-weight (VLBW) births.
- Reduce preterm births.
- Increase the proportion of pregnant women who receive early and adequate prenatal care.
- Increase abstinence from alcohol, cigarettes, and illicit drugs among pregnant women.
- Increase the proportion of pregnant women who attend a series of prepared childbirth classes.
- Increase the proportion of mothers who achieve a recommended weight gain during their pregnancies.
- Increase the proportion of women of childbearing potential with an intake of at least 400 μg of folic acid from fortified foods or dietary supplements.
- Reduce the proportion of women of childbearing potential who have low red blood cell folate concentrations.
- Increase the proportion of women delivering a live birth who received preconception care services and practiced key recommended preconception health behaviors.
- Reduce the proportion of persons aged 18–44 years who have impaired fecundity (i.e., a physical barrier preventing pregnancy or carrying a pregnancy to term).

- Reduce postpartum relapse of smoking among women who quit smoking during pregnancy.
- Increase the proportion of women giving birth who attend a postpartum care visit with a health worker.
- Increase the proportion of infants who are put to sleep on their backs.
- Increase the proportion of infants who are breast-fed.
- Increase the proportion of employers that have work-site lactation support programs.
- Reduce the proportion of breast-fed newborns who receive formula supplementation within the first 2 days of life.
- Increase the proportion of live births that occur in facilities that provide recommended care for lactating mothers and their babies.
- Reduce the occurrence of fetal alcohol syndrome.
- Reduce the proportion of children diagnosed with a disorder through newborn blood spot screening who experience developmental delay requiring special education services.
- Reduce the proportion of children with cerebral palsy born as LBW infants (less than 2,500 g).
- Reduce occurrence of neural tube defects.
- Increase the proportion of children with special health care needs who receive their care in family-centered, comprehensive, coordinated systems.
- Increase appropriate newborn blood-spot screening and follow-up testing.
- Increase the proportion of VLBW infants born at level III hospitals or subspecialty perinatal centers.

Healthy People 2020 objectives based on data from http://www.healthypeople.gov.

health topic area address a wide range of conditions, health behaviors, and health system indicators that affect the health, wellness, and quality of life of women, children, and families (USDHHS, 2015a).

Measuring health status is not a simple or convenient process. For example, some individuals with chronic illnesses do not see themselves as ill if they can control their condition through self-management. A traditional method used in this country to measure health is to examine mortality and morbidity data. Information is collected and analyzed to provide an objective description of the nation's health.

Mortality

Mortality is the incidence or number of individuals who have died over a specific period. This statistic is presented as rates per 100,000 and is calculated from a sample of death certificates. The National Center for Health Statistics, under the USDHHS, collects, analyzes, and disseminates the data on mortality rates in the United States.

Maternal Mortality

The **maternal mortality ratio** is the annual number of female deaths from any cause related to or aggravated by pregnancy or its management (excluding accidental or incidental causes) during pregnancy and childbirth or within 42 days of termination of pregnancy, irrespective of the duration and site of the pregnancy. It is reported as a ratio of deaths per 100,000 live births, for a specified year.

In the United States, the maternal mortality ratio is mixed depending on ethnic background. African American women suffer maternal mortality ratios three-to-fourfold increase when compared to those of any other ethnic group: about 35.6 of 100,000 African American mothers die due to childbirth, as compared with much lower rates in Whites (11.7), and women of other races (17.6) (Centers for Disease Control and Prevention [CDC], 2015a). The federal government has pledged to improve maternal–child care outcomes and thus reduce mortality ratios for women and children by endorsing the *Healthy People 2020* agenda, but the WHO (2015d) data show that the United States ranks 50th out of approximately 240 nations in the world for maternal mortality—with maternal mortality ratios higher than almost all European countries, as well as several countries in Asia and the Middle East. This statistic places the United States near the bottom of the top quartile of developed countries. For a country that spends more than any other country on health care and more on childbirth-related care than any other area of hospitalization—US $86 billion a year—this is a shockingly poor return on investment (International Center for Research on Women, 2015).

During the past several decades, mortality and morbidity have dramatically decreased as a result of an increased emphasis on hygiene, good nutrition, exercise, and prenatal care for all women. However, women are still experiencing complications at significant rates. The United States is one of the most medically and technologically advanced nations and has the highest per capita spending on health care in the world, but the maternal mortality rate has steadily increased over the years. The United States is one of only eight countries where maternal mortality is on the rise. The other countries include Afghanistan, Greece, Africa, and Central America (Kassebaum et al., 2014). Our current mortality rates indicate the need for improvement. For example:

- Two or three women die in the United States every day from pregnancy complications, and more than 30% of pregnant women (1.8 million women annually) experience some type of illness or injury during childbirth (Abel, 2015).
- The United States ranks 50th (in other words, below 49 other countries) in rates of maternal deaths (deaths per 100,000 live births) (WHO, 2015d).
- Most pregnancy-related complications are preventable. The top five leading causes of pregnancy-related mortality are embolism (20%), hemorrhage (17%), preeclampsia and eclampsia (16%), infection (13%), and cardiomyopathy (8%) (Chescheir, 2015).

The maternal mortality and morbidity rates for African American women have been three to four times higher than those for Whites (Creanga et al., 2015). This major racial disparity has persisted for more than 60 years, with African American women having at least a doubled risk of pregnancy-related death when compared with White women. This striking difference in the pregnancy-related mortality ratio is the largest disparity in the area of maternal and child health. Researchers do not entirely understand what accounts for this disparity, but some suspected causes of the higher maternal mortality rates for minority women include low socioeconomic status, limited or no insurance coverage, bias among health care providers (which may foster distrust), and quality of care available in the community. Language and legal barriers may also explain why some immigrant women do not receive good prenatal care. Lack of care

during pregnancy is a major factor contributing to a poor outcome. Prenatal care is well known to prevent complications of pregnancy and to support the birth of healthy infants, but not all women receive the same quality and quantity of health care during their pregnancy. Pregnancy-related mortality is on the rise in the United States. The *Healthy People 2020* goal for maternal deaths is 11.4 per 100,000 live births (USDHHS, 2015a). African American pregnant women had higher degrees of hypertension and lower hemoglobin levels on admission and had presented for prenatal care much later, on average, than White women or not at all (Creanga et al., 2015).

The Centers for Disease Control and Prevention (CDC) has noted that the disparity in maternal mortality rates between women of color and White women represents one of the largest racial disparities among public health indicators. Eliminating racial and ethnic disparities in maternal–child health care requires enhanced efforts at preventing disease, promoting health, and delivering appropriate and timely care (CDC, 2015a). The CDC has called for more research and monitoring to understand and address racial disparities, along with increased funding for prenatal and postpartum care. Research is needed to identify causes and to design initiatives to reduce these disparities, and the CDC is calling on Congress to expand programs to provide preconception and prenatal care to underserved women.

Fetal Mortality

The **fetal mortality rate** or fetal death rate refers to the spontaneous intrauterine death of a fetus at any time during pregnancy per 1,000 live births. Fetal deaths later in pregnancy >20 weeks of gestation are also referred to as stillbirths. Fetal mortality may be attributable to maternal factors (e.g., malnutrition, disease, or preterm cervical dilation) or fetal factors (e.g., chromosomal abnormalities or poor placental attachment).

Fetal mortality is a major, but often overlooked, public health problem. This refers to spontaneous intrauterine death at any time during pregnancy. The fetal mortality rate in the United States is 6.2 per 1,000 live births (CDC, 2015b). The goal of *Healthy People 2020* is to reduce it to 5.6 fetal deaths (USDHHS, 2015a). Much of the public concern regarding reproductive loss has concentrated on infant mortality, because less is known about fetal mortality. However, the impact of fetal mortality on families in the United States is considerable, because it provides an overall picture of the quality of maternal health and prenatal care.

Neonatal and Infant Mortality

The **neonatal mortality rate** is the number of infant deaths occurring in the first 28 days of life per 1,000 live births. The United States now ranks 41st in the world in terms of neonatal mortality, the death rate of infants less than 1 month old. The neonatal mortality rate is 4.5 per 1,000 live births (USDHHS, 2015b; World Bank, 2015). The goal of *Healthy People 2020* is to reduce it to 4.1 (USDHHS, 2015a). Each year the deaths of 2 million babies are linked to complications during birth or within the first month and the burden is inequitably carried by the poor. Evidence-based strategies are urgently needed to reduce the burden of intrapartum-related deaths (CDC, 2015c). The reliability of the neonatal mortality estimates depends on the accuracy and completeness of reporting and recording of births and deaths. Underreporting and misclassification are common, especially for deaths occurring early in life.

The perinatal mortality rate encompasses late and early neonatal mortalities and is defined as the number of stillbirths and deaths in the first week of life per 1,000 live births; it is also a useful health status indicator. Work is ongoing to improve estimates of stillbirth rates, a major component of perinatal mortality (WHO, 2015b). Perinatal mortality rate is a sum total of the following:

- Fetal mortality rate—the death of a fetus prior to expulsion or extraction from the mother. Fetal death is determined by no signs of life after birth.
- Neonatal mortality rate—the number of neonates dying before reaching 28 days of life, per 1,000 live births in a given year.

The **infant mortality rate** is the number of deaths occurring in the first 12 months of life. It is also documented as the number of deaths of infants younger than 1 year of age per 1,000 live births. Neonatal mortality and postneonatal mortality (covering the remaining 11 months of the first year of life) are reflected in the infant mortality rate. The infant mortality rate is used as an index of the general health of a country. Currently, about two thirds of infant deaths in the United States occur before 28 days, with the remaining third occurring in the postnatal period between 28 days and under 1 year (USDHHS, 2015a). Generally, this statistic is one of the most significant measures of maternal and child health. In the United States, the infant mortality rate is 6.17 (World Fact Book, 2015). *Healthy People 2020*'s goal is to reduce it to 6.0 (USDHHS, 2015a).

Despite the rapid decline in infant mortality for industrialized countries during the 21st century, the infant mortality rate in the United States has declined only marginally. Racial and ethnic disparities in infant mortality have persisted and increased, as have the percentages of preterm and low-birth-weight births. Infant mortality is a complex and multifactorial problem that has proved resistant to intervention efforts (McGill, 2015).

The infant mortality rate varies greatly from state to state as well as among ethnic groups. The United States has one of the highest gross national products in the world and is known for its technological capabilities,

the United States continues to lag behind in preserving infant's lives when compared with other industrialized countries (CDC, 2015d). The main causes of early infant death in this country include problems occurring at birth or shortly thereafter. These include prematurity, low birth weight, congenital anomalies, sudden infant death syndrome (SIDS), and respiratory distress syndrome (Oza et al., 2015).

Take Note!

African American and American Indian/Alaska Native infants have consistently had higher infant mortality rates than other ethnic groups (Kail & Cavanaugh, 2016).

Congenital anomalies remain the leading cause of infant mortality in the United States. Low birth weight and prematurity are major indicators of infant health and significant predictors of infant mortality (Wang et al., 2015). The high incidence of low birth weight (<2,500 g) in the United States is a significant reason why its infant mortality rate is higher than that of other countries (Redding et al., 2015).

After birth, other health promotion strategies can significantly improve an infant's health and chances of survival. Breast-feeding has been shown to reduce rates of infection in infants and to improve their long-term health (King et al., 2015). Emphasizing the importance of placing an infant on his or her back to sleep will reduce the incidence of SIDS. Encouraging mothers to join support groups to prevent postpartum depression and learn sound child-rearing practices will improve the health of both mothers and their infants.

Morbidity

Morbidity indicates a diseased state or condition. Many women enter their pregnancy with a chronic medical disease, an infection, or anemia or engage in lifestyle habits (smoking and drinking alcohol) that are detrimental to the well-being of the fetus. Any or all of these can lead to a poor pregnancy outcome.

Morbidity and Women

Women today face not only diseases of genetic origin but also diseases that arise from poor personal habits. Even though women represent 51% of the population, only recently have researchers and the medical community focused on their special health needs. A significant study identified an urgent need to improve women's access to health insurance and health care services, to place a stronger emphasis on prevention, and to invest in more research on women's health (National Women's

---

BOX 1.2

THE NATIONAL INDICATORS OF WOMEN'S HEALTH

- Lung cancer death rate
- Diabetes
- Heart disease death rate
- Binge drinking
- High school completion
- Poverty
- Wage gap
- Rate of acquired immunodeficiency syndrome (AIDS)
- Maternal mortality rate
- Rate of *Chlamydia* infection
- Breast cancer death rate
- Heart disease death rate
- Smoking
- Being overweight
- No physical activity during leisure time
- Eating five fruits and vegetables daily
- Colorectal screening
- Mammograms
- Pap smears
- First-trimester prenatal care
- Access to health insurance

Adapted from National Women's Law Center. (2010). *Making the grade on women's health: A national state-by-state report card.* Retrieved from http://hrc.nwlc.org/states/national-report-card

---

Law Center [NWLC], 2010). It identified 26 indicators of women's access to health care services, measuring the degree to which women receive preventive health care and engage in health-promoting activities (Box 1.2). The report card gave the nation an overall grade of "unsatisfactory," and not a single state received a grade of "satisfactory." As reported in the NWLC's *2010 National Report Card*, the nation has met several benchmarks since 2010: colorectal cancer screenings have increased; annual dental visits have increased; death rates from coronary heart disease have declined considerably; and a steady decline in the number of women who smoke and get mammograms. The nation missed many of the other benchmarks. Other substandard findings included the following:

- No state has focused enough attention on preventive measures, such as smoking cessation, exercise, nutrition, and screening for diseases.
- Too many women lack health insurance coverage: nationally, nearly one in five women has no health insurance.
- No state has adequately addressed women's health needs in the areas of reproductive health, mental health, and violence against women.
- Limited research has been done on health conditions that primarily affect women and that affect women differently than men (NWLC, 2010).

The passage of the **Affordable Care Act** (ACA) as well as *Healthy People 2020* hold great promise for women's health. The emphasis on access to preventive health care will hopefully make a positive impact on addressing the areas of deficiency identified in the *2010 Report Card*. It is essential that women take advantage of the new benefits, expansions, improvements included in the new law. Nurses have a critical role to play in monitoring the implementation of ACA to make sure all women receive the health care they need and deserve.

The health status of women all across the United States must be improved. Far too many states fail to meet the *Healthy People 2020's* goals for satisfactory health status, and states are only slowly grappling with policy changes that can make improvements in women's health. Since 2010, more states have made positive changes in their policies, but there is still a great distance to go. Much more needs to be done to improve access to health insurance and health care providers and services and to increase access to reproductive health services. Additionally, women need help attaining economic security, which, if achieved, would greatly improve their health and the health of their families. The NWLC report card brought to light problems and their possible solutions for creating a nation of healthy women, for the benefit of themselves, their families, and their communities. It is up to all women to advocate for improvement in their own health by writing a letter to their Congressional representatives demanding that they implement heath policies that promote all women's health. This political action is vital, since all women's health in the nation hangs in the balance.

Major Health Issues for Women

CARDIOVASCULAR DISEASECardiovascular disease (CVD) is the number one cause of death of women, regardless of racial or ethnic group. More than 500,000 women die annually in the United States of CVD—about one death per minute (Alexander et al., 2014). Women who have a heart attack are more likely than men to die. Heart attacks in women are often more difficult to diagnose than in men because of their vague and varied symptoms. Heart disease is still thought of as a "man's disease," and thus a heart attack may not be considered in the differential diagnosis when a woman presents to an emergency department.

Nurses need to look beyond the obvious "crushing chest pain" textbook symptom that heralds a heart attack in men. Symptoms may be atypical: dyspnea rather than chest pain. Causes of heart disease differ between men and women in several other ways—for example, menopause (associated with a significant rise in coronary events); history of preeclampsia; diabetes, high cholesterol levels, and left ventricular hypertrophy; smoking, including secondhand smoke; gestational hypertension; polycystic ovary syndrome; blood vessel inflammation and repeated episodes of weight loss and gain (increased coronary morbidity and mortality) (Manson & Bassuk, 2015). Nurses have a major role in empowering women to engage in a healthy-heart lifestyle to prevent them from becoming mortality statistics.

CANCER

Cancer is the second leading cause of death among women (American Cancer Society [ACS], 2015a). Women have a one-in-three lifetime risk of developing cancer, and one out of every four deaths is from cancer (Alexander et al., 2014). Although much attention is focused on cancer of the reproductive system, lung cancer is the number one killer of women (ACS, 2015b). This is largely the result of smoking and secondhand smoke. Lung cancer has no early symptoms, making early detection almost impossible. Thus, lung cancer has the lowest survival rate of any cancer: more than 90% of people who get lung cancer die of it (Islami et al., 2015).

Breast cancer occurs in one in every eight (12%) women in a lifetime. It was estimated that in 2015 about 231,840 new cases of invasive breast cancer would be diagnosed among women in the United States. An estimated 40,290 women were expected to die from the disease in 2015 (ACS, 2015c). White women get breast cancer at a higher rate than African American women, but African American women are more likely to get breast cancer before they are at age 40 and are more likely to die from it at any age. The causes of this inequality are complex and are thought to reflect social and economic disparities more than biologic differences associated with race. Socioeconomic disparities include inequalities in work, wealth, income, education, housing, and overall standard of living, as well as barriers to high-quality cancer prevention, early detection, and treatment services (ACS, 2015d).

Women living in North America have the highest rate of breast cancer in the world. As of 2015, there are over 3 million breast cancer survivors in the United States. It is the most common malignancy in women and second only to lung cancer as a cause of cancer mortality in women (ACS, 2015c). Although a positive family history of breast cancer, aging, and irregularities in the menstrual cycle at an early age are major risk factors, others risk factors include excess weight, not having children, oral contraceptive use, excessive alcohol consumption, a high-fat diet, and long-term use of hormone replacement therapy (ACS, 2015c). Breast cancer rates have dropped recently, possibly due to the decreased use of long-term hormone replacement therapy that occurred after the *Women's Health Initiative* report was released in 2002 and the *Million Women Study* in 2003 (Mirkin et al., 2015). However, early detection and treatment continue to offer the best chance for a cure, and reducing the risk of cancer by decreasing avoidable risks continues to be the best preventive plan.

PREGNANCY AND HEALTH ISSUES

Pregnant women are by no means immune to any of the above health issues. Many start a pregnancy with health conditions that might include hypertension, obesity, CVD, diabetes, autoimmune diseases, anemia, asthma, sexually transmitted infections (STIs), depression, or cancer. Although the majority of pregnant women are young and fairly healthy, the incidence of many chronic health issues in young women and childhood obesity is increasing secondary to the obesity epidemic in the United States. Obesity by itself increases the risk of blood clots, surgical births, preterm birth, macrosomia, diabetes, gestational hypertension, and postpartum infections (DeJoy & Bittner, 2015).

Women's health is a complex issue, and no single policy is going to change the overall dismal state ratings. Although progress in science and technology has helped reduce the incidence of and improve the survival rates for several diseases, women's health issues continue to have an impact on our society. By eliminating or decreasing some of the risk factors and causes of prevalent diseases and illnesses, society and science could minimize certain chronic health problems. Focusing on the causes and effects of particular illnesses could help resolve many women's health issues of today.

FACTORS AFFECTING MATERNAL, NEWBORN, AND WOMEN'S HEALTH

From conception, children are shaped by a myriad of factors such as genetics and the environment. As members of a family, they are also members of a specific population, community, culture, and society. As they learn and grow, they are affected by multiple, complex, and ever-changing influences around them. For example, dramatic demographic changes in the United States have led to shifts in majority and minority population groups. Globalization has led to an international focus on health. Access to and the types of health care available have changed due to modifications in health care delivery and financing. In addition, the United States is still grappling with issues such as immigration, poverty, homelessness, and violence. Prenatal care is important to monitor the pregnancy, detect and treat complications early, prevent diseases through immunization and good nutrition, and promote healthy lifestyles after childbirth. All of these services are needed for a healthy pregnancy outcome (McFarlane, 2015).

These factors may affect the person positively, promoting healthy growth and development, or negatively, increasing the person's health risks. Nurses, especially those working with women and their families, need to understand how these influences affect the quality of nursing care and health outcomes. They must examine the impact of these variables to gain the knowledge and skills needed to plan effective care, thereby achieving the best possible outcomes.

Family

The **family** is considered the basic social unit of our society. The way that families are defined has changed (Table 1.1). The United States Bureau of the Census (2015) defines family as a group of two or more people related by birth, marriage, or adoption and living together. Earlier definitions of family emphasized the legal ties or genetic relationships of people living in the same household with specific roles.

The family greatly influences the development and health of its members. For example, children learn health care activities, health beliefs, and health values from their family. The family's structure, the roles assumed by family members, and social changes that affect the family's life can influence the woman's and newborn's health status.

TABLE 1.1	EXAMPLES OF FAMILY STRUCTURES IN TODAY'S SOCIETY	
Nuclear family	Husband, wife, and children living in same household	May include natural or adopted children Once considered the traditional family structure; now less common due to increased divorce rates and child rearing by unmarried persons
Binuclear family	Child who is a member of two families due to joint custody; parenting is considered a "joint venture"	Always works better when the interests of the child are put first and above the parents' needs and desires
Single-parent family	One parent is responsible for care of children.	May result from death, divorce, desertion, birth outside marriage, or adoption. These families are likely to face challenges because of economic, social, and personal restraints; one person serves as the homemaker, caregiver, and financial provider.
Commuter family	Adults in the family live and work apart for professional or financial reasons, often leaving the daily care of children to one parent.	Similar to single-parent family
Step- or blended family	Adults with children from previous marriages or from the new marriage	May lead to family conflict due to different expectations on the part of the child and adults; they may have different views and practices related to child care and health
Extended family	Nuclear family and grandparents, cousins, aunts, and uncles	Need to identify the decision-maker and primary caretaker of the children Popular in some cultures, such as Hispanic and Asian cultures
LGBT family	Adults of the same sex living together with or without children	May face negative attitudes about their "different" lifestyle; are part of the American fabric. Two million children are being raised by LGBT parents. Public policy has not kept up with the changing reality of the American family.
Communal family	Group of people living together to raise children and manage household; unrelated by blood or marriage	May face negative attitudes about their "different" lifestyle Need to determine the decision-maker and caretaker of the children
Foster family	A temporary family for children who are placed away from their parents to ensure their emotional and physical well-being	May include the foster family's children and other foster children in the home Foster children are more likely to have unmet health needs and chronic health problems because they may have been in a variety of health systems.

TABLE 1.1	EXAMPLES OF FAMILY STRUCTURES IN TODAY'S SOCIETY (continued)	
Grandparents-as-parent families	Grandparents raising their grandchildren due to the inability or absence of the parents	May increase the risk for physical, financial, and emotional stress on older adults May lead to confusion and emotional stress for child if biologic parents are in and out of child's life
Adolescent families	Young parents who are still mastering the developmental tasks of their childhood	Are at greater risk for health problems in pregnancy and delivery; more likely to have premature infants, which then leads to risk of subsequent health and developmental problems Probably still need support from their family related to financial, emotional, and school issues

Adapted from Krueger, P. M., Jutte, D. P., Franzini, L., Elo, I., & Hayward, M. D. (2015). Family structure and multiple domains of child well-being in the United States: a cross-sectional study. *Population Health Metrics, 13*(1), 6; Edelman, C. L., & Mandle, C. L. (2014). *Health promotion throughout the lifespan* (8th ed.). St. Louis, MO: Mosby Elsevier; Brown, S. L., Manning, W. D., & Stykes, J. B. (2015). Family structure and child well-being: Integrating family complexity. *Journal of Marriage and Family, 77*(1), 177–190; and Dempsey, D. (2015). Familiarly queer? Same-sex relationships and family formation. In: G, Heard & D, Arunacha-lam (Eds.). *Family Formation in 21st Century Australia* (pp. 225–240). Netherlands: Springer.

Families are unique; every family has different views and requires distinct methods for support (Fig. 1.3).

Changes in Parental Roles Over Time

Parental roles have evolved over time due to social and economic changes as well as family changes. Traditionally, the role of a provider was assigned to the father and the mother performed the role of a nurturer. However, with more women in the workplace and more households with two parents working, today both parents are often the providers as well as the nurturers. Technological expansion has also played a part in affecting traditional roles, allowing some parents to work from home and therefore maintain the provider role while simultaneously fulfilling the nurturer and health manager roles. In addition to fathers taking on greater responsibilities related to household management, and infant and child care, the number of single-father parent families and grandparent families is increasing. One in three children born in the United States is to a single-parent family (Federal Interagency Forum on Child and Family Statistics [FIFCFS], 2015).

While mothers have services that aid their transition from the workplace into motherhood and then back into the workplace, fathers rarely have the same assistance. As fathers have begun to fill a more holistic role, society has realized that they have a tremendous impact on their children's lives starting at an early age. Therefore, it is important that men receive the same assistance as women during transitional periods, such as paternity time off from work and more flexible work schedules (FIFCFS, 2015). Providing assistive services will aid and empower men to be better parents in their children's lives.

Being a parent is one of the most challenging jobs a person will ever do. However, there is no manual that teaches how to be successful at it. Nurses must encourage involvement of both parents by inviting both mother and father to the maternity suites, learning their names, directing questions at them, and listening to their answers. By ensuring that both parents feel involved and important from the very first signs of pregnancy, during childbirth, and afterward, the building blocks can be laid with improved cognitive and socioemotional development of their children. Family well-being provides a foundation for positive parenting and child well-being (Newland, 2015).

Recall Sophia, the pregnant woman described at the beginning of the chapter. Identify the parental roles assumed by Sophia. How might these roles be different from those of her mother when she was Sophia's age?

Genetics

Genetics (the study of heredity and its variations) has implications for all stages of life and all types of diseases. The newborn's or infant's biologic traits, including gender, race, some behavioral traits, and the presence of certain diseases or illnesses are directly linked to genetic inheritance. New technologies in molecular biology and biochemistry have led to a better understanding of the mechanisms involved in hereditary transmission, including those associated with genetic disorders. These advances are leading to better diagnostic tests and better management options.

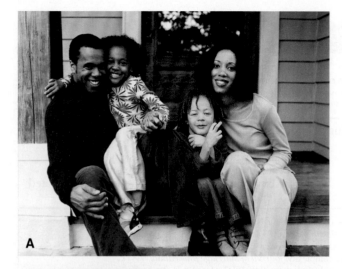

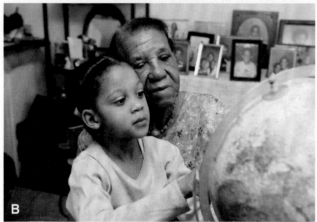

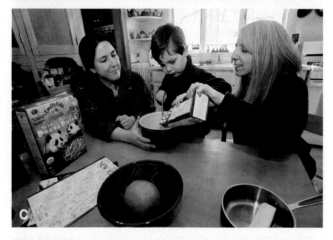

FIGURE 1.3 Nurses must take into account family dynamics when providing health care. There are many different family structures, and they influence the client's needs. **A.** The traditional nuclear family is composed of two parents and their biologic or adopted children. **B.** The extended family includes the nuclear family plus other family members, such as grandparents, aunts, uncles, and cousins. **C.** Gay and lesbian families comprise two people of the same sex sharing a committed relationship with or without children.

Gender

Gender is established when the sex chromosomes join. A person's gender can influence many aspects, such as physical characteristics and personal attributes, attitudes, and behaviors. Some diseases or illnesses are more common in one sex; for example, scoliosis is more common in females and color blindness in males (Snustad, 2015).

Race

Race refers to the physical features that distinguish members of a particular group, such as skin color, bone structure, or blood type. Some physical features that are normal in a particular race may be considered a sign of a disorder in other races. For example, epicanthic folds (the vertical folds of skin that partially or completely cover the inner canthi of the eye) are normal in Asian children, but may occur with Down syndrome or renal agenesis in other races. In addition, certain malformations and diseases are found more commonly in specific races. For example, sickle cell anemia occurs more often in African and Mediterranean population groups, and cystic fibrosis is seen more often in individuals from the Northwestern European population group (Donaldson et al., 2015).

Public awareness is important in educating couples at genetic risk about the benefits of screening programs and proactively seeking preconceptional genetic counseling to consider options that could include preimplantation genetic diagnosis (the use of in-vitro fertilization technology to screen for unaffected embryos). Preimplantation genetic diagnosis was developed as an alternative to prenatal diagnosis for couples with a family history of genetic disease (Cunningham, Goldsmith, & Skirton, 2015). The lack of engagement by ethnic minorities might simply reflect a lack of genetic awareness. Nurses can take the lead in assisting couples to gain the needed awareness that will empower them to make intelligent reproductive decisions.

Society

Society has a major impact on the health of women and their families. Major influences include social roles, socioeconomic status, the media, and the expanding global nature of society. Each of these may influence a person's self-concept, where he or she lives, the lifestyle he or she leads—and, thus, his or her health.

Social Roles

Society often prescribes specific patterns of behaviors: certain behaviors are permitted and others are prohibited. These social roles are often an important factor in the development of self-concept. Social roles influence a person's ideas about himself or herself. Social roles are generally carried out in groups with which the individual has intimate daily contact, such as the family, school, workplace, or peer groups.

Socioeconomic Status

Another dominant influence on health is a person's socioeconomic status, his or her relative position in society. This includes the family's economic, occupational, and educational levels. Low socioeconomic status typically has an adverse influence on an individual's health. Health care costs are continuing to rise, as are health insurance premiums. The family may not be able to afford food, health care, and housing; meals may be unbalanced, erratic, or insufficient. Housing may be overcrowded or have poor sanitation. Some families may not be able to afford or be aware of the importance of preventive care. As a result, they may be exposed to health risks such as lead poisoning or may not be immunized against communicable diseases.

The Media

Social networks and mass media have long influenced human behavior. Until recently, information exchange via various media was slow and limited. Today, given the 24-hour news cycle, information spreads like electronic wildfire. Although everyone is part of a social network, each person is only vaguely aware of his or her friends' friends and the ensuing global network to which all are connected electronically (Oeldorf-Hirsch & Sundar, 2015).

The mass media—the vehicles by which information reaches large numbers of people, e.g., television, the Internet, radio, movies, and newspapers—frequently cover health-related topics, and for some women can be leading sources of information about their health. The media can influence the behavior of women depending on the messages sent. One of the biggest influences is the advertisement of prescription medications on television. The frequent phrase at the end of the ad: "Ask your doctor if this medication is right for you" creates a powerful suggestion for the woman to request that specific medication when she visits her health care provider if her symptoms seem to match those portrayed in the ad.

Issues related to health promotion, contagion, disease diffusion, and general well-being are classic epidemiologic concerns that are addressed by social networks and mass media. Frequently, mass media depict a world in which unhealthy behaviors such as physical aggression, unprotected sex, smoking, and drinking are glamorous and risk free. These unrealistic messages can be detrimental to the health choices of young women. It is essential that nurses address these myths to dispel them.

POVERTY

Poverty is a measurement based on the specific monetary income of a family. The poverty threshold is the dollar amount that the United States Census Bureau uses to determine whether a family is living in poverty. If the individual's or family's income is below the threshold, then that person or family is said to be living in poverty.

Despite the many global economic gains that have been made during the past century, poverty continues to grow and the gap between rich and poor is widening. Major gaps continue to arise between the economic opportunities and status afforded to women and those offered to men. A disproportionate share of the burden of poverty rests on women's shoulders, and undermines their health. However, poverty, particularly for women, is more than monetary deficiency. Women continue to lag behind men in control of cash, credit, and collateral. Other forms of impoverishment may include deficiencies in literacy, education, skills, employment opportunities, mobility, and political representation, as well as pressures on time and energy linked to their responsibilities. These poverty factors may affect a woman's health (WHO, 2015c).

GLOBAL HEALTH FOR WOMEN

The struggle to ensure women's health worldwide is ongoing since a nation's health is directly related to maternal and child health. The poor state of maternal health in developing countries continues to go virtually unnoticed. Women throughout the world, particularly in Asia and Africa, continue to face enormous obstacles in their attempts to receive reproductive health services, including contraception, emergency obstetrical care, and safe abortion services (McFarlane, 2015).

Globally, an estimated 600,000 women die each year from pregnancy-related causes (United Nations International Children's Emergency Fund [UNICEF], 2015), but focusing only on pregnancy-related health issues provides an incomplete understanding of women's health within the global community. Approximately 800 women die every day from preventable causes related to pregnancy and childbirth, with 99% of these women dying in developing countries. Today, more than 50% of maternal deaths occur in just six countries: India, Nigeria, Pakistan, Afghanistan, Ethiopia, and Democratic Republic of the Congo (WHO, 2015d). In developing countries, the five major direct causes of maternal death are hemorrhage, sepsis, gestational hypertension, unsafe abortion, and obstructed labor. The four major direct causes of maternal death in the United States are hypertension (preeclampsia and eclampsia), hemorrhage, placenta previa, and abortions (WHO, 2015d). Women's health and well-being depend on many broader issues that are economic, political, and social in nature. These important factors are often ignored, but adverse effects of women's ill health cut across the economic layers of all societies, rich and poor.

Skewed perceptions, attitudes, and practices toward women persist around the world. They are not limited to the underdeveloped and developing worlds. Regrettably, women in developed countries also suffer from gender bias. A great variance in women's salaries compared with those of men and a reluctance to politically empower women are some of the examples. All over the world, major disparities remain between female and male access to education, employment, and salaries. Although women are the world's main food producers and their working hours are longer than those of men, women earn only 10% of the world's income and own less than 1% of property worldwide. Women comprise nearly two thirds of the world's 800 million illiterate adults. Even in regions with high rates of female literacy, women's wages continue to be lower than those of men, even for work of equal value. These discrepancies are not based on the issue of competence, but on bias (United Nations, 2016).

The world leaders who attend the Global Summit of Women in 2015 will agree to continue to promote gender equality and eliminate still-prevalent gender discrimination. They agreed to explore ways women can (1) reshape the business world, (2) reengineer communities, (3) redefine global leadership, (4) guarantee the free and equal right of women to own and inherit property, (5) recreate sustainable futures, (6) expand women's economic opportunities globally, and (7) restore peace worldwide (GlobeWomen, 2015).

Dramatic improvements in health have been achieved worldwide since the early 1990s. Moving forward will require collective global action—a daunting task given the current climate of global reproductive health politics and international economic insecurity. Even so, women have never shied away from a challenge. Global collaboration, policy action, resources, leadership, research, and evidence are needed to move forward to improve health for all women and their families.

Current successes could be explained by scientific advances delivered by health systems, economic growth, and expanded access to education and health services. However, ongoing poverty, low educational opportunities for girls, and poor public health decisions still prevent about a billion people in low-income and middle-income countries from fully sharing in these health gains.

Nevertheless, progress for women verses men has been slow. An example is the poor state of girls' health in India and China, the only two countries in the world where girls are more likely than boys to die before the age of 5. The poor progress in these countries can be explained by female infanticide and discrimination against girls when it comes to receiving vaccinations, medical care for acute illnesses, and adequate nutrition (WHO, 2015e).

Healthy People 2020's goal is to "improve public health and strengthen United States national security through global disease detection, response, prevention, and control strategies (USDHHS, 2015a)." The health of the United States population can be affected by public health threats or events around the world. As the world and its economies become increasingly globalized, including extensive international travel and commerce, it is essential to think about health in a global context. Rarely a week goes by without a headline about the emergence of an infectious disease or other health threat somewhere in the world. Globally, the rates of mortality from "lifestyle" conditions such as diabetes, obesity, heart disease, mental illness, substance abuse, and injuries are growing. The world community needs to work together to develop strategies to confront major health threats.

Improving women's health globally must be grounded in the principles of human rights and gender equality. Applied in a culturally sensitive manner, nurses must promote the empowerment of women in making their own health-related decisions to improve their overall health. A key to changing women's lifestyle behaviors and allowing them to make informed choices is for nurses to facilitate and partner with all women to access health information and increase their knowledge. Recognizing that all women are vital and equal members of society may finally lead to a long overdue reduction in worldwide maternal morbidity and mortality, decreased rates of human immunodeficiency virus/acquired immunodeficiency syndrome (HIV/AIDS) transmission, and an end to violence against women on a truly global scale.

HOMELESSNESS

Families with children are the fastest-growing segment of the homeless population. Homeless families commonly are victims of violence and may have mental health challenges. Homelessness occurs in large urban areas and midsize cities as well as suburban and rural areas.

Homelessness can have a negative impact on health and well-being in numerous ways, including:

- Mental health issues such as anxiety, depression, or aggressive behavior
- Chronic health problems and injuries
- Premature death and disability
- Nutritional deficiencies, affecting fetal growth and development
- Behaviors such as illegal substance use or unprotected sex with multiple partners
- Limited access to health care services such as preventive care, prenatal care, or dental care

Violence

Violence can occur in any setting and can involve anyone. Violence against women is a major public health concern with long-term health and social consequences—it affects thousands of lives and costs the health care system millions of dollars. Globally, 603 million women live in countries where intimate partner violence is not yet considered a crime. Up to 70% of women in the world report having experienced physical and/or sexual violence at some point in their lifetime (United Nations, 2016a). Violence affects families, women, and children of all ages, ethnic backgrounds, races, educational levels, and socioeconomic levels. Pregnancy is often a time when physical abuse starts or escalates, resulting in poor outcomes for the mother and the baby. The nurse is responsible for assessing for and following up on any abuse.

Violence in the home environment, known as intimate partner violence, affects many lives in the United States. The U.S. Bureau of Justice Office on Violence against Women (2015) estimates that over 1 million violent crimes are committed by former spouses, boyfriends, or girlfriends each year; about 85% of the victims are women. This violence is known as intimate partner abuse, family violence, wife beating, battering, marital abuse, or partner abuse, but regardless of the term used, its effects are widespread. Violence against women of any type can lead to a multitude of health consequences, including physical, reproductive, and psychological (Davies et al., 2015).

Nurses serve their clients best not by trying to rescue them, but by helping them build on their strengths and providing support, thereby empowering them to help themselves. All nurses need to include a screening tool like "RADAR" in every client visit (Bartlett Regional Hospital, n.d.; U.S. Prevention Services Task Force [USPSTF], 2015; Box 1.3).

Community

Community encompasses a broad range of concepts, from the nation where a person lives down to a particular neighborhood or group. The surrounding community affects many aspects of a person's health and general welfare. The quality of life within the community has a great influence on an individual's ability to develop and become a functional member of society. Community influences include the school, which is a community by itself, and peer groups. The support and assistance offered to women and their families from other areas of the community, such as school programs and community centers, can improve the individual's overall health and well-being.

Culture

Culture is a view of the world and a set of traditions that are used by a specific social group and are transmitted to the next generation. It plays a critical role with women and their families. A person's culture influences not only socialization but also his or her experiences related to health and specific health practices (Aggleton, Parker, & Thomas, 2015). Culture is a complex phenomenon involving many components, such as beliefs, values, language, time, personal space, and view of the world, all of which shape a person's actions and behavior. Individuals learn these patterns of cultural behaviors from their family and community through a process called *enculturation*, which involves acquiring knowledge and internalizing values. Culture is learned first in the family, then in school, and then in the community and other social organizations. Culture influences every aspect of development and is reflected in childbearing and child-rearing beliefs and practices designed to promote healthy adaptation (Galanti, 2015).

With today's changing demographic patterns, nurses must be able to assimilate cultural knowledge into their interventions, so they can care for culturally diverse women, children, and families. Nurses must be aware of the wide range of cultural traditions, values, and ethics. **Cultural competence** is the ability to apply knowledge about a client's culture so that the health care provided can be adapted to meet his or her needs. Cultural competence refers to the process by which individuals and systems respond respectfully and effectively to people of all cultures, languages, classes, races, ethnic backgrounds, disabilities, religions, genders, sexual orientation, and other diversity factors in a manner that recognizes, affirms, and values the worth of individuals, families, and communities, and protects and preserves the dignity of each. Nurses need to attain the knowledge, skills, and attitudes to provide effective care for diverse populations (Blanchet Garneau & Pepin, 2015). Nurses need to learn about general cultural groups, ethnicity, and health practices; how they affect women and their health; and the changing demographics of the population. This will help them view culture as a point of congruence rather than as a potential source of conflict with clients.

BOX 1.3

RADAR

R—Routinely screen every client for abuse.
A—Affirm feelings and assess abuse.
D—Document your findings.
A—Assess for your client's safety.
R—Review options and make referrals.

Adapted from Bartlett Regional Hospital. (n.d.). *Domestic violence assessment tool.* Retrieved from http://www.hospitalsoup.com/public/brhdvprotocol.pdf; U.S. Prevention Services Task Force [USPSTF]. (2015). *Screening for intimate partner violence and abuse of elderly and vulnerable adults: U.S. Prevention Services Task Force recommendation statement.* Available at: http://www.uspreventiveservicestaskforce.org/uspstf12/ipvelder/ipvelderfinalrs.htm; and Caring Unlimited.(2015). *Domestic abuse: Utilizing RADAR.* Available at: http://www.caring-unlimited.org/what-is-domestic-violence/for-service-providers/for-mental-health-and-substance-abuse-practitioners-social-workers/utilizing-radar

Cultural Groups

A society typically includes dominant and minority groups. The dominant group, often the largest group, is the group that has the greatest authority to control values and sanctions of the society (Phillips et al., 2015). As a result, the dominant or majority culture may have the largest impact on health. The minority cultural groups may remain in their own communities and maintain some of their traditions and values while mainstreaming into American society. A culture may contain many subcultures, and geographic differences also can occur; for example, Hispanics living in New York may be quite different from Hispanics living in Florida. Being aware of these differences is essential in providing culturally competent care. The more knowledge a nurse has about a specific culture, the more accurate and complete the cultural assessment will be. For example, if nurses are not aware that many Hispanics use traditional healers such as *curandros, masjistas, sobodoes, y(j)erberos,* and *esperititas,* they will not know how to ask specific and appropriate questions about the individual's use of these alternative practitioners and their therapies (Taber, Leyva, & Persoskie, 2015).

Nurses need to be aware of the health care values and practices that are passed along from one generation to the next. For example, a belief in folk healers relates to how the culture interprets illness and health. Some of these parts of the culture may have major influences on an individual's health. Table 1.2 highlights some major cultural groups and their common health beliefs and practices.

Take Note!

Nurses can have a lifelong influence on an individual's perceptions of health and use of health services. By understanding how a woman's and her family's culture influences their health practices, nurses can enhance the family's traditional practices, and different cultural practices can become sources of strength rather than areas of conflict.

Take Note!

The health status of a newborn may affect his or her long-term health and development.

Nutrition

Nutrition provides the body with the calories and nutrients required to sustain life and promote growth, as well as the essentials required to maintain health and prevent illness. Nutritional deficiencies or excesses are common problems in the United States, as evidenced by the persistent problem of iron-deficiency anemia and the increasing incidence of obesity (DeBruyne, Pinna, & Whitney, 2015). Inadequate food intake, social and cultural food practices or habits that may be nutritionally unsound, the availability of processed and nutritionally inadequate foods, lack of nutrition education in homes and schools, and the presence of illness that interferes with the ingestion, digestion, and absorption of food are factors that can affect an individual's nutrition.

At no other time of life is nutrition more important than during fetal development and infancy. Adequate nutrition is essential for tissue formation, neurologic development, bone growth, and overall long-term health. During pregnancy, a woman needs additional calories to support fetal growth and development as well as to support her own needs, and an adequate intake of folic acid is important to prevent neural tube defects (Fig. 1.4). Nutrition and its effects on health status are integrated throughout this text; see Chapter 11.

Lifestyle Choices

Lifestyle choices that affect an individual's health include eating; exercise; use of tobacco, drugs, or alcohol; and methods of coping with stress. Most health problems that arise today are due to an individual's lifestyle. Poor lifestyle choices made early in life can affect the quality of life as an individual ages. Also these poor choices affect the increasing incidence of chronic disease. The same concept of making poor choices can be applied to pregnant women and the health and well-being of the infant. Maintaining a healthy level of activity through exercise and hobbies is important for adults and children.

Environmental Exposure

Pregnant women are exposed to many and varied environmental chemicals. Scientific evidence documents that widespread exposure to environmental chemicals at levels that are encountered in daily life can have an adverse impact on reproductive and developmental health across the lifespan (Yin-Hsiu et al., 2015).

In utero, the fetus can be affected by the lack of maternal nutrition, environmental chemical exposures, maternal infections, or maternal use of alcohol, tobacco, and drugs. Nurses caring for pregnant women should be aware of the risks to the fetus posed by certain drugs, chemicals, and dietary agents, as well as maternal illnesses. These agents, known as teratogens, may be linked to preterm births and birth defects in children. Not all drugs or agents have fetal effects, however, and research is necessary to identify the correlations between teratogens and other variables.

Stress and Coping

Disasters such as the terrorist attacks of September 11, 2001, the killings at Columbine High School, Super

TABLE 1.2	BELIEFS AND PRACTICES OF SELECTED CULTURAL GROUPS
Cultural Group	**Beliefs and Practices Affecting Maternal and Children's Health**
African Americans	View of health as harmony with nature, illness as disruption in harmony Use of folk healing and home remedies common View of pregnancy as a state of wellness Emotional support during labor commonly from other women, primarily the woman's own mother Liberal use of oil on newborn's and infant's scalp and skin Belief in illnesses as natural (due to natural forces person hasn't protected self against) and unnatural (due to person or spirit) Illness commonly associated with pain Postpartum practices for the infant may include the use of a bellyband or a coin placed on top of the infant's umbilicus to prevent umbilical hernias Pain and suffering inevitable; relief achieved through prayers and laying on of hands
Asian Americans	Use of complementary modalities along with Western health care practices View of life as a cycle with everything connected to health Usually attended by a female relative and tend to be quiet and sedate during labor and birth Health viewed as a balance between the forces of yang and yin Illness is the disharmony of yin and yang Yang—energy outside of body where matter is dynamic, external, upward, ascending, and brilliant Yin—energy inside of body where matter is static, internal, downward, descending, dull, regressive, and hypoactive During postpartum, women don't expose themselves to cold air or bathe themselves for the first month to avoid exposure to illness Respect for authority emphasized Women are very modest and may insist on a female health care provider for maternity care View of pregnancy as a natural process and happy time for woman Little involvement of the father during labor; quiet, stoic appearance of woman during labor
Arab Americans	Women subordinate to men; young individuals subordinate to older persons Family loyalty is primary. Women value modesty and want their bodies covered during examinations. Procreation is regarded as the purpose of marriage, thus high fertility rates are favored. During labor, women openly express pain through facial expressions, verbalizations, and body movements. Mothers may be reluctant to bathe after childbirth because of beliefs that air gets into the mother and causes illness. Good health associated with eating properly, consuming nutritious foods, and fasting to cure disease Illness is due to inadequate diet, shifts in hot and cold, exposure of stomach while sleeping, emotional or spiritual distress, and "evil eye." Little emphasis on preventive care Breast-feeding often delayed for 2 to 3 days after birth. Cleanliness important for prayer
Hispanic Americans	Family is important: father is the source of strength, wisdom, and self-confidence; mother is the caretaker and decision-maker for health; children are persons who will continue the family and culture. During the period of *la cuerentena* (first 40 days after childbirth) women are thought to be susceptible to cold, so many will avoid taking showers, sitz baths, tub baths, washing their hair, or being exposed to cold air. Likely to be very vocal during labor by crying or frequently making loud screams Newborn protection from the "evil eye" Health as God's will, maintainable with a balance of hot and cold food intake Freedom from pain indicative of good health; pain tolerated stoically due to belief that it is God's will Folk medicine practices and prayers, herbal teas, and poultices for illness treatment

(continued)

TABLE 1.2	BELIEFS AND PRACTICES OF SELECTED CULTURAL GROUPS (continued)
Cultural Group	**Beliefs and Practices Affecting Maternal and Children's Health**
Native Americans	Place high value on family and tribe; respect for elders Family as an extended network providing care for newborns and children View of pregnancy as a normal and natural process; entire family may be present at birth Use of food to celebrate life events and in healing and religious ceremonies Health as harmony with nature; illness due to disharmony, evil spirits Restoration of physical, mental, and spiritual balance through healing ceremonies

Adapted from Edelman, C. L., & Mandle, C. L. (2014). *Health promotion throughout the lifespan* (8th ed.). St. Louis, MO: Mosby Elsevier; Krassen Covan, E. (2015). Maternal health practice: A mismatch of knowledge and expectations. *Health Care for Women International, 36*(1), 1–2; Vidaeff, A. C., Kerrigan, A. J., & Monga, M. (2015). Cross-cultural barriers to health care. *Southern Medical Journal, 108*(1), 1–4; Joshi, S. V., Reicherter, D., Pumariega, A. J., & Roberts, L. W. (2015). Multicultural and ethical considerations in American medicine. In: L. W. Roberts & D. Reicherter (Eds.). *Professionalism and ethics in medicine* (pp. 39–56). New York, NY: Springer; and Purnell, L. D. (2013). *Guide to culturally competent health care* (3rd ed.). Philadelphia, PA: F. A. Davis.

Storm Sandy in New Jersey, or Hurricane Katrina in New Orleans can have a significant impact on the well-being of women, children, and families. Stressors such as war, terrorism, violence, and natural disasters may decrease a person's coping ability. Exposure to traumatic events and violence may have long-term effects on an individual's psychosocial development and status.

Exposure to stress is not limited to disasters or traumatic events, however. Stress can also include areas such as inadequate finances, family crises, inadequate support systems, or domestic violence. Like disasters and traumatic events, the effects of these stressors can dramatically affect the health status of a woman or family.

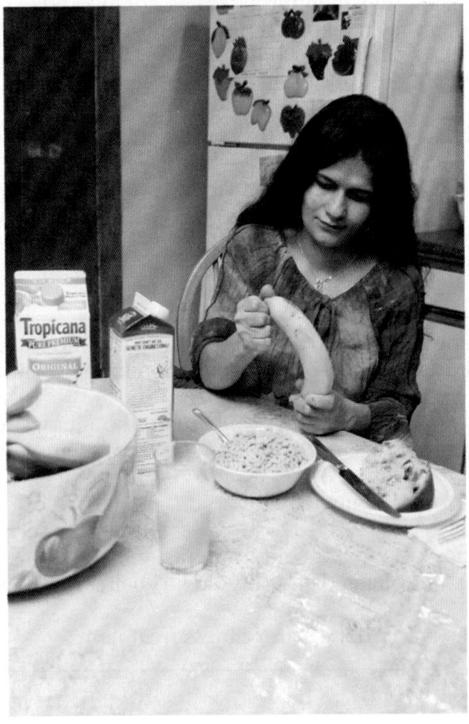

Recall Sophia, the 38-year-old pregnant woman who has come to the prenatal clinic for a visit. While talking with the nurse, Sophia mentions that her children are very involved in activities. She says, "My husband is busy at work, so I do most of the running around. Sometimes I feel like the people at the drive-through know me by name! My husband helps out on the weekends, but during the week, it's all me." What factors may be influencing Sophia's health? How might these factors be influencing the health of her family?

FIGURE 1.4 A pregnant client is eating a healthy meal to ensure adequate nutrition.

Health Care Cost Containment

The health care system functions within a market setting, offering goods and services that carry a cost to health care consumers and clients. There is no disagreement that health care costs have inflated beyond the pocketbooks of most Americans. The increase in costs has been attributed to such factors as technological advances, inflation, increased needs of a growing older adult population, longer life spans, and the cost of medical liability. The advent of managed care has led to a trend of attempting to reduce health care costs, but has not been very effective (Hall et al., 2015). The purpose of managed care is to achieve cost control by assigning set fees for services, monitoring the need for procedures such as tests and surgical operations, and stressing preventive care. One such mechanism is utilization review, which is employed to limit reimbursement of medical care that is determined to be medically necessary. These efforts have led to shorter hospital stays and increased awareness on the part of nurses about the costs of supplies and services. The overall challenge is to maintain the quality of care while reducing its cost. For example, if a pregnant woman with diabetes needs to go to an endocrinologist, she has very little choice except to purchase the services needed or go without care. In today's managed care environment, the woman will need to go through her primary health care provider or "gatekeeper" to receive a referral to a specialist. Often she must trust her primary provider to make that choice for her instead of making that decision on her own.

Although cost containment is important to restrain health care spending, such efforts should not reduce the quality or safety of care delivered. Preventive care (remember the old saying "an ounce of prevention is worth a pound of cure") has been shown to lower costs significantly. Mammograms, cervical cancer screenings, prenatal care, smoking cessation programs, and immunizations are a few examples of preventive care that yield positive outcomes and reduce overall health care costs. Using technological advances to diagnose and treat diseases early saves lives as well as money. Although the ACA expands insurance coverage to cover preventive screenings, there are still differences in availability of this coverage across many states (Sabik, Tarazi, & Bradley, 2015).

Nurses can be leaders in providing quality care within a limited-resource environment by emphasizing to their clients the importance of making healthy lifestyle and food choices, seeking early interventions for minor problems before they become major ones, and learning about health-related issues that affect them. Thus, they can select the best option for themselves and their families. Prevention services and health education are the cornerstones of delivering quality maternal, newborn, and women's health care.

Access to Health Care

The health care system continues to change. In the United States, changes in the health care system result from pressures coming from many directions. These changes reflect shifts in social and economic realities and the results of the biomedical and technological progress that has been made over the past several decades. The effects are felt by everyone who seeks health care in any form. The system of providing medical care in a high-tech environment has changed to providing health care in an environment with limited resources and access to services. Ways to allocate our limited health care resources continue to be the focus.

A major factor that affects access to care is health insurance. People without health insurance typically cannot afford to seek health care for maintenance and prevention interventions. The "working poor" may not earn enough money to afford health insurance or medical care, and part-time workers do not always receive health insurance benefits. In most states, a man and a woman of the same age and health status will be charged different

rates for exactly the same individual health insurance policy, a practice called *gender rating*. Women pay a much higher health insurance rate for the same coverage than do men in the United States—an inequality that has lessened with the full enactment of the ACA in 2014 (Starrs, 2015).

The ACA, which began fully in 2014, aims to make health insurance accessible to many Americans previously without health insurance. It obligates health insurance agencies to cover a wide range of preventive health services at no cost to the person. Ideally, in the future, people will start to look at their health care providers as partners in wellness, rather than providers who treat disease.

Preventive Care Focus

The emphasis on cost reduction has also led to an emphasis on preventive care and services. The ACA of 2014 has added preventive services for women. Research suggests that better access to preventive services can be maintained at a reasonable cost to the health care system, and that some services can lower the health care costs. For the ACA to be truly transformational for women's health, its promise to remove cost barriers to well-woman visits must be realized fully (Fitzgerald et al., 2015). Anticipatory guidance is vital during each health contact with women and their families. Education of the family includes everything from keeping the home safe to ways to prevent illness.

The Continuum of Care Emphasis

A *continuum of care* strategy is cost effective and provides efficient and effective services. This continuum extends from acute care settings such as hospitals to outpatient settings such as ambulatory care clinics, primary care offices, rehabilitative units, community care settings, long-term facilities, and homes. For example, a hospital stay is now integrated into a continuum that allows the client to complete therapy at home or at other community settings, while reentering the hospital for short periods for specific treatments or illnesses (Stanhope & Lancaster, 2014). The ACA offers provisions that the health care delivery system be person-centered with individual control; improves quality, and integrates care across settings and providers. It stresses expansion of community-based services and coordination of care while the person transitions from one setting to another to meet changing health care needs (Mansur & Thompson, 2015).

Improvements in Diagnosis and Treatments

Because of the tremendous improvements that have been made in technology and biomedicine, disorders and diseases are being diagnosed and treated earlier. The 1990s witnessed the establishment of a remarkable and productive connection between genetics and various pathophysiologic processes. For example, female fetuses with congenital adrenal hyperplasia, a genetic disorder resulting in a steroid enzyme deficiency that can lead to disfiguring anatomic abnormalities, are beginning to receive treatment before birth. In addition, many genetic defects are being identified so counseling and treatment may occur early. With these improved diagnoses and treatments, nurses may now be caring for individuals who have survived situations that once would have been fatal, who are living well beyond their life expectancy for a specific illness, or who are functioning with chronic disabilities (Dumas & Turner, 2015). For example, at one time, women with congenital heart disease did not live long enough to become pregnant. However, with new surgical techniques to correct the defects, many of these women survive and become pregnant, progressing through their pregnancy without significant problems.

Although positive and exciting, these advances and trends also pose new challenges for the health care community. For example, as health care for premature newborns improves and survival rates increase, the incidence of long-term chronic conditions such as respiratory airway dysfunction or developmental delays has also increased. As a result, nurses are faced with caring for clients at all stages along the health–illness continuum.

Empowerment of Health Care Consumers

As a result of the influence of managed care, the focus on prevention, a more educated population, and technological advances, individuals and families have taken on increased responsibility for their own health. Health care consumerism adds an important voice to the current United States health care system reform, as people become informed, proactive, and demand choices in the delivery of their health care. Health care consumers want to play a greater role in managing health and illness. Families want information about illnesses and they want to participate in making decisions about treatment options. As client advocates who value family-centered care, nurses are instrumental in promoting this empowerment. To do this, the nurse should respect the family's views and concerns, address all issues and concerns, consider the family members to be important participants, and always include the woman and her family in the decision-making process.

BARRIERS TO HEALTH CARE

Women are major consumers of health care services, in many cases arranging not only their own care but also that of family members. Compared with men, women

have more health problems, longer life spans, and more significant reproductive health needs (McFarlane, 2015). Access to care can be jeopardized by lower incomes and greater responsibilities (juggling work and family). Lack of finances or transportation, geographic misdistribution of health care providers, no babysitters, language or cultural barriers, inconvenient clinic hours, and the poor attitudes of health care workers often discourage clients from seeking health care (Tucker Edmonds, Mogul, & Shea, 2015).

Finances

The existence of financial barriers is one of the most important factors that limit care. Childbirth is the leading reason for hospitalization in the United States. For both private insurers and Medicaid, hospital maternity and newborn charges exceed those for any other condition. In United States hospitals, vaginal and cesarean births are costly. Many women have limited or no health insurance and cannot afford to pay for maternity care. Compared with other racial and ethnic groups, African American women tend to be younger, more likely to have a surgical birth, experience preterm births, to stay longer in the hospital, and to incur higher Medicaid costs. African American women experience a higher rate of adverse pregnancy outcomes than White or Hispanic women. Racial disparities in adverse pregnancy outcomes not only represent potential preventable human suffering, but also avoidable economic costs (Catov et al., 2015). Although Medicaid covers prenatal care in most states, the paperwork and enrollment process can be so overwhelming that many women do not register. Many families do not have health insurance, do not have enough insurance to cover the services they need, or cannot pay for services.

Transportation

Getting to and from appointments can be challenging for clients who do not drive or own a car or cannot use public transportation (if there is public transportation in the area). Prenatal care has the potential to improve perinatal outcomes and decrease health disparities, yet many women struggle with access to care. It can be difficult for these clients to attend all recommended prenatal health care visits, especially if they have other small children who must be taken along on a visit. These challenges can reduce the adherence to scheduled appointments and follow-up.

Language and Culture

Language is how people communicate with each other to increase their understanding or knowledge. If a health care worker cannot speak the same language as the client or does not have a trained interpreter available, a barrier is created. The client's complaints can be misinterpreted or ignored or their significance can be misconstrued. The language barrier might prevent the client from accessing the necessary care, such as prenatal care or preventive care.

Knowledge barriers (e.g., lack of understanding of the importance of prenatal care or child health promotion), low health literacy, gender attitudes, health beliefs, retention of information, and spiritual barriers (e.g., some forms of treatment are proscribed by religions) also pose barriers to receiving health care.

Low Health Literacy

Health literacy is defined as the degree to which individuals have the capacity to obtain, process, and understand basic health information and services needed to make appropriate health decisions (Health and Medicine Division (HMD), 2016). It also includes the ability to understand instructions on prescription drug bottles, appointment slips, education brochures, health care provider's directions, consent forms, and the ability to negotiate complex health care systems.

Vulnerable populations for low health literacy include older adults, immigrants, minorities, and low income populations. Low health literacy is a major source of economic inefficiency in the U.S. health system. It is estimated that the cost of it to the U.S. economy is approximately $106–238 billion annually (CDC, 2015f).

Low health literacy is associated with poor health outcomes, increased emergency room visits, higher morbidity and mortality rates, and less use of preventive health services. Nurses have the potential to impact and change these outcomes. Nurses can use screening tools to assess a client's health literacy in addition to identifying characteristics that indicate low health literacy. Having clients repeat the instructions verbally and having them demonstrate the specific treatment procedure needed for their continued care is essential. Simply handing a client a piece of paper with written instructions for a vital medication or treatment procedure is not advocating for that client (French, 2015).

Health Care Delivery System

The health care delivery system itself can create barriers. Fifty-eight percent of employed families with insurance are covered by some type of managed health care plan or health maintenance organization, but millions of Americans remain uninsured (Holden, Chen, & Dagher, 2015). This prospective payment system based on diagnosis-related groups limits the amounts of health care the family may receive. This also includes Medicaid reimbursements. As a result of cost-containment efforts, the trend is to discharge clients as soon as possible from the hospital and to deliver care in the home or through community-based services. Postpartum hospital stays are often shorter than 48 hours following a vaginal birth; thus, most postpartum care takes place in the home and the community. Home visits by nurses to provide support at home for mothers and infants is needed for high risk families to prevent health problems from becoming chronic with long-term effects (Aston et al., 2015). Although overall insurance plans may improve access to preventive services, they may limit access to specialty care, which greatly affects clients with chronic or long-term illnesses.

Clinic hours must meet the needs of the clients, not the health care providers who work there. Evening or weekend hours might be needed to meet the schedules of working clients. Clinic personnel should evaluate the availability and accessibility of the services they offer.

Unfortunately, some health care workers exhibit negative attitudes toward poor or culturally diverse families, and this could deter these clients from seeking health care. Long delays, hurried examinations, and rude comments by staff discourage clients from returning.

Consider This

I was a 17-year-old pregnant migrant worker needing prenatal care. Although my English wasn't good, I was able to show the receptionist my "big belly" and ask for services. All the receptionist seemed interested in was a Social Security number and health insurance—neither of which I had. She proceeded to ask me personal questions concerning who the father was and commented on how young I looked. The receptionist then "ordered" me in a loud voice to sit down and wait for an answer by someone in the back, but never contacted anyone that I could see. It seemed to me like all eyes were on me while I found an empty seat in the waiting room. After sitting there quietly for over an hour without any attention or answer, I left.

Thoughts: Why did she leave before receiving any health care service? What must she have been feeling during her wait? Would you come back to this clinic again? Why or why not?

LEGAL AND ETHICAL ISSUES IN MATERNAL, NEWBORN, AND WOMEN'S HEALTH CARE

Law and ethics are interrelated and affect all of nursing. Professional nurses must understand their scope of practice, standards of care, institutional or agency policies, and state laws. All nurses are responsible for knowing current information regarding ethics and laws related to their practice.

The AWHONN (2009) publishes their *Standards for Professional Nursing Practice in the Care of Women and Newborns*, which are summarized below:

- *Standard I: Assessment*—The RN collects health data about women and newborns in the context of women-centered and family-centered care.
- *Standard II: Diagnosis*—The RN formulates nursing diagnoses by analyzing assessment data to identify and differentiate normal physiologic and developmental transitions from pathophysiologic variations and other clinical issues.
- *Standard III: Outcomes Identification*—The RN individualizes expected outcomes for women and newborns.
- *Standard IV: Planning*—The RN develops a plan of care that includes interventions and alternatives to attain expected outcomes for women and newborns.
- *Standard V: Implementation*—The RN implements the interventions identified in the women's or newborn's plan of care.
- *Standard VI: Evaluation*—The RN evaluates the progress of women and newborns toward attainment of expected outcomes.
- *Standard VII: Quality of Practice*—The RN systematically evaluates and implements measures to improve the quality, safety, and effectiveness of nursing practice.
- *Standard VIII: Education*—The RN acquires and maintains knowledge and competencies that reflect current EBP.
- *Standard IX: Professional Practice Evaluation*—The RN evaluates his or her own nursing practice in relation to current evidence-based care information, professional standards and guidelines, statues, rules, and regulations.
- *Standard X: Ethics*—The RN's decisions and actions on behalf of women, fetuses, and newborns are determined in an ethical manner and guided by an ethical decision-making process.
- *Standard XI: Collegiality*—The RN interacts with and contributes to the professional development of peers, colleagues, and other health care providers.
- *Standard XII: Collaboration and Communication*—The RN collaborates and communicates with women, their families, the community, and other health care providers in providing safe care.
- *Standard XIII: Research*—The RN generates and/or integrates evidence to validate interprofessional knowledge in providing care to women and newborns.
- *Standard XIV: Resources and Technology*—The RN considers factors related to safety, effectiveness, technology, and expense in providing care to women and newborns.
- *Standard XV: Leadership*—The RN should serve as a role model, change agent, consultant, and mentor to all women, their families, and other health care professionals.

Several areas are of particular importance to the health care of women and their families. These include abortion, substance abuse, intrauterine therapy, maternal–fetal conflict, stem cell research, umbilical cord blood banking, informed consent, and confidentiality.

Abortion

Abortion has been a legal medical procedure in the United States for more than three decades, yet it continues to be a hotly debated and volatile legal, social, and political issue. It was an issue even before *Roe v. Wade,* the 1973 Supreme Court decision that legalized abortion. The Supreme Court ruled that a woman, in consultation with her health care provider, has a constitutionally protected right to have an abortion in early stages of pregnancy—that is, before viability—free from government interference. Nearly half of pregnancies among American women are unintended, and about 4 in 10 of these are terminated by abortion. Twenty-two percent of all pregnancies (excluding miscarriages) end in abortion (Guttmacher Institute, 2015).

Every time abortion is debated on the national level, the Hyde Amendment is cited. Named after its author, Rep Henry Hyde (R-Illinois), the Hyde Amendment places limits on federally funded abortions. By denying abortion coverage to low-income women on Medicaid, the Hyde Amendment has limited choices of low-income women regarding their reproductive rights.

Medical and surgical modalities are available to terminate a pregnancy, depending on how far the pregnancy has developed. A medical abortion by taking mifepristone and prostaglandins is well established and safe when performed as per guidelines with a success rate of up to 97%. A surgical intervention can be performed up to 14 weeks' gestation; a medical intervention can be performed up to 9 weeks' gestation (Hickey & Moore, 2015).

In September, 2000, the United States Food and Drug Administration approved mifepristone to be marketed in the United States as an alternative to surgical abortion. Medication abortion using mifepristone or a similar medication accounted for 38% of all nonhospital abortions, and about one quarter of abortions before 9 weeks' gestation (Guttmacher Institute, 2015). All women undergoing abortion need emotional support, a stable environment in which to recover, and nonjudgmental care throughout the process.

The issue of abortion separates people into two camps: pro-choice and pro-life. The pro-choice group supports the right of any woman to make decisions about her reproductive functions based on her own moral and ethical beliefs. The pro-life group feels strongly that abortion is murder and deprives the fetus of the basic right to life. Both sides will continue to debate this very emotional issue for years to come.

Abortion is a complex issue, and the controversy is not only in the public arena: many nurses struggle with the conflict between their personal convictions and their professional duty. Nurses are taught to be supportive client advocates and to interact with a nonjudgmental attitude under all circumstances even when personal and political views differ from those of their clients. With all the advances in abortion care, this points toward greater nursing involvement. Although this bodes well for woman-centered care, the burden on nurses is likely to increase incrementally. This may have an adverse effect on the affective attributes or emotions that those nurses possess (McLemore, Levi, & James, 2015).

Nurses need to clarify their personal values and beliefs on this issue and must be able to provide unbiased care before assuming responsibility for clients who might be in a position to consider abortion. Their decision to care for or refuse to care for such clients affects staff unity, influences staffing decisions, and challenges the ethical concept of duty (King et al., 2015).

The ANA's Code of Ethics for Nurses upholds the nurse's right to refuse to care for a client undergoing an abortion if the nurse ethically opposes the procedure (Fowler & Lachman, 2015). Nurses need to make their values and beliefs known to their managers before the situation occurs so that alternative staffing arrangements can be made. Open communication and acceptance of the personal beliefs of others can promote a comfortable working environment.

Substance Abuse

Substance abuse for any person is a problem, but when it involves a pregnant woman, substance abuse can cause preterm birth, placenta abruption, poor weight gain, low birth weight, stillbirth, spontaneous abortion, a variety of behavioral and cognitive problems in exposed children, and fetal injury, and thus has legal and ethical implications. Many state laws require evidence of prenatal drug exposure to be reported, which may lead to charges of negligence and child endangerment against the pregnant woman. It has been found that incarceration or threat of it has no effect in reducing cases of alcohol or drug abuse. Laws that criminalize drug use during pregnancy usually deter women from seeking prenatal care that can provide them access to appropriate counseling, referral, and monitoring (AWHONN, 2015). This punitive approach to fetal injury raises ethical and legal questions about the degree of government control that is appropriate in the interests of child safety. All pregnant women and women of childbearing age should be screened periodically for alcohol, tobacco, and prescription and illicit drug use. Nurses should employ a flexible approach to the care of women who have substance use problems, and they should encourage the use of all available community resources. Women should be counseled about the risks of preconception, antepartum, and postpartum substance abuse in a calm, nonjudgmental manner by nurses (AWHONN, 2015). Pregnant women who abuse substances should be afforded access to preventive, supportive, and recovery services that meet their special needs. The nurse can be instrumental in facilitation referral to community programs for both pregnant and postpartum women who can help ensure their full recovery and better lives for them and their children.

Intrauterine Therapy

Progress in prenatal diagnosis can lead to the diagnosis of severe fetal abnormalities, which previously would have resulted in a fatal outcome or the development of severe disability despite optimal postnatal care. Intrauterine therapy can now be offered in these selected cases and also in the treatment of fetal obstructive uropathy, intrauterine transfusions for fetal anemia, spina bifida repair, and stem cell transplantation. Intrauterine therapy is a procedure that involves opening the uterus during pregnancy, performing a surgery, and replacing the fetus in the uterus. Although the risks to the fetus and the mother are both great, fetal therapy may be used to correct anatomic lesions (Mathis, Raio, & Baud, 2015). Some argue that medical technology should not interfere with nature, and thus this intervention should not take place. Others argue that the surgical intervention improves the child's quality of life. For many people, these are the subjects of debate and intellectual discussion, but for nurses, these procedures may be part of their daily routine.

Nurses play an important supportive role in caring and advocating for clients and their families. As the use of technology grows, situations will surface more frequently that test a nurse's belief system. Encouraging open discussions to address emotional issues and differences of opinion among staff members is healthy and increases tolerance for differing points of view.

Maternal–Fetal Conflict

In maternity nursing, the ethical principles of beneficence and autonomy provide the fundamental framework that guides the management of all pregnant women. Because the fetus also needs to be considered, autonomy can become a complex issue giving rise to what is sometimes called *maternal–fetal conflict*.

Fetal care becomes problematic when what is required to benefit one member of the dyad will cause unacceptable harm to the other. Even when a fetal condition poses no health threat to the mother, caring for the fetal client will always carry some degree of risk to the mother, without direct therapeutic benefit for her. The ethical principles of beneficence (be of benefit) and nonmaleficence (do no harm) can come into conflict.

Because the clients are biologically linked, both, or neither, must be treated alike. It would be unethical to recommend fetal therapy as if it were medically indicated for both clients. Still, given a recommendation for fetal therapy, pregnant women, in most cases, will consent to treatment that promotes fetal health. When pregnant women refuse therapy, health care providers must remember that the ethical injunction against harming one client in order to benefit another is virtually absolute.

The use of court orders to force treatment on pregnant women raises many ethical concerns. Court orders force pregnant women to forfeit their autonomy in ways not required of competent men or nonpregnant women. There is an inconsistency in allowing competent adults to refuse therapy in all cases but pregnancy. The American Congress of Obstetricians and Gynecologists (ACOG) advocates counseling and education to convince a mother to follow her doctor's advice and condemns the use of coercion on a pregnant woman, because this violates the intent of the informed consent process. Faced with a continuing disagreement with a pregnant woman, a physician should turn to an institutional ethics committee. Resorting to the legal system is almost never justified (Campbell, 2015).

Stem Cell Research

The goal of stem cell research is the relief of human suffering, which ethically is good. Benefits of stem cell research include providing therapies for Parkinson's disease, regenerating diseased body tissues, repairing spinal cord injuries, and growing needed organs for transplant.

The therapeutic needs of sick clients, along with the potential benefits of that therapy must be balanced with ensuring rigorous scientific standards and effective consent procedures related to stem cell research. The ethical concerns surrounding stem cell research vary depending on the origin of the stem cells. Adult stem cells are cells found in adults and can replace old cells by reproducing new ones such as blood and liver cells. Bone marrow transplants are examples of the use of adult stem cells in medical therapy. Embryonic stem cells are derived from the inner cell mass of an early embryo. Stem cells, which can grow into any cell type in the body, have been touted as a potential cure for everything from type 1 diabetes to stroke. They are not without controversy, however; embryonic stem cells come from discarded human embryos, but they hold huge promise, too. The controversy is not about whether stem cells should be used, but rather what source of stem cells should be used, and how they are obtained (Devolder, 2015).

The controversy focuses on the use of embryonic stem cells, because the process of obtaining these cells results in the destruction of the embryo. Some people feel that the destruction of the human embryo constitutes the killing of a human being and reject this practice on religious grounds. Views about when life begins and whether the early embryo is considered a person with moral status are at the heart of the ethical deliberations related to the use of embryonic stem cells. Everyone has to decide on the basis of personal values and ethical background.

Umbilical Cord Blood Banking

Umbilical cord blood, the blood remaining in the umbilical cord at birth, can be collected at birth and be a source of stem cells for an individual in need of a bone marrow transplant later in life. The extraordinary scientific and technological advances of contemporary medicine constantly lead toward the introduction of new treatments. Umbilical cord blood is a potential vast source of primitive hematopoietic stem and progenitor cells available for clinical applications. Cord blood can be used as an alternative source for bone marrow transplantation and its use is developing into a new field of treatment for pediatric and adult clients presenting with hematologic disorders, immunologic defects, and specific genetic diseases (Meierrhenry et al., 2015).

Private banks were initially developed to store cord blood stem cells from newborns, for a fee, for potential future use by the same child or a family member if he or she developed disease later in life. Today, public cord blood banks store, for free, stem cells that can be used by anyone needing them, in a manner similar to the way public blood banks work. Umbilical cord banks are a central component, as the providers of umbilical cord tissue, in both medical treatment and scientific research with stem cells. But, whereas the creation of umbilical cord banks is seen as a successful practice, it is perceived as ethically risky by others.

Pregnant women should be aware that stem cells from cord blood cannot currently be used to treat inborn errors of metabolism or other genetic diseases in the same individual from which they were collected because the cord blood would have the same genetic mutation. Cord blood collected from a newborn who later develops childhood leukemia cannot be used to treat that leukemia for much the same reason.

The fact that private cord banks offer their services as "biologic insurance" in order to obtain informed consent from parents (by ensuring that the tissue that will be made available if their child needs it in the future) raises the issue of whether the consent is freely given or given under coercion. Another consideration that must be made in relation to privately owned cord banks has to do with the ownership of the stored umbilical cord. Conflicts between moral principles and economic interests (many physicians own private blood banks) cause dilemmas in the clinical practice of umbilical cord blood storage and use especially in privately owned banks (Guilcher, Fernandez, & Joffe, 2015).

Both ACOG (2012) and the American Academy of Pediatrics (AAP, 2010) have issued statements opposing the use of for-profit banks and criticizing their marketing tactics. Instead, they recommended that parents donate cord blood to public banks, which make it available for free to anyone who needs it. Globally, other organizations have done the same. Private umbilical cord blood banking raises a question of special legal regulation. This practice promises the safe storage of biologic material on the assumption that it may be useful, at a certain moment in future, for its own donor (or for a donor's close family member) for curing serious blood diseases (Elmoazzen & Holovati, 2015). Currently, it is recommended that delaying the clamping and cutting of the umbilical cord constitutes the best EBP. So, cord blood stem cell collection should not alter the timing of umbilical cord clamping. Nurses providing prenatal care to pregnant women need increased awareness and knowledge about options for storage, or "banking," of cord blood and tissue in order to present information to expectant parents that is accurate, evidence-based, and without bias.

Informed Consent

The purpose of **informed consent** in health care is to ensure that client autonomy is respected in decisions about their health care. It is an agreement by a client to undergo an operation or medical treatment or take part in a clinical trial after being informed of and understanding the risks involved. It is a legal document in all 50 states, and stems from the legal and ethical right an individual has to decide what is done to his or her body, and from the physician's ethical duty to make sure that individuals are involved in decisions about their own health care (Boyd, 2015).

The doctrine of informed consent protects clients' rights to voluntary consent or refusal of any medical treatment, procedure, or intervention based on information regarding the risks, benefits, and alternatives of care. This includes the provision of sufficient, evidence-based information to make a decision that reflects self-determination, autonomy, and control. Client consent or refusal is more than a legal doctrine to obtain a client's signature; it is a process of information exchange and involvement of clients in decision making (Grady, 2015).

Making informed choices during childbirth can be complex and multilayered. The process involves the integration of evidence-based information with individual health care needs, values, beliefs, and preferences. Thus, health care providers are obligated to adequately inform clients of planned procedures and to be assured of client permission prior to their performance. Client rights and autonomy need consideration because uninformed clients cannot make thoughtful decisions.

Four Key Components of Informed Consent

Informed consent has four key components: disclosure, comprehension, competency, and voluntariness (Cornock, 2015). It occurs prior to initiation of the procedure or specific care and addresses the legal and ethical requirements of informing the client about the procedure. The physician or the advanced practice nurse or the midwife is responsible for informing the client about the procedure and obtaining consent by providing a detailed description of the procedure or treatment, its potential risks and benefits, and alternative methods available. The nurse's responsibilities related to informed consent include the following:

1. Ensuring that the consent form is completed with signatures from the client
2. Serving as a witness to the signature process
3. Determining whether the client understands what she is signing by asking her pertinent questions
4. In certain states, mature minors and emancipated minors may consent to their own health care and certain health care may be provided to adolescents without parental notification, including contraception, pregnancy counseling, prenatal care, testing and treatment of STIs and communicable diseases (including HIV), substance abuse and mental illness counseling and treatment, and health care required as a result of a crime-related injury (Dickens & Cook, 2015).

Although laws vary from state to state, certain key elements are associated with informed consent (Box 1.4). Nurses need to be familiar with their specific state laws as well as the policies and procedures of the health care agencies where they work. Treating clients without

---

BOX 1.4

KEY ELEMENTS OF INFORMED CONSENT

- The decision maker must be of legal age in that state, with full civil rights, and must be competent (have the ability to make the decision).
- Information is presented in a manner that is simple, concise, and appropriate to the level of education and language of the individual responsible for making the decision.
- The decision must be voluntary, without coercion or force or under duress.
- There must be a witness to the process of informed consent.
- The witness must sign the consent form.

Adapted from US Department of Health and Human Services [USDHHS]. (2015). *Informed consent.* Available at: http://www.hhs.gov/ohrp/policy/consent/index.html; Nursing Midwifery Council. (2015). *The code: Professional standards of practice and behavior for nurses and midwives.* Retrieved from http://www.nmc-uk.org/Documents/NMC-Publications/revised-new-NMC-Code.pdf

obtaining proper consent may result in charges of assault, and the health care provider and/or facility may be held liable for any damages. Generally, only people over the age of majority (18 years of age) can legally provide consent for health care, except in the case of an emancipated minor (a person who is no longer subject to parental control, e.g., one who marries) (Arnold & Boggs, 2016).

Most care rendered in a health care setting is covered by the initial consent for treatment that is signed when the individual becomes a client at that office or clinic or by the consent to treatment signed on admission to a hospital or other inpatient facility. Certain procedures, however, may require a specific process of informed consent: major or minor surgery; invasive procedures such as amniocentesis or internal fetal monitoring; treatments placing the client at higher risk, such as chemotherapy or radiation therapy; procedures or treatments involving research; and photography involving the client.

Informed consent also rests on an assumption of competence (all adults are competent unless a court decides otherwise) and capacity (ability to understand alternatives and consequences of treatment and choose the best option). Nurses must use caution when determining the capacity of a client when the client has received medications that would alter his or her cognition ability to make decisions about care. Medications may need to be delayed or withheld temporarily to restore the client's capacity to make health care decisions.

If the client cannot provide consent, then the person closest to the client may give consent for emergency treatment. In an emergency, a verbal consent, via the telephone, may be obtained. Two witnesses must also be listening simultaneously and must sign the consent form, indicating that consent was received via the telephone. The ideal informed consent process would be achieved if a health care provider and a knowledgeable nurse collaborate for the client's good (Cornock, 2015).

Refusal of Medical Treatment

All clients have the right to refuse medical treatment, based on the American Hospital Association's Patient Care Partnership. Ideally, medical care without informed consent should be used only when the client's life is in danger. Clients may refuse treatment if it conflicts with their religious or cultural beliefs (Khoury, 2015). An example would be a Jehovah's Witness. Individuals of this faith have strong beliefs based on passages from the Bible that are interpreted as prohibiting the "consumption" of blood. Their beliefs prevent them from accepting transfusions of whole blood or its primary components. With recent advances and the use of biologic hemostats that aid coagulation and reduce blood loss, major surgery can be performed safely on a Jehovah's Witness who refuses a blood transfusion by utilizing these hemostats,

which decrease surgical blood loss (Carr, 2015). In these cases, it is important to educate the client and family about the importance of the recommended treatment without coercing or forcing the client to agree. Sometimes common ground may be reached between the family's religious or cultural beliefs and the health care team's recommendations. Communication and education are the keys in this situation.

Confidentiality

Nurses face particular challenge in respecting the confidentiality of clients in a world where information is quickly shared and where information about illness can be sensitive. Nurses have a duty of care toward clients. That duty includes maintaining privacy and confidentiality. With the establishment of the Health Insurance Portability and Accountability Act (HIPAA) of 1996, the confidentiality of health care information is now mandated by law. The primary intent of the law is to protect health insurance coverage for workers and their families when they change or lose jobs. Another aspect of the law requires the USDHHS to establish national standards for electronic transmission of health information. The HIPAA regulations were instituted to protect the privacy of individuals by safeguarding individually identifiable health care records, including those housed in electronic media. Protection of individual medical records extends not only to clinical health care sites but also to all ancillary health care providers, such as pharmacies, laboratories, and third-party payers. Each health care provider dealing with client health care data must provide for secure and limited access to the information (Price, 2015). For example, no information that clearly identifies a client can be on public display, including information on a client's chart. In maternal and newborn health care, information is shared only with the client, legal partner, parents, legal guardians, or individuals as established in writing by the client or the child's parents. This law promotes the security and privacy of health care and health information for all clients. Client information should always be kept confidential in the context of the state law, as well as the institution's policies.

Today, social media provide a rich source for errors to expose confidential client information. "Friending" clients on Facebook™, communicating about client care with identifiers, and posting inappropriate photos all lead to violations of HIPAA and/or employer policies resulting in discipline or termination of employment (Scruth et al., 2015).

Exceptions to confidentiality exist. For example, suspicion of physical or sexual abuse and injuries caused by a weapon or criminal act must be reported to the proper authorities. Abuse cases are reported to the appropriate welfare authorities, whereas criminal acts are reported to the police. The health care provider must also follow public health laws related to reporting certain infectious diseases to the local health department (e.g., tuberculosis, hepatitis, HIV, and other STIs). Finally, there is a duty to warn third parties when there is a specific threat to an identifiable person. There must be a balance between confidentiality and required disclosure. If health care information must be disclosed by law, the client must be informed that this will occur (Price, 2015).

IMPLICATIONS FOR NURSES

The health care system is intricately woven into the political and social structure of our society, and nurses should understand social, legal, and ethical health care issues so they can play an active role in meeting the health care needs of women and their families. Nurses are in a unique position because they are often the first contact clients have within health care systems. Nurses need to take a proactive role in advocating for and empowering their clients. For example, nurses can help women to increase control over the factors that affect health, thereby improving their health status. A woman may become empowered by developing skills not only to cope with her environment, but also to change it. Nurses can also assume this mentoring role with families, thus helping them to improve their overall health status and health outcomes.

Nurses must have a solid knowledge base about the factors affecting maternal, newborn, and women's health and barriers to health care. They can use this information to provide anticipatory guidance, health counseling, and teaching for women and their families. It also is useful in identifying high-risk groups so that interventions can be initiated early on, before problems occur.

When caring for women and their families, the nurse operates within the framework of the nursing process, which is applicable to all health care settings. Maternal, newborn, and women's health nursing is ever changing as globalization and its accompanying exchange of information expand. Nurses must remain up to date about new technologies and treatments and integrate high-quality, evidence-based interventions into the care they provide.

KEY CONCEPTS

- Maternal, newborn, and women's health nurses provide care using a philosophy that focuses on the family and the use of EBP in a case management environment to provide quality, cost-effective care.

- *Healthy People 2020* presents a national set of health goals and objectives for adults and children that focus on health promotion and disease prevention.

- One method to establish the aggregate health status of women and infants is with statistical data, such as mortality and morbidity rates.

- The infant mortality rate is the lowest in the history of the United States, but it is still higher than that of other industrialized countries. This high rate may be due to the number of low-birth-weight infants born in this country (CDC, 2015d).

- The family is considered the basic social unit of our society. The family greatly influences the development and health of its members because members learn health care activities, health beliefs, and health values from their family.

- Culture influences every aspect of development and is reflected in childbearing and child-rearing beliefs and practices designed to promote healthy adaptation.

- Other factors affecting the health of women and their families include health status and lifestyles, health care cost containment, improved diagnosis and treatment, and health care consumer empowerment. Finances, transportation, language, culture, and the health care delivery system can act as barriers to health care.

- Advances in science and technology have led to increased ethical dilemmas in health care.

- All clients have the right to refuse medical treatment based on the American Hospital Association's Patient Care Partnership.

- Nurses must be knowledgeable about the laws related to health care of women and their families in the state where they practice as well as the specific policies of their health care institution.

References and Recommended Readings

Abel, J. (2015). More women dying in childbirth in the U.S. than almost anywhere else. *Consumer Affairs*. Retrieved from http://www.consumeraffairs.com/news/more-women-dying-in-childbirth-in-the-us-than-almost-anywhere-else-050214.html

Aggleton, P., Parker, R., & Thomas, F. (2015). *Culture, health and sexuality: An introduction*. New York, NY: Taylor & Francis.

Alexander, L. L., LaRosa, J. H., Bader, H., & Garfield, S. (2014). *New dimensions in women's health* (5th ed.). Sudbury, MA: Jones & Bartlett.

American Academy of Pediatrics [AAP]. (2010). Policy statement: Children as hematopoietic stem cell donors. *Pediatrics, 125*, 392–404.

American Cancer Society [ACS]. (2015a). *Cancer facts for women*. Retrieved from http://www.cancer.org/Healthy/FindCancerEarly/WomensHealth/cancer-facts-for-women

American Cancer Society [ACS]. (2015b). *Lung cancer*. Retrieved from http://www.cancer.org/Cancer/LungCancer-Non-SmallCell/index

American Cancer Society [ACS]. (2015c). *Breast cancer facts and figures*. Retrieved from http://www.cancer.org/Research/CancerFacts-Figures/BreastCancerFactsFigures/index

American Cancer Society [ACS] (2015d) *Cancer facts and figures for African Americans*. Retrieved from http://www.cancer.org/acs/groups/content/@epidemiologysurveilance/documents/document/acspc-036921.pdf

American Congress of Obstetricians and Gynecologists [ACOG]. (2012). Committee opinion 399 reaffirmed: Umbilical cord blood banking. *Obstetrics & Gynecology, 111*(2), 475–477.

Arnold, E. C., & Boggs, K. U. (2016). *Interpersonal relationships: Professional communication skills for nurses* (7th ed.). St. Louis, MO: Elsevier.

Association of Women's Health, Obstetric and Neonatal Nurses [AWHONN]. (2009). *Standards for professional nursing practice in the care of women and newborns*. Washington, DC: Author.

Association of Women's Health, Obstetric and Neonatal Nurses [AWHONN]. (2015). Criminalization of pregnant women with substance use disorders. *Nursing for Women's Health, 19*(1), 93–95.

Aston, M., Price, S., Etowa, J., Vukic, A., Young, L., Hart, C., et al. (2015). The power of relationships: Exploring how public health nurses support mothers and families during postpartum home visits. *Journal of Family Nursing, 21*(1), 11–34.

Bartlett Regional Hospital. (n.d.). *Domestic violence assessment tool*. Retrieved from http://www.hospitalsoup.com/public/brhdvprotocol.pdf

Beal, J. A., Dalton, M. F., & Maloney, J. A. (2015). Should mother-baby rooming-in be the standard of care? *American Journal of Maternal Child Nursing, 40*(2), 74–75.

Blanchet Garneau, A., & Pepin, J. (2015). Cultural competence: A constructivist definition. *Journal of Transcultural Nursing, 26*(1), 9–15.

Boyd, K. (2015). The impossibility of informed consent?. *Journal of Medical Ethics, 41*(1), 44–47.

Campbell, A. V. (2015). The formative years: medical ethics comes of age. *Journal of Medical Ethics, 41*(1), 5–7.

Carr, C. (2015). *Beginning medical law*. New York, NY: Routledge.

Catov, J., Flint, M., Lee, M., Roberts, J., & Abatemarco, D. (2015). The relationship between race, inflammation and psychosocial factors among pregnant women. *Maternal & Child Health Journal, 19*(2), 401–409.

Centers for Disease Control and Prevention [CDC]. (2015a). *Pregnancy mortality surveillance system*. Atlanta: Author. Retrieved from www.cdc.gov/reproductivehealth/MaternalInfantHealth/PMSS.html#5

Centers for Disease Control and Prevention [CDC]. (2015b). *Fetal deaths*. Retrieved from http://www.cdc.gov/nchs/fetal_death.htm

Centers for Disease Control and Prevention [CDC]. (2015c). CDC grand rounds: Public health approaches to reducing U.S. infant mortality. *Morbidity and Mortality Weekly Report, 62*(31), 625–628.

Centers for Disease Control and Prevention [CDC]. (2015d). *QuickStats: Infant mortality rates*. Retrieved from http://www.cdc.gov/mmwr/preview/mmwrhtml/mm6026a6.htm

Centers for Disease Control and Prevention [CDC]. (2015f). *Health literacy: Accurate, accessible and actionable information for all*. Retrieved from http://www.cdc.gov/healthliteracy/index.html

Chescheir, N. C. (2015). Enough already! *Obstetrics & Gynecology, 125*(1), 2–4.

Clark, K., Beatty, S, & Reibel, T. (2015). Maternity care: A narrative overview of what women expect across their care continuum. *Midwifery 31*(4), 432–437.

Cornock, M. (2015). Clarifying consent. *Nursing Standard, 29*(21), 30.

Creanga, A. A., Berg, C. J., Syverson, C., Seed, K., Bruce, F. C., & Callaghan, W. M. (2015). Pregnancy-related mortality in the United States, 2006–2010. *Obstetrics & Gynecology, 125*(1), 5–12.

Cunningham, J., Goldsmith, L., & Skirton, H. (2015). The evidence base regarding the experiences of and attitudes to preimplantation genetic diagnosis in prospective parents. *Midwifery, 31*(2), 288–296.

Davies, L., Ford-Gilboe, M., Wilson, A., Varcoe, C., Wuest, J., Campbell, J., et al. (2015). Patterns of cumulative abuse among female survivors of intimate partner violence: Links to women's health and socioeconomic status. *Violence against Women, 21*(1), 30–48.

DeBruyne, L. K., Pinna, K., & Whitney, E. (2015). *Nutrition and diet therapy* (9th ed.). Boston, MA: CengageLearning.

DeJoy, S., & Bittner, K. (2015). Obesity stigma as a determinant of poor birth outcomes in women with high BMI: A conceptual framework. *Maternal & Child Health Journal, 19*(4), 693–699.

Denham, S. A., Eggenberger, S., Krumwiede, N., & Young, P. (2016). *Family-focused nursing care*. Philadelphia, PA: F.A. Davis.

Devolder, K. (2015). *The ethics of stem cell research*. Oxford, UK: Oxford University Press.

Dickens, B. M., & Cook, R. J. (2015). Types of consent in reproductive health care. *International Journal of Gynecology & Obstetrics, 128*(2), 181–184.

Donaldson, P., Daly, A., Ermini, L., & Bevitt, D. (2015). *Genetics of complex disease*. New York, NY: Taylor & Francis.

Dumas, A., & Turner, B. S. (2015). Introduction: Human longevity, utopia, and solidarity. *Sociological Quarterly, 56*(1), 1–17.

Elmoazzen, H., & Holovati, J. L. (2015). Cord blood clinical processing, cryopreservation, and storage. *Methods in Molecular Biology, 1257*, 369–379.

Federal Interagency Forum on Child and Family Statistics [FIFCFS]. (2015). *America's children: Key national indicators of well-being*. Retrieved from http://www.childstats.gov/index.asp

Fitzgerald, T., Glynn, A., Davenport, K., Waxman, J., & Johnson, P. A. (2015). Well-woman visits: Guidance and monitoring are key in this turning point for women's health. *Women's Health Issues, 25*(2), 89–90.

Fowler, M. D. & Lachman, V. (2015). Conscientious objection: When care collides with nurse's morals, ethics. *The American Nurse*. Retrieved from http://www.theamericannurse.org/index.php/2014/09/02/conscientious-objection/

French, K. S. (2015). Transforming nursing care through health literacy ACTS. *The Nursing Clinics of North America, 50*(1), 87–98.

Galanti, G. (2015). *Caring for patients from different cultures*. (5th ed.). Philadelphia, PA: University of Pennsylvania Press.

GlobeWomen. (2015). *2015 Global Summit of Women*. Retrieved from http://globewomen.org/globalsummit/

Grady, C. (2015). Enduring and emerging challenges of informed consent. *The New England Journal of Medicine, 372*(9), 855–862.

Guilcher, G. T., Fernandez, C. V., & Joffe, S. (2015). Are hybrid umbilical cord blood banks really the best of both worlds?. *Journal of Medical Ethics, 41*(3), 272–275.

GuttmacherInstitute. (2015). *Facts on inducted abortion in the United States*. Retrieved from http://www.guttmacher.org/pubs/fb_induced_abortion.html

Hain, D. J., & Kear, T. M. (2015). Using evidence-based practice to move beyond doing things the way we have always done them. *Nephrology Nursing Journal, 42*(1), 11–20.

Hall, J. P., Kurth, N. K., Chapman, S. C., & Shireman, T. I. (2015). Medicaid managed care: issues for beneficiaries with disabilities. *Disability and Health Journal, 8*(1), 130–135.

Hanrahan, K., Wagner, M., Matthews, G., Stewart, S., Dawson, C., Greiner, J., et al. (2015). Sacred cow gone to pasture: A systematic evaluation and integration of evidence-based practice. *Worldviews on Evidence-Based Nursing, 12*(1), 3–11.

Hickey, M., & Moore, P. (2015). Follow-up after medical abortion: does simple equal safe? *Lancet, 385*(9969), 669–670.

Holden, C. D., Chen, J., & Dagher, R. K. (2015). Preventive care utilization among the uninsured by race/ethnicity and income. *American Journal of Preventive Medicine, 48*(1), 13–21.

Health and Medicine Division (HMD). (2011). *The future of nursing: Leading change, advancing health*. Washington, DC: National Academies Press.

Health and Medicine Division (HMD). (2016). *Health literacy: Past, present, and future*. Retrieved from http://www.nationalacademies.org/hmd/Reports/2015/Health-Literacy-Past-Present-Future.aspx

International Center for Research on Women [ICRW]. (2015). *A price too high to bear: The costs of maternal mortality to families and communities*. Retrieved from http://www.icrw.org/publications/price-too-high-bear-costs-maternal-mortality-families-and-communities

Islami, F., Ward, E. M., Jacobs, E. J., Ma, J., Goding Sauer, A., Lortet-Tieulent, J., et al. (2015). Potentially preventable premature lung cancer deaths in the USA if overall population rates were reduced to those of educated whites in lower-risk states. *Cancer Causes & Control, 26*(3), 409–418.

Kail, R. V., & Cavanaugh, J. C. (2016). *Human development: A lifespan view* (7th ed.). Boston, MA: CengageLearning.

Kassebaum, N. J., Bertozzi-Villa, A., Coggeshall, M. S., Shackelford, K. A., Steiner, C., Heuton, K. R., et al. (2014). Global, regional, and national levels and causes of maternal mortality during 1990–2013: a systematic analysis for the Global Burden of Disease Study 2013. *Lancet, 384*(9947), 980–1004.

Khoury, B. S., Khoury J. N. (2015). Consent: a practical guide. *Australian Dental Journal, .60*(2), 138–142. Wiley Online Library.

Manson, J. E., & Bassuk, S. S. (2015). Biomarkers of cardiovascular disease risk in women. *Metabolism: Clinical and Experimental, 64*(3 Suppl 1), S33–S39.

Mansur, G., & Thompson, M. (2015). The benefit aftereffects of ACA—Accelerating toward a new health economy. *Benefits Quarterly, 31*(1), 26–31.

Mathis, J., Raio, L., & Baud, D. (2015). Fetal laser therapy: Applications in the management of fetal pathologies. *Prenatal diagnosis, 35*(7), 623–636. Wiley Online Library.

McFarlane, D. R. (2015). *Global population and reproductive health.* Burlington, MA: Jones & Bartlett Learning.

McGill, N. (2015). US life expectancy up, but chronic diseases are also, health rankings say. *Nation's Health, 45*(1), 6.

McLemore, M. R., Levi, A., & James, E. A. (2015). Recruitment and retention strategies for expert nurses in abortion care provision. *Contraception, 91*(6), 474–479.

Meierhenry, J. A., Ryzhuk, V., Miguelino, M. G., Lankford, L., Powell, J. S., Farmer, D., et al. (2015). Placenta as a source of stem cells for regenerative medicine. *Current Pathobiology Reports, 3*(1), 9–16.

Mintz, S. (2013). *Childbirth in early America.* Retrieved from http://www.digitalhistory.uh.edu/historyonline/childbirth.cfm

Mirkin, S., Archer, D. F., Pickar, J. H., & Komm, B. S. (2015). Recent advances help understand and improve the safety of menopausal therapies. *Menopause, 22*(3), 351–360.

National Women's Law Center. (2010). *Making the grade on women's health: A national state-by-state report card.* Retrieved from http://hrc.nwlc.org/states/national-report-card

Newland, L. A. (2015). Family well-being, parenting, and child well-being: Pathways to healthy adjustment. *Clinical Psychologist, 19*(1), 3–14.

Oeldorf-Hirsch, A., & Sundar, S. S. (2015). Posting, commenting, and tagging: Effects of sharing news stories on Facebook. *Computers in Human Behavior, 44* 240–249.

Oza, S., Lawn, J. E., Hogan, D. R., Mathers, C., & Cousens, S. N. (2015). Neonatal cause-of-death estimates for the early and late neonatal periods for 194 countries: 2000–2013. *Bulletin of the World Health Organization, 93*(1), 19–28.

Phillips, L. R., Salem, B. E., Jeffers, K. S., Kim, H., Ruiz, M. E., Salem, N., et al. (2015). Developing and proposing the ethno-cultural gerontological nursing model. *Journal of Transcultural Nursing, 26*(2), 118–128.

Price, B. (2015). Respecting patient confidentiality. *Nursing Standard, 29*(22), 50–57.

Rabor, F., Taghipour, A., & Najmabadi, K. (2015). Voices of mother's interaction with midwives in natural childbirth: A qualitative study. *Health, 7,* 153–160.

Redding, S., Conrey, E., Porter, K., Paulson, J., Hughes, K., & Redding, M. (2015). Pathways community care coordination in low birth weight prevention. *Maternal & Child Health Journal, 19*(3), 643–650.

Sabik, L. M., Tarazi, W. W., & Bradley, C. J. (2015). State Medicaid expansion decisions and disparities in women's cancer screening. *American Journal of Preventive Medicine, 48*(1), 98–103.

Scruth, E. A., Pugh, D. M., Adams, C. L., & Foss-Durant, A. M. (2015). Electronic and social media: The legal and ethical issues for healthcare. *Clinical Nurse Specialist, 29*(1), 8–11.

Simmons, W., Rothman, B. K., & Norman, B. M. (2013). *Laboring on: Birth in transition in the United States.* New York, NY: Routledge.

Snustad, D. P. (2015). *Principles of genetics* (7th ed.). Somerset, NJ: Wiley.

Stanhope, M., & Lancaster, J. (2014). *Community/public health nursing: Population-centered health care in the community* (9th ed.). St. Louis, MO: Mosby Elsevier.

Starrs, A. M. (2015). Safeguarding the ACA's gains for women. *Lancet, 385*(9962), 24–25.

Summers, N. (2016). *Fundamentals of case management practice: Skills for the human services* (5th ed.). Boston, MA: CengageLearning.

Taber, J., Leyva, B., & Persoskie, A. (2015). Why do people avoid medical care? A qualitative study using national data. *Journal of General Internal Medicine, 30*(3), 290–297.

Treadwell, J., Perez, R., Stubbs, D., McAllister, J. W., Stern, S., & Buzi, R. (2015). *Case management and care coordination: Supporting children and families to optimal outcomes.* New York, NY: Springer.

Tucker Edmonds, B., Mogul, M., & Shea, J. A. (2015a). Understanding low-income United Nations. *International Women's Day.* Retrieved from http://www.un.org/en/events/women/iwd/2011/un_high_commissioner_for_human_rights_message_2011.shtml

United Nations. (2016). *International Women's Day 2016.* Retrieved from http://www.unwomen.org/en/news/in-focus/international-womens-day

United Nations International Children's Emergency Fund [UNICEF]. (2015). *Maternal and newborn health: Challenges.* Retrieved from http://www.unicef.org/health/index_maternalhealth.html

United Nations International Children's Emergency Fund [UNICEF]. (2016). *Maternal and newborn health: Challenges.* Retrieved from http://www.unicef.org/search/search.php?q_en=maternal and newborn health&hits=10&type=Main&navigation= pageyear:2016

U.S. Bureau of Justice Office on Violence against Women. (2015). *Domestic violence.* Retrieved from http://www.ovw.usdoj.gov/domviolence.htm

U.S. Census Bureau. (2015). *American fact finder.* Retrieved from http://www.pobronson.com/factbook/pages/39.html

U.S. Department of Health & Human Services [USDHHS]. (2015a). *Healthy People 2020.* Retrieved from http://healthypeople.gov/2020/topicsobjectives2020/objectiveslist.aspx?topicId=26

U.S. Department of Health and Human Services, Health Resources and Services Administration, Maternal and Child Health Bureau. (2015b). *Child Health USA 2014.* Rockville, MD: U.S. Department of Health and Human Services.

U.S. Prevention Services Task Force [USPSTF]. (2015). *Screening for intimate partner violence and abuse of elderly and vulnerable adults.* Retrieved from http://www.uspreventiveservicestaskforce.org/uspstf12/ipvelder/ipvelderfinalrs.htm

Wang, Y., Liu, G., Canfield, M. A., Mai, C. T., Gilboa, S. M., Meyer, R. E., et al. (2015). Racial/ethnic differences in survival of United States children with birth defects: A population-based study. *The Journal of Pediatrics.* Retrieved from http://www.sciencedirect.com/science/article/pii/S0022347614011949

World Bank. (2015). *Mortality rate, neonatal (per 1000 live births).* Retrieved from http://data.worldbank.org/indicator/SH.DYN.NMRT

World Factbook. (2015). *Infant mortality rate.* Retrieved from https://www.cia.gov/library/publications/the-world-factbook/geos/us.html

World Health Organization [WHO]. (2015a). *Definition of health.* Retrieved from http://www.who.int/kobe_centre/about/faq/en/

World Health Organization [WHO]. (2015b). *Health status statistics.* Retrieved from http://www.who.int/healthinfo/statistics/indneonatalmortality/en

World Health Organization [WHO]. (2015c). *Women's health factsheet.* Retrieved from http://www.who.int/mediacentre/factsheets/fs334/en/index.html

World Health Organization [WHO]. (2015d). *Maternal mortality fact sheet.* Fact sheet No. 348. Retrieved from Http://www.who.int/mediacentre/factsheets/fs348/en/index.html.

World Health Organization [WHO]. (2015e). *Global health estimates summary tables: deaths by cause, age, and sex by various regional grouping.* Geneva: World Health Organization. Retrieved from http://www.who.int/healthinfo/global_burden_disease/en/.

Yin-Hsiu, C., Ferguson, K. K., Meeker, J. D., McElrath, T. F., & Mukherjee, B. (2015). Statistical methods for modeling repeated measures of maternal environmental exposure biomarkers during pregnancy in association with preterm birth. *Environmental Health: A Global Access Science Source, 14*(1), 146–171.

Young, D. (2014). It is better to light one candle than to curse the darkness: The legacy of Doris Haire. *Birth, 41,* 306–308.

MULTIPLE-CHOICE QUESTIONS

1. When preparing a presentation for a local woman's group on women's health problems, what would the nurse include as the number one cause of mortality for women in the United States?
   a. Breast cancer
   b. Childbirth complications
   c. Injury resulting from violence
   d. Heart disease

2. Which factor would most likely be responsible for a pregnant women's failure to receive adequate prenatal care in the United States?
   a. Belief that it is not necessary in a normal pregnancy
   b. Use of denial to cope with pregnancy
   c. Lack of health insurance to cover expenses
   d. Inability to trust traditional medical practices

3. When caring for an adolescent, in which instance must the nurse share information with the parents, no matter which state care is provided in?
   a. Pregnancy counseling
   b. Depression
   c. Contraception
   d. Tuberculosis

4. Client advocacy, utilization management, and coordination of care describe which of the following?
   a. Primary nursing care
   b. Case management
   c. Family-centered care
   d. Patient-focused care

5. Nurses in the United States working in maternity services need to have knowledge of a variety of cultures and be culturally competent in caring for women and their families because:
   a. All members of a specific culture are homogenous.
   b. Physiological differences exist among different cultures.
   c. Care can be individualized for different cultural preferences.
   d. Nondominant cultural groups are made up of new immigrants.

6. The nurse is preparing a class about homelessness. Which factors contribute to homelessness? Select all that apply.
   a. Decrease in the number of people living in poverty
   b. Unemployment
   c. Exposure to abuse or neglect
   d. Cutbacks in public welfare programs
   e. Establishment of community crisis centers

CRITICAL THINKING EXERCISES

1. As a nurse working in a federally funded low-income clinic offering women's health services, the nurse is becoming increasingly frustrated with the number of "no-shows" or appointments missed in your maternity clinic. Some clients come for their initial prenatal intake appointment and never come back. The nurse realizes that some just forget their appointments, but most don't even call to notify the clinic. Many of the clients are high risk and thus are jeopardizing their health and the health of their future child.
   a. What changes might be helpful to address this situation?
   b. Outline what the nurse might say at the next staff meeting to address the issue of clients making one clinic visit and then never returning.
   c. What strategies might the nurse use to improve attendance and notification?
   d. Describe what cultural and customer service techniques might be needed.

STUDY ACTIVITIES

1. Research a current policy, bill, or issue being debated on the community, state, or national level that pertains to the health and welfare of women or their families. Summarize the major facts and supporting and opposing arguments and prepare an oral report on your findings.

2. Within your clinical group, debate the following statement: should access to health care be a right or a privilege? Be able to back up your response.

3. Visit a local community health center that offers services to women from various cultures and their families. Interview the staff about any barriers to health care that they have identified. Investigate what the staff has done to minimize these barriers.

BRINGING IT ALL TOGETHER: CASE STUDY

Maize, a 64 year old Hispanic woman, presented to the Women's Clinic complaining about a vaginal discharge that was itchy and uncomfortable. Maize hadn't been to the clinic for years, since she had her last child decades ago. She never finished high school and was working locally as a motel housekeeper. She didn't have any health insurance, so tended to use home remedies to treat any health issue. Prior to her visit today, she had douched to attempt to treat this problem.

The health care provider examined Maize and prescribed vaginal suppositories for a yeast infection. Instructions were given to her verbally and in writing before she left. Maize shook her head in agreement that she understood the treatment regimen. A few days later the clinic nurse received a phone call from Maize stating that she would "just have to live with this condition because that medicine she got was "rank-tasting," it was making her gag when she attempted to swallow it, and she didn't think it was working!"

Go to thePoint **to find questions to consider about this case.**

2

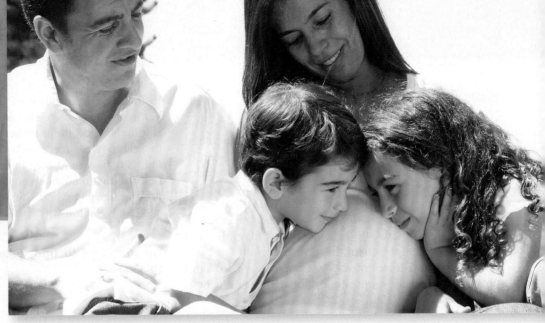

Family-Centered Community-Based Care

Learning Objectives

Upon completion of the chapter, you will be able to:

1. Define the key terms used in this chapter.
2. Examine the major components and key elements of family-centered community health care.
3. Explain the reasons for the increased emphasis on community-based care.
4. Differentiate community-based nursing from nursing in acute care settings.
5. Integrate the different levels of prevention in community-based nursing, providing examples of each.
6. Cite examples of cultural issues that may be faced when providing community-based nursing.
7. Describe the dynamic forces contributing to cultural diversity to adapt delivery of culturally competent care to women and their families.
8. Construct strategies for integrating elements of alternative/complementary therapies and scientific health care practice.
9. Identify the variety of settings where community-based care can be provided to women and their families.
10. Outline the various roles and functions assumed by the community health nurse.
11. Demonstrate the ability to use therapeutic communication skills when interacting with women and their families.
12. Evaluate the process of health teaching as it relates to women and their families.
13. Determine the importance of discharge planning and case management in providing community-based care.

Maria was home a few days after giving birth to her first child. She had just changed her newborn son and placed him on his stomach for a nap when the community health nurse arrived for a postpartum visit. Because the nurse did not speak Spanish and Maria did not speak English, a great deal of gesturing followed. After examining Maria, the nurse picked up Maria's son and placed him on his back in the crib. How might the nurse have prepared for this home visit? What message did the nurse convey in changing the newborn's position? What actions did the nurse take to decrease trust? What actions should she take to increase trust with this mother?

WOV

Words of Wisdom
To recognize diversity in others and respect it, nurses must first have some awareness of who they are.

INTRODUCTION

Women and their families receive most of their health care, both well and ill care, in the community setting. During the past several years, the health care delivery system has changed dramatically. Medicare's prospective payment system for hospitals, introduced in the United States in 1983, replaced cost reimbursement with a system of fixed rates that created incentives for hospitals to control costs. This focus on cost containment has meant that people are spending less time in the hospital. Clients are being discharged "sicker and quicker" from their hospital beds (Hansen, 2015). The health care system has responded by moving from reactive treatment strategies in hospitals to a proactive approach in the community. This has resulted in an increasing emphasis on health promotion and illness prevention within the community.

Nurses play an important role in the health and wellness of a community. They not only meet the health care needs of the individual but also go beyond that to implement interventions that affect the community as a whole. Nurses practice in a variety of settings within a community, such as clinics and physician offices, shelters, churches, health departments, community health centers, and homes. They promote the health of individuals, families, groups, communities, and populations and promote an environment that supports health.

This chapter describes the concepts of community and community-based nursing, addressing the varied settings where such care is provided to women and their families. The chapter also highlights the major roles and functions of community-based nurses, emphasizing their role as educators in health promotion and maintenance.

FAMILY-CENTERED CARE

Family-centered care refers to the collaborative partnership among the individual, family, and caregivers that exist to determine goals, share information, offer support, and formulate plans for health care. It is generally understood to be an approach in which clients and their families are considered integral components of the health care decision-making and delivery processes (McGurk, 2015; Pate & Andrews, 2015). Nursing support of the family can take many forms. For example, *informational support* is designed to provide supportive communication by making available understandable information to the family about their member's condition, treatment, development, and care; about their behavioral and emotional responses and needs; and about what to expect regarding their condition. *Emotional support* includes listening, exhibiting caring behaviors, and being concerned in ways that help the family cope with their member's illness and the other aspects of their lives that are affected by the illness. *Appraisal support*, also called *esteem support*, is conceptualized as enhancing, reinforcing, and

supporting the family role. Finally, *instrumental support* includes providing assistance of any kind, such as financial, time, labor, or environmental modifications. In short, nursing support to families includes providing a supportive relationship and ongoing information; helping maintain the family role by offering encouragement, affirmative comment, and appraisal; giving emotional support; and providing competent nursing care. To provide good-quality, family-centered care, nurses need adequate resources and appropriate education, as well as support from managers and other health care disciplines (Roberts, 2015).

The philosophy of family-centered care recognizes the family as the constant: the health of all the family members and their functional abilities influence the health of the client and other members of the family. The core concepts of family-centered care include:

- Providing dignity and respect for the client and family choices
- Sharing health care information that is meaningful and accurate
- Encouraging clients and their families to participate in decisions about their care
- Collaborating with clients, families, and other health care providers in the delivery of care (Nichols, Crow, & Balakas, 2015).

Family-centered care works well in all arenas of health care from preventive care to long-term care. Family-centered care enhances the confidence of all those involved about their skills and helps to prepare individuals for assuming responsibility for their own health care needs. It is vital for the nurse to assess how much knowledge the family already has about the client's health or illness. At the heart of family-centered care is a commitment to working with clients as partners, which is a shift from a "doing to and doing for" which was the mantra of the past.

Using a family-centered approach is associated with positive outcomes such as decreased anxiety, improved pain management, shorter recovery times, and enhanced confidence and problem-solving skills. Communication between the health care team and the family is also improved, leading to greater satisfaction for both health care providers and health care consumers (families). Parents should be involved in the care of and decision making for their newborn, and separations should be minimized. Their needs should be anticipated, respected, and addressed in the obstetrical unit. Open, clear, consistent information and communication should be maintained (Flagg, 2015). It is important for nurses to remain neutral to all they hear and see in order to enhance trust and maintain open communication lines with all family members. Nurses need to remember that the client is an expert about his or her own health; thus, nurses should work within the client's framework when planning health promotion interventions. Practicing true family-centered care may empower the family, strengthen family resources, and help the woman or child feel more secure throughout the process.

COMMUNITY-BASED CARE

Community may be defined as a specific group of people, often living in a defined geographic area, who share common interests, interact with each other, and function collectively within a defined social structure to address common concerns (Stanhope & Lancaster, 2014). The common features of a community may be common rights and privileges as members of a certain city or common ties of identity, values, norms, culture, language, or social support. Women are caregivers to children, parents, spouses, and neighbors and provide important social support in these roles.

A person can be a part of many communities during the course of daily life. Examples might include area of residence (home, apartment, shelter), gender, place of employment (organization or home), language spoken (Spanish, Chinese, English), educational background or student status, culture (Italian, African American, Indian), career (nurse, businesswoman, housewife), place of worship (church or synagogue), and community memberships (garden club, YMCA, support group, school PTA, youth organizations, athletic teams).

A **population** is a group of individuals who share personal or environmental characteristics. Typically the most common characteristic is geographic location. Populations are made up of human beings within complex social and physical environments. The betterment of human populations remains the goal of community-based nursing care. Examples of populations include nurses who work the night shift, older mothers having their first pregnancy, high risk infants, or Native Americans.

In community-based care, the community is the unit of service. The providers of care are concerned not only with the clients who present for service but also with the larger population of potential or at-risk clients.

Community Health Nursing

Community health nursing focuses on preventing illness and improving the health of populations and communities. Community health nurses work in geographically and culturally diverse settings. They address the current and potential health needs of a population or community. They promote and preserve the health of a population and are not limited to particular age groups or diagnoses. **Public health nursing** is a specialized area of community health nursing.

Epidemiology (the study of the causes, distribution, and control of disease in populations) can help determine the health and health needs of a population

and assist in planning health services. Community health nurses perform epidemiologic investigations to help analyze and develop health policy and community health initiatives. Community health initiatives can be focused on the community as a whole or a specific target population with specific needs. *Healthy People 2020: Improving the Health of Americans* is an example of a national health initiative that was developed using the epidemiologic process. *Healthy People* provides science-based, 10-year national objectives for improving the health of all Americans. *Healthy People 2020* ensures that health care professionals evaluate the individual as well as the community. It emphasizes the ever-present link between the individual's health and the health of the community (Lundy & Janes, 2016). *Healthy People 2020* identifies two major goals: to increase the quality of life and the life expectancy of individuals of all ages and to decrease health disparities among different populations. Relevant *Healthy People 2020* objectives are highlighted throughout this text, and *Healthy People 2020* is available online at http://www.healthypeople.gov. These objectives provide a tool for all health care providers to move from a focus on illness and cure to a focus on health promotion and illness prevention for entire populations.

The focus of health care initiatives today is on people and their needs, strengthening their abilities to shape their own lives. The emphasis has shifted away from dependence on health professionals toward personal involvement and personal responsibility, and this gives nurses the opportunity to interact with individuals in a variety of self-help roles. Nurses in the community can be the primary force in identifying the challenges and implementing changes in women's and newborn's health for the future.

Community-Based Nursing

In the past, the only community-based roles for nurses were community health nurses or public health nurses. This is now a subset of what is considered community-based nursing. The health needs of the society and consumer demand brought about community-based and community-focused services. The movement from an illness-oriented "cure" perspective in hospitals to a focus on health promotion and primary health care in community-based settings has dramatically changed employment opportunities for today's nurses. This shift in emphasis to primary care and outpatient treatment and management will likely continue. As a result, employment growth in a variety of community-based settings can be expected for properly educated nurses. With the worldwide strategic shift of health care delivery from secondary to primary care settings, more newly qualified nurses are working in primary care, making exposure to the variety of roles available to nurses essential for future workforce development (Clark & Paraska, 2015).

TABLE 2.1	COMMUNITY-BASED PRACTICE SETTINGS
Setting	Description
Ambulatory care settings	Physician's offices Health maintenance organizations (HMOs) Day surgery centers Freestanding urgent care centers Family planning clinics Mobile mammography centers
Health department services	Maternal/child health clinics Family planning clinics Sexually transmitted infection programs Immunization clinics Substance-abuse programs Jails and prisons
Home health care services	High-risk pregnancy/neonate care Maternal/child newborn care Skilled nursing care Hospice care
Long-term care	Skilled nursing facilities Nursing homes Hospices Assisted living
Other community-based settings	Parish nursing programs Summer camps Community-sponsored education programs School health programs Occupational health programs

The Bureau of Labor Statistics, U.S. Department of Labor, Occupational Employment Statistics (2015) found the following trends in registered nurse (RN) employment settings:

- Fifty-seven percent of RNs work in the hospital setting.
- Thirty-four percent work outside the hospital setting in community-based settings.
- The number of RNs employed in community-based settings has continued to grow largely due to an increase in nurses working in home health care and managed care organizations.

Community-based nursing settings include ambulatory care, home health care, occupational health, school health, and hospice settings (Table 2.1). Clinical practice within the community may also include case management, research, quality improvement, and discharge planning. Nurses with advanced practice and experience may be employed in areas of staff development, program development, and community education.

Community-Based Nursing Interventions

Nursing interventions involve any treatment that the nurse performs to enhance the client's outcome. Nursing practice in the community uses the nursing process and is similar to that in the acute care setting because assessing, performing procedures, administering medications, coordinating services and equipment, counseling clients and their families, and teaching about care are all part of the care administered by nurses in the community. Box 2.1 highlights the most common nursing interventions used in community-based nursing practice.

Community-Based Nursing Challenges

Despite the benefits achieved by caring for families in their own homes and communities, challenges also exist. Clients are being discharged from acute care facilities very early in their recovery course and present with more health care needs than in the past. As a result, nursing care and procedures in the home and community are becoming more complex and time consuming. Consider the example of a woman who develops a systemic infection, a pelvic abscess, and deep vein thrombosis in one leg after a cesarean birth and who is now being discharged from the hospital. The nurse's primary focus of care in this situation would be to administer heparin and antibiotics intravenously rather than educating her about child care and follow-up appointments. In the past, this

---

BOX 2.1

COMMUNITY-BASED NURSING INTERVENTIONS

- *Health screening*—Detecting unrecognized or preclinical illness among individuals so they can be referred for definitive diagnosis and treatment (e.g., mammogram or Pap smear, vision, and hearing checks).
- *Health education programs*—Assisting clients in making health-related decisions about self-care, use of health resources, and social health issues such as smoking bans and motorcycle helmet laws (e.g., childbirth education or breast self-examination, drug awareness programs).
- *Medication administration*—Preparing, giving, and evaluating the effectiveness of prescription and over-the-counter drugs (e.g., hormone therapy in menopausal women)
- *Telephone consultation*—Identifying the problem to be addressed; listening and providing support, information, or instruction; documenting advice/ instructions given to concerns raised by caller (e.g., consultation for a mother with a newborn with colic, interaction with a parent whose child has a fever or is vomiting).
- *Health system referral*—Passing along information about the location, services offered, and ways to contact agencies (e.g., referring a woman for a breast prosthesis after a mastectomy).
- *Instructional*—Teaching an individual or a group about a medication, disease process, lifestyle changes, community resources, or research findings concerning their environment (e.g., childbirth education class, basic life support classes for parents).
- *Nutritional counseling*—Demonstrating the direct relationship between nutrition and illness while focusing on the need for diet modification to promote wellness (e.g., Women, Infants, and Children [WIC] program; counselor interviewing a pregnant woman who has anemia).
- *Risk identification*—Recognizing personal or group characteristics that predispose people to develop a specific health problem, and modifying or eliminating them (e.g., genetic counseling of an older pregnant woman at risk for a Down syndrome infant; genetic screening of family members for cystic fibrosis or Huntington's disease).

Adapted from Murphy, J. W. (2015). *Community-based interventions.* New York, NY: Springer; and Lundy, K. S., & Janes, S. (2016). *Community health nursing: Caring for the public's health* (3rd ed.). Burlington, MA: Jones & Bartlett Learning.

---

difficult to spend the time needed while meeting the time restrictions dictated by their health care agencies. Nurses need to plan the tasks to be accomplished (Box 2.2).

Nurses working in the community have fewer resources available to them compared with the acute care setting. Decisions often have to be made in isolation. The nurse must possess excellent assessment skills and the ability to communicate effectively with the family to be successful in carrying out the appropriate plan of care. Nurses interested in working in community-based settings must be able to apply the nursing process in an environment that is less structured or controlled than that in acute care facilities. Nurses must be able to assimilate information well beyond the immediate physical and psychosocial needs of the client in a controlled acute care setting and deal with environmental threats, lifestyle choices, family issues, different cultural patterns, financial burdens, transportation problems, employment hazards, communication barriers, limited resources, and client acceptance and adherence to care regimens.

Although opportunities for employment in community-based settings are plentiful, many positions require a baccalaureate degree. Previous medical-surgical experience in an acute care setting is typically required by home health agencies because these nurses must function fairly independently within the home environment.

The nurse must also be familiar with and respectful of many different cultures and socioeconomic levels, remaining objective in dealing with such diversity and demonstrating an understanding of and appreciation for cultural differences. Interventions must be individualized to address the cultural, social, and economic diversity among clients in their own environment (Lundy & Janes, 2016).

The mission for all nurses is profound but simple: to treat with dignity and compassion every person who is in their care. Imagine for a moment what it would be like to be sick and not be able to communicate with your caregivers—to not understand what they are saying or to become greatly alarmed when you hear information in terms that are offensive or inappropriate in your culture. Quality care depends on quality communication, thus utilizing language interpreters can make a major difference in all situations (Purnell, 2015).

Shift in Responsibilities from Hospital-Based to Community-Based Nursing

Community care, especially home care, is a rapidly growing service in the United States (Adams, 2015). Community-based care has been shown to be a cost-effective method for providing care. An increase in disposable income and the increased longevity of individuals with chronic and debilitating health conditions have also contributed to the continued shift of health care to the community and home setting. Technology has advanced,

woman would have remained hospitalized for treatment, but home infusion therapy is now less costly and allows the client to be discharged sooner.

This demand on the nurse's time may limit the amount of time spent on prevention measures, education, and the family's psychosocial issues. More time may be needed to help families deal with these issues and concerns. With large client caseloads, nurses may find it

---

BOX 2.2

HOME CARE VISITATION PLANNING

- Review previous interventions to eliminate unsuccessful ones.
- Check previous home visit narrative to validate interventions.
- Communicate with previous nurse to ask questions and clarify.
- Formulate plan of interventions based on data received (e.g., client preference of IV placement or order of fluids).
- Prioritize client needs based on their potential to threaten the client's health status.
- Use Maslow's hierarchy of needs to set forth a plan of care.
- Address life-threatening physiologic issues first (e.g., an infectious process would take precedence over anorexia).
- Develop goals that reflect primary, secondary, and tertiary prevention levels.
- *Primary prevention*—Have the client consume adequate fluid intake to prevent dehydration.
- *Secondary prevention*—Administer drug therapy as prescribed to contain and treat an existing infectious process.
- *Tertiary prevention*—Instruct the stroke client how to exercise to minimize disability.
- Bear in mind the client's readiness to accept intervention and education.
- Ascertain the client's focus and how she sees her needs.
- Address client issues that might interfere with intervention (e.g., if the client is in pain, attempting to teach her about her care will be lost; her pain must be addressed first before she is ready to learn).
- Consider the timing of the visit to prevent interfering with other client activities.

- Schedule all visits at convenient times for the client if possible (e.g., if the client has a favorite soap opera to watch, attempt to schedule around that event if at all possible).
- Reschedule a home visit if a client event comes up suddenly.
- Be aware of nurse's safety in neighborhoods and take precautions to secure it.
- Outline nursing activities to be completed during the scheduled visit.
- Know the health care agency's policy and procedures for home visits.
- Consider the time line and other visits scheduled that day.
- Research evidence-based best practices to use in the home to validate your intervention decisions.
- Obtain necessary materials/supplies before making the visit.
- Assemble all equipment needed for any procedure in advance.
- Secure any equipment that might be needed if a problem occurs (e.g., bring additional IV tubing and a catheter to make sure the procedure can be carried out without delay).
- Determine criteria to be used to evaluate the effectiveness of the home visit.
- Revisit outcome goals to determine the effectiveness of the intervention.
- Assess the client's health status to validate improvement.
- Monitor changes in the client's behavior toward health promotion activities and disease prevention (e.g., verify/observe that the client demonstrates correct handwashing technique after instruction and reinforcement during the home care visit).

Adapted from de Chesnay, M., & Anderson, B. (2015). *Caring for the vulnerable* (4th ed.). Burlington, MA: Jones & Bartlett Learning; Lundy, K. S., & Janes, S. (2016). *Community health nursing: Caring for the public's health* (3rd ed.). Burlington, MA: Jones & Bartlett Learning; and Denham, S. A., Eggenberger, S., Young, P., & Krumwiede, N. (2015). *Family-focused nursing care.* Philadelphia, PA: F. A. Davis Company.

---

allowing for improved monitoring of clients in community settings and at home and also allowing complicated procedures to be done at home, such as intravenous administration of antibiotics and renal dialysis. There is a need to facilitate effective community-based care by extending the hospital and health care providers into the community by providing mobile access to information via a secure Internet. The design of future technologies to support complex health care in the home environment continues on the fast-track (Vizard, 2015).

Levels of Prevention in Community-Based Nursing

The concept of prevention is a key part of community-based nursing practice. The emphasis on health care delivery in community-based settings has moved beyond primary preventive health care (e.g., well-child checkups, routine physical examinations, prenatal care, and treatment of common acute illnesses) and now encompasses secondary and tertiary care.

PRIMARY PREVENTION

The concept of **primary prevention** involves preventing the disease or condition before it occurs through health promotion activities, environmental protection, and specific protection against disease or injury. Its focus is on **health promotion** to reduce the person's vulnerability to any illness by strengthening the person's capacity to withstand physical, emotional, and environmental stressors (Lundy & Janes, 2016).

Primary prevention encompasses a vast array of areas, including nutrition, good hygiene, sanitation, immunizations, protection from ultraviolet rays, genetic counseling, bicycle helmets, handrails on bathtubs, drug education for schoolchildren, adequate shelter, smoking cessation, family planning, and the use of seat belts (Stanhope & Lancaster, 2014). Prevention of disease is often difficult to put into practice. Among the challenges, the success of prevention is invisible in many cases, lacks drama, often requires persistent behavior change, and does not produce immediate results. The nurse's role is to help people change their lifestyle to move toward a state of optimal health and avoid illness. Nurses can address this by using evidence-based health promotion; identifying effective interventions built on research findings and applying them to improve the health and well-being of individuals, aggregates, and communities (Fig. 2.1).

Approximately 1/1,000 children in the United States are born each year with defects of the neural tube—the part of a growing fetus that will become the brain and spinal cord—which can cause severe mental and physical disability or death. It is the second most common major congenital anomaly worldwide (cardiac malformations are first). Neural tube defects (NTDs) are more common in Whites and Hispanics than African Americans (National Coalition for Health Professional Education in Genetics [NCHPEG], 2015). The prevention of NTDs is an example of primary prevention. The use of folic acid supplementation daily for 3 months before and 3 months after conception reduces the risk of first occurrence of NTD. American College of Obstetricians & Gynecologists [ACOG] (2013) recommends that all women be on a baseline dose of 400 µg of folic acid daily to prevent NTDs. Mandatory folic acid fortification for all pregnant women remains an effective public health intervention (Williams et al., 2015). Giving anticipatory guidance to parents with toddlers about poison prevention and safety during play is another example of primary prevention.

SECONDARY PREVENTION

Secondary prevention is the early detection and treatment of adverse health conditions. This level of prevention is aimed at halting the disease, thus shortening its duration and severity to get the person back to a normal state of functioning. Health screenings are the mainstay of secondary prevention. Pregnancy testing, blood pressure evaluations, cholesterol monitoring, fecal occult blood testing, breast examinations, mammography screening, hearing and vision examinations, and Papanicolaou (Pap) smears are examples of this level of prevention. Such interventions do not prevent the health problem but are intended for early detection and prompt treatment to prevent complications (Clark & Paraska, 2015).

A good example is osteoporosis, a common disease of the bones where one's body loses too much bone, makes too little bone, or both. Osteoporosis causes

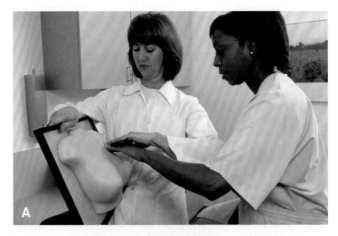

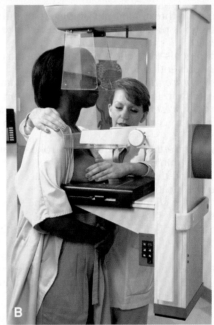

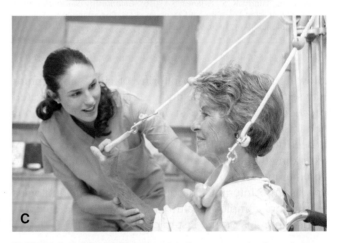

FIGURE 2.1 Levels of prevention in community-based nursing. **A.** At the primary prevention level, the nurse provides a woman with teaching about breast self-examination if high risk. **B.** At the secondary level of prevention, a woman undergoes a mammogram for early detection of breast problems. **C.** At the tertiary level of prevention, mastectomy after surgery, a nurse assists a client with her strength exercises.

significant morbidity and mortality in women. Its prevalence and costs to society are huge and its incidence is
rising as the population ages. Although osteoporosis is
preventable, it is a silent disease that does not become
apparent until a fracture occurs. Screening to identify
women at risk and instituting secondary prevention
pharmacotherapy will assist to reduce the incidence
of fractures and reduce mortality and morbidity. If the
health condition cannot be cured and further complications and disability arise, then the tertiary level of prevention is needed.

TERTIARY PREVENTION

Tertiary prevention is designed to reduce or limit the
progression of a permanent, irreversible disease or disability. The purpose of tertiary prevention is to restore
individuals to their maximum potential (Prince et al.,
2015). Tertiary intervention takes place only if the condition results in a permanent disability. Tertiary prevention
measures are supportive and restorative. For example,
tertiary prevention efforts would focus on minimizing
and managing the effects of a chronic illness such as
cerebrovascular disease or the chronic effects of sexually transmitted infections (STIs), e.g., herpes, human
immunodeficiency virus (HIV), and untreated syphilis.
Another example would involve working with women
who have suffered long-term consequences of violence.
Client education is the cornerstone of all disease management programs. The focus of the nurse would be to
maximize the woman's strengths through education, to
help her recover from the trauma and loss and to build
support systems.

The Nurse's Role in Community-Based Preventive Care

All health professionals have a special role in health promotion, health protection, and disease prevention. Much
of community nursing involves prevention, early identification, and prompt treatment of health problems and
monitoring for emerging threats that might lead to health
problems. Community-based nurses provide health care
for women and their families at all three levels of prevention. This care often involves advocating for services to
meet their needs.

Cultural Issues in Community-Based Nursing

The United States contains an ever-changing mix of
numerous, diverse cultural groups of people who arrive
daily from every corner of the world. The United States
has more immigrants than any other nation. The U.S.
Census Bureau (2015a) projects that the United States
foreign-born population will reach 78 million by 2060,
making up 19% of the total population.

Take Note!

More than one million immigrants come to the
United States each year, and more than half are
of childbearing age. Latin America accounts for more than
50% of immigrants to the United States. By the year 2050,
people of African, Asian, and Latino backgrounds will make
up one half of our population (U.S. Census Bureau, 2015b).

This growing diversity has significant implications
for the health care system. For years nurses have strug-
gled with the issues of providing optimal health care that
meets the needs of women and their families from various cultures and ethnic groups. In addition to displaying
competence in technical skills, nurses must also become
competent in caring for clients from diverse ethnic and
racial backgrounds. Adapting to different cultural beliefs
and practices requires flexibility and acceptance of others' viewpoints. Nurses must listen to clients and learn
about their beliefs about health and wellness. To provide culturally appropriate care to diverse populations,
nurses need to know, understand, and respect culturally
influenced health behaviors. Chapter 1 provides a more
detailed discussion of the impact of culture on the health
of women, children, and families.

Nurses must research and understand the cultural
characteristics, values, and beliefs of the various people
to whom they deliver care so that false assumptions and
stereotyping do not lead to insensitive care. Time orientation, personal space, family orientation (patriarchal,
matriarchal, or egalitarian), and language are important
cultural concepts. Although the location might be different in community-based care, these principles apply to
both inpatient and outpatient settings. Cultural competence and cultural adaptation are considered important
components of providing quality health care in multicultural societies. These include not only treatment of
disease, but also primary, secondary, and tertiary prevention measures by health care professionals, as well as
health promotion to all diverse cultures.

Culturally Competent Nursing Care

Cultural competence is defined as the knowledge,
willingness, and ability to adapt health care to enhance
its acceptability to and effectiveness with clients from
diverse cultures. Nurses need to possess an understanding of the perspectives, traditions, values, practices, and
family systems of culturally diverse individuals, families,
communities, and populations for whom they provide
care, as well as knowledge of the complex variables that
affect the achievement of health and well-being (Martin
et al., 2016). Cultural competence is a dynamic process
during which nurses obtain and then apply cultural information. Nurses must look at clients through their own
eyes and the eyes of clients and family members. Nurses

must develop nonjudgmental acceptance of cultural differences in clients, using diversity as a strength that empowers them to achieve mutually acceptable health care goals. Nurses must integrate their client's cultural beliefs and practices into health prescriptions to eliminate or mitigate health disparities and provide client satisfaction. Cultural competence is a dynamic, lifelong learning process. Understanding the process for assessing cultural patterns and factors that influence individual and group differences is critical in preventing overgeneralization and stereotyping (Purnell, 2015). This cultural awareness allows nurses to see the entire picture and improves the quality of care and health outcomes. Cultural competence does not appear suddenly; it must be developed through a series of steps (Box 2.3).

A level of cultural competence is needed by all nurses to increase their knowledge of diverse cultures, to change attitudes and values when working with clients of different cultures.

Cultural competence does not mean replacing one's own cultural identity with another, ignoring the variability within cultural groups, or even appreciating the cultures being served. Instead, nurses who are culturally competent show a respect for differences, an eagerness to learn, and a willingness to accept multiple views of the world. Much of the process of developing cultural competence involves a reexamination of nurses' values and the influence of these values on their beliefs, which affect attitudes and actions. At the core of both client centeredness and cultural competence is the importance of seeing the client as a unique person (Beard et al., 2015). It is important for all nurses to incorporate the client's traditional healing and health practices with conventional medicine by asking such questions as "Do you have treatment preferences you would like me to include in your care plan?" Some clients may prefer certain foods and/or drinks when they are ill. In addition, during fasting and religious seasons, diets may be different and need to be considered during the process of determining the appropriate course of treatment. Some clients may have a different idea about what is causing the illness. Spirituality, culture, and experience may have a significant role in the client's understanding and treatment of the illness.

Barriers to Cultural Competence

Barriers to cultural competence can be grouped into two categories: those related to providers and those related to systems. Illness is culturally shaped in the sense that how we perceive, experience, and cope with disease is based on our individual explanations of sickness. Awareness and appreciation of how this might be of influence—instead of mere knowledge about the cultural practices or beliefs of specific ethnic groups—help nurses deal effectively with cultural issues (Lundy & Janes, 2016).

BOX 2.3

STEPS TO DEVELOPING CULTURAL COMPETENCE

Cultural Awareness
- Become aware of, appreciate, and become sensitive to the values, beliefs, customs, and behaviors that have shaped one's own culture.
- Examine your own sociocultural heritage to gain personal insight.
- Recognize the influence of clients' cultures on their health status.
- Examine personal biases and prejudices toward other cultures.
- Become aware of differences in personal and clients' backgrounds.

Cultural Knowledge
- Apply knowledge of social and cultural factors across multiple backgrounds.
- Seek resources that increase your understanding of different sociocultural groups.
- Become familiar with culturally/ethnically diverse groups, worldviews, beliefs, practices, lifestyles, and problem-solving strategies.

Cultural Skills
- Apply relevant best evidence-based practices in providing culturally competent care.
- Learn how to perform a competent cultural assessment.
- Assess each client's unique cultural values, beliefs, and practices without depending solely on written facts about specific cultural groups.
- Advocate for social justice to eliminate health disparities in diverse populations.

Cultural Encounter
- Promote safe and quality outcomes of care for all diverse individuals.
- Adapt care practices and therapies to be consistent with client values and beliefs.
- Respect clients' sociocultural identity in a nonjudgmental manner when interacting.
- Learn key words or phases of clients' language to improve communication.
- Engage in cross-cultural interactions with people from culturally diverse backgrounds, such as attending religious services or ceremonies and participating in important family events.
- Participate in as many cultural encounters as possible to avoid cultural stereotyping.

Adapted from Waugh, E., Szafran, O., Triscott, J. C., & Parent, R. (2015). *Cultural competency skills for health professionals.* Alberta, Canada: Brush Education, Inc.; Purnell, L. D. (2015). *Culturally competent health care* (3rd ed.). Philadelphia, PA: F. A. Davis Company; and Martin, M. L., Heron, S., Moreno-Walton, L., & Jones, A. W. (2016). *Diversity and Inclusion in Quality Patient Care.* Switzerland: Springer International Publishers.

When a health care provider lacks knowledge of a client's cultural practices and beliefs or when the provider's beliefs differ from those of the client, the provider may be unprepared to respond when the client makes unexpected health care decisions. System-related barriers can occur if agencies that have not been designed for cultural diversity want all clients to conform to the established rules and regulations and attempt to fit everyone into the same mold.

Consider This

*O*ur medical mission took a team of nurse practitioners into the rural mountains of Guatemala to offer medical services to people who had never had any. One day, a distraught mother brought her 10-year-old daughter to the mission clinic, asking me if there was anything I could do about her daughter's right wrist. She had sustained a fracture a year ago and it had not healed properly. As I looked at the girl's malformed wrist, I asked if it had been splinted to help with alignment, knowing what the answer was going to be. The interpreter enlightened me by saying that this young girl would never marry and have children because of this injury. I appeared puzzled at the interpreter's prediction of this girl's future. It was later explained to me that if the girl could not make tortes from corn meal for her husband because of her wrist disability, she would not be worthy of becoming someone's wife and thus would probably live with her parents the rest of her life.

I reminded myself during the week of the medical mission not to impose my cultural values on the women for whom I was caring and to accept their cultural mores without judgment. These silent self-reminders served me well throughout the week, for I was open to learning about their lifestyles and customs.

Thoughts: *What must the young girl be feeling at the age of 10, being rejected for a disability that was not her fault? What might have happened if I had imposed my value system on this client? How effective would I have been in helping her if she did not feel accepted? This incident ripped my heart out, for this young girl will be deprived of a fulfilling family life based on a wrist disability. This is just another example of female suppression that happens all over the world—such a tragedy—and yet a part of their culture, on which nurses should not pass judgment.*

Use of Complementary and Alternative Medicine

The federal government formed the National Center for Complementary and Alternative Medicine (NCCAM) to conduct and support research and provide education and information on complementary and alternative medicine (CAM) to health care providers and the public.

The use of CAM is not unique to a specific ethnic or cultural group; interest in CAM therapies continues to grow nationwide and will affect care of many clients.

People from all walks of life and in all areas of the community use CAM. Overall, CAM use is seen more in women than men, and in people with higher educational levels. In the United States, approximately 40% of adults (about 4 in 10) and approximately 12% of children (about 1 in 9) are using some form of CAM. Prayer specifically for health reasons is the most commonly used CAM therapy (National Center for Complementary and Alternative Medicine [NCCAM], 2015). It is well known that CAM, including homeopathy, acupuncture, phytotherapy, and hydrotherapy, is also being used increasingly by midwives for childbirth (Hall, Griffiths, & McKenna, 2015).

Types of CAM

CAM includes diverse practices, products, and health care systems that are not currently considered to be part of conventional medicine (NCCAM, 2015). *Complementary* medicine is used together with conventional medicine, such as using aromatherapy to reduce discomfort after surgery or to reduce pain during a procedure or during early labor. *Alternative* medicine is used in place of conventional medicine, such as eating a special natural diet to control nausea and vomiting or to treat cancer instead of undergoing surgery, chemotherapy, or radiation that has been recommended by a conventional doctor. *Integrative* medicine combines mainstream medical therapies and CAM therapies for which there is some scientific evidence of safety and effectiveness (NCCAM, 2015).

INTEGRATIVE MEDICINE

Integrative medicine includes acupuncture, reflexology, therapeutic touch, meditation, yoga, massage, herbal therapies, nutritional supplements, homeopathy, naturopathic medicine, and many more used for the promotion of health and well-being (Treister-Goltzman & Peleg, 2015).

The philosophy of integrative medicine focuses on treating the whole person, not just the disease, and combines conventional Western medicine with complementary treatments. The goal is to treat the mind, body, and spirit all at the same time. History has taught us that in science, application of the results is never determined by a single study but, rather, by the weight of the evidence. Medicine rests on a foundation that begins with good clinical observations, case reports, and careful interpretations. Replication of these results by other scientists, which is the true hallmark of valid science, establishes whether those clinical observations are important and perhaps applicable. Although some of the therapies used are nonconventional, a guiding principle within integrative medicine is to use therapies that have some high-quality evidence to support them (King et al., 2015). The nurse should avoid judgment and encourage the family to research all evidence-based approaches that support healthy outcomes. Table 2.2 describes selected CAM therapies and treatments.

TABLE 2.2	SELECTED COMPLEMENTARY AND ALTERNATIVE THERAPIES
Therapy	**Description**
Aromatherapy	Use of essential oils to stimulate the sense of smell for balancing mind, body, and spirit
Homeopathy	Based on the theory of "like treats like"; helps restore the body's natural balance
Acupressure	Restoration of balance by pressing an appropriate point so self-healing capacities can take over
Feng shui (pronounced *fung shway*)	The Chinese art of placement. Objects are positioned in the environment to induce harmony with chi
Guided imagery	Use of consciously chosen positive and healing images along with deep relaxation to reduce stress and to help people cope
Reflexology	Use of deep massage on identified points of the foot or hand to scan and rebalance body parts that correspond with each point
Therapeutic touch	Balancing of energy by centering, invoking an intention to heal, and moving the hands from the head to the feet several inches from the skin
Herbal medicine	The therapeutic use of plants for healing and treating diseases and conditions
Spiritual healing	Praying, chanting, presence, laying on of hands, rituals, and meditation to assist in healing
Chiropractic therapy	Aimed at removing irritants to the nervous system to restore proper function (e.g., spinal manipulation done for musculoskeletal complaints)
Massage therapy	Therapeutic stroking or kneading of the body to decrease pain, produce relaxation, and/or to improve circulation to that body part

Adapted from Treister-Goltzman, Y., & Peleg, R. (2015). Trends in publications on complementary and alternative medicine in the medical literature. *Journal of Complementary & Integrative Medicine*. doi: 10.1515/jcim-2014-0055; Ernst, E. (2015). How nurses can be misled about complementary and alternative medicine. *Journal of Advanced Nursing*, 71(2), 235–236; Hall, H. G., Griffiths, D., & McKenna, L. G. (2015). Complementary and alternative medicine: Interaction and communication between midwives and women. *Women and Birth*. doi:10.1016/j.wombi.2014.12.003; and King, T. L., Brucker, M. C., Kriebs, J. M., Fahey, J. O., Gegor, C. L., & Varney, H. (2015). *Varney's midwifery* (5th ed.). Burlington, MA: Jones & Bartlett Learning.

Theories of CAM

The theoretic underpinnings of complementary and alternative health practices propose that health and illness are complex interactions of the mind, body, and spirit. It is then surmised that many aspects of clients' health experiences are not subject to traditional scientific methods. This field does not lend itself readily to scientific study or to investigation and therefore is not easily embraced by many hard-core scientists (Jaiswal et al., 2015). Much of what is considered to be alternative medicine comes from the Eastern world, folk medicine, and religious and spiritual practices. There is no unifying basic theory for the numerous treatments or modalities, except (as noted previously) that health and illness are considered to be complex interactions among the body, mind, and spirit.

Nursing Implications of CAM

Because of heightened interest in CAM and its widening use, anecdotal efficacy, and growing supporting research evidence, nurses need to be sensitive to and knowledgeable enough to answer many of the questions clients ask and to guide them in a safe, objective way (Ernst, 2015). Nurses have a unique opportunity to provide services that facilitate wholeness. They need to understand all aspects of CAM, including costs, client knowledge, and drug interactions, if they are to promote holistic strategies for clients and families.

The growing use of CAM during pregnancy and childbirth could be interpreted as a response by women regarding a need for autonomy and active participation in their health care. Studies have shown that massage, acupuncture, vitamins, and herbs are the most frequently applied CAM methods during pregnancy (Nursing & Midwifery Council, 2015).

Many clients who use CAM do not reveal this fact to their health care provider. Therefore, one of the nurse's most important roles during the assessment phase of the nursing process is to encourage clients to communicate their use of these therapies to eliminate the possibility of harmful interactions and contraindications with current medical therapies. When assessing clients, ask specific questions about any nonprescription medications they may be taking, including vitamins, minerals, or herbs. Clients should also be asked about any therapies they are taking that have not been ordered by their primary health care provider.

When caring for clients and their families who practice CAM, nurses need to:

- Be culturally sensitive to nontraditional treatments
- Acknowledge and respect different beliefs, attitudes, and lifestyles
- Keep an open mind, remembering that standard medical treatments do not work for all clients
- Accept CAM and integrate it if it brings comfort without harm
- Provide accurate information, not unsubstantiated opinions
- Advise clients how they can best monitor their condition using CAM
- Discourage practices only if they are harmful to the client's health
- Instruct the client to weigh the risks and benefits of CAM use
- Avoid confrontation when asking clients about CAM
- Be reflective, nonjudgmental, and open minded about CAM

The use of CAM is widespread, especially by women desiring to alleviate the nausea and vomiting of early pregnancy. Ginger lollipops or tea, Sea-Bands, and vitamin B_6 are frequently used to treat morning sickness (Brucker & King, 2016). Although these may not cause any ill effects during the pregnancy, most substances ingested cross the placenta and have the potential to reach the fetus, so nurses should stress to all pregnant women that they should be cautious when using CAM.

Women at risk for osteoporosis are seeking alternatives to hormone replacement therapy since the Women's Health Initiative study raised doubts about the benefit of estrogen. Some of the alternative therapies for osteoporosis include soy isoflavones, epimedium koreanum Nakai (herb) progesterone cream, magnet therapy, tai chi, and hip protectors (Mukhtar & Jackson, 2015). In addition, menopausal women may seek CAM therapies for hot flashes. Once again, despite many claims, most of these therapies have not undergone scientific testing and thus could place the woman at risk.

If clients are considering the use of or are using CAM therapies, suggest they check with their health care provider before taking any "natural" substance. Offer clients the following instructions:

- Keep in mind that "natural" does not necessarily mean "safe."
- Seek medical care when ill.
- Always inform the health care provider if you are taking herbs or other therapies.

- Be sure that any product package contains a list of all ingredients and amounts of each.
- Be aware that frequent or continual use of large doses of a CAM preparation is not advisable, and harm may result if therapies are mixed (e.g., vitamin E, garlic, and aspirin all have anticoagulant properties).
- Research CAM through resources such as books, websites, and articles (NCCAM, 2015).

All nurses, especially nurses working in the community, must educate themselves about the pros and cons of CAM and be prepared to discuss and help their clients make sense of it all. Expanding our consciousness by understanding and respecting diverse cultures and CAM will enable nurses to provide the best treatment for clients and their families receiving community-based care.

COMMUNITY-BASED NURSING CARE SETTINGS

Community-based nursing takes place in a variety of settings, including physicians' offices, clinics, health departments, urgent care centers, hospital outpatient centers, churches, shelters, and clients' homes. Nurses provide well care, episodic ill care, and chronic care. They work to promote, preserve, and improve the health of the women and their families in these settings.

Due to technological advances, cost containment, and shortened hospital stays, the home is a common care setting for women and families today. Home care is geared toward the needs of the client and family. Private-duty nursing care is used when more extensive care is needed; it may be delivered hourly (several hours per day) or on a full-time, live-in basis. Periodic nursing visits may be used for intermittent interventions, such as intravenous antibiotic administration, follow-up client teaching, and monitoring. The goals of nursing care in the home setting include promoting, restoring, and maintaining the health of the client.

Home care focuses on minimizing the effects of the illness or disability along with providing the client with the means to care for the illness or disability at home. Nurses in the home care setting are direct care providers, educators, advocates, and case managers.

Prenatal Care

Early, adequate prenatal care has long been associated with improved pregnancy outcomes (March of Dimes, 2015). Adequate prenatal care is a comprehensive process in which any problems associated with pregnancy are identified and treated. Basic components of prenatal care include early and continuing risk assessment, health promotion, medical and psychosocial interventions, and follow-up. Within the community setting, several services are available to provide health care for pregnant women (Box 2.4).

BOX 2.4

MATERNAL COMMUNITY HEALTH CARE SERVICES

- State public health prenatal clinics provide access to care based on a sliding-scale payment schedule is used or services may be paid for by Medicaid.
- Federally funded community clinics typically offer a variety of services, which may include prenatal, pediatric, adult health, and dental services. A sliding-scale payment schedule is used or Medicaid may cover costs.
- Hospital outpatient health care services offer maternal–child health services. Frequently they are associated with a teaching hospital in which medical school students, interns, and OB/GYN residents rotate through the clinic services to care for clients during their education process.
- Private OB/GYN offices are available for women with health insurance seeking care during their pregnancies. Some physicians in private practice will accept Medicaid clients as well as private clients.
- Community free clinics offer maternal–child services in some communities for women with limited economic resources (homeless, unemployed).
- Freestanding birth centers offer prenatal care for low-risk mothers as well as childbirth classes to educate couples regarding the birthing process. Most centers accept private insurance and Medicaid for reimbursement services.

- Midwifery services are available in many communities where midwives provide women's health services. They usually accept a multitude of payment plans ranging from private pay to health insurance to Medicaid for reimbursement purposes.
- WIC provides food, nutrition counseling, and access to health services for low-income women, infants, and children. WIC is a federally funded program and is administered by each state. All persons receiving Aid to Families with Dependent Children (AFDC), food stamps, or Medicaid are automatically eligible for WIC. An estimated 10 million people get WIC benefits monthly. WIC serves 53% of all infants born in the United States (USDA Food and Nutrition Service, 2015).
- Childbirth classes offer pregnant women and their partners a series of educational classes on childbirth preparation. Women attend them during their last trimester of pregnancy. Some classes are free and some have a fee.
- Local La Leche League groups provide mother-to-mother support for breast-feeding, nutrition, and infant care problem-solving strategies. All women who have an interest in breast-feeding are welcome to participate in the meetings, which are typically held in the home of a La Leche member.

Adapted from Community Health Network. (2015). *Maternity services.* Retrieved from http://www.ecommunity.com/ob; La Leche League. (2015). *Breastfeeding resources.* Retrieved from http://www.llli.org/resources.html; and USDA Food and Nutrition Service. (2015). *WIC fact sheet.* Retrieved from http://www.fns.usda.gov/wic/factsheets.htm

---

Not all women are aware of the community resources available to them. Most public health services are available for consultation, local hospitals have "hotlines" for questions, and public libraries have pregnancy-related resources as well as Internet access. Nurses can be a very helpful link to resources for all women regardless of their economic status.

Technologically advanced care has been shown to improve maternal and infant outcomes. Regionalized high-risk care, recommended by the American Academy of Pediatrics in the late 1970s, aimed to promote uniformity nationwide, covering the prenatal care of high-risk pregnancies and high-risk newborns. The advanced technology found in level III perinatal regional centers and community-based prenatal surveillance programs has resulted in better risk-adjusted mortality rates. Regionalized systems of perinatal care, along with telemedicine, are recommended to ensure that each mother and newborn achieves optimal outcomes. Telemedicine is when a health care provider uses interactive real-time audio and video telecommunications to deliver health services to a client at a site distant to the health care provider for the purpose of assessment, diagnosis, and treatment (Ivey et al., 2015). For example, fetal monitoring and ultrasound technology have traditionally been used in acute care settings to monitor the progress of many high-risk pregnancies. However, with the increased cost of hospital stays, many services were moved to outpatient facilities and into the home. The intent was to reduce health care costs and to monitor women with complications of pregnancy in the home rather than in the hospital. Examples of services offered in the home setting might include:

- Infusion therapy to treat infections or combat dehydration
- Hypertension monitoring for women with gestational hypertension
- Uterine monitoring for mothers who are at high risk for preterm labor
- Fetal monitoring to evaluate fetal well-being
- Portable ultrasound to perform a biophysical profile to assess fetal well-being

As a result, home care has the potential to produce cost savings compared with inpatient care.

Labor and Birth Care

Pregnancy involves numerous choices: cloth or disposable diapers, breast-feeding or bottle feeding, doctor or midwife, and where to give birth (at a birthing center, at home, or at a hospital). Deciding where to give birth depends on the woman's pregnancy risk status. For the pregnant woman who is at high risk as a result of medical or social factors, the hospital is considered the safest place for birth. Potential complications can be addressed because medical technology, skilled professionals, and neonatal services are available. For low-risk women, a freestanding birthing center or a home birth is an option.

The choice between a birthing center, home birth, or hospital depends on the woman's preferences, her risk status, her financial status, and her distance from a hospital. Some women choose an all-natural birth with no medications and no medical intervention, whereas others would feel more comfortable in a setting in which medications and trained staff are available if needed. Presenting the facts to women and allowing them to choose in collaboration with their health care provider is the nurse's role. Client safety is paramount, but at the same time nurses must protect the woman's right to select birth options. Nurses should promote family-centered care in all maternity settings (see Evidence-Based Practice 2.1).

Birthing Center

A birthing/childbirth center is a cross between a home birth setting and a hospital. Birthing centers offer a home-like setting but with proximity to a hospital in case of complications. Midwives often are the sole care providers in freestanding birthing centers, with obstetricians as backups in case of emergencies. Birthing centers usually have fewer restrictions and guidelines for families to follow and allow for more freedom in making decisions about labor. The rates of cesarean birth and the costs are much lower than those of a hospital. A study shows that midwife-led comprehensive care in a birthing center using the same medical guidelines as in standard care in hospitals reduced medical interventions without jeopardizing maternal and infant health (Arcia, 2015). The normal discharge time in birthing centers after childbirth is usually measured in hours (4 to 24 hours), not 24 to 48 hours, as is the case in hospitals.

Childbirth centers aim to provide a relaxing home environment and promote a "culture of normalcy." Pregnancy and childbirth are healthy, normal life events for most women. In birth centers, midwives and staff hold to the wellness model of birth, which means they provide

EVIDENCE-BASED PRACTICE 2.1

HOME BIRTH AFTER HOSPITAL BIRTH: WOMEN'S CHOICES AND REFLECTIONS

Women have been giving birth to newborns in the home setting since the beginning of time; giving birth in an institution has been the norm only since the early 20th century. The number of women in the United States choosing home birth is increasing. Little is known about women who choose home birth after having experienced hospital birth; therefore, the purpose of this research was to explore reasons why these women chose a home birth and their perceptions regarding both of their birth experiences.

STUDY

The research design was a qualitative description, whereby focus groups were conducted with women who had hospital births and subsequently choose a home birth and their perceptions regarding both birth experiences. Five focus groups were conducted (N = 20), recorded, and transcribed verbatim. Qualitative content analyses were applied to the women's narratives.

Findings

Five themes emerged from the focus group's narratives. (1) *Choices and empowerment*: With home birth, women felt they were given real choices rather than perceived choices, providing them feelings of power and control over their bodies. (2) *Interventions and interruptions*: Women believed interventions were done in the hospital

setting that were not beneficial to the birthing process, and there were numerous interruptions with their hospital births. (3) *Disrespect and dismissal*: Women believed during their hospital birth, providers were more focused on the laboring uterus than themselves; others were dismissed from their providers when choosing a home birth. (4) *Birth space*: Home birth provided a peaceful and calm environment surrounded by friends and family. (5) *Connection*: Women felt connected to their providers and family at home. Most women felt dissatisfied with their hospital birth that influenced their subsequent decision to choose a home birth for their next pregnancy.

Nursing Implications

This study brings forth several themes that influenced women to select a home birth verses a hospital birth. Many of the themes focus on the women's control of her own birth experience in the home setting verses the hospital setting that included unnecessary interventions and multiple interruptions that impacted the women's birth experience negatively. Nurses, working in labor and birth suites within hospitals, need to be aware of these five themes and work toward changing their birthing environments to make it a more positive experience. This study's findings can act as a catalyst toward change with additional focus group's comments done upon discharge. Collecting consumer's feedback is needed to continually meet their needs.

Adapted from Bernhard, C., Zielinski, R., Ackerson, K., & English, J. (2014). Home birth after hospital birth: Women's choices and reflections. *Journal of Midwifery & Women's Health*, 59(2), 160–166.

continuous, supportive care during which interventions are used only when medically necessary. Currently, the number of birth centers being established is on the rise. It is in these birth centers that midwives will learn about normalcy, building the skills needed to support women through labor, rather than managing labor. The current economic climate may result in more efficient use of resources, possibly normalizing birth (ACOG, 2015). The range of services for the expectant family often includes prenatal care, childbirth education, intrapartum care, and postpartum care, including home follow-up and family planning (Fig. 2.2). One of the hallmarks of the free-standing birthing center is that it can provide truly family-centered care by approaching pregnancy and birth as a natural family event and encouraging all family members to participate. Education is often provided by such centers, encouraging families to become informed and self-reliant in the care of themselves and their families (Sporek, 2015).

Birthing centers provide an alternative for women who are uncomfortable with a home birth but who do not want to give birth in a hospital. Advantages of birthing centers include a noninterventional approach to obstetric care, freedom to eat and move around during labor, ability to give birth in any position, and the right to have any number of family and friends attend the birth. Disadvantages are that some centers have rigid screening criteria, which may eliminate healthy mothers from using birth centers; many have rigid rules concerning transporting the mother to the hospital (e.g., prolonged labor and ruptured membranes); and many have no pediatrician on staff if the newborn has special needs after birth (Gardner, 2015).

Home Birth

Home births continue to constitute only a small percentage of all childbirths in the United States, in part

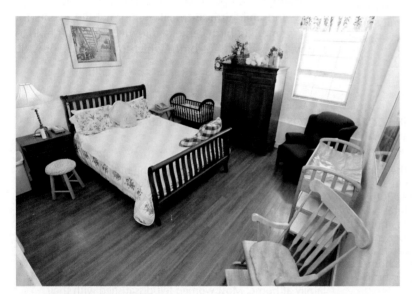

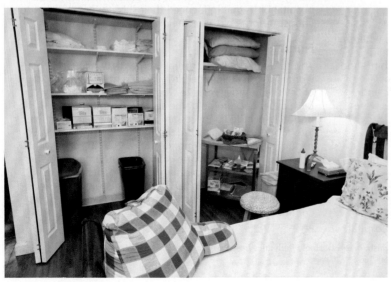

FIGURE 2.2 Birthing centers aim to provide a relaxing home-like environment and promote a culture of normality while offering a full range of health care services to the expectant family. (Photos by Gus Freedman.)

because of the concerns about safety. The literature is mixed regarding the safety of home births, but health care professionals should respect a woman's choice of birth settings, her right to choose, and her autonomy. Many women choose to have a home birth so it can be a family event. Feeling safe and in control can assist the birthing process because the woman feels more comfortable in her own surroundings and confident in her coping ability (Jokinen & Johnson, 2015).

For centuries women have been giving birth to babies in their home. Many women feel more comfortable and relaxed when giving birth in their own environment. Women who want no medical interventions and a very family-centered birth often choose to have a home birth. Home births are recommended for pregnant women who are considered to be at low risk for complications during labor and birth (ACOG, 2015). Home birth is advantageous because it:

* Is the least expensive
* Allows the woman to experience labor and birth in the privacy, comfort, and familiarity of home while surrounded by loved ones
* Permits the woman to maintain control over every aspect affecting her labor (e.g., positions, attire, and support people)
* Minimizes interference and unnecessary interventions, allowing labor to progress normally
* Provides continuous one-on-one care by the midwife throughout the childbirth process
* Promotes the development of a trusting relationship with the nurse midwife (American Pregnancy Association [APA], 2015)

A home birth does have some disadvantages, including the limited availability of pain medication and danger to the mother and baby if an emergency arises (e.g., placental abruption, uterine rupture, cord prolapse, or a distressed fetus). Delay in getting to the hospital could jeopardize the life of the child or the mother. A backup plan for a health care provider and nearby hospital on standby must be established should an emergency occur. The available evidence suggests that planned home birth is safe for women who are at low risk of complications and are cared for by appropriately qualified and AMCB-certified midwives with access to timely transfer to hospital if required (Grunebaum et al., 2015).

Postpartum and Newborn Care

Recent reforms in health care financing have reduced hospital stays significantly for new mothers. As a result, community-based nurses play a major role in extending care beyond the hospital setting. When new mothers are discharged from the hospital, most are still experiencing perineal discomfort and uterine cramping. They may still have pain from an episiotomy. They are fatigued

and may be constipated. They may feel uncertain about feeding and caring for their newborn. The prevalence of early postpartum mental health conditions is high also. Nurses are in prime position to identify mothers at risk. A recent study found that excessive infant crying problems, older age, lower educational levels, breastfeeding problems, and single first-time mothers with no partner support were predictors of maternal distress in the postpartum period (Aston et al., 2015). These new mothers need to be made aware of community resources such as telephone consultation by nurses, outpatient clinics, home visits, neighborhood mother's support groups, and online new parent forums.

Telephone Consultation

Many hospitals offer telephone consultation services by their maternity nurses. The discharged mother is given the phone number of the nursing unit on the day of discharge and is instructed to call if she has any questions or concerns. Because the nurses on the unit are familiar with her birth history and the newborn, they are in a good position to assist her in adjusting to her new role. Although this service is usually free, not all families recognize a problem early or use this valuable informational resource.

Outpatient Clinics

Outpatient clinics offer another community-based site where the childbearing family can obtain services. Usually the mother has received prenatal care before giving birth and thus has established some rapport with the nursing staff there. The clinic staff is usually willing to answer any questions she may have about her health or that of her newborn. Appointments usually include an examination of the mother and newborn and instructions about umbilical cord care, postpartum and infant care, and nutrition for both mother and infant.

Postpartum Home Visits

Home visits offer services similar to those offered at a scheduled clinic visit, but they also give the nurse an opportunity to assess the family's adaptation and dynamics and the home environment. During the past decade, hospital stays have averaged 24 to 48 hours or less for vaginal births and 72 to 96 hours for cesarean births (Centers for Disease Control and Prevention [CDC], 2015a). Federal legislation went into effect in 1998 that prohibited insurers from restricting hospital stays for mothers and newborns to less than 2 days for vaginal births or 4 days for cesarean births (CDC, 2015a). These shortened stays have reduced the time available for educating mothers about caring for themselves and their newborns. Home visiting programs in general seek to

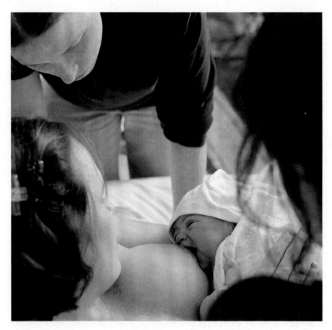

FIGURE 2.3 The nurse makes a postpartum home visit to assess the woman and her newborn. During the visit, the nurse assists the mother with breast-feeding.

promote child health/development, prevent child abuse/neglect, improve maternal well-being, and improve the parental capacity of mothers.

Postpartum care in the home environment usually includes:

- Monitoring the physical and emotional well-being of the family members (Fig. 2.3)
- Identifying potential or developing complications for the mother and newborn
- Assessing behaviors characteristic of postpartum depression
- Linking the family, as needed, to community social services and housing and governmental programs
- Reviewing of role adjustments and available community supports
- Contraception education and community locations to obtain it
- Bridging the gap between discharge and ambulatory follow-up for mothers and their newborns (Lundy & Janes, 2016)

The use of technology to complement home-based nursing care may enhance care. Technology in its many forms can help empower clients while they remain in the comfort of their own homes. Technology examples may include telephone conversations between clients and nurses to triage symptoms, provide advice, monitor vital signs, and provide guidance on use of medications; phone texting on health promotion; video conferencing; or local Internet-based support groups for sharing information with other new mothers (Vo et al., 2015).

Support Groups for New Mothers

Support groups for new mothers are typically local groups led by a facilitator with previous experience in motherhood, breast-feeding, and infant care. Usually they are composed of 6 to 12 mothers who share information on breast-feeding techniques, infant sleeping patterns, child care issues, body image issues, and how to integrate the new baby into the family unit. Support groups usually meet weekly and provide an avenue of support that encourages disclosure and provides contact with other new mothers experiencing the same journey and challenges.

Online Motherhood Forums and Blogs

Support groups in online communities provide an anonymous place to exchange information and advice. Previous research has suggested that these groups offer a safe, nonjudgmental forum for new mothers to share experiences and interact anonymously. They are seen as a safe, supportive space in which new mothers can better understand their new role of parenting. They offer a viable form of education for new parents, along with laughs, memories, deep thoughts and recollections of pre-motherhood days. Reasons for new mothers to seek out online blogs and forums include feelings of community or acceptance, the desire to be a good mother, for emotional support and the need for practical advice about parenting (Johnson, 2015).

High-Risk Newborn Home Care

With the reduced lengths of hospital stays, high-risk newborns are also being cared for in community settings. High-tech care once was provided only in the hospital. Now, however, the increasing cost of complex care and the influences of managed care have brought high-tech care into the home. Families have become health care systems by providing physical, emotional, social, and developmental home care for their technology-dependent infants. Suitable candidates for home care may include preterm infants who continue to need oxygen, low-birth-weight infants who need nutritional or hypercaloric formulas or adjunct feeding methods (e.g., tube feedings), or infants with hydrocephalus or cerebral palsy. Home care with prepared caregivers might contribute to earlier detection of significant residual/recurrent problems amenable to therapy. Studies suggest that improving home care for the high risk infant in the early months after discharge, a critical period for growth, has the potential to reduce incidences and burdens of their health care needs over the lifespan (Cheng et al., 2015). A wide range of equipment may be used, including mechanical ventilation, electronic apnea monitors, home oxygen equipment, intravenous infusion equipment, respiratory nebulizers, phototherapy, and suction equipment.

All family members must work together to provide 24-hour care. The parents must negotiate with insurers for reimbursement for durable medical equipment, must be able to troubleshoot equipment problems, and must be able to manage inventories of supplies and equipment. In addition, they must be able to assess the infant for problems; determine the problem; decide when to call the nurse, pharmacist, or physical therapist; and interpret and implement prescriptions. The use of technology in the home requires nurses to focus on the family home care system to provide total care to the infant.

Nurses can play a key role in assisting families by preparing them for and increasing their confidence in caring for their infants at home. This adaptation begins before discharge from the hospital. Family members are active participants in the transition-to-home plan. Recognition of parental needs and addressing each area in the discharge plan will ease the transition to home.

Assessment of the family's preparedness is essential. The following areas should be explored:

- *Parenting education*: Assess the family's knowledge of positioning and handling of their infant, nutrition, hygiene, elimination, growth and development, immunizations needed, and recognition of illnesses. Asking questions in a sensitive manner will assist the nurse in identifying knowledge deficiencies, so they can be reinforced in the nurse's teaching plan.
- *Postpartum care*: Determine the mother's concerns in areas of body image, weight loss, sleep/rest needs, discomfort, fatigue, and adjustment to her new role. Asking open-ended questions concerning these areas will help the nurse extract more information to include in the teaching plan. Targeting the mother's areas of concern will help the nurse focus on needed education to facilitate the mother's transition into her new role as a parent.
- *Support systems*: Assess physical and emotional support for the new mother by asking questions about the availability of her immediate family, other relatives, and significant others to provide help. If lacking, referrals may need to be made to community parenting programs, cooperative daycare, or other community resources needed to assist this family. Exploring these vital areas through sensitive questioning hopefully will convey the nurse's concern for the infant and family while obtaining a thorough assessment of the family's learning needs.

Once preparedness has been assessed, the nurse can intervene as necessary. For example, if the caretakers do not think they are prepared to maintain machinery, technology, medication, or developmental therapy, then the nurse can demonstrate the care to the family. The nurse provides instructions and hands-on experience in a supportive environment until the family's confidence increases. The nurse can also assist the family to anticipate the common problems that might occur (e.g., advising them to avoid running out of supplies, to have enough medication or special formula mixture to last throughout the weekend, and to keep backup batteries for powering machines or portable oxygen). The outcome of the preparedness assessment and intervention is that the safety of the infant is established and maintained.

Nursing for families who are using complex home care equipment requires caring for the infant and family members' physical and emotional well-being as well as providing solutions to problems they may encounter. Home health nurses need to identify, mobilize, and adapt a myriad of community resources to support the family in giving the best possible care in the home setting. Preparing families before hospital discharge, with home health nurses continuing and reinforcing that focus, will ease the burden of managing high-tech equipment in the home.

Women's Health Care

A woman's reproductive years span half her lifetime, on average. This is not a static period, but rather one that encompasses several significant stages. As her reproductive goals change, so do a woman's health care needs. Because of these changing needs, comprehensive community-centered care is critical.

Community-based women's health services have received increased emphasis during the past few decades simply because of economics. Women use more health care services than men, they make as many as 90% of health care decisions, and they represent the majority of the population (CDC, 2015b). Women spend 66 cents of every health care dollar, and seven of the ten most frequently performed surgeries in the United States are specific to women (Alexander et al., 2014). Examples of community-based women's health care services that can be freestanding or hospital based include:

- Screening centers that offer mammograms, Pap smears, bone density assessments, genetic counseling, ultrasound imaging, breast examinations, complete health risk appraisals, laboratory studies (complete blood count, cholesterol testing, thyroid testing, glucose testing for diabetes, follicle-stimulating hormone levels), and electrocardiograms
- Educational centers that provide women's health lectures, instruction on breast self-examinations and Pap smears, and computers for research
- Counseling centers that offer various support groups: genetics, psychotherapy, substance abuse, sexual assault, and domestic violence
- Wellness centers that offer stress reduction techniques, massage therapy, guided imagery, hypnosis, smoking cessation, weight reduction, tai chi, yoga, and women's fitness/exercise classes

- Alternative/wholeness healing centers that provide acupuncture, aromatherapy, biofeedback, therapeutic touch, facials, reflexology, and herbal remedies
- Retail centers that offer specialty equipment for rental and purchase, such as breast prostheses

Women have multiple choices regarding services, settings, and health care providers. In the past, most women received health care services from physicians such as obstetricians, gynecologists, and family physicians, but today nurse midwives and nurse practitioners are becoming more prevalent in providing well-woman care.

Nurses who work in community-based settings need to be familiar with the many health issues commonly encountered by women within their communities. All nurses who work with women of any age in community-based settings, including the workplace, schools, practitioners' offices, and clinics, should possess a thorough understanding of the scope of women's health care and should be prepared to intervene appropriately to prevent problems and to promote health.

ROLES AND FUNCTIONS OF THE COMMUNITY-BASED NURSE

Many nurses find the shift from acute care to community settings a challenge. With the shift in responsibilities from hospital care to community care, changes in nursing care have resulted. Nurses working in community-based settings share many of the same roles and responsibilities as their colleagues in acute care settings, but there are some differences. For example, in the community or home care setting the nurse will provide direct client care but will spend more time in the role of educator, communicator, and manager than the nurse in the acute care setting. In home care, the nurse will spend a significant amount of time in the supervisory or management role. Regardless of which setting (inpatient or outpatient) a nurse works in, principles of holistic care still apply universally.

Communicator

Effective therapeutic communication with women, children, and families is critical to the provision of quality nursing care. Client- and family-centered communication increases satisfaction with nursing care and aids in improving knowledge and health care skills (Arnold & Boggs, 2015). The significance of communication revolves around its effectiveness and the climate in which communication occurs. Trust, respect, and empathy are three factors needed to create and foster effective therapeutic communication among people.

Verbal and Nonverbal Communication

Nurses use verbal communication continuously throughout the day when interacting with their clients. Good verbal communication skills are necessary for excellent nursing assessment and teaching. Nonverbal communication, also referred to as body language, is composed of affective or expressive behavior, which can be demonstrated by attending to others and active listening. When clients and families feel they are being heard, trust and rapport are established.

Recall Maria, who recently was discharged from the hospital with her newborn son. How did the nurse communicate with Maria? Did the nurse's actions during the visit promote the development of trust between Maria and the nurse? What might have been done differently to foster trust?

Take Note!

People of all ages desire to be listened to without interruption (Bloomfield, 2015).

Active listening is critical to the communication process. Listening may uncover fears or concerns that the nurse may not have discovered through questioning. By not listening, critical information may be missed. Active listening is important in providing comprehensive nursing care. Research shows that exposure to an empathetic and active listening nurse has a calming and healing effect on clients (Arnold & Boggs, 2015). If the client or family senses that the nurse is not listening, they may be reluctant to share further information. During the interaction, determine whether the client's verbal communication is congruent with his or her nonverbal communication.

Communication With Families

When communicating with families, be honest. Families desire to be valued and should be equal partners in the health care team. Allow family members to verbalize concerns and questions. Explain the use of equipment and the correct sequence of procedures. Help the members understand the long-term as well as short-term effects of a health treatment.

Working With an Interpreter

Attempting to communicate with a family whose members do not speak English can be a highly frustrating situation for health care providers. Timely identification of a client's language needs at the first point of contact can facilitate the provision of language-appropriate services and contribute to quality of care, better outcomes, and client satisfaction (Kamimura et al., 2015). Interpreters are an invaluable aid and an essential component of client and family education. Working with an interpreter, whether in person or over the phone, requires coordination of efforts by both parties. This coordination is important so that both the family and the interpreter understand the information to be communicated. Working as a team, the nurse questions or informs and the interpreter conveys the information completely and accurately. *Healthy People 2020* also addresses the topic of language differences (see *Healthy People 2020*). In addition, many health care facilities subscribe to Language Line Services which is an on-demand interpretation company that provides telephone access to interpretation of 170 languages. Numerous other interpreters, translators, and language resources are available online.

HEALTHY PEOPLE *2020 • 2.1*

Objective ECBP-11 Increase the proportion of local health departments that have established culturally appropriate and linguistically competent community health promotion and disease prevention programs.

Nursing Significance

Work with professionals and individuals from various cultures to develop materials and programs for health promotion that are culturally competent. Ensure teaching materials are provided in the appropriate language.

Objective ECBP-10 Increase the number of community-based organizations (including local health departments, tribal health services, nongovernmental organizations, and state agencies) providing population-based primary prevention services in the following areas: injury, mental illness, tobacco use, substance abuse, unintended pregnancy, nutrition, and physical activity.

Nursing Significance

Educational and community-based programs play a key role in preventing disease and injury, improving and enhancing the quality of life. Education and community-based programs and strategies are designed to reach people outside of traditional health care settings. These settings may include schools, work sites, and health care agencies. Community health promotion activities are initiated by a health department or organization; organizers have a responsibility to engage the community. Realizing the vision of healthy people in healthy communities is possible only if the community, in its full cultural, social, and economic diversity, is an authentic partner in changing the conditions for health.

Healthy People objectives based on data from http://www.healthypeople.gov

---

HEALTHY PEOPLE *2020 • 2.2*

Objective HC/HIT-1 (Developmental) Improve the health literacy of the population.

Nursing Significance

Ideas about health and behaviors are shaped by communication, information, and technology. Health literacy is central to health care, public health, and the way our society views health. These processes make up the context and the ways professionals and the public search for, understand, and use health information, significantly impacting their health decisions and actions. Disparities in access to health information, services, and technology can result in lower usage rates of preventive services, less knowledge of chronic disease management, higher rates of hospitalization, and poorer reported health status. Thus, providing accurate, accessible, and actionable health information that is targeted or tailored to the individual client is essential.

Objective HC/HIT-2 Increase the proportion of persons who report that their health care providers have satisfactory communication skills.

Nursing Significance

Support shared decision making between clients and providers so that everyone buys into the treatment plan. Provide sound principles in the design of programs and interventions that result in healthier behaviors of the client and the family. Link the continuity of care within the community and at home to foster the best health outcomes.

Healthy People objectives based on data from http://www.healthypeople.gov.

Recall Maria, the woman with the newborn who is receiving home care. On the second visit to Maria's home, the nurse brought a Spanish-speaking interpreter who explained the reason for the "back to sleep" position and demonstrated to Maria several other useful positions for feeding and holding. Maria was smiling when the nurse left and asking when she would be back. What made the difference in their relationship during the second visit? What interventions demonstrate culturally competent care?

Communicating With Deaf Clients and Their Families

Nearly one in six Americans has hearing loss, and for those over the age of 65, the ratio climbs to one in three. By the end of this century, there will be approximately

360 million people around the world with some hearing disability. Studies show that deaf people have poorer health than those that hear normally, which is attributed to problems accessing health care and communicating with health care providers (Emond et al., 2015). Health care providers are under a duty to provide auxiliary aids and services to establish effective communication with their clients. Providing assistance to people with hearing impairments in health care settings is critically important because, without assistance through auxiliary aids and services, health service providers run the risk of not understanding the client's symptoms, misdiagnosing the client's health problem, and prescribing inadequate or even harmful treatment (Alselai & Alrashed, 2015).

Pregnant women who have hearing impairments are often neglected mostly because of a lack of understanding of how best to care for women with different communication needs. Nurses have a key role in exchanging information and taking the time to understand the needs of women with hearing impairments in order to act as an advocate and to help overcome the barriers that can be created by deafness. To fulfill this role, nurses need to have an understanding of the problems faced by women with hearing impairments and their partners when accessing maternity services (Velonaki et al., 2015).

For clients with hearing impairments, nurses should determine their desired method of communication: lip reading, American Sign Language (ASL), another method such as CART (Communication Access Real-time Translation) which can be viewed on a tablet, laptop, or smart phone, or some combination. If the nurse is not proficient in ASL and the client or family uses it, then an ASL interpreter must be available if another adult family member is not present for translation. According to federal law, deaf clients and deaf family members must be given the ability to communicate effectively with health care providers (Oliveira et al., 2015).

Direct Care Provider

The community-based nurse typically performs less direct physical care than the nurse in the acute care setting. Many times the nurse may observe the client or caregiver performing physical care tasks. Excellent assessment skills are especially important in the community care setting. The nurse often is functioning in an autonomous role, and after data collection, the community-based nurse will often decide whether to initiate, continue, alter, or end physical nursing care. Assessment extends beyond physical assessment of the client to include the environment and the community.

The nurse provides direct care to the perinatal client, beginning with the woman's first visit to the health care provider and extending through the pregnancy and birth. In addition, the nurse provides direct care involving the following areas:

- Contraception
- Abortion
- Infertility
- Screening for STIs
- Preconceptual risk assessment and care

Educator

As a result of shortened hospital stays and decreased admissions, providing client and family education is a key role for nurses in the community. Many times teaching begins in the community setting, especially the home. In the community-based setting, client teaching is often focused on assisting the client and family to achieve independence.

Regardless of the type of setting, nurses are in a unique position to help clients and families manage their own health care. Clients and families need to be knowledgeable about areas such as their condition, the health care management plan, and when and how to contact health care providers. With the limited time available in all health care arenas, nurses must focus on teaching goals and begin teaching at the earliest opportunity (Peter et al., 2015).

Take Note!

There is no prescription more valuable than knowledge (C. Everett Koop, MD, Former Surgeon General of the United States).

Client education occurs when nurses share information, knowledge, and skills with clients and families, thus empowering them to take responsibility for their health care. Through client education, clients and families can overcome feelings of powerlessness and helplessness and gain the confidence and capability to be active members in their plan of care.

Overall, client and family education allows clients and families to make informed decisions, ensures the presence of basic health care skills, promotes recognition of problem situations, promotes appropriate responses to problems, and allows for questions to be answered. When thorough and structured education begins in the hospital setting, it can carry over into the home setting, which can decrease hospital readmissions. An evidence-based discharge checklist describes the processes needed for a safe and optimal discharge and a recommended timeline of when to complete each step, starting on the first day of admission. A check list includes (1) indication for admission to the hospital; (2) primary care in the home; (3) medication safety; (4) follow-up plans; (5) home care referrals; (6) communication with community providers; and (7) client education (Coleman et al., 2015). It can play an important role in aiding bedside nurses to provide early formal education for clients and families being discharged home with a new device so that safe care can be achieved in the home setting (Ulin et al., 2015). Client and family education is a priority and is addressed in *Healthy People 2020*.

Take Note!

To cope effectively with illness, to understand and participate in decisions about treatment plans, and to maintain and improve health after treatment, clients and their families must have knowledge and skills relevant to their conditions (Joint Commission, 2015).

Steps of Client and Family Education

Client education is an integral component of nursing care. The steps of client and family education are similar to the steps of the nursing process: the nurse must assess, plan, implement, evaluate, and finally document education. Once the nurse achieves a level of comfort and experience with each of these steps, they blend together and become a harmonious daily part of nursing practice. Client education begins with the first client encounter and proceeds through discharge and beyond. Reassessment after each step or change in the process is critical to ensuring success.

INTERVENING TO ENHANCE LEARNING

Nurses are in an excellent position to foster an environment that is conducive to learning. For example, it is entirely appropriate to say to the client, "Many people have a problem reading and remembering the information on this paper (booklet, manual). Is this ever a problem for you?" Once a problem is acknowledged, the nurse is free to adjust verbal communication techniques and written materials to assist with learning and to communicate this need to the entire interdisciplinary health care team.

Nurses implement individualized teaching techniques based on the assessment information and identified goals. In general, the following techniques can facilitate learning:

- Slow down and repeat information often.
- Speak in conversational style using plain, nonmedical language.
- Break the information down and teach it in small, digestible bits using logical steps.
- Prioritize information and teach survival skills first.
- Use visuals, such as pictures, videos, and models.
- Teach using an interactive, hands-on approach.

If the client or family has poor health literacy skills, learning can be fostered by the use of pictures or illustrations, videos or audio tapes, or color coding (such as medication bottles or steps of a procedure). In addition, teaching can include a "backup" family member.

DOCUMENTING TEACHING AND LEARNING

Documenting client care and education is an imperative part of every nurse's professional practice and is the only means available to ensure that the educational plan and objectives have been completed. Documentation serves four main purposes:

1. First and foremost, the client's medical record serves as a communication tool that the entire interdisciplinary team can use to keep track of what the client and family have learned already and what learning still needs to occur.
2. Second, it serves to testify to the education the family has received if legal matters arise.
3. Third, it verifies standards set by the Joint Commission, Centers for Medicare and Medicaid Services, and other accrediting bodies that hold health care providers accountable for client education activities.
4. Finally, it informs third-party payers of the goods and services that were provided for reimbursement purposes.

Client and family education plays an essential role in promoting safe self-management practice. To ensure that clients and their families attain the required abilities, client and family education needs to be competency based. When developing and applying a competency-based education lesson/program, each nurse must identify essential competencies to be taught, optimal teaching methods, best method to evaluate achievement, and documentation of evidence that learning has taken place (Embo et al., 2015).

Discharge Planner and Case Manager

Because of the short length of stays in acute settings and the shift to community settings for clients with complex health needs, discharge planning and case management have become an important nursing role in the community (Stanhope & Lancaster, 2014). Discharge planning involves the development and implementation of a comprehensive plan for the safe discharge of a client from a health care facility and for continuing safe and effective care in the community and at home. Case management focuses on coordinating health care services while balancing quality and cost outcomes. Often clients requiring community-based care, especially home care, have complex medical needs that require an interdisciplinary team to meet their physical, psychosocial, medical, nursing, developmental, and education needs. The nurse plays an important role in initiating and maintaining the link between team members and the client to ensure that the client and family are receiving comprehensive, coordinated care.

Advocate and Resource Manager

Client advocate is another important role of the community-based nurse to ensure that the client's and family's needs are being met. Advocacy also helps ensure that the client and family have available to them appropriate resources and health care services. For example, the pregnant woman on bed rest at home may need help in caring for her other children, maintaining the household, or getting to her appointments. Women with complex medical needs may require financial assistance through Medicaid or Medicaid waivers (state-run programs that use federal and state money to pay for the health care of individuals with certain medical conditions). They may also need assistance in obtaining needed equipment, additional services, and transportation. Community-based nurses need a basic understanding of community, state, and federal resources to ensure that clients and their families have access to needed resources.

KEY CONCEPTS

- Family-centered care recognizes the concept of the family as the constant. The health and functional abilities of the family affect the health of the client and other members of the family. Family-centered care recognizes and respects family strengths and individuality, encourages referrals for family support, and facilitates collaboration. It ensures flexible, accessible, and responsive health care delivery while incorporating developmental needs and implementing policies to provide emotional and financial support to women and their families.

- Health care delivery has moved from acute care settings out into the community, with an emphasis on health promotion and illness prevention (Lundy & Janes, 2016). Community health nursing focuses on preventing health problems and improving the health of populations and communities, addressing the current and potential health needs of the population or community, and promoting and preserving the health of a population regardless of age or diagnosis. Community health nurses perform epidemiologic investigations to help analyze and develop health policy and community health initiatives.

- Community-based nurses focus on providing personal care to individuals and families in the community. They focus on promoting and preserving health as well as preventing disease or injury. They help women and their families cope with illness and disease. They focus on minimizing barriers to allow the client to develop to his or her full potential.

- Community-based nursing uses the nursing process in caring for clients in community settings and involves primary, secondary, and tertiary prevention levels. Nursing interventions in community-based settings include health screening, education, medication administration, telephone consultation, health system referral, instruction, nutritional counseling, and risk identification.

- Nurses working in the community need to develop cultural competence. Steps to gaining cultural competence include cultural self-awareness, cultural knowledge, cultural skills, and cultural encounters.

- Settings for community-based nursing including physicians' offices, clinics, health departments, urgent care centers, clients' homes, churches, and shelters (e.g., domestic violence shelters, homeless shelters, and disaster shelters). Nurses provide wellness care, episodic ill care, and chronic care to women and their families.

- Home health care situations have increased due to shorter hospital stays and cost containment measures along with an increase in the income and longevity of individuals with chronic and debilitating health conditions. Technology also has improved, which allows clients to be monitored and to undergo complicated procedures at home (Vizard, 2015).

- The roles and functions of the community-based nurse include communicator, direct care provider, educator, discharge planner and case manager, and advocate and resource manager.

- Open, honest communication is essential for community-based nurses. The use of an interpreter may be necessary to ensure effective communication. Maintaining confidentiality and providing privacy are key.

- A family's knowledge related to the client's health or illness is vital. Nurses working in the community play a major role in educating women and their families.

- Discharge planning provides a comprehensive plan for the safe discharge of a client from a health care facility and for continuing safe and effective care in the community. Case management focuses on coordinating health care services while balancing quality and costs. Discharge planning and case management contribute to improved transitions from the hospital to the community for women, their families, and the health care team.

- Community-based nurses act as resource managers to help ensure that the client and family have the necessary resources and appropriate health care services available to them.

References and Recommended Readings

Adams, J. H. (2015). The role of the clinical nurse specialist in home healthcare. *Home Healthcare Now, 33*(1), 44–48.

Alexander, L. L., LaRosa, J. H., Bader, H., & Garfield, S. (2014). *New dimensions in women's health* (6th ed.). Sudbury, MA: Jones & Bartlett.

Alselai, S. A., & Alrashed, A. M. (2015). Patient-nurses-relationship with in deaf and hard of hearing (D&HH) population. *Journal of Nursing and Health Science, 4*(1), 81–85.

American College of Obstetricians & Gynecologists [ACOG]. (2013). *Nutrition during pregnancy.* Retrieved from http://www.acog.org/~/media/For%20Patients/faq001.pdf?dmc=1&ts=20140104T0930145441

American College of Obstetricians & Gynecologists [ACOG]. (2015). Levels of maternal care. *American Journal of Obstetrics & Gynecology, 125*, 502–515.

American Pregnancy Association [APA]. (2015). *Home birth.* Retrieved from http://www.americanpregnancy.org/labornbirth/homebirth.html

Arcia, A. (2015). U.S. nulliparas' reasons for expected provider type and childbirth setting. *Journal of Perinatal Education, 24*(1), 61–72.

Arnold, E. C., & Boggs, K. U. (2015). *Interpersonal relationships: Professional communication skills for nurses* (7th ed.). St. Louis, MO: Elsevier Health Sciences.

Aston, M., Price, S., Etowa, J., Vukic, A., Young, L., Hart, C., et al. (2015). The power of relationships: Exploring how public health nurses support mothers and families during postpartum home visits. *Journal of Family Nursing, 21*(1), 11–34.

Beard, K. V., Gwanmesia, E., & Miranda-Diaz, G. (2015). Culturally competent care: Using the ESFT model in nursing. *American Journal of Nursing, 115*(6), 58–62. doi: 10.1097/01.NAJ.0000466326.99804.c4

Bloomfield, J., & Pegram, A. (2015). Care, compassion and communication. *Nursing Standard, 29*(25), 45–50.

Brucker, M. C., & King, T. L. (2016). *Pharmacology for women's health* (2nd ed.). Burlington, MA: Jones & Bartlett Learning.

Bureau of Labor Statistics, U.S. Department of Labor, Occupational Employment Statistics. (2015). *Work environment of registered nurses.* Retrieved from http://www.bls.gov/ooh/Healthcare/Registered-nurses.htm#tab-3

Centers for Disease Control and Prevention [CDC]. (2015a). *Hospital utilization.* Retrieved from http://www.cdc.gov/nchs/fastats/hospital.htm

Centers for Disease Control and Prevention [CDC]. (2015b). *New study profiles women's use of health care.* Retrieved from http://www.cdc.gov/nchs/pressroom/01news/newstudy.htm

Cheng, K. G., Hayes, G. R., Hirano, S. H., Nagel, M. S., & Baker, D. (2015). Challenges of integrating patient-centered data into clinical workflow for care of high-risk infants. *Personal and Ubiquitous Computing, 19*(1), 45–57.

Clark, C. C., & Paraska, K. K. (2015). *Health promotion for nurses: A practice guide.* Burlington, MA: Jones & Bartlett Learning.

Coleman, E. A., Roman, S. P., Hall, K. A., & Min, S. J. (2015). Enhancing the care transitions intervention protocol to better address the needs of family caregivers. *Journal for Healthcare Quality, 37*(1), 2–11.

Embo, M., Driessen, E., Valcke, M., & van der Vleuten, C. (2015). Integrating learning assessment and supervision in a competency framework for clinical workplace education. *Nurse Education Today, 35*(2), 341–346.

Emond, A., Ridd, M., Sutherland, H., Allsop, L., Alexander, A., & Kyle, J. (2015). Access to primary care affects the health of Deaf people. *British Journal of General Practice, 65*(631), 95–96.

Ernst, E. (2015). How nurses can be misled about complementary and alternative medicine. *Journal of Advanced Nursing, 71*(2), 235–236.

Flagg, A. J. (2015). The role of patient-centered care in nursing. *The Nursing Clinics of North America, 50*(1), 75–86.

Gardner, S. (2015). Choice of place of birth: Is it really that simple? *British Journal of Midwifery, 23*(1), 4.

Grünebaum, A., McCullough, L. B., Brent, R. L., Arabin, B., Levene, M. I., & Chervenak, F. A. (2015). Perinatal risks of planned home births in the United States. *American Journal of Obstetrics & Gynecology, 212*(3), 350.e1–e6.

Hall, H. G., Griffiths, D., & McKenna, L. G. (2015). Complementary and alternative medicine: Interaction and communication between midwives and women. *Women and Birth, 28*(2), 137–142.

Hansen, L. O. (2015). Passing beyond a wing and a prayer after hospital discharge. *Journal of General Internal Medicine, 30*(4), 390–391

Ivey, T. L., Hughes, D., Dajani, N. K., & Magann, E. F. (2015). Antenatal management of at-risk pregnancies from a distance. *Australian & New Zealand Journal of Obstetrics & Gynecology, 55*(1), 87–89.

Johnson, S. A. (2015). "Intimate mothering publics": comparing face-to-face support groups and Internet use for women seeking information and advice in the transition to first-time motherhood. *Culture, Health & Sexuality, 17*(2), 237–251.

Jokinen, M., & Johnson, G. (2015). Facilitate a home birth. *Midwives, 18*(1), 32–33.

Joint Commission on Accreditation of Healthcare Organizations. (2015). Joint Commission standards. Retrieved from http://www.jointcommission.org/Standards

Kamimura, A., Ashby, J., Myers, K., Nourian, M., & Christensen, N. (2015). Satisfaction with healthcare services among free clinic patients. *Journal of Community Health, 40*(1), 62–72.

King, T. L., Brucker, M. C., Kriebs, J. M., Fahey, J. O., Gegor, C. L., & Varney, H. (2015). *Varney's midwifery* (5th ed.). Burlington, MA: Jones & Bartlett Learning.

Lundy, K. S., & Janes, S. (2016) *Community health nursing: Caring for the public's health* (3rd ed.). Burlington, MA: Jones & Bartlett Learning.

March of Dimes. (2015). Prenatal care. Retrieved from http://www.marchofdimes.com/pregnancy/prenatalcare.html

Martin, M. L., Heron, S., Moreno-Walton, L., & Jones, A. W. (2016) *Diversity and Inclusion in Quality Patient Care.* Switzerland: Springer International Publishers.

McGurk, V. (2015). Person and family centered care. *Nursing Management—UK, 21*(10), 13.

Mukhtar, O., & Jackson, S. D. (2015). Drug therapies in older adults (part 1). *Clinical Medicine, 15*(1), 47–53.

National Center for Complementary and Alternative Medicine [NCCAM]. (2015). What is complementary and alternative medicine (CAM)? Retrieved from http://www.thenewmedicine.org/timeline/cam_use_in_america

National Coalition for Health Professional Education in Genetics [NCHPEG]. (2015). *Neural tube defects.* Retrieved from http://www.nchpeg.org/index.php?option=com_content&view=article&id=435

Nichols, K., Crow, K., & Balakas, K. (2015). Beyond implementation: Sustaining family-centered rounds. *MCN. The American Journal of Maternal Child Nursing, 40*(3), 145–152; quiz 11–12.

Nursing & Midwifery Council [NMC]. (2015). *Complementary and alternative therapies.* Retrieved from http://www.nmc-uk.org/Nurses-and-midwives/Regulation-in-practice/Regulation-in-Practice-Topics/Complementary-and-alternative-therapies/

Oliveira, Y. C., Coura, A. S., Costa, G. M., & França, I. S. (2015). Communication between health professionals-deaf people: an integrative review. *Journal of Nursing UFPE on line [JNUOL/DOI: 10.5205/01012007], 9*(2), 957–964.

Pate, M. D., & Andrews, M. F. (2015). Person- and family-centered care: A time for reflection. *AACN Advanced Critical Care, 26*(1), 10–12.

Peter, D., Robinson, P., Jordan, M., Lawrence, S., Casey, K., & Salas-Lopez, D. (2015). Reducing readmissions using teach-back: Enhancing patient and family education. *Journal of Nursing Administration, 45*(1), 35–42.

Prince, M. J., Fan, W., Yanfei, G., Gutierrez Robledo, L. M., O'Donnell, M., Sullivan, R., et al. (2015). The burden of disease in older people and implications for health policy and practice. *Lancet, 385*(9967), 549–562.

Purnell, L. D. (2015). *Culturally competent health care* (3rd ed.). Philadelphia, PA: F.A. Davis Company.

Roberts, B. (2015). Person and family centered care. *Creative Nursing, 21*(1), 63–64.

Sporek, P. E. (2015). Concrete midwifery. *British Journal of Midwifery, 23*(3), 227.

Stanhope, M., & Lancaster, J. (2014). *Public health nursing: Population-centered health car in the community* (9th ed.). St. Louis, MO: Mosby Elsevier.

Treister-Goltzman, Y., & Peleg, R. (2015). Trends in publications on complementary and alternative medicine in the medical literature. *Journal of Complementary & Integrative Medicine. 12*(2), 111–115. doi:10.1515/jcim-2014-0055

Ulin, K., Olsson, L. E., Wolf, A., & Ekman, I. (2015). Person-centered care – An approach that improves the discharge process. *European Journal of Cardiovascular Nursing.* pii: 1474515115569945. Date of Electronic Publication: 2015 Feb 3. Medline.

U.S. Census Bureau. (2015a). *Population profile of the United States*. Retrieved from http://www.census.gov/population/www/pop-profile/natproj.html

U.S. Census Bureau. (2015b). *How the Census Bureau measures the foreign-born population and immigration*. Retrieved fromhttp://blogs.census.gov/2013/09/05/how-the-census-bureau-measures-the-foreign-born-population-and-immigration/

U.S. Department of Health and Human Services. (2015). *Healthy People 2020*. Retrieved from http://healthypeople.gov/2020/topic-sobjectives2020/default.aspx

USDA Food and Nutrition Service. (2015). *WIC fact sheet*. Retrieved from http://www.fns.usda.gov/wic/factsheets.htm

Velonaki, V., Kampouroglou, G., Velonaki, M., Dimakopoulou, K., Sourtzi, P., & Kalokerinou, A. (2015). Nurses' knowledge, attitudes and behavior toward deaf patients. *Disability and Health Journal, 8*(1), 109–117.

Vizard, M. (2015). Harnessing technology for the improved management of diabetes and community-based care. *British Journal of Community Nursing, 20*(1), 26–27.

Vo, A., Shore, J., Waugh, M., Doarn, C. R., Richardson, J., Hathaway, O., et al. (2015). Meaningful use: A national framework for integrated telemedicine. *Telemedicine Journal and E-Health, 21*(5), 355–363.

Williams, J., Mai, C. T., Mulinare, J., Isenburg, J., Flood, T. J., Ethen, M., et al. (2015). Updated estimates of neural tube defects prevented by mandatory folic Acid fortification--United States, 1995–2011. *MMWR: Morbidity & Mortality Weekly Report, 64*(1), 1–5.

MULTIPLE-CHOICE QUESTIONS

1. A community-based nurse is involved in secondary prevention activities. Which activities might be included? Select all that apply.
   a. Fecal occult blood testing
   b. Hearing screening
   c. Smoking cessation program
   d. Cholesterol testing
   e. Hygiene program
   f. Pregnancy testing

2. A woman is to undergo a colonoscopy at a freestanding outpatient surgery center. Which would the nurse identify as a major disadvantage associated with this community-based setting?
   a. Increased risk for infection verses a hospital
   b. Increased health care costs verses a hospital
   c. Need to be transferred if complications arise
   d. Increased disruption of family functioning

3. When developing a teaching plan for a pregnant client with preterm labor who is to be discharged, what would the nurse do *first*?
   a. Decide which procedures and medications the client will need at home.
   b. Determine the client's learning needs and styles.
   c. Ask the client if she has ever had preterm labor before.
   d. Tell the client what the goals of the teaching session are.

4. Which action by a nurse would best demonstrate cultural competence?
   a. Being well versed in the customs and beliefs of his or her own culture
   b. Demonstrating an openness to the values and beliefs of other cultures
   c. Applying knowledge about various cultures in the practice setting
   d. Playing a role in establishing policies to address diverse cultures

5. Nurses working with an interpreter should emphasize the need for the interpreter to:
   a. Elaborate on the content being interpreted
   b. Clarify misinformation in their own words
   c. Paraphrase statements to reduce time
   d. Maintain confidentiality of content interpreted

6. Which factor would the nurse identify as being least likely to contribute to the rise in community-based care?
   a. Focus on illness-oriented curative care
   b. Rise in consumer disposable income
   c. Technological advances for home care
   d. Emphasis on primary care and treatment

CRITICAL THINKING EXERCISE

1. A 63-year-old woman from Saudi Arabia has become seriously ill while on a visit to the United States. It is projected that she will require a lengthy hospitalization. Describe the steps the nurse should take to communicate with and provide extensive health care teaching to this woman and her family.

2. A pregnant woman is discharged home from the hospital after admission due to preterm labor. The woman is to be on complete bed rest and will receive home health care through a local agency to assist her and her family and to monitor her health status. As the home health nurse assigned to this woman, what should your nursing assessment include?

STUDY ACTIVITIES

1. Shadow a nurse working in a community setting, such as a women's health clinic, birthing center, home care, or health department. Identify the role the nurse plays in the health of women and families in the setting and in the community.

2. Arrange for a visit to a community health center that offers services to various cultural groups. Interview the staff about the strategies used to overcome communication barriers and different health care practices for the women and their families in these groups.

3. Identify at least three community-based practice settings in which the nurse may practice family-centered care.

BRINGING IT ALL TOGETHER: CASE STUDY

The school nurse is becoming very distressed because of the high numbers of students she is seeing in the high school health clinic with sexually transmitted infections (STIs) recently. Just today, she saw a 14-year-old student experiencing pelvic pain secondary to an untreated gonorrhea infection. The nurse wants to initiate primary, secondary, and tertiary care interventions to address this problem.

Go to thePoint **to find questions to consider about this case.**

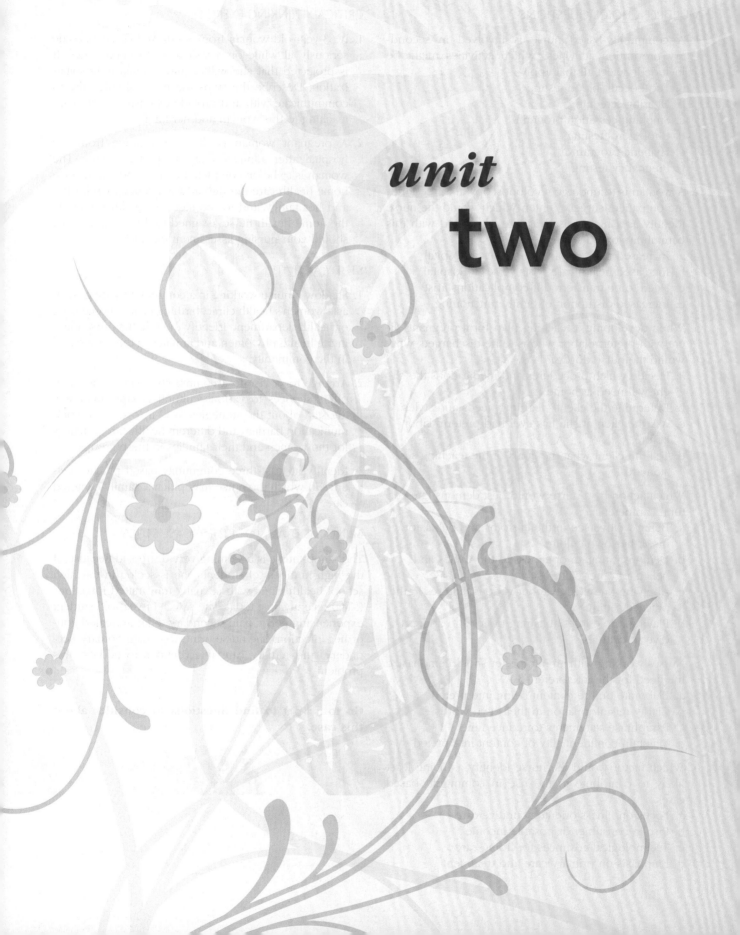

unit
two

Women's Health Throughout the Lifespan

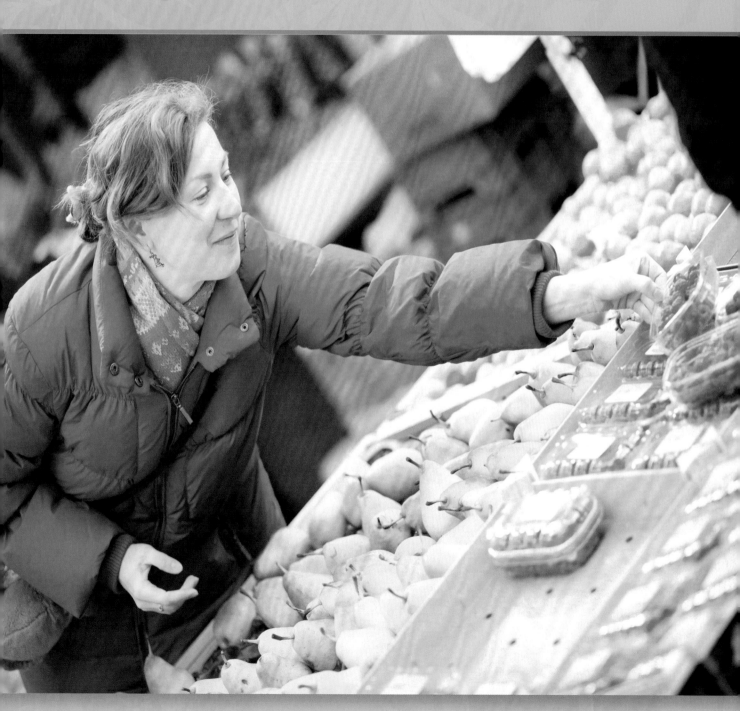

3

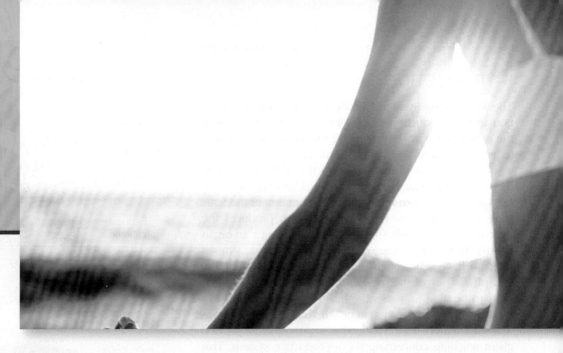

Anatomy and Physiology of the Reproductive Systems

Learning Objectives

Upon completion of the chapter, you will be able to:

1. Contrast the structure and function of the major external and internal female genital organs.
2. Outline the phases of the menstrual cycle, the dominant hormones involved, and the changes taking place in each phase.
3. Classify external and internal male reproductive structures and the function of each in hormonal regulation.

Linda, 49, started menstruating when she was 12 years old. Her menstrual periods have always been regular, but now she is experiencing irregular, heavier, and longer ones. She wonders if there is something wrong or if this is normal.

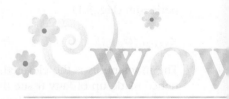

Words of Wisdom
All nurses should take care of and respect the human body, for it is a wondrous precision machine.

INTRODUCTION

The reproductive system is a collection of organs that function in the production of offspring. Scientists argue that the reproductive system is among the most important systems in the entire body. Without the ability to reproduce, a species dies. The female reproductive system produces the female reproductive cells (the eggs, or ova) and contains an organ (**uterus**) in which development of the fetus takes place; the male reproductive system produces the male reproductive cells (the sperm) and contains an organ (**penis**) that deposits the sperm within the female. Nurses need to have a thorough understanding of the anatomy and physiology of the male and female reproductive systems to be able to assess the health of these systems, to promote reproductive system health, to care for conditions that might affect the reproductive organs, and to provide client teaching concerning the reproductive system. This chapter reviews the female and male reproductive systems and the menstrual cycle as it relates to reproduction.

FEMALE REPRODUCTIVE ANATOMY AND PHYSIOLOGY

The female reproductive system is composed of both external and internal reproductive organs. It consists of the paired ovaries and oviducts, the uterus, the vagina, the external genitalia, and the mammary glands. All of these structures have evolved for the important functions of ovulation, fertilization of an ovum by a sperm, support of the developing embryo and fetus, and the birth and care of a newborn.

External Female Reproductive Organs

The external female reproductive organs collectively are called the **vulva** (which means "covering" in Latin). The vulva serves to protect the urethral and vaginal openings and is highly sensitive to touch to increase the female's pleasure during sexual arousal (Patton & Thibodeau, 2016). The structures that make up the vulva include the mons pubis, the labia majora and minora, the clitoris and prepuce, the structures within the vestibule, and the perineum (Fig. 3.1).

Mons Pubis

The mons pubis is the elevated, rounded, fleshy prominence made up of fatty tissue that overlays the symphysis pubis. The skin of this fatty tissue is covered with coarse, curly pubic hair after puberty. The mons pubis protects the symphysis pubis during sexual intercourse.

Labia

The labia majora (large lips), which are relatively large and fleshy, are comparable to the scrotum in males. The

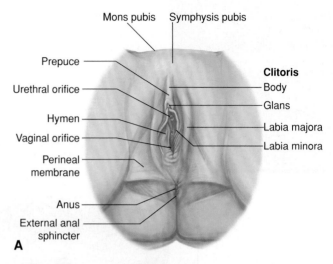

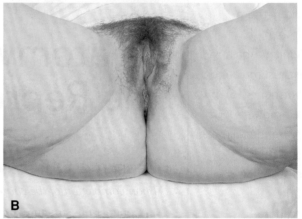

FIGURE 3.1 A. The external female reproductive organs. **B.** Normal appearance of external structures. (Photo by B. Proud.)

labia majora contain sweat and sebaceous (oil-secreting) glands; after puberty, they are covered with hair. Their function is to protect the vaginal opening and provide cushioning during sexual activity. The labia minora (small lips) are the delicate hairless inner folds of skin; they can be very small or up to 2 in wide. They lie just inside the labia majora and surround the openings to the vagina and urethra. The labia minora grow down from the anterior inner part of the labia majora on each side. These lips surround the vaginal opening and extend upward to form protection around both the clitoris and urethra. They are highly vascular and abundant in nerve supply. They lubricate the vulva, swell in response to stimulation, and are highly sensitive.

Clitoris and Prepuce

The clitoris is a small, cylindrical mass of erectile tissue and nerves. It is highly sensitive and is analogous to the head of the male's penis. Unlike the penis, however, the function of the clitoris is purely erogenous. Most of the components of the clitoris are buried under the skin and connective tissue of the vulva. It is located at the anterior junction of the labia minora. There are folds above and below the clitoris. The joining of the folds above the clitoris forms the prepuce, a hood-like covering over the clitoris; the junction below the clitoris forms the frenulum.

> **Take Note!**
> The hood-like covering over the clitoris is the site for female genital mutilation or cutting, which is a cultural ritual still practiced in some countries, including in the United States. It is internationally recognized as a human rights violation against women.

A rich supply of blood vessels gives the clitoris a pink color. Like the penis, the clitoris is very sensitive to touch, stimulation, and temperature and can become erect. For its small size, 9 to 11 cm, it has a generous blood and nerve supply. There are more free nerve endings of sensory reception located on the clitoris than on any other part of the body, and it is, unsurprisingly, the most erotically sensitive part of the genitalia for most females. Its function is sexual stimulation (Pauls, 2015).

> **Take Note!**
> The word clitoris is from the Greek word for "key"; in ancient times the clitoris was thought to be the key to a woman's sexuality.

Vestibule

The vestibule is an oval area enclosed by the labia minora laterally. It is inside the labia minora and outside of the hymen and is perforated by six openings. Opening into the vestibule are the urethra from the urinary bladder, the vagina, and two sets of glands. The opening to the vagina is called the introitus, and the half-moon–shaped area behind the opening is called the fourchette. Through tiny ducts beside the introitus, Bartholin's glands, when stimulated, secrete mucus that supplies lubrication for intercourse. Skene's glands are located on either side of the opening to the urethra. They secrete a small amount of mucus to keep the opening moist and lubricated for the passage of urine (Velkey et al., 2015).

The vaginal opening is surrounded by the hymen (maidenhead). The hymen is a tough, elastic, perforated, mucosa-covered tissue across the vaginal introitus. In a virgin, the hymen may completely cover the opening, but it usually encircles the opening like a tight ring. Because the degree of tightness varies among women, the hymen may tear at the first attempt at intercourse, or it may be so soft and pliable that no tearing occurs. In a woman who is not a virgin, the hymen usually appears as small tags of tissue surrounding the vaginal opening, but the

presence or absence of the hymen can neither confirm nor rule out sexual experience (Acien & Acien, 2015).

> **Take Note!**
> Heavy physical exertion, use of tampons, or injury to the area can alter the appearance of the hymen in girls and women who have not been sexually active.

Perineum

The perineum is the most posterior part of the external female reproductive organs. This external region is located between the vulva and the anus. It is made up of skin, muscle, and fascia. The perineum can become lacerated or incised during childbirth and may need to be repaired with sutures. Incising the perineum area to provide more space for the presenting part is called an episiotomy. Although still a common obstetric procedure, the use of episiotomy has decreased during the past 25 years. The procedure should be applied selectively rather than routinely. An episiotomy can add to postpartum discomfort and perineal trauma and can lead to fecal incontinence (King et al., 2015).

Internal Female Reproductive Organs

The internal female reproductive organs consist of the vagina, uterus, fallopian tubes, and ovaries (Fig. 3.2). These structures develop and function according to specific hormonal influences that affect fertility and childbearing.

Vagina

The **vagina** is a highly distensible canal situated in front of the rectum and behind the bladder. It is a tubular, fibromuscular organ lined with mucous membrane that lies in a series of transverse folds called rugae. The rugae allow for extreme dilation of the canal during labor and birth. The vagina is a canal that connects the external genitals (vulva) to the cervix. It receives the penis and the sperm ejaculated during sexual intercourse, and it serves as an exit passageway for menstrual blood and for the fetus during childbirth. The front and back walls normally touch each other so that there is no space in the vagina except when it is opened (e.g., during a pelvic examination or intercourse). In the adult, the vaginal cavity is 3 to 4 in long. Muscles that control its diameter surround the lower third of the vagina. The upper two thirds of the vagina lies above these muscles and can be stretched easily. During a woman's reproductive years, the mucosal lining of the vagina has a corrugated appearance and is resistant to bacterial colonization. Before puberty and after menopause (if the woman is not taking estrogen), the mucosa is smooth due to lower levels of estrogen (Farage, Miller, & Maibach, 2015).

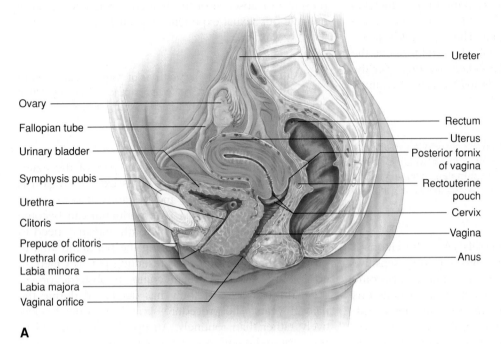

Ureter

Ovary

Fallopian tube

Urinary bladder

Symphysis pubis

Urethra

Clitoris

Prepuce of clitoris

Urethral orifice

Labia minora

Labia majora

Vaginal orifice

Rectum

Uterus

Posterior fornix of vagina

Rectouterine pouch

Cervix

Vagina

Anus

A

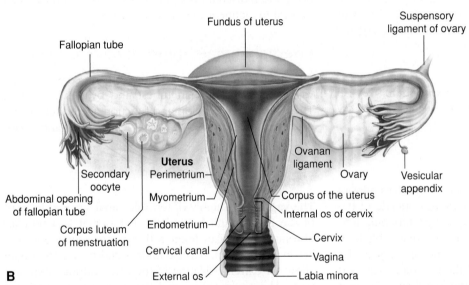

Fundus of uterus

Suspensory ligament of ovary

Fallopian tube

Secondary oocyte

Abdominal opening of fallopian tube

Corpus luteum of menstruation

Uterus
Perimetrium

Myometrium

Endometrium

Cervical canal

External os

Ovanan ligament

Ovary

Vesicular appendix

Corpus of the uterus

Internal os of cervix

Cervix

Vagina

Labia minora

B

FIGURE 3.2 The internal female reproductive organs. **A.** Lateral view. **B.** Anterior view. (Source: Anatomical Chart Company. [2001]. *Atlas of human anatomy.* Springhouse, PA: Springhouse.)

The vagina has an acidic environment, which protects it against ascending infections. Antibiotic therapy, douching, perineal hygiene sprays, and deodorants upset the acid balance within the vaginal environment and can predispose women to infections.

Uterus

The uterus is an inverted, pear-shaped muscular organ at the top of the vagina. It lies behind the bladder and in front of the rectum and is anchored in position by eight ligaments, although it is not firmly attached or adherent to any part of the skeleton. A full bladder tilts the uterus backward; a distended rectum tilts it forward. The uterus

alters its position by gravity or with change of posture, and is the size and shape of an inverted pear. It is the site of menstruation, receiving a fertilized ovum, development of the fetus during pregnancy, and contracting to help in the expulsion of the fetus and placenta. Before the first pregnancy, it measures approximately 3 in long, 2 in wide and 1 in thick. After a pregnancy, the uterus remains larger than before the pregnancy. After menopause, it becomes smaller and atrophies.

The uterine wall is relatively thick and composed of three layers: the **endometrium** (innermost layer), the myometrium (muscular middle layer), and the perimetrium (outer serosal layer that covers the body of the uterus). The endometrium is the mucosal layer that lines the uterine cavity in nonpregnant women. It varies in thickness from 0.5 to 5 mm and has an abundant supply of glands and blood vessels (Tambouret & Wilbur, 2015). The myometrium makes up the major portion of the uterus and is composed of smooth muscle linked by connective tissue with numerous elastic fibers. During pregnancy, the upper myometrium undergoes marked hypertrophy, but there is limited change in the cervical muscle content.

Anatomic subdivisions of the uterus include the convex portion above the uterine tubes (the fundus), the central portion (the corpus or body) between the fundus and the cervix, and the cervix, or neck, which opens into the vagina.

CERVIX

The **cervix,** the lower part of the uterus, is sometimes called the neck of the uterus. It opens into the vagina and has a channel that allows sperm to enter the uterus and menstrual discharge to exit. It is composed of fibrous connective tissue. During a pelvic examination, the part of the cervix that protrudes into the upper end of the vagina can be visualized. Like the vagina, this part of the cervix is covered by mucosa, which is smooth, firm, and doughnut shaped, with a visible central opening called the external os (Fig. 3.3). Before childbirth, the external cervical os is a small, regular, oval opening. After childbirth, the opening is converted into a transverse slit that resembles lips (Fig. 3.4). Except during menstruation or ovulation, the cervix is usually a good barrier against bacteria. The cervix has an alkaline environment, which protects the sperm from the acidic environment in the vagina.

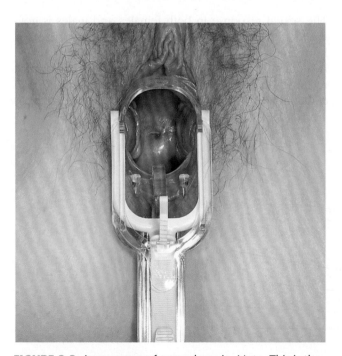

FIGURE 3.3 Appearance of normal cervix. Note: This is the cervix of a multipara female. (Photo by B. Proud.)

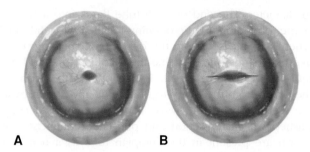

FIGURE 3.4 A. Nulliparous cervical os. **B.** Parous cervical os.

The canal or channel of the cervix is lined with mucus-secreting glands. This mucus is thick and impenetrable to sperm until just before the ovaries release an egg (ovulation). At ovulation, the consistency of the mucus changes so that sperm can swim through it, allowing fertilization. At the same time, the mucus-secreting glands of the cervix actually become able to store live sperm for 2 or 3 days. These sperm can later move up through the corpus and into the fallopian tubes to fertilize the egg; thus, intercourse 1 or 2 days before ovulation can lead to pregnancy. Because some women do not ovulate consistently, pregnancy can occur at varying times after the last menstrual period. During pregnancy the cervix is the vital mechanical barrier which resists compressive and tensile loads generated from a growing fetus. The channel in the cervix is too narrow for the fetus to pass through during pregnancy, but during labor it stretches to let the newborn through.

CORPUS

The corpus, or the main body of the uterus, is a highly muscular organ that enlarges to hold the fetus during pregnancy. The inner lining of the corpus (endometrium) undergoes cyclic changes as a result of the changing levels of hormones secreted by the ovaries: it is thickest during the part of the menstrual cycle in which a fertilized egg would be expected to enter the uterus and is thinnest just after menstruation. If fertilization does not take place during this cycle, most of the endometrium is shed and bleeding occurs, resulting in the monthly period. If fertilization does take place, the embryo attaches to the wall of the uterus, where it becomes embedded in the endometrium (about 1 week after fertilization); this process is called implantation (Patton & Thibodeau, 2015). Menstruation then ceases during the 40 weeks (280 days) of pregnancy. During labor, the muscular walls of the corpus contract to push the baby through the cervix and into the vagina.

Fallopian Tubes

The **fallopian tubes**, also known as oviducts, are hollow, cylindrical structures that extend 2 to 3 in from the upper edges of the uterus toward the ovaries. Each tube is about 7 to 10 cm long (4 in) and approximately 0.7 cm in diameter. The end of each tube flares into a funnel shape, providing a large opening for the egg to fall into when it is released from the ovary. Cilia (beating, hair-like extensions on cells) line the fallopian tube and the muscles in the tube's wall. The fallopian tubes convey the ovum from the ovary to the uterus and sperm from the uterus toward the ovary. This movement is accomplished via ciliary action and peristaltic contraction. If sperm are present in the fallopian tube as a result of sexual intercourse or artificial insemination, fertilization of the ovum can occur in the distal portion of the tube. If the egg is fertilized, it will divide over a period of 4 days while it moves slowly down the fallopian tube and into the uterus, where it implants into the uterine lining.

Ovaries

The **ovaries** are a set of paired glands resembling unshelled almonds that are the organs of gamete production in the female. They are set in the pelvic cavity below and to either side of the umbilicus. They are usually pearl colored, oblong, and have a lumpy surface. They are homologous to the testes. Each mature ovary weighs from 2 to 5 g and is about 4 cm long, 2 cm wide, and 1 cm thick (Jones & Lopez, 2014). The ovaries are not attached to the fallopian tubes but are suspended nearby from several ligaments, which help hold them in position. The development and the release of the ovum and the secretion of the hormones **estrogen** and **progesterone** are the two primary functions of the ovary. The ovaries link the reproductive system to the body's system of endocrine glands, as they produce the ova (eggs) and secrete, in cyclic fashion, the female sex hormones estrogen and progesterone. After an ovum matures, it passes into the fallopian tubes.

Breasts

The two mammary glands, or **breasts**, are accessory organs of the female reproductive system that are specialized to secrete milk following pregnancy. They overlie the pectoralis major muscles and extend from the second to the sixth ribs and from the sternum to the axilla. Each breast has a nipple located near the tip, which is surrounded by a circular area of pigmented skin called the areola. Each breast is composed of approximately 9 lobes (the number can range between 4 and 18), which contain glands (alveolar) and a duct (lactiferous) that leads to the nipple and opens to the outside (Fig. 3.5). The lobes are separated by dense connective and adipose tissues, which also help support the weight of the breasts (Kandeel, 2014).

During pregnancy, placental estrogen and progesterone stimulate the development of the mammary glands. Because of this hormonal activity, the breasts may double in size during pregnancy. At the same time, glandular tissue replaces the adipose tissue of the breasts.

Following childbirth and the expulsion of the placenta, levels of placental hormones (progesterone and lactogen) fall rapidly, and the action of prolactin (milk-producing hormone) is no longer inhibited. Prolactin stimulates the production of milk within a few days after childbirth, but in the interim, dark yellow fluid called colostrum is secreted. Colostrum contains more minerals and protein, but less sugar and fat, than mature breast milk. Colostrum secretion may continue for approximately a week after childbirth, with gradual conversion to mature milk. Colostrum is rich in maternal antibodies, especially immunoglobulin A (IgA), which offers protection for the newborn against enteric pathogens.

Female Sexual Response

The sexual response in both females and males is governed primarily by the nervous system rather than by hormones. The sexual response starts in a state of sexual neutrality, and the person's sexual desire is more of a reciprocal response than a spontaneous one (Housman & Odum 2016). The sexual cycle is usually thought of as

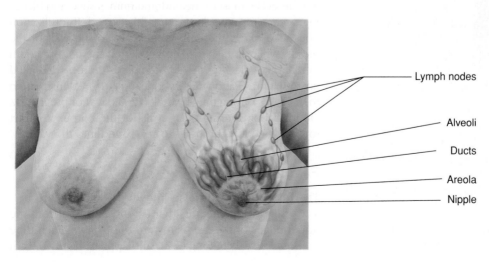

Lymph nodes

Alveoli

Ducts

Areola

Nipple

FIGURE 3.5 Anatomy of the breasts. (Photo by B. Proud.)

having five phases: desire, excitement, plateau, orgasm, and resolution:

1. *Desire:* Starts with a desire for sexual intimacy, also known as *libido.*
2. *Excitement:* Both men and women have a heightened sexual awareness. When a female is sexually aroused, her brain coordinates a patterned sexual response cycle consisting of increased heart rate, respiratory rate, blood pressure, and general level of excitement (Sherwood, 2016). With sexual stimulation, tissues in the clitoris and breasts and around the vaginal orifice fill with blood and the erectile tissues swell. At the same time, the vagina begins to expand and elongate to accommodate the penis. As part of the whole vasocongestive reaction, the labia majora and minor swell and darken. As sexual stimulation intensifies, the vestibular glands secrete mucus to moisten and lubricate the tissues to facilitate insertion of the penis. Hormones play an integral role in the female sexual response as well. Adequate estrogen and testosterone must be available for the brain to sense incoming arousal stimuli. Research indicates that estrogen preserves the vascular function of female sex organs and affects genital sensation. It also is believed to promote blood flow to these areas during stimulation. Testosterone is needed to stimulate sexual desire in women. Recent research findings also suggest that testosterone therapy improves sexual desire, arousal, orgasm frequency, and satisfaction in women (Davis, 2013).
3. *Plateau:* The heart rate, blood pressure, level of muscle tension, and respiration rate all increase. During this phase, the penile erection intensifies and the vagina constricts around the penis. Continued stimulation of the clitoris and penis with movement leads to the next phase of the sexual response—*orgasmic phase.*
4. *Orgasm:* Women experience rhythmic contractions of the pelvic muscles and vaginal walls. In men, ejaculation occurs during the *orgasmic phase* and both sexes experience a peak of sexual pleasure at orgasm. Typically the woman feels warm and relaxed after an orgasm. Within a short time after orgasm, the two physiologic mechanisms that created the sexual response, vasocongestion and muscle contraction, rapidly dissipate. The orgasmic experience varies from person to person and from time to time in the same person. Orgasm is an intense sensation of pleasure achieved by stimulation of erogenous zones. Women do not have a refractory period after each orgasm and can, therefore, experience multiple orgasms. Clitoral sexual response and the female orgasm are not affected by aging (Minkin, 2016). Some orgasms are intense, some are quiet, and some are gentle (Wheatley & Puts, 2015). At the completion of the sexual episode, the brain and body return to an unaroused state, which is termed *sexual resolution*. During this phase, the heart rate, blood pressure, and respirations slow; the muscles relax. Frequently, fatigue sets in for both people.

THE FEMALE REPRODUCTIVE CYCLE

The female reproductive cycle is a complex process that encompasses an intricate series of chemical secretions and reactions to produce the ultimate potential for fertility and birth. The female reproductive cycle is a general term that includes the ovarian cycle, the endometrial (uterine) cycle, the hormonal changes that regulate them, and the cyclical changes in the breasts. The endometrium, ovaries, pituitary gland, and hypothalamus are all involved in the cyclic changes that help to prepare the body for fertilization. Absence of fertilization results in menstruation, the monthly shedding of the uterine lining. **Menstruation** (shedding of the endometrium) marks the beginning and end of the monthly cycle. Menopause is the naturally occurring cessation of menstrual cycles.

The menstrual cycle results from a functional hypothalamic–pituitary–ovarian axis and a precise sequencing of hormones that lead to ovulation. The ovarian cycle, during which ovulation occurs, and the endometrial cycle, during which menstruation occurs, are divided at midcycle by ovulation. **Ovulation** occurs when the ovum is released from its follicle; after leaving the ovary, the ovum enters the fallopian tube and journeys toward the uterus. If sperm fertilize the ovum during its journey, pregnancy occurs (Fig. 3.6).

Ovarian Cycle

The ovarian cycle is the series of events associated with a developing oocyte (ovum or egg) within the ovaries. Whereas men manufacture sperm daily, often into advanced age, women are born with a single lifetime supply of ova that are released from the ovaries gradually throughout the childbearing years. In the female ovary, 1 million oocytes are present at birth, and about 200,000 to 400,000 follicles are still present at puberty. Typically, a woman ovulates one oocyte per month over an approximately 40-year reproductive lifespan. This accounts for the loss of 400 to 500 follicles. By age 35 she will have fewer than 100,000 follicles, and, by menopause, her follicular supply will be nearly depleted (Jones & Lopez, 2014). The ovarian cycle begins when the follicular cells (ovum and surrounding cells) swell and the maturation process starts. The maturing follicle at this stage is called a graafian follicle. The ovary raises many follicles monthly, but usually only one follicle matures to reach ovulation. The ovarian cycle consists of three phases: the follicular phase, ovulation, and the luteal phase.

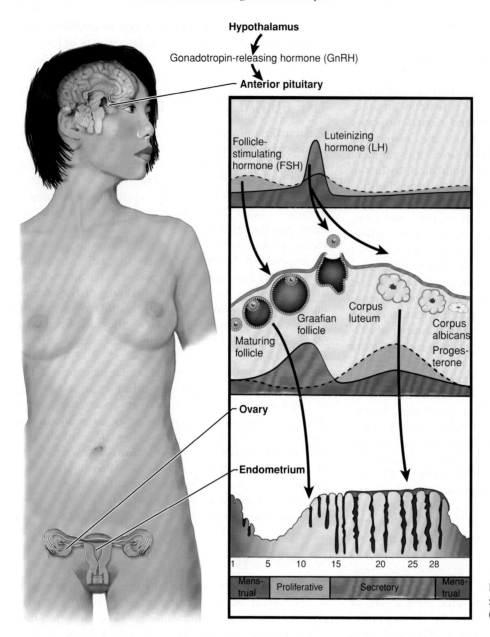

FIGURE 3.6 Menstrual cycle summary based on a 28-day (average) menstrual cycle.

Follicular Phase

This phase is so named because it is when the follicles in the ovary grow and form a mature egg. The goal of this phase is to produce an ovum for fertilization. This phase starts on day 1 of the menstrual cycle and continues until ovulation, approximately 10 to 14 days later. The follicular phase is not consistent in duration because of the time variations in follicular development. These variations account for the differences in menstrual cycle lengths (Sherwood, 2016). The hypothalamus is the initiator of this phase. Increasing levels of estrogen secreted from the maturing follicular cells and the continued growth of the dominant follicle cell induce proliferation of the endometrium and myometrium. This thickening of the uterine lining supports an implanted ovum if pregnancy occurs.

Prompted by the hypothalamus, the pituitary gland releases **follicle-stimulating hormone** (FSH), which stimulates the ovary to produce 5 to 20 immature follicles. Each follicle houses an immature oocyte or egg. The follicle that is targeted to mature fully will soon rupture and expel a mature oocyte in the process of ovulation. A surge in **luteinizing hormone** (LH) from the anterior pituitary gland is actually responsible for affecting the final development and subsequent rupture of the mature follicle.

Ovulation

At ovulation, a mature follicle ruptures in response to a surge of LH, releasing a mature oocyte (ovum). No one single event causes ovulation. This usually occurs on day 14 in a 28-day cycle. When ovulation occurs, there is a drop in estrogen. Typically ovulation takes place approximately 10 to 12 hours after the LH peak and 24 to 36 hours after estrogen levels peak (King et al., 2015). The distal ends of the fallopian tubes become active near the time of ovulation and create currents that help carry the ovum into the uterus. The life span of the ovum is only about 24 hours; unless it meets a sperm on its journey within that time, it will die.

During ovulation, the cervix produces thin, clear, stretchy, slippery mucus that is designed to capture the man's sperm, nourish it, and help the sperm travel up through the cervix to meet the ovum for fertilization. Ovulation symptoms also include vaginal spotting, an increase in vaginal discharge giving the woman a "feeling of wetness," an increased libido leading to more desire to be intimate, a slight rise in basal body temperature, and lower abdominal cramping.

The one constant, whether a women's cycle is 28 days or 120 days, is that ovulation takes place 14 days before menstruation (Housman & Odum, 2016).

 Take Note!

About one in five women can feel a pain on one side of the abdomen around the time the egg is released. This midcycle pain is called mittelschmerz.

Luteal Phase

The luteal phase begins at ovulation and lasts until the menstrual phase of the next cycle. It typically occurs on days 15 through 28 of a 28-day cycle. After the follicle ruptures as it releases the egg, it closes and forms a corpus luteum. The corpus luteum secretes increasing amounts of the hormone progesterone, which interacts with the endometrium to prepare it for implantation. At the beginning of the luteal phase, progesterone induces the endometrial glands to secrete glycogen, mucus, and other substances. These glands become tortuous and have large lumens due to increased secretory activity. The progesterone secreted by the corpus luteum causes the temperature of the body to rise slightly until the start of the next period. A significant increase in temperature, usually 0.5° to 1°F, is generally seen within a day or two after ovulation has occurred; the temperature remains elevated until 3 days before the onset on the next menstruation (Housman & Odum, 2016). This rise in temperature can be plotted on a graph and gives an indication of when ovulation has occurred. In the absence of fertilization, the corpus luteum begins to degenerate and consequently ovarian hormone levels decrease. As estrogen and progesterone levels decrease, the endometrium undergoes involution. In a 28-day cycle, menstruation then begins approximately 14 days after ovulation in the absence of pregnancy. FSH and LH are generally at their lowest levels during the luteal phase and highest during the follicular phase.

Endometrial (Uterine) Cycle

The endometrial (uterine) cycle occurs in response to cyclic hormonal changes. The four phases of the endometrial cycle are the proliferative phase, secretory phase, ischemic phase, and menstrual phase.

Proliferative Phase

The proliferative phase of the endometrial cycle corresponds to the follicular phase of the ovarian cycle. It starts with enlargement of the endometrial glands in response to increasing amounts of estrogen. The blood vessels become dilated and the endometrium increases in thickness dramatically from 0.5 to 5 mm in height and increases eightfold in thickness in preparation for implantation of the fertilized ovum (Oyelowo & Johnson, 2016). Cervical mucus becomes thin, clear, stretchy, and more alkaline, making it more favorable to sperm to enhance the opportunity for fertilization. The proliferative phase starts on about day 5 of the menstrual cycle and lasts to the time of ovulation. This phase depends on estrogen stimulation resulting from ovarian follicles, and this phase coincides with the follicular phase of the ovarian cycle.

Secretory Phase

The secretory phase begins at ovulation to about 3 days before the next menstrual period. Under the influence of progesterone released by the corpus luteum after ovulation, the endometrium becomes thickened and more vascular (growth of the spiral arteries) and glandular (secretion of more glycogen and lipids). These dramatic changes are all in preparation for implantation, if it were to occur. This phase typically lasts from day 15 (after ovulation) to day 28 and coincides with the luteal phase of the ovarian cycle. In the absence of fertilization by day 23 of the menstrual cycle, the corpus luteum begins to degenerate and consequently ovarian hormone levels decrease. As estrogen and progesterone levels decrease, the endometrium undergoes involution.

 Concept Mastery Alert

Proliferative Versus Secretory Phases of the Uterine Cycle

During the proliferative phase, the ovarian follicles are producing increased amounts of estrogen, and the endometrium prepares for possible fertilization with pronounced growth. The secretory phase begins at time of ovulation. If the ovum is not fertilized, then the corpus luteum degenerates and hormone levels fall, ultimately resulting in menstruation.

Ischemic Phase

If fertilization does not occur, the ischemic phase begins. Estrogen and progesterone levels drop sharply during this phase as the corpus luteum starts to degenerate. Changes in the endometrium occur with spasm of the arterioles, resulting in ischemia of the basal layer. The ischemia leads to shedding of the endometrium down to the basal layer, and menstrual flow begins.

Menstrual Phase

The menstrual phase begins as the spiral arteries rupture secondary to ischemia, releasing blood into the uterus, and the sloughing of the endometrial lining begins. If fertilization does not take place, the corpus luteum degenerates. As a result, both estrogen and progesterone levels fall and the thickened endometrial lining sloughs away from the uterine wall and passes out via the vagina. The beginning of the menstrual flow marks the end of one menstrual cycle and the start of a new one. Most women report menstrual bleeding for an average of 3 to 7 days. The amount of menstrual flow varies, but averages 1 ounce or a range of approximately 2/3 to 2 2/3 ounces in volume per cycle (Thornhill & Gangestad, 2015).

Menstruation

Menstruation is a term derived from the Latin word *mensis*, meaning "month." It is the normal, predictable physiologic process whereby the inner lining of the uterus (endometrium) is expelled by the body. Typically, this occurs monthly. Menstruation has many effects on girls and women, including emotional and self-image issues. In the United States, the average age at **menarche** (the start of menstruation in females) is 12.8 years, with a range between 8 and 18. Genetics is the most important factor in determining the age at which menarche starts, but geographic location, nutrition, weight, general health, nutrition, cultural and social practices, the girl's educational level, attitude, family environment, and beliefs are also important (Krieger et al., 2015).

Pubertal events preceding the first menses have an orderly progression: Thelarche, the development of breast buds; adrenarche, the appearance of pubic and then axillary hair, followed by a growth spurt; and menarche (occurring about 2 years after the start of breast development). In healthy pubertal girls, the menstrual period varies in flow heaviness and may remain irregular in occurrence for up to 2 years following menarche. After that time, the regular menstrual cycle should be established. Most women will experience 300 to 400 menstrual cycles within their lifetime (King et al., 2015). Normal, regular menstrual cycles vary in frequency and blood loss (Kandeel, 2014). Irregular menses can be associated with irregular ovulation, polycystic ovary syndrome, type 2 diabetes, weather conditions, stress, disease, and hormonal imbalances (Senie, 2014).

Think back to Linda, who was introduced at the beginning of the chapter. What questions might need to be asked to assess her condition? What laboratory work might be anticipated to validate her heavier flow?

Although menstruation is a normal process, various world cultures have taken a wide variety of attitudes toward it, seeing it as everything from a sacred time to an unclean time. Folk culture surrounding menstrual-related matters has considerable implications for symptom expression and treatment-seeking behavior. Recent research findings imply the need for education to help adolescent girls manage menstrual symptoms and increase awareness of the benefit of treating them. Given that menstrual-related information comes from mothers, family, and social culture, negative attitudes toward their monthly cycles can be formed in young impressionable girls. Nurses, through formal instruction, can help young girls in shaping good menstrual attitudes and a more positive image of this natural physiologic process (Clark & Paraska, 2014).

Take Note!

Knowledge about menstruation has increased significantly and attitudes have changed. What was once discussed only behind closed doors is discussed openly today.

Consider This

We had been married for 2 years when my husband and I decided to start a family. I began thinking back to my high school biology class and tried to remember about ovulation and what to look for. I also used the Internet to find the answers I was seeking. As I was reading, it all started to come into place. During ovulation, a woman's cervical mucus increases and she experiences a wet sensation for several days midcycle. The mucus also becomes stretchable during this time. In addition, body temperature rises slightly and then falls if no conception takes place. Armed with this knowledge, I began to check my temperature daily before arising and began to monitor the consistency of my cervical mucus. I figured that monitoring these two signs of ovulation could help me discover the best time to conceive. After 6 months of trying without results, I wondered what I was doing wrong. Did I really understand my body's reproductive activity?

Thoughts: *What additional suggestions might the nurse offer this woman in her journey to conception? What community resources might be available to assist this couple? How does knowledge of the reproductive system help nurses take care of couples who are trying to become pregnant?*

Menstrual Cycle Hormones

The menstrual cycle involves a complex interaction of hormones. The predominant hormones include gonadotropin-releasing hormone, FSH, LH, estrogen, progesterone, and prostaglandins. Box 3.1 summarizes menstrual cycle hormones.

Gonadotropin-Releasing Hormone

Gonadotropin-releasing hormone (GnRH) is secreted from the hypothalamus in a pulsatile manner throughout the reproductive cycle. It pulsates slowly during the follicular phase and increases during the luteal phase. GnRH induces the release of FSH and LH to assist with ovulation.

Follicle-Stimulating Hormone

FSH is secreted by the anterior pituitary gland and is primarily responsible for the maturation of the ovarian follicle. FSH secretion is highest and most important during the first week of the follicular phase of the reproductive cycle.

Luteinizing Hormone

LH is secreted by the anterior pituitary gland and is required for both the final maturation of preovulatory follicles and luteinization of the ruptured follicle. As a result, estrogen production declines and progesterone secretion continues. Thus, estrogen levels fall a day before ovulation, and progesterone levels begin to rise.

Estrogen

Estrogen is secreted by the ovaries and is crucial for the development and maturation of the follicle. Estrogen is predominant at the end of the proliferative phase, directly preceding ovulation. After ovulation, estrogen levels drop sharply as progesterone dominates. In the endometrial cycle, estrogen induces proliferation of the endometrial glands. Estrogen also causes the uterus to increase in size and weight because of increased glycogen, amino acids, electrolytes, and water. Blood supply is expanded as well.

Progesterone

Progesterone is secreted by the corpus luteum. Progesterone levels increase just before ovulation and peak 5 to 7 days after ovulation. During the luteal phase, progesterone induces swelling and increased secretion of the endometrium. This hormone is often called the hormone of pregnancy because of its calming effect (reduces uterine contractions) on the uterus, allowing pregnancy to be maintained.

Prostaglandins

Prostaglandins are primary mediators of the body's inflammatory processes and are essential for the normal physiologic function of the female reproductive system. They are a closely related group of oxygenated fatty acids that are produced by the endometrium, with a variety of effects throughout the body. Although they have regulatory effects and are sometimes called hormones, prostaglandins are not technically hormones because they are produced by all tissues rather than by special glands (Jones & Lopez, 2014). Prostaglandins increase during follicular maturation and play a key role in ovulation by freeing the ovum inside the graafian follicle. Large amounts of prostaglandins are found in menstrual blood. Current research suggests that the pathogenesis of menstrual cramps/pain is due to prostaglandin F2a (PGF2a), a potent myometrial stimulant and vasoconstrictor, in the secretory endometrium. Elevated prostaglandin levels are found in the endometrial fluid of women with dysmenorrhea (painful menses) and correlates well with their degree of pain. Nonsteroidal anti-inflammatory drugs have been introduced as the primary choice of treatment for menstrual cramps (Nguyen et al., 2015).

Perimenopause

Perimenopause or menopausal transition and menopause are biologic markers of the transition from young adulthood to middle age. Neither of these is a symptom or disease, but rather a natural maturing of the reproductive system.

During the perimenopausal years (2 to 8 years prior to menopause), women may experience physical changes associated with decreasing estrogen levels, which may include vasomotor symptoms of hot flashes, irregular menstrual cycles, sleep disruptions, forgetfulness, irritability, mood disturbances, weight gain and bloating, irregular menses, headaches, decreased vaginal lubrication, night sweats, fatigue, vaginal atrophy, and depression (McNamara, Batur, & DeSapri, 2015). Vasomotor symptoms (hot flashes and night sweats) are the most common complaints for which women seek treatment. Several therapies can be considered to help manage these complaints. Choosing an appropriate treatment approach for the management of these symptoms requires careful assessment of the risk/benefit ratio of each alternative, as well as individual client preference (Schuiling & Likis, 2016).

Menopause

Menopause is a universal and irreversible part of the overall aging process involving a woman's reproductive system, after which she no longer menstruates. This naturally occurring phase of every woman's life marks the end of her childbearing capacity. The average age of natural menopause—defined as 1 year without a menstrual period—is 50 to 51 years old (Alexander et al., 2014). This period is frequently termed the *climacteric* or *perimenopause*, but mostly recently the *menopausal transition* has been used (Hoyt & Falconi, 2015). As the average life expectancy for women increases, the number of women reaching and living in menopause has escalated. Most women can expect to spend more than one third of their lives beyond menopause. It is usually marked by atrophy of the breasts, uterus, fallopian tubes, and ovaries (Crawford, 2015).

Many women pass through menopause without untoward symptoms. These women remain active and in good health with little interruption of their daily routines. Other women experience vasomotor symptoms, which give rise to sensations of heat, cold, sweating, headache, insomnia, and irritability. A recent study found that women experiencing menopausal symptoms reported significantly lower health-related quality of life and significantly high work impairment when compared to women without menopausal symptoms (Coney, 2015).

Until recently, hormone therapy was the mainstay of menopause pharmacotherapy, but with the recent results of the Women's Health Initiative trial and the Heart and Estrogen Replacement Study (HERS), the use of hormone therapy has become controversial. Many women have turned to nontraditional remedies to manage their menopausal symptoms. Common complementary and alternative medicine (CAM) remedies used for the treatment of menopausal symptoms include black cohosh, dong quai, St John's wort, hops, wild yam, ginseng, evening primrose

oil, exercise, and acupuncture. Evidence supporting the efficacy and safety of most CAM for relief of menopausal symptoms is limited and most of the reports of efficacy do not support use of them (Wicks & Mahady, 2015). Nurses can play a major role in assisting menopausal women by educating and counseling them about the multitude of options available for disease prevention and treatments for menopausal symptoms during this time of change in their lives. Menopause should be an opportunity for women to strive for a healthy, long life, and nurses can help to make this opportunity a reality. (See Chapter 4 for more information about menopause.)

Recall Linda, who was experiencing changes in her menstrual patterns. Which hormones might be changing, and which systems might they affect? What approach should the nurse take to enlighten Linda about what is happening to her?

MALE REPRODUCTIVE ANATOMY AND PHYSIOLOGY

The male reproductive system, like that of the female, consists of those organs that facilitate reproduction. The male organs are specialized to produce and maintain the male sex cells, or sperm; to transport them, along with supporting fluids, to the female reproductive system; and to secrete the male hormone testosterone. The organs of the male reproductive system include the penis, scrotum, two **testes** (where sperm cells and testosterone are made), and accessory organs (epididymis, vas deferens, seminal vesicles, ejaculatory duct, urethra, bulbourethral glands, and prostate gland).

External Male Reproductive Organs

The penis and the scrotum form the external genitalia in the male (Fig. 3.7).

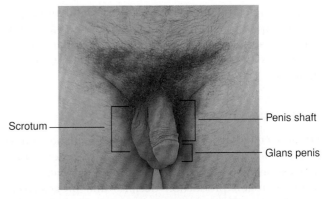

FIGURE 3.7 The external male reproductive organs. (Photo by B. Proud.)

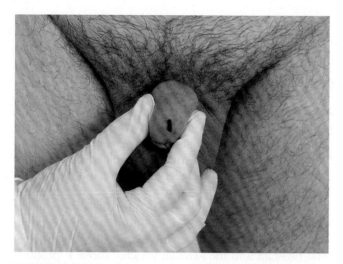

FIGURE 3.8 The urinary meatus. (Photo by B. Proud.)

Penis

The penis is the organ for copulation and serves as the outlet for both sperm and urine. The penis becomes engorged with blood during sexual arousal and is inserted into the female vagina during intercourse. The skin of the penis is thin, with no hairs. The prepuce (foreskin) is a circular fold of skin that extends over the glans unless it is removed by circumcision shortly after birth. The urinary meatus, located at the tip of the penis, serves as the external opening to the urethra (Fig. 3.8). The penis is composed mostly of erectile tissue. Most of the body of the penis consists of three cylindrical spaces

(sinuses) of erectile tissue. The two larger ones, the corpora cavernosa, are side by side. The third sinus, the corpus spongiosum, surrounds the urethra. Erection results when nerve impulses from the autonomic nervous system dilate the arteries of the penis, allowing arterial blood to flow into the erectile tissues of the organ.

Scrotum

The scrotum is the thin-skinned sac that surrounds and protects the testes. The scrotum also acts as a climate-control system for the testes, because they need to be slightly cooler than body temperature to allow normal sperm development. The scrotum is covered with hair starting in puberty. The cremaster muscles in the scrotal wall relax or contract to allow the testes to hang farther from the body to cool or to be pulled closer to the body for warmth or protection (Patton & Thibodeau, 2015). A medial septum divides the scrotum into two chambers, each of which encloses a testis.

Internal Male Reproductive Organs

The internal structures include the testes, the ductal system, and accessory glands (Fig. 3.9).

Testes

The testes are oval bodies in the size of large olives that lie in the scrotum; usually the left testis hangs a

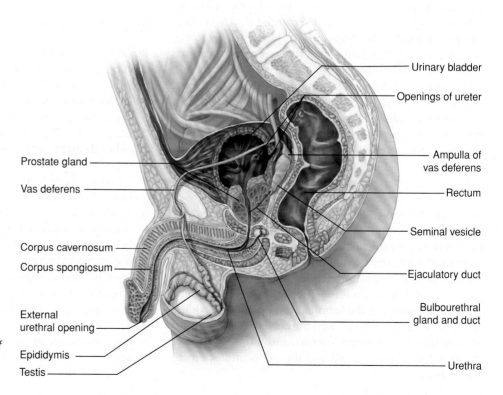

FIGURE 3.9 Lateral view of the internal male reproductive organs. (Source: Anatomical Chart Company. [2001]. *Atlas of human anatomy*. Springhouse, PA: Springhouse.)

Prostate gland

Vas deferens

Corpus cavernosum

Corpus spongiosum

External
urethral opening

Epididymis

Testis

Urinary bladder

Openings of ureter

Ampulla of
vas deferens

Rectum

Seminal vesicle

Ejaculatory duct

Bulbourethral
gland and duct

Urethra

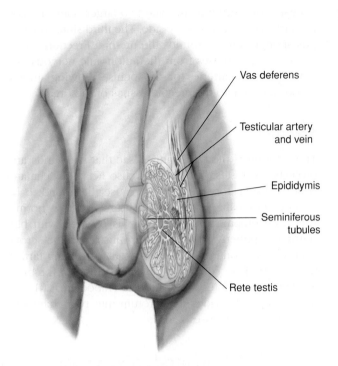

Vas deferens

Testicular artery and vein

Epididymis

Seminiferous tubules

Rete testis

FIGURE 3.10   Internal structures of a testis.

little lower than the right one. These two nut-like structures are analogous to ovaries in the female and two testes are present in males. The testes have two functions: producing sperm and synthesizing testosterone (the primary male sex hormone). Sperm is produced in the seminiferous tubules of the testes. Similar to the female reproductive system, the anterior pituitary releases the gonadotropins, FSH and LH. These hormones stimulate the testes to produce testosterone, which assists in maintaining spermatogenesis, increases sperm production by the seminiferous tubules, and stimulates production of seminal fluid (Jones & Lopez, 2014). The epididymis, which lies against the testes, is a coiled tube almost 20 ft long. It collects sperm from the testes and provides the space and environment for sperm to mature (Fig. 3.10).

The Ductal System

The vas deferens is a cord-like duct that transports sperm from the epididymis. One such duct travels from each testis up to the back of the prostate and enters the urethra to form the ejaculatory ducts. Other structures, such as blood vessels and nerves, also travel along with each vas deferens and together form the spermatic cord. The urethra is the terminal duct of the reproductive and urinary systems, serving as a passageway for semen (fluid containing sperm) and urine. It passes through the prostate gland and the penis and opens to the outside.

Accessory Glands

The seminal vesicles, which produce nutrient seminal fluid, and the prostate gland, which produces alkaline prostatic fluid, are both connected to the ejaculatory duct leading into the urethra. The paired seminal vesicles are convoluted pouch-like structures lying posterior to, and at the base of, the urinary bladder in front of the rectum. They secrete an alkaline fluid that contains fructose and prostaglandins. The fructose supplies energy to the sperm on its journey to meet the ovum, and the prostaglandins assist in sperm mobility.

The prostate gland lies just under the bladder in the pelvis and surrounds the middle portion of the urethra. Usually the size of a walnut, this gland enlarges with age. The prostate and the seminal vesicles above it produce fluid that nourishes the sperm. This fluid provides most of the volume of semen, the secretion in which sperm are expelled during ejaculation. Other fluid that makes up the semen comes from the vas deferens and from mucous glands in the head of the penis.

The bulbourethral glands (Cowper's glands) are two small structures about the size of peas, located inferior to the prostate gland. They are composed of several tubes whose epithelial linings secrete a mucus-like fluid. It is released in response to sexual stimulation and lubricates the head of the penis in preparation for sexual intercourse, in addition, neutralizes the acidity of the urethra to protect sperm during their journey out of the body during ejaculation. Their existence is said to be constant, but they gradually diminish in size with advancing age.

Male Sexual Response

Regardless of the type of sexual stimulation, the physiologic response in both men and women is similar and usually follows a five-phase pattern, as described earlier:
1. *Desire:* Starts with a desire for sexual intimacy. This can also be termed libido.
2. *Excitement:* The man experiences sexual arousal with either thoughts or physical sexual stimuli which cause specific changes such as the heart beating faster, blood pressure rising, the testicles enlarging and more blood flowing into the penis, creating an erection.
3. *Plateau:* It is the phase between excitement and orgasm in which the head of the penis enlarges and becomes more purplish in color; the glands secrete semen into the urethra; and it is challenging to stop from having an orgasm.
4. *Orgasm:* It is a total body response. The tension that built up during the previous two phases is released. It triggers a series of muscle spasms in the legs, stomach, arms, back, and penis. The feelings are intense and pleasurable. Ejaculation of semen occurs at this time.

5. *Resolution:* The body returns to the physiologic non-stimulated state. The blood flows out of the penis and erection ceases; an overall feeling of relaxation ensues, and the testes and scrotum return to their normal size (Housman & Odum, 2016).

Sexual behavior involves the participation of autonomic and somatic nerves and the integration of numerous spinal sites in the central nervous system (CNS). The penile portion of the process that leads to erections represents only a single component. Penile erections are an integration of complex physiologic processes involving the CNS, peripheral nervous system, and hormonal and vascular systems (Sherwood, 2016). With sexual stimulation, the arteries leading to the penis dilate and increase blood flow into erectile tissues. At the same time, the erectile tissue compresses the veins of the penis, reducing blood flow away from the penis. Blood accumulates, causing the penis to swell and elongate and producing an erection. As in women, the culmination of sexual stimulation is an orgasm, a pleasurable feeling of physiologic and psychological release.

Orgasm is accompanied by emission (movement of sperm from the testes and fluids from the accessory glands) into the urethra, where the sperm and fluids are mixed to form semen. As the urethra fills with semen, the base of the erect penis contracts, this increases pressure. This pressure forces the semen through the urethra to the outside (ejaculation). During ejaculation, the ducts of the testes, epididymis, and vas deferens contract and cause expulsion of sperm into the urethra, where the sperm mixes with the seminal and prostatic fluids. These substances, together with mucus secreted by accessory glands, form the semen, which is discharged from the urethra.

KEY CONCEPTS

- The female reproductive system produces the female reproductive cells (the eggs, or ova) and contains an organ (uterus) where the fetus develops. The male reproductive system produces the male reproductive cells (the sperm) and contains an organ (penis) that deposits the sperm within the female.

- The internal female reproductive organs consist of the vagina, the uterus, the fallopian tubes, and the ovaries. The external female reproductive organs make up the vulva. These include the mons pubis, the labia majora and minora, the clitoris and prepuce, structures within the vestibule, and the perineum.

- The breasts are accessory organs of the female reproductive system that are specialized to secrete milk following pregnancy.

- The main function of the reproductive cycle is to stimulate growth of a follicle to release an egg and prepare a site for implantation if fertilization occurs.

- Menstruation, the monthly shedding of the uterine lining, marks the beginning and end of the cycle if fertilization does not occur.

- The ovarian cycle is the series of events associated with a developing oocyte (ovum or egg) within the ovaries.

- At ovulation, a mature follicle ruptures in response to a surge of LH, releasing a mature oocyte (ovum).

- The endometrial cycle is divided into four phases: the follicular or proliferative phase, the luteal or secretory phase, the ischemic phase, and the menstrual phase.

- The menstrual cycle involves a complex interaction of hormones. The predominant hormones are gonadotropin-releasing hormone (GnRH), FSH, LH, estrogen, progesterone, and prostaglandins.

- The organs of the male reproductive system include the penis, scrotum, two testes (where sperm cells and testosterone are made), and accessory organs (epididymis, vas deferens, seminal vesicles, ejaculatory ducts, urethra, bulbourethral glands, and prostate gland).

References and Recommended Readings

Acién, M., & Acién, P. (2015). Normal embryological development of the female genital tract. In *Female genital tract congenital malformations* (pp. 3–14). London: Springer.

Alexander, L. L., LaRosa, J. H., Bader, H., & Garfield, S. (2014). *New dimensions in women's health* (6th ed.). Sudbury, MA: Jones and Bartlett.

Clark, C. C., & Paraska, K. K. (2014). *Health promotion for nurses: A practical guide.* Burlington, MA: Jones & Bartlett Learning.

Coney, P. (2015). Menopause. *eMedicine.* Retrieved from http://emedicine.medscape.com/article/264088-overview

Crawford, S. L. (2015). What should women expect after stopping hormone therapy? *Menopause, 22*(4), 367–368.

Davis, S. R. (2013). Androgen therapy in women, beyond libido. *Climacteric, 16,* 18–24.

Farage, M. A., Miller, K. W., & Maibach, H. I. (2015). Postmenopausal vulva and vagina. In *Skin, mucosa and menopause* (pp. 385–395). Heidelberg, Berlin: Springer.

Housman, J., & Odum, M. (2016). *Alters & Schiff's essential concepts for healthy living* (7th ed.). Burlington, MA: Jones & Bartlett Learning.

Hoyt, L. T., & Falconi, A. (2015). Puberty and perimenopause: Reproductive transitions and their implications for women's health. *Social Science & Medicine, 132,* 103–112.

Jones, R. E., & Lopez, K. H. (2014). *Human reproductive biology* (4th ed.). Waltham, MA: Elsevier.

Kandeel, F. (2014). *Female reproductive and sexual medicine.* New York, NY: Springer.

King, T. L., Brucker, M. C., Kriebs, J. M., Fahey, J. O., Gegor, C. L., & Varney, H. (2015). *Varney's midwifery* (5th ed.). Burlington, MA: Jones & Bartlett Learning.

Krieger, N., Kiang, M. V., Kosheleva, A., Waterman, P. D., Chen, J. T., & Beckfield, J. (2015). Age at menarche: 50-year socioeconomic trends among US-born black and white women. *American Journal of Public Health, 105*(2), 388–397.

McNamara, M., Batur, P., & DeSapri, K. T. (2015). Perimenopause. *Annals of Internal Medicine, 162*(3), ITC1–ITC1.

Minkin, M. J. (2016). Sexual health and relationships after age 60. *Maturitus, 83,* 27–32. Doi: 10.1016/j.maturitas.2015.10.004

Nguyen, A. M., Humphrey, L., Kitchen, H., Rehman, T., & Norquist, J. M. (2015). A qualitative study to develop a patient-reported outcome for dysmenorrhea. *Quality of Life Research, 24*(1), 181–191.

Oyelowo, T., & Johnson, J. L. B. (2016). *A guide to women's health* (2nd ed.). Burlington, MA: Jones & Bartlett Learning.

Patton, K. T., & Thibodeau, G. A. (2015). *Anatomy & physiology* (9th ed.). St. Louis, MO: Mosby Elsevier.

Patton, K. T., & Thibodeau, G. A. (2016). *The human body in health and disease* (6th ed.). St. Louis, MO: Mosby Elsevier.

Pauls, R. N. (2015). Anatomy of the clitoris and the female sexual response. *Clinical Anatomy, 28*(3), 376–384.

Senie, R. T. (2014). *Epidemiology of women's health*. Burlington, MA: Jones & Bartlett Learning.

Schuiling, K. D., & Likis, F. E. (2016). *Women's gynecologic health* (3rd ed.). Burlington, MA: Jones and Bartlett Learning.

Sherwood, L. (2016). *Human physiology: From cells to systems* (9th ed.). Boston, MA: Cengage Learning.

Tambouret, R. H., & Wilbur, D. C. (2015). Normal histology and cytology of the endocervix and endometrium. In *Glandular lesions of the uterine cervix* (pp. 25–40). New York, NY: Springer.

Thornhill, R., & Gangestad, S. W. (2015). The functional design and phylogeny of women's sexuality. In T. K. Shackelford, & R. D. Hansen (Eds.), *The evolution of sexuality* (pp. 149–184). Switzerland: Springer International Publishing.

Velkey, J. M., Hall, A. H., & Robboy, S. J. (2015). Normal vulva: Embryology, anatomy, and histology. In *Vulvar pathology* (pp. 3–17). New York, NY: Springer.

Wheatley, J. R., & Puts, D. A. (2015). Evolutionary science of female orgasm. In *The evolution of sexuality* (pp. 123–148). Springer International Publishing.

Wicks, S. M., & Mahady, G. B. (2015). Herbal and complementary medicines used for women's health. In *Medicines for women* (pp. 373–399). Switzerland: Springer International Publishing.

MULTIPLE-CHOICE QUESTIONS

1. The predominant anterior pituitary hormones that orchestrate the menstrual cycle include:
   a. Thyroid-stimulating hormone (TSH)
   b. Follicle-stimulating hormone (FSH)
   c. Corticotropin-releasing hormone (CRH)
   d. Gonadotropin-releasing hormone (GnRH)

2. Which glands are located on either side of the female urethra and secrete mucus to keep the opening moist and lubricated for urination?
   a. Cowper's
   b. Bartholin's
   c. Skene's
   d. Seminal

3. What event occurs during the proliferative phase of the menstrual cycle?
   a. Menstrual flow starts
   b. Endometrium thickens
   c. Ovulation occurs
   d. Progesterone secretion peaks

4. Which hormone is produced in high levels to prepare the endometrium for implantation just after ovulation by the corpus luteum?
   a. Estrogen
   b. Prostaglandins
   c. Prolactin
   d. Progesterone

5. Sperm maturation and storage in the male reproductive system occur in the:
   a. Testes
   b. Vas deferens
   c. Epididymis
   d. Seminal vesicles

6. The nurse is preparing to teach a class to a group of middle-aged women regarding the most common vasomotor symptoms experienced during menopause and possible modalities of treatment available. Common vasomotor symptoms would include which of the following?
   a. Chronic fatigue and confusion
   b. Forgetfulness and irritability
   c. Night sweats and hot flashes
   d. Decrease in sexual response and appetite

CRITICAL THINKING EXERCISE

1. The school nurse was asked to speak to a 10th-grade biology class about menstruation. The teacher felt that the students did not understand this monthly event and wanted to dispel some myths about it. After the nurse explains the factors influencing the menses, one girl asks, "Could someone get pregnant if she had sex during her period?"

   a. How should the nurse respond to this question?
   b. What factor regarding the menstrual cycle was not clarified?
   c. What additional topics might this question lead to that might be discussed?

STUDY ACTIVITIES

1. Should sex education be taught in public schools, and if so, what topics should be addressed? Debate the pros and cons of teaching this and then outline which topics should be covered.

2. Respond to the following as a topic sentence: "When I was growing up, talking about sexual matters with my parents was … because…. Now the situation is …?"

3. List the predominant hormones and their function in the menstrual cycle.

4. The ovarian cycle describes the series of events associated with the development of the _____ within the ovaries.

5. Sperm cells and the male hormone testosterone are made in which of the following structures? Select all that apply.
   a. Vas deferens
   b. Penis
   c. Scrotum
   d. Ejaculatory ducts
   e. Prostate gland
   f. Testes
   g. Seminiferous tubules
   h. Bulbourethral glands

BRINGING IT ALL TOGETHER: CASE STUDY

A 53-year-old woman came to see her women's health nurse practitioner for her annual examination. She had a hysterectomy 20 years ago for a prolapsed uterus and has been healthy up until now. She had a long list of symptoms that had been bothering her, but until recently just chalked them up to the aging process. She told the nurse practitioner that she was experiencing insomnia, weight gain around her middle despite not consuming additional calories, painful intercourse, and hot flashes that were increasing in frequency throughout the day and night. She had been taking black cohosh for these distressing symptoms for the past several months, but was not getting any relief. She was concerned that something awful was wrong with her since this natural herb was not reducing her symptoms and they seemed to be getting worse.

Go to thePoint **to find questions to consider about this case.**

4

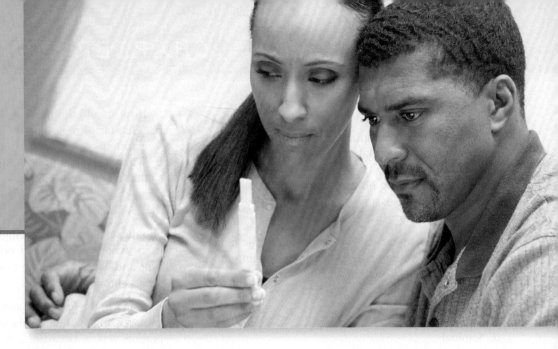

Common Reproductive Issues

Learning Objectives

Upon completion of the chapter, you will be able to:

1. Examine common reproductive concerns in terms of symptoms, diagnostic tests, and appropriate interventions.

2. Identify risk factors and outline appropriate client education needed in common reproductive disorders.

3. Compare and contrast the various contraceptive methods available and their overall effectiveness.

4. Analyze the physiologic and psychological aspects of menopausal transition.

5. Delineate the nursing management needed for women experiencing common reproductive disorders.

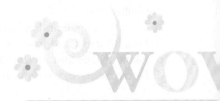

Words of Wisdom
When women bare their souls to us, we must respond without judgment.

Izzy, a 27-year-old, presents to her health care provider complaining of progressive severe pelvic pain associated with her monthly periods. She has to take off work and "dope up" with pills to endure the pain. In addition, she has been trying to conceive for over a year without any luck.

INTRODUCTION

Good health throughout the life cycle begins with the individual. Women today can expect to live well into their 80s and need to be proactive in maintaining their own quality of life. Women need to take steps to reduce their risk of disease and need to become active partners with their health care professional to identify problems early, when treatment may be most successful (Teaching Guidelines 4.1). Nurses can assist women in maintaining their quality of life by helping them to become more attuned to their body and its clues and can use the assessment period as an opportunity for teaching and counseling. Nurses are in a prime position to offer information that provides women with the tools needed to maintain a healthy lifestyle and assist in altering behaviors that may cause harm or illness.

Teaching Guidelines 4.1

TIPS FOR BEING AN ACTIVE PARTNER IN MANAGING YOUR HEALTH

- Become an informed consumer. Read, ask, and search.
- Know your family history and know factors that put you at high risk.
- Maintain a healthy lifestyle and let moderation be your guide.
- Schedule regular medical checkups and screenings for early detection.
- Ask your health care provider for a full explanation of any treatment.
- Seek a second medical opinion if you feel you need more information.
- Know when to seek medical care by being aware of disease symptoms.

Common reproductive issues addressed in this chapter that nurses might encounter in caring for women include menstrual disorders, infertility, contraception, abortion, and the menopausal transition.

MENSTRUAL DISORDERS

Many women sail through their monthly menstrual cycles with little or no concern. With few symptoms to worry about, their menses are like clockwork, starting and stopping at nearly the same times every month. For others, the menstrual cycle causes physical and emotional symptoms that initiate visits to their health care provider for consultation. The following menstruation-related conditions will be discussed in this section: amenorrhea, dysmenorrhea, abnormal uterine bleeding (AUB), premenstrual syndrome (PMS), premenstrual dysphoric disorder (PMDD), and endometriosis. To gain an understanding of menstrual disorders, nurses should know the terms used to describe them (Box 4.1).

BOX 4.1

MENSTRUAL DISORDER VOCABULARY

- *meno* = menstrual related
- *metro* = time
- *oligo* = few
- *a* = without, none or lack of
- *rhagia* = excess or abnormal
- *dys* = not or pain
- *rhea* = flow

Amenorrhea

Amenorrhea simply means absence of menses. Amenorrhea is normal in prepubertal, pregnant, postpartum, and postmenopausal females. The uterus, endometrial lining, ovaries, pituitary, and hypothalamus must function properly and in harmony for a menstrual cycle to occur. The two categories of amenorrhea are primary and secondary amenorrhea. Primary amenorrhea is defined as either the:

1. absence of menses by age 14, with absence of growth and development of secondary sexual characteristics; or
2. absence of menses by age 16, with normal development of secondary sexual characteristics (Schuiling & Likis, 2016).

Ninety-eight percent of girls living in the United States menstruate by age 15 (Krieger et al., 2015). Findings of recent studies indicate that age at menarche has overall declined since the twentieth century (King et al., 2015). Once menarche has occurred, cycles may take up to 2 years to become regular, ovulatory cycles. Secondary amenorrhea is the absence of regular menses for three cycles or irregular menses for 6 months in women who have previously menstruated regularly.

Nurses need to consider the causes of amenorrhea as occurring in one of the four anatomical areas: outflow area of the uterus and vagina, the ovaries, the pituitary gland, or the central nervous system. Outflow area problems are obstructive in nature and can be found on physical exam, whereas ovarian, pituitary, and central nervous system problems involve disruptions in the hypothalamic–pituitary–ovarian axis that controls the neuroendocrine processes required for a normal menstrual cycle and are generally found through laboratory analysis (King et al., 2015).

Etiology

Primary amenorrhea has multiple causes:
- Extreme weight gain or loss
- Congenital abnormalities of the reproductive system
- Stress from a major life event
- Excessive exercise
- Eating disorders (anorexia nervosa or bulimia)
- Cushing disease
- Polycystic ovary syndrome

- Hypothyroidism
- Turner syndrome—defective development of the gonads (ovary or testes)
- Imperforate hymen
- Chronic illness—diabetes, thyroid disease, depression
- Pregnancy
- Cystic fibrosis
- Congenital heart disease (cyanotic)
- Ovarian or adrenal tumors
- Causes of secondary amenorrhea can include:
- Pregnancy
- Breast-feeding
- Emotional stress
- Pituitary, ovarian, or adrenal tumors
- Depression
- Hyperthyroid or hypothyroid conditions
- Malnutrition
- Hyperprolactinemia
- Rapid weight gain or loss
- Chemotherapy or radiation therapy to the pelvic area
- Vigorous exercise, such as long-distance running
- Kidney failure
- Colitis
- Chemotherapy, irradiation
- Use of tranquilizers or antidepressants
- Postpartum pituitary necrosis (Sheehan syndrome)
- Early menopause (Kovanci & Schutt, 2015).

Therapeutic Management

Therapeutic intervention depends on the cause of the amenorrhea. The treatment of primary amenorrhea involves the correction of any underlying disorders and estrogen replacement therapy to stimulate the development of secondary sexual characteristics (Moses, 2015a). If a pituitary tumor is the cause, it might be treated with drug therapy, surgical resection, or radiation therapy. Surgery might be needed to correct any structural abnormalities of the genital tract. Dopamine agonists are effective in treating hyperprolactinemia. In most cases, this treatment restores normal ovarian endocrine function and ovulation (Goswami, 2015). Therapeutic interventions for secondary amenorrhea can include:

- cyclic progesterone, when the cause is anovulation, or **oral contraceptives** (OCs);
- bromocriptine to treat hyperprolactinemia;
- nutritional counseling to address anorexia, bulimia, or obesity;
- gonadotropin-releasing hormone (GnRH), when the cause is hypothalamic failure;
- thyroid hormone replacement, when the cause is hypothyroidism (Creatsas & Creatsa, 2015).

Nursing Assessment

Nursing assessment for the young girl or woman experiencing amenorrhea includes a thorough health history, physical examination, and several laboratory and diagnostic tests of selected hormone levels to help to identify an underlying cause.

HEALTH HISTORY AND PHYSICAL EXAMINATION

A thorough history and physical examination are needed to determine the etiology. The history should include questions about the women's menstrual history; past illnesses; hospitalizations and surgeries; obstetric history; use of prescription and over-the-counter drugs; recent or past lifestyle changes; and history of present illness, with an assessment of any body changes.

The physical examination should begin with an overall assessment of the woman's nutritional status and general health. A sensitive and gentle approach to the pelvic examination is critical in young women. Height, weight, and body mass index (BMI) should be taken, along with vital signs. Hypothermia, bradycardia, hypotension, and reduced subcutaneous fat may be observed in women with anorexia nervosa. Facial hair and acne might be evidence of androgen excess secondary to a tumor. The presence or absence of axillary and pubic hair may indicate adrenal and ovarian hyposecretion or delayed puberty. A general physical examination may uncover unexpected findings that are indirectly related to amenorrhea. For example, hepatosplenomegaly, which may suggest a chronic systemic disease or an enlarged thyroid gland, might point to a thyroid disorder as well as a reason for amenorrhea (Tharpe, Farley, & Jordan, 2016). Examination of the breasts also deserves careful attention because breast development is a reliable indicator of estrogen production. The Tanner stages of breast development should be noted also. The Tanner stages include:

- Stage I—Papilla elevation only
- Stage II—Breast buds palpable and areolae enlarge ~11 years old
- Stage III—Elevation of breast contour; areolae enlarge ~12 years old
- Stage IV—Areolae forms secondary mound on the breast ~13 years old
- Stage V—Adult breast contour; areola recesses to breast contour (Moses, 2015b)

Information gained from the history and physical exam clearly can exclude certain diagnostic possibilities, but first impressions also can be deceiving and lead to errors in judgment. A methodical, systematic approach to identify the etiology of amenorrhea is the best.

LABORATORY AND DIAGNOSTIC TESTS

Common laboratory tests that might be ordered to determine the cause of amenorrhea include:

- karyotype (might be positive for Turner syndrome);
- ultrasound to detect ovarian cysts;
- quantitative human chorionic gonadotropin (hCG) test to rule out pregnancy;
- thyroid function studies to determine thyroid disorder;

- prolactin level (an elevated level might indicate a pituitary tumor);
- follicle-stimulating hormone (FSH) level (an elevated level might indicate ovarian failure);
- luteinizing hormone (LH) level (an elevated level might indicate gonadal dysfunction);
- 17-ketosteroids (an elevated level might indicate an adrenal tumor) (Pagana, Pagana, & Pagana, 2015).

Nursing Management

Counseling and education are primary interventions and appropriate nursing roles. Address the diverse causes of amenorrhea, the relationship to sexual identity, possible infertility, and the possibility of a tumor or a life-threatening disease. Evidence is mounting that loss of menstrual regularity is a risk factor for later development of osteoporosis and hip fractures, so treatment to restore regular menstrual cycles is essential (Carlson, 2015). In addition, inform the woman about the purpose of each diagnostic test, how it is performed, and when the results will be available to discuss with her. Listening sensitively, interviewing, and presenting treatment options are paramount to gain the woman's cooperation and understanding.

Nutritional counseling is also vital in managing this disorder, especially if the woman has findings suggestive of an eating disorder. The relation between eating disorders and menstrual dysfunction has been identified in research studies. Careful evaluation of menstrual status is warranted for all women with eating disorders. Timely intervention is important because shorter duration of illness is associated with improved outcomes (Golden et al., 2015). Although not all causes can be addressed by making lifestyle changes, emphasize maintaining a healthy lifestyle (Teaching Guidelines 4.2).

Teaching Guidelines 4.2

TIPS FOR MAINTAINING A HEALTHY LIFESTYLE

- Balance energy expenditure with energy intake to maintain ideal weight range.
- Modify your diet to maintain ideal weight to avoid becoming over weight.
- Avoid excessive use of alcohol and mood-altering or sedative drugs.
- Avoid cigarette smoking to prevent cardiovascular disease and lung cancer.
- Identify areas of emotional stress and seek assistance to resolve them.
- Balance work, recreation, and rest to reduce anxiety and stress in life.
- Maintain a positive outlook regarding the diagnosis and prognosis.
- Participate in ongoing care to monitor any medical conditions.

- Maintain bone density through:
  - Calcium intake (1,200 to 1,600 mg daily)
  - Vitamin D (600 to 1,000 International Units/daily)
  - Weight-bearing exercise (30 min or more daily)
  - Hormone therapy (HT) for low risk women

Adapted from Centers for Disease Control and Prevention. (2015a). *Healthy eating for a healthy weight*. Retrieved from http://www.cdc.gov/healthyweight/healthy_eating/; and Housman, J., & Odum, M. (2016). *Alters & Schiff's essential concepts for healthy living* (7th ed.). Burlington, MA: Jones & Bartlett Learning.

Dysmenorrhea

Dysmenorrhea refers to painful menstruation and is a common problem in adolescence. This condition has also been termed *cyclic perimenstrual pain*. Usually pain starts along with the start of bleeding and lasts for 48 to 72 hours (Creatsas & Creatsa, 2015). The term *dysmenorrhea* is derived from the Greek words *dys*, meaning "difficult, painful, or abnormal," and *rrhea*, meaning "flow." Based on results of large epidemiologic studies, it is estimated that it may affect more than half of menstruating women. It is the leading cause of absenteeism of work and school, and has adverse effects on the quality of life of young women (Joshi et al., 2015). Another recent research study linked early smoking (<13 years old) to an increased risk for developing chronic dysmenorrhea (Weinberger, Smith, Allen, et al., 2015). Uterine contractions occur during all periods, but in some women these cramps can be frequent and very intense. It has a major impact on women's quality of life, work productivity, and health care utilization. Dysmenorrhea is classified as primary (spasmodic) or secondary (congestive) (Calis et al., 2015).

Etiology

Primary dysmenorrhea refers to painful menstrual bleedings in the absence of any detectable underlying pathology. It is caused by increased prostaglandin production by the endometrium in an ovulatory cycle. This hormone causes contraction of the uterus, and levels tend to be higher in women with severe menstrual pain than women who experience mild or no menstrual pain. Dysmenorrhea is caused by an excess of prostaglandin production. These levels are highest during the first 2 days of menses, when symptoms peak (Maurice & Rosenzweig, 2015). This results in increased rhythmic uterine contractions from vasoconstriction of the small vessels of the uterine wall. This condition usually begins within a few years of the onset of ovulatory cycles at menarche.

Secondary dysmenorrhea is painful menstruation due to pelvic or uterine pathology. It may be caused by endometriosis, adenomyosis, fibroids, pelvic infection, an intrauterine system, cervical stenosis, or congenital uterine or vaginal abnormalities. Adenomyosis involves the ingrowth of the endometrium into the uterine musculature. Endometriosis involves ectopic implantation of endometrial tissue in other parts of the pelvis. It occurs most commonly in the third or fourth decade of life and affects 10% of women of reproductive age. The pain tends to get worse, rather than better, over time (American College of Obstetricians & Gynecologists [ACOG], 2015a). **Endometriosis** is the most common cause of secondary dysmenorrhea and is associated with pain beyond menstruation, dyspareunia, low back pain, heavy or irregular bleeding, bloating, nausea and vomiting, and infertility (ACOG, 2015a). Treatment is directed toward removing the underlying pathology.

Think back to Izzy from the chapter opener. Is her pelvic pain complaint a common one with women?

Therapeutic Management

The goal of treatment is to provide adequate pain relief to allow the woman to perform her usual activities. Current treatment is mainly based on surgery and ovarian suppressive agents (OCs, progestins, GnRh antagonist, levonorgestrel-releasing intrauterine system, and androgenic agents). Hormonal treatment is often associated with unwanted side effects and recurrence of symptoms when stopped. Severe dysmenorrhea can be distressing, adversely affecting social and occupational activities. Treatments vary from over-the-counter remedies to hormonal control. However, for some women satisfactory pain relief is difficult to achieve, and increasingly they seek alternative options. Complementary therapies such as acupuncture (needles are used to stimulate certain points of the body to balance the flow of energy within the body) and acupressure (the use of fingers and hands to stimulate acupoints and maintains the balance of energy) are gaining popularity and the evidence base for their use is growing (Wicks & Mahady, 2015).

Therapeutic intervention is directed toward pain relief and building coping strategies that will promote a productive lifestyle. General measures for management include client education and reassurance. Treatment is supportive and should be guided by individual needs. Treatment measures usually include treating infections if present; suppressing the endometrium if endometriosis is suspected by administering low-dose OCs; administering prostaglandin inhibitors to reduce the pain; administering Depo-Provera to suppress ovulation, which thins the endometrial lining of the uterus with subsequent reduction of fluid contents of the uterus during menses; and initiating lifestyle changes (Schuiling & Likis, 2016). Table 4.1 lists selected treatment options for dysmenorrhea.

Nursing Assessment

As with any gynecologic complaint, a thorough focused history and physical examination are needed to make the diagnosis of primary or secondary dysmenorrhea. In primary dysmenorrhea, the history usually reveals the typical cramping pain with menstruation, and the physical examination is completely normal. In secondary dysmenorrhea, the history discloses cramping pain starting after 25 years old with a pelvic abnormality, a history of infertility, heavy menstrual flow, irregular cycles, and little response to nonsteroidal anti-inflammatory drugs (NSAIDs), OCs, or both (Elnashar, 2015).

HEALTH HISTORY AND CLINICAL MANIFESTATIONS

Note the past medical history, including any chronic illnesses and family history of gynecologic concerns. Determine medication and substance use, such as prescription medications, contraceptives, anabolic steroids, tobacco, and marijuana, cocaine, or other illegal drugs. A detailed sexual history is essential to assess for inflammation and scarring (adhesions) secondary to pelvic inflammatory disease (PID). Women with a previous history of PID, sexually transmitted infections (STIs), low consumption of fruits and vegetables, depression, high stress level, multiple sexual partners, or unprotected sex are at increased risk (Tharpe et al., 2016).

During the initial interview, the nurse might ask some of the following questions to assess the woman's history of dysmenorrhea:

- At what age did your menstrual cycles start?
- Have your cycles always been painful, or did the pain start recently?
- When in your cycle do you experience the pain?
- How would you describe the pain you feel?
- Are you sexually active?
- What impact does your cycle have on your physical and social activity?
- When was the first day of your last menstrual cycle?
- Was the flow of your last menstrual cycle a normal amount for you?
- Do your cycles tend to be heavy or last longer than 5 days?
- Are your cycles generally regular and predictable?
- What have you done to relieve your discomfort? Is it effective?
- Has there been a progression of symptom severity?
- Do you have any other symptoms?

Assess for clinical manifestations of dysmenorrhea. Affected women experience sharp, intermittent spasms of pain, usually in the suprapubic area. Pain may radiate to the back of the legs or the lower back. Pain usually develops within hours of the start of menstruation and peaks as the flow becomes heaviest during the first day or two of the cycle (King et al., 2015). Systemic symptoms of nausea, vomiting, diarrhea, fatigue, fever, headache, or dizziness are fairly common. Explore the history for physical symptoms of bloating, water retention, weight gain, headache, muscle aches, abdominal pain, food cravings, or breast tenderness.

TABLE 4.1	TREATMENT OPTIONS FOR DYSMENORRHEA		
Therapy Options		**Dosage**	**Comments**
Nonsteroidal anti-inflammatory agents (NSAIDs)			NSAIDS prevent prostaglandin synthesis by inhibiting COX-1 and COX-2 conversion, reducing cramping.
Ibuprofen (Advil, Motrin, Midol)		400–800 mg TID	Take with meals. Do not take with aspirin.
Naproxen (Anaprox, Naprelan, Naprosyn, Aleve)		250–500 mg TID	Avoid alcohol. Watch for signs of GI bleeding. Same as above.
Hormonal contraceptives			Decrease prostaglandin synthesis; second-line treatment.
Low-dose oral contraceptives		Taken daily—extended cycle formulas (84 d on, 7 d off)	Take active pills for an extended time to reduce number of monthly cycles.
Depo-medroxyprogesterone (DMPA), Depo-Provera		150 mg IM every 12 wks	Within 9–12 mo of DMPA therapy, 75% of women will experience amenorrhea.
Levonorgestrel-releasing IUS (Mirena)		Inserted into uterine cavity and may remain for up to 5 yrs	Inhibits ovulation and decreases thickness of endometrium. Inhibits uterine contractions and reduces pain from menstrual cramps.
Selective estrogen receptor modulators (SERMS)		Used for women not responding to NSAIDS and oral contraceptives; dosage is individualized	Adverse effects include hot flashes, nausea and vomiting, and risk of thromboembolism.
Raloxifene hydrochloride (Evista); tamoxifen citrate (Nolvadex)			Research is needed to validate effectiveness, doses, side effects, and contradictions.
Complementary therapies Thiamine (vitamin B) Vitamin E (tocopherols) Magnesium Omega-3 fatty acids (fish oil)			Gives sense of control over life.
Lifestyle changes Daily exercise Limited salty foods Weight loss Smoking cessation Relaxation techniques			

Adapted from Calis, K. A., Popat, V., Dang, D. K., & Kalantaridou, S. N. (2015). Dysmenorrhea. eMedicine. Retrieved from http://emedicine.medscape.com/article/253812-overview; King, T. L., Brucker, M. C., Kriebs, J. M., Fahey, J. O., Gegor, C. L., & Varney, H. (2015). *Varney's midwifery* (5th ed.). Burlington, MA: Jones and Bartlett Learning; Schuiling, K. D., & Likis, F. E. (2016). *Women's gynecologic health* (3rd ed.). Burlington, MA: Jones & Bartlett Learning.

PHYSICAL EXAMINATION

The physical examination performed by the health care provider centers on the bimanual pelvic examination. This examination is done during the nonmenstrual phase of the cycle. Explain to the woman how it is to be performed, especially if it is her first pelvic examination. Prepare the woman in the examining room by offering her a cover gown to put on and covering her lap with a privacy sheet on the examination table. Remain in the examining room throughout the examination to assist the health care provider with any procedures or specimens and to offer the woman reassurance.

LABORATORY AND DIAGNOSTIC TESTS

Common diagnostic tests that may be ordered to determine the cause of dysmenorrhea can include:
- complete blood count to rule out anemia;
- urinalysis to rule out a bladder infection;
- pregnancy test (hCG level) to rule out pregnancy;
- cervical culture to exclude STI;
- erythrocyte sedimentation rate to detect an inflammatory process;
- stool guaiac test to exclude gastrointestinal bleeding or disorders;
- pelvic and/or vaginal ultrasound to detect pelvic masses or cysts;
- diagnostic laparoscopy and/or laparotomy to visualize pathology that may account for the symptoms (Tharpe et al., 2016).

What diagnostic tests might be ordered to diagnose Izzy's pelvic pain?

Nursing Management

Educating the client about the normal events of the menstrual cycle and the etiology of her pain is paramount in achieving a successful outcome. Explaining the normal menstrual cycle will teach the woman the correct terms to use, so she can communicate her symptoms more accurately and will help dispel myths. Provide the woman with monthly graphs or charts to record menses, the onset of pain, the timing of medication, relief afforded, and coping strategies used. This involves the woman in her care and provides objective information so that therapy can be modified if necessary.

The nurse should explain in detail the dosing regimen and the side effects of the medication therapy selected. Commonly prescribed drugs include NSAIDs such as ibuprofen (Motrin, Advil) or naproxen (Naprosyn). These drugs alleviate dysmenorrhea symptoms by decreasing intrauterine pressure and inhibiting prostaglandin synthesis, thus reducing pain (Skidmore-Roth, 2015). The primary goal of NSAID therapy of dysmenorrhea is to preempt the production of prostaglandins; thus starting the medication prophylactically and using sufficient doses to maximally suppress prostaglandin production are essential. If pain relief is not achieved in two to four cycles, a low-dose combination OC may be initiated. Client teaching and counseling should include information about how to take pills, side effects, and danger signs to watch for.

Encourage the woman to apply a heating pad or warm compress to alleviate menstrual cramps. Additional lifestyle changes that the woman can make to restore some sense of control and active participation in her care are listed in Teaching Guidelines 4.3.

Teaching Guidelines 4.3
TIPS FOR MANAGING DYSMENORRHEA

- Exercise to increase endorphins and suppress prostaglandin release.
- Limit salty foods to prevent fluid retention.
- Increase water consumption to serve as a natural diuretic.
- Increase fiber intake with fruits and vegetables to prevent constipation.
- Use heating pads or warm baths to increase comfort.
- Take warm showers to promote relaxation.
- Sip on warm beverages, such as decaffeinated green tea.
- Keep legs elevated while lying down or lie on side with knees bent.
- Use stress management techniques to reduce emotional stress.
- Practice relaxation techniques to enhance ability to cope with pain.
- Stop smoking and decrease alcohol use which causes vasoconstriction.

Adapted from Calis, K. A., Popat, V., Dang, D. K., & Kalantaridou, S. N. (2015). Dysmenorrhea. *EMedicine.* Retrieved from http://emedicine.medscape.com/article/253812-overview; Smith, R. P., & Kaunitz, A. M. (2015). Painful menstrual periods: Beyond the basics. *UpToDate.* Retrieved from http://www.uptodate.com/contents/painful-menstrual-periods-dysmenorrhea-beyond-the-basics; and ACOG. (2015d). Dysmenorrhea: Painful periods. FAQ046. Retrieved from www.acog.org/~/media/For Patients/faq046.ashx

Abnormal Uterine Bleeding

Disturbances of menstrual bleeding manifest in a wide range of presentations. *AUB* is the umbrella term used to describe any deviation from normal menstruation or from a normal menstrual cycle pattern. It can occur in women of any age. The key characteristics are regularity, frequency, volume or heaviness of flow, and duration of flow, but each of these may exhibit considerable variability.

AUB is a disorder that occurs most frequently in women at the beginning and end of their reproductive years. AUB is defined as a painless endometrial bleeding that is prolonged, excessive, and irregular, and not attributed to any underlying structural or systemic disease (Creatsas & Creatsa, 2015). It is frequently associated with anovulatory cycles, which are common for the first year after menarche and is associated with immaturity of the hypothalamic–pituitary–ovarian axis. It also occurs later in life as women approach menopause and experience irregular menstrual cycles.

The pathophysiology of AUB is related to a hormone disturbance. With anovulation, estrogen levels rise as usual in the early phase of the menstrual cycle. In the absence of ovulation, a corpus luteum never forms and progesterone is not produced. The endometrium moves into a hyperproliferative state, ultimately outgrowing its estrogen supply. This leads to irregular sloughing of the endometrium and excessive bleeding (King et al., 2015). If the bleeding is heavy enough and frequent enough, anemia can result. AUB is similar to several other types of uterine bleeding disorders and sometimes overlaps these conditions. They include:

- menorrhagia (abnormally long, heavy periods, prolonged bleeding);
- oligomenorrhea (bleeding occurs at intervals of more than 35 days);
- metrorrhagia (bleeding between periods, irregular bleeding);
- menometrorrhagia (excessive uterine bleeding at and between menstrual periods);
- polymenorrhea (too frequent periods).

Etiology

The possible causes of AUB may include:
- Adenomyosis
- Pregnancy
- Hormonal imbalance
- Fibroid tumors (see Chapter 7)
- Endometrial polyps or cancer
- Endometriosis
- Intrauterine systems (IUS)
- Polycystic ovary syndrome
- Morbid obesity
- Adnomyosis
- Steroid therapy
- Hypothyroidism
- Blood dyscrasias/clotting disorder
- Malignancy and hyperplasia
- Uterine polyps

Therapeutic Management

Treatment of AUB depends on the cause of the bleeding, the age of the client, and whether or not she desires future fertility. When known, the underlying cause of the disorder is treated. Otherwise, the goal of treatment is to normalize the bleeding, correct the anemia, prevent or

diagnose early cancer, and restore quality of life (Schuiling & Likis, 2016).

Treatment options for AUB include combined OCs, progestogens, NSAIDS, tranexamic acid (antifibrinolytic), GnRH analogs, Danazol, and Levonorgestrel = releasing intrauterine system (LNG IUS) (Bitzer et al., 2015).

Management of AUB might include medical care with pharmacotherapy or insertion of a hormone-secreting intrauterine system. OCs are used for cycle regulation as well as for contraception. They help prevent the risks associated with prolonged, unopposed estrogen stimulation of the endometrium. NSAIDS and progestin therapy (progesterone-releasing IUS [Mirena] or Depo-Provera) decrease menstrual blood loss significantly (Skidmore-Roth, 2015). The drug categories used in the treatment of AUB are the following:
- *Estrogens*: cause vasospasm of the uterine arteries to decrease bleeding
- *Progestins*: used to stabilize an estrogen-primed endometrium
- *OCs*: regulate the cycle and suppress the endometrium
- *NSAIDs:* inhibit prostaglandins in ovulatory menstrual cycles
- *Progesterone-releasing IUSs*: suppress endometrial growth
- *Androgens*: create a high-androgen/low-estrogen environment that inhibits endometrial growth
- *Antifibrinolytic drugs*: (tranexamic acid) prevent fibrin degradation to reduce bleeding
- *Iron replacement therapy*: replenish iron stores lost during heavy bleeding

If the client does not respond to medical therapy, surgical intervention might include dilation and curettage (D&C), endometrial ablation, uterine artery embolization, or hysterectomy. Surgery should be considered in women for whom medical treatment has failed, cannot be tolerated, or is contraindicated (Kho & Mathur, 2015). Endometrial ablation is an alternative to hysterectomy, but both would be for the woman no longer desiring fertility as both procedures can cause infertility. Techniques used for ablation include laser, electrosurgery excision procedure, freezing, heated fluid infusion, or thermal balloon ablation. Most women will have reduced menstrual flow following endometrial ablation, and up to half will stop having periods. Younger women are less likely than older women to respond to endometrial ablation. Recent scientific evidence supports that up to one quarter of clients treated with endometrial ablation require repeat ablation or subsequent hysterectomy to stop AUB. Hysterectomy should be considered a last resort for AUB (ACOG, 2015b).

Nursing Assessment

A thorough history should be taken to differentiate between AUB and other conditions that might cause vaginal bleeding, such as pregnancy and pregnancy-related conditions (abruptio placentae, ectopic pregnancy, abortion, or placenta previa); systemic conditions such as Cushing disease, blood dyscrasias, liver disease, renal disease, or thyroid disease; and genital tract pathology such as infections, tumors, or trauma (Schuiling & Likis, 2016).

Assess for clinical manifestations of AUB, which commonly include vaginal bleeding between periods, irregular menstrual cycles (usually less than 28 days between cycles), infertility, mood swings, hot flashes, vaginal tenderness, variable menstrual flow ranging from scanty to profuse, obesity, acne, stress, anorexia, thyroid disease, and diabetes. Signs of polycystic ovary syndrome might be present, because it is associated with unopposed estrogen stimulation, elevated androgen levels, and insulin resistance, and is a common cause of anovulation (Tharpe et al., 2016).

Measure orthostatic blood pressure and orthostatic pulse; a drop in pressure or pulse rate may occur with anemia. The health care provider, with the nurse assisting, performs a pelvic examination to identify any structural abnormalities.

Common diagnostic/lab tests that may be ordered to determine the cause of AUB include:
- Complete blood count to detect anemia
- Prothrombin time to detect blood dyscrasias
- Pregnancy test to rule out a spontaneous abortion or ectopic pregnancy
- Thyroid-stimulating hormone level to screen for hypothyroidism
- Transvaginal ultrasound to measure endometrium
- Pelvic ultrasound to view any structural abnormalities
- Endometrial biopsy to check for intrauterine pathology
- D&C for diagnostic evaluation

Nursing Management

Educate the client about normal menstrual cycles and the possible reasons for her abnormal pattern. Inform the woman about treatment options. Do not simply encourage the woman to "live with it." Instruct the client about any prescribed medications and potential side effects. For example, if high-dose estrogens are prescribed, the woman may experience nausea. Teach her to take antiemetics as prescribed and encourage her to eat small, frequent meals to alleviate nausea. Adequate follow-up and evaluation are essential for women who do not respond to medical management. See Nursing Care Plan 4.1: Overview of a Woman With Abnormal Uterine Bleeding.

Concept Mastery Alert

Treatments for Premenstrual Syndrome

Possible treatment options for PMS include reduction of caffeine intake, vitamin and mineral supplements, diuretic therapy, and NSAIDs. Medication therapy that has been found to be helpful for clients with PMS are antidepressants and anxiolytics. Other medications that are used are diuretics and NSAIDs.

Take Note!

Complications such as infertility can result from lack of ovulation, severe anemia can result secondary to prolonged or heavy menses, depression and embarrassment may be secondary to the irregular and heavy bleeding, and endometrial cancer can occur associated with prolonged buildup of the endometrial lining without menstrual bleeding (Hoyt & Falconi, 2015).

Premenstrual Syndrome

PMS describes a constellation of recurrent symptoms that occur during the luteal phase or last half of the menstrual cycle and resolve with the onset of menstruation. A majority of women in their reproductive years' experience a variety of premenstrual symptoms that can alter their behavior and well-being. Women have between 400 and 500 menstrual cycles over their reproductive years, and since premenstrual distress symptoms peak during 4 to 7 days prior to menses, consistently symptomatic women may spend up to 10 years of their lives in a state of compromised physical functioning and/or psychological well-being; thus it would constitute a major health problem for women (Tacani et al., 2015). The American College of Obstetricians and Gynecologists (ACOG) defines PMS as "the cyclic occurrence of symptoms that are sufficiently severe to interfere with some aspects of life, and that appear with consistent and predictable relationship to menses" (ACOG, 2015c). A woman experiencing PMS may have a wide variety of seemingly unrelated symptoms; for that reason, it is difficult to define and more challenging to diagnose. PMS affects millions of women during their reproductive years. Approximately 80% of women will experience cyclic fluctuations in mood, sleep, and sense of well-being, related to their menstrual cycles (King et al., 2015). The exact cause of PMS is not known. It is thought to be related to the interaction between hormonal events and neurotransmitter function, specifically serotonin. Not all women respond to serotonin reuptake inhibitors (SSRIs; Prozac, Paxil, Zoloft), however, which implies that other mechanisms may be involved (Skidmore-Roth, 2015).

As defined by the American Psychiatric Association, PMDD is a more severe variant of PMS affecting 5% to 8% of premenopausal women. Experts compare the difference between PMS and PMDD to the difference between a mild tension headache and a migraine. Risk factors identified that predispose to PMS/PMDD are age between 25 and 35 years, a psychiatric history, a family history of PMDD, unhealthy living habits, and stressful life events (Santamaria & Lago, 2015). PMDD markedly interferes with work, school, social activities, and relationships with others.

Therapeutic Management

Treatment of PMS is often frustrating for both clients and health care providers. Clinical outcomes can be expected

Overview of a Woman with Abnormal Uterine Bleeding

Stacy, a 52-year-old obese woman, comes to her gynecologist with the complaint of heavy erratic bleeding. Her periods were fairly regular until about 4 months ago, and since that time they have been unpredictable, excessive, and prolonged. Stacy reports she is tired all the time, can't sleep, and feels "out of sorts" and anxious. She is fearful she has cancer.

NURSING DIAGNOSIS: Fear related to current signs and symptoms possibly indicating a life-threatening condition

Outcome Identification and Evaluation

The client will acknowledge her fears as evidenced by statements made that fear and anxiety have been lessened after explanation of diagnosis.

Interventions: *Reducing Fear and Anxiety*

- Distinguish between anxiety and fear to determine appropriate interventions.
- Check complete blood count and assess for possible anemia secondary to excessive bleeding to determine if fatigue is contributing to anxiety and fear. Fatigue occurs because the oxygen-carrying capacity of the blood is reduced.
- Reassure client that symptoms can be managed to help address her current concerns.
- Provide client with factual information and explain what to expect to assist client with identifying fears and help her to cope with her condition.

- Provide symptom management to reduce concerns associated with the cause of bleeding.
- Teach client about early manifestations of fear and anxiety to aid in prompt recognition and to minimize escalation of anxiety.
- Assess client's use of coping strategies in the past and reinforce use of effective ones to help control anxiety and fear.
- Instruct client in relaxation methods, such as deep-breathing exercises and imagery, to provide her with additional methods for controlling anxiety and fear.

NURSING DIAGNOSIS: Deficient knowledge related to menopausal transition and its management

Outcome Identification and Evaluation

The client will demonstrate understanding of her symptoms as evidenced by making health-promoting lifestyle choices, verbalizing appropriate health care practices, and adhering to measures and complying with therapy.

Interventions: *Providing Client Education*

- Assess client's understanding of menopausal transition and its treatment to provide a baseline for teaching and developing a plan of care.
- Review instructions about prescribed procedures and recommendations for self-care, frequently obtaining feedback from the client to validate adequate understanding of information.
- Outline link between anovulatory cycles and excessive buildup of uterine lining in menopausal transition women to assist client in understanding the etiology of her bleeding.
- Provide written material with pictures to promote learning and help client visualize what is occurring to her body during menopausal transition.
- Inform client about the availability of community resources and make appropriate referrals as needed to provide additional education and support.
- Document details of teaching and learning to allow for continuity of care and further education, if needed.

to improve as a result of recent consensus on the diagnostic criteria for PMS and PMDD, data from clinical trials, and the availability of evidence-based clinical guidelines.

The management of PMS or PMDD requires a multidimensional approach because these conditions are not likely to have a single cause, and they appear to affect multiple systems within a woman's body; therefore, they are not likely to be amenable to treatment with a single therapy (Naeimi, 2015). To reduce the negative impact of premenstrual disorders on a woman's life education, along with reassurance and anticipatory guidance, is needed for women to feel they have some control over their condition.

Take Note!

Because there are no diagnostic tests that can reliably determine the existence of PMS or PMDD, the woman herself must decide that she needs help during this time of the month. The woman must embrace multiple therapies and become an active participant in her treatment plan to find the best level of symptom relief.

Therapeutic interventions for PMS and PMDD address the symptoms because the exact cause of this condition is still unknown. Treatments may include vitamin supplements, diet changes, exercise, lifestyle changes, and medications (Box 4.2). Medications used in treating PMDD may include antidepressant and anti-anxiety drugs, diuretics, anti-inflammatory medications, analgesics, synthetic androgen agents, OCs, or GnRH agonists to regulate menses. Unlike the approach to the treatment of depression, antidepressants need not be given daily but can be effective when used cyclically, only in the luteal phase, or even limited to the duration of the monthly symptoms.

COMPLEMENTARY AND ALTERNATIVE THERAPIES

No single treatment is universally recognized as effective, and many clients often turn to therapeutic approaches outside of conventional medicine. Many women use dietary supplements and herbal remedies for their menstrual health and treating their bleeding disorders, although there has been little research to demonstrate their efficacy. Alternative treatments for treating PMDD include calcium supplementation, vitex agnus castus (chaste tree berry), hypericum perforatum (St. John's wort), and cognitive/behavioral/relaxation therapies (Wicks & Mahady, 2015). Some other alternative therapies include the use of yoga, magnesium, vitamin B$_6$, evening primrose oil, vitex agnus castus, ginkgo biloba, viburnum, dandelion, stinging nettle, burdock, raspberry leaf, and skullcap (Tremellen & Pearce, 2015). Although research has not validated the efficacy of these alternative therapies, it is important for the nurse to be aware of the alternative products that many women choose to use.

BOX 4.2

TREATMENT OPTIONS FOR PMS AND PMDD

- Lifestyle changes
- Reduce stress
- Exercise three to five times each week
- Eat a balanced diet and increase water intake
- Decrease caffeine intake
- Stop smoking and limit the intake of alcohol
- Attend a PMS/women's support group
- Vitamin and mineral supplements
- Multivitamin daily
- Vitamin E, 400 units daily
- Calcium, 1,200 to 1,600 mg daily
- Magnesium, 200 to 400 mg daily
- Medications
- NSAIDs taken a week prior to menses
- OCs (low dose)
- Antidepressants (SSRIs)
- Anxiolytics (taken during luteal phase)
- Diuretics to remove excess fluid
- Progestins
- GnRH agonists
- Danazol (androgen hormone inhibits estrogen production)

Adapted from Walsh, S., Ismaili, E., Naheed, B., & O'Brien, S. (2015). Diagnosis, pathophysiology and management of premenstrual syndrome. *The Obstetrician & Gynaecologist.* DOI:10.1111/tog.12180; King, T. L., Brucker, M. C., Kriebs, J. M., Fahey, J. O., Gegor, C. L., & Varney, H. (2015) *Varney's midwifery.* Burlington, MA: Jones & Bartlett Learning; and Htay, T. T., & Aung, K. (2015). Premenstrual dysphoric disorder. *eMedicine.* Retrieved from http://emedicine.medscape.com/article/293257-overview

---

Nursing Assessment

Although little consensus exists in the medical literature and among researchers about what constitutes PMS and PMDD, the physical and psychological symptoms are very real. The extent to which the symptoms debilitate or incapacitate a woman is highly variable.

More than 150 symptoms are assigned to PMS, but irritability, food cravings, mood swings, tearfulness, depression, sleep disturbances, headache, back pain, fatigue, bloating, edema of the face, abdominal area, and extremities, tension, and dysphoria (a profound state of unease and anxiety) are the most prominent and consistently described (Tacani et al., 2015). To establish the diagnosis of PMS, elicit a description of cyclic symptoms occurring before the woman's menstrual period. The woman should chart her symptoms daily for two cycles. These data will help demonstrate symptoms clustering around the luteal phase of ovulation, with resolution after bleeding starts. Ask the woman to bring her list of symptoms to the next appointment. Symptoms can be categorized using the following:

- **A**—*anxiety*: difficulty sleeping, tenseness, mood swings, and clumsiness
- **C**—craving: cravings for sweets, salty foods, chocolate

- **D**—depression: feelings of low self-esteem, anger, easily upset
- **H**—hydration: weight gain, abdominal bloating, breast tenderness
- **O**—other: hot flashes or cold sweats, nausea, change in bowel habits, aches or pains, dysmenorrhea, acne breakout (Naeimi, 2015).

The ACOG diagnostic criteria for PMS consist of having at least one of the following affective and somatic symptoms during the 5 days before menses in each of the three previous cycles:
- Affective symptoms: depression, angry outbursts, irritability, anxiety
- Somatic symptoms: breast tenderness, abdominal bloating, edema, headache
- Symptoms relieved from days 4 to 13 of the menstrual cycle (ACOG, 2015c).

In PMDD, the main symptoms are mood disorders such as depression, anxiety, tension, and persistent anger or irritability. Physical symptoms such as headache, joint and muscle pain, lack of energy, bloating, and breast tenderness are also present (Htay, 2015). It is estimated that up to 75% of reproductive-age women experience premenstrual symptoms that meet the ACOG criteria for PMS and up to 5% meet the diagnostic criteria for PMDD (Pearlstein, 2015).

According to the American Psychiatric Association, a woman must have at least five of the typical symptoms to be diagnosed with PMDD (Pearlstein, 2015). These must occur during the week before and a few days after the onset of menstruation and must include one or more of the first four symptoms:
- Affective lability: sadness, tearfulness, irritability
- Anxiety and tension
- Persistent or marked anger or irritability
- Depressed mood, feelings of hopelessness
- Difficulty concentrating
- Sleep difficulties
- Increased or decreased appetite
- Increased or decreased sexual desire
- Chronic fatigue
- Headache
- Constipation or diarrhea
- Breast swelling and tenderness (Htay, 2015).

Nursing Management

Educate the client about the management of PMS or PMDD. Advise her that lifestyle changes often result in significant symptom improvement without pharmacotherapy. Encourage women to eat a balanced diet that includes nutrient-rich foods to avoid hypoglycemia and associated mood swings. Encourage all women to participate in aerobic exercise three times a week to promote a sense of well-being, decrease fatigue, and reduce stress.

Administer calcium (1,200 to 1,600 mg/day), magnesium (400 to 800 mg/day), and vitamin B$_6$ (50 to 100 mg/day) as prescribed. In some studies, these nutrients have been shown to decrease the intensity of PMS symptoms. NSAIDs may be useful for painful physical symptoms and spironolactone (Aldactone) may help with bloating and water retention. Herbs such as vitex agnus castus (chaste tree berry), evening primrose, and SAM-e (a dietary supplement used to enhance mood) may be recommended; although not harmful, not all herbs have enough clinical or research evidence to document their safety or efficacy. Nutritional treatments include a diet low in salt, alcohol, caffeine, and sugar (Schuiling & Likis, 2016).

A recent research study proposes calcium (1,600 mg/day) and vitamin D (400 International Units/day) supplementation in adolescents and women in an effort to prevent PMS, but further research using a larger population needs to be conducted to validate this (Santamaria & Lago, 2015).

Explain to your client the relationship between cyclic estrogen fluctuation and changes in levels of serotonin levels, and how the different management strategies help maintains serotonin levels, thus improving symptoms. It is important to rule out other conditions that might cause erratic or dysphoric behavior. If the initial treatment regimen does not work, explain to the woman that she should return for further testing. Behavioral counseling and stress management might help women regain control during these stressful periods. Reassuring the woman that support and help are available through many community resources/support groups can be instrumental in her acceptance of this monthly disorder. Nurses can be a very calming force for many women experiencing PMS or PMDD. A holistic approach, including lifestyle modifications, pharmacotherapy, herbal therapies, and cognitive behavioral therapy, is most beneficial for symptom reduction, improvement in daily functioning, and quality of life. See Evidence-Based Practice 4.1.

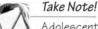 **Take Note!**

Adolescents and women who experience more extensive emotional symptoms with PMS should be evaluated for PMDD, because they may require antidepressant therapy.

Endometriosis

Endometriosis is one of the most common gynecologic diseases, affecting more than 6 million women in the United States, about 10% of the adult women population (Kapoor et al., 2015). In this condition, for unknown reasons bits of functioning endometrial tissue are located outside of their normal site, the uterine cavity. This endometrial tissue is commonly found attached to the ovaries, fallopian tubes, the outer surface of the uterus, the bowels, the area between the vagina and the rectum

EVIDENCE-BASED PRACTICE 4.1 THE EFFECT OF WHEAT GERM EXTRACT ON PREMENSTRUAL SYNDROME SYMPTOMS

STUDY

PMS is one of the most common disorders in women and impairs work and social relationships. Several treatment modalities have been proposed including herbal medicines. Herbal medicines are among the most common treatments because they are economical, safe, noninvasive, and have fewer side effects than do traditional medicines. Wheat germ contains magnesium, zinc, calcium, selenium, potassium, phosphorus, chromium, and vitamins A, E, C, B12, B6, Niacin, folic acid. Considering the properties of wheat germ, this study aimed to determine the effects of wheat germ extract on the symptoms of PMS.

Findings

This triple-blind clinical trial was conducted on 84 women that completed daily records regarding their symptoms for two consecutive months while taking 400 mg capsules of wheat germ extract or placebo three times a day from day 16 until day 5 of the next menstrual cycle. The study found that wheat germ significantly reduced the severity of physical symptoms (64%), psychological symptoms (66%), and general symptoms (65%) when compared to the placebo group within the first month of treatment. No complications were observed in either group.

Nursing Implications

Based on the study results, it seems that using wheat germ extract reduces the severity of general, psychological and physical symptoms of PMS in women that take it during their mid-cycle. Given the positive effects of taking B6 and E, calcium, and magnesium in previous studies to reduce the symptoms of PMS, it makes sense that wheat germ which contains all of the compounds listed would help relieve PMS symptoms. Nurses can suggest using nontraditional modalities to women that request them and cite this study's results to validate them.

Adapted from Ataollahi, M., Akbari, S. A. A., Mojab, F., & Alavi Majd, H. (2015). The effect of wheat germ extract on premenstrual syndrome symptoms. *Iranian Journal of Pharmaceutical Research: IJPR, 14*(1), 159–166.

(rectovaginal septum), and the pelvic side wall (Fig. 4.1). The places where the tissue attaches are called implants, or lesions. Endometrial tissue found outside the uterus responds to hormones released during the menstrual cycle in the same way as endometrial lining within the uterus.

At the beginning of the menstrual cycle, when the lining of the uterus is shed and menstrual bleeding begins, these abnormally located implants swell and bleed also. In short, the woman with endometriosis experiences several "mini-periods" throughout her abdomen, wherever this endometrial tissue exists. In addition to cyclic bleeding outside the uterus, scarring, and adhesion formation throughout the pelvis occurs. Symptoms begin as early as adolescence and typically settle after menopause.

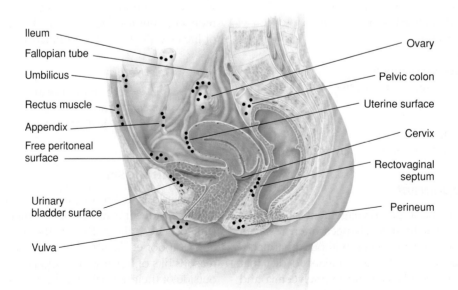

FIGURE 4.1 Common sites of endometriosis formation. (Asset provided by Anatomical Chart Co.)

Think back to Izzy, with her progressive pelvic pain and infertility concerns. After a pelvic examination, her health care provider suspects she has endometriosis.

Etiology and Risk Factors

It is not currently known why endometrial tissue becomes transplanted and grows in other parts of the body. Several theories exist, but to date none has been scientifically proven. However, several factors that increase a woman's risk of developing endometriosis have been identified:

- The aging process
- Family history of endometriosis in a first-degree relative
- Short menstrual cycle (less than 28 days)
- Long menstrual flow (more than 1 week)
- High dietary fat consumption
- Young age of menarche (younger than 12)
- Few (one or two) or no pregnancies (Johnson, Reid, & Hunter, 2015).

Therapeutic Management

Therapeutic management of the client with endometriosis needs to take into consideration the following factors:

severity of symptoms, desire for fertility, degree of disease, and the client's therapy goals. The aim of therapy is to suppress levels of estrogen and progesterone, which cause the endometrium to grow. Current treatment of endometriosis is mainly based on surgery and ovarian suppressive agents (OCs, progestins, GnRh agonist and androgenic agents). Approximately only half of women with endometriosis experience pain relief from existing medial or surgical treatments (NICHD, 2015). Treatment can include surgical removal of ectopic endometrial tissue or medications such as NSAIDs, OCs, Depo-Provera, synthetic testosterone, GnRH agonists, etc. Also, alternative therapies may be used, including acupuncture and supplements of vitamins, minerals, and fish oil (Elnashar, 2015). These interventions may control symptoms initially, but many have significant adverse effects and limits on duration of therapy (Table 4.2).

Nursing Assessment

Nurses encounter women with endometriosis in a variety of settings: community health settings, schools, clinics, day surgical centers, and hospitals. Health care professionals must not trivialize or dismiss the concerns of these women, because early recognition is essential to preserve fertility. The diversity of presenting symptoms and a low index of suspicion contribute to women with

TABLE 4.2	TREATMENT OPTIONS FOR ENDOMETRIOSIS
Therapy Options	**Comment**
Surgical intervention	
Conservative surgery	Removal of implants/lesions using laser, cautery, or small surgical instruments. This intervention will reduce pain and allows pregnancy to occur in the future.
Definitive surgery	Abdominal hysterectomy, with or without bilateral salpingo-oophorectomy. Will eliminate pain but will leave a woman unable to become pregnant in the future.
Medication therapy	
NSAIDs	First-line treatment to reduce pain; taken early when premenstrual symptoms are first felt
Oral contraceptives	Suppresses cyclic hormonal response of the endometrial tissue
Progestogens	Used to cast off the endometrial cells and thus destroy them
Antiestrogens	Suppresses a woman's production of estrogen, thus stopping the menstrual cycle and preventing further growth of endometrium
Gonadotropin-releasing hormone analogues (GnRH-a)	Suppresses endometriosis by creating a temporary pseudomenopause

Adapted from Kapoor, D. W., Alderman, E., Hiraoka, M. K., & Davila, G. W. (2015). Endometriosis. eMedicine. Retrieved from http://emedicine.medscape.com/article/271899-overview; Elnashar, A. (2015). Emerging treatment of endometriosis. *Middle East Fertility Society Journal.* doi:10.1016/j.mefs.2014.12.002. Retrieved from http://www.sciencedirect.com/science/article/pii/S1110569014200562; King, T. L., Brucker, M. C., Kriebs, J. M., Fahey, J. O., Gegor, C. L., & Varney, H. (2015). *Varney's midwifery* (5th ed.). Burlington, MA: Jones and Bartlett Learning.

endometriosis falling through the cracks and not being diagnosed promptly.

HEALTH HISTORY

Obtain a health history and elicit a description of signs and symptoms to determine risk factors. Endometriosis is often asymptomatic, but it can be a severe and debilitating condition. It typically is chronic and progressive. Ask specifically about menarche, history of menstrual problems, details of pregnancies, and difficulties with conception. Assess the client for clinical manifestations, which include:

- Infertility
- Back pain
- Pain before and during menstrual periods
- Pain during or after sexual intercourse
- Painful urination
- Depression
- Fatigue
- Painful bowel movements
- Chronic pelvic pain
- Hypermenorrhea (heavy menses)
- Pelvic adhesions
- Irregular and more frequent menses
- Premenstrual vaginal spotting (Schuiling & Likis, 2016)

The two most common symptoms are infertility and pelvic pain. Endometriosis occurs in 38% of infertile women and in 71% to 87% of women with chronic pelvic pain (Kapoor et al., 2015). About 30% to 40% of women with this condition are infertile, making it one of the top three causes of female infertility (Brown & Farquhar, 2015).

What are the two most common symptoms experienced by women with endometriosis? Is Izzy's profile typical? As a nurse, what would be your role in Izzy's continued workup?

PHYSICAL EXAMINATION AND LABORATORY AND DIAGNOSTIC TESTS

The pelvic examination typically correlates with the extent of the endometriosis. The usual finding is nonspecific pelvic tenderness. The hallmark finding is the presence of tender nodular masses on the uterosacral ligaments, the posterior uterus, or the posterior cul-de-sac. The only definitive diagnosis is the one made during surgery (Signorile & Baldi, 2015).

After a thorough history and a pelvic examination, the health care provider may suspect endometriosis, but the only certain method of diagnosing it is by seeing it. Pelvic or transvaginal ultrasound is used to assess pelvic organ structures. However, a laparoscopy is needed to diagnose endometriosis. Laparoscopy is the direct visualization of the internal organs with a lighted instrument

BOX 4.3

ORGANIZATIONS AND WEB RESOURCES TO ASSIST THE CLIENT WITH ENDOMETRIOSIS

- American College of Obstetricians and Gynecologists (ACOG)
  http://www.acog.org
  e-mail: resources@acog.org
- American Society of Reproductive Medicine
  http://www.asrm.org
  e-mail: asrm@asrm.org
- Center for Endometriosis Care
  http://www. centerforendo.com
- Endometriosis Association
  http://www.endometriosisassn.org
  http://www.KillerCramps.org
- Endometriosis Association support groups
  e-mail: support@endometriosisassn.org
- National Institute of Child Health and Human Development Information Resource Center
  http://www.nichd.nih.gov
  e-mail: NICHDClearinghouse@ mail.nih.gov
- National Women's Health Information Center (U.S. Department of Health and Human Services)
  http://www.4women.gov

inserted through an abdominal incision. A tissue biopsy of the suspected implant taken at the same time and examined microscopically confirms the diagnosis.

Nurses can play a role by offering a thorough explanation of the condition and explaining why tests are needed to diagnose endometriosis. The nurse can set up appointments for imaging studies and laparoscopy.

Nursing Management

In addition to the interventions outlined above, the nurse should encourage the client to adopt healthy lifestyle habits with respect to diet, exercise, sleep, and stress management. Referrals to support groups and Internet resources can help the woman to understand this condition and to cope with chronic pain. A number of organizations provide information about the diagnosis and treatment of endometriosis and offer support to women and their families. Nurses are uniquely situated to improve client outcomes by assisting women to make informed treatment decisions. A prompt diagnosis ensures appropriate care (Box 4.3).

INFERTILITY

Infertility is defined as the inability to conceive a child after 1 year of regular sexual intercourse unprotected by contraception (RESOLVE, 2015). Secondary infertility is the inability to conceive after a previous pregnancy. Many people take the ability to conceive and produce a child for granted, but infertility affects more than 6 million Americans, or up to 20% of the reproductive-age population and as many 186 million people worldwide, according to the American Society for Reproductive Medicine (ASRM, 2015). Infertility is a widespread problem that has an emotional, social, and economic impact on couples. Although male infertility contributes to more than half of all causes, infertility remains a woman's social burden. It affects relationships, leads to tension and anger between partners, and can result in severe sexual dysfunction and breakdown of the relationship. Nurses must recognize infertility and understand its causes and treatment options so that they can help couples understand the possibilities as well as the limitations of current therapies. Nurses have a central role in supporting couples through these stressful treatments. Couples will frequently confide in their nurse and can gain great benefit from a sympathetic and sensible discussion. Recent studies have found that women wish to be treated with respect and dignity and given appropriate information and support. Infertility was once considered a disorder of inconvenience, but it is now classified as a disease in the United States Regulatory Americans with Disabilities Act (Turchi, 2015). Women want their distress recognized and they want to feel cared for and to have confidence in health care providers in situations where outcomes are uncertain. The caring aspect of professional nursing is an essential component of meeting the special needs of these couples (Whitman, 2015). Prevention of infertility through education should also be incorporated into any client–nurse interaction.

After completing several diagnostic tests, Izzy is diagnosed with endometriosis. She asks you about her chances of becoming pregnant and becoming pain-free. What treatment options would you explain to Izzy? What information can you give about her future childbearing ability?

Cultural Considerations

Infertility is not only a physiologic problem, but is one that can initiate a life crisis that is experienced with psychological, familial, social, and cultural consequences. Cross-culturally, the expectation for couples to reproduce is an accepted norm and the inability to conceive may be considered a violation of this cultural norm. In this context, infertility represents a crisis for the couple. The manner in which different cultures, ethnic groups, and religious groups perceive and manage infertility may be very different. For example, many African Americans believe that assisted reproductive techniques are unnatural and that they remove the spiritual or divine nature of creation from conception. For this reason, they may seek spiritual rather than medical assistance when trying to conceive. The Hispanic culture believes that children

validate the marriage, so families are typically large. Like the African-American culture, Hispanics are very spiritual and may consider infertility a test of faith and seek spiritual counseling. Disappointing one's spouse is of greater concern to African-American women, whereas avoiding the stigmatization of infertility is of greatest concern to Asian-American women (Inhorn & Patrizio, 2015).

Religion often influences cultural factors and for this reason may also be considered when pursuing treatment for infertility. In the Orthodox Jewish religion, procreation is considered to be a "mitzvah," a commandment to have children. However, even Orthodox Jews accept the use of contraceptives to prevent conception when it is not desired. Conservative and Reform Jews put no restrictions on contraception. Roman Catholics have a very restrictive view on the use of assisted reproductive technologies since in their view procreation cannot be separated from the relationship between parents. Thus, God wants human life to begin through the "conjugal act" and not artificially. Most religious teachings speak to the significance of procreation, thus infertility can impact the self and relational identities of the couple wishing to

Consider This

We had been married for 3 years and wanted to start a family, but much to our dismay nothing happened after a year of trying. I had some irregular periods and was finally diagnosed with endometriosis and put on Clomid for three cycles. After that time without achieving a pregnancy, I went to a fertility expert. The doctor lasered the misplaced endometriosis tissue, sent carbon dioxide through my tubes to make sure they were patent, and put me back on Clomid, but still with no luck. Finally, 2 years later, we were put on an in vitro fertilization (IVF) waiting list and prayed we would have the money for the procedure when we were chosen. By then I felt a failure as a woman. We then decided that it was more important for us to be parents than it was for me to be pregnant, so we considered adoption. We tried for another year without any results.

We went to the adoption agency to fill out the paperwork for the process to begin. Our blood was taken and we waited for an hour, wondering the whole time why it was taking so long for the results. The nurse finally appeared and handed a piece of paper to me with the word "positive" written on it. I started to cry tears of joy, for a pregnancy had started and our long journey of infertility was finally ending.

Thoughts: *For many women the dream of having a child is not easily realized. Infertility can affect self-esteem, disrupt relationships, and result in depression. This couple experienced many years of frustration in trying to have a family. What help can be offered to couples during this time? What can be said to comfort the woman who feels she is a failure?*

become parents. Therefore, the risk is present for both a crisis of identity and of faith (Dombo & Flood, 2015). Nurses must be cognizant of the client's cultural and religious background and how it may dictate which, if any, reproductive treatment options are chosen. Nurses need to include this awareness in their counseling of infertile couples.

Etiology and Risk Factors

Reproduction requires the interaction of the female and the male reproductive tracts, which involves (1) the release of a normal preovulatory oocyte, (2) the production of adequate spermatozoa, (3) the normal transport of the gametes to the ampullary portion of the fallopian tube (where fertilization takes place), and (4) the subsequent transport of the cleaving embryo into the endometrial cavity for implantation and development (Puscheck & Woodward, 2015).

Multiple known and unknown factors affect fertility. Female-factor infertility is detected in about 40% of cases, and male-factor infertility in about 40% of cases. The remaining 20% fall into a category of combined (both male and female factors) or unexplained infertility. In women, ovarian dysfunction (40%) and tubal/pelvic pathology (40%) are the primary contributing factors to infertility (ASRM, 2015).

Risk factors for infertility in women include:
- Overweight or underweight (can disrupt hormone function)
- Hormonal imbalances leading to irregular ovulation
- Uterine fibroids
- Tubal blockages
- Cervical stenosis
- Reduced oocyte quality
- Chromosomal abnormalities
- Congenital anomalies of the uterus
- Immune system disorders
- Chronic illnesses such as diabetes, thyroid disease, asthma
- STIs
- Ectopic pregnancy
- Age older than 27
- Endometriosis
- Turner syndrome
- Eating disorders
- History of PID
- Smoking and alcohol consumption
- Multiple miscarriages
- Menstrual abnormalities
- Exposure to chemotherapeutic agents
- Psychological stress (Senie, 2014)

Risk factors for infertility in men include:
- Exposure to toxic substances (lead, mercury, x-rays, chemotherapy)
- Cigarette or marijuana smoke
- Heavy alcohol consumption
- Use of prescription drugs for ulcers or psoriasis
- Exposure of the genitals to high temperatures (hot tubs or saunas)
- Hernia repair
- Obesity is associated with decreased sperm quality
- Cushing syndrome
- Frequent long-distance cycling or running
- STIs
- Undescended testicles (cryptorchidism)
- Mumps after puberty (Puscheck & Woodward, 2015)

Therapeutic Management

As noted earlier, the main causes of infertility are female factor (anovulation, tubal damage, endometriosis, and ovarian failure), male factor (low or absent numbers of motile sperm in the ejaculate, and erectile dysfunction), or unexplained infertility (Jin, 2015). The test results are presented to the couple and different treatment options are suggested. The majority of infertility cases are treated with drugs or surgery. Treatment options include lifestyle changes, such as weight loss, and smoking cessation; taking clomiphene to promote ovulation; hormone injections to promote ovulation; intrauterine insemination; and *in vitro* fertilization. Various ovulation-enhancement drugs and timed intercourse might be used for the woman with ovulation problems. The woman should understand a drug's benefits and side effects before consenting to take it. Depending on the type of drug used and the dosage, some women may experience multiple births. If the woman's reproductive organs are damaged, surgery can be done to repair them. Still other couples might opt for the hi-tech approaches of artificial insemination (Fig. 4.2), IVF (Fig. 4.3), and egg donation, or they may contract for a gestational carrier or surrogate (Jin, 2015). Table 4.3 lists selected treatment options for infertility.

Nursing Assessment

Infertile couples are under tremendous pressure and often keep the problem a secret, considering it to be very personal. Couples are often beset by feelings of inadequacy and guilt, and many are subject to pressures from both family and friends. As the problem becomes more chronic, they may begin to blame one another, with consequent marital discord. Seeking help is often a very difficult step for them, and it may take a lot of courage to discuss something about which they feel deeply embarrassed or upset. The nurse working in this specialty setting must be aware of the conflict and problems couples present with and must be very sensitive to their needs.

A full medical history should be taken from both partners, along with a physical examination. The data

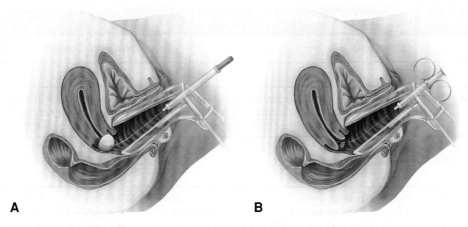

FIGURE 4.2 Artificial insemination. Sperm are deposited next to the cervix (**A**) or injected directly into the uterine cavity (**B**).

needed for the infertility evaluation are very sensitive and of a personal nature, so the nurse must use very professional interviewing skills.

Infertility has numerous causes and contributing factors, so it is important to use the process of elimination, determining what problems do not exist to better comprehend the problems that do exist. At the first visit, a plan of investigation is outlined and a complete health history is taken. This first visit forces many couples to confront the reality that their desired pregnancy may not occur naturally. Alleviate some of the anxiety associated with diagnostic testing by explaining the timing and reasons for each test.

Assessing Male Factors

The initial screening evaluation for the male partner should include a reproductive history and a semen analysis. From the male perspective, three things must happen for conception to take place: the number of sperm must be adequate; those sperm must be healthy and mature; and the sperm must be able to penetrate and fertilize the egg. Normal males have more than 20 million sperm per milliliter with greater than 50% motility (World Health Organization [WHO], 2015). Semen analysis is the most important indicator of male fertility. The man should abstain from sexual activity for 24 to 48 hours before giving the sample. For a semen examination, the man is asked to produce a specimen by ejaculating into a specimen container and delivering it to the laboratory for analysis within 1 to 2 hours. When the specimen is brought to the laboratory, it is analyzed for volume, viscosity, number of sperm, sperm viability, motility, and sperm shape. If semen parameters are normal, no further male evaluation is necessary (Puscheck & Woodward, 2015).

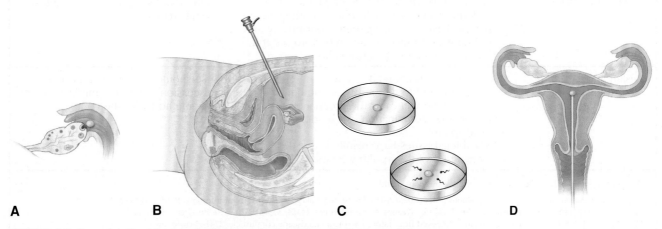

FIGURE 4.3 Steps involved in vitro fertilization. **A.** Ovulation. **B.** Capture of the ova (done here intra-abdominally). **C.** Fertilization of ova and growth in culture medium. **D.** Insertion of fertilized ova into uterus.

TABLE 4.3	SELECTED TREATMENT OPTIONS FOR INFERTILITY	
Procedure	Comments	Nursing Considerations
Fertility drugs		
Clomiphene citrate (Clomid)	A nonsteroidal synthetic antiestrogen used to induce ovulation. Clomid is typically discontinued after three cycles of use.	Nurse can advise the couple to have intercourse every other day for 1 wk starting after day 5 of medication.
Human menopausal gonadotropin (HMG); Pergonal	Induces ovulation by direct stimulation of ovarian follicle	Same as above
Artificial insemination	The insertion of a prepared semen sample into the cervical os or intrauterine cavityEnables sperm to be deposited closer to improve chances of conception.Husband or donor sperm can be used.	Nurse needs to advise couple that the procedure might need to be repeated if not successful the first time.
*Assisted reproductive technologies**		
In vitro fertilization (IVF)	Oocytes are fertilized in the lab and transferred to the uterus. Usually indicated for tubal obstruction, endometriosis, pelvic adhesions, and low sperm counts	Nurse advises woman to take medication to stimulate ovulation so the mature ovum can be retrieved by needle aspiration.
Gamete intrafallopian transfer (GIFT)	Oocytes and sperm are combined and immediately placed in the fallopian tube so fertilization can occur naturally. Requires laparoscopy and general anesthesia, which increases risk	Nurse needs to inform couple of risks and have consent signed.
Intracytoplasmic sperm injection (ICSI)	One sperm is injected into the cytoplasm of the oocyte to fertilize it. Indicated for male factor infertility.	Nurse needs to inform the male that sperm will be aspirated by a needle through the skin into the epididymis.
Donor oocytes or sperm	Eggs or sperm are retrieved from a donor and the eggs are inseminated; resulting embryos are transferred via IVF. Recommended for women older than 40 yrs and those with poor-quality eggs.	Nurse needs to support couple in their ethical/religious discussions prior to deciding.
Preimplantation genetic diagnosis (PGD)	Used to identify genetic defects in embryos created through IVF before pregnancy. This is done specifically when one or both genetic parents have a known genetic abnormality and testing is performed on an embryo to see if it also carries a genetic abnormality.	Nurse should inform couple about this option and support them until test results return.
Gestational carrier (surrogacy)	Laboratory fertilization takes place and embryos are transferred to the uterus of another woman, who will carry the pregnancy. Or intrauterine insemination can be done with the male sperm. Medical-legal issues have resulted over the "true ownership" of the resulting infant.	Nurse should encourage an open discussion regarding implications of this method with the couple.

*When other options have been exhausted, these are considered.

Adapted from American Society for Reproductive Medicine. (2015). Frequently asked questions about infertility. Retrieved from http://www.asrm.org/detail.aspx?id=2322; Jin, J. (2015). Treatments for infertility. *JAMA*, 313(3), 320--320; Puscheck, E. E., & Woodward, T. L. (2015). Infertility. eMedicine. Retrieved from http://emedicine.medscape.com/article/274143-overview

A recent study shows that social strain and stress are highest among couples without a clear etiology for their infertility. These findings highlight the clinically significant negative sexual, personal, and social strains of a perceived infertility diagnosis for men (Cavallini, 2015). Nurses need to be very cognizant of this impact on males and address it.

The physical examination routinely includes:
- assessment for appropriate male sexual characteristics, such as body hair distribution, development of the Adam's apple, and muscle development;
- examination of the penis, scrotum, testicles, epididymis, and vas deferens for abnormalities (e.g., nodules, irregularities, varicocele);
- assessment for normal development of external genitalia (small testicles);
- performance of a digital internal examination of the prostate to check for tenderness or swelling (Dohle, 2015).

Assessing Female Factors

The initial assessment of the woman should include a thorough history of factors associated with ovulation and the pelvic organs. Diagnostic tests to determine female infertility may include:
- Assessment of ovarian function
- Ovulation predictor kits used midcycle
- Urinary LH level
- Clomiphene citrate challenge test
- Assessment of pelvic organs
- Papanicolaou (Pap) smear to rule out cervical cancer or inflammation
- Cervical culture to rule out any STIs
- Ultrasound to assess pelvic structures
- Hysterosalpingography to visualize structural defects
- Laparoscopy to visualize pelvic structures and diagnose endometriosis (Dadhich, Ramasamy, & Lipshultz, 2015)

Laboratory and Diagnostic Testing

The diagnostic procedures that should be done during an infertility workup should be guided by the couple's history. They generally proceed from less to more invasive tests.

HOME OVULATION PREDICTOR KITS
Home ovulation predictor kits contain monoclonal antibodies specific for LH and use the ELISA test to determine the amount of LH present in the urine. A significant color change from baseline indicates the LH surge and presumably the most fertile day of the month for the woman.

CLOMIPHENE CITRATE CHALLENGE TEST
The clomiphene citrate challenge test is used to assess a woman's ovarian reserve (ability of her eggs to become fertilized). FSH levels are drawn on cycle day 3 and on cycle day 10 after the woman has taken 100 mg clomiphene citrate on cycle days 5 through 9. If the FSH level is greater than 15, the result is considered abnormal and the likelihood of conception with her own eggs is very low (Schuiling & Likis, 2016).

HYSTEROSALPINGOGRAPHY
Hystersalpingography is the gold standard in assessing patency (being open and unobstructed) of the fallopian tubes. Fallopian tube obstruction is among the most common causes of female factor infertility. Ultrasonography and magnetic resonance imaging (MRI) are used in this assessment. In hysterosalpingography, 3 to 10 mL of an opaque contrast medium is slowly injected through a catheter into the endocervical canal so that the uterus and tubes can be visualized during fluoroscopy and radiography. If the fallopian tubes are patent, the dye will ascend upward to distend the uterus and the tubes and will spill out into the peritoneal cavity (Fig. 4.4) (Hemingway & Trew, 2015).

LAPAROSCOPY
A laparoscopy is usually performed early in the menstrual cycle. It is not part of the routine infertility evaluation. It is used when abnormalities are found on the ultrasound or the hysterosalpingogram. Because of the added risks of surgery, the need for anesthesia, and operative costs, it is only used when clearly indicated. During the procedure, an endoscope is inserted through a small incision in the anterior abdominal wall. Visualization of the peritoneal cavity in an infertile woman may reveal endometriosis, pelvic adhesions, tubal occlusion, fibroids, or polycystic ovaries (Kodaman, 2015).

Nursing Management

Nurses play an important role in the care of infertile couples. They are pivotal educators about preventive health care. A number of potentially modifiable risk factors are

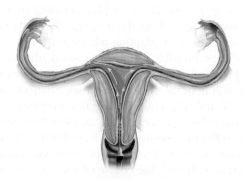

FIGURE 4.4 Insertion of a dye for a hysterosalpingogram. The contrast dye outlines the uterus and fallopian tubes on an x-ray to demonstrate patency.

associated with the development of impaired fertility in women, and women need to be aware of these risks to institute change. The nurse is most effective when he or she offers care and treatment in a professional manner and regards the couple as valued and respected individuals. The nurse must be respectful of and mindful that many women may seek spiritual help for their infertility issues in addition to traditional medical modalities (King et al., 2015). The nurse's focus must encompass the whole person, not just the results of the various infertility studies. Throughout the entire process, the nurse's role is to provide information, anticipatory guidance, stress management, and counseling. The couple's emotional distress is usually very high, and the nurse must be able to recognize that anxiety and provide emotional support. The nurse may need to refer couples to a reproductive endocrinologist or surgeon, depending on the problem identified.

There is no absolute way to prevent infertility per se because so many factors are involved in conception. Nurses can be instrumental in educating men and women about the factors that contribute to infertility. The nurse can also outline the risks and benefits of treatments so that the couple can make an informed decision. As couples struggle with infertility, they frequently turn to nurses for empathy, counseling, and support. By understanding the struggles and lived experiences of women and couples experiencing infertility, the nurse can tailor his/her approach to better meet their needs so that the pregnancy and birth experience of these women are healing, transformative, and positive.

With advances in genetics and reproductive medicine also come a myriad of ethical, social, and cultural issues that will affect the couple's decisions. With this in mind, provide an opportunity for the couple to make informed decisions in a nondirective, nonjudgmental environment. It is important to encourage couples to remain optimistic throughout investigation and treatment. Through the use of advocacy and anticipatory guidance, assist and support couples through the diagnosis and treatment of infertility (Ying & Loke, 2015).

Finances and insurance coverage often dictate the choice of treatment. Help couples decipher their insurance coverage and help them weigh the costs of various procedures by explaining what each will provide in terms of their infertility problems. Assisting them to make a priority list of diagnostic tests and potential treatment options will help the couple plan their financial strategy.

Many infertile couples are not prepared for the emotional roller coaster of grief and loss that accompanies infertility treatments. Financial concerns and coping as a couple are two major areas of stress when treatment is undertaken. During the course of what may be months or even years of infertility care, it is essential to develop a holistic approach to nursing care. Stress management and anxiety reduction need to be addressed, and referral

---

to a peer support group such as RESOLVE might be in order (Box 4.4).

CONTRACEPTION

Contraception is any method that prevents conception or childbirth, including OCs, sterilization of the female, and the male condom, which are the most popular methods in the United States (Alan Guttmacher Institute, 2015a). Additional types of contraceptives are discussed later in this chapter.

In the United States, there are approximately 68 million women in their childbearing years (between the ages of 15 and 44), and throughout those years a variety of contraceptive methods may be used. Studies have shown that 98% of sexually active women in the United States admit to having used at least one form of contraception; however, despite the widespread use of contraceptives, almost half of all pregnancies in the United States are unintended, accounting for a higher unintended pregnancy rate than any other Western county (Centers for Disease Control and Prevention [CDC], 2015b). As outlined in the United Nations Population Fund (UNFPA) *State of the World Population 2014 Report*, over 7 billion people inhabit the earth now and over 80 million people are added to the world each year, more than half of whom are unintended.

In addition to unwanted pregnancies, which can result in abortion, some contraceptives also help prevent transmission of STIs and human immune deficiency virus (HIV). The UNFPA report also shows that about 50,000 people in the United States become infected with HIV every year. Much of this suffering could be prevented by access to and consistent use of safe, efficient, appropriate, modern contraception for everyone who wants it, as well as proper education regarding benefits and instructions for use (UNFPA, 2015). In addition, climate change (extreme temperature changes and rising ocean levels) will interact with population growth in ways that put additional stress on already weak health systems and will exacerbate vulnerability to the adverse health effects of climate change. The damage done to the environment by modern society is perhaps one of the most inequitable health risks of our time (UNFPA 2015).

Today, the voluntary control of fertility is of vital importance to modern society. From a global perspective, countries currently face a crisis of rapid population growth that has begun to threaten human survival. At the present rate, the population of the world will double in 40 years; in several of the more socioeconomically disadvantaged countries, populations will double in less than 20 years (UNFPA 2015).

Types of Contraceptive Methods

Contraceptive methods can be divided into four types: behavioral methods, barrier methods, hormonal methods, and permanent methods. Women must decide which method is appropriate for them to meet their changing contraceptive needs throughout their life cycles. Nurses can educate and assist women during this selection process. This part of the chapter will outline the most common birth control methods available.

In an era when many women wish to delay pregnancy and avoid STIs, choices are difficult. Numerous methods of contraception are available today, and many more will be offered in the near future. The ideal contraceptive method for many women would have the following characteristics: ease of use, safety, effectiveness, minimal side effects, "naturalness," nonhormonal method, and immediate reversibility (Samra-Latif & Wood, 2015). Currently, no one contraceptive method offers everything. Box 4.5 outlines the contraceptive methods available today. Table 4.4 provides a detailed summary of each type, including information on failure rates, advantages, disadvantages, STI protection, and danger signs.

(text continues on page 110)

HEALTHY PEOPLE 2020 • 4.1

Objective	Nursing Significance
FP-1 Increase the proportion of pregnancies that are intended.	Would reduce number of unplanned pregnancies and girls not finishing their education. This would in turn reduce the number of single parents on state financial assistance.
FP-2 Reduce the proportion of females experiencing pregnancy despite use of a reversible contraceptive method.	Awareness of contraceptive methods and accessibility brings about better compliance and prevention of unintended pregnancies.
FP-3 Increase the proportion of publicly funded family planning clinics that offer the full range of FDA-approved methods of contraception, including emergency contraception, on site.	Would increase accessibility to contraception and prevent unintended pregnancies.
FP-7 Increase the proportion of sexually active persons who received reproductive health services.	Accessibility of reproductive resources can offer pregnancy prevention and preventive education.

Healthy People objectives based on data from http://www.healthypeople.gov

BOX 4.5

OUTLINE OF CONTRACEPTIVE METHODS

Reversible Methods
- Behavioral
  - Abstinence
  - Fertility awareness–based methods (FAMs)
  - Withdrawal (coitus interruptus)
  - Lactational amenorrhea method (LAM)
- Barrier
  - Condom (male and female)
  - Diaphragm
  - Cervical cap
  - Sponge
- Hormonal
  - OC
  - Injectable contraceptive
  - Transdermal patch
  - Vaginal ring
  - Implantable contraceptive
  - Intrauterine contraceptive
  - Emergency contraceptive

Permanent Methods
- Tubal ligation or Essure for women
- Vasectomy for men

TABLE 4.4 SUMMARY OF CONTRACEPTIVE METHODS

Type	Description	Failure Rate	Pros	Cons	STI Protection	Danger Signs	Comments
Abstinence	Refrain from sexual activity	None	Costs nothing	Difficult to maintain	100%	None	Must be joint couple decision.
Fertility awareness–based methods	Refrain from sex during fertile period	25%	No side effects; acceptable to most religious groups	High failure rate with incorrect use	None	None	Requires high level of couple commitment.
Withdrawal (coitus interruptus)	Man withdraws before ejaculation	27%	Involves no devices and is always available	Requires considerable self-control by the man	None	None	Places woman in trusting and dependent role.
Lactational amenorrhea method (LAM)	Uses lactational infertility for protection from pregnancy	1%–2% chance of pregnancy in first 6 mo	No cost; not coitus linked	Temporary method; effective for only 6 mo after giving birth	None	None	Mother must breast-feed infant on demand without supplementation for 6 mo.
Male condom	Thin sheath placed over an erect penis, blocking sperm	15%	Widely available; low cost; physiologically safe	Decreased sensation for man; interferes with sexual spontaneity; breakage risk	Provides protection against STIs	Latex allergy	Couple must be instructed on proper use of condom.
Female condom	Polyurethane sheath inserted vaginally to block sperm	21%	Use controlled by woman; eliminates postcoital drainage of semen	Expensive for frequent use; cumbersome; noisy during sex act; for single use only	Provides protection against STIs	Allergy to polyurethane	Couple must be instructed on proper use of condom.
Diaphragm with spermicide	Shallow latex cup with spring mechanism in its rim to hold it in place in the vagina	16%	Does not use hormone; considered medically safe; provides some protection against cervical cancer	Requires accurate fitting by health care professional; increase in UTIs	None	Allergy to latex, rubber, polyurethane, or spermicide Report symptoms of toxic shock syndrome May become dislodged in female superior position	Woman must be taught to insert and remove diaphragm correctly.

Method	Description	Effectiveness	Advantages	STI Protection	Disadvantages	Side Effects	Nursing Considerations
Cervical cap with spermicide	Soft cup-shaped latex device that fits over base of cervix	24%	No use of hormones; provides continuous protection while in place	None	Requires accurate fitting by health care professional; odor may occur if left in too long	Irritation, allergic reaction; abnormal Pap test; risk of toxic shock syndrome	Instructions on insertion and removal must be understood by client.
Sponge with spermicide	Disk-shaped polyurethane device containing a spermicide that is activated by wetting it with water	25%	Offers immediate and continuous protection for 24 hr; OTC	None	Can fall out of vagina with voiding; is not form fitting in the vagina	Irritation, allergic reactions; toxic shock syndrome can occur if sponge left in too long	Caution woman not to leave sponge in beyond 24 hr.
Oral contraceptives (combination)	A pill that suppresses ovulation by combined action of estrogen and progestin	8%	Easy to use; high rate of effectiveness; protection against ovarian and endometrial cancer	None	User must remember to take pill daily; possible undesirable side effects; high cost for some women; prescription needed	Dizziness, nausea, mood changes, high blood pressure, blood clots, heart attacks, strokes	Each woman must be assessed thoroughly to make sure she is not a smoker and does not have a history of thromboembolic disease.
Oral contraceptives (progestin-only minipills)	A pill containing only progestin that thickens cervical mucus to prevent sperm from penetrating	8%	No estrogen-related side effects; may be used by lactating women; may be used by women with history of thrombophlebitis	None	Must be taken with meticulous accuracy; may cause irregular bleeding; less effective than combination pills	Irregular bleeding, weight gain, increased incidence of ectopic pregnancy	Women should be screened for history of functional ovarian cysts, previous ectopic pregnancy, and hyperlipidemia prior to giving prescription.
Patch (Ortho Evra)	Transdermal patch that releases estrogen and progestin into circulation	8%	Easy system to remember; very effective	None	May cause skin irritation where it is placed; may fall off and not be noticed and thus provide no protection	Less effective in women weighing more than 200 pounds	Instruct woman to apply patch every week for 3 wks and then not to wear one during week 4.

(continued)

TABLE 4.4 | E SUMMARY OF CONTRACEPTIVE METHODS (continued)

Type	Description	Failure Rate	Pros	Cons	STI Protection	Danger Signs	Comments
Ring (NuvaRing)	Vaginal contraceptive ring about 2 inches in diameter that is inserted into the vagina; releases estrogen and progestin	8%	Easy system to remember; very effective	May cause a vaginal discharge; can be expelled without noticing and not offer protection	None	Similar to oral contraceptives	Instruct woman to use a backup method if ring is expelled and remains out for more than 3 hr.
Depo-Provera injection	An injectable progestin that inhibits ovulation	3%	Long duration of action (3 mo); highly effective; estrogen-free; may be used by smokers; can be used by lactating women	Menstrual irregularities; return visit needed every 12 wks; weight gain, headaches, depression; return to fertility delayed up to 12 mo	None	If depression is a problem, this method may increase the depression.	Inform woman that fertility is delayed after stopping the injections.
Implant (Nexplanon)	A time-release implant (one rod) of levonorgestrel for 3 yrs	0.05%	Long duration of action; low dose of hormones; reversible; estrogen-free	Irregular bleeding; weight gain; breast tenderness; headaches; difficulty in removal	None	If bleeding is heavy, anemia may occur.	Before insertion, assess woman to make sure she is aware that this method will produce about 3 years of infertility.
Intrauterine contraceptives (IUCs)	A T-shaped device inserted into the uterus that releases copper or progesterone or levonorgestrel	1%	It is immediately and highly effective; allows for sexual spontaneity; can be used during lactation; return to fertility not impaired; requires no motivation by the user after insertion	Insertion requires a skilled professional; menstrual irregularities; prolonged amenorrhea; can be unknowingly expelled; may increase the risk of pelvic infection; user must regularly check string for placement; no protection against STIs; delay of fertility after discontinuing for possibly 6–12 mo	None	Cramps, bleeding, pelvic inflammatory disease; infertility; perforation of the uterus	Instruct woman how to locate string to check monthly for placement.

Postcoital emergency contraceptives (ECs)	Combination of levonorgestrel-only pills; combined estrogen and progestin pills; or the copper IUS inserted within 72 hr after unprotected intercourse	80%	Provides a last chance to prevent a pregnancy	Risk of ectopic pregnancy if EC fails	None	Nausea, vomiting, abdominal pain, fatigue, headache	Inform woman that ECs do not interrupt an established pregnancy, and the sooner they are taken the more effective they are.
Permanent sterilization							
Male	Sealing, tying, or cutting the vas deferens	<1%	One-time decision provides permanent sterility; short recovery time; low long-term risks	Procedures are difficult to reverse; initial cost may be high; chance of regret; some pain/discomfort after procedures	None for both	Postoperative complications: pain, bleeding, infection	Counsel both as to permanence of procedure and urge them to think it through prior to signing consent.
Female	Fallopian tubes are blocked to prevent conception	<1%					

Adapted from Raymond, E. G., & Cleland, K. (2015). Emergency contraception. *New England Journal of Medicine, 372*(14), 1342–1348; King, T. L., Brucker, M. C., Kriebs, J. M., Fahey, J. O., Gegor, C. L., & Varney, H. (2015). *Varney's midwifery.* Burlington, MA: Jones & Bartlett Learning; Ilic, K. (2015). Emergency contraception. In *Medicines for women* (pp. 203–225). Springer International Publishing; Samra-Latif, O. M., & Wood, E. (2015). Contraception. eMedicine. Retrieved from http://emedicine.medscape.com/article/258507-overview; Schuiling, K. D., & Likis, F. E. (2016). *Women's gynecologic health* (3rd ed.). Burlington, MA: Jones & Bartlett Learning.

Sexual Abstinence

Sexual abstinence (not having vaginal or anal intercourse) is one of the least expensive forms of contraception and has been used for thousands of years. Basically, pregnancy cannot occur if sperm is kept out of the vagina. It also reduces the risk of contracting HIV/AIDS and other STIs, unless body fluids are exchanged through oral sex; however, some infections, like herpes and human papilloma virus (HPV), can be passed by skin-to-skin contact. Dental dams can be used to prevent transmission, however. There are many pleasurable options for sex play without intercourse ("outercourse"), such as kissing, masturbation, erotic massage, sexual fantasy, sex toys such as vibrators, and oral sex.

Many people have strong feelings about abstinence based on religious and moral beliefs. There are many good and personal reasons to choose abstinence. For some it is a way of life, whereas for others it is a temporary choice. Some people choose sexual abstinence because they want to:

- wait until they are older;
- wait for a long-term relationship;
- avoid pregnancy or STIs;
- relieve feelings of depression or anxiety;
- follow religious or cultural expectations.

Fertility Awareness–Based Methods

Fertility awareness refers to any natural contraceptive method that does not require hormones, pharmaceutical compounds, physical barriers, or surgery to prevent pregnancy. FAMs use physical signs and symptoms that change with hormone fluctuations throughout a woman's menstrual cycle to predict a woman's fertility. Ovulation occurs on one day during each menstrual cycle, and the several days preceding ovulation are when intercourse is most likely to result in pregnancy. Collectively, the potentially fertile days up to and including the day of ovulation are called the "fertile window." Awareness of fertility is a better fertility-producing method than contraceptives. Less than 1% of women in the United States who use contraception employ these methods (King et al., 2015). The unifying theme of FAMs is that a woman can reduce her chance of pregnancy by abstaining from coitus or using barrier methods during times of fertility. These methods require couples to take an active role in preventing pregnancy through their sexual behaviors and women need to have regular menstrual cycles for it to be effective. Couples agree to practice certain techniques, use calculations, and be observant of the "fertile" and the "safe" periods in a monthly menstrual cycle. Using these methods for birth control requires a strong commitment from both partners. The normal physiologic changes caused by hormonal fluctuations during

the menstrual cycle can be observed and charted. This information can then be used to avoid or promote pregnancy. Fertility awareness methods rely on the following assumptions:

- A single ovum is released from the ovary 14 days before the next menstrual period. It lives approximately 24 hours.
- Women using this method must have regular menstrual cycles for it to be effective.
- Sperm can live up to 5 days after intercourse. The "unsafe period" during the menstrual cycle is thus approximately 6 days: 3 days before and 3 days after ovulation. Because body changes start to occur before ovulation, the woman can become aware of them and not have intercourse on these days or use another method to prevent pregnancy.
- The exact time of ovulation cannot be determined, so 2 to 3 days are added to the beginning and end to avoid pregnancy.

Techniques used to determine fertility include the cervical mucus ovulation method, the basal body temperature (BBT) method, the symptothermal method, standard day's method, and two-day method (Everett, 2014). Fertility awareness methods are moderately effective but are very unforgiving if not carried out as prescribed. Fertility awareness can be used in combination with coital abstinence or barrier methods during fertile days if pregnancy is not desired.

CERVICAL MUCUS OVULATION METHOD

Cervical mucus is a jellylike vaginal discharge that comes from the cervix. The **cervical mucus ovulation method** is used to assess the character of the cervical mucus. Cervical mucus changes in consistency during the menstrual cycle and plays a vital role in fertilization of the egg. Studies conducted by the WHO indicate that 93% of women, regardless of their education level, are capable of identifying and distinguishing fertile and infertile cervical secretions (Planned Parenthood, 2015a). In the days preceding ovulation, fertile cervical mucus helps draw sperm up and into the fallopian tubes, where fertilization usually takes place. It also helps maintain the survival of sperm. As ovulation approaches, the mucus becomes more abundant, clear, slippery, and smooth; it can be stretched between two fingers without breaking. Under the influence of estrogen, this mucus looks like egg whites. It is called *spinnbarkeit* mucus (Fig. 4.5). After ovulation, the cervical mucus becomes thick and dry under the influence of progesterone.

The cervical position can also be assessed to confirm changes in the cervical mucus at ovulation. Near ovulation, the cervix feels soft and is high/deep in the vagina, the os is slightly open, and the cervical mucus is copious and slippery (Bieber et al, 2015). This method works

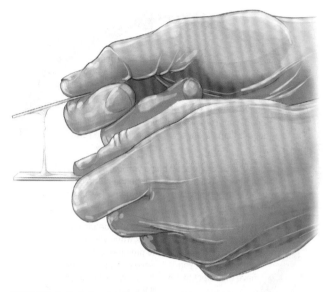

FIGURE 4.5 Spinnbarkeit mucus is cervical mucus that can stretch a distance before breaking.

because the woman becomes aware of her body changes that accompany ovulation. When she notices them, she abstains from sexual intercourse or uses another method to prevent pregnancy. Each woman is an individual, so each woman's unsafe time of the month is unique and thus must be individually assessed and determined.

BASAL BODY TEMPERATURE METHOD

The **BBT** refers to the lowest temperature reached on awakening. The woman takes her temperature orally before rising and records it on a chart. Preovulation temperatures are suppressed by estrogen, whereas postovulation temperatures are increased under the influence of heat-inducing progesterone. Temperatures typically rise within a day or two after ovulation and remain elevated for approximately 2 weeks (at which point bleeding usually begins). If using this method by itself, the woman should avoid unprotected intercourse until the BBT has been elevated for 3 days. Nurses should instruct women using the BBT method that it is important to keep in mind that illness and any drugs, including alcohol, can raise their body temperature and give a false reading. Other fertility awareness methods should be used along with BBT for better results (Fig. 4.6).

SYMPTOTHERMAL METHOD

The **symptothermal method** relies on a combination of techniques to recognize ovulation, including BBT, cervical mucus changes, alterations in the position and firmness of the cervix, and other symptoms of ovulation, such as increased libido, *mittelschmerz* (midcycle, lower abdominal pain at ovulation), pelvic fullness or tenderness, and breast tenderness (Planned Parenthood, 2015a). Combining all these predictors increases the

Basal body temperature

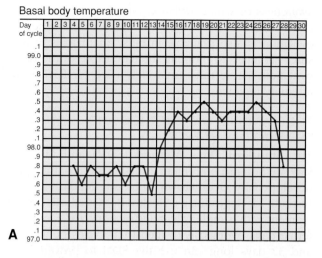

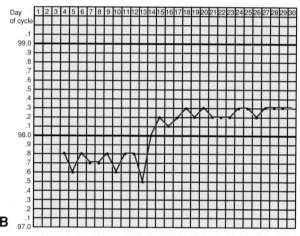

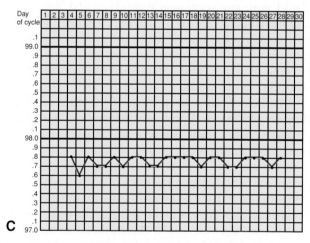

FIGURE 4.6 Basal body temperature graph. **A.** The woman's temperature dips slightly at midpoint in the menstrual cycle, then rises sharply, an indication of ovulation. Toward the end of the cycle (the 24th day), her temperature begins to decline, indicating that progesterone levels are falling and that she did not conceive. **B.** The woman's temperature rises at the midpoint in the cycle and remains at that elevated level past the time of her normal menstrual flow, suggesting that pregnancy has occurred. **C.** There is no preovulatory dip and no rise of temperature anywhere during the cycle. This is the typical pattern of a woman who does not ovulate.

awareness of when ovulation occurs and increases the effectiveness of this method. A home predictor test for ovulation is also available in most pharmacies. It measures LH levels to pinpoint the day before or the day of ovulation. These tests are widely used for fertility and infertility regimens.

THE STANDARD DAYS METHOD AND THE TWO-DAY METHOD

The **Standard Days Method** (SDM) and the Two-Day Method are both natural methods of contraception developed by Georgetown University Medical Center's Institute for Reproductive Health. Both methods provide women with simple, clear instructions for identifying fertile days. Women with menstrual cycles between 26 and 32 days long can use the SDM to prevent pregnancy by avoiding unprotected intercourse on days 8 through 19 of their cycles. Most SDM users utilize a visual aid—CycleBeads—to assist their correct use of SDM. An international clinical trial of the SDM showed that the method is more than 95% effective when used correctly (Wright, Iqteit, & Hardee, 2015). SDM identifies the 12-day "fertile window" of a woman's menstrual cycle. These 12 days takes into account the life span of the women's egg (about 24 hours) and the viability of the sperm (about 5 days) as well as the variation in the actual timing of ovulation from one cycle to another. For the Two-Day Method, women observe the presence or absence of cervical secretions by examining toilet paper or underwear or by monitoring their physical sensations. Every day, the woman asks two simple questions: "Did I note any secretions yesterday?" and "Did I note any secretions today?" If the answer to either question is yes, she considers herself fertile and avoids unprotected intercourse. If the answers are no, she is unlikely to become pregnant from unprotected intercourse on that day (King et al., 2015).

To help women keep track of the days on which they should avoid unprotected intercourse, a string of 32 color-coded beads (CycleBeads) is used, with each bead representing a day of the menstrual cycle. Starting with the red bead, which represents the first day of her menstrual period, the woman moves a small rubber ring one bead each day. The brown beads are the days when pregnancy is unlikely, and the white beads represent her fertile days (Stanford, 2015). This method has been used in underdeveloped countries for women with limited educational resources (Fig. 4.7).

Withdrawal (Coitus Interruptus)

In **coitus interruptus**, also known as withdrawal, a man controls his ejaculation during sexual intercourse and ejaculates outside the vagina. It is better known colloquially as "pulling out in time" or "being careful."

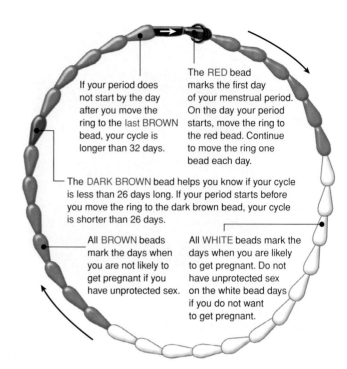

FIGURE 4.7 CycleBeads help women use the Standard Days Method.

It is one of the oldest and most widely used means of preventing pregnancy in the world and also one of the least effective methods in preventing pregnancy (Creatsas, 2015). The problem with this method is that the first few drops of the true ejaculate contain the greatest concentration of sperm, and if some pre-ejaculatory fluid escapes from the urethra before orgasm, conception may result. This method requires that the woman rely solely on the cooperation and judgment of the man. Nurses might wish to discuss emergency contraceptives be available with this couple or use a more effective method of contraception.

Lactational Amenorrhea Method

The **LAM** is an effective temporary method of contraception used by breast-feeding mothers. It relies on physiologic changes associated with breast-feeding for contraception. Continuous breast-feeding usually can postpone ovulation and thus prevent pregnancy. Breast-feeding stimulates the hormone prolactin, which is necessary for milk production, and also inhibits the release of another hormone, gonadotropin, which is necessary for ovulation.

Breast-feeding as a contraceptive method can be fairly effective for up to 6 months after giving birth only if:
- a woman has not had a period since she gave birth;
- infant is younger than 6 months of age;

- the woman breast-feeds her baby at least six times daily on both breasts;
- she breast-feeds her baby "on demand" at least every 4 hours;
- a woman does not substitute other foods for a breast-milk meal;
- nighttime feedings are provided at least every 6 hours.

Also, pumping or manual expression of milk may reduce effectiveness. Do not rely on this method after 6 months (Planned Parenthood, 2015a).

Nurses can help couples to make a decision about family planning options available in the postpartum period by discussing the advantages and disadvantages of each, taking into consideration the demands of the postpartum period. The options they may consider include lactational amenorrhea, combined oral contraception, implants, intrauterine systems, injectable methods, barrier methods, emergency contraception, and sterilization (Hughes, 2015).

Barrier Methods

Barrier contraceptives are forms of birth control that prevent pregnancy by preventing the sperm from reaching the ovum. Mechanical barriers include condoms, diaphragms, cervical caps, and sponges. These devices are placed over the penis or cervix to physically obstruct the passage of sperm through the cervix. Chemical barriers called spermicides may be used along with mechanical barrier devices. They come in creams, jellies, foam, suppositories, and vaginal films. They chemically destroy the sperm in the vagina. These contraceptives are called barrier methods because they not only provide a physical barrier for sperm, but also protect against STIs. Since the HIV/AIDS epidemic started in the early 1980s, these methods have become extremely popular. Progress has been made in society's reaction to condom use as a disease prevention device now and not just as a contraceptive (Haddad, Philpott-Jones, & Schonfeld, 2015).

Many of these barrier methods contain latex. Allergy to latex was first recognized in the late 1970s, and since then it has become a major health concern, with increasing numbers of people affected. According to the American Academy of Allergy, Asthma and Immunology (AAAAI) (2015), 6% of the general population, 10% of health care workers, and 50% of spina bifida clients are sensitive to natural rubber latex. Health care workers in both the medical and dental environments, as well as specific groups of individuals including those with spina bifida, myelodysplasia, and food allergies (banana, kiwi, avocado, and others), are at increased risk of sensitization (Kim, 2015). Teaching Guidelines 4.4 provides tips for individuals with latex allergy.

Teaching Guidelines 4.4
TIPS FOR INDIVIDUALS ALLERGIC TO LATEX

Symptoms of latex allergy include:
- Skin rash, itching, hives.
- Itching or burning eyes.
- Swollen mucous membranes in the genitals.
- Shortness of breath, difficulty breathing, wheezing.
- Anaphylactic shock.
- Use of or contact with latex condoms, cervical caps, and diaphragms is contraindicated for men and women with a latex allergy.
- If the female partner is allergic to latex, have the male partner apply a natural condom over the latex one.
- If the male partner experiences penile irritation after condom use, try different brands or place the latex condom over a natural condom.
- Use polyurethane condoms rather than latex ones.
- Use female condoms; they are made of polyurethane.
- Switch to another birth control method that isn't made with latex, such as OCs, intrauterine systems, Depo-Provera, fertility awareness, and other nonbarrier methods. However, these methods do not protect against STIs.

Adapted from American Academy of Allergy, Asthma and Immunology. (2015). Latex allergy: Tips to remember. Retrieved from http://www.aaaai.org/conditions-and-treatments/library/allergy-library/latex-allergy.aspx; Kim, J. S. (2015). Latex allergy. In *Allergy and clinical immunology* (pp. 288–293). Chichester: John Wiley & Sons. doi: 10.1002/9781118609125.ch32; and Occupational Health and Safety Administration. (2015). Latex allergy. Retrieved from http://www.osha.gov/SLTC/latexallergy

CONDOMS

Condoms are barrier methods of contraceptives made for both males and females. The male condom is made from latex or polyurethane or natural membrane and may be coated with spermicide. Male condoms are available in many colors, textures, sizes, shapes, and thicknesses. When used correctly, the male condom is put on over an erect penis before it enters the vagina and is worn throughout sexual intercourse (Fig. 4.8). It serves as a barrier to pregnancy by trapping seminal fluid and sperm and offers protection against STIs. Condoms are not perfect barriers, however, because breakage and slippage can occur. Emergency postcoital contraception may need to be sought to prevent a pregnancy. In addition, the nonlatex condoms have a higher risk of pregnancy and STIs than latex condoms (Everett, 2014).

The female condom is a polyurethane pouch inserted into the vagina. It consists of an outer and inner ring that is inserted vaginally and held in place by the pubic bone. Some women complain that the female condom is cumbersome to use and makes noise during

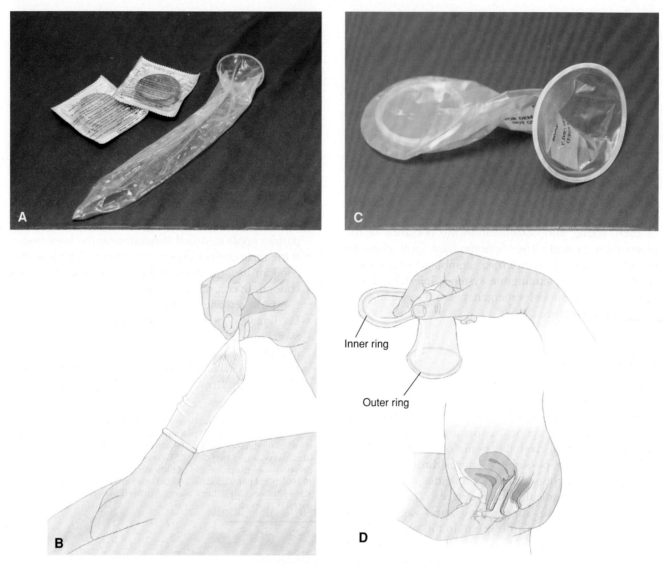

FIGURE 4.8 **A.** Male condom. **B.** Applying a male condom. Leaving space at the tip helps to ensure the condom will not break with ejaculation. **C.** The female condom. **D.** Insertion technique.

intercourse. Female condoms are readily available, are inexpensive, and can be carried inconspicuously by the woman. The female condom was the first woman-controlled method that offered protection against pregnancy and some STIs. Nurses can play a key role in educating clients on how to initiate and maintain use of the female condom, an underused method for HIV/STI and pregnancy prevention in the United States. Providing a brief education session along with free samples would go a long way to promote increased use of this device to prevent STIs transmission as well as pregnancy (Boyd et al., 2015).

DIAPHRAGM

The **diaphragm** is a soft latex dome surrounded by a metal spring. Used in conjunction with a spermicidal jelly

or cream, it is inserted into the vagina to cover the cervix (Fig. 4.9). The diaphragm may be inserted up to 4 hours before intercourse but must be left in place for at least 6 hours afterwards. Diaphragms are available in a range of sizes and styles. The diaphragm is available only by prescription and must be professionally fitted by a health care provider. Women may need to be refitted with a different-sized diaphragm after pregnancy, abdominal or pelvic surgery, or weight loss or gain of 10 pounds or more. As a general rule, diaphragms should be replaced every 1 to 2 years. Recently, a single-size diaphragm used with contraceptive jelly was introduced and studied for its effectiveness. The single-size diaphragm was deemed safe and as effective as a standard individually fitted one based on a population sample of >400 women that participated in the research study (Schwartz et al., 2015).

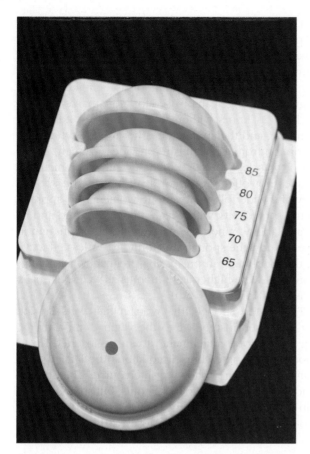

FIGURE 4.9 Sample diaphragm used for measuring.

The diaphragm provides both a physical and chemical barrier to sperm (Tharpe et al., 2016).

Diaphragms are user-controlled, nonhormonal methods that are needed only at the time of intercourse, but they are not effective unless used correctly. Women need to receive thorough instruction about diaphragm use and should practice putting one in and taking it out before they leave the health care office (Fig. 4.10).

Results of a two-year multisite study indicate that the effectiveness rates of the SILCS single-size, contoured diaphragm are similar to those of traditional diaphragms, but they also provide a long-term controlled release of the lead candidate anti-HIV microbicide dapivirine. This would make it a new multipurpose prevention device (Schwartz et al., 2015). The biggest difference with this new device is that since it is a single size, a pelvic exam to assess size is not required, and it also releases an anti-HIV microbicide that potentially is capable of preventing HIV transmission. Most women in the study were able to correctly insert, remove, and check correct position of the device by simply using the instructions (Schwartz et al., 2015).

CERVICAL CAP

The **cervical cap** is smaller than the diaphragm and covers only the cervix; it is held in place by suction. Caps

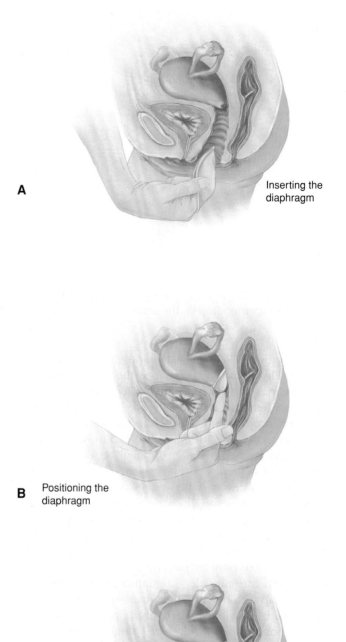

A Inserting the diaphragm

B Positioning the diaphragm

C Removing the diaphragm

FIGURE 4.10 Application of a diaphragm. **A.** To insert, fold the diaphragm in half, separate the labia with one hand, then insert upwards and back into the vagina. **B.** To position, make certain the diaphragm securely covers the cervix. **C.** To remove, hook a finger over the top of the rim and bring the diaphragm down and out.

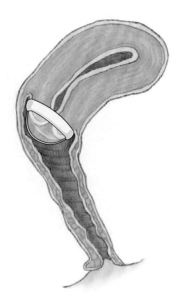

FIGURE 4.11 A cervical cap is placed over the cervix and used with a spermicidal jelly, the same as a diaphragm.

are made from silicone or latex and are used with spermicide (Fig. 4.11). The FemCap is the only cervical cap device currently available in the United States and comes in three sizes (Planned Parenthood, 2016). The cap may be inserted up to 36 hours before intercourse and provides protection for 48 hours. The cap must be kept in the vagina for 6 hours after the final act of intercourse and should be replaced every year of use. A refitting may also be necessary when a woman experiences pregnancy, abortion, or weight changes. The dome of the cap is filled about one third full with spermicide. Spermicide should not be applied to the rim because it might interfere with the seal that must form around the cervix. The cap is available only by prescription and must be fitted by a health care provider. Contraindications to use of a cervical cap include cervical cancer, recent urinary tract infection, latex allergy, pelvic-organ prolapse, and history of toxic shock syndrome. Using the cervical cap during menstruation may increase the risk of toxic shock syndrome and, therefore, should be avoided (Schuiling & Likis, 2016).

CONTRACEPTIVE SPONGE

The **contraceptive sponge** is a nonhormonal, non-prescription device that includes both a barrier and a spermicide. When it was removed from the market in 1995, it was the most popular OTC female contraceptive in America (Everett, 2014). The manufacturer, Wyeth, stopped making the sponge rather than upgrade its manufacturing plant after the Food and Drug Administration (FDA) found deficiencies, but the device's effectiveness and safety were never questioned. After receiving reapproval from the FDA in 2009, the contraceptive sponge is once again being marketed to women.

The contraceptive sponge is a soft concave device that prevents pregnancy by covering the cervix and releasing spermicide. The sponge, made of polyurethane saturated with nonoxynol-9 (1,000 mg), releases 125 mg of the spermicide over 24 hours of use. Unlike the diaphragm, the sponge can be used for more than one coital act within 24 hours without the insertion of additional spermicide, and the sponge does not require fitting or a prescription from a health care provider (Zieman, 2015). While it was less effective than several other methods and does not offer protection against STIs, the sponge achieved a wide following among women who appreciated the spontaneity with which it could be used and its easy availability. When compared with the diaphragm in a recent study, the sponge was found to be less effective than the diaphragm in preventing pregnancy. Discontinuation rates were higher at 12 months as well (Sharma & Walmsley, 2015).

To use the sponge, the woman first wets it with water, and then inserts it into the vagina with a finger, using a cord loop attachment. It can be inserted up to 24 hours before intercourse and should be left in place for at least 6 hours following intercourse. The sponge provides protection for up to 12 hours, but should not be left in for more than 30 hours after insertion to avoid the risk of toxic shock syndrome (Moses, 2015c).

Hormonal Methods

Several options are available to women who want long-term but not permanent protection against pregnancy. These methods of contraception work by altering the hormones within a woman's body. They rely on estrogen and progestin or progestin alone to prevent ovulation. When used consistently, these methods are a reliable way to prevent pregnancy. Hormonal methods include OCs, injectables, implants, vaginal rings, and transdermal patches.

ORAL CONTRACEPTIVES

As early as 1937, scientists recognized that the injection of progesterone inhibited ovulation in rabbits and provided contraception. The first hormonal pill, called *Enovid*, was approved by the FDA in May 1960. It contained high levels of estrogen to prevent ovulation. Since that time, it has evolved through gradual lowering of estrogen and is now combined with many different progestins. Breakthrough bleeding was reported in early clinical trials in women, and the role of estrogen in cycle control was launched. This established the rationale for modern-combination OCs that contains both estrogen and progesterone (Stewart & Black, 2015).

Development of hormonal contraception marked a revolutionary step in social change that has improved the lives of women and families worldwide. Since the first OC was introduced, hormonal contraception has

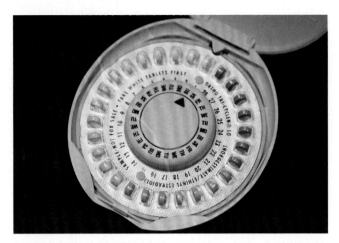

FIGURE 4.12 Oral contraceptive.

undergone various stages of advancement. Today, OC regimens are safer and more tolerable, with equal or improved efficacy, than the early formulations. Incremental decreases in the estrogen dosage helped to alleviate some of the unwanted side effects of the pill (Craik & Melvin, 2015). Today, over 30-combination OCs are available in the United States. The most notable change in over 50 years of OC improvement has been the lowering of the estrogen dose to as low as 10 mcg and the introduction of new progestins.

Oral contraception is the most popular method of nonsurgical contraception, used by approximately 25 million women in the United States (Fig. 4.12) (Samra-Latif & Wood, 2015). Unlike the original OCs that women took decades ago, the new low-dose forms carry fewer health risks.

OC, although most commonly prescribed for contraception, has long been used in the management of a wide range of conditions and has many health benefits, such as:

- reduced incidence of ovarian and endometrial cancer;
- prevention and treatment of endometriosis;
- decreased incidence of acne and hirsutism;
- decreased incidence of ectopic pregnancy;
- decreased incidence of acute PID and possible protection against PID;
- reduced incidence of fibrocystic breast disease;
- decreased perimenopausal symptoms;
- reduced risk of developing uterine fibroids;
- maintenance of bone mineral density;
- improvement in asthmatic symptoms;
- delayed onset of multiple sclerosis and arthritis;
- increased menstrual cycle regularity;
- lower incidence of colorectal cancer;
- decreased number of pregnancy-related deaths by preventing pregnancy;
- reduced iron-deficiency anemia by treating menorrhagia;
- reduced incidence of dysmenorrhea (Evans & Sutton, 2015).

OCs work primarily by suppressing ovulation by adding estrogen and progesterone to a woman's body, thus mimicking pregnancy. This hormonal level stifles GnRH, which in turn suppresses FSH and LH and thus inhibits ovulation. Cervical mucus also thickens, which hinders sperm transport into the uterus. Implantation is inhibited by suppression of the maturation of the endometrium and alterations of uterine secretions (Everett, 2014).

The combination pills are prescribed as monophasic pills, which deliver fixed dosages of estrogen and progestin, or as multiphasic ones. Multiphasic pills (e.g., biphasic and triphasic OCs) alter the amount of progestin and estrogen within each cycle. To maintain adequate hormonal levels for contraception and enhance adherence to the regimen, OCs should be taken at the same time daily.

OCs that contain progestin are sometimes called mini-pills. Progestin-only pills (POPs) have both advantages and disadvantages when compared with combined pills. The pill-taking regimen is simple and fixed; no pill color changes or days without pill-taking occur. These pills are appropriate for women who cannot take estrogen in combined OCs, for example, a woman older than 35 years who smokes cigarettes. They are prescribed for women who cannot take estrogen at all. These OCs work primarily by thickening the cervical mucus to prevent penetration of the sperm and make the endometrium unfavorable for implantation. POPs must be taken at a certain time every 24 hours. Breakthrough bleeding and a higher risk of pregnancy have made these OCs less popular than combination OCs (Craik & Melvin, 2015).

Extended OC regimens have been used for the management of menstrual disorders and endometriosis for years but now are attracting wider attention. Surveys asking women about their willingness to reduce their menstrual cycles from 12 to 4 annually were returned with a resounding "yes!" (Zorbas, Economopoulos, & Vlahos, 2015). Research has confirmed that the extended use of active OC pills carries the same safety profile as the conventional 28-day regimens. OCs taken continuously or in long cycles offer benefits with regard to menstrual symptoms and the recurrence of symptoms related to endometriosis (Zieman, 2015). The extended regimen consists of 84 consecutive days of active combination pills, followed by 7 days of placebos. The woman has four withdrawal-bleeding episodes a year. Seasonale and Seasonique, a combination OC, is on the market for women who choose to reduce the number of periods that they have. In 2009, the makers of Seasonique came out with LoSeasonique. LoSeasonique consists of 84 orange tablets containing 0.1 mg levonorgestrel and 0.02 mg ethinyl estradiol and 7 yellow tablets containing 0.01 mg ethinyl estradiol. The risk profile is similar to those of its sister products, Seasonale and Seasonique; however, the risk of unplanned breakthrough bleeding is increased (Samra-Latif & Wood, 2015).

Lybrel was the first FDA-approved OC with 365-day combination dosing. It contains a low combined daily dose of the hormones levonorgestrel and ethinyl estradiol (90 and 20 mcg, respectively). It provides women with more hormonal exposure on a yearly basis (13 additional weeks of hormone intake per year) than conventional cyclic OCs that contain the same strength of synthetic estrogens and similar strength of progestins (Samra-Latif & Wood, 2015). There is no physiologic requirement for cyclic hormonal withdrawal bleeds while taking OCs (Skidmore-Roth, 2015).

A growing body of evidence indicates that over-the-counter access to OC pills is safe and effective and that women are interested in obtaining pills this way. With half of all pregnancies being unintended—a figure that has remained unchanged for decades—innovation is needed to address this statistic. Although an over-the-counter contraceptive pill may sound revolutionary in the United States, over-the-counter access is already a reality in more than 100 countries and has been for decades. ACOG supports over-the-counter access to contraceptive pills, but numerous social and professional groups oppose it (Foster et al., 2015). Even after ACOG's support, women will probably not be seeing an over-the-counter OC product on the local pharmacy shelf any time soon, despite its cost-effectiveness and impact on reduction in unintended pregnancies.

The balance between the benefits and the risks of OCs must be determined for each woman when she is being assessed for this type of contraceptive. It is a highly effective contraceptive when taken properly but can aggravate many medical conditions, especially in women who smoke. Comparison Chart 4.1 lists advantages and disadvantages of OCs. A thorough history and pelvic examination, including a Pap smear, are not required before the medication is prescribed, but a regular medical follow-up is advised. Women should also be counseled that the effectiveness of OCs is decreased when the woman is taking antibiotics; thus, the woman will need to use an alternative or secondary method during this period to prevent pregnancy.

Nurses need to provide OC users with a great deal of education before they leave the health care facility. They need to be able to identify early signs and symptoms that might indicate a problem.

Take Note!

The mnemonic "ACHES" can help women remember the early warning signs that necessitate a return to the health care provider (Box 4.6).

COMPARISON CHART 4.1	ADVANTAGES AND DISADVANTAGES OF ORAL CONTRACEPTIVES
Advantages	**Disadvantages**
Regulate and shorten menstrual cycle	Offer no protection against STIs
Decrease severe cramping and bleeding	Pose slightly increased risk of breast cancer
Reduce anemia	
Reduce ovarian and colorectal cancer risk	Modest risk for venous thrombosis and pulmonary emboli
Decrease benign breast disease	Increased risk for migraine headaches
Reduce risk of endometrial cancer, colorectal cancer, and ovarian cancer	
Improve acne and reduces incidence of menstrual headaches	Increased risk for myocardial infarction, stroke, and hypertension for women who smoke
Minimize perimenopausal symptoms	May increase risk of depression
Decrease incidence of rheumatoid arthritis	User must remember to take pill daily
Improve PMS symptoms	High cost for some women
Protect against loss of bone density and reduces risk of osteoporosis	

Adapted from Jick, S. (2015). Oral contraceptives and the risk of venous thromboembolism. In *Medicines for Women* (pp. 181–201). Springer International Publishing; Zieman, M. (2015). *Managing contraception on the go* (13th ed.). New York: Ardnet Media; and Everett, S. (2014). *Handbook of contraception and sexual health* (3rd ed.). New York: Routledge.

EARLY SIGNS OF COMPLICATIONS FOR USERS OF ORAL CONTRACEPTIVES

- A = Abdominal pain may indicate liver or gallbladder problems.
- C = Chest pain or shortness of breath may indicate a pulmonary embolus.
- H = Headaches may indicate hypertension or impending stroke.
- E = Eye problems may indicate hypertension or an attack.
- S = Severe leg pain may indicate a thromboembolic event.

Adapted from Everett, S. (2014). *Handbook of contraception and sexual health* (3rd ed.). New York: Routledge.

INJECTABLE CONTRACEPTIVE

Injectable contraception includes progestin-only and combination estrogen and progestin agents that provide safe and highly effective birth control for up to three months. Injectable agents are widely available and play an important role in family planning worldwide. They offer a discrete, convenient, reversible, and noncoital-dependent method of birth control.

Depo-Provera is the trade name for an intramuscular injectable of a progesterone-only contraceptive given every 12 weeks which contains 150 mg/1 mL. Depo-subQ Pronera is a lower-dose injectable given subcutaneously delivering 104 mg/0.65 mL every 12 weeks. They are the only injectable agents available in the United States. Depo-Provera works by suppressing ovulation and the production of FSH and LH by the pituitary gland, by increasing the viscosity of cervical mucus and causing endometrial atrophy. A single injection of 150 mg into the buttocks acts like other progestin-only products to prevent pregnancy for 3 months at a time (Fig. 4.13). The primary side effect of Depo-Provera is menstrual cycle disturbance.

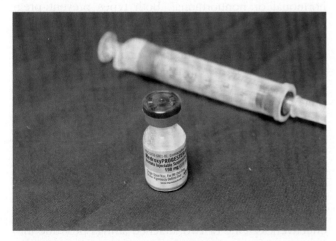

FIGURE 4.13 Injectable contraceptive.

Recent clinical studies have raised concerns about whether Depo-Provera reduces bone mineral density. This evidence has prompted the manufacturer and the FDA to issue a warning about the long-term use (>2 years) of Depo-Provera and bone loss (Wolfe & Cansino, 2015). It is not entirely clear if this loss in bone mineral density (BMD) is reversible because there have not been any long-term prospective studies in current and past users. It is highly recommended that bone density scans be done while on Depo-Provera (Curtis, 2014).

TRANSDERMAL PATCHES

Transdermal delivery of contraceptive hormones avoids hepatic first-pass metabolism, allowing a lower total hormone dose when compared to that of oral products that are metabolized in the liver. A **transdermal patch**, Ortho Evra, is available in the United States. It is a matchbox-sized patch containing hormones that are absorbed through the skin when placed on the lower abdomen, upper outer arm, buttocks, or upper torso (avoiding the breasts). The patch is applied weekly for 3 weeks, followed by a patch-free week during which withdrawal bleeding occurs. The patch delivers continuous levels of progesterone and estrogen. Transdermal absorption allows the drug to enter the bloodstream directly, avoiding rapid inactivation in the liver known as first-pass metabolism. Because estrogen and progesterone are metabolized by liver enzymes, avoiding first-pass metabolism was thought to reduce adverse effects. However, recent evidence suggests that the risk of venous thrombosis and embolism is increased with the patch and the risk of skin burns occurring if undergoing an MRI, but still less than the risk of venous thromboembolism during pregnancy (Nelson, 2015). Additional studies are under way to understand the clinical significance of these latest findings, but in the interim nurses need to focus on ongoing risk assessment and should be prepared to discuss current research findings with clients.

Adherence to the regimen of combination contraceptive patch use has been shown to be significantly greater than adherence with OCs. In addition, research suggests that overweight and obese women with weights exceeding 198 pounds should be advised of the potentially decreased effectiveness of the patch and increase incidence of venous thromboembolism and weight gain (Pocius & Dutton, 2015). The patch provides combination HT with a side-effect profile similar to that of OCs (Fig. 4.14).

VAGINAL RINGS

Approved in 2001 by the FDA, the **vaginal ring** contains both estrogen and progesterone hormones. The contraceptive vaginal ring, NuvaRing, is a flexible, soft, transparent ring that is inserted by the user for a 3-week period of continuous use followed by a ring-free week

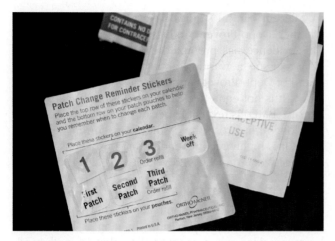

FIGURE 4.14 Transdermal patch.

to allow withdrawal bleeding (Fig. 4.15). Ethinyl estradiol and etonogestrel are rapidly absorbed through the vaginal epithelium and result in a steady serum concentration. Because the hormones are released directly into the vagina, a lower daily dose of hormones is required in comparison with OC doses. Studies have demonstrated that the efficacy and safety of the ring are equivalent to those of OCs. Clients report being highly satisfied with the vaginal ring and report fewer systemic side effects than do OC users. The ring provides effective cycle control as well as symptom relief for women with menorrhagia, dysmenorrhea, and polycystic ovarian syndrome. Reported problems associated with the use of vaginal rings include erosion of vaginal wall, ring expulsion, interference with coitus, unpleasant ring odor, and premature discontinuation due to vaginal discomfort (Khan & Krupanidhi, 2015). The ring can be inserted by the woman and does not have to be fitted. The woman compresses the ring and inserts it into the vagina, behind the pubic bone, as far back as possible, but precise placement is not critical. The hormones are absorbed through

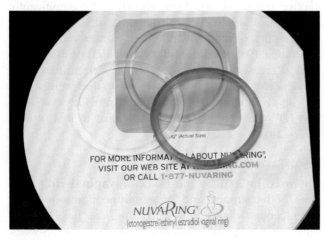

FIGURE 4.15 Vaginal ring.

the vaginal mucosa. It is left in place for 3 weeks and then removed and discarded. Effectiveness and adverse events are similar to those seen with combination OCs. Clients need to be counseled regarding timely insertion of the ring and what to do in case of accidental expulsion. Recent studies suggest that a vaginal ring containing etonogestrel and ethinyl estradiol used in an extended regimen is a safe contraceptive method that offers good cycle control and can be an option for women who have gastric intolerance or other side effects when using oral hormonal contraceptives (King et al., 2015).

IMPLANTABLE CONTRACEPTIVES

The **implant** is a subdermal time-release method that delivers synthetic progestin that inhibits ovulation. Once in place, it delivers 3 years of continuous, highly effective contraception. Like POPs, implants act by inhibiting ovulation and thickening cervical mucus, so sperm cannot penetrate. A single-rod progestin implant (Nexplanon) is currently available in the United States. Nexplanon is 4 cm long and 2 mm in diameter, and contains 68 mg of the hormone progestin. The implant is radio-opaque and is over 99% effective (King et al., 2015). The side effects are also similar to those of POPs: irregular bleeding, headaches, weight gain, breast tenderness, and depression. Fertility is restored quickly after it is removed. Implants require a minor surgical procedure for both insertion and removal. The implants do not offer any protection against STIs.

Hormonal side effects are not exclusive to implants but tend to be a problem with all hormonal contraceptives. Preinsertion counseling by the nurse is essential to prepare the woman for any such side effects. Expert counseling should cover the one side effect most likely to cause discontinuation: initial irregular bleeding and the possibility of amenorrhea with longer use (Craik & Rowlands, 2015).

INTRAUTERINE CONTRACEPTIVES

Intrauterine contraceptives are classified as either hormonal or nonhormonal. Both types prevent pregnancy via inhibition of sperm mobility and sperm viability and change the speed of transport of the ovum in the fallopian tube. An intrauterine contraceptive (IUC) is a small plastic T-shaped object that is placed inside the uterus to provide contraception (Fig. 4.16). It prevents pregnancy by making the endometrium of the uterus hostile to implantation of a fertilized ovum by causing a nonspecific inflammatory reaction and inhibiting sperm and ovum from meeting (Wildemeersch & Jandi, 2015). The hormonal IUC will make monthly periods lighter, shorter, and less painful, making this a useful method for women with heavy, painful periods. The implants contain either copper or progesterone to enhance their effectiveness. One or two attached strings protrude into the vagina so that the user can check for placement.

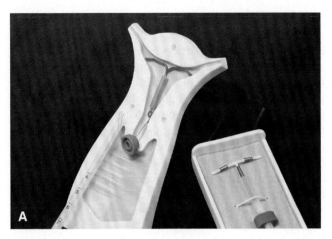 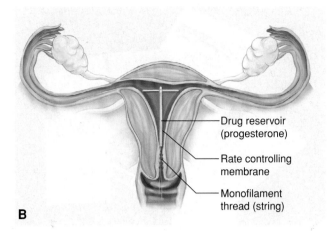

Drug reservoir (progesterone)

Rate controlling membrane

Monofilament thread (string)

FIGURE 4.16 **A.** Intrauterine contraceptive. **B.** An IUC in place in the uterus.

Currently three IUCs are available in the United States: the copper ParaGard-TCu-380A, the levonorgestrel-releasing intrauterine system (LNG-IUS) marketed as Mirena, and another LNG-IUD marketed as Skyla. The ParaGard-TCu-380A is approved for 10 years of use and is nonhormonal. Its mechanism of action is based on the release of copper ions, which alone are spermicidal. Additionally, the device causes an inflammatory action leading to a hostile uterine environment. The TCu-380A is also approved for use as emergency contraception. Mirena provides intrauterine conception for 5 years, but has been shown to be effective for as long as 7 years. Skyla has been approved for 3 years of pregnancy prevention. Both devices release a low dose of progestin causing thinning of the endometrium and thickening of cervical mucus, which inhibits sperm entry into the upper genital tract. Their use results in a major reduction in menstrual flow and dysmenorrhea, suggesting that they are viable alternative to hysterectomy and endometrial ablation in women with menorrhagia (Atkin et al., 2015). An advantage of these hormonally impregnated intra-uterine systems is that they are relatively maintenance-free: users must consciously discontinue using them to become pregnant rather than making a daily decision to avoid conception (Alan Guttmacher Institute, 2015a).

The IUCs provide a safe, highly effective, long-lasting, yet reversible method of contraception. Expanding access to intrauterine contraception is an important measure to reduce the rate of unintended pregnancy in the United States. Nurses should consider including them in their discussion to appropriate candidates, including women who are nulliparous, adolescent, immediately postpartum, or postabortion, and those who desire emergency contraception, and as an alternative to permanent sterilization. Limitations barriers to obtaining intrauterine contraception such as requiring cervical cancer screening before insertion, routine testing for gonorrhea and chlamydial infection in low-risk women, or scheduling insertion only during menses are unnecessary. IUC

insertion can take place on any day of the menstrual cycle, if absence of pregnancy is confirmed (Cheng & Van Leuven, 2015). Box 4.7 highlights the warning signs of the potential complications of IUCs.

EMERGENCY CONTRACEPTION

Unplanned pregnancy is a major health, economic, and social issue for women. Approximately one third of all unplanned pregnancies end in abortion (CDC, 2015b). Using an emergency contraceptive provides a woman a second chance to prevent an unintended pregnancy. **Emergency contraception** (EC) reduces the risk of pregnancy after unprotected intercourse or contraceptive failure such as condom breakage (Raymond & Cleland, 2015). It is used within 72 hours of unprotected intercourse to prevent pregnancy. The sooner ECs are taken, the more effective they are. They reduce the risk of pregnancy for a single act of unprotected sex by almost 80% (Samra-Latif & Wood, 2015). The methods available in the United States are POPs, Plan B One-Step (Fig. 4.17), Next Choice, Next Choice One Dose; combined estrogen and progestin pills, or insertion of a copper-releasing intrauterine system up to 7 days after unprotected intercourse. Ulipristal acetate (marketed as Ella) is a selective

---

BOX 4.7

WARNINGS FOR INTRAUTERINE SYSTEM USERS OF POTENTIAL COMPLICATIONS

• P = Period late, pregnancy, abnormal spotting or bleeding
• A = Abdominal pain, pain with intercourse
• I = Infection exposure, abnormal vaginal discharge
• N = Not feeling well, fever, chills
• S = String length shorter or longer or missing

Adapted from King, T. L., Brucker, M. C., Kriebs, J. M., Fahey, J. O., Gegor, C. L., & Varney, H. (2015). *Varney's midwifery*. Burlington, MA: Jones & Bartlett Learning.

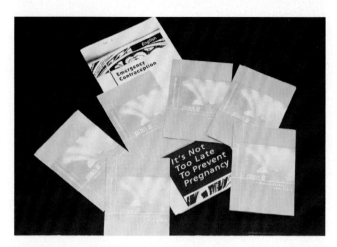

FIGURE 4.17 Emergency contraceptive kit.

progesterone receptor modulator that, when taken as a single 30-mg dose, is a new, safe, and effective emergency contraceptive that can be used from the first day and up to 5 days following unprotected intercourse. The older progesterone-only emergency contraceptive, levonorgestrel, is taken as two 0.75-mg pills 12 hours apart (Next Choice®; Watson Pharmaceuticals Inc., Morristown, NJ, USA) or as a single 1.5-mg pill (Plan B One-Step™; Watson Pharmaceuticals Inc.), and is approved for only 72 hours after unprotected intercourse (Mulligan, 2015).

Access to emergency contraceptives has been controversial for minors. Prior to 2013, the pills were available by prescription only, and even when approved for nonprescription status, access was restricted based on age. In 2013, several judicial courts and the FDA ruled in favor of nonprescription access to EC by all women regardless of age. At this time, the federal government has not appealed these rulings, but many states have placed restrictions on access of EC (Casey & Isaacs, 2015). The only contraindication to the use of any of the four EC methods is a known pregnancy as defined as implantation.

Although access to EC has increased with nonprescription status and approval of Plan B One-Step without age restrictions, many barriers remain in public awareness and unintended pregnancies continue to rise. Because of the lack of awareness of EC and the politics surrounding it, EC is not used as widely as would be warranted by the incidence of unprotected coitus. Nurses need to educate their female clients to bring about increased awareness of this second chance method. Table 4.5 lists recommended oral medication and intrauterine regimens.

Prime points to stress concerning ECs are the following:
- ECs do not offer any protection against STIs or future pregnancies.
- ECs should not be used in place of a regular birth control method, because they are less effective.
- ECs may delay the next menses, so evaluation for pregnancy is needed if menses does not occur within three weeks after EC use
- Report any severe abdominal pain to health care provider immediately.
- ECs are regular birth control pills given at a higher dose.
- ECs are contraindicated during pregnancy (Ilic, 2015).

 Take Note!

Contrary to popular belief, ECs do not induce abortion and are not related to mifepristone or RU-486, the so-called abortion pill approved by the FDA in 2000.

Mifepristone chemically induces abortion by blocking the body's progesterone receptors, which are necessary for pregnancy maintenance. ECs simply prevent embryo creation and uterine implantation from occurring in the first place. There is no evidence that ECs have any effect on an already implanted ovum. The side effects are nausea and vomiting.

TABLE 4.5	EMERGENCY POSTCOITAL CONTRACEPTION OPTIONS	
Product	Dosage (Within 72 Hr)	Comments
Combined estrogen and progestin pills (Yuzpe regimen)	OCSs are taken in various formulations to prevent conception.	Interfere with the cascade of events that result in ovulation and fertilization
Plan B One-Step	1.5 mg pill taken	Can cause nausea and vomiting
Intrauterine		
Copper-bearing IUS (ParaGard-TCu-380A)	Inserted within 5 d after unprotected sexual episode	Can be left in for long-term contraception (10 yrs)

Adapted from King, T. L., Brucker, M. C., Kriebs, J. M., Fahey, J. O., Gegor, C. L., & Varney, H. (2015). *Varney's midwifery*. Burlington, MA: Jones &Bartlett Learning; Ilic, K. (2015). Emergency contraception. In *Medicines for Women* (pp. 203–225). Springer International Publishing.

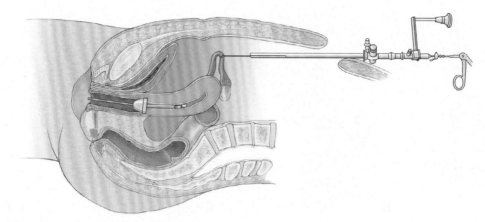

FIGURE 4.18 Laparoscopy for tubal sterilization.

Sterilization

Sterilization is a permanent, safe, and highly effective method of contraception for those who are certain they do not want any or any more children. Vasectomy is the only highly reliable form of male contraception. Approximately 600,000 tubal occlusions and 200,000 vasectomies are performed in the United States annually and over 220 million worldwide (ACOG, 2013). It is the most widely used method of family planning in the world in both developed and developing countries. Sterilization refers to surgical procedures intended to render the person infertile. Laparoscopic, abdominal, and hysteroscopic methods of female sterilization are available in the United States, with most of these procedures performed outside the hospital. Sterilization is a safe and effective form of permanent birth control. In the United States, it is still the second most commonly used form of contraception overall and is the most frequently used method among married women and among women over 30 years of age (McKay & Schunmann, 2015). More women than men undergo surgical sterilization. According to the CDC (2015b), approximately 18% of women undergo female sterilization in comparison with 7% of men in the United States. Sterilization should be considered a permanent end to fertility because reversal surgery is difficult, expensive, and not always successful. Because these methods are intended to be irreversible, all couples should be appropriately counseled about the permanency of sterilization and the availability of highly effective, long-acting, reversible methods of contraception before their decision is made.

TUBAL LIGATION

Tubal ligation, the sterilization procedure for women, can be performed postpartum, after an abortion, or as an interval procedure unrelated to pregnancy. Mini-laparotomies and laparoscopies are the two most common techniques. In the laparoscopy procedure, the abdomen is filled with carbon dioxide gas so that the abdominal wall balloons away from the tubes to provide a view of the fallopian tubes. They are grasped and sealed with a cauterizing instrument or with rings, bands, or clips, or cut and tied (Fig. 4.18).

ESSURE

Essure is a nonsurgical, nonhormonal, permanent birth control method that is 99% effective. This method is for women who desire no more children as it is a permanent method of birth control. It offers several advantages over a conventional tubal ligation: general anesthesia and incisions are not needed, thereby increasing safety, lowering costs, and improving access to sterilization. A tiny coil (Essure) is introduced and released into the fallopian tubes through the cervix. The coil promotes tissue growth in the fallopian tubes, and over a period of 3 months, this growth blocks the tubes. The build-up of tissue creates a barrier that keeps sperm from the reaching the ovum, thus preventing conception (Thurkow, 2015). This less-invasive technique uses a hysteroscopy under local anesthesia in an office setting. Sterilization does not occur immediately after this procedure, so women must be educated to use additional contraception for 3 months until permanent tubal occlusion is verified.

VASECTOMY

Male sterilization is accomplished with a surgical procedure known as a **vasectomy**. More than 500,000 men have a vasectomy performed in the United States each year (Mcfarlane, 2015). It is usually performed under local anesthesia in a urologist's office, and most men can return to work and normal activities in a day or two. The procedure involves making a small incision into the scrotum and cutting the vas deferens, which carries sperm from the testes to the penis (Fig. 4.19). Complications from vasectomy are rare and minor in nature. Immediate risks include infection, hematoma, and pain. After vasectomy, semen no longer contains sperm. This is not immediate, though, and the man must submit semen specimens for analysis 8 to 16 weeks after a vasectomy

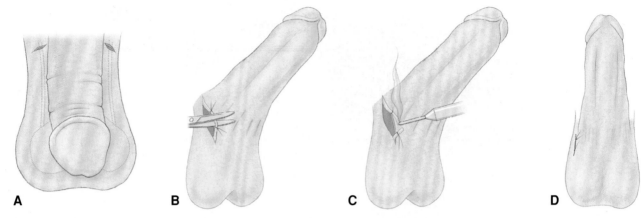

FIGURE 4.19 Vasectomy. **A.** Site of vasectomy incisions. **B.** The vas deferens is cut with surgical scissors. **C.** Cut ends of the vas deferens are cauterized to ensure blockage of the passage of sperm. **D.** Final skin suture.

until two specimens show that no sperm is present. When the specimen shows azoospermia, the man's sterility is confirmed (Whitaker, 2015).

Nursing Management of the Woman Choosing a Contraceptive Method

The choice of a contraceptive method is a very personal one involving many factors. What makes a woman choose one contraceptive method over another? In making contraceptive choices, couples must balance their sexual lives, their reproductive goals, and each partner's health and safety. The search for a choice that satisfies all three objectives is challenging. A method that works for a sexually active teenage girl may not meet her needs later in life. Several considerations influence a person's choice of contraceptives:

• Motivation
• Cost
• Cultural and religious beliefs (Box 4.8)
• Convenience
• Effectiveness
• Side effects
• Desire for children in the future
• Safety of the method
• Comfort level with sexuality
• Protection from STIs
• Interference with spontaneity

If a contraceptive is to be effective, the woman must understand how it works, must be able to use it correctly and consistently, and must be comfortable and confident with it. If a client cannot adhere to taking a pill daily, consider a method used once a week (transdermal patches), once every 3 weeks (transvaginal ring), or once every 3 months (Depo-Provera injection). Another option may be a progesterone IUC that lasts 3 to 5 years and reduces menstrual flow significantly.

Regardless of which method is chosen, the client's needs should be paramount in the discussion. The nurse can educate clients about which methods are available and their advantages and disadvantages, efficacy, cost, and safety. Knowledge of contraceptive effectiveness is crucial to making an informed choice. The couple has to comprehend the pros and cons of the contraceptive methods being considered. Choice may be influenced by understanding the likelihood of pregnancy with each method and factors that influence effectiveness. Counseling can help the woman choose a contraceptive

BOX 4.8

SELECTED RELIGIOUS CHOICES FOR FAMILY PLANNING AND ABORTION

• Roman Catholic—Abstinence and natural family planning; no abortion
• Judaism (Orthodox)—Family planning and abortion accepted in first trimester. Conservative and Reform Judaism accept both family planning and abortion.
• Islam—Family planning accepted; abortion only for serious reasons
• Protestant Christianity—Firmly in favor of family planning; mixed on abortion
• Buddhism—Long experience with family planning and abortion
• Hinduism—Accept both family planning and abortion
• Native American religions—Accept both family planning and abortion
• Chinese religions—Taoism and Confucianism accept both

Adapted from McFarland, M. R., & Wehbe-Alamah, H. B. (2015). *Leininger's cultural care diversity and universality: A worldwide nursing theory* (3rd ed.). Burlington, MA: Jones & Bartlett Learning; and McFarlane, D. R. (2015). *Global population and reproductive health.* Burlington, MA: Jones & Bartlett Learning.

method that is efficacious and fits her preferences and lifestyle.

Nursing Assessment

When assessing which contraceptive method might meet the client's needs, the nurse might ask the following:
- Do your religious beliefs interfere with any methods?
- Will this method interfere with your sexual pleasure?
- Are you aware of the various methods currently available?
- Is cost a major consideration, or does your insurance cover it?
- Does your partner influence which method you choose?
- Are you in a stable, monogamous relationship?
- Have you heard anything troubling about any of the methods?
- How comfortable are you touching your own body?
- What are your future plans for having children?

Although deciding on a contraceptive is a very personal decision between a woman and her partner, nurses can assist in this process by performing a complete health history and physical examination, and by educating the woman and her partner about necessary laboratory and diagnostic testing. Areas of focus during the nursing assessment are as follows:
- Medical history: smoking status, cancer of reproductive tract, diabetes mellitus, migraines, hypertension, thromboembolic disorder, allergies, risk factors for cardiovascular disease (CVD)
- Family history: cancer, CVD, hypertension, stroke, diabetes
- OB/GYN history: menstrual disorders, current contraceptive, previous STIs, PID, vaginitis, sexual activity
- Personal history: use of tampons and female hygiene products, plans for childbearing, comfort with touching herself, number of sexual partners and their involvement in the decision
- Physical examination: height, weight, blood pressure, breast examination, thyroid palpation, pelvic examination
- Diagnostic testing: urinalysis, complete blood count, Pap smear, wet mount to check for STIs, HIV/AIDS tests, lipid profile, glucose level

Figure 4.20 shows an example of a family planning flow record that can be used during the assessment. After collecting the assessment data above, consider the medical factors to help decide if the woman is a candidate for all methods or whether some should be eliminated. For example, if she reports she has multiple sex partners and a history of pelvic infections, she would not be a good candidate for an intrauterine contraceptive. Barrier methods (male or female condoms) of contraception might be recommended to this client to offer protection against STIs.

Nursing Diagnoses

A few nursing diagnoses that might be appropriate based on the nurse's assessment during the decision-making process include:
- Deficient knowledge related to:
  - methods available
  - side effects/safety
  - correct use of method chosen
  - previous myths believed
- Risk for infection related to:
  - unprotected sexual intercourse
  - past history of STIs
  - methods offering protection

Nursing diagnoses applicable to the contraceptive would be:
- Health-seeking behaviors related to:
  - perceived need for limiting number of children
  - overall health relative to contraceptives
- Risk for ineffective health maintenance related to:
  - not being familiar with the various contraceptive methods
  - being unaware of high-risk sexual behavior leading to STIs
- Fear related to:
  - not understanding the correct procedure to use
  - unintended pregnancy occurring if not used correctly
  - general health concerning the long-term side effects

Nursing Interventions

Contraception is an important issue for all couples, and the method used should be decided by the woman and her partner jointly. Facilitate this process by establishing a trusting relationship with the client and by providing unbiased, accurate information about all methods available. As a nurse, reflect honestly on your feelings about contraceptives while allowing the client's feelings to be paramount. Be aware of the practical issues involved in contraceptive use, and avoid making assumptions, making decisions on the woman's behalf, and making judgments about her and her situation. To do so, it is important to keep up to date on the latest methods available and convey this information to clients. Encourage female clients to take control of their lives by sharing information that allows them to plan their futures.

The following guidelines are helpful in counseling and educating the client or couple about contraceptives:
- Encourage the client/couple to participate in choosing a method.
- Provide client education. The client/couple must become informed users before the method is chosen. Education should be targeted to the client's level so it is understood. Provide step-by-step teaching and an

FAMILY PLANNING FLOW (VISIT) RECORD

Name:_____
ID #:_____
Date of Birth:_____

	Date:			Date:	
Current Method					
Reason for Visit					
LMP					
SUBJECTIVE DATA	Pt.	Comments		Pt.	Comments
Severe headaches					
Depression					
Visual abnormalities					
Dyspnea/chest pain					
Breast changes					
SBE					
Abdominal pain					
Nausea and vomiting					
Dysuria/frequency					
Menstrual irregularities					
Vaginal discharge/infections					
Leg pain					
Surgery, injury, infections, or serious illness since last visit					
Allergic reaction					
Pregnancy plans					
Other					
OBJECTIVE DATA	Weight	B.P.		Weight	B.P.
Other					
Lab					
ASSESSMENT					
Check here if assessment continues on progress notes	O			O	
PLAN					
Type of contraceptive given					
COUNSELING/EDUCATION					
Next appointment					
SIGNATURE/TITLE					
SIGNATURE/TITLE					

O = normal   ✓ = abnormal

FIGURE 4.20 Family planning flow (visit) record.

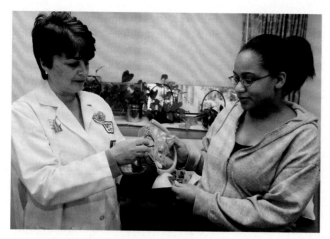

FIGURE 4.21 The nurse demonstrates insertion of a vaginal ring during client teaching.

opportunity for practice for certain methods (cervical caps, diaphragms, vaginal rings, and condoms). See Teaching Guidelines 4.5 and Figure 4.21.

- Obtain written informed consents, which are needed for intrauterine contraceptives, implants, abortion, or sterilization. Informed consent implies that the client is making a knowledgeable, voluntary choice; has received complete information about the method, including the risks; and is free to change her mind before using the method or having the procedure (Schuiling & Likis, 2016).
- Discuss contraindications for all selected contraceptives.
- Consider the client's cultural and religious beliefs when providing care.
- Address myths and misperceptions about the methods under consideration in your initial discussion of contraceptives.

Teaching Guidelines 4.5

TIPS FOR THE USE OF CERVICAL CAPS, DIAPHRAGMS, VAGINAL RINGS, AND CONDOMS

Cervical Cap Insertion/Removal Technique

- It is important to be involved in the fitting process.
- To insert the cap, pinch the sides together, compress the cap dome, insert into the vagina, and place over the cervix.
- Use one finger to feel around the entire circumference to make sure there are no gaps between the cap rim and the cervix.
- After a minute or two, pinch the dome and tug gently to check for evidence of suction. The cap should resist the tug and not slide off easily.
- To remove the cap, press the index finger against the rim and tip the cap slightly to break the suction. Gently pull out the cap.

- The woman should practice inserting and removing the cervical cap three times to validate her proficiency with this device.

Client Teaching and Counseling Regarding the Cervical Cap

- Fill the dome of the cap up about one third full with spermicide cream or jelly. Do not apply spermicide to the rim, since it may interfere with the seal.
- Wait approximately 30 minutes after insertion before engaging in sexual intercourse to be sure that a seal has formed between the rim and the cervix.
- Leave the cervical cap in place for a minimum of 6 hours after sexual intercourse. It can be left in place for up to 48 hours without additional spermicide being added.
- Do not use during menses due to the potential for toxic shock syndrome. Use an alternative method such as condoms during this time.
- Replace the cervical cap after each year of use.
- Inspect the cervical cap prior to insertion for cracks, holes, or tears.
- After using the cervical cap, wash it with soap and water, dry thoroughly, and store in its container.

Diaphragm Insertion/Removal Technique

- Always empty the bladder prior to inserting the diaphragm.
- Inspect diaphragm for holes or tears by holding it up to a light source, or fill it with water and check for a leak.
- Place approximately a tablespoon of spermicidal jelly or cream in the dome and around the rim of the diaphragm.
- The diaphragm can be inserted up to 6 hours prior to intercourse.
- Select the position that is most comfortable for insertion:
  - Squatting
  - Leg up, raising the nondominant leg up on a low stool
  - Reclining position, lying on back in bed
  - Sitting forward on the edge of a chair
- Hold the diaphragm between the thumb and fingers and compress it to form a "figure-eight" shape.
- Insert the diaphragm into the vagina, directing it downward as far as it will go.
- Tuck the front rim of the diaphragm behind the pubic bone so that the rubber hugs the front wall of the vagina.
- Feel for the cervix through the diaphragm to make sure it is properly placed.
- To remove the diaphragm, insert the finger up and over the top side and move slightly to the side, breaking the suction.
- Pull the diaphragm down and out of the vagina.

Client Teaching and Counseling Regarding the Diaphragm

- Avoid the use of oil-based products, such as baby oil, because they may weaken the rubber.
- Wash the diaphragm with soap and water after use and dry thoroughly.
- Place the diaphragm back into the storage case.
- The diaphragm may need to be refitted after weight loss or gain or childbirth.
- Diaphragms should not be used by women with latex allergies.

Vaginal Ring Insertion/Removal Technique and Counseling

- Each ring is used for one menstrual cycle, which consists of 3 weeks of continuous use followed by a ring-free week to allow for menses.
- No fitting is necessary—one size fits all.
- The ring is compressed and inserted into the vagina, behind the pubic bone, as far back as possible.
- Precision placement is not essential.
- Backup contraception is needed for 7 days if the ring is expelled for more than 3 hours during the 3-week period of continuous use.
- The vaginal ring is left in place for 3 weeks, then removed and discarded.
- The vaginal ring is not recommended for women with uterine prolapse or lack of vaginal muscle tone (Schuiling & Likis, 2016).

Male Condom Insertion/Removal Technique and Counseling

- Always keep the condom in its original package until ready to use.
- Store in a cool, dry place.
- Spermicidal condoms should be used if available.
- Check expiration date before using.
- Use a new condom for each sexual act.
- Condom is placed over the erect penis prior to insertion.
- Place condom on the head of the penis and unroll it down the shaft.
- Leave a half-inch of empty space at the end to collect ejaculate.
- Avoid use of oil-based products, because they may cause breakage.
- After intercourse, remove the condom while the penis is still erect.
- Discard condom after use.

Female Condom Insertion/Removal Technique and Counseling

- Practice wearing and inserting prior to first use with sexual intercourse.
- Condom can be inserted up to 8 hours before intercourse.
- Condom is intended for one-time use.

- It can be purchased over the counter—one size fits all.
- Avoid wearing rings to prevent tears; long fingernails can also cause tears.
- Spermicidal lubricant can be used if desired.
- Insert the inner ring high in the vagina, against the cervix.
- Place the outer ring on the outside of the vagina.
- Make sure the erect penis is placed inside the female condom.
- Remove the condom after intercourse. Avoid spilling the ejaculate.

Education and Counseling of women using Injectable Contraceptives

- Consume a diet high in calcium and vitamin D to prevent bone mineral loss.
- Know the conditions that need to be reported to the health care provider:
  - Significant headaches
  - Menorrhagia
  - Depression
  - Severe abdominal pain
- Awareness of any infection present at injection site.

It is also important to clear up common misconceptions about contraception and pregnancy. Clearing up misconceptions will permit new learning to take hold and a better client response to whichever methods are explored and ultimately selected. Some common misconceptions include:

- Breast-feeding protects against pregnancy.
- Pregnancy can be avoided if the male partner "pulls out" before he ejaculates.
- Pregnancy cannot occur during menses.
- Douching after sex will prevent pregnancy.
- Pregnancy will not happen during the first sexual experience.
- Taking birth control pills protects against STIs.
- The woman is too old to get pregnant.
- If female orgasm is not reached, conception is not likely.
- Irregular menstruation prevents pregnancy.

When discussing in detail each method of birth control, focus on specific information for each method outlined. Include information such as how this particular method works to prevent pregnancy under normal circumstances of use; the noncontraceptive benefits to overall health; advantages and disadvantages of all methods; the cost involved for each particular method; danger signs that need to be reported to the health care provider; and the required frequency of office visits needed for the particular method.

In addition, outline factors that place the client at risk for method failure. Contraceptives can fail for any

TABLE 4.6	CONTRACEPTIVE PROBLEMS AND EDUCATIONAL NEEDS

Contraceptive Failure

Problem	Client Education Needed
Not following instructions for use of contraceptive correctly	Take pill the same time every day. Use condoms properly and check condition before using. Make sure diaphragm or cervical cap covers cervix completely. Check IUD for placement monthly.
Inconsistent use of contraceptive	Contraceptives must be used regularly to achieve maximum effectiveness. All it takes is one unprotected act of sexual intercourse to become pregnant. Two to 5% of condoms will break or tear during use.
Condom broke during sex	Check expiration date. Store condoms properly. Use only a water-based lubricant. Watch for tears caused by long fingernails. Use spermicides to decrease possibility of pregnancy. Seek emergency postcoital conception.
Use of antibiotics or other herbs taken with OCs	Use alternative methods during the antibiotic therapy, plus 7 additional days. Implement on day 1 of taking antibiotics.
Belief that you can't get pregnant during menses or that it is safe "just this one-time"	It may be possible to become pregnant on almost any day of the menstrual cycle.

of many reasons. Use Table 4.6 to provide client education concerning a few of the reasons for contraceptive failure. Help clients who have chosen abstinence or fertility awareness methods to define the sexual activities in which they do or do not want to participate. This helps them set sexual limits or boundaries. Help them to develop communication and negotiation skills that will allow them to be successful. Supporting, encouraging, and respecting a couple's choice of abstinence is vital for nurses.

After clients have chosen a method of contraception, it is important to address the following:

- Emphasize that a second method to use as a backup is always needed.
- Provide both oral and written instructions on the method chosen.
- Discuss the need for STI protection if not using a barrier method.
- Inform the client about the availability of ECs.

Steady progress in contraception research has been achieved over the past several years. Hormonal and nonhormonal contraceptives have improved women's lives by reducing different health conditions that contribute to morbidity. However, the contraceptives available today are not suitable to all users, and the need to expand contraceptive choices still exists. It is hoped that the introduction of newer methods in the near future with additional health benefits will continue to help women and couples meet their family planning needs.

ABORTION

Abortion is defined as the expulsion of an embryo or fetus before it is viable (Alexander et al., 2014). Abortion can be a medical or surgical procedure. The purpose of abortion is to terminate a pregnancy. More than 40% of all women will end a pregnancy by abortion at some time in their reproductive lives. Both in the United States and globally, more than one fifth of all known pregnancies end in abortion (McFarlane, 2015). Surgical abortion is the most common procedure performed in the United States (approximately 1.3 million annually) and might be the most common surgical procedure in the world (Alan Guttmacher Institute, 2015b). Both medical and surgical abortions are safe and legal in the United States; an abortion is considered a woman's constitutional right based on the fundamental right to privacy. Eighty-nine percent of abortions occur in the first 12 weeks of pregnancy (Alan Guttmacher Institute, 2015b).

Since the landmark U.S. Supreme Court decision *Roe v. Wade* legalized abortion in 1973, debate has continued over how and when abortions are provided.

Every state has laws regulating some aspects of the provision of abortion, and many have passed restrictions such as parental consent or notification requirements, mandated counseling and waiting periods, and limits on funding for abortion. Each state addresses these matters independently, and the laws that are passed or enforced are legislative decisions and a function of the political system. Although opponents of abortion continue to be very much a part of the current debates, recently they have refocused their attention on "regulation legislation" among the states to reduce the number of abortions not medically necessary (Kreitzer, 2015).

Surgical Abortion

Two types of surgical abortion are available: vacuum aspiration or dilation, and evacuation (D&C). Method selection is based on gestational age. It is an ambulatory procedure done under local anesthesia. The cervix is dilated prior to surgery and then the products of conception are removed by suction evacuation. The uterus may gently be scraped by curettage to make sure that it is empty. The entire procedure lasts about 10 minutes. The overall risk of complications is less than 1% for surgical termination (Upadhyay et al., 2015).The major risks and complications in the first trimester are infection, retained tissue or hemorrhage, uterine perforation, retained products of conception, or cervical tear (Udoh et al., 2015). For women whose blood is Rh negative, *RhoGAM* is indicated prior to start of either medical or surgical termination.

Medical Abortion

Medical abortions are achieved through administration of medication either vaginally or orally. The administration of medication occurs in the clinic or doctor's office, may require two to four office visits, and costs between $300 and $800 (Planned Parenthood, 2015b). Three drugs are currently used to terminate a pregnancy during the first trimester. The first drug is methotrexate (an antineoplastic agent; Rheumatrex) followed by misoprostol (a prostaglandin agent; Cytotec) given as a vaginal suppository or in oral form 3 to 7 days later. Methotrexate induces abortion because of its toxicity to trophoblastic tissue, the growing embryo. Misoprostol works by causing uterine contractions, which helps to expel the products of conception. This method is 90% to 98% successful in completing an abortion (Patil & Edelman, 2015).

The second drug used to induce first-trimester abortions involves using mifepristone (a progesterone antagonist; Mifeprex, RU-486) followed 48 hours later by misoprostol (a prostaglandin agent), which causes contractions of the uterus and expulsion of the uterine contents. Currently, the most widely used method of medication abortion in the United States is the administration of mifepristone in conjunction with misoprostol. Another frequent method used includes the combination of methotrexate with misoprostol (Schuiling & Likis, 2016). Mifepristone, the generic name for RU-486, is sold under the brand names Mifeprex and Early Option. Mifepristone is an antiprogestin and blocks the action of progesterone, which is necessary for the maintenance of the pregnancy. This method is 95% effective when used within 49 days after the last menstrual cycle (Patil & Edelman, 2015).

Another drug frequently used is misoprostol (Cytotec), which is a prostaglandin analog that softens the cervix and causes uterine contractions, which results in the expulsion of uterine contents. There is no standard protocol for use of misoprostol (Cytotec) alone for termination of early pregnancy, and it is not FDA-approved for this purpose (King et al., 2015). Complications of medical abortions include incomplete expulsion of uterine contents, uterine infection, and heavy bleeding (Ganatra, Guest, & Berer, 2015).

The assessment of the woman with an unintended pregnancy should be performed with cautious sensitivity. It is essential to explore the women's feelings about pregnancy before congratulating or consoling her. The encounter should be guided by the feelings of the client, not by the assumptions and values of the nurse.

Abortion is a very emotional, deeply personal issue. Give support and accurate information. If for personal, religious, or ethical reasons you feel unable to actively participate in the care of a woman undergoing an abortion, you still have the professional responsibility to ensure that the woman receives the nursing care and help she requires. This may necessitate a transfer to another area or a staffing reassignment. Nurses must keep in mind that all women have the right to have access to unbiased, factual information about available reproductive health choices, whether they seek to end or start a pregnancy, from which they can then make informed decisions about their own reproductive health.

MENOPAUSAL TRANSITION

Menopause is a natural process that occurs in all women's lives as part of normal aging. *Meno* is derived from the Greek word for "month," and *pause* is derived from the Greek word for "pause" or "halt." Menopause is the technical term for a point in time at which menses and fertility cease (King et al., 2015). The change of life. The end of fertility. The beginning of freedom. Whatever people call it, menopause is a unique and personal experience for every woman. The term **menopausal transition** refers to the transition from a woman's reproductive phase of her life to her final menstrual period. This period is also referred to as *perimenopause*. It is the end of her menstruation and childbearing capacity. The average age of natural menopause—defined as 1 year without a menstrual period—is 51.4 years old. The average age of natural menopause has remained constant for the last several hundred years despite improvements in nutrition and health care (Alexander et al., 2014). With current female life expectancy at 84 years, this event comes in the middle of a woman's adult life. Many women go through the menopausal transition with few or no symptoms, while some have significant or even disabling symptoms.

 Take Note!
Humans are virtually the only species to outlive their reproductive capacities.

Menopause signals the end of an era for many women. It concludes their ability to reproduce, and some women find advancing age, altered roles, and these physiologic changes to be overwhelming events that may precipitate depression and anxiety (Woods & Mitchell, 2015). Menopause does not happen in isolation. Midlife is often experienced as a time of change and reflection. Change happens in many arenas: children are leaving or returning home, employment pressures intensify as career moves or decisions are required, older adult parents require more care or the death of a parent may have a major impact, and partners are retrenching or undergoing their own midlife crises. Women must negotiate all these changes in addition to menopause. Managing these stressful changes can be very challenging for many women as they make the transition into midlife.

A woman is born with approximately 2 million ova, but only about 400 ever mature fully to be released during the menstrual cycle. The absolute number of ova in the ovary is a major determinant of fertility. Over the course of her premenopausal life there is a steady decline in the number of immature ova (Wood, 2015). No one understands this depletion, but it does not occur in isolation. Maturing ova are surrounded by follicles that produce two major hormones: estrogen, in the form of estradiol, and progesterone. The cyclic maturation of the ovum is directed by the hypothalamus. The hypothalamus triggers a cascade of neurohormones, which act through the pituitary and the ovaries as a pulse generator for reproduction. This hypothalamic–pituitary–ovarian axis begins to break down long before there is any sign that menopause is imminent. Some scientists believe that the pulse generator in the hypothalamus simply degenerates; others speculate that the ovary becomes more resistant to the pituitary hormone FSH and simply shuts down (Schuiling & Likis, 2016). The final act in this well-orchestrated process is amenorrhea.

As menopause approaches, more and more of the menstrual cycles become anovulatory. This period of time, usually 2 to 8 years before cessation of menstruation, is termed *perimenopause* (McNamara, Batur, & DeSapri, 2015). In perimenopause, the ovaries begin

to fail, producing irregular and missed periods and an occasional hot flash. When menopause finally appears, viable ova are gone. Estrogen levels plummet by 90%, and estrone, produced in fat cells, replaces estradiol as the body's main form of estrogen. The major hormone produced by the ovaries during the reproductive years is estradiol; the estrogen found in postmenopausal women is estrone. Estradiol is much more biologically active than estrone (Hoyt & Falconi, 2015). In addition, testosterone levels decrease with menopause.

Menopausal transition, with its dramatic decline in estrogen, affects not only the reproductive organs, but also other body systems:
- Brain: hot flashes, disturbed sleep, mood and memory problems
- Cardiovascular: lower levels of high-density lipoprotein (HDL) and increased risk of CVD
- Skeletal: rapid loss of bone density that increases the risk of osteoporosis
- Breasts: replacement of duct and glandular tissues by fat
- Genitourinary: vaginal dryness, stress incontinence, cystitis
- Gastrointestinal: less absorption of calcium from food, increasing the risk for fractures
- Integumentary: dry, thin skin and decreased collagen levels
- Body shape: more abdominal fat; waist size that swells relative to hips

Therapeutic Management

Menopausal transition should be managed individually. In the past, despite the wide diversity of symptoms and risks, the traditional reaction was to reach for the one-size-fits-all therapy: HT. Today the medical community is changing its thinking in light of the Women's Health Initiative (WHI) study and the Heart and Estrogen/Progestin Replacement Study Follow-Up (HERS II), which reported that long-term HT increased the risks of heart attacks, strokes, and breast cancer; in short, the overall health risks of HT exceeded the benefits (Kyvernitakis et al., 2015). In addition, HT did not protect against the development of coronary artery disease (CAD), nor did it prevent the progression of CAD, as it was previously touted to do.

A recent research finding examined the timing of HT in relation to CAD in women and it found that the earlier initiation of HT was associated with less CAD in women with natural but not surgical menopause. A Cochrane Review study found that HT in postmenopausal women overall, had little benefit in CAD prevention, but caused an increase in the risk of stroke and venous thromboembolic events (Boardman et al., 2015). As expected, the fallout from this study and others forced practitioners to re-evaluate their usual therapies and tailor treatment to each client's history, needs, and risk factors. A current study, however, shows that the incidence of fractures among menopausal transition and postmenopausal women increased significantly in the 3 years after publication of the WHI and HERS II results. This trend followed a decline in the use of HT, concurrent with an increase in the use of other bone-modifying agents (Bakour & Williamson, 2015). There is considerable evidence that estrogen or HT reduces the risk of postmenopausal osteoporotic fracture of both the spine and hip (Mirkin et al., 2015).

A number of treatment options are available, but factors in the client's history should be the driving force when determining therapy. Women need to educate themselves about the latest research findings and collaborate with their health care provider on the right menopause therapy. The following factors should be considered in management:

- The risk/benefit ratio is highest in younger women who begin HT not long after menopause.
- HT is approved for two indications: relief of vasomotor symptoms and prevention of osteoporosis.
- Research suggests that HT may be beneficial for preventing diabetes, improving mood, or avoiding urinary tract problems.
- Using HT long beyond menopause carries increased risks, which, for some women, may be outweighed by the benefits (Bakour & Williamson, 2015).

Many women consider nonhormonal therapies such as bisphosphonates and selective estrogen receptor modulators (SERMs). Consider weight-bearing exercises, calcium, vitamin D, smoking cessation, and avoidance of alcohol to treat or prevent osteoporosis. Annual breast examinations and mammograms are essential. Local estrogen creams can be used for vaginal atrophy. Consider herbal therapies for symptoms, although none have been validated by rigorous research studies (Ismail et al., 2015).

ACOG recently revised guidelines on treating menopausal symptoms. Their recommendations include systemic HT, with estrogen or estrogen plus progestin, is the most effective approach for treating vasomotor symptoms; the lowest effective dose for the shortest duration is the best regimen; thromboembolic disease and breast cancer are risks for combined systemic HT; and local estrogen therapy is advised for isolated atrophic vaginal symptoms (2014).

Although numerous symptoms have been attributed to menopause (Box 4.9), some of them are more closely related to the aging process than to estrogen deficiency. A few of the more common menopausal conditions and their management are discussed next.

Managing Hot Flashes and Night Sweats

The emergence of hot flashes and night sweats (also known as vasomotor symptoms) coincides with a

---

BOX 4.9

COMMON SYMPTOMS OF MENOPAUSE
- Hot flashes or flushes of the head and neck
- Dryness in the eyes and vagina
- Personality changes
- Anxiety and/or depression
- Loss of libido
- Decreased lubrication
- Weight gain and water retention
- Night sweats
- Atrophic changes—loss of elasticity of vaginal tissues
- Fatigue
- Irritability
- Poor self-esteem
- Insomnia
- Stress incontinence
- Heart palpitations

Adapted from Coney, P. (2015). Menopause. *Emedicine*. Retrieved from http://emedicine.medscape.com/article/264088-overview; Kessenich, C. R. (2015). Inevitable menopause. *Nursing Spectrum*. Retrieved from http://ce.nurse.com/ce232-60/Inevitable-Menopause; and Schuiling, K. D. & Likis, F. E. (2016). *Women's gynecologic health* (3rd ed.). Burlington, MA: Jones & Bartlett Learning.

---

period in life that is also marked by dynamic changes in hormone and reproductive function that interconnect with the aging process, changes in metabolism, lifestyle behaviors, and overall health (Wood, 2015). Hot flashes and night sweats are classic signs of estrogen deficiency and the predominant complaint of perimenopausal women. A hot flash is a transient and sudden sensation of warmth that spreads over the body, particularly the neck, face, and chest. Hot flashes are caused by vasomotor instability. This instability causes inappropriate peripheral vasodilation of superficial blood vessels, which gives the sensation of heat. Nearly 85% of menopausal women experience them (Alexander et al., 2014). Hot flashes are an early and acute sign of estrogen deficiency. These flashes can be mild or extreme and can last from 2 to 30 minutes and may occur as frequently as every hour to several times per week. On average, women experience hot flashes for a period of 6 months to 2 years, but the symptoms may last up to 10 years or more. Severe vasomotor symptoms can have a significant and detrimental effect on quality of life. Factors that trigger vasomotor symptoms include caffeine and alcohol consumption, intake of hot drinks and spicy foods, hot environment, depression, stress, and anxiety (Avis et al., 2015).

Many options are available for treating hot flashes. Treatment must be based on symptom severity, the client's medical history, and the client's values and concerns. Although the gold standard in the treatment of hot flashes is estrogen, this is not recommended for all women who have high risk factors in their history.

TRADITIONAL THERAPIES FOR THE MANAGEMENT OF HOT FLASHES

The following are traditional therapies for the management of hot flashes:

- Pharmacologic options
- HT unless contraindicated
- Androgen therapy (potentiates estrogen)
- Estrogen and androgen combinations
- Progestin therapy (Depo-Provera injection every 3 months)
- Clonidine (central alpha-adrenergic agonist) weekly patch
- Neurontin (antiseizure) decreased hot flashes
- Propranolol (beta-adrenergic blocker)
- Brisdelle: FDA approved nonhormonal medication
- Short-term sleep aids: Ambien, Dalmane
- Gabapentin (Neurontin): antiseizure drug
- SSRIs: venlafaxine (Effexor) and paroxetine (Paxil) have shown promise (King & Brucker, 2016)

COMPLEMENTARY AND ALTERNATIVE THERAPIES FOR MANAGEMENT OF HOT FLASHES

Many women are choosing alternative treatments for managing menopausal symptoms. Bioidentical hormones have the ability to bind to receptors in the human body and function in the same way as a woman's natural hormones. They simulate three estrogens (estradiol, estriol, and estrone), as well as progesterone, testosterone, dehydroepiandrosterone (DHEA), thyroxine, and cortisol. Bioidentical hormones are not, however, natural hormones. The estrogens are derived via a chemical process from soybeans (*Glycine max*) and progesterone from Mexican yam (*dioscorea villosa*). As with conventional hormones, however, bioidentical hormones are available only with a physician's prescription and through a pharmacy. Because of their natural origin, women perceive that alternative treatments are safer. The interest in phytoestrogens came about because of the low prevalence of hot flashes in Asian women, which was attributed to their diet being rich in phytoestrogens. Recent studies have found that black cohosh, multibotanical herbs, and increased soy intake do not reduce the frequency or severity of menopausal hot flashes or night sweats.

Other remedies for easing menopausal symptoms might include red clover, motherwort, ginseng, sarsaparilla root, valerian root, L-tryptophan, calcium-magnesium, and kelp tablets (Ismail et al., 2015). Again, research thus far has been skeptical about their efficacy, but many women report they ease their symptoms and their use has skyrocketed. Although some benefits may accrue from their use, evidence of the efficacy of alternative products in menopause is largely anecdotal. Small, preliminary clinical trials might demonstrate the safety of some of the nonpharmacologic products. Nurses should be aware of the purported action of these agents as well as any adverse effects or drug interactions.

The following are lifestyle changes and CAM therapies for the treatment of hot flashes:

- Lifestyle changes
- Lower room temperature; use fans
- Wear clothing in layers for easy removal
- Limit caffeine and alcohol intake
- Drink 8 to 10 glasses of water daily
- Stop smoking or cut back
- Avoid hot drinks and spicy food
- Take calcium (1,200 to 1,600 mg) and vitamin D (400 to 600 International Units)
- Exercise daily, but not just before bedtime
- Maintain a healthy weight
- Identify stressors and learn to manage them
- Keep a diary to identify triggers of hot flashes
- Phytoestrogens: isoflavones, ligands, coumetrols
- Black cohosh
- Chamomile: mild sedative to alleviate insomnia
- Unopposed transdermal progesterone
- Compounded bioidentical hormones
- Try relaxation techniques, deep breathing, and meditation
- Acupuncture may reduce the frequency of hot flashes
- Vitamin E: 100 mg daily
- Dehydroepiandrosterone (DHEA)
- Chaste tree berry (vitex): balances progesterone and estrogen
- Dong quai: acts as a form of phytoestrogen
- Ginseng: purported to improve memory
- St. John's wort: reduces depression and fatigue
- Wild yam: treats menopausal symptoms
- Valerian root: induces sleep and relaxation (Wood, 2015)

Managing Urogenital Changes

Menopausal transition can be a physically and emotionally challenging time for women. In addition to the psychological burden of leaving behind the reproductive phase of life and the stigma of an aging body, sexual difficulties resulting from urogenital changes plague most women but are frequently not addressed. Sexual desire is affected by endocrine and psychosocial factors. Menopausal hormonal changes are relevant to the causes of sexual dysfunction during reproductive aging. The frequency of sexual intercourse declines as women enter midlife. Whereas partner availability and function probably play a role, menopausal symptoms, such as vaginal dryness, are also present (Comhaire & Depypere, 2015).

Vaginal atrophy occurs during menopause because of declining estrogen levels. These changes include thinning of the vaginal walls, an increase in pH, irritation, increased susceptibility to infection, **dyspareunia** (difficult or painful sexual intercourse), loss of lubrication with intercourse, vaginal dryness, and a decrease in sexual desire related to these changes. Decreased estrogen levels can also influence a woman's sexual function as well. Delayed clitoral reaction, decreased vaginal lubrication, diminished circulatory response during sexual stimulation, and reduced contractions during orgasm have all been linked to low estrogen levels (Coney, 2015).

Management of these changes might include the use of estrogen vaginal tablets (Vagifem) or Premarin cream; Estring, an estrogen-releasing vaginal ring that lasts for months; testosterone patches; and over-the-counter moisturizers and lubricants (Astroglide) (King et al., 2015). A positive outlook on sexuality and a supportive partner are also needed to make the sexual experience enjoyable and fulfilling. Nurses can improve the sexual health and quality of life in menopausal women by educating them about their symptoms and offering them choices about managing them.

Take Note!

Sexual health is an important aspect of the human experience. By keeping an open mind, listening to women, and providing evidence-based treatment options, the nurse can help improve quality of life for menopausal women.

Preventing and Managing Osteoporosis

Osteoporosis has been recognized as a significant worldwide public health problem. As the world's population ages, both in the United States and internationally, the prevalence of osteoporosis is expected to increase significantly. **Osteoporosis** is the state of diminished bone density. This disorder is a systemic skeletal disease characterized by low bone mass and microarchitectural deterioration of bone tissue with a consequent increase in bone fragility and susceptibility to fracture (National Osteoporosis Foundation [(NOF], 2015a).

According to recent information from NOF (2015a), osteoporosis is a major medical problem that affects 10 million women and 2 million men in the United States. An additional 34 million Americans have low bone mass. Each year, an estimated 1.5 million individuals in the United States experience a fragility fracture secondary to osteoporosis, resulting in an annual cost of ⊠18 billion. By 2025, experts predict that osteoporosis will be responsible for approximately 3 million fractures and ⊠26 billion in costs each year (NOF, 2015a). With the rapidly aging population, the problem of osteoporosis is now reaching epidemic proportions. Seventy-five million baby boomers are entering the stage in their lives when they are most at risk for osteoporosis. One half of all women and one third of all men will sustain a fragility fracture during their lifetimes. Osteoporosis continues to be underdiagnosed and undertreated because it is often not recognized until the first fracture occurs.

Women are greatly affected by osteoporosis after menopause. Osteoporosis is a condition in which bone

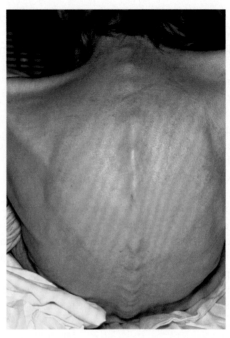

FIGURE 4.22 Skeletal changes associated with osteoporosis. (John Radcliffe Hospital/Photo Researcher Inc.)

mass declines to such an extent that fractures occur with minimal trauma. Bone loss begins in the third or fourth decade of a woman's life and accelerates rapidly after menopause (Alexander et al., 2014). This condition puts many women into long-term care, with a resulting loss of independence. Figure 4.22 shows the skeletal changes associated with osteoporosis.

Most women with osteoporosis do not know they have the disease until they sustain a fracture, usually of the wrist or hip. Risk factors include:
• Increasing age
• Postmenopausal status without hormone replacement
• Small, thin-boned frame
• Low bone mineral density
• White or Asian with small bone frame
• Impaired eyesight that would increase risk of falling
• Rheumatoid arthritis
• Family history of osteoporosis
• Sedentary lifestyle
• History of treatment with:
  • Antacids with aluminum
  • Heparin
  • Long-term use of steroids > 3 months
  • Thyroid replacement drugs
• Smoking and consuming alcohol
• Low calcium and vitamin D intake
• Excessive amounts of caffeine
• Personal history of nontraumatic fracture
• Anorexia nervosa or bulimia (NOF, 2015a)

Currently, no method exists for directly measuring bone mass. Instead a BMD measurement is used. BMD is a two-dimensional measurement of the average content of mineral in a section of bone. BMD evaluations are made at the hip, femoral neck, and spine. There is a significant relationship between BMD and fracture: as BMD is reduced, the risk of fracture increases (Sullivan et al., 2015). Screening tests to measure bone density are not good predictors for young women who might be at risk for developing this condition. Dual-energy x-ray absorptiometry (DXA or DEXA) is a screening test that calculates the mineral content of the bone at the spine and hip. It is highly accurate, fast, and relatively inexpensive. The dual energy x-ray absorptiometry scan (DEXA scan) is the gold standard radiologic method for identifying osteoporosis through measuring BMD (U.S. Preventive Services Task Force, 2015).

Hip fracture is the most devastating of the fragility fractures secondary to osteoporosis. A number of medical, social, and economic consequences follow a hip fracture. Of women older than 50 years, on average, 24% die within the first year after hip fracture (Wang et al., 2015). The concern surrounding osteoporosis is not the rate of fracture alone but also the potential for lifelong disability secondary to fracture. The incidence of hip fracture is estimated to double by the year 2025 and nearly double again by 2050. For women, this is a projected 240% increase (NOF, 2015a).

The best management for this painful, crippling, and potentially fatal disease is prevention.

Women can modify many risk factors by doing the following:
- Engage in daily weight-bearing exercise, such as walking to increase osteoblast activity.
- Increase calcium and vitamin D intake.
- Avoid smoking and excessive alcohol (more than two drinks per day).
- Discuss bone health with a health care provider.
- When appropriate, have a bone density test and take medication if needed (NOF, 2015b).

Medications that can help in preventing and managing osteoporosis include:
- HT (Premarin)
- SERMs (raloxifene [Evista])
- Calcium and vitamin D supplements (Tums)
- Estrogen agonist/antagonist [SERM] (Evista)
- Bisphosphonates (Actonel, Fosamax, Boniva, or Reclast)
- Parathyroid hormone (Forteo)
- Calcitonin (Miacalcin) (King & Brucker, 2016)

Preventing and Managing Cardiovascular Disease

Despite the dramatic decrease in annual CVD mortality and total cardiovascular mortality for American women each year since 2000, CVD remains the number-one killer of women, accounting for one in three deaths in the United States. This is likely due to increased rates of obesity, sedentary lifestyle, diabetes, and high cholesterol levels (Chomistek et al., 2015). More women die from heart disease and stroke than the next five causes of death combined, including breast cancer. Half a million women die annually in the United States of CVD, with strokes accounting for about 20% of the deaths (Alexander et al., 2014). This translates into approximately one death every minute. While men's mortality from CVD has decreased since the 1980s, women's mortality from CVD has climbed. This has resulted in a sex-related CVD mortality gap, with women having higher mortality than men since 1984. Contributing to this female-majority CVD mortality gap is a lack of awareness among women and their physicians of the risk for CVD. Awareness campaigns, such as the Heart Truth and the Red Dress symbol, appear to have improved recognition of CVD risk in women. Further, female-specific guidelines have been developed to prevent and reduce CVD in women. Though the current understanding of the role of menopause in CVD is controversial, studies suggest that menopause does not exacerbate CVD independent of aging, and HT is not effective for secondary prevention of CVD (Hale & Shufelt, 2015).

For the first half of a woman's life, estrogen seems to be a protective substance for the cardiovascular system by smoothing, relaxing, and dilating blood vessels. It even helps boost HDL and lower low-density lipoprotein (LDL) levels, helping to keep the arteries clean from plaque accumulation. But when estrogen levels plummet as women age and experience menopause, the incidence of CVD increases dramatically. Women are more likely to have atypical cardiovascular symptoms compared with men. This may lead to a delayed or misdiagnosis of CAD and suboptimal treatment. These symptoms may include:
- A – Angina (chest pain)
- B – Breathlessness
- C – Chronic fatigue
- D – Dizziness
- E – Edema of hands and feet
- F – Fluttering of the heart
- G – Gastric upset
- H – Heavy pain in back and shoulders

Menopause is not the only factor that increases a woman's risk for CVD. Lifestyle and medical history factors such as the following play a major role:
- Smoking
- Obesity
- High-fat diet
- Sedentary lifestyle
- High cholesterol levels
- Family history of CVD
- Hypertension
- Apple-shaped body
- Diabetes

Two of the major risk factors for coronary heart disease are hypertension and dyslipidemia. Both are modifiable and can be prevented by lifestyle changes and, if needed, controlled by medication. This is why prevention is essential. In addition, women who experience early menopause lose the protection afforded by endogenous estrogen to the cardiac system and are at greater risk for more extensive atherosclerosis. Major preventive strategies include a healthy diet, increased activity, exercise, smoking cessation, decreased alcohol intake, and weight reduction.

Nurses, particularly those caring for women during their reproductive years, are uniquely positioned to provide education and support for women's long-term cardiovascular health. Raising awareness of heart disease in women is an essential role for nurses. The good news is that CVD is largely preventable. Because CVD is a chronic disease that develops over time, primary prevention lifestyle modification interventions are most effective if initiated before the development of overt disease. Stressing the importance of lifestyle modifications must begin early in life and should be reinforced from the beginning of a young woman's reproductive years through menopause. Nurses are in an ideal position to teach the importance of good nutrition, healthy weight, and daily exercise before CVD becomes clinically evident.

Nursing Assessment

Menopausal transition is a universal and irreversible part of the overall aging process involving a woman's reproductive system. Although not a disease state, menopausal transition does place women at greater risk for the development of many conditions of aging. Nurses can help the woman become aware of her risk for postmenopausal diseases, as well as strategies to prevent them. The nurse can be instrumental in assessing risk factors and planning interventions in collaboration with the client. These might include:

- Screening for osteoporosis, CVD, and cancer risk
- Assessment of blood pressure to identify hypertension
- Blood cholesterol test to identify hyperlipidemia risk
- Mammogram to find a cancerous lesion
- Pap smear to identify cervical cancer
- Pelvic examination to identify endometrial cancer or masses
- Digital rectal examination to assess for colon cancer
- Bone density testing as a baseline at menopause to identify osteopenia (low bone mass), which might lead to osteoporosis
- Assessing lifestyle to plan strategies to prevent chronic conditions:
- Dietary intake of fat, cholesterol, and sodium
- Weight management
- Calcium intake

- Use of tobacco, alcohol, and caffeine
- Amount and type of daily exercise routines

Nursing Management

There is no "magic bullet" in managing menopause. Nurses can counsel women about their risks and help them to prevent disease and debilitating conditions with specific health maintenance education. Women should make their own decisions, but the nurse should make sure they are armed with the facts to do so intelligently. Nurses can offer a thorough explanation of the menopausal process, including the latest research findings, to help women understand and make decisions about this inevitable event.

If the woman decides to use HT to control her menopausal symptoms, after being thoroughly educated, she will need frequent reassessment. There are no hard-and-fast rules that apply to meeting a woman's individual needs. The nurse can provide realistic expectations of the therapy to reduce the woman's anxiety and concern.

It is also useful to emphasize the value of friends to gain support and share information and resources. Often just talking about emotional difficulties such as the death of a parent or problematic relationships helps solve problems. It also shows the woman that her emotional responses are valid.

Healthy lifestyles and stress management techniques are vital to health and longevity, and it is important to keep these on the client's agenda when discussing menopause (North American Menopause Society, 2015). Evidence-based interventions include lifestyle modifications, risk management therapies, and preventive drug interventions, such as the following:

- Participate actively in maintaining health.
- Exercise regularly to prevent CVD and osteoporosis.
- Take supplemental calcium and eat appropriately to prevent osteoporosis.
- Stop smoking to prevent lung and heart disease.
- Reduce caffeine and alcohol intake to prevent osteoporosis.
- Monitor blood pressure, lipids, and diabetes (drug therapy management).
- Use low-dose aspirin to prevent blood clots.
- Reduce dietary intake of fat, cholesterol, and sodium to prevent CVD.
- Maintain a healthy weight for body frame.
- Perform breast self-examinations for breast awareness.
- Control stress to prevent depression (Worel & Hayman, 2015).

These life approaches may seem low-tech, but they can stave off menopause-related complications such as CVD, osteoporosis, and depression. These tips for healthy living work well, but the client needs to be motivated to stick with them.

KEY CONCEPTS

- Establishing good health habits and avoiding risky behaviors early in life will prevent chronic conditions later in life.

- PMS has more than 150 symptoms, and at least 2 different syndromes have been recognized: PMS and PMDD.

- Endometriosis is a condition in which bits of functioning endometrial tissue are located outside their normal site, the uterine cavity.

- Infertility is a widespread problem that has an emotional, social, and economic impact on couples.

- More than half of all unintended pregnancies occur in women who report using some method of birth control during the month of conception.

- Hormonal methods include OCs, injectables, implants, vaginal rings, and transdermal patches.

- Recent studies have shown that the extension of active extended cycle OC pills carries the same safety profile as the conventional 28-day regimens (Zieman, 2015).

- Currently three intrauterine contraceptives are available in the United States: the copper ParaGard-TCu-380A, the levonorgestrel-releasing intrauterine system (LNG-IUS) marketed as Mirena and another LNG-IUD marketed as Skyla (King et al., 2015).

- OCs, sterilization, and male condoms are the most popular methods of contraception in the United States and worldwide (Alan Guttmacher Institute, 2015a).

- Menopause, with a dramatic decline in estrogen levels, affects not only the reproductive organs but also other body systems.

- Most women with osteoporosis do not know they have the disease until they sustain a fracture, usually of the wrist or hip (NOF, 2015a).

- Half a million women die annually in the United States of CVDs, with strokes accounting for about 20% of the deaths (Alexander et al., 2014).

- Nurses should aim to have a holistic approach to the sexual health of women from menarche through menopause.

References and Recommended Readings

Alan Guttmacher Institute. (2015a). *Facts on contraceptive use*. Retrieved from http://www.guttmacher.org/pubs/fb_contr_use.html

Alan Guttmacher Institute. (2015b). *Facts on induced abortion in the United States*. Retrieved from http://www.guttmacher.org/pubs/fb_induced_abortion.html

Alexander, L. L., LaRosa, J. H., Bader, H., & Garfield, S. (2014). *New dimensions in women's health* (6th ed.). Sudbury, MA: Jones & Bartlett.

American College of Obstetricians & Gynecologists (ACOG) (2013). ACOG Practice bulletin no. 133: Benefits and risks of sterilization. *Obstetrics & Gynecology, 121*(2 Pt 1), 392–404. doi: http://10.0.4.73/01.AOG.0000426425.33845.b2

American Academy of Allergy, Asthma and Immunolog. (2015). *Latex allergy: Tips to remember*. Retrieved from http://www.aaaai.org/conditions-and-treatments/library/allergy-library/latex-allergy.aspx

American College of Obstetricians & Gynecologists. (2015a). *Dysmenorrhea: Painful periods*. Retrieved from https://www.acog.org/-/media/For-Patients/faq046.pdf?dmc=1&ts=20150312T1116116502

American College of Obstetricians & Gynecologists. (2015b). *Management of acute abnormal uterine bleeding with ovarian dysfunction*. Retrieved from http://contemporaryobgyn.modernmedicine.com/contemporary-obgyn/content/tags/abnormal-uterine-bleeding/acog-guidelines-glance-bulletin-aub-o-much?page=full

American College of Obstetricians & Gynecologists. (2015c). *Premenstrual syndrome*. Retrieved from http://www.acog.org/Search.aspx?Keyword=PMS

American College of Obstetricians & Gynecologists. (2015d). *Dysmenorrhea: Painful periods*. FAQ046. Retrieved from www.acog.org/~/media/ForPatients/faq046.ashx

American Society for Reproductive Medicine. (2015). *Frequently asked questions about infertility*. Retrieved from http://www.asrm.org/Patients/faqs.html

Ataollahi, M., Akbari, S. A. A., Mojab, F., & Alavi Majd, H. (2015). The effect of wheat germ extract on premenstrual syndrome symptoms. *Iranian Journal of Pharmaceutical Research : IJPR, 14*(1), 159–166.

Atkin, K., Beal, M. W., Long-Middleton, E., & Roncari, D. (2015). Long-acting reversible contraceptives for teenagers: Primary care recommendations. *The Nurse Practitioner, 40*(3), 38–46.

Avis, N. E., Crawford, S. L., Greendale, G., Bromberger, J. T., Everson-Rose, S. A., Gold, E. B., et al. (2015). Duration of menopausal vasomotor symptoms over the menopause transition. *JAMA Internal Medicine, 175*(4), 531–539.

Bakour, S. H., & Williamson, J. (2015). Latest evidence on using hormone replacement therapy in the menopause. *Obstetrician & Gynecologist, 17*(1), 20–28.

Bieber, E. J., Sanfilippo, J. S., Horowitz, I. R., & Shafi, M.I (2015). *Clinical gynecology* (2nd ed.). Cambridge: Cambridge University Press.

Bitzer, J., Heikinheimo, O., Nelson, A. L., Calaf-Alsina, J., & Fraser, I. S. (2015). Medical management of heavy menstrual bleeding: A comprehensive review of the literature. *Obstetrical & Gynecological Survey, 70*(2), 115–130.

Boardman, H. M. P, Hartley, L., Eisinga, A., Main, C., Roqué i Figuls, M., Bonfill Cosp, X., et al. (2015). Hormone therapy for preventing cardiovascular disease in post-menopausal women. *Cochrane Database of Systematic Reviews*, (3), CD002229. doi: 10.1002/14651858.CD002229.pub4

Boyd, K., Perkins, P., Lawrence, K., Sutherland, J., & Blake, K. (2015). The female condom: Knowledge, image, and power. *Journal of Black Sexuality and Relationships, 1*(3), 97–112.

Brown, J., & Farquhar, C. (2015). An overview of treatments for endometriosis. *JAMA, 313*(3), 296–297.

Calis, K. A., Popat, V., Dang, D. K., & Kalantaridou, S. N. (2015). Dysmenorrhea. *eMedicine*. Retrieved from http://emedicine.medscape.com/article/253812-overview

Carlson, J. L. (2015). The menstrual cycle. In C. M. Gordon & M. S. LeBoff (Eds.), *The Female Athlete Triad* (pp. 29–38). Philadelphia, PA: Springer Publishers.

Casey, F., & Isaacs, C. (2015). Are we getting the word out about emergency contraception? *Contemporary OB/GYN, 60*(2), 18–19.

Cavallini, G. (2015). General therapeutic approach to male infertility. In G. Cavallini & G. Beretta (Eds.), *Clinical Management of Male Infertility* (pp. 33–39). Switzerland: Springer International Publishing.

Centers for Disease Control and Prevention. (2015a). *Healthy eating for a healthy weight*. Retrieved from http://www.cdc.gov/healthy-weight/healthy_eating/

Centers for Disease Control and Prevention. (2015b). *Contraceptive use*. National Center for Health Statistics. Retrieved from http://www.cdc.gov/women/natstat/reprhlth.htm#contraception

Cheng, S. C. J., & Van Leuven, K. A. (2015). Intrauterine contraception and the facts for college health. *The Journal for Nurse Practitioners*, *11*(4), 417–423.

Chomistek, A. K., Chiuve, S. E., Eliassen, A. H., Mukamal, K. J., Willett, W. C., & Rimm, E. B. (2015). Healthy lifestyle in the primordial prevention of cardiovascular disease among young women. *Journal of the American College of Cardiology*, *65*(1), 43–51.

Comhaire, F. H., & Depypere, H. T. (2015). Hormones, herbal preparations and nutraceuticals for a better life after the menopause: Part I. *Climacteric*, *18*(3):364–371. doi: 10.3109/13697137.2014.985646.

Coney, P. (2015) Menopause. *Emedicine*. Retrieved from http://emedicine.medscape.com/article/264088-overview

Craik, J., & Rowlands, S. (2015). Contraceptive devices for women: Implants, intrauterine devices and other products. In Mira Harrison-Woolrych (Ed.), *Medicines for Women* (pp. 227–270). Switzerland: Springer International Publishing.

Craik, J., & Melvin, L. (2015). Oral contraceptives: Benefits and risks. In *Medicines for Women* (pp. 141–180). Springer International Publishing.

Creatsas, G. K. (2015). Prevention of adolescent pregnancies. In Bart C. J. M. Fauser & A. R. Genazzani (Eds.), *Frontiers in gynecological endocrinology* (pp. 41–45). Switzerland: Springer International Publishing.

Creatsas, G. K., & Creatsa, M. (2015). Disorders of the menstrual cycle during adolescence. In Bart C. J. M. Fauser & A. R. Genazzani (Eds.), *Frontiers in Gynecological Endocrinology* (pp. 3–9). Switzerland: Springer International Publishing.

Curtis , K. M. (2014). U.S. selected practice recommendations for contraceptive use, 2013. *MMWR Recommendations & Reports*, *62*(5), 1–61.

Dadhich, P., Ramasamy, R., & Lipshultz, L. I. (2015). The male infertility office visit. *The Italian Journal of Urology and Nephrology*. Retrieved from http://europepmc.org/abstract/med/25604696

Dohle, G. R. (2015). Male factors in couple's infertility. In V. Mirone (Ed.), *Clinical Uro-Andrology* (pp. 197–201). Berlin Heidelberg: Springer Publishers.

Dombo, E. A., & Flood, M. (2015). Spirituality infertility counseling. In S. N. Covington (Ed.), *Fertility Counseling* (Vol. *11*, pp. 74–85), Cambridge: Cambridge University Press.

Elnashar, A. (2015). Emerging treatment of endometriosis. *Middle East Fertility Society Journal*. Retrieved from http://www.sciencedirect.com/science/article/pii/S1110569014200562

Evans, G., & Sutton, E. L. (2015). Oral contraception. *Medical Clinics of North America*, *99*(3), 479–503.

Everett, S. (2014). *Handbook of contraception and sexual health* (3rd ed.). New York: Routledge.

Foster, D. G., Biggs, M. A., Phillips, K. A., Grindlay, K., & Grossman, D. (2015). Potential public sector cost-savings from over-the-counter access to oral contraceptives. *Contraception*. doi: http://dx.doi.org/10.1016/j.contraception.2015.01.010

Ganatra, B., Guest, P., & Berer, M. (2015). Expanding access to medical abortion: challenges and opportunities. *Reproductive Health Matters*, *22*(44), 1–3.

Golden, N. H., Katzman, D. K., Sawyer, S. M., Ornstein, R. M., Rome, E. S., Garber, A. K., et al. (2015). Update on the medical management of eating disorders in adolescents. *Journal of Adolescent Health*, *56*(4), 370–375.

Goswami, D. (2015). Primary ovarian insufficiency: The paradox of menopause in young women. *MAMC Journal of Medical Sciences*, *1*(1), 3–5.

Haddad, L. B., Philpott-Jones, S., & Schonfeld, T. (2015). Contraception and prevention of HIV transmission: A potential conflict of public health principles. *Journal of Family Planning and Reproductive Health Care*, *41*(1), 20–23.

Hale, G. E., & Shufelt, C. L. (2015). Hormone therapy in menopause: An update on cardiovascular disease considerations. *Trends in Cardiovascular Medicine*. doi:10.1016/j.tcm.2015.01.008

Hemingway, A. P., & Trew, G. H. (2015). Hysterosalpingography. In G. F. Grimbizis, R. Campo, B. C. Tarlatzis, & S. Gordts (Eds.), *Female genital tract congenital malformations* (pp. 49–61). London: Springer Publishers.

Housman, J., & Odum, M. (2016) *Alters & Schiff's essential concepts for healthy living* (7th ed.). Burlington, MA: Jones & Bartlett Learning.

Hoyt, L. T., & Falconi, A. (2015). Puberty and perimenopause: Reproductive transitions and their implications for women's health. *Social Science & Medicine*, *132*, 103–112.

Htay, T. T. (2015). Premenstrual dysphoric disorder. *eMedicine*. Retrieved from http://emedicine.medscape.com/article/293257-overview

Hughes, H. (2015). Postpartum contraception. *Journal of Family Health Care*, *19*(1), 9–10.

Ilic, K. (2015). Emergency contraception. In M. Harrison-Woolrych (Ed.), *Medicines for women* (pp. 203–225). Switzerland: Springer.

Inhorn, M. C., & Patrizio, P. (2015). Infertility around the globe: New thinking on gender, reproductive technologies and global movements in the 21st century. *Human Reproduction Update*. doi: 10.1093/humupd/dmv016

Ismail, R., Taylor-Swanson, L., Thomas, A., Schnall, J. G., Cray, L., Mitchell, E. S., et al. (2015). Effects of herbal preparations on symptom clusters during the menopausal transition. *Climacteric*, *18*(1), 11–28.

Jick, S. (2015). Oral contraceptives and the risk of venous thromboembolism. In M. Harrison-Woolrych (Ed.), *Medicines for Women* (pp. 181–201). Switzerland: Springer International Publishing.

Jin, J. (2015). Treatments for infertility. *JAMA*, *313*(3), 320–320.

Johnston, J. L., Reid, H., & Hunter, D. (2015). Diagnosing endometriosis in primary care: clinical update. *British Journal of General Practice*, *65*(631), 101–102.

Joshi, T., Kural, M. R., Agrawal, D. P., Noor, N. N., & Patil, A. (2015). Primary dysmenorrhea and its effect on quality of life in young girls. *International Journal of Medical Science and Public Health*, *4*(3), 381–385.

Kapoor, D. W., Alderman, E., Hiraoka, M. K., & Davila, G. W. (2015) Endometriosis. *eMedicine*. Retrieved from http://emedicine.medscape.com/article/271899-overview

Khan, A. B., & Krupanidhi, C. S. C. (2015). A review on vaginal drug delivery system. *RGUHS Journal of Pharmaceutical Sciences*, *4*(4), 142–147.

Kessenich, C. R. (2015). Inevitable menopause. *Nursing Spectrum*. Retrieved from http://ce.nurse.com/ce232-60/Inevitable-Menopause

Kho, C. L., & Mathur, M. (2015). Uterine artery embolization for acute dysfunctional uterine bleeding with failed medical therapy: A novel approach to management. *BMJ Case Reports*, *2015*. doi:10.1136/bcr-2014-204446

Kim, J. S. (2015). Latex allergy. In H. A. Sampson (Ed.), *Allergy and clinical immunology* (pp. 288–293), Chichester: John Wiley & Sons.

King, T. L., & Brucker, M. C. (2016). *Pharmacology for women's health* (2nd ed.). Sudbury, MA: Jones & Bartlett Learning.

King, T. L., Brucker, M. C., Kriebs, J. M., Fahey, J. O., Gegor, C. L., & Varney, H. (2015). *Varney's midwifery*. Burlington, MA: Jones & Bartlett Learning.

Kodaman, P. H. (2015). Current strategies for endometriosis management. *Obstetrics and Gynecology Clinics of North America*, *42*(1), 87–101.

Kovanci, E., & Schutt, A. K. (2015). Premature ovarian failure: Clinical presentation and treatment. *Obstetrics and Gynecology Clinics of North America*, *42*(1), 153–161.

Kreitzer, R. J. (2015). Politics and morality in state abortion policy. *State Politics & Policy Quarterly*. doi:1532440014561868.

Krieger, N., Kiang, M. V., Kosheleva, A., Waterman, P. D., Chen, J. T., & Beckfield, J. (2015), Age at menarche: 50-Year socioeconomic trends among US-born Black and White women. *American Journal of Public Health*, *105*(2), 388–397.

Kyvernitakis, I., Kostev, K., Hars, O., Albert, U., & Hadji, P. (2015). Discontinuation rates of menopausal hormone therapy among postmenopausal women in the post-WHI Study ERA. *Climacteric* *18*(5), 1–22.

Maurice, J. M., & Rosenzweig, B. A. (2015). Acute gynecologic pelvic pain. In J. A. Myers, K. W. Millikan & T. J. Saclarides (Eds.), *Common surgical diseases* (pp. 319–322). New York: Springer Publishers.

McFarland, M. R., & Wehbe-Alamah, H. B. (2015) *Leininger's cultural care diversity and universality: A worldwide nursing theory* (3rd ed.). Burlington, MA: Jones & Bartlett Learning.

McFarlane, D. R. (2015). *Global population and reproductive health*. Burlington, MA: Jones & Bartlett Learning.

McKay, R., & Schunmann, C. (2015). Male and female sterilization. *Obstetrics, Gynecology & Reproductive Medicine*. doi: http://dx.doi.org/10.1016/j.ogrm.2015.02.004

McNamara, M., Batur, P., & DeSapri, K. T. (2015). In the clinic. Perimenopause. *Annals of Internal Medicine*, *162*(3), ITC1–ITC15.

Mirkin, S., Archer, D. F., Pickar, J. H., & Komm, B. S. (2015). Recent advances help understand and improve the safety of menopausal therapies. *Menopause (10723714)*, *22*(3), 351–360.

Moses, S. (2015a) Primary amenorrhea. *Family Practice Notebook*. Retrieved from http://www.fpnotebook.com/gyn/Menses/PrmryAmnrh.htm

Moses, S. (2015b) Female Tanner stage. *Family Practice Notebook*. Retrieved from http://www.fpnotebook.com/endo/exam/fmltnrstg.htm

Moses, S. (2015c) Contraceptive sponge. *Family Practice Notebook*. Retrieved from http://www.fpnotebook.com/gyn/contraception/CntrcptvSpng.htm

Mulligan, K. (2015). Access to emergency contraception and its impact on fertility and sexual behavior. *Health Economics*. doi:10.1002/hec.3163

Naeimi, N. (2015) The prevalence and symptoms of premenstrual syndrome under examination. *Journal of Biosciences and Medicines*, *3*, 1–8.

National Institute of Child Health and Human Development. (2015). Endometriosis. (NIH Pub. No. 02–2413). Retrieved from http://www.nichd.nih.gov/publications/pubs/endometriosis

National Osteoporosis Foundation. (2015a). *Osteoporosis: Fast facts*. Retrieved from http://www.nof.org/osteoporosis/diseasefacts.htm

National Osteoporosis Foundation. (2015b). *Steps to prevent osteoporosis*. Retrieved from http://www.nof.org/prevention/index.htm

Nelson, A. L. (2015). Transdermal contraception methods: Today's patches and new options on the horizon. *Expert Opinion on Pharmacotherapy*, *16*(6), 863–873

North American Menopause Society. (2015). *Staying healthy at menopause and beyond*. Retrieved from http://www.menopause.org/for-women/menopauseflashes/staying-healthy-at-menopause-and-beyond

Occupational Health and Safety Administration. (2015). *Latex allergy*. Retrieved from http://www.osha.gov/SLTC/latexallergy

Pagana, K. D., Pagana, T. J., & Pagana, T. N. (2015). *Mosby's diagnostic and laboratory test reference* (12th ed.). St. Louis, MO: Elsevier Mosby.

Patil, E., & Edelman, A. (2015). Medical abortion: Use of mifepristone and misoprostol in first and second trimesters of pregnancy. *Current Obstetrics and Gynecology Reports*, *4*(1), 69–78.

Pearlstein, T. (2015) Depressive disorders: Premenstrual dysphoric disorder. In *Psychiatry* (4th ed.). Chichester: John Wiley & Sons. doi: 10.1002/9781118753378.ch51

Planned Parenthood. (2015a). *Fertility awareness-based methods*. Retrieved from http://www.plannedparenthood.org/health-topics/birth-control/fertility-awareness-4217.htm

Planned Parenthood. (2015b). *The abortion pill*. Retrieved from http://m.plannedparenthood.org/mt/www.plannedparenthood.org/health-topics/abortion/abortion-pill-medication-abortion-4354.asp

Planned Parenthood. (2016). *Cervical cap (FemCap)*. Retrieved from https://www.plannedparenthood.org/learn/birth-control/cervical-cap

Pocius, K. D., & Dutton, C. R. (2015). Update on hormonal contraception and obesity. *Current Obstetrics and Gynecology Reports*, *4*, 61–68.

Puscheck, E. E., & Woodward, T. L. (2015). Infertility. *eMedicine*. Retrieved from http://emedicine.medscape.com/article/274143-overview

Raymond, E. G., & Cleland, K. (2015). Emergency contraception. *New England Journal of Medicine*, *372*(14), 1342–1348

RESOLVE (National Infertility Association). (2015). *What is infertility?* Retrieved from http://www.resolve.org/infertility-overview/what-is-infertility

Samra-Latif, O. M., & Wood, E. (2015). Contraception. *eMedicine*. Retrieved from http://emedicine.medscape.com/article/258507-overview

Santamaría, M., & Lago, I. (2015). Premenstrual experience premenstrual syndrome and dysphoric disorder. In M. Saenza-Herrero (Ed.), *Psychopathology in women* (pp. 423–449). Switzerland: Springer International Publishing.

Schuiling, K. D., & Likis, F. E. (2016) *Women's gynecologic health* (4th ed.). Burlington, MA: Jones & Bartlett Learning.

Schwartz, J. L., Weiner, D. H., Lai, J. J., Frezieres, R. G., Creinin, M. D., Archer, D. F., et al. (2015). Contraceptive efficacy, safety, fit, and acceptability of a single-size diaphragm developed with end-user input. *Obstetrics & Gynecology*, *125*(4), 895–903.

Senie, R. T. (2014). *Epidemiology of women's health*. Burlington, MA: Jones & Bartlett Learning.

Sharma, M., & Walmsley, S. (2015). Contraceptive options for HIV-positive women: Making evidence-based, patient-centered decisions. *HIV Medicine*. doi: 10.1111/hiv.12221

Signorile, P. G., & Baldi, A. (2015). New evidence in endometriosis. *The International Journal of Biochemistry & Cell Biology*, *60*, 19–22.

Skidmore-Roth, L. (2015). *Mosby's 2015 nursing drug reference* (28th ed.). St. Louis, MO: Elsevier Mosby.

Smith, R. P., & Kaunitz, A. M. (2015). Treatment of primary dysmenorrhea in adult women. *UpToDate*. Retreved from http://www.uptodate.com/contents/treatment-of-primary-dysmenorrhea-in-adult-women

Stanford, J. B. (2015). Revisiting the fertile window. *Fertility and Sterility*. doi:10.1016/j.fertnstert.2015.02.015

Stewart, M., & Black, K. (2015). Choosing a combined oral contraceptive pill. *Australian Prescriber*, *38*(1), 6–11.

Sullivan, S. D., Lehman, A., Thomas, F., Johnson, K. C., Jackson, R., Wactawski-Wende, J., et al. (2015). Effects of self-reported age at nonsurgical menopause on time to first fracture and bone mineral density in the Women's Health Initiative Observational Study. *Menopause (New York, N.Y.)*. [Serial on the Internet. Retrieved from MEDLINE.

Tacani, P. M., Ribeiro, D. O., Barros Guimarães, B. E., Machado, A. P., & Tacani, R. E. (2015). Characterization of symptoms and edema distribution in premenstrual syndrome. *International Journal of Women's Health*, *7*, 297–303.

Tharpe, N. L., Farley, C. L., & Jordan, R. G. (2016). *Clinical practice guidelines for midwifery & women's health* (5th ed.). Burlington, MA: Jones & Bartlett Learning.

Thurkow, A. L. (2015). Hysteroscopic sterilization. In O. Istre (Ed.), *Minimally invasive gynecological surgery* (pp. 49–59). Berlin Heidelberg: Springer.

Tremellen, K., & Pearce, K. (2015). *Nutrition, fertility, and human reproductive function*. Boca Raton, FL: CRC Press Taylor & Francis Group.

Turchi, P. (2015). Prevalence, definition, and classification of infertility. In G. Cavallini & G. Beretta (Ed.), *Clinical management of male infertility* (pp. 5–11). Switzerland: Springer International Publishing.

Udoh A., Effa E. E., Oduwole O., Okusanya B. O., Okafo O., & Iya J. (2015) Antibiotics for treating septic abortion. *Cochrane Database of Systematic Reviews*, *2015*(2), CD011528. doi: 10.1002/14651858.CD011528

United Nations Population Fund. (2015). *The state of the world population 2014 report*. Retrieved from http://www.unfpa.org/swp#ref_state-of-world-population-2014

Upadhyay, U. D., Desai, S., Zlidar, V., Weitz, T. A., Grossman, D., Anderson, P., et al. (2015). Incidence of emergency department visits and complications after abortion. *Obstetrics & Gynecology*, *125*(1), 175–183.

U.S. Preventive Services Task Force. (2015). Screening for osteoporosis: Recommendation statement. *The Journal of Family Practice*, *62*(5), 249–252; *83*(10), 1197–1200.

Walsh, S., Ismaili, E., Naheed, B., & O'Brien, S. (2015). Diagnosis, pathophysiology and management of premenstrual syndrome. *The Obstetrician & Gynaecologist*. doi:10.1111/tog.12180

Wang, Q., Chen, D., Cheng, S. M., Nicholson, P., Alen, M., & Cheng, S. (2015). Growth and aging of proximal femoral bone: a study with women spanning three generations. *Journal of Bone and Mineral Research: The Official Journal of the American Society for Bone and Mineral Research*, *30*(3), 528–534.

Weinberger, A. H., Smith, P. H., Allen, S. S., Cosgrove, K. P., Saladin, M. E., Gray, K. M., et al. (2015). Systematic and meta-analytic review of research examining the impact of menstrual cycle phase and ovarian hormones on smoking and cessation. *Nicotine & Tobacco Research*, *17*(4), 407–421.

Whitaker, T. (2015). Vasectomy. In A. L. Halverson & D. C. Borgstrom (Eds.), *Advanced surgical techniques for rural surgeons* (pp. 251–254). New York: Springer.

Whitman, M. (2015). Patient education: What worries the patient most? *Nursing2015*, *45*(1), 52–54.

Wicks, S. M., & Mahady, G. B. (2015). Herbal and complementary medicines used for women's health. In M. Harrison-Woolrych (Ed.), *Medicines for women* (pp. 373–399). Switzerland: Springer International Publishing.

Wildemeersch, D., & Jandi, S. (2015). Intrauterine device quo vadis? Why intrauterine device use should be revisited particularly in nulliparous women? *Open Access Journal of Contraception, 6*, 1–12.

Wolfe, K., & Cansino, C. (2015). Injectable contraception: Current practices and future trends. *Current Obstetrics and Gynecology Reports, 4*(1), 26–36.

Wood, D. (2015). Inevitable menopause. *Nurse.Com Nursing Spectrum (Philadelphia Tri-State), 24*(3), 26–31.

Woods, N. F., & Mitchell, E. S. (2015). The menopausal transition and women's health. In M. A. Farage, K. W. Miller, N. F. Woods, & H. I. Maibach (Eds.), *Skin, Mucosa and Menopause* (pp. 433–452). Berlin Heidelberg: Springer.

Worel, J. N., & Hayman, L. L. (2015). Cardiovascular disease prevention in women: Reducing the major threat to women's health. *Journal of Cardiovascular Nursing, 30*(1), 5–7.

World Health Organization. (2015). Infertility in developing countries. *Reproductive Health*. Retrieved from http://www.who.int/reproductive-health/infertility/index.htm

Wright, K., Iqteit, H., & Hardee, K. (2015) *Standard Days Method of contraception: Evidence on use, implementation, and scale-up.* Working Paper, The Evidence Project. Washington, DC: Population Council.

Ying, L. Y., & Loke, A. Y. (2015). An analysis of the concept of partnership in the couples undergoing infertility treatment. *Journal of Sex & Marital Therapy.* doi:10.1080/0092623X.2015.1010676

Zieman, M. (2015). *Managing contraception on the go* (13th ed.). New York: Ardnet Media

Zorbas, K. A., Economopoulos, K. P., & Vlahos, N. F. (2015). Continuous versus cyclic oral contraceptives for the treatment of endometriosis: a systematic review. *Archives of Gynecology and Obstetrics,* 1–7. doi: 10.1007/s00404-015-3641-1

MULTIPLE-CHOICE QUESTIONS

1. A couple is considered infertile after how many months of trying to conceive?
   a. 6 months
   b. 12 months
   c. 18 months
   d. 24 months

2. A couple reports that their condom broke while they were having sexual intercourse last night. What would you advise to prevent pregnancy?
   a. Inject a spermicidal agent into the woman's vagina immediately.
   b. Obtain emergency contraceptives and take them immediately.
   c. Douche with a solution of vinegar and hot water tonight.
   d. Take a strong laxative now and again at bedtime.

3. Which of the following combination contraceptives has been approved for extended continuous use?
   a. Seasonale
   b. Triphasil
   c. Ortho Evra
   d. Mirena

4. Which of the following measures helps prevent osteoporosis?
   a. Supplementing with iron
   b. Sleeping 8 hours nightly
   c. Eating lean meats only
   d. Walking daily

5. Which of the following activities will increase a woman's risk of cardiovascular disease if she is taking oral contraceptives?
   a. Eating a high-fiber diet
   b. Smoking cigarettes
   c. Taking daily multivitamins
   d. Drinking alcohol

6. The nurse is preparing to teach a class to a group of middle aged women regarding the most common vasomotor symptoms experienced during menopause and possible modalities of treatment available. Which of the following would be a vasomotor symptom experienced by menopausal women?
   a. Weight gain
   b. Bone density
   c. Hot flashes
   d. Heart disease

7. Throughout life, a woman's most proactive activity to promote her health would be to engage in:
   a. consistent exercise
   b. socialization with friends
   c. quality quiet time with herself
   d. consuming water

8. What comment by a woman would indicate that a diaphragm is not the best contraceptive device for her?
   a. "My husband says it is my job to keep from getting pregnant."
   b. "I have a hard time remembering to take my vitamins daily."
   c. "Hormones cause cancer and I don't want to take them."
   d. "I am not comfortable touching myself down there."

9. The most common cause of menstrual abnormality in a reproductive-age woman is:
   a. ectopic pregnancy
   b. coagulopathy
   c. carcinoma
   d. anovulation

CRITICAL THINKING EXERCISE

1. Ms. London, age 25, comes to your family planning clinic requesting to have an IUC inserted because "birth control pills give you cancer." In reviewing her history, you note she has been into the STI clinic three times in the past year with vaginal infections and was hospitalized for PID last month. When you question her about her sexual history, she reports having sex with multiple partners and not always using protection.
   a. Is an IUC the most appropriate method for her? Why or why not?
   b. What myths/misperceptions will you address in your counseling session?
   c. Outline the safer sex discussion you plan to have with her.

STUDY ACTIVITIES

1. Develop a teaching plan for an adolescent with PMS and dysmenorrhea.

2. Arrange to shadow a nurse working in family planning for the morning. What questions does the nurse ask to ascertain the kind of family planning method that is right for each woman? What teaching goes along with each method? What follow-up care is needed? Share your findings with your classmates during a clinical conference.

3. Surf the Internet and locate three resources for infertile couples to consult that provide support and resources.

4. Sterilization is the most prevalent method of contraception used by married couples in the United States. Contact a local urologist and gynecologist to learn about the procedure involved and the cost of a male and female sterilization. Which procedure poses less risk to the person and costs less?

5. Take a field trip to a local drugstore to check out the variety and costs of male and female condoms. How many different brands did you find? What was the range of costs?

6. Noncontraceptive benefits of combined oral contraceptives include which of the following? Select all that apply.
   a. Protection against ovarian cancer
   b. Protection against endometrial cancer
   c. Protection against breast cancer
   d. Reduction in incidence of ectopic pregnancy
   e. Prevention of functional ovarian cysts
   f. Reduction in deep venous thrombosis
   g. Reduction in the risk of colorectal cancer

BRINGING IT ALL TOGETHER: CASE STUDY

L. H. is a 66-year-old White female who presents to the Women's Health Primary Care Clinic for her annual gynecologic examination. She states that she is fairly healthy with no active medical conditions other than hypertension controlled with medication. She is postmenopausal and feels she is doing well, but has a few questions and concerns. Her primary concern is that she is bothered by vaginal dryness and pain with sexual intercourse. Over-the-counter lubricants and moisturizers have not been useful. She never took HT since her hot flashes were not severe, but asks if she should start taking it now to reduce her vaginal dryness.

Go to thePoint **to find questions to consider about this case.**

5

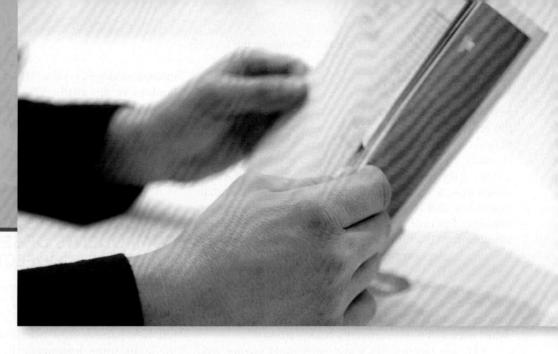

Sexually Transmitted Infections

Learning Objectives

Upon completion of the chapter, you will be able to:

1. Evaluate the spread and control of sexually transmitted infections.

2. Identify risk factors and outline appropriate client education needed in common sexually transmitted infections.

3. Describe how contraceptives can play a role in the prevention of sexually transmitted infections.

4. Analyze the physiologic and psychological aspects of sexually transmitted infections.

5. Outline the nursing management needed for women with sexually transmitted infections.

Sandy, a 19-year-old girl, couldn't imagine what these "things" were that appeared "down there" in her genital area last week. She was too embarrassed to tell anyone, so she stopped by the college health service today to find out what they were.

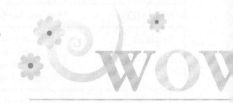

Words of Wisdom
Unconditional self-acceptance in clients is the core to reducing risky behavior and fostering peace of mind.

INTRODUCTION

Sexually transmitted infections (STIs) are infections of the reproductive tract caused by microorganisms transmitted through vaginal, anal, or oral sexual intercourse (Centers for Disease Control and Prevention [CDC], 2015a). STIs are a significant health challenge globally which pose a serious threat not only to women's sexual health but also to the general health and well-being of millions of people worldwide (see Box 5.1 for STI classification). STIs constitute an epidemic of tremendous magnitude. An estimated 65 million people live with an incurable STI, 18,000 die from acquired immune deficiency syndrome (AIDS) annually, and another 20 million are newly infected each year (CDC, 2015a). The incidence of STIs continues to rise and costs the United States over $18 billion annually (CDC, 2015a).

STIs are biologically sexist, presenting greater risk and causing more complications among women than among men. Women are diagnosed with two thirds of the estimated 20 million new cases of STIs annually in the United States. After only a single exposure, women are twice as likely as men to acquire infections from pathogens that cause gonorrhea, chlamydial infection, hepatitis B, and syphilis. Every day, more than one million people are newly infected with STIs that can lead to morbidity, mortality, and an increased risk of human immunodeficiency virus (HIV) acquisition (Fernández-Romero et al., 2015). STIs may contribute to cervical cancer, infertility, ectopic pregnancy, chronic pelvic pain, and death. Certain infections can be transmitted in utero to the fetus or during childbirth to the newborn (Table 5.1).

Additional information on therapeutic management of STIs can be found in Chapter 20.

CULTURAL AND PSYCHOLOGICAL COMPONENTS OF SEXUALLY TRANSMITTED INFECTIONS

Nurses should always address a woman's psychosocial well-being whenever a diagnosis of any STI is given. The woman may be afraid or embarrassed to tell her partner and ask him or her to seek treatment. In some instances, the woman may be afraid that telling her partner may place her in danger of escalating abuse. The nurse can empathize with the woman's feelings and suggest specific ways of talking with partners that will help decrease her anxiety and assist in efforts to control infection (Reidy et al., 2016). Nurses implementing STI prevention strategies must also acknowledge the possible role of violence in increasing women's risk as a barrier to practicing safer sex. Research suggests a strong association

TABLE 5.1	SEXUALLY TRANSMITTED INFECTIONS AND EFFECTS ON THE FETUS OR NEWBORN	
STI	**Effects on Fetus or Newborn**	
Chlamydia	Can be infected during delivery Eye infections (neonatal conjunctivitis), pneumonia, low birth weight, preterm birth, stillbirth	
Gonorrhea	Can be infected during delivery Rhinitis, vaginitis, urethritis, inflammation of sites of fetal monitoring, chorioamnionitis, preterm birth, IUGR Ophthalmia neonatorum can lead to blindness and sepsis (including arthritis and meningitis).	
Genital herpes	Contamination can occur during birth. Intellectual disability, blindness, seizures, premature birth, low birth weight, death	
HIV/AIDS	Preterm birth, low birth weight, HIV positive status, intrauterine fetal death, miscarriage	
Syphilis	Can be passed in utero Can result in fetal or infant death Congenital syphilis symptoms include skin ulcers, rashes, fever, weakened or hoarse cry, swollen liver and spleen, jaundice and anemia, various deformations.	
Trichomoniasis	Premature rupture of membranes, preterm birth, low birth weight	
Genital warts	May develop warts in throat (laryngeal papillomatosis); uncommon but life threatening	

Adapted from Burnett, E., Loucks, T. L., & Lindsay, M. (2015). Perinatal outcomes in HIV positive women with concomitant sexually transmitted infections. *Infectious Diseases in Obstetrics & Gynecology*. doi: 10.1155/2015/5084822015(508482; Centers for Disease Control and Prevention [CDC]. (2015s). *HIV among pregnant women, infants, and children*. Retrieved from http://www.cdc.gov/hiv/risk/gender/pregnantwomen/facts/; and Anderson, B., & Cu-Uvin, S. (2015). HIV and pregnancy. *UpToDate*. Retrieved from http://www.uptodate.com/contents/hiv-and-pregnancy-beyond-the-basics.

CDC CLASSIFICATION OF SEXUALLY TRANSMITTED INFECTIONS

- Infections characterized by vaginal discharge
  - Vulvovaginal candidiasis
  - Trichomoniasis
  - Bacterial vaginosis
- Infections characterized by cervicitis
  - Chlamydia
  - Gonorrhea
- Infections characterized by genital ulcers
  - Genital herpes simplex
  - Syphilis
- Vaccine-preventable STIs
  - Hepatitis A
  - Hepatitis B
  - Human papillomavirus (HPV)
- Ectoparasitic infections
  - Pediculosis pubis
  - Scabies

Adapted from Centers for Disease Control and Prevention [CDC]. (2015k). *STD treatment guidelines*. Retrieved from http://www.cdc.gov/std/treatment/2010/default.htm.

BOX 5.2

SEXUALLY TRANSMITTED INFECTIONS IN DIVERSE CULTURES

Cultural adaptation is an important step in the process of implementing health promotion interventions that, having been proven to be effective in one culture, are being applied in another. Nurses working with women from diverse cultures need to be cognizant of effective methods of STI prevention.

In a recent CDC study, greater prevention intervention efficacy was observed in studies that specifically targeted females of different cultures that used gender- or culture-specific materials, used female deliverers, addressed empowerment issues, provided skills training in condom use and negotiation of safer sex, and used role-playing to teach negotiation skills. The incidence of STIs was reduced significantly (Thomas et al., 2015). To truly maximize the impact of behavioral interventions and risk reduction programs, nurses must adjust for social and cultural differences within any diverse population group for which they care.

Racial minorities continue to face severe disparities in all reportable STIs, but African Americans are the group most affected. Gonorrhea rates among African Americans are higher than those for any other racial or ethnic group and 15 times higher than that of Whites (Kraft et al., 2015). Nurses cannot ignore the glaring racial disparities in rates of STIs. Research has shown that socioeconomic barriers to quality health care and higher overall prevalence of STIs within minority communities contribute to this pervasive threat. It is imperative that the health care team work together to improve access to effective STI prevention and treatment services in local communities for those who need it the most. By adopting a multicultural approach to the control of STIs, nurses can address specific cultural attitudes and behaviors that may impact exposure to STIs and intervene to reduce them.

---

between intimate partner violence and STIs. Both need to be addressed to reduce the spread of STIs. Even brief interventions in the health care settings are not only feasible but also potentially lifesaving for women experiencing violence in their lives (Durevall & Lindskog, 2015).

STIs know no gender, class, racial, ethnic, or social barriers—all individuals are vulnerable if exposed to the infectious organism. The problem of STIs has still not been tackled adequately on a global scale, and until this is done, numbers worldwide will continue to increase. Nurses working with women from diverse cultures need to be cognizant of effective methods of STI prevention (Box 5.2).

Given the high value some cultures place on virginity and fidelity, a diagnosis of an STI can be devastating to the woman and her family. Even to suggest a test for STIs can appear inappropriate or offensive. When a client must be screened for STIs, explaining the need carefully and not revealing to other family members that testing has occurred are essential. By adopting a multicultural approach to the control of STIs, nurses can address specific cultural and religious attitudes and behaviors that influence exposure to STIs (Thomas et al., 2015). To maximize the impact of behavioral interventions and risk reduction programs, the nurse must adjust for social and cultural differences within all diverse populations. Nurses play a crucial role in supporting women from diverse cultures within sexual health services and as trusted health care providers in a range of settings.

SEXUALLY TRANSMITTED INFECTIONS AND ADOLESCENTS

STIs occur disproportionately in adolescents. An estimated two thirds of all STIs occur among persons under the age of 25. Forty-seven percent of high school students report having been sexually active. These data reinforce existing recommendations for sexual health education and STI prevention targeting adolescents before sexual debut (Liu et al., 2015).

Risk Factors

Because of biologic and behavioral factors, adolescents are at particularly high risk for acquiring STIs and for the serious, long-term, potentially life-altering sequelae that can develop from undiagnosed, untreated infections. Each year 5 million cases of STIs occur among teenagers

(CDC, 2015a). In the United States, teens who are sexually active experience high rates of STIs, and some groups are at higher risk, including African American youths, abused youths, homeless youths, young men having sex with men, and lesbian, gay, bisexual, and transgendered (LGBT) youths. High-risk factors in adolescents include having multiple or new sexual partners and not using condoms for any number of reasons. Inexperience with condoms also can lead to more condom accidents, such as breakage caused by storage in a hot environment, opening packages with teeth, using long fingernails to put condoms on, slippage if the wrong size condom is used, or failure to hold the condom while withdrawing. Furthermore, some adolescents are unwilling to disclose their sexual activity. If symptoms of an STI develop, they may misperceive them as normal, consequently delaying medical treatment. Untreated STIs can cause pelvic inflammatory disease (PID, which can lead to infertility), adverse pregnancy outcomes, and anogenital and cervical cancers. In addition, the presence of other STIs increases the likelihood of both transmitting and acquiring HIV (Smith, 2015).

Take Note!

It is estimated that before graduating from high school, 25% of adolescents will contract an STI (CDC, 2015a).

Biologic and behavioral factors place teenagers at high risk. Female adolescents are more susceptible to STIs than males due to their anatomy. During adolescence and young adulthood, women's columnar epithelial cells are especially sensitive to invasion by sexually transmitted organisms, such as chlamydia and gonococci, because they extend out over the vaginal surface of the cervix, where they are unprotected by cervical mucus; these cells recede to a more protected location as women age. Behaviorally, adolescents and young adults tend to think they are invincible and deny the risks of their behavior. This risky behavior exposes them to STIs and HIV/AIDS. Adolescents frequently have unprotected intercourse, they engage in partnerships of limited duration, and they face many obstacles that prevent them from using the health care system.

Healthy People 2020 Objective

Healthy People 2020 (U.S. Department of Health & Human Services [USDHHS], 2010) provides science-based, 10-year national objectives for improving the health of all people in the United States. For three decades, *Healthy People* has established benchmarks and monitored progress over time. One specific *Healthy People 2020* goal that applies to this chapter is to promote healthy sexual behaviors, strengthen community

capacity, and increase access to quality services to prevent STIs and their complications.

An important feature of *Healthy People 2020* is its emphasis on responsibility. People need to accept responsibility for their lifestyle choices and behaviors. This personal responsibility is especially important for sexually active adolescents because they contract the highest rate of STIs as a result of making poor choices. Chlamydial and gonorrheal infections are the two most commonly reported bacterial STIs in the United States, and their prevalence is highest among females aged 15 to 24. Human papillomavirus (HPV) infection, trichomoniasis, and herpes simplex virus (HSV) infections are also common in adolescents (Jones, 2015). The *Healthy People 2020* objective, "Increase the proportion of sexually active persons aged 15 to 19 years who use condoms to both effectively prevent pregnancy and provide barrier protection against disease," addresses this personal responsibility focus (USDHHS, 2010).

Healthy People 2020's emphasis on personal responsibility gives adolescents a role in the quality of their lives and the length of healthy life they may have by making the right choices and engaging in nonrisky behaviors.

Nursing Assessment

Many health care providers fail to assess adolescent sexual behavior and STI risks, to screen for asymptomatic infection during clinic visits, or to counsel adolescents on STI risk reduction. Nurses need to remember that they play a key role in the detection, prevention, and treatment of STIs in adolescents. All states allow adolescents to give consent to confidential STI testing and treatment. Table 5.2 discusses the clinical manifestations of common STIs in adolescents.

Nursing Management

Prevention of STIs among adolescents is critical. Health care providers have a unique opportunity to provide counseling and education to their clients. Adolescents are less willing to be open to nurses and less likely to return for care if they are uncertain about confidentiality. Nurses working with adolescents need to convey their willingness to discuss sexual habits, and any interactions with clients need to be direct and nonjudgmental.

Nurses can provide effective guidance and promote sexual health so that primary or repeat infections can be avoided. Adolescents bear disproportionate burdens when it comes to STIs, so education is needed to help them protect their reproductive futures. Specific actions to take include the following:

- Encourage the client to complete antibiotic prescriptions (specific management for each type of STI is discussed below).

(text continues on page 151)

TABLE 5.2 COMMON SEXUALLY TRANSMITTED INFECTIONS

Disease	Causative Organism	Transmission Mode	Diagnostic Testing	Female Symptoms	Male Symptoms	Treatment
Chlamydia Curable STI Seen frequently among sexually active adolescents and young adults Sexually active adolescents should be screened at least annually.	*Chlamydia trachomatis* (bacteria)	Vaginal, anal, oral sex, and by childbirth	Culture fluid from urethral swabs in males or endocervical swabs for females and conjunctival secretions in neonates	May be asymptomatic Dysuria Vaginal discharge (mucus or pus) Endocervicitis May lead to pelvic inflammatory disease, ectopic pregnancy, and infertility Can cause inflammation of the rectum and lining of the eye (conjunctivitis) Can infect the throat from oral sexual contact with an infected partner	May be asymptomatic Dysuria Penile discharge (mucus or pus) Urethral tingling May lead to epididymitis (inflammation of the epididymis, the tubular structure that connects the testicle with the vas deferens) and sterility Can cause inflammation of the rectum and lining of the eye (conjunctivitis) Can infect the throat from oral sexual contact with an infected partner	Azithromycin (Zithromax) Doxycycline (Vibramycin) Erythromycin (EES) Ofloxacin (Floxin) Sexual partners need evaluation, testing, and treatment also.
Gonorrhea Curable STI Client is often co-infected with *Chlamydia trachomatis*	*Neisseria gonorrhoeae* (bacteria)	Vaginal, anal, oral sex, and by childbirth	Staining samples directly for the bacterium, detection of bacterial genes or DNA in urine, and growing the bacteria in laboratory cultures More than one test may be used	May be asymptomatic or no recognizable symptoms until serious complications such as pelvic inflammatory disease Dysuria Urinary frequency Vaginal discharge (yellow, foul) Dyspareunia Endocervicitis Arthritis	Most produce symptoms but can be asymptomatic Dysuria Penile discharge (pus) Arthritis May lead to epididymitis and sterility Symptoms of rectal infection include discharge, anal itching, and occasional painful bowel movements with fresh blood.	Usually a single dose of one of the following: Cefixime (Suprax) Ciprofloxacin (Cipro) Ceftriaxone (Rocephin) Ofloxacin (Floxin) Levofloxacin (Levaquin) **No Floxin or Cipro if <18 years or pregnant!**

(continued)

TABLE 5.2 COMMON SEXUALLY TRANSMITTED INFECTIONS (continued)

Disease	Causative Organism	Transmission Mode	Diagnostic Testing	Female Symptoms	Male Symptoms	Treatment
				May lead to pelvic inflammatory disease, ectopic pregnancy, and infertility. Symptoms of rectal infection include discharge, anal itching, and occasional painful bowel movements with fresh blood.		Azithromycin (Zithromax) Doxycycline (Vibramycin) Usually will be treated for co-infection with chlamydia, so a combination is given (e.g., ceftriaxone and doxycycline). Sexual partners need evaluation, testing, and treatment also.
Genital herpes Lifelong recurrent viral disease Most people have not been diagnosed. There is no cure.	Herpes simplex virus II (HSV II)	Having sexual contact (vaginal, oral, or anal) with someone who is shedding the herpes virus either during an outbreak or during a period with no symptoms Can be transmitted through close skin-to-skin contact	Visual inspection and symptoms or culture Virologic and type-specific serologic tests can tell if herpes simplex virus II is present but does not confirm genital herpes, though most providers will assume a positive HSV II means genital herpes. IgG/IgM antibody testing is also done.	Blister-like genital lesions Dysuria Fever, headache, muscle aches	Blister-like genital lesions Dysuria Fever, headache, muscle aches	Acyclovir (Zovirax) Other antivirals DOES NOT CURE, just controls symptoms Sexual partners benefit from evaluation and counseling. If symptomatic, they need treatment. If asymptomatic, offer testing and education.
Syphilis	*Treponema pallidum* (spirochete bacteria)	Sexual contact with an infected person	Blood tests Venereal Disease Research Laboratory (VDRL), Rapid Plasma Reagin (RPR), and treponemal tests (e.g.,	Disease is divided into four stages: *Primary infection* • Chancre on place of entrance of bacteria (usually vulva or vagina but can develop in other parts of the body)	Disease is divided into four stages: *Primary infection* • Chancre on place of entrance of bacteria (usually on penis but can develop in other parts of the body)	Penicillin G inj. (if penicillin allergy, doxycycline or erythromycin) Azithromycin; Rocephin, Cipro Sexual partners need evaluation and testing.

Disease	Cause	Transmission	Diagnosis	Signs & Symptoms (Female)	Signs & Symptoms (Male)	Treatment
			fluorescent treponemal antibody absorbed [FTA-ABS] can lead to a presumptive diagnosis. Dark-field examination and direct fluorescent antibody tests of lesion exudate or tissue provide definitive diagnosis of early syphilis.	*Secondary infection* • Maculopapular rash (hands & feet) • Sore throat • Lymphadenopathy • Flu-like symptoms*Latent infection* • No symptoms • No longer contagious • Many people if not treated will suffer no further signs and symptoms. Some people will go on to develop tertiary or late syphilis. *Tertiary infections* • Tumors of skin, bones & liver • CNS symptoms • CV symptoms • Usually not reversible at this stage	*Secondary, latent, and tertiary infections* All similar to female symptoms	
Trichomoniasis	*Trichomonas vaginalis* (protozoan)	Vaginal intercourse with an infected partner; May be picked up from direct genital contact with damp or moist objects, such as towels, wet clothing, or a toilet seat	Microscopic evaluation of vaginal secretions or culture	Many women have symptoms but some may be asymptomatic. Dysuria Urinary frequency Vaginal discharge (yellow, green, or gray & foul odor) Dyspareunia Irritation or itching of genital area	Most infected men are asymptomatic. Dysuria Penile discharge (watery, white)	Metronidazole (Flagyl) Sexual partners need evaluation, testing, and treatment also.

(continued)

TABLE 5.2 COMMON SEXUALLY TRANSMITTED INFECTIONS (continued)

Disease	Causative Organism	Transmission Mode	Diagnostic Testing	Female Symptoms	Male Symptoms	Treatment
Genital Warts (condylomata acuminata) One of the most common STIs in the United States Could lead to cancers of the cervix, vulva, vagina, anus, or penis No cure; warts can be removed but virus remains	Human papillomavirus	Vaginal, anal, or oral sex with an infected partner	Visual inspection Abnormal Pap smear may indicate cervical infection of HPV.	Wart-like lesions that are soft, moist, or flesh colored and appear on the vulva and cervix and inside and surrounding the vagina and anus Sometimes appear in clusters that resemble cauliflower-like bumps, and are either raised or flat, small or large	Wart-like lesions that are soft, moist, or flesh colored and appear on the scrotum or penis Sometimes appear in clusters that resemble cauliflower-like bumps, and are either raised or flat, small or large	May disappear without treatment Treatment is aimed at removing the lesions rather than HPV itself No optimal treatment has been identified, but there are several ways to treat them depending on size and location. Most methods rely on chemical or physical destruction of the lesion: Imiquimod cream 20% Podophyllin antimitotic solution 0.5% Podofilox solution 5% 5-Fluorouracil cream Trichloroacetic acid (TCA) Small warts can be removed by: • Freezing (cryosurgery) • Burning (electrocautery) • Laser treatment Large warts that have not responded to treatment may be removed surgically.

Adapted from Centers for Disease Control and Prevention [CDC]. (2015k). *STD treatment guidelines*. Retrieved from http://www.cdc.gov/std/treatment/2010/default.htm; and King, T. L., Brucker, M. C., Kriebs, J. M., Fahey, J. O., Gegor, C. L., & Varney, H. (2015). *Varney's midwifery* (5th ed.). Burlington, MA: Jones & Bartlett Learning.

HEALTHY PEOPLE *2020 • 5.1*

Healthy People 2020 STI Objectives	Nursing Significance
STD-1 Reduce the proportion of young adults with *Chlamydia trachomatis* infections.	Provide confidential care to all young females.
STD-3 Increase the proportion of sexually active females aged 21 to 24 years enrolled in Medicaid plans that are screened for genital *Chlamydia* infections during the measurement year.	Assess for sexual behaviors and STI risks during clinic visits; take every opportunity to educate on risks of STIs and risk reduction.
STD-4 Increase the proportion of sexually active females aged 21 to 24 years and under enrolled in commercial health insurance plans that are screened for genital *Chlamydia* infections during the measurement year.	Be direct and nonjudgmental and tailor your approach to the client.
STD-6 Reduce gonorrhea rates.	Encourage women to minimize their lifetime number of sexual partners.
STD-7 Reduce sustained domestic transmission of primary and secondary syphilis.	Educate about the importance of correct and consistent condom use.
STD-9 (Developmental) Reduce the proportion of females with human papillomavirus (HPV) infection.	
STD-10 Reduce the proportion of young adults with genital herpes infection due to herpes simplex type 2.	

Healthy People objectives based on data from http://www.healthypeople.gov.

- Adapt the style and content of any message to the client's developmental level.
- Identify risk factors and risk behaviors and guide the client to develop specific individualized actions of prevention.
- Teach adolescents about their sexual development to foster understanding of their bodily changes—the role of hormones and the emotions they are experiencing.
- Encourage adolescents to postpone initiation of sexual intercourse for as long as possible, but if they choose to have sexual intercourse, explain the necessity of using barrier methods, such as male and female condoms (Teaching Guidelines 5.1). For teens who have already

had sexual intercourse, the clinician can encourage abstinence at this point. If adolescents are sexually active, they should be directed to teen clinics, and contraceptive options should be explained. In areas where specialized teen clinics are not available, nurses should feel comfortable discussing sexuality, safety, and contraception with teens. Encourage adolescents to minimize their lifetime number of sexual partners, to use barrier methods consistently and correctly, and to be aware of the connection between drug and alcohol use and the incorrect use of barrier methods. Table 5.3 discusses barriers to condom use and means to overcome them.

HEALTHY PEOPLE *2020 • 5.2*

Healthy People 2020 STIs & Adolescents	Nursing Significance
STD-1 Reduce the proportion of adolescents with *Chlamydia trachomatis* infections.	Educate adolescents that abstinence is the only way to completely avoid contracting sexually transmitted infections.
STD-3 Increase the proportion of sexually active adolescents enrolled in Medicaid plans that are screened for genital *Chlamydia* infections during the measurement year.	Encourage adolescents to postpone initiation of sexual intercourse for as long as possible. For teens who have already had sexual intercourse, encourage abstinence at this point.
STD-4 Increase the proportion of adolescents enrolled in commercial health insurance plans that are screened for genital *Chlamydia* infections during the measurement year.	Encourage adolescents to minimize their lifetime number of sexual partners.
STD-5 Reduce the proportion of adolescents who have ever required treatment for pelvic inflammatory disease (PID).	Encourage adolescents always to use condoms if participating in any sexual act.
	Provide an open and confidential environment so that adolescents will report symptoms and seek treatment earlier.

Healthy People objectives based on data from http://www.healthypeople.gov.

TABLE 5.3	CANADIAN GUIDELINES: BARRIERS TO CONDOM USE AND MEANS TO OVERCOME THEM
Perceived Barrier	**Intervention Strategy**
Decreases sexual pleasure (sensation) Note: Often perceived by those who have never used a condom	• Encourage client to try. • Put a drop of water-based lubricant or saliva inside the tip of the condom or on the glans of the penis before putting on the condom. • Try a thinner latex condom or a different brand or more lubrication.
Decreases spontaneity of sexual activity	• Incorporate condom use into foreplay. • Remind client that peace of mind may enhance pleasure for self and partner.
Embarrassing, juvenile, "unmanly"	• Remind client that it is "manly" to protect himself and others.
Poor fit (too small or too big, slips off, uncomfortable)	• Smaller and larger condoms are available.
Requires prompt withdrawal after ejaculation	• Reinforce the protective nature of prompt withdrawal and suggest substituting other postcoital sexual activities.
Fear of breakage may lead to less vigorous sexual activity.	• With prolonged intercourse, lubricant wears off and the condom begins to rub. Have a water-soluble lubricant available to reapply.
Nonpenetrative sexual activity	• Condoms have been advocated for use during fellatio; unlubricated condoms may prove best for this purpose due to the taste of the lubricant. • Other barriers, such as dental dams or an unlubricated condom, can be cut down the middle to form a barrier; these have been advocated for use during certain forms of nonpenetrative sexual activity (e.g., cunnilingus and anolingual sex).
Allergy to latex	• Polyurethane male and female condoms are available. • A natural skin condom can be used together with a latex condom to protect the man or woman from contact with latex.

Adapted from Public Health Agency of Canada. (2015). *Canadian guidelines on sexually transmitted infections.* Retrieved from http://www.phac-aspc.gc.ca/std-mts/sti-its/pdf/401mts-prisencharge-eng.pdf.

Teaching Guidelines 5.1
PROPER CONDOM USE

• Use latex condoms to create a mechanical barrier for STIs and pregnancy
• Use a new condom with each act of sexual intercourse. Never reuse a condom.
• Handle condoms with care to prevent damage from sharp objects such as fingernails and teeth.
• Ensure condom has been stored in a cool, dry place away from direct sunlight. Do not store condoms in wallet or automobile or anywhere they would be exposed to extreme temperatures.
• Do not use a condom if it appears brittle, sticky, or discolored. These are signs of aging.
• Put condom on before any genital contact because sperm is present in preejaculate fluid.
• Put condom on when penis is erect. Ensure it is placed so it will readily unroll.
• Hold the tip of the condom while unrolling. Ensure there is a space at the tip for semen to collect, but make sure no air is trapped in the tip.
• Ensure adequate lubrication during intercourse. If external lubricants are used, use only water-based lubricants such as K-Y jelly with latex condoms. Oil-based or petroleum-based lubricants, such as body lotion, massage oil, or cooking oil, can weaken latex condoms.
• Withdraw while penis is still erect, and hold condom firmly against base of penis.

Adapted from Kimberlin, D. W. (Ed.). (2015). *Red Book Online: Report of the committee on infectious diseases* (30th ed.). Retrieved from http://redbook.solutions.aap.org/; and Public Health Agency of Canada. (2015). *Canadian guidelines on sexually transmitted infections.* Retrieved from http://www.phac-aspc.gc.ca/std-mts/sti-its/pdf/401mts-prisencharge-eng.pdf.

Think back to Sandy, who was introduced at the beginning of the chapter. How should the nurse handle Sandy's anxious state? What specific questions should the nurse ask Sandy to determine the source of the possible infection in her genital area?

INFECTIONS CHARACTERIZED BY VAGINAL DISCHARGE

Vaginitis is a generic term that means inflammation and infection of the vagina. Vaginitis has hundreds of causes, but more often than not the cause is infection by one of three organisms:

* *Candida*, a fungus
* *Trichomonas*, a protozoan
* *Gardnerella*, a bacterium

The complex balance of microbiologic organisms in the vagina is a key element in the maintenance of health. Subtle shifts in the vaginal environment may allow organisms with pathologic potential to proliferate, causing infectious symptoms.

The nurse's role in managing vaginitis is one of primary prevention and education to limit recurrences of these infections. Primary prevention begins with changing the sexual behaviors that place women at risk for infection. In addition to assessing women for the common signs and symptoms and risk factors, the nurse can help women to avoid vaginitis or to prevent a recurrence by teaching them to take the precautions highlighted in Teaching Guidelines 5.2.

Teaching Guidelines 5.2
PREVENTING VAGINITIS

* Avoid douching to prevent altering the vaginal environment.
* Use condoms to avoid spreading the organism.
* Avoid tights, nylon underpants, and tight clothes.
* Wipe from front to back after using the toilet.
* Wash only with hypoallergenic bar soaps; avoid using liquid soaps or body washes.
* Avoid powders, bubble baths, and perfumed vaginal sprays.
* Wear clean cotton underpants.
* Change out of wet bathing suits as soon as possible.
* Become familiar with the signs and symptoms of vaginitis.
* Choose to lead a healthy lifestyle.

Genital/Vulvovaginal Candidiasis

Genital/vulvovaginal candidiasis (VVC) is one of the most common causes of vaginal discharge. It is also referred to as yeast, monilia, and a fungal infection. It is not considered an STI because *Candida* is a normal constituent in the vagina and becomes pathologic only when the vaginal environment becomes altered. An estimated 75% of women will have at least one episode of VVC, and 40% to 50% will have two or more episodes in their lifetime (CDC, 2015b).

Therapeutic Management

Treatment of candidiasis includes one of the following medications:

* Miconazole (Monistat) cream or suppository
* Clotrimazole (Mycelex) tablet or cream
* Terconazole (Terazol) cream or intravaginal suppository
* Fluconazole (Diflucan) oral tablet (Prabhu & Gardella, 2015).

Most of the above medications are used intravaginally in the form of a cream, tablet, or suppositories for 3 to 7 days. If fluconazole (Diflucan) is prescribed, a 150-mg oral tablet is taken as a single dose.

Topical azole preparations are effective in the treatment of VVC, relieving symptoms and producing negative cultures in 80% to 90% of women who complete therapy (CDC, 2015b). If VVC is not treated effectively during pregnancy, the newborn can develop an oral infection known as thrush during the birth process; that infection must be treated with a local azole preparation after birth.

Nursing Assessment

Assess the client's health history for predisposing factors for VVC, which include:

* Pregnancy
* Use of oral contraceptives with high estrogen content
* Use of broad-spectrum antibiotics
* Diabetes mellitus
* Obesity
* Use of steroid and immunosuppressive drugs
* HIV infection
* Wearing tight, restrictive clothes and nylon underpants
* Trauma to vaginal mucosa from chemical irritants or douching

Assess the client for clinical manifestations of genital/vulvovaginal candidiasis. Typical symptoms, which can worsen just before menses, include:

* Pruritus
* Vaginal discharge (thick, white, curd-like)
* Vaginal soreness
* Vulvar burning
* Erythema in the vulvovaginal area
* Dyspareunia
* External dysuria

Figure 5.1 shows the typical appearance of VVC.

Speculum examination will reveal white plaques on the vaginal walls. The vaginal pH remains within normal range. Definitive diagnosis is made by a wet smear, which reveals the filamentous hyphae and

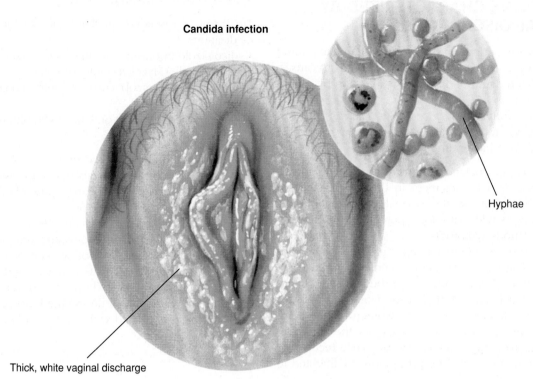

Candida infection

Hyphae

Thick, white vaginal discharge

FIGURE 5.1 Vulvovaginal candidiasis. (Asset provided by Anatomical Chart Co.)

spores characteristic of a fungus when viewed under a microscope.

Nursing Management

Teach the following preventive measures to women with frequent VVC infections:

- Reduce dietary intake of simple sugars and soda.
- Wear white, 100% cotton underpants.
- Avoid wearing tight pants or exercise clothes with spandex.
- Shower rather than taking tub baths.
- Wash with a mild, unscented soap and dry the genitals gently.
- Avoid the use of bubble baths or scented bath products.
- Wash underwear in unscented laundry detergent and hot water.
- Dry underwear in a hot dryer to kill the yeast that clings to the fabric.
- Remove wet bathing suits promptly.
- Practice good body hygiene.
- Avoid vaginal sprays/deodorants.
- Avoid wearing pantyhose (or cut out the crotch to allow air circulation).
- Use white, unscented toilet paper and wipe from front to back.

- Avoid douching (which washes away protective vaginal mucus).
- Avoid the use of superabsorbent tampons (use pads instead).

Trichomoniasis

Trichomoniasis is another common vaginal infection that causes a discharge, but is not always sexually transmitted. The organism can live on damp/wet surfaces and poorly cleaned/maintained hot tubs and drains. The woman may be markedly symptomatic or asymptomatic. Men are asymptomatic carriers. Although this infection is localized, there is increasing evidence of preterm birth, premature rupture of membranes, low-birth-weight infants, postpartum endometritis, and infertility in women with this vaginitis. The high prevalence of this infection worldwide and frequency of co-infection with other STIs make trichomoniasis a compelling public health concern. Notably, research has shown that infection with trichomoniasis increases the risk of HIV transmission in both men and women (Smith & Ramos, 2015). *Trichomonas vaginalis* is an ovoid, single-cell protozoan parasite that can be observed under the microscope making a jerky swaying motion. In the United States, an estimated 3.7 million people have the infection, but only about 30% develop any symptoms of trichomoniasis. Infection is more common in women than in men, and older women are more likely than younger women to have been infected (CDC, 2015c).

Therapeutic Management

A single 2-g dose of oral metronidazole (Flagyl) or tinidazole (Tindamax) for both partners is a common treatment for this infection. Sex partners of women with trichomoniasis should be treated to avoid recurrence of infection.

Nursing Assessment

Assess the client for clinical manifestations of trichomoniasis, which include:
- A heavy yellow/green or gray frothy or bubbly discharge
- Vaginal pruritus and vulvar soreness
- Dyspareunia
- A cervix that may bleed on contact
- Dysuria
  - Vaginal odor, described as foul
  - Vaginal or vulvar erythema
- Petechiae on the cervix

Figure 5.2 shows the typical appearance of trichomoniasis.

The diagnosis is confirmed when a motile flagellated trichomonad is visualized under the microscope. In addition, a vaginal pH of greater than 4.5 is a typical finding. U.S. Food and Drug Administration (FDA)-approved tests for trichomoniasis in women include the OSOM Trichomonas Rapid Test (Genzyme Diagnostics, Cambridge, MA), an immunochromatographic capillary flow dipstick technology, and the Affirm VPIII (Becton Dickinson, San Jose, CA), a nucleic acid probe test that evaluates for *T. vaginalis*, *Gardnerella vaginalis*, and *Candida albicans*. Each of these tests, which are performed on vaginal secretions, has a sensitivity of >83% and a specificity of >97%. Both tests are considered point-of-care diagnostics (CDC, 2015c).

Nursing Management

Instruct clients to avoid sex until they and their sex partners are cured (i.e., when therapy has been completed and both partners are symptom-free) and also to avoid consuming alcohol during treatment because mixing the medications and alcohol causes severe nausea and vomiting (CDC, 2015c). In addition, it is important to provide information regarding infection cause and transmission, effects on reproductive organs and future fertility, and the need for partner notification and treatment. Follow-up testing is not indicated if symptoms resolve with treatment. See Evidence-Based Practice 5.1 for interventions for trichomoniasis in pregnancy.

Bacterial Vaginosis

A third common infection of the vagina is bacterial vaginosis (BV) caused by the gram-negative bacillus *G. vaginalis*. It is the most prevalent cause of vaginal discharge

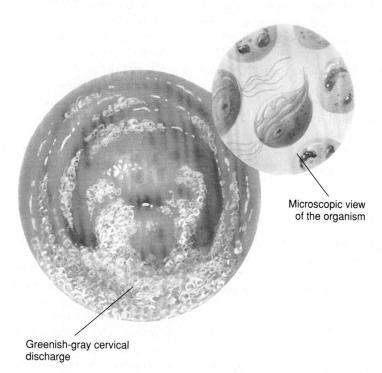

Microscopic view
of the organism

Greenish-gray cervical
discharge

FIGURE 5.2 Trichomoniasis. (Asset provided by Anatomical Chart Co.)

EVIDENCE-BASED PRACTICE 5.1   ADOLESCENT PATIENT PREFERENCES SURROUNDING PARTNER NOTIFICATION FOR SEXUALLY TRANSMITTED INFECTIONS

STUDY

A sexually transmitted epidemic exists among adolescents. Important barriers to addressing the sexually transmitted infection (STI) epidemic among adolescents are the inadequate partner notification of positive STI results and insufficient rates of partner testing and treatment. However, adolescent attitudes regarding partner notification and treatment are not well understood. The objective of this study was to qualitatively explore the barriers to and preferences for partner notification and treatment among adolescent males and females tested for STIs in an emergency department (ED) setting and to explore the acceptability of ED personnel notifying their sexual partners. This was a descriptive, qualitative study in which a convenience sample of 40 adolescents (18 females, 22 males) 14 to 21 years of age who presented to either adult or pediatric EDs with STI-related complaints participated. Data were analyzed using framework analysis.

Findings

Barriers to partner notification included fear of retaliation or loss of the relationship, lack of understanding of or

concern for the consequences associated with an STI, and social stigma and embarrassment. Participants reported two primary barriers to their partners obtaining STI testing and treatment: lack of transportation to the health care site and the partner's fear of STI-positive test results. Most participants were agreeable with a health care provider notifying their sexual partners of the STI exposure by phone.

Nursing Implications

Since several barriers exist to addressing the STI epidemic among adolescents, nurses can intervene by assisting partner notification and treatment to reduce spread. Adolescents may lack the communication skills and developmental maturity to address a difficult topic such as STIs with their partners. Partner notification of STI exposures is essential to reduce the rates of STIs among adolescents. Nurses can help in this endeavor by participating in the STI notification process to prevent further spread and reduction of future complications.

Adapted from Reed, J. L., Huppert, J. S., Gillespie, G. L., Taylor, R. G., Holland, C. K., Alessandrini, E. A., et al. (2015). Adolescent patient preferences surrounding partner notification and treatment for sexually transmitted infections. *Academic Emergency Medicine*, *22*(1), 61–66.

or malodor, but up to 50% of women are asymptomatic. BV is a sexually associated infection characterized by alterations in vaginal flora in which lactobacilli in the vagina are replaced with high concentrations of anaerobic bacteria. BV was named so because bacteria are the etiologic agents and an associated inflammatory response is lacking. The bacterial imbalance is associated with sexual contact, but is not usually spread through sex. The cause of the microbial alteration is not fully understood but is associated with having multiple sex partners, douching, and lack of vaginal lactobacilli (CDC, 2015d). Research suggests that BV is associated with preterm labor, premature rupture of membranes, chorioamnionitis, postpartum endometritis, and PID (CDC, 2015d).

Therapeutic Management

Treatment for BV includes oral metronidazole (Flagyl) or clindamycin (Cleocin) cream. Treatment of the male partner has not been beneficial in preventing recurrence because sexual transmission of BV has not been proven (CDC, 2015d).

Nursing Assessment

Assess the client for clinical manifestations of BV. Primary symptoms are a thin, white homogeneous vaginal

discharge and a characteristic "stale fish" odor, often recognized only after sexual intercourse. Figure 5.3 shows the typical appearance of BV.

To diagnose BV, three of the following four criteria must be met:

- Thin, grayish white homogeneous vaginal discharge which adheres to the vaginal mucosa
- Vaginal pH > 4.5
- Positive "whiff test" (secretion is mixed with a drop of 10% potassium hydroxide on a slide, producing a characteristic stale fishy odor)
- A pH greater than 4.5
- The presence of clue cells on wet-mount examination (CDC, 2015d).

Nursing Management

The nurse's role is one of primary prevention and education to limit recurrences of these infections. Primary prevention begins with changing hygiene behaviors that place women at risk for infection. In addition to assessing women for common signs, symptoms, and risk factors (recent antibiotic use, decreased estrogen production, douching, and sexual activity with a new partner), the nurse can help women to avoid vaginitis or to prevent a recurrence by teaching them to take the precautions highlighted in Teaching Guidelines 5.2.

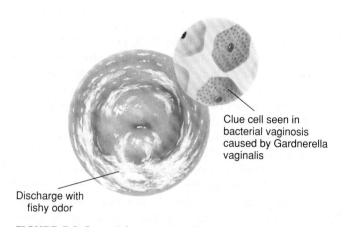
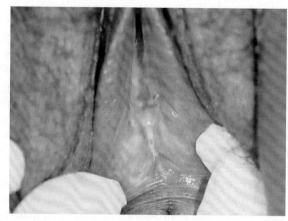

Clue cell seen in bacterial vaginosis caused by Gardnerella vaginalis

Discharge with fishy odor

FIGURE 5.3 Bacterial vaginosis. (Illustration provided by Anatomical Chart Co. Photograph from Sweet, R. L., & Gibbs, R. S. [2005]. *Atlas of infectious diseases of the female genital tract.* Philadelphia, PA: Lippincott Williams & Wilkins.)

INFECTIONS CHARACTERIZED BY CERVICITIS

Cervicitis is a catchall term that implies the presence of inflammation or infection of the cervix. It is used to describe everything from symptomless erosions to an inflamed cervix that bleeds on contact and produces quantities of purulent discharge containing organisms not ordinarily found in the vagina. Cervicitis is usually caused by gonorrhea or chlamydia, as well as almost any pathogenic bacterial agent and a number of viruses. The treatment of cervicitis involves the appropriate therapy for the specific organism that has caused it.

Chlamydia

Chlamydia is the most commonly reported bacterial STI in the United States. The CDC (2015e) estimates that over 3 million new cases occur each year; the highest predictor for the infection is age. The highest rates of infection are among those aged 15 to 19, mainly because their sexual relations are often unplanned and are sometimes the result of rape, and typically happen before they have the experience and skills to protect themselves. The rates are highest among this group regardless of demographics or location (CDC, 2015e). The young have the most to lose from acquiring STIs, because they will suffer the consequences the longest and might not reach their full reproductive potential. The most common risk factors associated with chlamydia are age >25 years, recent change in sexual partner or multiple sexual partners, poor socioeconomic conditions, exchange of sex for money, non-White race, single status, and lack of use of barrier contraception (Qureshi, 2015).

Asymptomatic infection is common among both men (50%) and women (70%). Men primarily develop urethritis. In women, chlamydia is linked with cervicitis, acute urethral syndrome, salpingitis, chronic pelvic pain, dysuria, stillbirth, ectopic pregnancy, PID, and infertility (Simmons, 2015). Chlamydia causes half of the 1 million recognized cases of PID in the United States each year, and treatment costs run over $800 million yearly. The CDC recommends yearly chlamydia testing of all sexually active women aged 25 or younger, older women with risk factors for chlamydial infections (those who have a new sex partner or multiple sex partners), and all pregnant women (CDC, 2015e).

Chlamydia trachomatis is the bacterium that causes chlamydia. It is an intracellular parasite that cannot produce its own energy and depends on the host for survival. It is often difficult to detect, and this can pose problems for women due to the long-term consequences of untreated infection. Untreated chlamydia has been linked to increased incidence and severity of sequelae, such as PID and infertility in women. After a single chlamydial infection, the risk of developing PID is estimated to be approximately 20% to 50% %, and the risk of developing tubal infertility is estimated to be approximately 10% to 20% (Amoako & Balen, 2015). Moreover, lack of treatment provides more opportunity for the infection to be transmitted to sexual partners. An estimated 100,000 pregnant women are affected by this STI. When untreated, chlamydia is associated with premature rupture of membranes, preterm labor, and postpartum endometritis (Collins, 2015). Newborns delivered to infected mothers may develop conjunctivitis, which occurs in 1% to 12% of all newborns. Ophthalmia neonatorum is an acute mucopurulent conjunctivitis occurring in the first month of birth. It is essentially an infection acquired during vaginal delivery. The most frequent infectious agents involved in are *C. trachomatis* and *Neisseria gonorrhoeae* (Moore & MacDonald, 2015).

Therapeutic Management

Antibiotics are usually used in treating this STI. The CDC treatment options for chlamydia include doxycycline (Vibramycin) 100 mg orally twice a day for 7 days or azithromycin (Zithromax) 1 g orally in a single dose. Because of the common co-infection of chlamydia and gonorrhea, a combination regimen of ceftriaxone (Rocephin) with doxycycline or azithromycin is prescribed frequently (CDC, 2015e). Additional CDC guidelines for client management include annual screening of all sexually active women aged 20 to 25 years, screening of all high-risk people, and treatment with antibiotics effective against both gonorrhea and chlamydia for anyone diagnosed with a gonococcal infection (CDC, 2015e).

Except in pregnant women, test-of-cure (repeat testing 3 to 4 weeks after completing therapy) is not recommended for women treated with the recommended or alterative regimens, unless therapeutic adherence is in question, symptoms persist, or reinfection is suspected. Pregnant women should be retested in 3 to 6 months after the initial infection, preferably in the third trimester, because of an increased risk for reinfection (King et al., 2015).

Nursing Assessment

Assess the health history for significant risk factors for chlamydia, which may include:
- Being an adolescent
- Having multiple sex partners
- Having a new sex partner
- Engaging in sex without using a barrier contraceptive (condom)
- Using oral contraceptives
- Being pregnant
- Having a history of another STI (Schuiling & Likis, 2016).

Assess the client for clinical manifestations of chlamydia. The majority of women (70%) are asymptomatic (CDC, 2015e). If the client is symptomatic, clinical manifestations include:
- Mucopurulent vaginal discharge
- Urethritis
- Bartholinitis
- Endometritis
- Salpingitis
- Dysfunctional uterine bleeding

The diagnosis can be made by urine testing or swab specimens collected from the endocervix or vagina. Culture, direct immunofluorescence, enzyme immunoassay, or nucleic acid amplification methods by polymerase chain reaction or ligase chain reaction (DNA probe, such as GenProbe or Pace2) are highly sensitive and specific when used on urethral and cervicovaginal swabs. They can also be used with good sensitivity and specificity on first-void urine specimens (King et al., 2015). The chain reaction tests are the most sensitive and cost-effective. Because the majority of chlamydia cases are asymptomatic, the CDC recommends screening of all women with a new sex partner and annual screening for women 25 years and younger (CDC, 2015e).

Chlamydia is an important preventable cause of infertility and other adverse reproductive health outcomes. Effective prevention interventions are available to reduce the burden of chlamydia and its sequelae, but they are underutilized. Although many prevention programs are available, improvements can be made in raising awareness about chlamydia, increasing screening coverage, and enhancing partner services. In addition, nurses can focus their efforts on reaching disproportionately affected racial/ethnic groups. To break the cycle of chlamydia transmission in the United States, health care providers should encourage annual chlamydia screening for all sexually active females less than 25 years old, maximize use of effective partner treatment services, and rescreen infected females and males 3 months after treatment (CDC, 2015e).

Gonorrhea

Gonorrhea is a serious and potentially very severe bacterial infection. It is the second most commonly reported infection in the United States and globally is an urgent problem because it is now capable of rapidly developing resistance to multiple antibiotic classes. Gonorrhea is highly contagious and is a reportable infection to the health department authorities. Gonorrhea increases the risk for PID, infertility, ectopic pregnancy, and HIV acquisition and transmission (CDC, 2015f). It is rapidly becoming more and more resistant to cure. In the United States, over 820,000 new gonorrhea infections occur annually, with 570,000 of them occurring among young people 15 to 24 years old (CDC, 2015f). In common with all other STIs, it is an equal-opportunity infection—no one is immune to it, regardless of race, creed, gender, age, or sexual preference.

The cause of gonorrhea is an aerobic gram-negative intracellular diplococcus, *N. gonorrhoeae*. The site of infection is the columnar epithelium of the endocervix. Gonorrhea is almost exclusively transmitted by sexual activity. In pregnant women, gonorrhea is associated with chorioamnionitis, premature labor, premature rupture of membranes, and postpartum endometritis (Piszczek, Jean, & Khaliq, 2015). It can also be transmitted to the newborn in the form of ophthalmia neonatorum during birth by direct contact with gonococcal organisms in the cervix. Ophthalmia neonatorum is highly contagious and, if untreated, leads to blindness in the newborn.

Therapeutic Management

Gonorrhea can be cured with the right treatment. CDC now recommends dual therapy (i.e., using two drugs) as the treatment for gonorrhea. Dual drug therapy is recommended to prevent drug resistance, and is also effective against chlamydia. The treatment of choice for uncomplicated gonococcal infections is a single intramuscular dose of ceftriaxone (Rocephin) 250 mg plus a single dose of azithromycin 1 g orally or doxycycline 100 mg orally twice a day for 7 days (Kohlhoff & Hammerschlag, 2015; Wong, 2015). Pregnant women should not be treated with quinolones or tetracyclines. Pregnant women with a positive test for gonorrhea should be treated with the same recommended dual therapy as above (CDC, 2015f). To prevent gonococcal ophthalmia neonatorum, a prophylactic agent should be instilled into the eyes of all newborns; this procedure is required by law in most states. Erythromycin or tetracycline ophthalmic ointment in a single application is recommended (CDC, 2015f). With use of recommended treatment, follow-up testing to document eradication of gonorrhea is no longer recommended. Instead, rescreening in 3 months to identify reinfection is suggested (CDC, 2015f).

Nursing Assessment

Assess the client's health history for risk factors, which may include low socioeconomic status, living in an urban area, single status, inconsistent use of barrier contraceptives, age under 25 years old, and multiple sex partners. Assess the client for clinical manifestations of gonorrhea, keeping in mind that 70% of women infected with gonorrhea are totally symptom-free (Wong, 2015). Because women are so frequently asymptomatic, they are regarded as a major factor in the spread of gonorrhea. If symptoms are present, they might include:

- Abnormal vaginal discharge
- Dysuria
- Cervicitis
- Abnormal vaginal bleeding
- Bartholin's abscess
- Enlarged lymph nodes locally
- PID
- Neonatal conjunctivitis in newborns
- Mild sore throat (for pharyngeal gonorrhea)
- Rectal infection (itching, soreness, bleeding, discharge)
- Perihepatitis (King et al., 2015).

Sometimes a local gonorrheal infection is self-limiting (there is no further spread), but usually the organism ascends upward through the endocervical canal to the endometrium of the uterus, further on to the fallopian tubes, and out into the peritoneal cavity. When the peritoneum and the ovaries become involved, the condition is known as PID (discussed later in this chapter). The scarring to the fallopian tubes is permanent. This

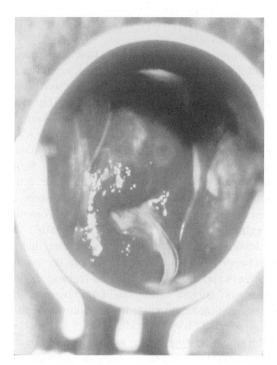

FIGURE 5.4 Gonorrhea. (From Gorbach, S. L., et al. [2004]. *Infectious diseases.* Philadelphia, PA: Lippincott Williams & Wilkins.)

damage is a major cause of infertility and is a possible contributing factor in ectopic pregnancy (Heller, 2015).

If gonorrhea remains untreated, it can enter the bloodstream and produce a disseminated gonococcal infection. This severe form of infection can invade the joints (arthritis), the heart (endocarditis), the brain (meningitis), and the liver (toxic hepatitis). Figure 5.4 shows the typical appearance of gonorrhea.

The CDC recommends screening for all women at risk for gonorrhea. Pregnant women should be screened at the first prenatal visit and again at 36 weeks of gestation. Nucleic acid hybridization tests (GenProbe) are used for diagnosis. Any woman suspected of having gonorrhea should be tested for chlamydia also because co-infection (45%) is extremely common (CDC, 2015f).

Nursing Management of Chlamydia and Gonorrhea

The prevalence of chlamydia and gonorrhea is increasing dramatically, and these infections can have long-term effects on people's lives. Sexual health is an important part of a person's physical and mental health, and nurses have a professional obligation to address it. Be particularly sensitive when addressing STIs because women are often embarrassed, feel guilty or angry, or may even be fearful of outcomes related to telling partners about the diagnosis (see earlier section on the cultural and psychological impacts of STI diagnosis). There is still a social stigma attached to STIs, so women need to be reassured about confidentiality.

The nurse's knowledge about chlamydia and gonorrhea should include treatment strategies, referral sources, and preventive measures. The nurse should be skilled at client education and counseling and be comfortable talking with, and advising, women diagnosed with these infections. Provide education about risk factors for these infections. High-risk groups include single women, women younger than 25 years old, African American women, women with a history of STIs, those with new or multiple sex partners, those with inconsistent use of barrier contraception, and women living in communities with high infection rates (Comkornruecha, 2013). Assessment involves taking a health history that includes a comprehensive sexual history. Ask about the number of sex partners and the use of safer sex techniques. Review previous and current symptoms. Emphasize the importance of seeking treatment and informing sex partners. The four-level P-LI-SS-IT model (Box 5.3) can be used to determine interventions for various women because it can be adapted to the nurse's level of knowledge, skill, and experience. Of utmost importance is the willingness to listen and show interest and respect in a nonjudgmental manner.

In addition to meeting the health needs of women with chlamydia and gonorrhea, the nurse is responsible for educating the public about the increasing incidence of these infections. This information should include high-risk behaviors associated with these infections, signs and symptoms, and the treatment modalities available. Stress that both of these STIs can lead to infertility and long-term sequelae. Teach safer sex practices to people in nonmonogamous relationships. Know the physical and psychosocial responses to these STIs to prevent transmission and the disabling consequences. Nurses must also inform their pregnant clients that they should avoid quinolones or tetracyclines to prevent risks associated with irreversible tooth discoloration and enamel hypoplasia in the newborn (Kohlhoff & Hammerschlag, 2015).

 Take Note!

If the epidemic of chlamydia and gonorrhea is to be halted, nurses must take a major front-line role now.

INFECTIONS CHARACTERIZED BY GENITAL ULCERS

In the United States, the majority of young, sexually active clients who have genital ulcers have genital herpes, syphilis, or chancroid. The frequency of each condition differs by geographic area and client population; however, genital herpes is the most prevalent of these diseases (CDC, 2015g). More than one of these diseases can be present in a client who has genital ulcers. All three of these diseases have been associated with an increased risk for HIV infection. Not all genital ulcers are caused by STIs.

Genital Herpes Simplex

Genital herpes is a recurrent, lifelong viral infection that has the potential for transmission throughout the lifespan. The CDC (2015h) estimates that one out of six people in the United States have genital HSV infection, with 776,000 people getting new cases annually. About 22% of pregnant women are infected with HSV. The most devastating consequence of maternal genital herpes is neonatal herpes disease, which occurs in approximately 1 in 3,200 births in the US and has a high mortality rate (James & Kimberlin, 2015).

Genital herpes is more common among females (1 out of 5) than males (1 out of 9) in part due to prolonged contact with semen during vaginal intercourse. Two serotypes of HSV have been identified: HSV-1 and HSV-2. HSV-1 is associated mainly with oral herpes (commonly called cold sores and fever blisters) and HSV-2 is mainly associated with genital herpes, both types can cause outbreaks in either location. Approximately 80% of individuals infected with genital herpes are asymptomatic and unaware of being infected with the virus (Leone, 2015).

HSV is transmitted by contact of mucous membranes or breaks in the skin with visible or nonvisible lesions. Most genital herpes infections are transmitted by individuals unaware that they have an infection. Many have mild or unrecognized infections but still shed the

---

BOX 5.3

THE P-LI-SS-IT MODEL

P Permission—gives the woman permission to talk about her experience

LI Limited Information—information given to the woman about STIs
- Factual information to dispel myths about STIs
- Specific measures to prevent transmission
- Ways to reveal information to her partners
- Physical consequences if the infections are untreated

SS Specific Suggestions—an attempt to help women change their behavior to prevent recurrence and prevent further transmission of the STI

IT Intensive Therapy—involves referring the woman or couple for appropriate treatment elsewhere based on their life circumstances

Adapted from Annon, J. S. (1976). The PLISSIT model: A proposed conceptual scheme for the behavioral treatment of sexual problems. *Journal of Sex Education Therapy, 2,* 1–15.

herpes virus intermittently. HSV is transmitted primarily by direct contact with an infected individual who is shedding the virus. Kissing, sexual contact (including oral sex), and vaginal delivery are means of transmission.

Having sex with an infected partner places the individual at risk for contracting HSV. After the primary outbreak, the virus remains dormant in the nerve cells for a lifetime, resulting in periodic recurrent outbreaks. Recurrent genital herpes outbreaks are triggered by precipitating factors such as emotional stress, menses, ultraviolet light exposure, illness, surgery, fatigue, genital trauma, immunosuppression, and sexual intercourse, but more than half of recurrences occur without a precipitating cause. Immunocompromised women have more frequent and more severe recurrent outbreaks than normal hosts. A genital herpes infection during pregnancy can cause a spontaneous abortion, preterm labor, microcephaly, low-birth-weight infant, microophthalmia, chorioretinitis, and/or neonatal HSV infection (Silasi et al., 2015).

Living with genital herpes can be difficult due to the erratic, recurrent nature of the infection, the location of the lesions, the unknown causes of the recurrences, and the lack of a cure. Upon diagnosis, clients have important concerns related not to the physical nature of the disease but to the social consequences, including transmission and the impact on their sex life. Furthermore, the stigma associated with this infection may affect the individual's feelings about herself and her interaction with partners. Potential psychosocial consequences may include emotional distress, isolation, fear of rejection by a partner, fear of transmission of the disease, loss of confidence, and altered interpersonal relationships (Alexander et al., 2014).

Along with the increase in the incidence of genital herpes has been an increase in neonatal HSV infections, which are associated with a high incidence of mortality and morbidity. The risk of neonatal infection with a primary maternal outbreak is between 30% and 50%; it is less than 1% with a recurrent maternal infection (CDC, 2015h).

Therapeutic Management

No cure exists, but antiviral drug therapy helps to reduce or suppress symptoms, shedding, and recurrent episodes. Advances in treatment with acyclovir (Zovirax) 400 mg orally three times daily for 7 to 10 days, famciclovir (Famvir) 250 mg orally three times daily for 7 to 10 days, or valacyclovir (Valtrex) 1 g orally twice daily for 7 to 10 days have resulted in an improved quality of life for those infected with HSV. However, these drugs neither eradicate latent virus nor affect the risk, frequency, or severity of recurrences after the drug is discontinued (CDC, 2015h). Suppressive therapy is recommended for individuals with six or more recurrences per year. The

natural course of the disease is for recurrences to be less frequent over time. The safety of antiviral therapy has not been established during pregnancy.

Therapeutic management also includes counseling regarding the natural history of the disease, the risk of sexual and perinatal transmission, and the use of methods to prevent further spread. The following guidelines can help the nurse when delivering information in a time-limited environment: (1) Use all available client reading materials; (2) have another knowledgeable staff member in the office who can spend extra time with women who need it; (3) refer clients to good and accurate websites such as the American Social Health Association website (refer to for additional information); (4) know the phone numbers of herpes support groups in your area; (5) educate the client to abstain from all sexual activity until HSV lesions resolve; (6) use good hand hygiene to prevent spread; (7) educate that there is no cure, and that practicing safer sex (using condoms and dental dams) with every sex act is essential to prevent transmission; and (8) encourage all clients to inform their current sex partners that they have genital herpes and to inform future partners before initiating a sexual relationship. Finally, many experts recommend a sympathetic, nonjudgmental approach. The nurse can state in clear terms that having herpes does not change the core of the person or make the person less worthwhile (Myers et al., 2015).

Nursing Assessment

Assess the woman for risk factors, which may include having unprotected sexual intercourse, multiple sexual partners, lower socioeconomic status, a history of STIs, and increasing age (Moses, 2015). Assess the client for clinical manifestations of HSV. Clinical manifestations can be divided into the primary episode and recurrent infections. The first or primary episode is usually the most severe, with a prolonged period of viral shedding. Primary HSV is a systemic disease characterized by multiple painful vesicular lesions, mucopurulent discharge, superinfection with candida, fever, chills, malaise, dysuria, headache, genital irritation, inguinal tenderness, and lymphadenopathy. The lesions in the primary herpes episode are frequently located on the vulva, vagina, and perineal areas. The vesicles will open and weep and finally crust over, dry, and disappear without scar formation (Fig. 5.5). This viral shedding process usually takes up to 2 weeks to complete.

Recurrent infection episodes may occur five to eight times per year and are usually much milder with fewer lesions and shorter in duration than the primary one. Tingling, itching, pain, unilateral genital lesions, and a more rapid resolution of lesions are characteristics of recurrent infections. Recurrent herpes is a localized disease characterized by typical HSV lesions at the site of

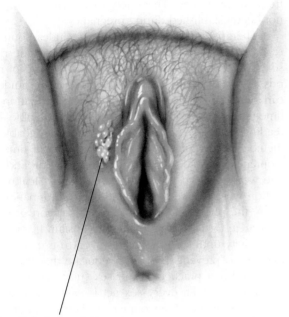

Herpetic lesions on labia majora

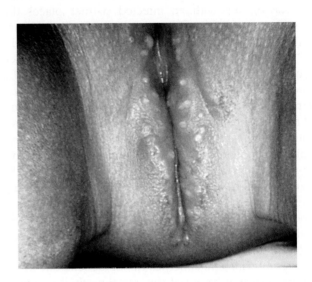

FIGURE 5.5 Genital herpes simplex. (Illustration provided by Anatomical Chart Co. Photograph courtesy of Stephen Ludwig, MD.)

initial viral entry. Recurrent herpes lesions are fewer in number and less painful and resolve more rapidly (King et al., 2015).

Diagnosis of HSV is often based on clinical signs and symptoms and is confirmed by viral culture of fluid from the vesicles. The IgG/IgM antibody testing is frequently done for screening purposes. Papanicolaou (Pap) smears are an insensitive and nonspecific diagnostic test for HSV and should not be relied on for diagnosis. The women should be tested for all common STIs, especially if she has a new sexual partner. Ideally, the woman will initiate an open conversation with her sexual partner about the risk of transmission and the need for safer sexual practices.

Syphilis

Syphilis is a complex, curable bacterial infection caused by the spirochete *Treponema pallidum*. It is often thought to be a disease of the past, largely eradicated in modern America, but its incidence is on the rise in certain populations (gay men, bisexual men, men having sex with men, and women of color living in the South). It is estimated that 12 million people globally are infected annually (Ramsey, 2015). It is a serious systemic disease that can lead to disability and death if untreated. Syphilis has a complex life cycle during which episodes of active clinical disease are punctuated with periods of latency. About 2.1 million pregnant women have active syphilis every year. Congenital syphilis can occur

when an infected mother directly infects her fetus. Without screening and treatment, 69% of these women will have an adverse outcome to their pregnancy (Angoori, 2015). Rates of syphilis in the United States are increasing, especially among young adults and African Americans in urban areas and in the South (CDC, 2015i). The World Health Organization (WHO, 2015d) estimates that the rates of maternal syphilis and subsequent neonatal mortality and morbidity easily exceed that of other neonatal infections, especially among lower socioeconomic classes, aboriginal and African American cultures, and sex trade workers. It continues to be one of the most important STIs both because of its biologic effect on HIV acquisition and transmission and because of its impact on infant health (Tipple & Taylor, 2015). All pregnant women should be screened for syphilis infection at their first prenatal visit and repeated in the third trimester For women in high-risk groups, repeat serology testing may be necessary in the third trimester and at birth (CDC, 2015j).

The syphilis spirochete rapidly penetrates intact mucous membranes or microscopic lesions in the skin and within hours enters the lymphatic system and bloodstream to produce a systemic infection long before the appearance of a primary lesion. The site of entry may be vaginal, rectal, or oral (Klein, McLaud, & Rogers, 2015). The syphilis spirochete can cross the placenta after 9 weeks of gestation. One out of every 10,000 infants born in the United States has congenital syphilis (CDC, 2015i). Maternal infection consequences for the newborn include spontaneous abortion, low birth weight, prematurity, stillbirth, intrauterine growth restriction, and multisystem failure of the heart, lungs, spleen, liver, and pancreas, as well as structural bone damage, nervous system involvement, and intellectual disability (Chen et al., 2015).

Therapeutic Management

Fortunately, an effective treatment is available for syphilis. Single-dose therapy is preferred for ease of use of azithromycin (Zithromax, Z-Pak) 1 g orally once, or ceftriaxone (Rocephin) 250 mg IM once or ciprofloxacin (Cipro) 500 mg orally twice a day for three days, or erythromycin base 500 mg orally three times a day for seven days can be prescribed. Ciprofloxacin is contraindicated for pregnant and lactating women. Penicillin G benzathine 2.4 million units IM weekly for 3 weeks can also be used for treatment, but client adherence can be challenging (King et al., 2015). The preparations used, the dosage, and the length of treatment depend on the stage and clinical manifestations of disease (CDC, 2015j). Other medications, such as doxycycline, are available if the client is allergic to penicillin.

Women should be reevaluated at 6 and 12 months after treatment for primary or secondary syphilis with additional serologic testing. Women with latent syphilis should be followed clinically and serologically at 6, 12, and 24 months (Lawrence et al., 2015).

 Concept Mastery Alert

Syphilis Transmission in Pregnancy

Although some sexually transmitted infections such as gonorrhea and the herpes virus are transmitted to the newborn by the birth canal, syphilis is transmitted through the placenta at any time during the pregnancy. This means the fetus is at risk during the entire pregnancy, unless the mother is diagnosed and properly treated.

Nursing Assessment

Syphilis has many nonspecific signs and symptoms that may be overlooked by the health care provider, or may simply be indistinguishable from other more common diseases. Regrettably, undiagnosed and untreated syphilis may lead to life-threatening complications such as hepatitis, stroke, and nervous system damage (Klein et al., 2015). Assess the client for any clinical manifestations of syphilis. If untreated, syphilis is a lifelong infection progressing in orderly staging. The five stages of syphilis infection are (1) primary, (2) secondary, (3) early latent, (4) late latent, and (5) tertiary. The primary, secondary, and early latent stages are considered the most infectious: the estimated risk of per person transmission

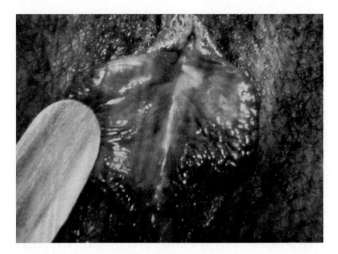

FIGURE 5.6 Chancre of primary syphilis. (From Sweet, R. L., & Gibbs, R. S. [2005]. *Atlas of infectious diseases of the female genital tract.* Philadelphia, PA: Lippincott Williams & Wilkins.)

is 60%. Furthermore, in these stages, the fetus is at higher risk of acquiring maternal infections Klein et al., 2015).

Primary syphilis is characterized by a chancre (painless ulcer) at the site of bacterial entry that will disappear within 1 to 6 weeks without intervention (Fig. 5.6). Motile spirochetes are present on dark-field examination of ulcer exudate. In addition, painless bilateral adenopathy is present during this highly infectious period. The client is highly infectious whenever chancres are present. If left untreated, the infection progresses to the secondary stage.

Secondary syphilis appears 2 to 6 months after the initial exposure and is manifested by flu-like symptoms and a maculopapular rash of the trunk, palms, and soles. Alopecia and adenopathy are both common during this stage. In addition to rashes, secondary syphilis may present with symptoms of fever, pharyngitis, weight loss, and fatigue (Peterman et al., 2015). The secondary stage of syphilis lasts about 2 years. Once the secondary stage subsides, the latency periods (early and late) begin. These stages are characterized by the absence of any clinical manifestations of disease, although the serology is positive. This stage can last as long as 20 years. If not treated, *tertiary* or *late syphilis* occurs, with life-threatening heart disease and neurologic disease that slowly destroys the heart, with inflammation of the aorta, eyes, brain, central nervous system, and skin.

Clients with a diagnosis of HIV or another STI should be screened for syphilis, and all pregnant women should be screened at their first prenatal visit. Serologic testing for syphilis is evaluated by using both nontreponemal and treponemal tests. Nontreponemal tests measure immunoglobulin M (IgM) and immunoglobulin G (IgG). Although these tests are less specific, they are commonly used for primary screening because they are rapid to perform and inexpensive. The most commonly used nontreponemal tests are the rapid plasma regain (RPR) and the Venereal Disease Research Laboratory (VDRL) tests. Treponemal tests detect treponema-specific immunoglobulin A (IgA), IgM, and IgG antibodies, giving these tests a greater accuracy. Current treponemal tests include the EIA, fluorescent treponemal antibody absorption (FTA-ABS), *T. pallidum* agglutination assay (TPPA), and *T. pallidum* hemagglutination assay (TPHA) (Schuiling & Likis, 2016).

A presumptive diagnosis can be made by using two serologic tests:

- Nontreponemal tests (VDRL and RPR)
- Treponemal tests (FTA-ABS and TP-PA). Dark-field microscopic examinations and direct fluorescent antibody tests of lesion exudate or tissue are the definitive methods for diagnosing early syphilis (CDC, 2015k).

Nursing Management of Herpes and Syphilis

Genital ulcers from either herpes or syphilis can be devastating to women, and the nurse can be instrumental in helping her through this difficult time. Referral to a support group may be helpful. Address the psychosocial aspects of these STIs with women by discussing appropriate coping skills, acceptance of the lifelong nature of the condition (herpes), and options for treatment and rehabilitation. Nurses can help to ameliorate the misery, morbidity, and mortality associated with STIs through safe, accurate, sensitive, and supportive care. Teaching Guidelines 5.3 highlights appropriate teaching points for the client with genital ulcers.

Teaching Guidelines 5.3
CARING FOR GENITAL ULCERS

- Abstain from intercourse during the prodromal period and when lesions are present.
- Wash hands with soap and water after touching lesions to avoid autoinoculation.
- Use comfort measures such as wearing nonconstricting clothes, wearing cotton underwear, urinating in water if urination is painful, taking lukewarm sitz baths, and air-drying lesions with a hair dryer on low heat.
- Avoid extremes of temperature such as ice packs or hot pads to the genital area as well as application of steroid creams, sprays, or gels.
- Use condoms with all new or noninfected partners.
- Inform health care professionals of your condition.

Pelvic Inflammatory Disease

PID is a common and serious reproductive health disorder in which rates remain unacceptably high among adolescent girls and young adult women in the United States. It refers to an inflammatory state of the upper female genital tract and nearby structures. The fallopian tubes, ovaries, or peritoneum may be involved and endometriosis may also be present. PID results from an ascending polymicrobial infection of the upper female reproductive tract, frequently caused by untreated chlamydia or gonorrhea (Fig. 5.7). Annually, in the United States, the CDC (2015l) estimates that more than one million women experience an episode of acute PID. Up to 10% to 15% of these women may become infertile as a result of PID. A large proportion of the ectopic pregnancies, pelvic abscess formations, and chronic pelvic pain that occur every year is due to the consequences of PID (CDC, 2015l). It is a serious health problem in the United States, costing an estimated ☒10 billion annually in terms of hospitalizations and surgical procedures (Gilbert, 2015). All sexually active women are at risk for PID, but common risk factors include age less than 25 years, residence in an inner city, multiple sexual partners, sex with a new partner, insertion of an intrauterine contraceptive (IUC) within the past 6 weeks, vaginal douching, history of STI in the woman or her partner, lack of barrier contraceptive use, and a previous episode of PID. Women of African or African Caribbean ethnicity also have a higher reported prevalence of the condition (Simmons, 2015). Complications include fibrosis, scarring, loss of tubal function, ectopic pregnancy, pelvic abscess, infertility, recurrent or chronic episodes of the disease, chronic abdominal pain, pelvic adhesions, and depression (Simmons, 2015). Because of the seriousness of the complications of PID, an accurate diagnosis is critical.

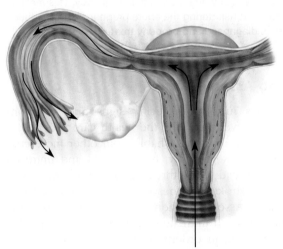

Spread of gonorrhea or chlamydia

FIGURE 5.7 Pelvic inflammatory disease. Chlamydia or gonorrhea spreads up the vagina into the uterus and then to the fallopian tubes and ovaries.

Therapeutic Management

Broad-spectrum antibiotic therapy is generally required to cover chlamydia, gonorrhea, and/or any anaerobic infection. The current CDC recommendation (Blank, 2015) is: ceftriaxone 250 mg in a single injection plus doxycycline 100 mg twice a day for 14 days with or without metronidazole 500 mg orally, twice a day for 14 days, or cefoxitin 2 g intramuscularly in a single dose and probenecid 1 g orally administered concurrently in a single dose plus doxycycline 100 mg orally twice a day for 14 days with or without metronidazole 500 mg orally twice a day for 14 days. PID in pregnancy is uncommon, but a combination of cefotaxime, azithromycin, and metronidazole for 14 days may be used. Tetracyclines and quinolones should be avoided during pregnancy (King et al., 2015). The client is treated on an ambulatory basis with a single-dose injectable antibiotic or is hospitalized and given antibiotics intravenously. The decision to hospitalize a woman is based on clinical judgment and the severity of her symptoms (e.g., severely ill with high fever, a tubo-ovarian abscess is suspected, the woman is immunocompromised or presents with protracted vomiting). Treatment then includes intravenous antibiotics, increased oral fluids to improve hydration, bed rest, and pain management. Follow-up is needed to validate that the infectious process has disappeared to prevent the development of chronic pelvic pain.

Nursing Assessment

Nursing assessment of the woman with PID involves a complete health history and assessment of clinical manifestations, physical examination, and laboratory and diagnostic testing.

HEALTH HISTORY AND CLINICAL MANIFESTATIONS

Explore the client's current and past medical health history for risk factors for PID, which may include:

- Adolescence or young adulthood
- Non-White female
- Having multiple sex partners
- Early onset of sexual activity
- History of PID or STI
- Sexual intercourse at an early age
- Alcohol or drug use
- Having intercourse with a partner who has untreated urethritis
- Recent insertion of an IUC
- Nulliparity
- Cigarette smoking
- Recent termination of pregnancy
- Lack of consistent condom use
- Lack of contraceptive use
- Douching
- Prostitution

Assess the client for clinical manifestations of PID, keeping in mind that, because of the wide variety of clinical manifestations of PID, clinical diagnosis can be challenging. To reduce the risk of missed diagnosis, the CDC has established criteria for the diagnosis of PID. Minimal criteria (all must be present) are lower abdominal tenderness, adnexal tenderness, and cervical motion tenderness. Additional supportive criteria that support a diagnosis of PID are:

- Abnormal cervical or vaginal mucopurulent discharge
- Oral temperature above 101°F (38.3°C)
- Cervical motion tenderness
- Elevated erythrocyte sedimentation rate (inflammatory process)
- Elevated C-reactive protein level (inflammatory process)
- *N. gonorrhoeae* or *C. trachomatis* infection documented (causative bacterial organism)
- White blood cells on saline vaginal smear
- Prolonged or increased menstrual bleeding
- Dysmenorrhea
- Dysuria
- Acute lower abdominal pain
- Painful sexual intercourse
- Nausea
- Vomiting (CDC, 2015l).

PHYSICAL EXAMINATION AND LABORATORY AND DIAGNOSTIC TESTS

Inspect the client for presence of fever (usually over 101°F [38.3°C]) or vaginal discharge. Palpate the abdomen, noting tenderness over the uterus or ovaries. Laparoscopy is the current criterion standard for the diagnosis of PID. No single test is highly specific or sensitive for the disease, but certain laboratory studies that can be used to support the diagnosis include the erythrocyte sedimentation rate, C-reactive protein, and chlamydial and gonococcal DNA probes and cultures (Simmons, 2015).

Nursing Management

If the woman with PID is hospitalized, maintain hydration via intravenous fluids if necessary and administer analgesics as needed for pain. Semi-Fowler's positioning facilitates pelvic drainage. A key element to treatment of PID is education to prevent recurrence. Depending on the clinical setting (hospital or community clinic) where the nurse encounters the woman diagnosed with PID, a risk assessment should be done to ascertain what interventions are appropriate to prevent a recurrence. To gain the woman's cooperation, explain the various diagnostic tests needed. Discuss the implications of PID and the risk factors for the infection; her sexual partner should be included if possible. Sexual counseling should include practicing safer sex, limiting the number of sexual partners, using barrier contraceptives consistently, avoiding vaginal douching, considering another contraceptive method if she has an IUC and has multiple sexual partners, and completing the course of antibiotics prescribed (Shepherd, 2015). Explain the serious sequelae that may occur if the condition is not treated or if the woman does not adhere to the treatment plan. Ask the woman to have her partner go for evaluation and treatment to prevent a repeat infection. Provide nonjudgmental support while stressing the importance of barrier contraceptive methods and follow-up care. Teaching Guidelines 5.4 gives further information related to PID prevention.

Teaching Guidelines 5.4
PREVENTING PELVIC INFLAMMATORY DISEASE

- Advise sexually active girls and women to insist their partners use condoms.
- Discourage routine vaginal douching, as this may lead to bacterial overgrowth.
- Encourage regular STI screening.
- Emphasize the importance of having each sexual partner receive antibiotic treatment.

VACCINE-PREVENTABLE STIs

Some STIs can be effectively prevented through preexposure vaccination. Vaccines are under development or are undergoing clinical trials for certain STIs, including HIV and HSV. However, the only vaccines currently available are for prevention of hepatitis A, hepatitis B, and HPV infection. Vaccination efforts focus largely on integrating the use of these available vaccines into STI prevention and treatment activities (CDC, 2015g).

Human Papillomavirus

HPV is the most common viral infection in the United States. HPV is so common that nearly all sexually active men and women will get at least one type of HPV at some point in their lives (CDC, 2015m). Genital warts or condylomata (Greek for "warts") are caused by HPV. Conservative estimates suggest that in the United States, approximately 79 million people have productive HPV infection, and 14 million Americans acquire it annually (CDC, 2015m). Clinical studies have confirmed that HPV is the cause of essentially all cases of cervical cancer, which is the fourth most common cancer in women in the United States, following lung, breast, and colorectal cancer. Every year in the United States, over 12,000 women are diagnosed with cervical cancer, and about 4,000 women die from this disease. About 1% of sexually active men and women in the United States have genital warts at any given time (American Cancer Society [ACS], 2015). HPV-mediated oncogenesis is responsible for up to 95% of cervical squamous cell carcinomas and nearly all preinvasive cervical neoplasms (CDC, 2015m). More than 40 types of HPV can infect the genital tract. Types 16, 18, 31, 35, 39, 45, 51, 52, 58, 59, and 68 are associated with cervical dysplasia and may contribute to the development of anal, cervical, penile, and cancers (ACS, 2015). HPV is most prevalent in young women between the ages of 20 and 24 years, followed closely by the 15- to 19-year-old age group (Gearhart, Randall, Buckley, & Buckley, 2016).

Take Note!

The lifetime risk of HPV infection is estimated to be as high as 50% in sexually active individuals.

Nursing Assessment

Nursing assessment of the woman with HPV involves a complete health history and assessment of clinical manifestations, physical examination, and laboratory and diagnostic testing. A woman with HPV lesions may have symptoms such as profuse, irritating vaginal discharge, itching, dyspareunia, or bleeding after intercourse. She may also report 'bumps' on her labia. Physical inspection of the external genitalia is important whenever HPV lesions are suspected or seen.

HEALTH HISTORY AND CLINICAL MANIFESTATIONS

Assess the client's health history for risk factors for HPV, which include having multiple sex partners, age (15 to 25 years), sex with a male who has had multiple sexual partners, and first intercourse at age 16 or younger (Mohanty & Ghosh, 2015). Risk factors contributing to the development of cervical cancer include smoking, few or no screenings for cervical cancer, multiple sex partners, immunosuppressed state, long-term contraceptive use (more than 2 years), co-infection with another STI, pregnancy, nutritional deficiencies, and early onset of sexual activity (Gearhart, Higgins, Randall, & Buckley, 2016).

Assess the client for clinical manifestations of HPV. Most HPV infections are asymptomatic, unrecognized, or subclinical. Visible genital warts usually are caused by HPV types 6 or 11. In addition to the external genitalia, genital warts can occur on the cervix and in the vagina, urethra, anus, and mouth. Depending on the size and location, genital warts can be painful, friable (easily pulverized or crumbled), and pruritic (itching), although most are typically asymptomatic (Fig. 5.8). The strains of HPV associated with genital warts are considered low risk for development of cervical cancer, but other HPV types (16, 18, 31, 33, and 35) have been strongly associated with cervical cancer (CDC, 2015m).

These regular Pap smears will detect the cellular changes associated with HPV. The FDA has recently approved an HPV test as a follow-up for women who have an ambiguous Pap test. In addition, this HPV test may be a helpful addition to the Pap test for general screening of women aged 30 and over. The HPV test is a diagnostic test that can determine the specific HPV strain, which is useful in discriminating between low-risk and high-risk HPV types. A specimen for testing can be obtained with a fluid-phase collection system such as Thin Prep. The HPV test can identify 13 of the high-risk types of HPV associated with the development of cervical cancer and can detect high-risk types of HPV even before there are any conclusive visible changes to the cervical cells. If the test is positive for the high-risk types of HPV, the woman should be referred for colposcopy, which is a visual examination of the cervix using magnification and simple staining solutions such as acetic acid and Lugol's solution. It is sometimes accompanied by a biopsy to confirm a cervical abnormality (Decker, McLachlin, & Lotocki, 2015).

Upon physical examination, it is determined that Sandy has genital warts. The nurse finds out that Sandy engaged in high-risk behavior with a stranger she "hooked up" with recently at college. She couldn't imagine that he would give her an STI because "he looked so clean-cut." She wonders how she could possibly have genital warts. What information should be given to Sandy about STIs in general? What specific information about HPV should be stressed?

Therapeutic Management

There is currently no medical treatment or cure for HPV. Instead, therapeutic management focuses heavily on prevention through the use of the HPV vaccine and education and on the treatment of lesions and warts caused by HPV. The FDA has approved three HPV vaccines to prevent cervical cancer: Cervarix, Gardasil, and Gardasil 9.

The CDC's Advisory Committee on Immunization Practices (ACIP) has recommended the vaccine for routine administration to 11- and 12-year-old girls and boys. This recommendation has created a firestorm from many parents feeling that such a vaccine would give young women a false sense of security and lead to promiscuity. Nurses may encounter parental resistance and will need to present the facts to parents about the effectiveness of the vaccines and prevention of cervical cancer. The ACIP also endorses the use of a HPV vaccine for girls and boys as young as age 9 and recommends that women between the ages of 13 and 26 receive the vaccination

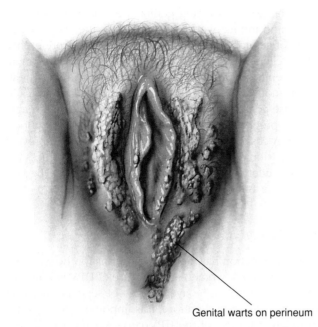

Genital warts on perineum

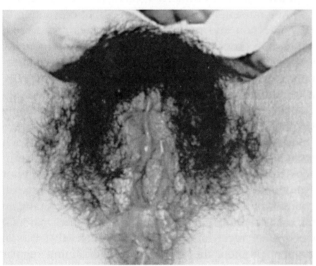

FIGURE 5.8 Genital warts. (Illustration provided by Anatomical Chart Co. Photograph from Gorbach, S. L., et al. [2004]. *Infectious diseases*. Philadelphia, PA: Lippincott Williams & Wilkins.)

PHYSICAL EXAMINATION AND LABORATORY AND DIAGNOSTIC TESTS

Clinically, visible warts are diagnosed by inspection. The warts are fleshy papules with a warty, granular surface. Lesions can grow very large during pregnancy, affecting urination, defecation, mobility, and descent of the fetus (CDC, 2015m). Large lesions, which may resemble cauliflowers, exist in coalesced clusters and bleed easily.

Pap smears now are performed every 3 to 5 years for low-risk women. This current standard of care, calling for less frequent cervical cancer screening than in the past, makes it critical for women to understand when they are to have them and follow through to get them.

series, which consists of three injections over 6 months. All three are prophylactic HPV vaccines designed primarily for cervical cancer prevention. Cervarix is effective against HPV-16, -18, -31, -33, and -45, the five most common cancer-causing types, including most causes of adenocarcinoma for which we cannot screen adequately. Gardasil is effective against HPV-16, -18, and -31, three common squamous cell cancer-causing types. In addition, Gardasil is effective against HPV-6 and -11, causes of genital warts and respiratory papillomatosis. The most important determinant of vaccine impact to reduce cervical cancer is its duration of efficacy. To date, Cervarix's efficacy is proven for 6.4 years and Gardasil's for 5 years (CDC, 2015n). Gardasil 9 is effective against HPV types 6, 11, 16, 18, 31, 33, 45, 52, and 58. According to the FDA, the new vaccine (Gardasil 9) can potentially prevent about 90% of cervical, vulvar, vaginal, and anal cancers (Gearhart, Higgins, Randall, & Buckley, 2016). Prophylactic HPV vaccines are safe, well tolerated, and highly efficacious in preventing persistent infections and cervical diseases associated with vaccine-HPV types among young females. However, long-term efficacy and safety need to be addressed in the future (Castle & Schmeler, 2015).

The vaccine is administered intramuscularly in three separate 0.5-mL doses. The first dose may be given to any individual 9 to 26 years old prior to infection with HPV. The second dose is administered 2 months after the first, and the third dose is given 6 months after the initial dose. The deltoid region of the upper arm or anterolateral area of the thigh may be used. The most common vaccine side effects include pain, fainting, redness, and swelling at the injection site; fatigue; headache; muscle and joint aches; and gastrointestinal distress. Serious adverse events reported to the CDC include blood clots occurring in the heart, lungs, or legs, Guillain–Barré syndrome, and less than 30 deaths (CDC, 2015n). Most client profiles had risk factors that may have attributed to these adverse events and not to the vaccine alone (CDC, 2015n).

If the woman does not receive primary prevention with the vaccine, then secondary prevention would focus on education about the importance of receiving regular Pap smears and, for women over age 30, including an HPV test to determine whether the woman has a latent high-risk virus that could lead to precancerous cervical changes. Finally, treatment options for precancerous cervical lesions or genital warts caused by HPV are numerous and may include:

- Topical trichloroacetic acid (TCA) 80% to 90%
- Liquid nitrogen cryotherapy
- Topical imiquimod 5% cream (Aldara)
- Topical podophyllin 10% to 25%
- Laser carbon dioxide vaporization
- Client-applied Podofilox 0.5% solution or gel
- Simple surgical excision
- Loop electrosurgical excisional procedure (LEEP)
- Intralesional interferon therapy (King et al., 2015)

The goal of treating genital warts is to remove the warts and induce wart-free periods for the client. Treatment of genital warts should be guided by the preference of the client and available resources. No single treatment has been found to be ideal for all clients, and most treatment modalities appear to have comparable efficacy. Because genital warts can proliferate and become friable during pregnancy, they should be removed using a local agent. A cesarean birth is not indicated solely to prevent transmission of HPV infection to the newborn, unless the pelvic outlet is obstructed by warts (Gearhart, Higgins, Randall, & Buckley, 2016).

Nursing Management

An HPV infection has many implications for the woman's health, but most women are unaware of HPV and its role in cervical cancer. The average age of sexual debut is in early adolescence; therefore, it is important to target this population for use of the HPV/cervical cancer vaccine.

Key nursing roles are teaching about prevention of HPV infection and promotion of vaccines and screening tests in order to reduce the morbidity and mortality associated with cervical cancer caused by HPV infection. Teach all women that the only way to prevent HPV is to refrain from any genital contact with another individual. Although the effect of condoms in preventing HPV infection is unknown, latex condom use has been associated with a lower rate of cervical cancer. Teach women about the link between HPV and cervical cancer. Explain that, in most cases, there are no signs or symptoms of infection with HPV. Strongly encourage all young women between the ages of 9 and 26 (and in the case of young girls between 9 and 18, their parents) to consider receiving the vaccine against HPV. For all women, promote the importance of obtaining regular Pap smears and, for women over age 30, suggest an HPV test to rule out the presence of a latent high-risk strain of HPV.

Education and counseling are important aspects of managing women who have genital warts. Teach the woman that:

- Even after genital warts are removed, HPV still remains and viral shedding will continue.
- The likelihood of transmission to future partners and the duration of infectivity after treatment for genital warts are unknown.
- The recurrence of genital warts within the first few months after treatment is common and usually indicates recurrence rather than reinfection (CDC, 2015m).

In the absence of major national health policy mandates, a multilevel, multifaceted approach will be needed to achieve high rates of HPV vaccination in the United States. Nurses need to focus on the education of their clients regarding indications of HPV vaccination and work on approaches to communicating most effectively with parents about the safety and benefits of vaccination and the risks associated with not vaccinating their children.

Sandy is being treated for HPV and is anxious for her "things" to disappear and never return. What education is needed to prevent further transmission from Sandy to any future sexual partners?

Hepatitis A and B

Hepatitis is an acute, systemic, viral infection that can be transmitted sexually. The viruses associated with hepatitis or inflammation of the liver are hepatitis A, B, C, D, E, and G. Hepatitis A is an inflammation of the liver caused by infection with the hepatitis A virus (HAV). Hepatitis A is highly contagious and spreads primarily through the fecal–oral route from person-to-person or by ingesting contaminated food or water. Hepatitis A can also be transmitted through sexual intercourse. Person-to-person transmission through the fecal–oral route (i.e., ingestion of something that has been contaminated with the feces of an infected person) is the primary means of HAV transmission in the United States (CDC, 2015o). Most infections result from close personal contact with an infected household member or sex partner. A HAV infection produces a self-limited disease that does not result in chronic infection or chronic liver disease, but it can be easily passed on to others within the same household.

The hepatitis B virus (HBV) is transmitted by infected body fluids through saliva, blood serum, semen, menstrual blood, and vaginal secretions, and through activities that involve percutaneous (i.e., puncture through the skin) or mucosal contact with infectious blood or body fluids (e.g., semen, saliva). Transmission also occurs via having sex with an infected partner; injection-drug use that involves sharing needles, syringes, or drug-preparation equipment; birth to an infected mother; contact with the blood or open sores of an infected person; needle sticks or sharp instrument exposures; or sharing items such as razors or sharing toothbrushes with an infected person. HBV is not spread through food or water, sharing eating utensils, breast-feeding, skin-to-skin contact, coughing, or sneezing (CDC, 2015p).

The WHO estimates that globally about 2 billion people have been infected with HBV and that more than 240 million have chronic (long-term) liver infections as a result. Worldwide, hepatitis B has the highest death rate (780,000 annually) of any STI except HIV (WHO, 2015a). Risk factors for infection include having multiple sex partners, engaging in unprotected receptive anal intercourse, and having a history of other STIs (CDC, 2015p). The most effective means to prevent the transmission

of hepatitis A or B is preexposure immunization. Vaccines are available for the prevention of HAV and HBV, both of which can be transmitted sexually. Every person seeking treatment for an STI should be considered a candidate for HBV vaccination, and some individuals (e.g., men who have sex with men, and injection-drug users) should be considered for HAV vaccination (CDC, 2015p).

Therapeutic Management

Unlike other STIs, HAV and HBV are preventable through immunization. HAV is usually self-limiting and does not result in chronic infection. HBV can result in serious, permanent liver damage. Treatment is generally supportive. No specific treatment for acute HBV infection exists.

Nursing Assessment

Assess the client for clinical manifestations of hepatitis A and B. Hepatitis A produces flu-like symptoms with malaise, fatigue, anorexia, nausea, pruritus, fever, and upper right quadrant pain. Symptoms of hepatitis B are similar to those of hepatitis A, but with less fever and skin involvement. The diagnosis of hepatitis A cannot be made based on clinical manifestations alone and requires serologic testing. The presence of IgM antibody to HAV is diagnostic of acute HAV infection. Hepatitis B is detected by a blood test that looks for antibodies and proteins produced by the virus and are positively diagnosed by the presence of hepatitis B surface antigen (HBsAg) (Pyrsopoulos & Reddy, 2015).

Nursing Management

Nurses should encourage all women to be screened for hepatitis when they have their annual Pap smear, or sooner if high-risk behavior is identified. Nurses should also encourage women to undergo HBV screening at their first prenatal visit and repeat screening in the last trimester for women with high-risk behaviors to comply with USPSTF (2015) recommendations. Nurses can also explain that hepatitis B vaccine is given to all infants after birth in most hospitals. The vaccination consists of a series of three injections given within 6 months. The vaccine has been shown to be safe and well tolerated by most recipients (CDC, 2015p). Hepatitis A vaccine is strongly encouraged for children between 12 and 23 months of age; persons 1 year of age and older traveling to countries with a high prevalence of hepatitis A, such as Central or South America, Mexico, Asia, Africa, and eastern Europe; men who have sex with men; persons who use street drugs; and persons with chronic liver disease (CDC, 2015o). For others, hepatitis A vaccine series (two doses 6 months apart) may be started whenever a person is at risk for infection.

Hepatitis C

Hepatitis C is an infection caused by the hepatitis C virus (HCV) that attacks the liver and leads to inflammation. It is estimated that about 3% of the world's population has been infected with HCV and that there are more than 170 million chronic carriers who are at risk for developing liver cirrhosis and/or liver cancer (WHO, 2015e). Although HCV is not usually transmitted sexually, it deserves a brief mention here because injection-drug use by women places them at risk for it. HCV-infected pregnant women have a 2% to 8% risk of viral transmission to their newborn, but the mechanism and timing of mother-to-fetus transmission are not fully understood. Although the typical transmission of HCV is not sexual, it can be transmitted sexually. Those with the virus are instructed to refrain from unprotected sexual activity. Women at high risk include those with a history of injection-drug use, health care workers, and those with a history of blood transfusion before 1992 (Dhawan, 2015). The prevalence of HCV infection in pregnant women is approximately 1%. The majority of infected women are not aware they have HCV because they are not clinically ill. Perinatal transmission of HCV is relatively rare, except in women who are immunocompromised (e.g., have HIV/AIDS). A timely diagnosis of HIV and HCV is needed to start treatment, with the best option is to treat HCV before pregnancy (Snijdewind et al., 2015).

Hepatitis infections continue to be an important public health challenge. These viruses impact the entire age spectrum from newborns to the older population. Nurses from all disciplines may, therefore, encounter hepatitis-infected clients. As such, all nurses have a unique opportunity to prevent new infections through client education and improve health outcomes for those already infected.

ZIKA VIRUS DISEASE

Zika virus is transmitted to humans primarily through the bite of an infected *Aedes* species mosquito during the daytime. The most common symptoms of Zika are fever, rash, headaches, bone pains, joint tenderness, and conjunctivitis. The illness is typically mild with symptoms lasting for several days to a week after being bitten. Up to 80% of people infected with the virus have no symptoms (CDC, 2016). The virus is in the Caribbean as well as parts of Central and South America. The virus has been reported to be spread through blood transfusions, sexual contact and can also be passed from a pregnant woman to her fetus and has been linked to a serious birth defect of the brain termed microcephaly. The CDC, WHO, and other scientific organizations are working to understand this possible link.

In 2016 the World Health Organization declared Zika virus a public health emergency of international concern. The CDC recommends abstaining from oral, anal,

or vaginal sexual contact with anyone who has traveled to areas with active infections. Pregnant women are also discouraged from traveling to regions with active infections (2016). At this time, there is no vaccine given to prevent Zika, or anti-viral medication to treat the infection. Prevention measures would include better housing construction, use insect repellents, wear long-sleeved shirts and pants, regular use of air conditioning, use of window screens, avoid traveling to mosquito-infested areas, and state and local mosquito control efforts.

ECTOPARASITIC INFECTIONS

Ectoparasites are a common cause of skin rash and pruritus throughout the world, affecting persons of all ages, races, and socioeconomic groups. Overcrowding, global traveling, immigration, delayed diagnosis and treatment, and poor public education contribute to the prevalence of ectoparasites in both industrial and nonindustrial nations. Approximately 300 million ectoparasitic cases are reported worldwide each year (CDC, 2015g). These infections include infestations of scabies and pubic lice. Because these parasites are easily passed from one person to another during sexual intimacy, clients should be assessed for them when receiving care for other STIs.

Scabies is an intensely pruritic dermatitis caused by a mite. The worldwide prevalence has been estimated at about 100 million cases annually (Monsel & Chosidow, 2015). In general, transmission occurs by direct skin-to-skin contact. The female mite burrows under the skin and deposits eggs, which hatch. The lesions start as a small papule that reddens, erodes, and sometimes crusts. Diagnosis is based on history and appearance of linear burrows in the webs of the fingers, on the elbows, in the axillae, buttocks, and the genitalia (Mutasim, 2015). Aggressive infestation can occur in immunodeficient, debilitated, or malnourished people, but healthy people do not usually suffer sequelae. Scabies treatment includes topical administration of a scabicidal agent (e.g., permethrin, crotamiton, or ivermectin), as well as an antibiotic if a secondary infection is present.

Lice are parasitic insects that can be found on people's head, body or pubic areas. Clients with pediculosis pubis (pubic louse) usually seek treatment because of the pruritus, because of a rash brought on by skin irritation from scratching, or because they notice lice or nits in their pubic hair, axillary hair, abdominal and thigh hair, and sometimes in the eyebrows, eyelashes, and beards. Infestation is usually asymptomatic until after a week or so, when bites cause pruritus and secondary infections from scratching (Fig. 5.9). Diagnosis is based on history and the presence of nits (small, shiny, yellow, oval, dewdrop-like eggs) affixed to hair shafts or lice (a yellowish, oval, wingless insect) (Guenther & Maguiness, 2015).

Treatment has two aspects: medication and environmental control measures. Medications used include

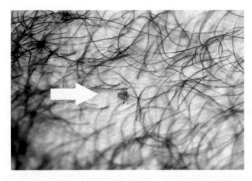

FIGURE 5.9 Pubic lice. A small brown living crab louse is seen at the base of hairs (*arrow*). (From Goodheart, H. [2009]. *Goodheart's photoguide of common skin disorders.* Philadelphia, PA: Lippincott Williams & Wilkins.)

topical anti-louse agents such as permethrin shampoos, malathion, spinosad, or ivermectin. Bedding and clothing should be washed in hot water and dried using a hot setting on the dryer; dry cleaning or sealing clothes in plastic bags for 2 weeks to decontaminate them. Sexual partners should also be treated, as well as family members who live in close contact with the infected person.

Nursing care of a woman infested with lice or scabies involves a three-tiered approach: eradicating the infestation with medication, removing nits, and preventing spread or recurrence by managing the environment. The CDC recommends regimens using pyrethrins and permethrins. Frequently, a combination of malathion or ivermectin is also added. Nurses should provide education about these products (Teaching Guidelines 5.5). The nurse can follow these same guidelines to prevent the health care facility from becoming infested.

Teaching Guidelines 5.5
TREATING AND MINIMIZING THE SPREAD OF SCABIES AND PUBIC LICE

- Use the medication according to the manufacturer's instructions.
- Remove nits with a fine-toothed nit comb.
- Do not share any personal items with others or accept items from others.
- Treat objects, clothing, and bedding and wash them in hot water.
- Meticulously vacuum carpets to prevent a recurrence of infestation.

HUMAN IMMUNODEFICIENCY VIRUS

Many advances have been made in the prevention of HIV transmission and management of HIV/AIDS since the virus was discovered in the early 1980s. Since that time, AIDS has claimed more than 40 million lives (WHO, 2015b). One of the most important discoveries has been antiretroviral

treatment, which can halt the replication of the virus and ease symptoms, turning AIDS into a chronic condition instead of a rapidly terminal illness. Despite advances, HIV remains a major public health challenge today.

Globally, an estimated 35 million people are infected or living with HIV, of which 22.5 million are in sub-Saharan Africa. In addition, of the 2.5 million children in the world estimated to be living with HIV, 2.3 million are in sub-Saharan Africa (WHO, 2015b).

In the United States, an estimated 1.2 million people currently live with HIV, with almost one in six unaware of their infections. An estimated 50,000 new HIV infections occur annually; typically, every 10 minutes a person in the United States becomes infected with HIV (CDC, 2015q). In terms of epidemiology, fatality rate, and its social, legal, ethical, and political aspects, HIV/AIDS is a public health crisis and has generated more concern than any other infectious disease in modern medical history. The course of HIV infection is characterized primarily by latency. Unfortunately, profound immune suppression eventually develops and the illness is lethal. More than 650,000 people have died of AIDS in the United States since the 1980s (CDC, 2015q).

HIV/AIDS continues to outpace the science, financing, prevention, and treatment efforts of the past quarter century. The economic impact of HIV/AIDS presents huge challenges. While the causality between poverty and HIV is not clear, it is certain that HIV pushes households and individuals into poverty. While many illnesses create catastrophic expenditures that can result in poverty, HIV/AIDS is among the worst because its victims are ill for a prolonged period of time before they die, and many are the chief household income earners. According to the WHO, the lower a person's socioeconomic status is, the worse the health outcomes for them. An intervention to address this issue is to help women's vocational development and economic empowerment since the illness exists for years (Conyers et al., 2015). To date, there is no cure for this fatal viral infection.

The HIV virus is transmitted by intimate sexual contact; by sharing needles for intravenous drug use; from mother to fetus during pregnancy or breast-feeding; and by transfusion of blood or blood products. Men who have sex with men represent the largest proportion of new infections, followed by men and women infected through heterosexual sex (CDC, 2015q). Among racial/ethnic groups in the United States, African Americans are at the highest risk of acquiring HIV/AIDS, and account for 45% of new HIV infections. The African American community continues to be ravaged by HIV/AIDS infection, despite the marked expenditures utilized to reduce incidence among this cohort. Efforts to produce culturally appropriate programs that work continue to elude officials, and HIV/AIDS has become pandemic within this racial/ethnic group. More awareness of HIV/AIDS using media campaigns is needed to reduce risky behaviors (Nunn et al., 2015).

The number of women with HIV infection and AIDS has been increasing steadily worldwide. Today, women account for one in four (25%) new HIV infections in the United States. Women of color have been especially hard hit and represent the majority of women living with the disease and newly infected ones. Most women are infected through heterosexual sex (Kaiser Family Foundation, 2015). The WHO estimates that over 25 million women are living with HIV/AIDS worldwide, accounting for approximately 50% of the 40 million adults living with HIV/AIDS (CDC, 2015r). HIV disproportionately affects African American and Hispanic women: together they represent less than 25% of all women in the United States; yet they account for more than 82% of AIDS cases among women (CDC, 2015r). African American women in this country suffer disproportionately from the HIV/AIDS epidemic, as they acquire new HIV infections at nearly 15 times the rate of White women (CDC, 2015r). Women are particularly vulnerable to heterosexual transmission of HIV as a result of substantial mucosal exposure to seminal fluids. This biologic fact amplifies the risk of HIV transmission when coupled with the high prevalence of nonconsensual sex, sex without condoms, and the unknown and/or high-risk behaviors of their partners (CDC, 2015r). Therefore, the face of HIV/AIDS is becoming the face of young women. That shift will ultimately exacerbate the incidence of HIV because women spread it not only through sex, but also through nursing and childbirth.

AIDS is a breakdown in the immune function caused by HIV, a retrovirus. A sufficient quantity of viruses must be transferred to infect a person. The virus cannot live long outside the human body; it cannot be transmitted via tears or sweat. The HIV infection is associated with continued activation of immune system and is the driving force behind CD4 T cell depletion and progression to AIDS. The infected person develops opportunistic infections or malignancies that become fatal. Progression from HIV infection to AIDS occurs at a median of 11 years after infection (Bharaj & Chahar, 2015). HIV transmission modalities include the following:

- Sexual intercourse with an infected partner unprotected by condoms
- Blood transfusions from infected donors or organ transplants from infected donors
- Needle sticks from contaminated sharps or sharing needles with infected people
- Mother-to-infant during pregnancy, childbirth or breastfeeding

More than 30 years have passed since HIV/AIDS began to affect our society. Since then, 50 million people have been infected by the virus, with AIDS being the fourth leading cause of death globally (CDC, 2015q). The morbidity and mortality of HIV continue to hold the attention of the medical community. While there has been a dramatic improvement in both morbidity and mortality with the use of highly active antiretroviral therapy, the incidence of HIV infection continues to rise.

Take Note!

More than 90% of individuals infected with HIV worldwide do not know they are infected and, thus, are at risk of spreading it sexually to others (CDC, 2015q).

The fetal and neonatal effects of acquiring HIV through perinatal transmission are devastating and eventually fatal. An infected mother can transmit HIV infection to her newborn before or during birth and through breast-feeding. Most cases of mother-to-child HIV transmission, the cause of more than 90% of pediatric-acquired infections worldwide, occur late in pregnancy or during delivery. Transmission rates vary from 25% in untreated non–breast-feeding populations in industrialized countries to about 40% among untreated breast-feeding populations in developing countries (Castel, Magnus, & Greenberg, 2015). Despite the dramatic reduction in perinatal transmission, hundreds of infants will be born infected with HIV.

HIV and Adolescents

The effects of HIV and AIDS on adolescents and young adults is of increasing concern, but it is difficult to get accurate data because of the varying ways in which this population seeks health care services. Some adolescents continue to receive care through pediatricians and adult services, but many do not have access to health care. HIV infections are increasing in adolescents and young adults aged 13 to 24 years. Approximately 25% of cases of STIs reported in the United States each year are among teenagers. More than two million adolescents between the ages of ten and nineteen are living with HIV, and many do not receive the care and support they need to stay in good health. This is particularly significant because the risk of HIV transmission increases substantially if either partner is infected with an STI (WHO, 2015c). At least one adolescent in the United States is infected with HIV each hour. Since it takes an average of 11 years for AIDS symptoms to appear when HIV is left untreated, it is obvious that many adults with AIDS were infected as adolescents.

Nurses can play a key role in preventing and controlling HIV infection by promoting risk reduction counseling and offering routine HIV testing to adolescents. Most sexually active youth do not feel that they are at risk for contracting HIV and have never been tested. Obtaining a sexual history and creating an atmosphere that promotes nonjudgmental risk counseling is a key component of the adolescent visit. In light of increasing numbers of people with HIV/AIDS and missed opportunities for HIV testing, the CDC (2015q) recommends universal and routine HIV testing for all clients seen in health care settings who are 13 to 64 years of age.

Clinical Manifestations

HIV infection undergoes three distinct phases: acute seroconversion, asymptomatic infection, and then progression to AIDS. When a person is initially infected with HIV, he or she goes through an acute primary infection period for about 3 weeks. The HIV viral load drops rapidly because the host's immune system works well to fight this initial infection. The onset of the acute primary infection occurs 2 to 6 weeks after exposure. Symptoms include fever, pharyngitis, rash, and myalgia. Most people do not associate this flu-like condition with HIV infection. After initial exposure, there is a period of 3 to 12 months before seroconversion. The person is considered infectious during this time.

After the acute phase, the infected person becomes asymptomatic, but the HIV virus begins to replicate. Even though there are no symptoms, the immune system runs down. A normal person has a CD4 T-cell count of 450 to 1,200 cells per microliter. When the CD4 T-cell count reaches 200 or less, the person is considered to have AIDS. The immune system begins a constant battle to fight this viral invasion, but over time it falls behind. A viral reservoir occurs in T cells that can store various stages of the virus. The onset and severity of the disease correlate directly with the viral load: the more HIV virus that is present, the worse the person will feel. As profound immunosuppression begins to occur, an opportunistic infection will occur, qualifying the person for the diagnosis of AIDS. As of now, AIDS will eventually develop in everyone who is HIV positive.

The WHO now recommends earlier initiation of antiretroviral therapy (ART) for adults and adolescents, the delivery of more client-friendly ART drugs, and prolonged use of ART drugs to reduce the risk of mother-to-child transmission of HIV. ART should be started when the CD4 counts are below 350 cells/microliter. Further recommendations include initiation of ART irrespective of CD4 cell count or clinical stage for people co-infected with active tuberculosis or hepatitis B with severe liver disease, pregnant women in serodiscordant partnerships, and children under 5 years of age (Bennett & Gilroy, 2015).

Diagnosis

Several types of tests are approved to detect HIV. These tests are designed to detect antigens, antibodies, or RNA. The enzyme-linked immunosorbent assay (ELISA) is used as the initial screening test to determine presence of the HIV virus. When ELISA generates a positive result, a confirmation test (Western blot test) is then performed. In addition, several point-of-care or rapid antibody tests are available. Two categories of screening methods are currently used: rapid HIV tests and confirmatory tests. The rapid tests allow for screening at the point-of-care and quick results. Five rapid HIV tests that are FDA approved include: (1) OraQuick Advance HIV tests (whole blood used); (2) Uni-Gold Recombigen HIV test (whole blood used); (3) Reveal G-3 Rapid HIV Antibody test (serum or plasma used); (4) Multispot (serum or plasma used); and (5) Clearview Stat-Pak and complete

(whole blood used). A positive result is followed up with one of two confirmatory tests: Western blot (WB) or immunofluorescence (IFA) (Shafiee et al., 2015).

Quick tests for HIV produce results in 10 to 20 minutes and also lower the health care worker's risk of occupational exposure by eliminating the need to draw blood. The CDC's Advancing HIV Prevention initiative, launched in 2003, has made increased testing a national priority. The CDC recommends HIV screening of all US residents aged 13 to 64 years in all health care settings (CDC, 2015r).

Fewer than half of adults between the ages of 18 and 64 have ever had an HIV test, according to the CDC. The agency estimates that one fourth of the million HIV-infected people in the United States do not know they are infected. This means they are not receiving treatment that can prolong their lives, and they may be unknowingly infecting others. In addition, even when people do get tested, one in three fails to return to the testing site to learn their results when there is a 2-week wait. The CDC hopes that the new "one-stop" approach to HIV testing will change that pattern.

People who are infected with HIV but not aware of it are not able to take advantage of the therapies that can keep them healthy and extend their lives, nor do they have the knowledge to protect their sex or drug-use partners from becoming infected. Knowing whether one is positive or negative for HIV confers great benefits in healthy decision-making.

Rapid point-of-service HIV tests are becoming powerful screening tools in various health care settings because they offer the opportunity to not only screen for HIV, but also to educate the person regarding risk factors, and discuss their test results—all in one clinical visit. Most use a fingerstick drop of blood or a swab of saliva taken from the mouth. Results are typically ready within 10 to 20 minutes. If the confirmation test (WB or IFA) is positive, the person is infected with HIV and is capable of transmitting the virus to others. HIV antibody is detectable in at least 95% of people within 3 months after infection (CDC, 2015q).

Therapeutic Management

The goals of HIV drug therapy are as follows:
- Decrease the HIV viral load below the level of detection.
- Restore the body's ability to fight off pathogens.
- Improve the client's quality of life.
- Reduce HIV morbidity and mortality (Bennett & Gilroy, 2015).

Highly active antiretroviral therapy (HAART), which combines at least three antiretroviral drugs, has dramatically improved the prognosis of HIV/AIDS. Often treatment begins with combination HAART at the time of the first infection, when the person's immune system is still intact. The current HAART standard is a triple combination therapy, but some clients may be given a fourth or fifth agent.

Current therapy to prevent the transmission of HIV to the newborn includes a three-part regimen:

1. The mother takes an oral antiretroviral agent at 14 to 34 weeks of gestation; it is continued throughout pregnancy.
2. During labor, an antiretroviral agent is administered intravenously until delivery.
3. An antiretroviral syrup is administered to the infant within 12 hours after birth.

Dramatic new treatment advances with antiretroviral medications have turned a disease that used to be a death sentence into a chronic, manageable one for individuals who live in countries where ART is available. Despite these advances in treatment, however, only a minority of HIV-positive people in the United States who take antiretroviral medications are receiving the full benefits because they are not adhering to the prescribed regimen. Successful ART requires nearly perfect adherence to a complex medication regimen; less-than-perfect adherence leads to drug resistance (King et al., 2015).

Adherence is difficult because of the complexity of the regimen and the lifelong duration of treatment. A typical antiretroviral regimen may consist of three or more medications taken twice daily. Adherence is made even more difficult because of the unpleasant side effects, such as nausea and diarrhea. Women in early pregnancy already experience these, and the antiretroviral medication only exacerbates them.

Nursing Management

Nurses can play a major role in caring for the HIV-positive woman by helping her accept the possibility of a shortened life span, cope with others' reactions to a stigmatizing illness, and develop strategies to maintain her physical and emotional health. Educate the woman about changes she can make in her behavior to prevent spreading HIV to others, and refer her to appropriate community resources such as HIV medical care services, substance abuse services, mental health services, and social services. See Nursing Care Plan 5.1: Overview of the Woman Who Is HIV Positive.

Providing Education About Drug Therapy

The goal of antiretroviral therapy is to suppress viral replication so that the viral load becomes undetectable by diagnostic tests. This is done to preserve immune function and delay disease progression but is a challenge because of the side effects of nausea and vomiting, diarrhea, altered taste, anorexia, flatulence, constipation, headaches, anemia, and fatigue. Although not everyone experiences all of the side effects, the majority do have some of them. Current research has not documented the long-term safety of exposure of the fetus to antiretroviral agents during pregnancy, but collection of data is ongoing.

Help to reduce the development of drug resistance and thus treatment failure by identifying the barriers to adherence; identifying these barriers can help the woman to overcome them. Some of the common barriers exist because the woman:

- Does not understand the link between drug resistance and nonadherence
- Fears revealing her HIV status by being seen taking medication
- Has not adjusted emotionally to the HIV diagnosis
- Does not understand the dosing regimen or schedule
- Experiences unpleasant side effects frequently
- Feels anxious or depressed (Dubin, 2015)

Educate the woman about the prescribed drug therapy and stress that it is very important to take the regimen as prescribed. Offer suggestions about how to cope with anorexia, nausea, and vomiting by:

- Separating the intake of food and fluids
- Eating dry crackers upon arising
- Eating six small meals daily
- Using high-protein supplements (Boost, Ensure) to provide quick and easy protein and calories
- Eating "comfort foods," which may appeal when other foods do not

Promoting Adherence to Therapy

Remaining adherent to drug therapy is a huge challenge for many HIV-infected people. Adherence becomes difficult when the same pills that are supposed to thwart the disease are making the person sick. Nausea and diarrhea are just two of the possible side effects. It is often difficult to increase the client's quality of life when so much oral medication is required. The combination medication therapy is challenging for many people, and staying compliant over a period of years is extremely difficult. Stress the importance of taking the prescribed antiretroviral drug therapies by explaining that they help prevent replication of the retroviruses and subsequent progression of the disease and also decrease the risk of perinatal transmission of HIV. In addition, provide written materials describing diet, exercise, medications, and signs and symptoms of complications and opportunistic infections. Reinforce this information at each visit.

Preventing HIV Infection

Despite the available information about HIV infection and AIDS, it causes great anxiety and fear of the unknown. It is vital to take a leadership role in educating the public about risky behaviors in the fight to control this disease. The core of HIV prevention is to reduce the number of sexual contacts and to use condoms. This is all good advice for many women, but some simply do not have the economic and social power or choices or control over their lives to put that advice into practice. Recognize that fact, and address the factors that will give

Overview of the Woman Who is HIV Positive

Annie, a 28-year-old African American woman, is HIV-positive. She acquired HIV through unprotected sexual contact. She has been inconsistent in taking her antiretroviral medications and presents today stating she is tired and does not feel well.

NURSING DIAGNOSIS: Risk for infection related to positive HIV status and inconsistent adherence to antiretroviral therapy regimen

Outcome Identification and Evaluation

The client will remain free of opportunistic infections as evidenced by temperature within acceptable parameters and absence of signs and symptoms of opportunistic infections.

Interventions: *Minimizing the Risk of Opportunistic Infections*

- Assess CD4 count and viral loads *to determine disease progression* (CD4 counts <500/L and viral loads >10,000 copies/L = increased risk for opportunistic infections).
- Assess complete blood count *to identify presence of infection* (>10,000 cells/mm^3 may indicate infection).
- Assess oral cavity and mucous membranes for painful white patches in mouth *to evaluate for possible fungal infection.*
- Teach client to monitor for general signs and symptoms of infections, such as fever, weakness, and fatigue, *to ensure early identification.*
- Provide information explaining the importance of avoiding people with infections when possible *to minimize risk of exposure to infections.*

- Teach importance of keeping appointments so her CD4 count and viral load can be monitored *to alert the health care provider about her immune system status.*
- Instruct her to reduce her exposure to infections via:
  - Meticulous hand hygiene
  - Thorough cooking of meats, eggs, and vegetables
  - Wearing shoes at all times, especially when outdoors
- Encourage a balance of rest with activity throughout the day *to prevent overexertion.*
- Stress importance of maintaining prescribed antiretroviral drug therapies *to prevent disease progression and resistance.*
- If necessary, refer Annie to a nutritionist to help her understand what constitutes a well-balanced diet with supplements *to promote health and ward off infection.*

NURSING DIAGNOSIS: Deficient knowledge related to HIV infection and possible complications

Outcome Identification and Evaluation

The client will demonstrate increased understanding of HIV infection as evidenced by verbalizing appropriate health care practices and adhering to therapy and reduce her risk of further exposure and reduce risk of disease progression.

Interventions: *Providing Client Education*

- Assess her understanding of HIV and its treatment *to provide a baseline for teaching.*
- Establish trust and be honest with Annie; encourage her to talk about her fears and the impact of the disease *to provide an outlet for her concerns.* Encourage her to discuss reasons for her nonadherence to therapy.
- Provide a nonjudgmental, accessible, confidential, and culturally sensitive approach *to promote Annie's self-esteem and allow her to feel that she is a priority.*
- Explain measures, including safer sex practices and birth control options, to prevent disease transmission; determine her willingness to practice safer sex to protect others *to determine further teaching needs.*
- Discuss the signs and symptoms of disease progression and potential opportunistic infections *to promote early detection for prompt intervention.*
- Outline with the client the availability of community resources and make appropriate referrals as needed *to provide additional education and support.*
- Encourage Annie to keep scheduled appointments *to ensure follow-up and allow early detection of potential problems.*

women more control over their lives by providing antici-patory guidance, giving ample opportunities to practice negotiation techniques and refusal skills in a safe envi-ronment, and encouraging the use of female condoms to protect against this deadly virus. Prevention is the key to reversing the current infection trends.

Providing Care During Pregnancy and Childbirth

Voluntary counseling and HIV testing should be offered to all pregnant women as early in the pregnancy as pos-sible to identify HIV-infected women so that treatment can be initiated early. Once a pregnant woman is identified as being HIV positive, she should be informed about the risk for perinatal infection. Current evidence indicates that in the absence of antiretroviral medications, 25% of infants born to HIV-infected mothers will become infected with HIV (CDC, 2015q). If women do receive a combination of antiretroviral therapies during pregnancy, however, the risk of HIV transmission to the newborn drops below 2% (Castel, Magnus, & Greenberg, 2015). In addition, HIV can be spread to the infant through breast-feeding, and thus all HIV-infected pregnant women should be counseled to avoid breast-feeding and use formula instead. A recent maternal infection with HIV may raise the risk of transmis-sion through breast-feeding to twice that of a woman with earlier established infection, probably as a result of the high viral load associated with recent infection (Koletzko, 2015).

In addition, the woman needs instructions on ways to enhance her immune system by following these guide-lines during pregnancy:
- Getting adequate sleep each night (7 to 9 hours)
- Avoiding infections (e.g., staying out of crowds, good hand hygiene)
- Decreasing stress in her life
- Consuming adequate protein and vitamins
- Increasing her fluid intake to 2 liters daily to stay hydrated
- Planning rest periods throughout the day to prevent fatigue

As said earlier, despite the dramatic reduction in perinatal transmission, hundreds of infants will be born infected with HIV. The birth of each infected infant is a missed prevention opportunity. To minimize perina-tal HIV transmission, identify HIV infection in women, preferably before pregnancy; provide information about disease prevention; and encourage HIV-infected women to follow the prescribed drug therapy.

Providing Appropriate Referrals

The HIV-infected woman may have difficulty coping with the normal activities of daily living because she has less energy and decreased physical endurance. She may be overwhelmed by the financial burdens of medical and drug therapies, the emotional responses

to a life-threatening condition, and, if she is pregnant, concern about her infant's future. A case management approach is needed to deal with the complexity of her needs during this time. Be an empathetic listener and make appropriate referrals for nutritional services, coun-seling, homemaker services, spiritual care, and local sup-port groups. Many community-based organizations have developed programs to address the numerous issues regarding HIV/AIDS. The national AIDS hotline (1-800-342-AIDS) is a good resource. Table 5.4 provides a sum-mary of the perinatal effects of STIs during pregnancy.

PREVENTING SEXUALLY TRANSMITTED INFECTIONS

Education about safer sex practices—and the resulting increase in the use of condoms—can play a vital role in reducing STI rates all over the world. Clearly, knowledge and prevention are the best defenses against STIs. The prevention and control of STIs is based on the following concepts (American College of Obstetricians & Gynecol-ogists [ACOG], 2015; U.S. FDA, 2015):
1. Education and counseling of persons at risk about safer sexual behavior
2. Recommending immunizations that prevent Hepatitis B and HPV preexposure
3. Educating people that latex condoms offer some pro-tection and reduce risk of transmission
4. Identifying asymptomatic infected individuals and symptomatic individuals unlikely to seek diagnosis and treatment
5. Effectively diagnosing and treating infected individuals
6. Evaluating, treating, and counseling sex partners of people who are infected with an STI

Nurses play an integral role in identifying and pre-venting STIs. They have a unique opportunity to educate the public about this serious public health issue by com-municating the methods of transmission and symptoms associated with each condition, tracking the updated CDC treatment guidelines, and offering clients strategic preventive measures to reduce the spread of STIs. Nurses have a huge role to play to ensure all women are well educated about STIs by informing them how these infec-tions are transmitted, symptoms, risk factors, potential for adverse effects, screening, and treatment recommen-dations. Armed with this knowledge, women can make fully informed decisions about accepting screening and adhering to treatment and follow-up advice.

It is not easy to discuss STI prevention when globally we are failing at it. Knowledge exists on how to prevent every single route of transmission, but the incidence of STIs continues to climb. Challenges to prevention of STIs include lack of resources and difficulty in changing the behaviors that contribute to their spread. Regardless of the challenging factors involved, nurses must continue to

TABLE 5.4	MATERNAL AND FETAL EFFECTS FROM SEXUALLY TRANSMITTED INFECTIONS	
STI	**Maternal Effects**	**Fetal Effects**
Candidiasis	Resistant to treatment during pregnancy; uncomfortable localized genital itching and discharge	Can acquire thrush in the mouth during birthing process if mother infected
Trichomoniasis	Has been implicated in causing the premature rupture of membranes (PROM) and preterm births	Risk of prematurity
Bacterial vaginosis	Increases risk for spontaneous abortion, PROM, chorioamnionitis, postpartum endometritis, and preterm labor	Risk of neonatal sepsis
Chlamydia	Postpartum endometritis, PROM, and preterm birth	Conjunctivitis, which can lead to blindness; low birth weight; and pneumonitis
Gonorrhea	Chorioamnionitis, preterm birth, PROM, intrauterine growth restriction (IUGR), and postpartum sepsis	Eye infection (*gonococcal ophthalmia*), which can cause blindness
Genital herpes	Spontaneous abortion, intrauterine infection, preterm labor, PROM, and IUGR	Birth anomalies and transplacental infection
Syphilis	Spontaneous abortion, preterm birth, and stillbirth	Congenital syphilis, leading to multisystem organ failure and structural damage, and intellectual disability
Human papillomavirus (HPV)	May cause dystocia if large lesions	None known
Hepatitis B	May cause preterm birth; can be transmitted to fetus if active in last trimester	Can become chronic carrier of hepatitis B, which may lead to liver cancer or cirrhosis
HIV	Fatigue, nausea, and weight loss	Transmission can occur transplacentally, during childbirth or through breast milk

Adapted from Centers for Disease Control and Prevention [CDC]. (20145j). *STD & pregnancy – CDC fact sheet*. Retrieved from http://www.cdc.gov/std/pregnancy/stdfact-pregnancy.htm; King, T. L., Brucker, M. C., Kriebs, J. M., Fahey, J. O., Gegor, C. L., & Varney, H. (2015). *Varney's midwifery* (5th ed.). Burlington, MA: Jones & Bartlett Learning; and Schuiling, K. D., &Likis, F. (2016). *Women's gynecologic health* (3rd ed.). Burlington, MA: Jones & Bartlett Learning.

educate and to meet the needs of all women to promote their sexual health. Successful treatment and prevention of STIs is impossible without education. Successful teaching approaches include giving clear, accurate messages that are age appropriate and culturally sensitive.

Primary prevention strategies include educating all women, especially adolescents, regarding the risk of early sexual activity, the number of sexual partners, and STIs. Sexual abstinence is ideal but often not practiced; therefore, the use of barrier contraception (condoms) should be encouraged (see Teaching Guidelines 5.1).

Secondary prevention involves the need for annual pelvic examinations with Pap smears for all sexually active women, regardless of age. Many women with STIs are asymptomatic, so regular screening examinations are paramount for early detection. Understanding the relationship between poor socioeconomic conditions and poor patterns of sexual and reproductive self-care is significant in disease prevention and health promotion strategies.

Every successful form of prevention requires a change in behavior. The nursing role in teaching and rendering quality health care is invaluable evidence that the key to reducing the spread of STIs is through behavioral change. Nurses working in these specialty areas have a responsibility to educate themselves, their clients, their families, and the community about STIs and to provide compassionate and supportive care to clients. Some strategies nurses can use to prevent the spread of STIs are detailed in Box 5.4.

Behavior Modification

Research validates that changing behaviors does result in a decrease in new STI infections, but it must encompass all

SELECTED NURSING STRATEGIES TO PREVENT THE SPREAD OF SEXUALLY TRANSMITTED INFECTIONS

- Provide basic information about STI transmission.
- Outline safer sexual behaviors for people at risk for STIs.
- Refer clients to appropriate community resources to reduce risk.
- Screen asymptomatic persons with STIs.
- Identify barriers to STI testing and remove them.
- Offer pre-exposure immunizations for vaccine-preventable STIs.
- Respond honestly about testing results and options available.
- Counsel and treat sexual partners of persons with STIs.
- Educate school administrators, parents, and teens about STIs.
- Support youth development activities to reduce sexual risk-taking.
- Promote the use of barrier methods (condoms, diaphragms) to prevent the spread of STIs.
- Assist clients to gain skills in negotiating safer sex.
- Discuss reducing the number of sexual partners to reduce risk.

Consider This

I was thinking of my carefree college days, when the most important thing was having an active sorority life and meeting guys. I had been raised by very strict parents and was never allowed to date under their watch. Since I attended an out-of-state college, I figured that my parents' outdated advice and rules no longer applied. Abruptly, my thoughts of the past were interrupted by the HIV counselor asking about my feelings concerning my positive diagnosis. What was there to say at this point? I had a lot of fun but never dreamed it would haunt me for the rest of my life, which was going to be shortened considerably now. I only wish I could turn back the hands of time and listen to my parents' advice, which somehow doesn't seem so outdated now.

Thoughts: *All of us have thought back on our lives to better times and wondered how our lives would have changed if we had made better choices or gone down another path. It is a pity that we have only one chance to make good, sound decisions at times. What would you have changed in your life if given a second chance? Can you still make a change for the better now?*

levels—governments, community organizations, schools, churches, parents, and individuals (WHO, 2015d). Education must address the following: ways to prevent becoming infected; condom promotion; target vulnerable populations such as adolescents, sex workers, men who have sex with men, and people who inject drugs; ways to prevent transmitting infection; symptoms of STIs; and treatment. At this point in the STI epidemic, nurses do not have time to debate the relative merits of prevention versus treatment: both are underused and underfunded, and one leads to the other. But being serious about prevention and focusing on the strategies outlined above will bring about a positive change on everyone's part.

Contraception

The spread of STIs could be prevented by access to safe, efficient, appropriate barrier contraceptives. The consistent and correct use of condoms plays an important role in preventing the spread of STIs. Nurses can play an important role in helping women to identify their risk of STIs and to adopt preventive measures through the dual protection that contraceptives offer. Traditionally, family planning and STI services have been separate entities. Family planning services have addressed a woman's need for contraception without considering her or her partner's risk of STIs; meanwhile, STI services have been heavily slanted toward men while ignoring their contraceptive needs.

Many women are at significant risk for unintended pregnancy and STIs; yet with this separation of services,

there is limited evaluation of whether they need dual protection—that is, concurrent protection from STIs and unintended pregnancy. This lack of integration of services represents a missed opportunity to identify many at-risk women and to offer them counseling on dual protection. Nurses can play a key role in influencing clients to initiate and maintain use of the female condom, an underused method for STI and pregnancy prevention (Alexander et al., 2015).

Nurses can expand their scopes in either setting by discussing dual protection by use of a male or female condom alone or by use of a condom along with a non-barrier contraceptive. Because barrier methods are not the most effective means of fertility control, they have not been typically recommended as a method alone for dual protection. Unfortunately, the most effective pregnancy prevention methods—sterilization, hormonal methods, and intrauterine systems—do not protect against STIs. Dual-method use protects against STIs and pregnancy.

KEY CONCEPTS

- Avoiding risky sexual behaviors may preserve fertility and prevent chronic conditions later in life.
- An estimated 65 million people live with an incurable sexually transmitted infection (STI), and another 15 million are infected each year (CDC, 2015a).
- The most reliable way to avoid transmission of STIs is to abstain from sexual intercourse (i.e., oral, vaginal,

or anal sex) or to be in a long-term, mutually monogamous relationship with an uninfected partner.

○ Barrier methods of contraception are recommended because they increase protection from contact with urethral discharge, mucosal secretions, and lesions of the cervix or penis.

○ The high rate of asymptomatic transmission of STIs calls for teaching high-risk women the nature of transmission and how to recognize infections.

○ Nurses should practice good hand hygiene and follow standard precautions to protect themselves and their clients from STIs.

○ Nurses are in an important position to promote the sexual health of all women. Nurses should make their clients and the community aware of the perinatal implications and lifelong sequelae of STIs.

References and Recommended Readings

Alexander, K. A., Jemmott, L. S., Teitelman, A. M., & D'Antonio, P. (2015). Addressing sexual health behavior during emerging adulthood: A critical review of the literature. *Journal of Clinical Nursing, 24,* 4–18.

Alexander, L. L., LaRosa, J. H., Bader, H., & Garfield, S. (2014). *New dimensions in women's health* (6th ed.). Sudbury, MA: Jones & Bartlett.

American Cancer Society [ACS]. (2015). *HPV vaccine information for clinicians—Fact sheet.* Retrieved from http://www.cancer.org/Cancer/CervicalCancer/DetailedGuide/cervical-cancer-key-statistics

American College of Obstetricians & Gynecologists [ACOG] (2015). *How to prevent sexually transmitted infections.* Retrieved from http://www.acog.org/-/media/For-Patients/faq009.pdf?dmc=1&ts=20150428T1518040649

Amoako, A. A., & Balen, A. H. (2015). Female infertility: Diagnosis and management. In F. Bandeira, H. Gharib, A. Golbert, L. Griz & M. Faria (Eds.), *Endocrinology and diabetes* (pp. 123–131). London: Springer Publishers.

Anderson, B., & Cu-Uvin, S. (2015). HIV and pregnancy. *UpToDate.* Retrieved from http://www.uptodate.com/contents/hiv-and-pregnancy-beyond-the-basics

Angoori, G. R. (2015). Early congenital syphilis. *Indian Journal of Pediatric Dermatology, 16*(2), 75–77.

Annon, J. S. (1976). The PLISSIT model: A proposed conceptual scheme for the behavioral treatment of sexual problems. *Journal of Sex Education Therapy, 2,* 1–15.

Barry, M., Kauffman, C. L., Wilson, B. B., Rozen, E., & Rosh, A. J. (2015). Scabies. *eMedicine.* Retrieved from http://emedicine.medscape.com/article/1109204-overview

Bennett, N. J., & Gilroy, S. A. (2015). HIV disease. *eMedicine.* Retrieved from http://emedicine.medscape.com/article/211316-overview

Bharaj, P., & Chahar, H. S. (2015). Immune activation and HIV pathogenesis: Implications for therapy. *Journal of Antivirals and Antiretrovirals, 7,* 15–21.

Blank, J. (2015). Pelvic inflammatory diseases. In T. J. Saclarides, J. A. Myers, & K. W. Millikan (Eds.), *Common surgical diseases* (pp. 327–329). New York, NY: Springer Publishers.

Burnett, E., Loucks, T. L., & Lindsay, M. (2015). Perinatal outcomes in HIV positive women with concomitant sexually transmitted infections. *Infectious Diseases in Obstetrics & Gynecology.* doi: 10.1155/2015/508482

Castel, A. D., Magnus, M., & Greenberg, A. E. (2015). Update on the epidemiology and prevention of HIV/AIDS in the USA. *Current Epidemiology Reports, 2,* 110–119.

Castle, P. E., & Schmeler, K. M. (2015). HPV vaccination: For women of all ages? *The Lancet, 384*(9961), 2178–2180.

Centers for Disease Control and Prevention [CDC]. (2015a). *STD data and statistics.* Retrieved from http://www.cdc.gov/std/stats

Centers for Disease Control and Prevention [CDC]. (2015b). *Genital vulvovaginal candidiasis (VVC).* Retrieved from http://www.cdc.gov/fungal/candidiasis/genital/

Centers for Disease Control and Prevention [CDC]. (2015c). *Trichomoniasis.* Retrieved from http://www.cdc.gov/std/trichomonas/

Centers for Disease Control and Prevention [CDC]. (2015d). *Bacterial vaginosis.* Retrieved from http://www.cdc.gov/Std/BV/default.htm

Centers for Disease Control and Prevention [CDC]. (2015e). *Chlamydia.* Retrieved from http://www.cdc.gov/std/chlamydia/default.htm

Centers for Disease Control and Prevention [CDC]. (2015f). *Gonorrhea.* Retrieved from http://www.cdc.gov/std/gonorrhea/STDFact-gonorrhea-detailed.htm

Centers for Disease Control and Prevention [CDC]. (2015g). *Sexually transmitted diseases.* Retrieved from http://www.cdc.gov/std/default.htm

Centers for Disease Control and prevention [CDC]. (2015h). *Genital herpes – CDC fact sheet.* Retrieved from http://www.cdc.gov/std/herpes/stdfact-herpes.htm

Centers for Disease Control and Prevention [CDC]. (2015i). *Syphilis – CDC fact sheet.* Retrieved from http://www.cdc.gov/sTD/syphilis/STDFact-Syphilis-detailed.htm

Centers for Disease Control and Prevention [CDC]. (2015j). *STD & pregnancy – CDC fact sheet.* Retrieved from http://www.cdc.gov/std/pregnancy/stdfact-pregnancy.htm

Centers for Disease Control and Prevention [CDC]. (2015k). *STD treatment guidelines.* Retrieved from http://www.cdc.gov/std/treatment/2010/default.htm

Centers for Disease Control and Prevention [CDC]. (2015l). *Pelvic inflammatory disease (PID) – CDC fact sheet.* Retrieved from http://www.cdc.gov/std/pid/STDFact-PID.htm

Centers for Disease Control and Prevention [CDC]. (2015m). *Human papillomavirus (HPV).* Retrieved from http://www.cdc.gov/hpv/

Centers for Disease Control and Prevention [CDC]. (2015n). *HPV vaccines.* Retrieved from http://www.cdc.gov/vaccines/hcp/vis/vis-statements/hpv-gardasil.html

Centers for Disease Control and Prevention [CDC]. (2015o). *Hepatitis A inform information for health professionals.* Retrieved from http://www.cdc.gov/hepatitis/HAV/HAVfaq.htm#A2

Centers for Disease Control and prevention [CDC]. (2015p). *Hepatitis B information for health professionals.* Retrieved from http://www.cdc.gov/hepatitis/HBV/HBVfaq.htm

Centers for Disease Control and Prevention [CDC]. (2015q). *HIV/AIDS.* Retrieved from http://www.cdc.gov/hiv/basics/index.html

Centers for Disease Control and Prevention [CDC]. (2015r). *HIV among women.* Retrieved from http://www.cdc.gov/hiv/risk/gender/women/facts/index.html

Centers for Disease Control and Prevention [CDC]. (2015s). *HIV among pregnant women, infants, and children.* Retrieved from http://www.cdc.gov/hiv/risk/gender/pregnantwomen/facts/

Centers for Disease Control and Prevention [CDC]. (2016). *Zika virus.* Retrieved from http://www.cdc.gov/zika/pregnancy/protect-yourself.html

Chen, M. Y., Klausner, J. D., Fairley, C. K., Guy, R., Wilson, D., & Donovan, B. (2015). Syphilis: A fresh look at an old foe. *Sexual Health, 12*(2), 93–95.

Comkornruecha, M. (2013). Gonococcal infections. *Pediatrics in Review, 34*(5), 228–234.

Collins, B. (2015). *Updated researches in chlamydia.* New Delhi: M L Books International.

Conyers, L. M., Chiu, Y. C., Shamburger-Rousseau, A., Johnson, V., & Misrok, M. (2015). Common threads: An integrated HIV prevention and vocational development intervention for African American women living with HIV/AIDS. *Journal of Health Disparities Research and Practice, 7*(7), 9. Retrieved from http://digitalscholarship.unlv.edu/jhdrp/vol7/iss7/9

Decker, K. M., McLachlin, C. M., & Lotocki, R. (2015). Performance measures related to colposcopy for Canadian cervical cancer screening programs: Identifying areas for improvement. *Journal of Obstetrics & Gynecology Canada, 37*(3), 245–251.

Dhawan, V. K. (2015). Hepatitus C. *eMedicine.* Retrieved from http://emedicine.medscape.com/article/177792-overview

Dubin, J. (2015). Rapid testing for HIV. *eMedicine.* Retrieved from http://emedicine.medscape.com/article/783434-overview

Durevall, D., & Lindskog, A. (2015). Intimate partner violence and HIV infection in sub-Saharan Africa. *World Development, 72,* 27–42.

Fernández-Romero, J. A., Deal, C., Herold, B. C., Schiller, J., Patton, D., Zydowsky, T., et al. (2015). Multipurpose prevention technologies: The future of HIV and STI protection. *Trends in Microbiology, 23*(7), 429–436 (Open Access).

Gearhart, P. A., Higgins, R. V., Randall, T. C. & Buckley, R. M. (2016). Human papillomavirus. *eMedicine*. Retrieved from http://emedicine.medscape.com/article/219110-overview

Gearhart, P. A., Randall, T. C., & Buckley, R. M. (2015). Human papillomavirus. *eMedicine*. Retrieved from http://emedicine.medscape.com/article/219110-overview

Gilbert, L. (2015). Update on pelvic inflammatory disease. *Pathology--Journal of the RCPA, 47*, S49.

Guenther, L. C., & Maguiness, S. (2015). Pediculosis and pthiriasis. *eMedicine*. Retrieved from http://emedicine.medscape.com/article/225013-overview

Heller, D. S. (2015). Diseases of the fallopian tube. In *OB-GYN pathology for the clinician* (pp. 135–145). Switzerland: Springer International Publishing.

James, S. H., & Kimberlin, D. W. (2015). Quantitative herpes simplex virus concentrations in neonatal infection. *The Journal of Pediatrics, 166*(4), 793–795.

Jones, E. (2015). *Sexually transmitted infections*. New Delhi: M L Books International.

Kaiser Family Foundation. (2015). *Women and HIV/AIDS in the United States*. Retrieved from http://kff.org/hivaids/fact-sheet/women-and-hivaids-in-the-united-states/

King, T. L., Brucker, M. C., Kriebs, J. M., Fahey, J. O., Gegor, C. L., & Varney, H. (2015). *Varney's midwifery* (5th ed.). Burlington, MA: Jones & Bartlett Learning.

Klein, J., Mclaud, M., & Rogers, D. (2015). Syphilis on the rise: Diagnosis, treatment, and prevention. *The Journal for Nurse Practitioners, 11*(1), 49–55.

Kohlhoff, S. A., & Hammerschlag, M. R. (2015). Treatment of chlamydial infections: 2014 update. *Expert Opinion on Pharmacotherapy, 16*(2), 205–212.

Koletzko, B., et al. (Eds.). (2015). *Pediatric nutrition in practice. World review of nutrition & dietetics* (vol. *113*, pp. 173–177). Switzerland: Karger Medical and Scientific Publishers.

Kraft, J. M., Whiteman, M. K., Carter, M. W., Snead, M. C., DiClemente, R. J., Murray, C. C., et al. (2015). Identifying psychosocial and social correlates of sexually transmitted diseases among Black female teenagers. *Sexually Transmitted Diseases, 42*(4), 192–197.

Lawrence, D., Cresswell, F., Whetham, J., & Fisher, M. (2015). Syphilis treatment in the presence of HIV: The debate goes on. *Current Opinion in Infectious Diseases, 28*(1), 44–52.

Leone, P. (2015). Expert commentary: Genital herpes transmission. *Herpes, 11*(2), 48–49.

Liu, G., Hariri, S., Bradley, H., Gottlieb, S. L., Leichliter, J. S., & Markowitz, L. E. (2015). Trends and patterns of sexual behaviors among adolescents and adults aged 14 to 59 years, United States. *Sexually Transmitted Diseases, 42*(1), 20–26.

Mohanty, G., & Ghosh, S. N. (2015). Risk factors for cancer of cervix, status of screening and methods for its detection. *Archives of Gynecology and Obstetrics, 291*(2), 247–249.

Monsel, G., & Chosidow, O. (2015). 24 Scabies, lice, and myiasis. In D. Schlossberg (Ed.), *Clinical infectious disease* (2nd ed., Chapter 24). Cambridge, UK: Cambridge University Press.

Moore, D. L., & MacDonald, N. E. (2015). Preventing ophthalmia neonatorum. *Pediatrics & Child Health, 20*(2), 93–96.

Moses, S. (2015). Genital herpes. *Family Practice Notebook*. Retrieved from http://www.fpnotebook.com/ID/STD/GntlHrps.htm

Mutasim, D. F. (Ed.) (2015). Generalized pruritus. In *Practical skin pathology* (pp. 125–129). Switzerland: Springer International Publishing.

Myers, J. L., Buhi, E. R., Marhefka, S., Daley, E., & Dedrick, R. (2015). Associations between individual and relationship characteristics and genital herpes disclosure. *Journal of Health Psychology*. doi: 1359105315575039

Nunn, A., Sanders, J., Carson, L., Thomas, G., Cornwall, A., Towey, C., et al. (2015). African American community leaders' policy recommendations for reducing racial disparities in HIV infection, treatment, and care results from a community-based participatory research project in Philadelphia, Pennsylvania. *Health Promotion Practice, 16*(1), 91–100.

Peterman, T. A., Su, J., Bernstein, K. T., & Weinstock, H. (2015). Syphilis in the United States: On the rise? *Expert Review of Anti-Infective Therapy, 13*(2), 161–168.

Pickering, L. K. (Ed.). (2014). *Red book: AAP report of the Committee on Infectious Diseases*. Retrieved from http://aapredbook.aappublications.org/site/about/Pediatrics-2014-Pickering-898-906.pdf

Piszczek, J., Jean, R. S., & Khaliq, Y. (2015). Gonorrhea treatment update for an increasingly resistant organism. *Canadian Pharmacists Journal/Revue des Pharmaciens du Canada, 148*(2), 82–89.

Prabhu, A., & Gardella, C. (2015). Common vaginal and vulvar disorders. *Medical Clinics of North America, 99*(3), 553–574.

Public Health Agency of Canada. (2015). Canadian guidelines on sexually transmitted infections. Retrieved from http://www.phac-aspc.gc.ca/std-mts/sti-its/pdf/401mts-prisencharge-eng.pdf

Pyrsopoulos, N. T., & Reddy, K. R. (2015). Hepatitis B. *eMedicine*. Retrieved from http://emedicine.medscape.com/article/177632-overview

Qureshi, S. (2015). Chlamydia genitourinary infections. *eMedicine*. Retrieved from http://emedicine.medscape.com/article/214823-overview#aw2aab6b2b3

Ramsey, P. S. (2015). Editorial commentary: Post-syphilotherapy titers in pregnancy. *Clinical Infectious Diseases, 60*(5), 691–692.

Reed, J. L., Huppert, J. S., Gillespie, G. L., Taylor, R. G., Holland, C. K., Alessandrini, E. A., et al. (2015). Adolescent patient preferences surrounding partner notification and treatment for sexually transmitted infections. *Academic Emergency Medicine, 22*(1), 61–66.

Reidy, D. E., Brookmeyer, K. A., Gentile, B., Berke, D. S., & Zeichner, A. (2016). Gender role discrepancy stress, high-risk sexual behavior, and sexually transmitted disease. *Archives of Sexual Behavior, 45*(2), 459–465. doi: 10.1007/s10508-014-0413-0.

Schuiling, K. D., & Likis, F. (2016). *Women's gynecologic health* (3rd ed.). Burlington, MA: Jones & Bartlett Learning.

Shafiee, H., Wang, S., Inci, F., Toy, M., Henrich, T. J., Kuritzkes, D. R., et al. (2015). Emerging technologies for point-of-care management of HIV infection. *Annual Review of Medicine, 66*, 387–405.

Shepherd, S. M. (2015). Pelvic inflammatory disease. *eMedicine*. Retrieved from http://emedicine.medscape.com/article/256448-overview

Silasi, M., Cardenas, I., Kwon, J. Y., Racicot, K., Aldo, P., & Mor, G. (2015). Viral infections during pregnancy. *American Journal of Reproductive Immunology, 73*, 199–213.

Simmons, S. (2015). Understanding pelvic inflammatory disease. *Nursing, 45*(2), 65–66.

Smith, H. (2015). Sexually transmitted infections. *Professional Nursing Today, 18*(1), 29–32.

Smith, D.S., & Ramos, N. (2015). Trichomoniasis. *eMedicine*. Retrieved from http://emedicine.medscape.com/article/230617-overview

Snijdewind, I. J., Smit, C., Schutten, M., Nellen, F. J., Kroon, F. P., Reiss, P., et al. (2015). Low mother-to-child-transmission rate of Hepatitis C virus in cART treated HIV-1 infected mothers. *Journal of Clinical Virology, 68*, 11–15.

Thomas, T. L., Yarandi, H. N., Dalmida, S. G., Frados, A., & Klienert, K. (2015). Cross-cultural differences and sexual risk behavior of emerging adults. *Journal of Transcultural Nursing, 26*(1), 64–72.

Tipple, C., & Taylor, G. P. (2015). Syphilis testing, typing, and treatment follow-up: A new era for an old disease. *Current Opinion in Infectious Diseases, 28*(1), 53–60.

U.S. Department of Health and Human Services [USDHHS]. (2010). *Healthy people 2020*. Retrieved from http://www.healthypeople.gov/2020/topicsobjectives2020/default.aspx

U.S. Food and Drug Administration [FDA]. (2015). *Condoms and sexually transmitted diseases*. Retrieved from http://www.fda.gov/ForPatients/Illness/HIVAIDS/ucm126372.htm

U.S. Preventive Services Task Force [USPSTF]. (2015). *USPSTF recommendations*. Retrieved from http://www.uspreventiveservicestaskforce.org/uspstf12/hepb/hepbfinalresplan.htm

Wong, B. (2015). Gonorrhea. *eMedicine*. Retrieved from http://emedicine.medscape.com/article/218059-overview

World Health Organization [WHO]. (2015a). *Hepatitis B*. Retrieved from http://www.who.int/mediacentre/factsheets/fs204/en/

World Health Organization [WHO]. (2015b). *HIV/AIDS*. Retrieved from http://www.who.int/hiv/en/

World Health Organization [WHO]. (2015c). *Adolescents falling through the gaps in HIV services*. Retrieved from http://www.who.int/mediacentre/news/releases/2013/hiv-adolescents-20131125/en/

World Health Organization [WHO]. (2015d). *Sexually transmitted infections (STIs)*. Retrieved from http://www.who.int/mediacentre/factsheets/fs110/en/

World Health Organization [WHO]. (2015e). *Hepatitus C*. Retrieved from http://www.who.int/mediacentre/factsheets/fs164/en/

World Health Organization [WHO]. (2016). *Zika virus*. Retrieved from http://www.who.int/mediacentre/factsheets/zika/en/

MULTIPLE CHOICE QUESTIONS

1. The nurse's primary role related to sexually transmitted infections is:
   a. Case reporting of partners
   b. Detection and education
   c. Sexual counseling
   d. Diagnosis and treatment

2. A 16-year-old teen comes to the clinic for routine care and is diagnosed with gonorrhea. The teen asks the nurse why she needs treatment for this since she has no symptoms. The nurse should explain that possible complications of lack of treatment could result in:
   a. Sterility, birth defects, and miscarriage
   b. The need for future births by cesarean section
   c. Skin rashes and hearing loss
   d. Disseminated systemic infections

3. Which of the following contraceptive methods offers protection against sexually transmitted infections (STIs)?
   a. Oral contraceptives
   b. Withdrawal
   c. Latex condom
   d. Intrauterine contraceptive (IUC)

4. In teaching about human immunodeficiency virus (HIV) transmission, the nurse explains that the virus cannot be transmitted by:
   a. Shaking hands
   b. Sharing drug needles
   c. Sexual intercourse
   d. Breast-feeding

5. A woman with human papilloma virus (HPV) is likely to present with which nursing assessment finding?
   a. Profuse, pus-filled vaginal discharge
   b. Clusters of genital warts
   c. Single painless ulcer
   d. Multiple vesicles on genitalia

6. The nurse's discharge teaching plan for the woman with pelvic inflammatory disease (PID) should reinforce which of the following potentially life-threatening complications?
   a. Involuntary infertility
   b. Chronic pelvic pain
   c. Depression
   d. Ectopic pregnancy

7. To confirm a finding of primary syphilis, the nurse would observe which of the following on the external genitalia?
   a. A highly variable skin rash
   b. A yellow–green vaginal discharge
   c. A nontender, indurated ulcer
   d. A localized gumma formation

CRITICAL THINKING EXERCISES

1. Sally, age 17, comes to the teen clinic saying that she is in pain and has some "crud" between her legs. The nurse takes her into the examining room and questions her about her symptoms. Sally states she had numerous genital bumps that had been filled with fluid, then ruptured and turned into ulcers with crusts. In addition, she has pain on urination and overall body pain. Sally says she had unprotected sex with several men when she was drunk at a party a few weeks back, but she thought they were "clean."
   a. What STI would the nurse suspect?
   b. The nurse should give immediate consideration to which of Sally's complaints?
   c. What should be the goal of the nurse in teaching Sally about STIs?

STUDY ACTIVITIES

1. Go to the CDC web site and select a specific STI of interest. Educate yourself about one specific STI thoroughly and share your expertise with your clinical group.

2. Contact your local health department and request current statistics regarding three STIs. Ask them to compare the current number of cases reported to last year's report. Has the number of STIs increased or decreased? What may be some of the reasons for the change in the number of cases reported?

3. Request permission to attend a local STI clinic to shadow a nurse for a few hours. Describe the nurse's counseling role with clients and what specific information is emphasized to clients.

4. Two common STIs that appear together and are commonly treated together regardless of identification of the secondary one are _____ and

   _____.

5. Genital warts can be treated with which of the following? Select all that apply.
   a. Penicillin
   b. Podophyllin
   c. Imiquimod
   d. Cryotherapy
   e. Antiretroviral therapy
   f. Acyclovir

CHAPTER WORKSHEET

BRINGING IT ALL TOGETHER: CASE STUDY

Grace, a 25-year-old college student, came back upset from her annual gynecologic appointment at the college health center. The results from her pap smear were "abnormal" and she would need further testing to rule out cervical cancer. She had heard about cervical cancer but did not think it could happen to someone of her age, so she looked for some information on the Internet. What she found surprised and worried her. She learned that each year approximately 13,000 new cases of cervical cancer are found and that over 4,000 women die of the disease. This is twice as many as die of HIV/AIDS. She also learned that 93% of cervical cancers are caused by a virus.

Go to thePoint **to find questions to consider about this case.**

6

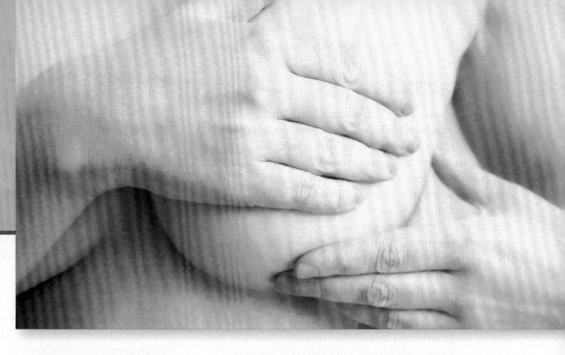

Disorders of the Breasts

Learning Objectives

Upon completion of the chapter, you will be able to:

1. Identify the incidence, risk factors, screening methods, and treatment modalities for benign breast conditions.

2. Appraise reasons behind breast augmentation including the potential benefits and risks.

3. Outline preventive strategies for breast cancer through lifestyle changes and health screening.

4. Analyze the incidence, risk factors, treatment modalities, and nursing considerations related to breast cancer.

5. Develop an educational plan to teach BSE to a group of high-risk women.

Nancy hasn't been able to sleep well since she felt the lump in her left breast over a month ago, just after her 60th birthday. She knows she is at high risk because her mother died of breast cancer, but she can't bring herself to have it checked out.

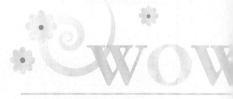

Words of Wisdom
Focus on reducing fear, anxiety, pain, and loneliness in all women diagnosed with a breast disorder.

INTRODUCTION

The breasts are modified sweat glands, lying over the pectoralis major muscles of the chest wall. Physiologically, the breast is an organ specialized for milk formation to nourish their offspring. Each breast extends approximately from the second to the sixth rib. The female breasts are closely linked to womanhood in American culture. Women's breasts act as physical markers for transitions from one stage of life to another, and although the primary function of the breasts is lactation, they are perceived as a symbol of beauty and sexuality.

This chapter discusses assessments, screening procedures, and management of specific benign and malignant breast disorders. Nurses play a key role in helping women maintain breast health by providing education and screening. A good working knowledge of early detection techniques, diagnosis, and treatment options is essential.

BENIGN BREAST DISORDERS

A benign breast disorder is any noncancerous breast abnormality. Though not life-threatening, benign disorders can cause pain and discomfort, and they account for a large number of visits to primary care providers. Fully understanding benign breast disorders should enable the nurse to appropriately evaluate symptoms, determine which breast lesions require treatment, and identify women who are at increased risk for breast cancer.

Depending on the type of benign breast disorder, treatment might or might not be necessary. Although these disorders are benign, the emotional trauma women experience is phenomenal. Fear, anxiety, disbelief, helplessness, and depression are just a few of the reactions that a woman may have when she discovers a lump in her breast. Many women believe that all lumps are cancerous, but actually more than 80% of the lumps discovered are benign and need no treatment (Alexander et al., 2014). Patience, support, and education are essential components of nursing care.

The most commonly encountered benign breast disorders in women include fibrocystic changes of the breasts, fibroadenomas, and mastitis. Although these breast disorders are considered benign, fibrocystic changes of the breasts carry a cancer risk, with prolific masses and hyperplastic changes occurring within the breasts. Generally speaking, fibroadenomas and mastitis carry little cancer risk (Seetharam & Rodrigues, 2015). Table 6.1 summarizes benign breast conditions.

Fibrocystic Breast Changes

Fibrocystic breast changes, also known as *benign breast disease* (BBD), represent a variety of changes in the glandular and structural tissues of the breast. Because this condition affects 50% to 60% of all women at some point, it is more accurately defined as a "change" rather than a "disease." Fibrocystic changes are caused by an overgrowth of fibrous tissues in the connective tissues supporting the breasts. This is frequently accompanied by the presence of fluid-filled cysts, which contribute to the lumpy feeling experienced by women. In contrast

TABLE 6.1	SUMMARY OF BENIGN BREAST DISORDERS				
Breast Condition	Nipple Discharge	Site	Characteristics/ Age of Client	Tenderness	Diagnosis and Treatment
Fibrocystic breast changes	+ or −	Bilateral; upper outer quadrant	Round, smooth Several lesions Cyclic, palpable 30–50 yrs old	+	Aspiration and biopsy; Limit caffeine; ibuprofen; supportive bra
Fibroadenomas	−	Unilateral; nipple area or upper outer quadrant	Round, firm, movable Palpable, rubbery Well delineated Single lesion 15–30 yrs old	−	Mammogram; "Watchful waiting" Aspiration and biopsy; Surgical excision
Mastitis	−	Unilateral; outer quadrant	Wedge shaped Warmth, redness Swelling Nipple cracked Breast engorged	+	Antibiotics; Warm shower; Supportive bra; Breast-feeding; Increase fluids

Adapted from Alexander, L. L., LaRosa, J. H., Bader, H., & Garfield, S. (2014). *New dimensions in women's health* (6th ed.). Sudbury, MA: Jones & Bartlett; American Cancer Society [ACS]. (2015a). *Non-cancerous breast conditions.* Retrieved from http://www.cancer.org/Healthy/FindCancerEarly/WomensHealth/Non-CancerousBreastConditions/non-cancerous-breast-conditions-fibrocystic-changes; and Bope, E. T., & Kellerman, R. D. (2015). *Conn's current therapy 2015.* Philadelphia, PA: Saunders Elsevier.

to malignant breast lesions, the cysts that develop move freely when palpated and symptoms decline after menopause when levels of estrogen and progesterone drop (Sabel, 2015). Fibrocystic changes do not increase the risk of breast cancer for most women except when the breast biopsy shows "atypia" or abnormal breast cells. The cause for concern for many women with fibrocystic changes is that breast examinations and mammography become more difficult to interpret with multiple cysts present, and early cancerous lesions may occasionally be overlooked (American Cancer Society [ACS], 2015a).

Fibrocystic breast changes are most common in women between the ages of 20 and 50. The condition is rare in postmenopausal women not taking hormone replacement therapy (HRT). According to the ACS (2015a), fibrocystic breast changes affect at least half of all women at some point in their lives and are the most common breast disorder today.

Therapeutic Management

Management of the symptoms of fibrocystic breast changes begins with self-care. For some women, diet and lifestyle changes help to reduce discomfort. Other options include wearing a supportive bra, taking over-the-counter pain relievers, and limiting salt consumption which can cause fluid retention (Files, Allen, & Pruthi, 2015). In severe cases drugs, including bromocriptine, tamoxifen, or danazol, can be used to reduce the influence of estrogen on breast tissue. However, several undesirable side effects, including masculinization, have been documented. Aspiration or surgical removal of breast lumps will reduce pain and swelling by removing the space-occupying mass.

Nursing Assessment

Nursing assessment consists of a health history, physical examination, and laboratory and diagnostic tests.

HEALTH HISTORY

Ask the woman about common clinical manifestations, which include lumpy, tender breasts, particularly during the week before menses. Changes in breast tissue produce pain by nerve irritation from edema in connective tissue and by fibrosis from nerve pinching. The pain is cyclic and frequently dissipates after the onset of menses. The pain is described as a dull, aching feeling of fullness. Masses or nodularities usually appear in both breasts and are often found in the upper outer quadrants. Some women also experience spontaneous clear to yellow nipple discharge when the breast is squeezed or manipulated.

PHYSICAL EXAMINATION

It is best to examine a woman's breast a week after menses, when swelling has subsided. The breast exam is performed using the Triple Touch Method in which the

health care provider uses the pads of the middle three fingers and makes dime-sized overlapping circles to feel the breast tissue with three levels of pressure: light, medium, and firm (Jarvis, 2015). Observe the breasts for fibrosis, or thickening of the normal breast tissues, which occurs in the early stages. Cysts form in the later stages and feel like multiple, smooth, well-delineated tiny pebbles or bumpy oatmeal under the skin (Fig. 6.1). On physical examination of the breasts, a few characteristics might be helpful in differentiating a cyst from a cancerous lesion. Cancerous lesions typically are fixed and painless and may cause skin retraction (pulling). Cysts tend to be mobile and tender and do not cause skin retraction in the surrounding tissue.

LABORATORY AND DIAGNOSTIC TESTS

Mammography can be helpful in distinguishing fibrocystic changes from breast cancer. Ultrasound is a useful adjunct to mammography for breast evaluation because it helps to differentiate a cystic mass from a solid one (Dixon & Macaskill, 2015). Ultrasound produces images of the breasts by sending sound waves through a gel applied to the breasts. Fine-needle aspiration biopsy can also be done to differentiate a solid tumor, cyst, or malignancy. A fine-needle aspiration biopsy uses a thin needle guided by ultrasound to the mass. In a method called stereotactic needle biopsy, a computer maps the exact location of the mass using mammograms taken from two angles, and the map is used to guide the needle.

Nursing Management

A nurse caring for a woman with fibrocystic breast changes can teach her about the condition, provide tips for self-care (Teaching Guidelines 6.1), suggest lifestyle changes, and demonstrate how to perform monthly breast self-examination (BSE) after her menses to monitor the changes. Nursing Care Plan 6.1 presents a plan of care for a woman with fibrocystic breast changes.

Teaching Guidelines 6.1
RELIEVING SYMPTOMS OF FIBROCYSTIC BREAST CHANGES

- Wear an extra-supportive bra to prevent undue strain on the ligaments of the breasts to reduce discomfort.
- Take oral contraceptives, as recommended by a health care practitioner, to stabilize the monthly hormonal levels.
- Eat a low-fat diet rich in fruits, vegetables, and grains to maintain a healthy nutritional lifestyle and ideal weight.
- Apply heat to the breasts to help reduce pain via vasodilation of vessels.
- Take diuretics, as recommended by a health care practitioner, to counteract fluid retention and swelling of the breasts.

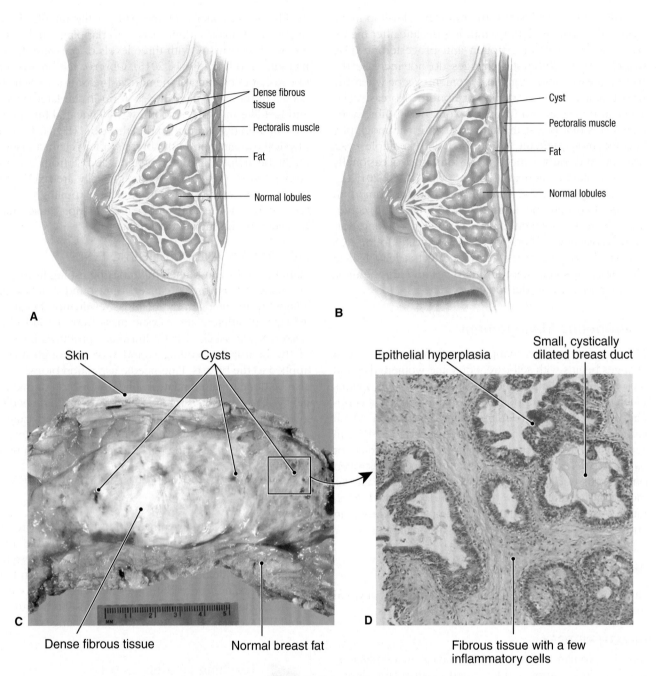

FIGURE 6.1 **A.** Fibrocystic breast changes. **B.** Breast cysts. **C.** This gross study shows that most of the abnormal tissue is fibrous. Cysts are relatively inconspicuous in this example. **D.** The microscopic study shows dense fibrous tissue containing dilated ducts lined by hyperplastic epithelium. (Images A & B are from The Anatomical Chart Company [2006]. *Atlas of Pathophysiology*. Springhouse, PA: Springhouse Corporation. Images C & D courtesy of McConnell, Thomas H. [2014]. *The Nature of Disease Pathology for the Health Professions*, 2nd edition. Philadelphia, PA: Lippincott Williams & Wilkins.)

- Reduce salt intake to reduce fluid retention and swelling in the breasts.
- Take over-the-counter medications, such as acetylsalicylic acid (Aspirin) or ibuprofen (Motrin, Advil, Nuprin), to reduce inflammation and discomfort.
- Use thiamine and vitamin E therapy. This has been found helpful for some women, but research has failed to demonstrate a direct benefit from either therapy.

- Take medications as prescribed (e.g., bromocriptine, tamoxifen, or danazol).
- Discuss the possibility of aspiration or surgical removal of breast lumps with a health care practitioner.
- Avoid caffeinated drinks (coffee, tea, soda) which tend to trigger breast discomfort.

Overview of the Woman with Fibrocystic Breast Changes

Sheree Rollins is a 37-year-old woman who comes to the clinic for her routine checkup. During the examination, she says, "Sometimes my breasts feel so heavy and they ache a lot. I noticed a couple of lumpy areas in my breast last week just before I got my period. Is this normal? Now they feel like they're almost gone. Should I be worried?" Clinical breast examination reveals two small (pea-sized), mobile, slightly tender nodules in each breast bilaterally. No skin retraction noted. Previous mammogram revealed fibrocystic breast changes.

NURSING DIAGNOSIS: Pain related to changes in breast tissue

Outcome Identification and Evaluation

The client will demonstrate a decrease in breast pain as evidenced by a pain rating of 1 or 2 on a pain rating scale of 0 to 10 and statements that pain is lessened.

Interventions: *Relieving Pain*

- Ask client to rate her pain using a numeric pain rating scale to establish a baseline.
- Discuss with client any measures used to relieve pain to determine effectiveness of the measures.
- Encourage use of a supportive bra to aid in reducing discomfort.
- Instruct client in use of over-the-counter analgesics to promote pain relief.

- Advise the client to apply warm compresses or allow warm water from the shower to flow over her breasts to promote vasodilation and subsequent pain relief.
- Tell client to reduce her intake of salt to reduce risk of fluid retention and swelling leading to increased pain.

NURSING DIAGNOSIS: Deficient knowledge related to fibrocystic breast changes and appropriate care measures

Outcome Identification and Evaluation

The client will verbalize understanding of condition as evidenced by statements about the cause of breast changes and appropriate choices for lifestyle changes, and demonstration of self-care measures.

Interventions: *Providing Client Education*

- Assess client's knowledge of fibrocystic breast changes to establish a baseline for teaching.
- Explain the role of monthly hormonal level changes and describe the signs and symptoms to promote understanding of this condition.
- Teach the client how to perform breast self-examination after her menstrual period to monitor for changes.
- Encourage client to report any changes promptly to ensure early detection of problems.
- Suggest client speak with her primary care provider about the use of oral contraceptives to help stabilize monthly hormonal levels.
- Review lifestyle choices, such as eating a low-fat diet rich in fruits, vegetables, and grains, and adhering to screening recommendations to promote health.
- Discuss measures for pain relief to minimize discomfort associated with breast changes.

Fibroadenomas

Fibroadenomas are common benign solid breast tumors that occur in about 25% of all women and account for up to half of all breast biopsies. They are the most common mass in women aged 15 to 25 years (Seetharam & Rodrigues, 2015). They are considered hyperplastic lesions associated with an aberration of normal development and involution rather than a neoplasm. Fibroadenomas can be stimulated by external estrogen, progesterone, lactation, and pregnancy (Schuiling & Likis, 2016). They are composed of both fibrous and glandular tissue that feels round or oval, firm, rubbery and smooth, and is mobile and may be tender. They are usually unilateral, but may present in both breasts (Alexander et al., 2014). Giant fibroadenomas account for approximately 4% of cases. These masses are frequently larger than 5 cm and occur most often in pregnant or lactating women. These large lesions may regress in size once hormonal stimulation subsides (Janardhan, Venkateshwar, & Rao, 2015). Fibroadenomas are rarely associated with cancer.

Therapeutic Management

Treatment may include a period of "watchful waiting" because many fibroadenomas stop growing or shrink on their own without any treatment. Other growths may need to be surgically removed if they do not regress or if they remain unchanged. Cryoablation, an alternative to surgery, can also be used to remove a tumor. In this procedure, extremely cold gas is piped into the tumor using ultrasound guidance. The tumor freezes and dies. The current trend is toward a more conservative approach to treatment after careful evaluation and continued monitoring.

Nursing Assessment

Ask the woman about clinical manifestations of fibroadenomas. These lumps are felt as firm, rubbery, well-circumscribed, freely mobile nodules that might or might not be tender when palpated.

Breast fibroadenomas are usually detected incidentally during clinical or self-examinations and are usually located in the upper outer quadrant of the breast; more than one may be present (Fig. 6.2). Several other breast lesions have similar characteristics, so every woman with a breast mass should be evaluated to exclude cancer. A clinical breast examination by a health care provider is critical. In addition, diagnostic studies include imaging studies (mammography, ultrasound, or both) and some form of biopsy, most often a fine-needle aspiration, core needle biopsy, or stereotactic needle biopsy. The core needle biopsy removes a small cylinder of tissue from the breast mass, more than the fine-needle aspiration biopsy. If additional tissue needs to be evaluated, the

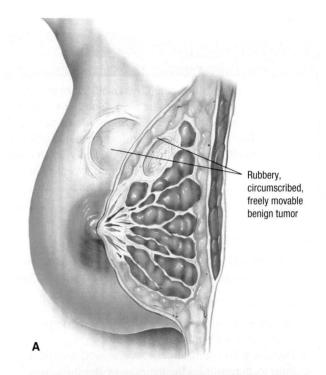

Rubbery, circumscribed, freely movable benign tumor

A

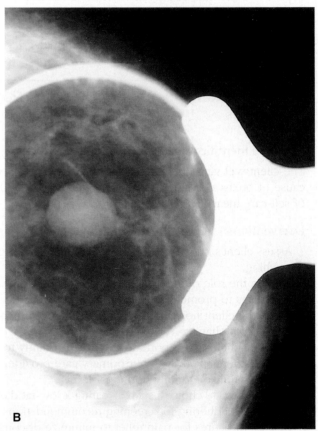

B

FIGURE 6.2 A. Fibroadenoma. (Asset provided by Anatomical Chart Co.) **B.** Spot compression view of a smoothly marinated mass proven to represent a fibroadenoma. Ultrasonography demonstrated a solid mass.

advanced breast biopsy instrument (ABBI) is used. This instrument removes a larger cylinder of tissue for examination by using a rotating circular knife. The ABBI procedure removes more tissue than any of the other methods except a surgical biopsy (ACS, 2015a).

Nursing Management

The nurse should urge the client to return for reevaluation in 6 months, perform monthly BSEs, and return annually for a clinical breast examination. Recent studies suggest that women with high breast density and proliferative benign breast disease are at very high risk for future breast cancer. Women with low breast density are at low risk, regardless of their benign pathologic diagnosis (Slanetz, Freer, & Birdwell, 2015). This is all the more reason for women to have close monitoring over time.

Mastitis

Mastitis is an infection or inflammation of the connective tissue in the breast that occurs primarily in lactating or engorged women. The prevalence of it in breast-feeding women may be as high as 33% (Faguy, 2015). Mastitis is divided into lactational or nonlactational types. The usual causative organisms for lactational mastitis are *Staphylococcus aureus*, *Hemophilus influenzae*, and hemophilus and streptococcus species, the source of which is the baby's flora. Lactating mastitis typically occurs in the first two to three weeks of lactation, but can occur at any stage of lactation. One or more of the ducts drain poorly or become blocked, resulting in bacterial growth in the retained milk (Pluchinotta, 2015). The only evidence-based predisposing factor that may lead to mastitis is the development of milk stasis. However, other associated factors include damaged or cracked nipples, especially those colonized with *Staphylococcus aureus*; irregular or missed feedings; failing to allow the infant to empty one breast completely before moving on to the next breast; poor latch and transfer of milk; illness of mother or infant; oversupply; a tight bra; blocked nipple pore or duct; being primiparous women; and maternal stress and fatigue (Miller & Kennedy, 2015).

Nonlactational mastitis can be caused by duct ectasia, which occurs when the milk ducts become congested with secretions and debris, resulting in periductal inflammation. It may be divided into central (periareolar) and peripheral breast lesions. Periareolar infections consist of active inflammation around nondilated subareolar breast ducts—a condition termed periductal mastitis. Peripheral nonlactating breast abscesses are less common than periareolar abscesses and are often associated with an underlying condition such as diabetes, rheumatoid arthritis, steroid treatment, granulomatous lobular mastitis, and trauma (Faguy, 2015). Women with these types of abscesses present with greenish nipple discharge, nipple retraction, and noncyclical pain.

Therapeutic Management

Effective milk removal, pain medication, and antibiotic therapy have been the mainstays of treatment. Management of both types of mastitis involves the use of oral antibiotics (usually a penicillinase-resistant penicillin or cephalosporin), warm compresses to the inflamed area of the breast, continued breast-feeding, and acetaminophen (Tylenol) for pain and fever (King et al., 2015).

Nursing Assessment

Assess the client's health history for risk factors for mastitis, which include poor hand hygiene ductal abnormalities, nipple cracks and fissures, lowered maternal defenses due to fatigue, tight clothing, poor support of pendulous breasts, failure to empty the breasts properly while breast-feeding, or missing breast-feedings.

The diagnosis of mastitis is made clinically on the basis of a localized, unilateral area of erythema with associated fever. Assess the client for clinical manifestations of mastitis, which include flu-like symptoms of malaise, nausea, headache, leukocytosis, fever, fatigue, and chills. Physical examination of the breasts reveals increased warmth, swollen area of one breast, redness, tenderness, and swelling. The nipple is usually cracked or abraded and the breast is distended with milk (Fig. 6.3). In a lactating woman, severe engorgement can be differentiated from mastitis because engorgement is bilateral with general involvement of the whole breast. Ultrasound scans can be undertaken to differentiate between the types of mastitis or abscesses, but typically the diagnosis is made based on history and examination.

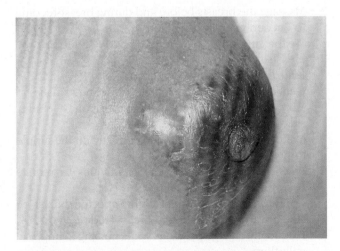

FIGURE 6.3 Mastitis. (From Sweet, R. L., & Gibbs, R. S. [2009]. *Infectious diseases of the female genital tract.* Philadelphia, PA: Lippincott Williams & Wilkins.)

Nursing Management

Teach the woman about the etiology of mastitis and encourage her to continue to breast-feed, emphasizing that it is safe for her infant to do so. Stress to all breast-feeding mothers to check for medication safety before taking it. Drugs administered to mothers can accumulate in the bodies of their infants and can alter infant's bowel flora, causing diarrhea. Mothers should be warned about this to reduce their anxiety. Once it has been declared safe to do so, the nurse should urge them to take the medication as prescribed until completed. Continued emptying of the breast or pumping improves the outcome, decreases the duration of symptoms, and decreases the incidence of breast abscess. Thus, continued breast-feeding is recommended in the presence of mastitis (King et al., 2015).

Although 80% of breast biopsy results prove to be benign, increased surveillance is necessary because of the risk of cancer development. The recommended follow-up schedule is imaging (mammography or ultrasound) and a clinical breast exam by a surgeon at 6, 12, and 24 months after a benign breast biopsy finding (Tharpe, Farley, & Jordan, 2016). Instructions for the woman with mastitis are detailed in Teaching Guidelines 6.2.

Teaching Guidelines 6.2
CARING FOR MASTITIS

- Take medications as prescribed to reduce inflammation and infection.
- Continue breast-feeding, as tolerated to keep the milk flowing.
- Begin feeding on most affected breast to allow it to be emptied first.
- Massage the breasts before and during breast-feeding to encourage milk extraction.
- Wear a supportive bra 24 hours a day to support the breasts for comfort.
- Increase fluid intake to stay hydrated.
- Gentle massage toward nipple several times daily.
- Vary the infants breast-feeding position – cradle, side-lying, football and belly to belly
- Make sure infant is positioned correctly on the nipple to prevent discomfort.
- Practice good hand hygiene techniques to reduce risk of bacterial transfer.
- Apply warm compresses to the affected breast or take a warm shower before breast-feeding.
- Frequently change positions while nursing to improve milk flow.
- Get adequate rest and nutrition to support or improve the immune system.

- Instruct to contact their health care provider if fever returns, chills, or worsening symptoms.

Adapted from American Cancer Society [ACS]. (2015a). *Non-cancerous breast conditions*. Retrieved from http://www.cancer.org/healthy/findcancerearly/womenshealth/non-cancerousbreastconditions/non-cancerous-breast-conditions-intro; King, T. L., Brucker, M. C., Kriebs, J. M., Fahey, J. O., Gegor, C. L., & Varney, H. (2015). *Varney's midwifery* (5th ed.), Berlington, MA: Jones & Bartlett Learning; and Tharpe, N. L., Farley, C. L., & Jordan, R. G. (2016). *Clinical practice guidelines for midwifery & women's health*. (4th ed.), Burlington, MA: Jones & Bartlett Learning.

MALIGNANT BREAST DISORDER

Breast cancer is a neoplastic disease in which normal body cells are transformed into malignant ones (National Cancer Institute ([NCI], 2015a). It is the most common cancer in women and the second leading cause of cancer deaths (lung cancer is first) among American women. Breast cancer accounts for one of every three cancers diagnosed in the United States (ACS, 2015a). A new case is discovered every 2 minutes. It is estimated that 1 out of every 8 women will develop the disease at some time during her life, and the mortality rate of those with breast cancer is 1 in 36 (NCI, 2015a).

Over 200,000 cases of invasive breast cancer are diagnosed in the United States each year (ACS, 2015a). Breast cancer can also affect men, but only 1% of all individuals diagnosed with breast cancer annually are men. About 2000 men are diagnosed with breast cancer annually, with about a 1 in 4 mortality rate (Khan, Allerton, & Petitt, 2015). Because men are not routinely screened for

Consider This

It was pouring down rain and I was driving alone along dark wet streets to my 8 AM appointment for a breast ultrasound. I recently had my annual mammogram and the radiologist thought he saw something suspicious on my right breast. I was on my way to confirm or refute his suspicions, and I couldn't keep focused on the road ahead. For the past few days I had been a basket case, fearing the worst. I was playing in my mind, what I would do if...? What changes would I make in my life and how would I react when told? I have been through such personal turmoil since that doctor announced he wanted "more tests."

Thoughts: *This woman is worrying and is emotionally devastated before she even has a conclusive diagnosis. Is this a typical reaction to a breast disorder? Why do women fear the worst? Many women use denial to mask their feelings and hope against hope the doctor made a mistake or misread their mammogram. How would you react if you or your sister, girlfriend, or mother were confronted with a breast disorder?*

breast cancer, the diagnosis is often delayed. The most common clinical manifestation of male breast cancer is a painless, firm, subareolar breast mass. Any suspicious breast mass in a male should undergo diagnostic biopsy. If a malignancy is diagnosed, typical treatment is mastectomy with assessment of the axillary nodes.

The cause of breast cancer, while not well understood, is thought to be a complex interaction between environmental, genetic, and hormonal factors. Breast cancer is a progressive rather than a systemic disease, meaning that most cancers grow from small size with low metastatic potential to larger size and greater metastatic potential. Tumor stage, size, and lymph node involvement are major predictors of metastatic potential (Arora et al., 2015).

Pathophysiology

Cancer is not just one disease, but rather a group of diseases that result from unregulated cell growth. Without regulation, cells divide and grow uncontrollably until they eventually form a tumor. Extensive research has determined that all cancer is the result of changes in DNA or chromosome structure that cause the mutation of specific genes. Most genetic mutations that cause cancer are acquired sporadically, which means they occur by chance and are not necessarily due to inherited mutations (Shannon & Chittenden, 2015). Cancer development is thought to be clonal in nature, which means that each cell is derived from another cell. If one cell develops a mutation, any daughter cell derived from that cell will have that same mutation, and this process continues until a malignant tumor forms.

Breast cancer starts in the epithelial cells that line the mammary ducts within the breast. The growth rate depends on hormonal influences, mainly estrogen and progesterone. The two major categories of breast cancer are noninvasive and invasive. Noninvasive, or in situ, breast cancers are those that have not extended beyond their duct, lobule, or point of origin into the surrounding breast tissue. Conversely, invasive (infiltrating) breast cancers have extended into the surrounding breast tissue, with the potential to metastasize. Many researchers believe that most invasive cancers probably originate as noninvasive cancers (Cuzick & Thorat, 2015).

Breast cancer is considered to be a highly variable disease. While the process of metastasis is a complex and poorly understood phenomenon, there is evidence to suggest that new vascularization of the tumor plays an important role in the biologic aggressiveness of breast cancer (Toi et al., 2015). Breast cancer metastasizes widely and to almost all organs of the body, but primarily to the bone, lungs, lymph nodes, liver, and brain. The first sites of metastases are usually local or regional, involving the chest wall or axillary supraclavicular lymph nodes or bone (ACS, 2015a).

Invasive Ductal Carcinoma

By far the most common breast cancer is invasive ductal carcinoma, which represents 85% of all cases (ACS, 2015c). Carcinoma is a malignant tumor that occurs in epithelial tissue; it tends to infiltrate and give rise to metastases. The incidence of this cancer peaks in the sixth decade of life (>60 years old). It spreads rapidly to axillary and other lymph nodes, even while small. Infiltrating ductal carcinoma may take various histologic forms—well differentiated and slow growing, poorly differentiated and infiltrating, or highly malignant and undifferentiated with numerous metastases. This common type of breast cancer starts in the ducts, breaks through the duct wall, and invades the fatty breast tissue. This type of cancer accounts for 75% of all breast cancers (Stopeck, Chalasani, & Thompson, 2015).

Invasive Lobular Carcinoma

Invasive lobular carcinomas, which originate in the terminal lobular units of breast ducts, account for 10% of all cases of breast cancer. The peak incidence is in women aged 40 to 50 years old. It presents as an area of ill-defined thickening rather than a palpable mass. The tumor is frequently located in the upper outer quadrant of the breast, and by the time it is discovered the prognosis is usually poor (Selvi, 2015).

Other Invasive Carcinomas

Other invasive types of cancer include tubular carcinoma (29%), which is fairly uncommon and typically occurs in women aged 55 and older. Colloid carcinoma (2% to 4%) occurs in women 60 to 70 years of age and is characterized by the presence of large pools of mucus interspersed with small islands of tumor cells. Medullary carcinoma accounts for 5% to 7% of malignant breast tumors; it occurs frequently in younger women (<50 years of age) and grows into large tumor masses. Inflammatory breast cancer (<4%) often presents with skin edema, redness, and warmth and is associated with a poor prognosis. Paget's disease (2% to 4%) originates in the nipple and typically occurs with invasive ductal carcinoma (Bope & Kellerman, 2015).

Staging of Breast Cancer

Breast cancers are classified into three stages based on:
1. Tumor size
2. Extent of lymph node involvement
3. Evidence of metastasis

The purposes of tumor staging are to determine the probability that the tumor has metastasized, to decide on an appropriate course of therapy, and to assess the

TABLE 6.2	STAGING OF BREAST CANCER
Stage	**Characteristics**
0	In situ, early type of breast cancer
I	Localized tumor <1 inch in diameter
II	Tumor 1–2 inches in diameter; spread to axillary lymph nodes
III	Tumor 2 inches or larger; spread to other lymph nodes and tissues
IV	Cancer has metastasized to other body organs

Adapted from American Cancer Society [ACS]. (2015h). *How is breast cancer staged?* Retrieved from http://www.cancer.org/Cancer/BreastCancer/DetailedGuide/breast-cancer-staging.

client's prognosis. Table 6.2 gives details and characteristics of each stage (also Fig. 6.4). The overall 10-year survival rate for a woman with stage I breast cancer is 80% to 90%; for a woman with stage II, it is about 50%. The outlook is not as good for women with stage III or IV disease (Alexander et al., 2014).

There is no completely accurate way to know whether the cancer has micrometastasized to distant organs, but certain tests can help determine if the cancer has spread. A bone scan can be performed to assess the bones. Magnetic resonance imaging (MRI) can be used to detect metastases to the liver, abdominal cavity, lungs, or brain.

Risk Factors

An estimated 80% of women in whom breast cancer develops have no documented risk factors (Bope & Kellerman, 2015). Breast cancer is thought to develop in response to a number of related factors: aging; gender (99% of cases occur in women, delayed childbearing or never bearing children, genetic influences); BRCA1 and BRCA2 genetic mutations; history of receiving ionizing radiation; high breast density; postmenopausal obesity; family history of cancer; hormonal factors such as early menarche <12 years, late menopause >50 years, first term pregnancy >30 to 35 years of age; HRT with estrogen plus progestin; and ingestion of two drinks or more alcohol each day (ACS, 2015b). Other factors might contribute to breast cancer but have not been scientifically proven.

In 1970, the lifetime risk for developing breast cancer was 1 in 10; since then, the risk has gradually risen (NCI, 2015b). This slight increase in incidence might be explained in a variety of ways: better detection and screening tools are available, which have identified more cases; women are living to an older age, when their risk increases; and lifestyle changes in American women (having their first pregnancy at an older age, having fewer children, and using hormonal therapy to treat the symptoms of menopause) might have produced the higher numbers. Age is a significant risk factor. Because rates of breast cancer increase with age, estimates of risk at specific ages are more meaningful than estimates of lifetime risk. The estimated chances of a woman being diagnosed with breast cancer between the ages of 30 and 70 are detailed in Table 6.3.

Risk factors for breast cancer can be divided into those that cannot be changed (nonmodifiable risk factors) and those that can be changed (modifiable risk factors). Nonmodifiable risk factors (ACS, 2015b) are:
- Gender (female)
- Aging (>50 years old)
- Genetic mutations (BRCA1 and BRCA2 genes)
- Personal history of ovarian or colon cancer
- Increased breast density increases the risk three- to fivefold
- Family history of breast cancer
- Personal history of breast cancer (three- to fourfold increase in risk for recurrence)
- Race/Ethnicity (higher in White women, but African-American women are more likely to die of it)

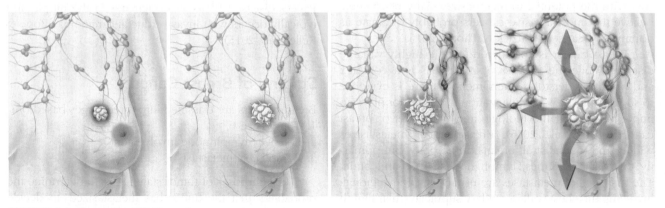

FIGURE 6.4 Stages I to IV of breast cancer.

TABLE 6.3	ESTIMATED RISK OF BREAST CANCER AT SPECIFIC AGES
Ages 30–39	1 out of 233
Ages 40–49	1 out of 69
Ages 50–59	1 out of 42
Ages 60–69	1 out of 29

Adapted from American Cancer Society [ACS]. (2015i). *How many women get breast cancer?* Retrieved from http://www.cancer.org/cancer/breastcancer/overviewguide/breast-cancer-overview-key-statistics.

- Previous abnormal breast biopsy (atypical hyperplasia)
- Exposure to chest radiation (radiation damages DNA)
- Previous breast radiation (12 times normal risk)
- Early menarche (<12 years old) or late onset of menopause (>55 years old), which represents increased estrogen exposure over the lifetime
- Modifiable risk factors related to lifestyle choices (ACS, 2015b) include:
- Not having children at all or not having children until after age 30—this increases the risk of breast cancer by not reducing the number of menstrual cycles
- Postmenopausal use of estrogens and progestins—the Women's Health Initiative study (2002) reported increased risks with long-term (>5 years) use of HRT
- Failing to breast-feed for up to a year after pregnancy—increases the risk of breast cancer because it does not reduce the total number of lifetime menstrual cycles
- Alcohol consumption—boosts the level of estrogen in the bloodstream
- Smoking—exposure to carcinogenic agents found in cigarettes
- Obesity and consumption of high-fat diet—fat cells produce and store estrogen, so more fat cells create higher estrogen levels
- Sedentary lifestyle and lack of physical exercise—increases body fat, which houses estrogen

Breast cancer incidence rates are higher in non-Hispanic White women compared with African-American women for most age groups. However, African-American women have a higher incidence rate before 40 years of age and are more likely to die from breast cancer at every age (ACS, 2015b). Some of that gap is because of social factors such as poverty and restricted access to health care. Some studies have also found genetic differences in the type of breast cancer that develops in African-American and White women. Little is known, however, about whether other risk factors have a different impact in women of different races. A new study's findings suggest that the risk factors are similar in both races (ACS, 2015b).

The presence of risk factors, especially several of them, calls for careful ongoing monitoring and evaluation to promote early detection. Even though risk factors are important considerations, many women with newly diagnosed breast cancer have no known risk factors. Although routine mammography and self-examination are prudent for high-risk women, these precautions may become lifesavers for early detection of cancerous lesions.

Consuming a low-fat diet with plenty of fruits, vegetables, legumes, and whole grains can provide all the vitamins and nutrients our bodies need and has been shown to significantly reduce the risk of developing many types of cancer. A plant-based diet can also reduce cancer recurrence: high-fiber, low-fat diets rich in fruits and vegetables, avoiding sugared beverages and calorie dense foods, and processed meats reduces breast cancer recurrence (Catsburg et al., 2015). They studied the effectiveness of a high-vegetable, low-fat diet, aimed at markedly raising circulating carotenoid concentrations from food sources, in reducing additional breast cancer events and early death in women with early-stage invasive breast cancer. It is a prescription for cancer prevention that has only positive side effects—lower cholesterol, weight loss, and a lower risk of heart disease. Adherence to a plant-based diet that limits red meat intake may be associated with reduced risk of breast cancer, particularly in postmenopausal women (Catsburg et al., 2015).

Screening for breast cancer begins with a routine history and physical exam. Nurses should take every opportunity to educate and emphasize the goal of breast cancer screening: early detection reduces mortality. Screening also includes a BSE, clinical breast exam, and mammography.

Diagnosis

Many studies can be performed to make an accurate diagnosis of a malignant breast lump. Diagnostic tests include:
- Diagnostic mammography or digital mammography
- Magnetic resonance mammography (MRM)
- Fine-needle aspiration
- Stereotactic needle-guided biopsy
- Sentinel lymph node biopsy
- Hormone receptor status
- Infrared thermal imaging
- DNA ploidy status
- Cell proliferative indices
- HER-2/neu genetic marker (Han et al., 2015)

Mammography

Mammography has become an accepted screening procedure that is sanctioned by most cancer organizations and is paid for annually by most health insurance agencies. Mammography serves a twofold purpose: to screen and to diagnose. Mammography involves taking x-ray pictures of a bare breast while it is compressed between two plastic plates. This procedure is a screening tool used to identify and characterize a breast mass and to detect an early malignancy. It remains the gold standard screening method for women at average risk for breast cancer. It is relatively inexpensive, requires only a low dose of radiation, and reliably identifies malignant tumors, especially those that are too small to feel. It can also be used to investigate breast lumps and other symptoms. A screening mammogram typically consists of four views, two per breast (Fig. 6.5). It can detect lesions as small as 0.5 cm (the average size of a tumor detected by a woman practicing occasional BSE is approximately 2.5 cm) (Rifkin & Lazris, 2015).

A diagnostic mammogram is performed when a woman has suspicious clinical findings on a breast examination or an abnormality has been found on a screening mammogram. A diagnostic mammogram uses additional views of the affected breast as well as magnification views. Diagnostic mammography provides the radiologist with additional detail to render a more

specific diagnosis. Currently, digital mammography is being used to diagnose breast lesions.

Most women find the 10-minute mammography procedure uncomfortable but not painful. Teaching Guidelines 6.3 offers tips for a client to follow before she undergoes this procedure.

Teaching Guidelines 6.3
PREPARING FOR A SCREENING MAMMOGRAM

- Schedule the procedure just after menses, when breasts are less tender.
- Do not use deodorant or powder on the day of the procedure, because they can appear on the x-ray film as calcium spots.
- Acetaminophen (Tylenol) or acetylsalicylic acid (aspirin) can relieve any discomfort after the procedure.
- Remove all jewelry from around your neck, because the metal can cause distortions on the film image.
- Select a facility that is accredited by the American College of Radiology to ensure appropriate credentialed staff.

The U.S. Preventive Services Task Force (USPSTF) changed its recommendations for breast cancer screening in 2009, resulting in considerable controversy. The USPSTF now recommends biennial screening mammography for women aged 50 to 74 years. Previously, women 40 years and older were advised to start screening mammography. They stated that the decision to start regular, biennial screening mammography before the age of 50 years should be an individual one and take client context into account, including the client's values regarding specific benefits and harms. In addition, the USPSTF concluded that the current evidence is insufficient to assess the additional benefits and harms of screening mammography in women 75 years or older. Finally, the USPSTF recommended against teaching BSE because scientific evidence does not support this practice as a valid screening method for women since its sensitivity ranges from 12% to 41%, lower than that of the clinical breast exam done by a health care provider and mammography, and it is age-dependent. The USPSTF is currently updating their breast cancer screening recommendation guidelines and may return to every 1 to 2 years for women age 40 or older for diagnostic mammograms (USPSTF, 2015).

The American Cancer Society (ACS) has different guidelines for women with no symptoms or family history of breast cancer than the USPSTF. They still recommend annual mammograms and clinical breast exams for women starting at age 40 and do not recommend stopping them at any age. They also recommend a clinical breast exam about every three years for women in

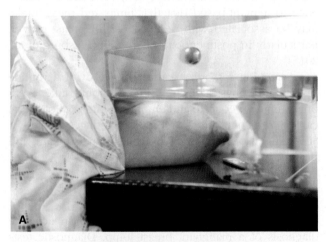
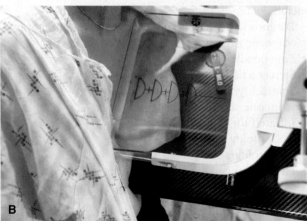

FIGURE 6.5 Mammography. **A.** A top-to-bottom view of the breast. **B.** A side view of the breast.

their 20s and 30s and every year for women >40. BSE is an option for women starting in their 20s (ACS, 2015d).

The American Congress of Obstetricians and Gynecologists (ACOG) recommends that mammography screening be offered annually to women beginning at age 40. Previous ACOG guidelines recommended mammograms every 1 to 2 years starting at age 40 and annually beginning at age 50. ACOG continues to recommend annual clinical breast exams (CBEs) for women aged 40 and older, and every 1 to 3 years for women aged 20 to 39. Additionally, it encourages breast self-awareness for women ages 20 and older (ACOG, 2015).

This conflicting information can be confusing to women trying to make decisions about breast cancer screening. Nurses can present the latest evidence-based research to help women make informed decisions based on their age, overall health status, and family history of cancer. (See Table 6.4 for a helpful outline.) There really isn't any clear direction given to women by the authoritative agencies; they in essence leave the decision up to the woman and her health care provider. The associated risk is delay in detecting a breast lesion early when it could be treated and her life saved.

Magnetic Resonance Mammography

MRM is a relatively new procedure that might allow for earlier detection because it can detect smaller lesions and provide finer detail. MRM is a highly accurate (>90% sensitivity for invasive carcinoma) but costly tool. Contrast infusion is used to evaluate the rate at which the dye initially enters the breast tissue. The basis of the high sensitivity of MRM is the tumor angiogenesis (vessel growth) that accompanies a majority of breast cancers, even early ones. Malignant lesions tend to exhibit increased enhancement within the first 2 minutes (Bhatti et al. 2015). Currently MRM is used as a complement to mammography and CBE because it is expensive, but recent research findings report that it is more accurate than mammography for size assessment of breast lesions (Poulos, 2015).

Fine-Needle Aspiration Biopsy or Core Biopsy

Fine-needle aspiration biopsy is done to identify a solid tumor, cyst, or malignancy. It is a simple office procedure that can be performed with or without anesthesia. A small (23 to 27-gauge) needle connected to a 10-mL or larger syringe is inserted into the breast mass and suction is applied to withdraw the contents. The aspirate is then sent to the cytology laboratory to be evaluated for abnormal cells.

A core needle biopsy is much like a fine needle biopsy except that a larger needle is used to withdraw small cylinders or cores of tissue from the abnormal area of the breast. It takes longer than the fine needle biopsy, but more tissue is sampled to be tested.

TABLE 6.4	SCREENING RECOMMENDATIONS FROM USPSTF, ACS, AND ACOG
The U.S. Preventive Services Task Force	In 2009, the USPSTF changed its recommendations for breast cancer screening for women with no symptoms or no family history of breast cancer. Previously they advised screening mammography for women aged 40 years and older. Updated recommendations include biennial screening mammography for women aged 50 to 74 years, and no breast self-examination (BSE) since scientific evidence does not support this practice as a valid screening method for women because its sensitivity ranges from 12% to 41%, which is lower than that of the clinical breast exam done by a health professional and mammography, and it is age dependent. The previous recommendations are now under review (2015). The USPSTF states that a woman's decision to start regular, biennial screening mammography before the age of 50 years should be an individual one and take client context into account, including the client's values regarding specific benefits and harms. The USPSTF also reports that current evidence is insufficient to assess the additional benefits and harmful aspects of screening mammography in women 75 years or older (USPSTF, 2015).
The American Cancer Society	Guidelines from the ACS differ from those of the USPSTF for women with no symptoms or no family history of breast cancer. The ACS still recommends annual mammograms and clinical breast exams for women starting at age 40 and do not recommend stopping them at any age. They suggest that BSEs can be optional for women from age 20 onward (ACS, 2015d).
The American Congress of Obstetricians and Gynecologists	The ACOG recommends screening mammograms be offered annually to women beginning at age 40. Previous guidelines recommended a mammogram every 1 to 2 years starting at age 40 and annually beginning at age 50. Clinical breast exams are still recommended every year, but BSEs are optional and not strongly recommended (ACOG, 2015).

Stereotactic Needle-Guided Biopsy

This diagnostic tool is used to target and identify mammographically detected nonpalpable lesions in the breast. This procedure is less expensive than an excisional biopsy. The procedure takes place in a specially equipped room and generally takes about an hour. Women are required to lie prone and must be able to remain still for approximately 20 minutes while the biopsy is taken. When proper placement of the breast mass is confirmed by digital mammograms, the breast is locally anesthetized and a spring-loaded biopsy gun is used to obtain two or three core biopsy tissue samples. After the procedure is finished, the biopsy area is cleaned and a sterile dressing is applied.

Sentinel Lymph Node Biopsy

The status of the axillary lymph nodes is an important prognostic indicator in early-stage breast cancer. The presence or absence of malignant cells in lymph nodes is highly significant: the more lymph nodes involved and the more aggressive the cancer, the more powerful chemotherapy will have to be, both in terms of the toxicity of drugs and the duration of treatment (Tsujimoto, 2015). With a sentinel lymph node biopsy, the clinician can determine whether breast cancer has spread to the axillary lymph nodes without having to do a traditional axillary lymph node dissection. Experience has shown that the lymph ducts of the breast typically drain to one lymph node first before draining through the rest of the lymph nodes under the arm. The first lymph node is called the sentinel lymph node.

This procedure can be performed under local anesthesia. A radioactive blue dye is injected 2 hours before the biopsy to identify the afferent sentinel lymph node. The surgeon usually removes one to three nodes and sends them to the pathologist to determine whether cancer cells are present. The sentinel lymph node biopsy is usually performed before a lumpectomy to make sure the cancer has not spread. Removing only the sentinel lymph node can allow women with breast cancer to avoid many of the side effects (lymphedema) associated with a traditional axillary lymph node dissection. This procedure is associated with less morbidity compared to the axillary lymph node dissection, which results in more accurate staging, better axillary tumor control and improved survival. It is considered a standard of care for initial evaluation of metastatic spread to the axillary lymph node chain (Chatterjee, Serniak, & Czerniecki, 2015).

Hormone Receptor Status

Normal breast epithelium has hormone receptors and responds specifically to the stimulatory effects of estrogen and progesterone. Most breast cancers retain estrogen receptors, and for those tumors estrogen will retain proliferative control over the malignant cells. It is therefore, useful to know the hormone receptor status of the cancer to predict which women will respond to hormone manipulation. Hormone receptor status reveals whether the tumor is stimulated to grow by estrogen and progesterone. Postmenopausal women tend to be ER+; premenopausal women tend to be ER− (Kalinsky et al., 2015). To determine hormone receptor status, a sample of breast cancer tissue obtained during a biopsy or a tumor removed surgically during a lumpectomy or mastectomy is examined by a cytologist.

Therapeutic Management

Women diagnosed with breast cancer have many treatments available to them. Generally, treatments fall into two categories: local and systemic. Local treatments are surgery and radiation therapy. Effective systemic treatments include chemotherapy, hormonal therapy, and immunotherapy (Evidence-Based Practice 6.1).

Treatment plans are based on multiple factors, with the primary factors being whether the cancer is invasive or noninvasive, the tumor's size and grade, the number of cancerous axillary lymph nodes, the hormone receptor status, and the ability to obtain clear surgical margins (ACS, 2015e). A combination of surgical options and adjunctive therapy is often recommended.

Another consideration in making decisions about a treatment plan is genetic testing for BRCA1 and BRCA2 genetic mutations. This genetic testing became available in 1995 and can pinpoint women who have a significantly increased risk for breast, ovarian cancer, and contralateral breast cancer: individuals with BRCA1 and BRCA2 mutations have a 75% lifetime risk of breast cancer and a 30% lifetime risk of ovarian cancer. Most cases of breast and ovarian cancer are sporadic in nature, but approximately 10% of breast and ovarian cancers are thought to result from genetic inheritance (Li et al., 2015). DNA (from a blood or saliva sample) is needed for mutation testing. The sample is sent to a laboratory for analysis. It usually takes about a month to get the results back. Testing positive for a BRCA1 or BRCA2 mutation can significantly alter health care decisions. In some cases, before genetic testing was available, lumpectomy with radiation, or mastectomy was the treatment most often recommended. However, if the woman is found to have a BRCA1 mutation, she is most likely to be offered the option of bilateral prophylactic mastectomy and possible bilateral oophorectomy. A recent study found that current evidence does not support worse breast cancer survival of BRCA1/2 mutation carriers in the adjuvant setting; differences if any are likely to be small when compared to non BRCA 1/2 mutation carriers (van den Broek et al., 2015).

Discovery of mutations in the breast and ovarian cancer susceptibility genes BRCA1 and BRCA2 can have

EVIDENCE-BASED PRACTICE 6.1

COMBINATION (SEVERAL DRUGS AT A TIME) VERSUS SEQUENTIAL CHEMOTHERAPY (SAME DRUG GIVEN ONE AFTER THE OTHER) FOR METASTATIC BREAST CANCER

STUDY

Combination chemotherapy can cause greater tumor cell kill if the drug dose is not compromised, while sequential single agent chemotherapy may allow for greater dose intensity and treatment time, potentially meaning greater benefit from each single agent. In addition, sequentially using single agents might cause less toxicity and impairment of quality of life, but it is not known whether this might compromise survival time. The purpose of this study was to assess the effect of combination chemotherapy compared to the same drugs given sequentially in women with metastatic breast cancer.

Findings

Randomized controlled trials of combination chemotherapy compared to the same drugs used sequentially in women with metastatic breast cancer in the first-, second-, or third-line setting were selected. Twelve trials reporting on nine treatment comparisons (2317 patients randomized) were identified. The findings concluded that sequential single agent chemotherapy has a positive effect on progression-free survival, whereas combination chemotherapy has a higher response rate and a higher

risk of febrile neutropenia in metastatic breast cancer. There was no difference in overall survival time between these treatment strategies, but when drugs were given one at a time, there was more time before the tumors grew back again. However, combination chemotherapy caused tumors to shrink more. Generally this study supports the recommendations by international guidelines to use sequential monotherapy unless there is rapid disease progression.

Nursing Implications

Although not entirely conclusive in its findings, nurses need to be aware of this study's findings to be able to counsel women when both therapies are being considered. This study suggests that accurate information about both therapies is needed for all women with metastatic breast cancer, for them to make an informed decision. Nurses need to remember that metastatic breast cancer is not currently curable, but can be effectively treated with chemotherapy. Average survival is about two years, but many women live much longer. The type of therapy chosen should take into consideration optimizing survival, minimizing side effects, and quality of life.

Adapted from Dear, R. F., McGeechan, K, Jenkins, M. C., Barratt, A., Tattersall, M. H. N, & Wilcken, N. (2015). Combination versus sequential single agent chemotherapy for metastatic breast cancer. *Cochrane Database of Systematic Reviews, 2013* (3), Art. No.: CD008792. DOI: 10.1002/14651858.CD008792.pub2.

emotional consequences for both the tested individual and his or her relatives.

Severe psychological distress can occur as a result of genetic testing. Their distress relates to family cancer history, relationships, coping strategies, communication patterns, and mutation status (Wevers et al., 2015). Nurses might find it useful to explore these issues in order to prepare clients before BRCA1/BRCA2 testing and to support them through shifts in family dynamics after disclosure of results. Also, many women perceive their breasts as intrinsic to their femininity, self-esteem, and sexuality, and the risk of losing a breast can provoke extreme anxiety (Alexander et al., 2014). Nurses need to address the physical, emotional, and spiritual needs of the women they care for, as well as their families, since this mutation is inherited in an autosomal dominant fashion. Nurses should identify the woman's personal coping style which has an impact on her likelihood of experiencing distress after her diagnosis. Women who are emotionally expressive and/or have a "fighting spirit" usually experience lower levels of emotional distress. Based on Mendelian genetics, women with BRCA1 and BRCA2 mutations have a 5- to 20-fold increased risk of developing breast and ovarian cancer (Caple & Schub, 2015).

Surgical Options

Generally, the first treatment option for a woman diagnosed with breast cancer is surgery. A few women with tumors larger than 5 cm or inflammatory breast cancer may undergo neoadjuvant chemotherapy or radiotherapy to shrink the tumor before surgical removal is attempted (Debled et al., 2015). The surgical options depend on the type and extent of cancer. The choices are typically either breast-conserving surgery (lumpectomy with radiation) or mastectomy with or without reconstruction. The overall survival rate with lumpectomy and radiation is about the same as that with modified radical mastectomy (ACS, 2015f). Research has shown that the survival rates in women who have had mastectomies versus those who have undergone breast-conserving surgery followed by radiation are the same. However, lumpectomy may not be an option for some women, including those:

- Who have two or more cancer sites that cannot be removed through one incision
- Whose surgery will not result in a clean margin of tissue
- Who have active connective tissue conditions (lupus or scleroderma) that make body tissues especially sensitive to the side effects of radiation

- Who have had previous radiation to the affected breast
- Whose tumors are larger than 5 cm (2 inches) (National Comprehensive Cancer Network [NCCN], 2015).

These decisions are made jointly between the woman and her surgeon. If mastectomy is chosen, because of either tumor characteristics or client preference, then discussion needs to include breast reconstruction and regional lymph node biopsy versus sentinel lymph node biopsy. The mastectomy techniques are a simple mastectomy with sentinel node biopsy or a radical mastectomy with regional node biopsy. Removal of numerous lymph nodes places the client at high risk for lymphedema.

BREAST-CONSERVING SURGERY

Breast-conserving surgery, the least invasive procedure, is the wide local excision (or lumpectomy) of the tumor along with a 1-cm margin of normal tissue. A lumpectomy is often used for early-stage localized tumors. The goal of breast-conserving surgery is to remove the suspicious mass along with tissue free of malignant cells to prevent recurrence. The results are less drastic and emotionally less scarring than having a mastectomy to the woman. Women undergoing breast-conserving therapy receive radiation after lumpectomy with the goal of eradicating residual microscopic cancer cells to limit locoregional recurrence. In women who do not require adjuvant chemotherapy, radiation therapy typically begins 2 to 4 weeks after surgery to allow healing of the lumpectomy incision site. Radiation is administered to the entire breast at daily doses over a period of several weeks (Corradini et al., 2015).

A sentinel lymph node biopsy may also be performed since the lymph nodes draining the breast are located primarily in the axilla. Theoretically, if breast cancer is to metastasize to other parts of the body, it will probably do so via the lymphatic system. If malignant cells are found in the nodes, more aggressive systemic treatment may be needed.

MASTECTOMY

A simple mastectomy is the removal of all breast tissue, the nipple, and the areola. The axillary nodes and pectoral muscles are spared. This procedure would be used for a large tumor or multiple tumors that have not metastasized to adjacent structures or the lymph system.

A modified radical mastectomy is another surgical option; conducive to breast reconstruction and results in greater mobility and less lymphedema (Alexander et al., 2014). This procedure involves removal of breast tissue, and a few positive axillary nodes. Breast-conserving surgeries do not increase the future risk of death from recurrent disease when compared mastectomy (Schuiling & Likis 2016).

In conjunction with the mastectomy, lymph node surgery (removal of underarm nodes) may need to be done to reduce the risk of distant metastasis and improve a woman's chance of long-term survival. For women with a positive sentinel node biopsy, 10 to 20 underarm lymph nodes may need to be removed. Complications associated with axillary lymph node surgery include nerve damage during surgery, causing temporary numbness down the upper aspect of the arm; seroma formation (fluid build-up) followed by wound infection; restrictions in arm mobility (some women need physiotherapy); and lymphedema (swelling related to the lymph glands). In many women lymphedema can be avoided by:

- Avoiding using the affected arm for drawing blood, inserting intravenous lines, or measuring blood pressure (can cause trauma and possible infection)
- Seeking medical care immediately if the affected arm swells
- Wearing gloves when engaging in activities such as gardening that might cause injury
- Wearing a well-fitted compression sleeve to promote drainage return

Women having mastectomies must decide whether to have further surgery to reconstruct the breast. If the woman decides to have reconstructive surgery, it ideally is performed immediately after the mastectomy. The woman must also determine whether she wants the surgeon to use saline implants or natural tissue from her abdomen (TRAM flap method) or back (LAT flap method).

If reconstructive surgery is desired, the ultimate decision regarding the method will be determined by the woman's anatomy (e.g., is there sufficient fat and muscle to permit natural reconstruction?) and her overall health status. Both procedures require a prolonged recovery period.

Some women opt for no reconstruction, and many of them choose to wear breast prostheses. Some prostheses are worn in the bra cup and others fit against the skin or into special pockets created into clothing.

Whether to have reconstructive surgery is an individual and very complex decision. Each woman must be presented with all of the options and then allowed to decide. The nurse can play an important role here by presenting the facts to the woman so that she can make an intelligent decision to meet her unique situation. Breast reconstruction surgery can help restore the look and feel of the breast after a mastectomy. Performed by a plastic surgeon, breast reconstruction can be done immediately after the mastectomy or at a later date. Breast reconstruction can be done with breast implants (filled with saline or silicone); natural tissue flaps (using skin fat and muscle from your own body); or a combination of both. Side effects or complications include risk of rupture, hardening of the tissues around the implant, infection, and pain. Nurses need to educate the woman about these potential problems and make sure they

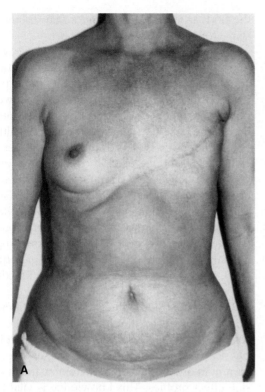 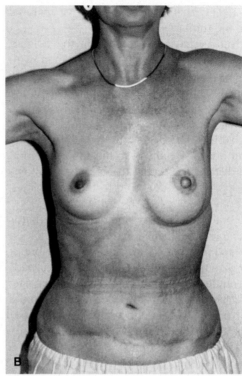

FIGURE 6.6 Before and after photos of postmastectomy and reconstruction.

understand before consenting to breast reconstruction. See Figure 6.6 for examples of pre- and postmastectomy and reconstruction.

BREAST AUGMENTATION

Breast augmentation is a common surgical procedure with women undergoing it with implants for a variety of reasons ranging from aesthetic to reconstructive surgery following a mastectomy. Saline-filled or silicone-filled implants are used in cosmetic enhancement and reconstructive surgeries. The exact anatomical placement of breast implants can vary, but the location typically is subglandular (over the pectoral muscle) or subpectoral (under the muscle). Breast implants are not lifetime devices, but most are guaranteed for approximately 10 years in case of rupture. Breast augmentation with implants is not without risks. Potential complications include capsular contracture, rippling, implant rupture, infection, or hematoma. Capsular contraction occurs when scar tissue forms, contracts, and hardens around the implant. Rippling most often occurs when wrinkles form in the implant or as a complication of contracture (Mugea, 2015).

Breast examination in women with reconstructive surgery is done exactly the same way as for natural breasts. Breasts with implants in place usually feel firmer than normal breast tissue on palpation due to the formation of a fibrotic band or capsule around the implant. If implants are used, press firmly inward at the edges of the implant to feel the ribs beneath.

Adjunctive Therapy

Adjunctive therapy is supportive or additional therapy that is recommended after surgery. Adjunctive therapies include local therapy such as radiation therapy and systemic therapies using chemotherapy, hormonal therapy, and immunotherapy.

RADIATION THERAPY

Radiation therapy (also called radiotherapy) uses high-energy rays to destroy cancer cells that might have been left behind in the breast, chest wall, or underarm area after a tumor has been removed surgically. Usually serial radiation doses are given 5 days a week to the tumor site for 6 to 8 weeks postoperatively. Each treatment takes only a few minutes, but the dose is cumulative. Women undergoing breast-conserving therapy receive radiation to the entire breast after lumpectomy with the goal of eradicating residual microscopic cancer cells to reduce the chance of recurrence (Chu et al., 2015).

Side Effects. Side effects of traditional radiation therapy include inflammation, local edema, anorexia, swelling, and heaviness in the breast; sunburn-like skin changes in the treated area; and fatigue. Changes to the breast tissue and skin usually resolve in about a year in most women (Lara et al., 2015). This type of therapy can be given several ways: external beam radiation, which delivers a carefully focused dose of radiation from a machine outside the body, or internal radiation, in which tiny pellets that contain radioactive material are placed into the tumor.

Several advances have taken place in the field of radiation oncology for the treatment of women with early-stage breast cancer that assist in reducing the side effects. The treatment position for external radiation has changed from supine to prone, with the arm on the affected side raised above the head, so that the treated breast hangs dependently through the opening of the treatment board. Treatment in the prone position improves dose distribution within the breast and allows for a decrease in the dose delivered to the heart, lung, chest wall, and other breast (NCCN, 2015).

High-dose brachytherapy is another advance that is an alternative to traditional radiation treatment. A balloon catheter is used to insert radioactive seeds into the breast after the tumor has been removed surgically. The seeds deliver a concentrated dose directly to the operative site; this is important because most cancer recurrences in the breast occur at or near the lumpectomy site (Chang et al., 2015). This allows a high dose of radiation to be delivered to a small target volume with a minimal dose to the surrounding normal tissue. This procedure takes 4 to 5 days as opposed to the 4 to 6 weeks that traditional radiation therapy takes; it also eliminates the need to delay radiation therapy to allow for wound healing. Brachytherapy is now used as a primary radiation treatment after breast-conserving surgery in selected women as an alternative to whole breast irradiation (Guinot et al., 2015). Side effects of brachytherapy include redness or discharge around catheters, fever, and infection. Daily cleansing of the catheter insertion site with a mild soap and application of an antibiotic ointment will minimize the risk of infection.

Intensity-modulated radiation therapy (IMRT) offers still another new approach to the delivery of treatment to reduce the dose within the target area while sparing surrounding normal structures. A computed tomography scan is used to create a three-dimensional model of the breast. Based on this model, a series of intensity-modulated beams is produced to the desired dose distribution to reduce radiation exposure to underlying structures. Acute toxicity is thus minimized (Muralidhar, Soubhagya, & Ahmed, 2015). Research is ongoing to evaluate the impact of all of these advances in radiation therapy.

CHEMOTHERAPY

Chemotherapy refers to the use of drugs that are toxic to all cells and interfere with a cell's ability to reproduce. They are particularly effective against malignant cells but affect all rapidly dividing cells, especially those of the skin, the hair follicles, the mouth, the gastrointestinal tract, and the bone marrow. Breast cancer is a systemic disease in which micrometastases are already present in other organs by the time the breast cancer is diagnosed. Chemotherapeutic agents perform a systemic "sweep" of

the body to reduce the chances that distant tumors will start growing.

Chemotherapy may be indicated for women with tumors larger than 1 cm, positive lymph nodes, or cancer of an aggressive type. Chemotherapy is prescribed in cycles, with each period of treatment followed by a rest period. Treatment typically lasts 3 to 6 months, depending on the dose used and the woman's health status.

Different classes of drugs affect different aspects of cell division and are used in combinations or "cocktails." The most active and commonly used chemotherapeutic agents for breast cancer include alkylating agents, anthracyclines, antimetabolites, and vinca alkaloids. Fifty or more chemotherapeutic agents can be used to treat breast cancer; however, a combination drug approach appears to be more effective than a single drug treatment (ACS, 2015g). Refer to Evidence-Based Practice 6.1.

Side Effects. Side effects of chemotherapy depend on the agents used, the intensity of dosage, the dosage schedule, the type and extent of cancer, and the client's physical and emotional status. Nurses need to remain current in order to accommodate new treatments and the side effect profiles. This knowledge is vital to providing evidence-based care for breast cancer women receiving these treatments (Bourdeanu & Lui, 2015). However, typical side effects include nausea and vomiting, diarrhea or constipation, hair loss, weight loss, stomatitis, fatigue, and immunosuppression. The most serious is bone marrow suppression (myelosuppression). This causes an increased risk of infection, bleeding, and a reduced red blood cell count, which can lead to anemia. Treatment of the side effects can generally be addressed through appropriate support medications such as antinausea drugs. In addition, growth-stimulating factors, such as epoetin alfa (Procrit) and filgrastim (Neupogen), help keep blood counts from dropping too low. Counts that are too low would stop or delay the use of chemotherapy.

An aggressive systemic option, when other treatments have failed or when there is a strong possibility of relapse or metastatic disease, is high-dose chemotherapy with bone marrow and/or stem cell transplant. This therapy involves the withdrawal of bone marrow before the administration of toxic levels of chemotherapeutic agents. The marrow is frozen and then returned to the client after the high-dose chemotherapy is finished. Clinical trials are still researching this experimental therapy (King et al., 2015).

HORMONAL THERAPY

One of estrogen's normal functions is to stimulate the growth and division of healthy cells in the breasts. However, in some women with breast cancer, this normal function contributes to the growth and division of cancer cells.

The objective of endocrine therapy is to block or counter the effect of estrogen. Estrogen plays a central role in the pathogenesis of cancer, and treatment with estrogen deprivation has proven to be effective. Approximately two-thirds of women diagnosed with early-stage breast cancer have hormone-sensitive disease (estrogen receptor positive and/or progesterone receptor positive), and adjuvant hormone therapy play an essential role in reducing the risk of recurrence and improving survival (Gradishar, 2015). Several different drug classes are used to interfere or block estrogen receptors. They include selective estrogen receptor modulators (SERMs), estrogen receptor down-regulators, aromatase inhibitors, luteinizing hormone-releasing hormone, progestin, and biologic response modifiers (King et al., 2015). Current recommendations for most women with ER+ breast cancer are to take a hormone-like medication—known as a SERM antiestrogenic agent—daily for up to 5 years after initial treatment. Certain areas in the female body (breasts, uterus, ovaries, skin, vagina, and brain) contain specialized cells called hormone receptors that allow estrogen to enter the cell and stimulate it to divide. SERMs enter these same receptors and act like keys, turning off the signal for growth inside the cell (King et al., 2015). The best-known SERM is tamoxifen (Nolvadex, 20 mg daily for 5 years). Although it works well in preventing further spread of cancer, it is also associated with an increased incidence of endometrial cancer, pulmonary embolus, deep vein thrombosis, hot flashes, vaginal discharge and bleeding, stroke, and cataract formation (Jager et al., 2015).

Another SERM is the anti-osteoporosis drug raloxifene (Evista), which has shown promising results. It has antiestrogen effects on the breast and uterus. In recent studies involving postmenopausal women at high risk for breast cancer, raloxifene worked as well as tamoxifen in preventing breast cancer, but with fewer serious adverse effects. Both drugs cut the cancer risk in half (Bevers, 2015). It was originally marketed solely for the prevention and treatment of osteoporosis but is now used as adjunctive breast cancer therapy.

Another class of endocrine agents, aromatase inhibitors, works by inhibiting the conversion of androgens to estrogens. Aromatase inhibitors include letrozole (Femara, 2.5 mg daily), exemestane (Aromasin, 25 mg daily), and anastrozole (Arimidex, 1 mg daily for 5 years), all of which are taken orally. These are usually given to women with advanced breast cancer. In recent clinical studies in postmenopausal women with breast cancer, third-generation aromatase inhibitors were shown to be superior to tamoxifen for the treatment of metastatic disease (Bevers, 2015).

Side Effects. The side effects associated with these endocrine therapies include hot flashes, bone pain, bone thinning, insomnia, weight gain, depression, fatigue,

nausea, cough, dyspnea, and headache (Breast Cancer Organization, 2015). Women with hormone-sensitive cancers can live for long periods without any intervention other than hormonal manipulation, but quality-of-life issues need to be addressed in the balance between treatment and side effects.

IMMUNOTHERAPY

Immunotherapy, used as an adjunct to surgery, represents an attempt to stimulate the body's natural defenses to recognize and attack cancer cells. Trastuzumab (Herceptin, 2- to 4-mg/kg intravenous infusion) is the first monoclonal antibody approved for breast cancer (NCCN, 2015). Some tumors produce excessive amounts of HER-2/neu protein, which regulates cancer cell growth. Breast cancers that overexpress the HER-2/neu protein are associated with a more aggressive form of disease and a poorer prognosis. Trastuzumab blocks the effect of this protein to inhibit the growth of cancer cells. It can be used alone or in combination with other chemotherapy to treat clients with metastatic breast disease. Although immunotherapy has shown some promise against the fight against cancer, recent data suggests that greater success will be achieved by combining it with other therapies, such as radiation (Leavy, 2015).

 Concept Mastery Alert

Tamoxifen Versus Trastuzumab in Breast Cancer Treatment

Tamoxifen is a selective estrogen receptor modulator used to prevent further spread of breast cancer in women with ER-positive breast cancer. Trastuzumab is a monoclonal antibody used in the treatment of breast cancer and is considered immunotherapy.

Side Effects. Adverse effects of trastuzumab include cardiac toxicity, vascular thrombosis, hepatic failure, fever, chills, nausea, vomiting, and pain with first infusion (Skidmore-Roth, 2015).

NURSING PROCESS FOR THE CLIENT WITH BREAST CANCER

When a woman is diagnosed with breast cancer, she faces treatment that may alter her body shape, may make her feel unwell, and may not carry a certainty of cure. Nurses can support women from the time of diagnosis, through the treatments, and through follow-up after the surgical and adjunctive treatments have been completed. Allowing clients the time to ask questions and to discuss any necessary preparations for treatment is critical. As our understanding of breast disorders keeps improving, treatments continue to change.

Although the goal of treatment remains improved survival, increasing emphasis is being focused on prevention. Breast cancer prevention measures focus on evaluating and reducing risk factors. Approaches for reducing breast cancer risk include lifestyle modifications (diet and physical exercise), chemoprevention (SERMs & AIs), and prophylactic surgery (bilateral salpingoopjorectomy & bilateral prophylactic mastectomy) (Euhus & Diaz, 2015). Nurses can have an impact on early detection of breast disorders, treatment, and symptom management. Women with a cancer diagnosis often experience negative emotions and nurses' empathic response can help alleviate their distress (Alexander et al., 2014). A nurse who is involved in the woman's treatment plan from the beginning can effectively offer support throughout the whole experience.

Teamwork is important in breast screening and caring for women with breast disorders. Treatment is often fragmented between the hospital and community treatment centers, which can be emotionally traumatic for the woman and her family. The advances being made in the diagnosis and treatment of breast disorders mean that guidelines are constantly changing, requiring all health care providers to keep up to date. Informed nurses can provide support and information and, most importantly, continuity of care for the woman undergoing treatment for a breast problem.

The nurse plays a particularly important role in providing psychological support and self-care teaching to clients with breast cancer. Nurses can influence both physical and emotional recovery, which are both important aspects of care that help in improving the woman's quality of life and the ability to survive. The nurse's role should extend beyond helping clients; spreading the word in the community about screening and prevention is a big part in the ongoing fight against cancer. The community should see nurses as both educators and valued sources of credible information. This role will help improve clinical outcomes while achieving high levels of client satisfaction.

Despite the new guidelines issued by various governmental agencies regarding BSEs, a CBE done by a professional health care provider is essential for good breast health for all women. See Box 6.1 for additional information.

Remember Nancy from the chapter opener? Is her response typical of many women upon discovering a lump in their breast? Nancy confides her discovery of the lump and her worries to you. What advice would you give her?

ASSESSMENT

Early breast cancer has no symptoms. The earliest sign of breast cancer is often an abnormality seen on a screening mammogram before the woman or the health care provider feels it. A healthy, asymptomatic presentation is typical. However, symptoms may include a lump in the breast that is usually nontender, fixed, and hard with irregular borders. In the woman presenting with a breast disorder, take a thorough history of the problem and explore the woman's risk factors for breast cancer. Assess the woman for clinical manifestations of breast cancer, such as changes in breast appearance and contour, which become apparent with advancing breast cancer (ACS, 2015d). These changes include:

- Continued and persistent changes in the breast
- A lump or thickening in one breast
- Persistent nipple irritation
- Unusual breast swelling or asymmetry
- A lump or swelling in the axilla
- Changes in skin color or texture
- Nipple retraction, tenderness, or discharge

Complete a breast examination to validate the clinical manifestations and findings of the health history and risk factor assessment. The CBE involves both inspection and palpation (Box 6.1). Helpful characteristics in evaluating palpable breast masses are described in Table 6.5. If a lump can be palpated, the cancer has been there for quite some time.

Be cognizant of the impact that breast cancer has on a woman's emotional state, coping ability, and quality of life. Women may experience sadness, vulnerability, loss of control, alteration of body image and integrity, anger, the illness's impact on relationships, fear of mortality, the need to reprioritize her life, and guilt as a result of having breast cancer. However, despite potential negative outcomes, many women have a positive outlook for their future and adapt to treatment modalities with a good quality of life (Kleban & Glaser, 2015). Closely monitor clients for their psychosocial adjustment to diagnosis and treatment and be able to identify those who need further psychological intervention. By giving practical advice, the nurse can help the woman adjust to her altered body image and to accept the changes in her life.

Because family members play a significant role in supporting women through breast cancer diagnosis and treatment, assess the emotional distress of both partners during the course of treatment and, if needed, make a referral for psychological counseling. By identifying interpersonal strains, negative psychosocial side effects of cancer treatment can be minimized.

NURSING DIAGNOSIS

Appropriate nursing diagnoses for a woman with a diagnosis of breast cancer might include:

- Disturbed body image related to:
  - Loss of body part (breast)
  - Loss of femininity
  - Loss of hair due to chemotherapy

BOX 6.1

CLINICAL BREAST EXAMINATION BY HEALTH CARE PROVIDER

If the woman is deemed high risk, the nurse would then teach the woman to perform a BSE to enhance breast awareness.

Purpose: To Assess Breasts for Abnormal Findings

• Inspect the breast for size, symmetry, and skin texture and color. It is common for the left breast to be slightly larger than the right. Inspect the nipples and areola. Ask the client to sit at the edge of the examination table, with her arms resting at her sides.

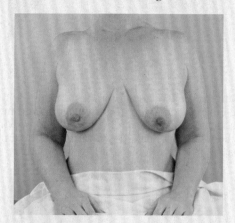

• Inspect the breast for masses, retraction, dimpling, or ecchymosis.
• The client places her hands on her hips.

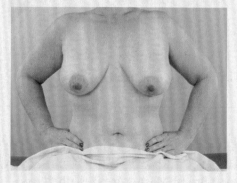

• She then raises her arms over her head so the axillae can also be inspected.

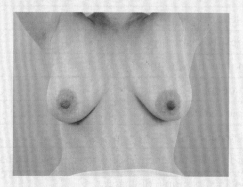

• The client then stands, places her hands on her hips, and leans forward.

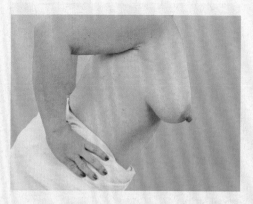

• Palpate the breasts using the pads of your first three fingers and make a rotary motion on the breast. Assist the client into a supine position with her arms above her head. Place a pillow or towel under the client's head to help spread the breasts. Three patterns might be used to palpate the breasts:

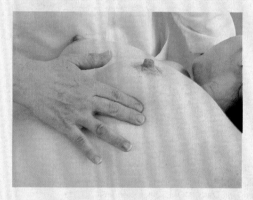

1. Spiral

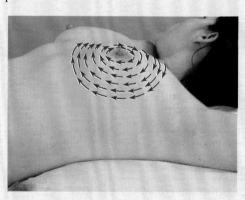

(continues on Page 204)

CLINICAL BREAST EXAMINATION BY HEALTH CARE PROVIDER (continued)

2. Pie-shaped wedges

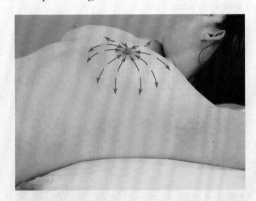

3. Vertical strip

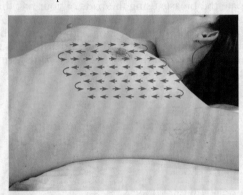

• Compress the nipple gently between the thumb and index finger to evaluate for masses and squeeze to check for any discharge.

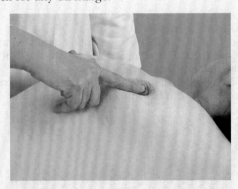

• Palpate the axillary area for any tenderness or lymph node enlargement. Have the client sit up and move to the edge of the examination table. While supporting the client's arm, palpate downward from the armpit, palpating toward the ribs just below the breast.

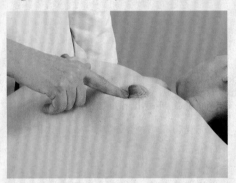

Adapted from Ball, J. W., Dains, J. E., Flynn, J. A., Soloman, B. S., & Stewart, R. W. (2015). *Seidel's guide to physical examination* (8th ed.). St. Louis, MO: Elsevier Saunders.

TABLE 6.5 | **CHARACTERISTICS OF BENIGN VERSUS MALIGNANT BREAST MASSES**

Benign Breast Masses Are Described As	Malignant Breast Masses Are Described As
• Frequently painful	• Hard to palpation
• Firm, rubbery mass	• Painless
• Bilateral masses	• Irregularly shaped (poorly delineated)
• Induced nipple discharge	• Immobile, fixed to the chest wall
• Regular margins (clearly delineated)	• Skin dimpling
• No skin dimpling	• Nipple retraction
• No nipple retraction	• Unilateral mass
• Mobile, not affixed to the chest wall	• Bloody, serosanguineous, or serous nipple discharge
• No bloody discharge	• Spontaneous nipple discharge

- Fear related to:
  - Diagnosis of cancer
  - Prognosis of disease
- Deficient knowledge related to:
  - Cancer treatment options
  - Reconstructive surgery decisions
  - Breast self-examination

NURSING INTERVENTIONS

Offer information, support, and perioperative care to women diagnosed with breast cancer who are undergoing treatment. Implement health promotion and disease prevention strategies to minimize the risk for developing breast cancer and to promote optimal outcomes.

Remember Nancy, who discovered a breast lump? You offer to go with her to the doctor. After a full examination and several diagnostic tests, the results come back positive for breast cancer. What treatment options does Nancy have, and what factors need to be considered in selecting those options?

Providing Client Education

Help the woman and her partner to prioritize the voluminous amount of information given to them so that they can make informed decisions. Explain all treatment options in detail so the client and her family understand them. By preparing an individualized packet of information and reviewing it with the woman and her partner (if applicable), the nurse can help the woman understand her specific type of cancer, the diagnostic studies and treatment options she may choose, and the goals of treatment. For example, nurses play an important role in educating women about the use of endocrine therapies, observing women's experiences with treatment, and communicating those observations to their primary health care providers to make dosage adjustments, in addition to contributing to the knowledge base of endocrine therapy in the treatment of breast cancer.

Providing information is a central role of the nurse in caring for the woman with a diagnosis of breast cancer. This information can be given via telephone counseling, one-to-one contact, and pamphlets. Telephone counseling with women and their partners may be an effective method to improve symptom management and quality of life. Educate women on living with risk, maintaining quality of life, and participating in support groups (Strayer & Schub, 2014).

Providing Emotional Support

The diagnosis of cancer affects all aspects of life for a woman and her family. The threatening nature of the disease and feelings of uncertainty about the future can lead to anxiety and stress. Address the woman's need for:

- Information about diagnosis and treatment
- Physical care while undergoing treatments
- Contact with supportive people
- Education about disease, options, and prevention measures
- Discussion and support by a caring, competent nurse

Reassure the client and her family that the diagnosis of breast cancer does not necessarily mean imminent death, a decrease in attractiveness, or diminished sexuality. Encourage the woman to express her fears and worries. Be available to listen and address the woman's concerns in an open manner to help her toward recovery. All aspects of care must include sensitivity to the client's personal efforts to cope and heal. Some women will become involved in organizations or charities that support cancer research; they may participate in breast cancer walks to raise awareness or become a *Reach to Recovery* volunteer to help others. Each woman copes in her own personal manner, and all of these efforts can be positive motivators for her own healing.

To help women cope with the diagnosis of breast cancer, the ACS launched *Reach to Recovery* more than 30 years ago. Specially trained breast cancer survivors give women and their families' opportunities to express their feelings, verbalize their fears, and get answers. Recovery volunteers can also, when appropriate, provide a temporary breast form and give information on types of permanent prostheses, as well as lists of where those items are available in the community. Most importantly, *Reach to Recovery* volunteers offer understanding, support, and hope through face-to-face visits or by telephone; they are proof that people can survive breast cancer and live productive lives. National contact information is 1-800-ACS-2345.

Providing Postoperative Care

For the woman who has had surgery to remove a malignant breast lump or an entire breast, excellent postoperative nursing care is crucial. Tell the woman what to expect in terms of symptoms and when they usually occur during treatment and after surgery. This allows women to anticipate these symptoms and proactively employ management strategies to improve their cancer experience. Postoperative care includes immediate postoperative care, pain management, care of the affected arm, wound care, mobility care, respiratory care, emotional care, referrals, and educational needs.

Immediate Postoperative Care

Assess the client's respiratory status by auscultating the lungs and observing the breathing pattern. Assess circulation; note vital signs, skin color, and skin temperature. Observe the client's neurologic status by evaluating the level of alertness and orientation. Monitor the wound for amount and color of drainage. Monitor the intravenous lines for patency, correct fluid, and rate. Assess the drainage tube for amount, color, and consistency of drainage.

Pain Management

Provide analgesics as needed. Reassure the woman that her pain will be controlled. Teach the woman how to communicate her pain intensity on a scale of 0 to 10, with 10 being the worst pain imaginable. Assess the client's pain level frequently and anticipate pain before assisting the woman to ambulate.

Affected Arm Care

Elevate the affected arm on a pillow to promote lymph drainage. Make sure that no treatments are performed on the affected arm, including laboratory draws, intravenous lines, blood pressures, and so on. Place a sign above the bed to warn others not to touch the affected arm.

Wound Care

Observe the wound often and empty drainage reservoirs as needed. Tell the client to report any evidence of infection early, such as fever, chills, or any area of redness or inflammation along the incision line. Also tell the client to report any increase in drainage, foul odor, or separation at the incision site.

Mobility Care

Perform active range-of-motion and arm exercises as ordered. Encourage self-care activities for successful rehabilitation. Perform dressing and drainage care; explain the care during the procedure.

Respiratory Care

Assist with turning, coughing, and deep breathing every 2 hours. Explain that this helps to expand collapsed alveoli in the lungs, promotes faster clearance of inhalation agents from the body, and prevents postoperative pneumonia and atelectasis.

Emotional Care and Referrals

Encourage the client to participate in her care. Assess her coping strategies preoperatively. Explain possible body image concerns after discharge. Promote the ACS web sites, which provide the latest cancer therapy news. Encourage the client to attend local support groups for breast cancer survivors, such as *Reach to Recovery*.

Educational Needs

Provide follow-up information about adjunctive therapy. Explain that radiation therapy may start within weeks postoperatively. Discuss chemotherapy, its side effects and cycles, home care during treatment, and future monitoring strategies. Explain hormonal therapy, including antiestrogens or aromatase inhibitors. Teach progressive arm exercises to minimize lymphedema. Explain that ongoing surveillance is needed to detect recurrence of cancer or a new primary site and that the client will typically see the health care provider every 6 months.

> Nancy underwent a mastectomy with radiation and chemotherapy. What follow-up care is needed? How can the nurse assist Nancy to cope with her uncertain future? What community resources might help her?

IMPLEMENTING HEALTH PROMOTION AND DISEASE PREVENTION STRATEGIES

In the past, most women assumed that there was little they could do to reduce their risk of developing breast cancer, but since the 1970s significant advances have been made in the diagnosis and treatment of breast cancer. Mortality rates have decreased since 1990, particularly in women <50 years old. The declining incidence of breast cancer and lower mortality rates have been attributed to early detection, improved treatment, and research (Sestak & Cuzick, 2015). However, research has found that the choices women make concerning breast cancer screening, diet, exercise, and other health practices have a profound impact on cancer risk. In the fight against cancer, nurses often assume a variety of roles, such as educator, counselor, advocate, and role model. Nurses can offer education about the following:

- Prevention
- Early detection
- Screening
- Dispelling myths and fears
- Self-examination techniques if needed
- Individual risk status and strategies for risk reduction

It is important to be knowledgeable about the most current evidence-based practices and cognizant of how the media presents this information. Offer prevention strategies within the context of a woman's life. Factors such as lifestyle choices, economic status, and multiple roles need to be taken into consideration when counseling women. Advocate for healthy lifestyles and making sound choices to prevent cancer. Nurses, like all health care providers, should offer guidance from a comprehensive perspective that acknowledges the unique needs of each individual. Nurses need to not only be proficient in the postoperative physical care of clients who undergo mastectomy but also demonstrate advanced skills related to the educational needs of clients and their families and to ensure care is delivered in a manner that is client-centered and individualized. Nurses require advanced skills to meet the social and psychological care needs of the woman and her family during this major life event (Fallowfield & Jenkins, 2015).

Breast cancer is a frightening experience for all women but is particularly burdensome on African-American women, ranking second among the cause of cancer deaths in them. Although the incidence of breast cancer is highest in White women, African-American women have a higher breast cancer mortality rate at every age and a lower survival rate than any other racial or ethnic group. Statistics indicate that the gap is widening (ACS, 2015e).

Like a black cloud hanging over their heads, with little regard for any victim, breast cancer stalks women everywhere they go. Many women are left with new health risks and lingering effects associated with treatment (e.g., limited mobility, memory problems, low social activity, and support). Many have a close friend or relative who is battling the disease; many have watched their mothers and sisters die of this dreaded disease. Those with risk factors live with even greater anxiety and fear. No woman wants to hear those chilling words: "The biopsy is positive. You have breast cancer." Provide women with information about detection and risk factors, inform them about the new ACS screening guidelines, instruct them on BSE, and outline dietary changes that might reduce their risk of breast cancer.

Awareness is the first step toward a change in habits. Raising the level of awareness about breast cancer is of paramount importance, and nurses can play an important role in health promotion, disease prevention, and education.

Breast Cancer Screening

The three components of early detection are BSE, CBE, and mammography. The ACS (2015d) has issued breast cancer screening guidelines that, for the first time, offer specific guidance for the women and greater clarification of the role of breast examinations (see Table 6.4). ACS screening guidelines are revised about every 5 years to include new scientific findings and developments.

Women are exposed to multiple sources of cancer prevention information, and much of it may not be sound. Discuss the benefits, risks, and potential limitations of BSE, CBE, and mammography with each woman and tailor the information to her specific risk factors (ACS, 2015b). Based on the new guidelines, make clinical judgments as to the appropriateness of recommending BSE, and reevaluate the need to teach the procedure to all women; the focus might instead be on encouraging regular mammograms (depending, of course, on the woman's individual risk factors).

Breast Self-Examination

BSE is a technique that enables a woman to detect any changes in her breasts. BSEs, once thought essential for early breast cancer detection, are now considered optional. Instead, breast awareness is stressed. Breast awareness refers to a woman being familiar with the normal consistency of both breasts and the underlying tissue. This emphasis is now on awareness of breast changes, not just discovery of cancer. Research has shown that BSE plays a small role in detecting breast cancer compared with self-awareness. However, doing BSE is one way for a woman to know how her breasts normally feel so that she can notice any changes that do occur (ACS, 2015d).

If appropriate, there are two steps to conducting a BSE: visual inspection and tactile palpation. The visual part should be done in three separate positions: with the arms up behind the head, with the arms down at the sides, and bending forward. Instruct the woman to look for:
* Changes in shape, size, contour, or symmetry
* Skin discoloration or dimpling, bumps/lumps
* Sores or scaly skin
* Discharge or puckering of the nipple

In the second part, the tactile examination, the health care provider feels the woman's breasts in one of three specific patterns: spiral, pie-shaped wedges, or a vertical strip (up and down). When using any of the three patterns, the woman should use a circular rubbing motion (in dime-sized circles) without lifting the fingers. The examiner checks not only the breasts but also between the breast and the axilla, the axilla itself, and the area above the breast up to the clavicle and across the shoulder. The pads of the three middle fingers on the right hand are used to assess the left breast; the pads of the three middle fingers on the left hand are used to assess the right breast. Instruct the woman to use three different degrees of pressure:
* Light (move the skin without moving the tissue underneath)
* Medium (midway into the tissue)
* Hard (down to the ribs)

Nutrition

Nutrition plays a critical role in health promotion and disease prevention. Cancer is considered to be a chronic disease that may be influenced at many stages by nutrition. These factors may affect prevention, progression, and treatment of the disease (Shrivastava, Shrivastava, & Ramasamy, 2015). Being overweight or obese is a risk factor for breast cancer in postmenopausal women. Excess body weight has been linked to an increased risk of postmenopausal breast cancer, and growing evidence also suggests that obesity is associated with poor prognosis in women diagnosed with early-stage breast cancer. Dozens of studies demonstrate that women who are overweight or obese at the time of breast cancer diagnosis are at increased risk of cancer recurrence and death compared with leaner women, and some evidence suggests that women who gain weight after breast cancer diagnosis may also be at increased risk of poor outcomes (Wright et al., 2015). *Healthy People 2020* identified being overweight or obese as one of the 10 leading health indicators and a major health concern (U.S. Department of Health and Human Services, 2010). Almost 65% of women over the age of 20 years are overweight; of these, 33.4% are obese (Carlson, 2015). A Mediterranean diet high in fruits, vegetables, and high-fiber carbohydrates and low in animal fat seems to offer protection against breast cancer as well as weight control. Women who followed these dietary guidelines decreased their risk of breast cancer. In addition, substantial evidence has shown that obesity, as measured by body mass index (BMI) is linked to breast cancer outcomes and greater mortality risks (Chan & Norat, 2015).

The Women's Health Initiative Dietary Modification Trial (Brasky et al., 2015) was designed to study a low-fat diet, a nutritional approach to prevention of chronic diseases. It found a marginally statistically significant reduction in breast cancer incidence among women in the low-fat dietary pattern group, and also disproved that 'heart healthy eating' prevented future cardiac events in women.

The American Institute for Cancer Research, which conducts extensive research, made the following recommendations to reduce a woman's risk for developing breast cancer:

• Engaging in daily moderate exercise and weekly vigorous physical activity
• Consuming at least five servings of fruits and vegetables daily
• Not smoking or using any tobacco products
• Keeping a maximum BMI of 25 and limiting weight gain to no more than 11 pounds since age 18
• Consuming seven or more daily portions of complex carbohydrates, such as whole grains and cereals
• Limiting intake of processed foods and refined sugar
• Limiting consumption of energy-dense foods and sugary drinks

• Avoiding use of dietary supplements which are unlikely to improve prognosis
• Restricting red meat intake to approximately 3 ounces daily
• Limiting intake of fatty foods, particularly those of animal origin
• Restricting intake of salted foods and use of salt in cooking (Swisher et al., 2015).

The medical community is also starting to study the role of phytochemicals in health. The unique geographic variability of breast cancer around the world and the low rate of breast cancer in Asia compared with Western countries prompted this interest. This area of research appears hopeful for women seeking to prevent breast cancer as well as those recovering from it. Although the mechanism is not clear, certain foods demonstrate anticancer properties and boost the immune system. Phytochemical-rich foods include:

• Green tea and herbal teas
• Garlic
• Whole grains and legumes
• Onions and leeks
• Soybeans and soy products
• Tomato products (cooked tomatoes)
• Fruits (citrus, apricots, pumpkin, berries)
• Green leafy vegetables (spinach, collards, romaine)
• Colorful vegetables (carrots, squash, tomatoes)
• Cruciferous vegetables (broccoli, cabbage, cauliflower)
• Flax seeds (Bahadoran, Karimi, & Abedini, 2015).

Adopt a holistic approach when addressing the nutritional needs of women with breast cancer. Incorporate nutritional assessment into the general overall assessment of all women. Culturally sensitive nutritional assessment tools need to be developed and used to enhance this process. Providing examples of appropriate foods associated with the woman's current dietary habits, relating current health status to nutritional intake, and placing proposed modifications within a realistic personal framework may increase a woman's willingness to incorporate needed changes in her nutritional behavior. Be able to interpret research results and stay up to date on nutritional influences so that you can transmit this key information to the public.

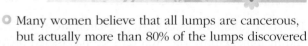

KEY CONCEPTS

○ Many women believe that all lumps are cancerous, but actually more than 80% of the lumps discovered are benign and need no treatment (Alexander et al., 2014).

○ The most commonly encountered benign breast disorders in women include fibrocystic breasts, fibroadenomas, and mastitis (Bope & Kellerman, 2015).

- Current research suggests that women with fibrocystic breast disease or other benign breast conditions are more likely to develop breast cancer later only if a breast biopsy shows "atypia" or abnormal breast cells (ACS, 2015a).

- Fibroadenomas are common benign solid breast tumors that can be stimulated by external estrogen, progesterone, lactation, and pregnancy.

- Mastitis is an infection of the connective tissue in the breast that occurs primarily in lactating or engorged women; it is divided into lactational or nonlactational types.

- Management of both types of mastitis involves the use of oral antibiotics (usually a penicillinase-resistant penicillin or cephalosporin) and acetaminophen (Tylenol) for pain and fever (Miller & Kennedy, 2015).

- Breast cancer is the most common cancer in women and the second leading cause of cancer deaths (lung cancer is first) among American women (ACS, 2015a).

- Breast cancer metastasizes widely and to almost all organs of the body, but primarily to the bone, lungs, lymph nodes, liver, and brain.

- The etiology of breast cancer is unknown, but the disease is thought to develop in response to a number of related factors: aging, delayed childbearing or never bearing children, high breast density, family history of cancer, late menopause, obesity, and hormonal factors.

- Breast cancer treatments fall into two categories: local and systemic. Local treatments are surgery and radiation therapy. Effective systemic treatments include chemotherapy, hormonal therapy, and immunotherapy.

- Women commonly perceive their breasts as intrinsic to their femininity, self-esteem, and sexuality, and the risk of losing a breast can provoke extreme anxiety.

- Nurses can influence both physical and emotional recovery, which are both important aspects of care that help in improving the woman's quality of life and the ability to survive.

- Providing up-to-date information and emotional support are central roles of the nurse in caring for the woman with a diagnosis of breast cancer.

References and Recommended Readings

American Cancer Society [ACS]. (2015b). *Risk factors for breast cancer*. Retrieved from http://www.cancer.org/cancer/breastcancer/detailedguide/breast-cancer-risk-factors

American Cancer Society [ACS]. (2015c). *Types of breast cancer*. Retrieved: http://www.cancer.org/cancer/breastcancer/detailedguide/breast-cancer-breast-cancer-types

American Cancer Society [ACS]. (2015d). *Guidelines for the early detection of breast cancer*. Retrieved from http://www.cancer.org/healthy/findcancerearly/cancerscreeningguidelines/american-cancer-society-guidelines-for-the-early-detection-of-cancer

American Cancer Society [ACS]. (2015e). *Cancer Facts & Figures*. Retrieved from http://www.cancer.org/acs/groups/content/@epidemiologysurveilance/documents/document/acspc-036845.pdf

American Cancer Society [ACS]. (2015f). *How is breast cancer treated?* Retrieved from http://www.cancer.org/cancer/breastcancer/detailedguide/breast-cancer-treating-surgery

American Cancer Society [ACS]. (2015g). *Chemotherapy for breast cancer*. Retrieved from http://www.cancer.org/cancer/breastcancer/detailedguide/breast-cancer-treating-chemotherapy

American Congress of Obstetricians and Gynecologists [ACOG]. (2015). Annual mammograms now recommended for women beginning at age 40. Retrieved from http://www.acog.org/About%20ACOG/News%20Room/News%20Releases/2011/Annual%20Mammograms%20Now%20Recommended%20for%20Women%20Beginning%20at%20Age%2040.aspx

Arora, R., Schmitt, D., Karanam, B., Tan, M., Yates, C., & Dean-Colomb, W. (2015). Inhibition of the Warburg effect with a natural compound reveals a novel measurement for determining the metastatic potential of breast cancers. *Oncotarget, 6*(2), 662–678.

Bahadoran, Z., Karimi, Z., & Abedini, S. (2015). Healthy dietary patterns and the risk of breast cancer: A review of current data. *American Journal of Life Sciences, 3*(2-1), 1–5.

Bevers, T. B. (2015). Breast cancer risk reduction therapy: The low-hanging fruit. *Journal of the National Comprehensive Cancer Network, 13*(4), 376–378.

Bhatti, L., Hoang, J. K., Dale, B. M., & Bashir, M. R. (2015). Advanced magnetic resonance techniques: 3 T. *Radiologic Clinics of North America, 53*(3), 441–455.

Bourdeanu, L., & Liu, E. A. (2015). Systemic treatment for breast cancer: chemotherapy and biotherapy agents. In *Seminars in Oncology Nursing*. WB Saunders. doi:10.1016/j.soncn.2015.02.003

Brasky, T. M., Rodabough, R. J., Liu, J., Kurta, M. L., Wise, L. A., Orchard, T. S., et al. (2015). Long-chain ω-3 fatty acid intake and endometrial cancer risk in the Women's Health Initiative. *The American Journal of Clinical Nutrition, 101*(4), 824–834.

Breast Cancer Organization. (2015). *Hormonal therapy side effects*. Retrieved from http://www.breastcancer.org/treatment/hormonal/comp_chart

Caple, C., & Schub, T. (2015). Breast cancer: Psychological adjustment. *CINAHL Information systems*. (Online 4/17/15) *Evidence-based Care Sheet*. Retrieved from http://web.b.ebscohost.com.ezproxy.net.ucf.edu/ehost/pdfviewer/pdfviewer?sid=415529de-e3be-4ada-b09e-fde7fd22ec97%40sessionmgr111&vid=33&hid=118

Catsburg, C., Kim, R. S., Kirsh, V. A., Soskolne, C. L., Kreiger, N., & Rohan, T. E. (2015). Dietary patterns and breast cancer risk: a study in 2 cohorts. *The American Journal of Clinical Nutrition, 101*(4), 817–823.

Chan, D. S., & Norat, T. (2015). Obesity and breast cancer: Not only a risk factor of the disease. *Current Treatment Options in Oncology, 16*(5), 1–17.

Chang, Z., Craciunescu, O., Xu, X., Steffey, B., Meltsner, S., Cai, J., et al. (2015). Evaluating radiation-induced changes with diffusion weighted imaging in patients with gynecologic cancers treated with combined external beam radiation radiotherapy and high-dose-rate brachytherapy: Initial results. *Brachytherapy, 14*, S75–S76.

Chatterjee, A., Serniak, N., & Czerniecki, B. J. (2015). Sentinel lymph node biopsy in breast cancer: A work in progress. *The Cancer Journal, 21*(1), 7–10.

Chu, Q. D., Caldito, G., Miller, J. K., & Townsend, B. (2015). Postmastectomy radiation for N2/N3 breast cancer: Factors associated with low compliance rate. *Journal of the American College of Surgeons, 220*(4), 659–669.

Carlson, R. H. (2015). Obesity and breast cancer: Research update. *Oncology Times, 37*(9), 33.

Corradini, S., Niyazi, M., Niemoeller, O. M., Li, M., Roeder, F., Eckel, R., et al. (2015). Adjuvant radiotherapy after breast conserving surgery – A comparative effectiveness research study. *Radiotherapy & Oncology, 114*(1), 28–34.

Cuzick, J., & Thorat, M. (2015). PG 6.02 Preventing invasive breast cancer in women at high risk based on benign/in situ pathology. *The Breast, 24,* S11.

Debled, M., MacGrogan, G., Breton-Callu, C., Ferron, S., Hurtevent, G., Fournier, M., et al. (2015). Surgery following neoadjuvant chemotherapy for HER2-positive locally advanced breast cancer. Time to reconsider the standard attitude. *European Journal of Cancer, 51*(6), 697–704.

Dixon, J. M., & Macaskill, E. J. (2015). Management of benign breast disease. In *Breast disease* (pp. 51–77). New York, NY: Springer Publishers.

Euhus, D. M., & Diaz, J. (2015). Breast cancer prevention. *The Breast Journal, 21*(1), 76–81.

Faguy, K. (2015). Breast disorders in pregnant and lactating women. *Radiologic Technology, 86*(4), 419M–438M.

Fallowfield, L., & Jenkins, V. (2015). Psychosocial/Survivorship issues in breast cancer: are we doing better? *Journal of the National Cancer Institute, 107*(1), 335.

Files, J. A., Allen, S. V., & Pruthi, S. (2015). Management of breast pain. In *Breast disease* (pp. 79–91). New York, NY: Springer Publishers.

Gradishar, W. J. (2015). Adjuvant therapy for breast cancer: Hormonal therapy. In *Breast disease* (pp. 353–362). New York, NY: Springer Publishers.

Guinot, J. L., Baixauli-Perez, C., Soler, P., Tortajada, M. I., Moreno, A., Santos, M. A., et al. (2015). High-dose-rate brachytherapy boost effect on local tumor control in young women with breast cancer. *International Journal of Radiation Oncology Biology Physics, 91*(1), 165–171.

Han, F., Shi, G., Liang, C., Wang, L., & Li, K. (2015). A simple and efficient method for breast cancer diagnosis based on infrared thermal imaging. *Cell Biochemistry and Biophysics, 71*(1), 491–498.

Jager, N. G., Linn, S. C., Schellens, J. H., & Beijnen, J. H. (2015). Tailored tamoxifen treatment for breast cancer patients: a perspective. *Clinical Breast Cancer, 15*(4), 241–244.

Janardhan, J., Venkateshwar, P., & Rao, K.S. (2015). Giant fibroadenoma of the breast: Conservative surgery. *International Archives of Integrated Medicine. 2*(4), 156–160.

Jarvis, C. (2015). *Physical examination & health assessment* (7th ed.), St. Louis, MO: Elsevier Health Sciences.

Kalinsky, K., Mayer, J. A., Xu, X., Pham, T., Wong, K. L., Villarin, E., et al. (2015). Correlation of hormone receptor status between circulating tumor cells, primary tumor, and metastasis in breast cancer patients. *Clinical and Translational Oncology, 17*(7), 539–546.

Khan, M. H., Allerton, R., & Pettit, L. (2015). Hormone therapy for male breast cancer. *Clinical Breast Cancer,* (Online 2/7/15). doi:10.1016/j.clbc.2015.01.007

King, T. L., Brucker, M. C., Kriebs, J. M., Fahey, J. O., Gegor, C. L., & Varney, H. (2015). *Varney's midwifery.* (5th ed.), Berlington, MA: Jones & Bartlett Learning.

Kleban, R., & Glaser, S. (2015). The many dimensions of breast cancer: Determining the scope of needed services. *Handbook of oncology social work: Psychosocial care for people with cancer* (pp. 93–99). New York, NY: Oxford University press.

Lara, P. C., López-Peñalver, J. J., Farias, V. A., Ruiz-Ruiz, M. C., Oliver, F. J., & Ruiz de Almodóvar, J. M. (2015). Direct and bystander radiation effects: A biophysical model and clinical perspectives. *Cancer Letters, 356*(1), 5–16.

Leavy, O. (2015). Immunotherapy: A triple blow for cancer. *Nature Reviews Cancer. 15*(5), 258–259.

Li, J., Holm, J., Bergh, J., Eriksson, M., Darabi, H., Lindström, L. S., et al. (2015). Breast cancer genetic risk profile is differentially associated with interval and screen-detected breast cancers. *Annals of Oncology, 26*(3), 517–522.

Miller, A.C., & Kennedy, C. (2015). Breast abscess and masses. *eMedicine.* Retrieved from http://emedicine.medscape.com/article/781116-overview#a0104

Mills, S. (2013). Performing a clinical breast exam. *Nursing, 43*(9), 68.

Mugea, T. T. (2015). Complications of breast augmentation. In *Aesthetic surgery of the breast* (pp. 425–512). Berlin Heidelberg: Springer.

Muralidhar, K. R., Soubhagya, B., & Ahmed, S. (2015). Intensity modulated radiotherapy versus volumetric modulated arc therapy in breast cancer: A comparative dosimetric analysis. *International Journal of Cancer Therapy and Oncology, 3*(2), 1–6.

National Cancer Institute [NCI]. (2015a). *Breast cancer.* Retrieved from http://www.cancer.gov/cancertopics/types/breast

National Cancer Institute [NCI]. (2015b). Probability of breast cancer in American women. Retrieved from http://www.cancer.gov/cancer-topics/factsheet/detection/probability-breast-cancer

National Comprehensive Cancer Network [NCCN]. (2015). *Breast cancer treatment guidelines: NCCN patient guidelines.* Retrieved from http://www.nccn.org/patients/patient_gls/_english/_breast/5_treatment.asp

Pluchinotta, A. M. (2015). Inflammatory diseases of the breast. In *The Outpatient Breast Clinic* (pp. 169–195). Springer International Publishing.

Poulos, A. (2015). Diagnostic breast imaging: Mammography, sonography, magnetic resonance imaging, and interventional procedures. *Journal of Medical Radiation Sciences, 62*(1), 86–87.

Rifkin, E., & Lazris, A. (2015). Breast cancer screening: Mammograms. In *Interpreting Health Benefits and Risks* (pp. 33–41). Springer International Publishing.

Sabel, M. S. (2015). Overview of benign breast disease. *UpToDate.* Retrieved from http://www.uptodate.com/contents/overview-of-benign-breast-disease

Schuiling, K. D., & Likis, F.E. (2016). *Women's gynecological health* (3rd ed.), Burlington, MA: Jones & Bartlett Learning.

Seetharam, P., & Rodrigues, G. (2015). Benign breast disorders: An insight with a detailed literature review. *Webmed Central Breast, 6*(1).

Sestak, I., & Cuzick, J. (2015). Update on breast cancer risk prediction and prevention. *Current Opinion in Obstetrics and Gynecology, 27*(1), 92–97.

Selvi, R. (2015). Invasive lobular carcinoma. In *Breast diseases* (pp. 281–286). India: Springer Publishers.

Shannon, K. M., & Chittenden, A. (2015). Breast cancer genetics and risk assessment. In *Breast cancer screening and diagnosis* (pp. 1–21). New York, NY: Springer Publishers.

Shrivastava, S. R., Shrivastava, P. S., & Ramasamy, J. (2015). Assessing the contribution of dietary factors in breast cancer. *Clinical Cancer Investigation Journal, 4*(1), 1–5.

Skidmore-Roth, L. (2015)). *Mosby's 2015 nursing drug reference* (28th ed.), St. Louis, MO: Elsevier Health Science.

Slanetz, P. J., Freer, P. E., & Birdwell, R. L. (2015). Breast-density legislation—Practical considerations. *New England Journal of Medicine, 372*(7), 593–595.

Stopeck, A. T., Chalasani, P., & Thompson, P. A. (2015). Breast cancer. *EMedicine.* Retrieved from http://emedicine.medscape.com/article/1947145-overview

Strayer, D. A., & Schub, T. (2014). Breast cancer. *Published by CINAHL Information Systems,* Full Text, EBSCOhost

Swisher, A. K., Abraham, J., Bonner, D., Gilleland, D., Hobbs, G., Kurian, S., et al. (2015). Exercise and dietary advice intervention for survivors of triple-negative breast cancer: effects on body fat, physical function, quality of life, and adipokine profile. *Supportive Care in Cancer, 23*(10), 2995–3003.

Toi, M., Winer, E.P., Benson, J.R., & Klimberg, S. (2015). *Personalized treatment of breast cancer.* Japan: Springer Publishers.

Tsujimoto, M. (2015). Recent advances in sentinel node biopsy in breast surgery. *Breast Cancer, 22*(3), 211.DOI: 10.1007/s12282-015-0601-3

U.S. Department of Health and Human Services. (2015). *Healthy people 2020.* Retrieved from http://www.healthypeople.gov/2020/topicsobjectives2020/default.aspx

U.S. Preventive Services Task Force [USPSTF]. (2015). *Screening for breast cancer.* Retrieved from http://www.uspreventiveservicestask-force.org/breastcancer.htm

van den Broek, A. J., Schmidt, M. K., van 't Veer, L. J., Tollenaar, R. M., & van Leeuwen, F. E. (2015). Worse breast cancer prognosis of BRCA1/BRCA2 mutation carriers: What's the evidence? A systematic review with meta-analysis. *PLoS ONE, 10*(3), 1–29.

Wevers, M. R., Ausems, M. M., Verhoef, S., Bleiker, E. A., Hahn, D. E., Brouwer, T., et al. (2015). Does rapid genetic counseling and testing in newly diagnosed breast cancer patients cause additional psychosocial distress? Results from a randomized clinical trial. *Genetics in Medicine: Official Journal of the American College of Medical Genetics, 18*(2), 137–144.

Wright, C. E., Harvie, M., Howell, A., Evans, D. G., Hulbert-Williams, N., & Donnelly, L. S. (2015). Beliefs about weight and breast cancer: an interview study with high risk women following a 12 month weight loss intervention. *Hereditary Cancer in Clinical Practice, 13* (1), 1.

Writing Group for the Women's Health Initiative Investigators (2002). Women's Health Initiative Study. *JAMA, 288*(3), 321–333.

MULTIPLE-CHOICE QUESTIONS

1. Breast self-examinations involve both touching of breast tissue and:
   a. Palpation of cervical lymph nodes
   b. Firm squeezing of both breast nipples
   c. Visualizing both breasts for any change
   d. A mammogram to evaluate breast tissue

2. Which of the following is the strongest risk factor for breast cancer?
   a. Advancing age and being female
   b. High number of children
   c. Genetic mutations in BRCA1 and BRCA2 genes
   d. Family history of colon cancer

3. A biopsy procedure that traces radioisotopes and blue dye from the tumor site through the lymphatic system into the axillary nodes is:
   a. Stereotactic biopsy
   b. Sentinel node biopsy
   c. Axillary dissection biopsy
   d. Advanced breast biopsy

4. The most serious potential adverse reaction from chemotherapy is:
   a. Thrombocytopenia
   b. Deep vein thrombosis
   c. Alopecia
   d. Myelosuppression

5. What suggestion would be helpful for the client experiencing painful fibrocystic breast changes?
   a. Increase her caffeine intake.
   b. Take a mild analgesic when needed.
   c. Reduce her intake of leafy vegetables.
   d. Wear a bra bigger than she needs.

6. A postoperative mastectomy client should be referred to which of the following organizations for assistance upon discharge from the hospital?
   a. National Organization for Women (NOW)
   b. Food and Drug Administration (FDA)
   c. March of Dimes Foundation (MDF)
   d. Reach to Recovery (RTR)

7. Breast cancer that is localized is referred to as
   a. Primary
   b. In situ
   c. Metastasized
   d. Localized

8. A 25-year-old woman presents with an asymptomatic breast mass. Which of the following is true concerning her diagnosis and treatment?
   a. All breast masses should be considered premalignant

   b. The breast mass should be surgically removed immediately
   c. Ultrasound is typically used to determine the diagnosis
   d. Since it is asymptomatic, just reassurance is needed now

CRITICAL THINKING EXERCISE

1. Mrs. Gordon, 48, presents to the women's community clinic where you work as a nurse. She is very upset and crying. She tells you that she found lumps in her breast: "I know that it's cancer and I will die." When you ask her about her problem, she says she does not check her breasts monthly and hasn't had a mammogram for years because "they're too expensive." She also describes the intermittent pain she experiences.
   a. What specific questions would you ask this client to get a clearer picture?
   b. What education is needed for this client regarding breast health?
   c. What community referrals are needed to meet this client's future needs?

2. Ruth Davis, 51, stops in at the urgent care facility with an anxious look on her face. She tells the nurse practitioner that she has green discharge coming from her right breast and discomfort intermittently. She can't understand how this would happen since she hasn't previously had any nipple discharge or pain.
   a. What benign breast condition might the nurse practitioner suspect based on her description?
   b. What specific information should the nurse practitioner give Mrs. Davis about duct ectasia?
   c. The typical treatment of this benign breast condition would include what?

STUDY ACTIVITIES

1. Discuss with a group of women what their breasts symbolize to them and to society. Do they symbolize something different to each one?

2. When a woman experiences a breast disorder, what feelings might she be experiencing and how can a nurse help her sort them out?

3. Interview a woman who has fibrocystic breast changes and find out how she manages this condition.

4. An infection of the breast connective tissue that frequently occurs in the lactating woman is
   _____.

CHAPTER WORKSHEET

BRINGING IT ALL TOGETHER: CASE STUDY

A 67-year-old obese woman presents to her internist after several years' absence a right breast mass that she felt 4 weeks ago that seems to be getting larger. She also has recently noticed a 10-pound weight loss over the past 6 months and occasional right upper quadrant discomfort. She also states that she has been feeling tired over the last several months, but rationalized it as 'old age' catching up with her.

ASSESSMENT

She has a family history of breast and colon cancer in her immediate family and both of her parents died from these (mother from breast cancer and father from colon cancer). Her aunt also had breast cancer, but is in remission now after treatment. She can't remember when the last time she had a pap smear or mammogram. She admits that she does not keep up with her health check-ups, since she babysits for her grandchildren and has difficulty scheduling them. She confesses that her diet hasn't been what it should be, since her grandchildren prefer fast food and sodas for meals, rather than home cooked ones. Thus, she gives into them and eats what they want.

Go to thePoint **to find questions to consider about this case.**

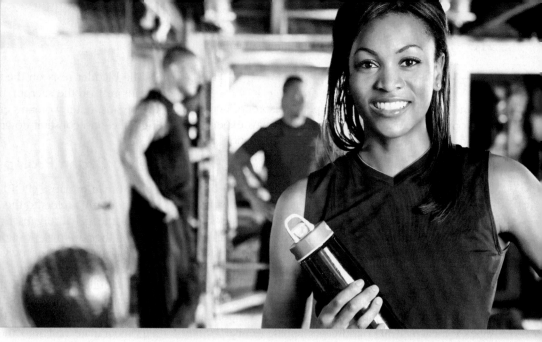

7

Benign Disorders of the Female Reproductive Tract

Learning Objectives

Upon completion of the chapter, you will be able to:

1. Characterize the major pelvic relaxation disorders in terms of etiology, management, and nursing interventions.

2. Outline the nursing management needed for the most common benign reproductive disorders in women.

3. Evaluate urinary incontinence in terms of pathology, clinical manifestations, treatment options, and effect on quality of life.

4. Compare the various benign growths in terms of their symptoms and management.

5. Analyze the emotional impact of polycystic ovarian syndrome and the nurse's role as a counselor, educator, and advocate.

Liz, a 26-year-old, overweight woman, presented to the clinic with hirsutism and facial acne and told the nurse that she was concerned about her irregular menstrual periods. She also said that recently the hair on top of her head seemed to be falling out. What diagnostic tests might the nurse anticipate with this client? How can the nurse prepare Liz for them?

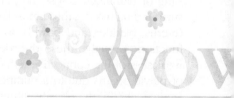

Words of Wisdom
Women can influence their aging process by making wise lifestyle choices early on.

INTRODUCTION

The incidence of several benign pelvic disorders increases as women age. For instance, women may experience pelvic floor disorders related to pelvic relaxation or urinary incontinence. These disorders generally develop after years of wear and tear on the muscles and tissues that support the pelvic floor—such as that which occurs with childbearing, chronic coughing, straining, surgery, or simply aging. In addition to pelvic floor disorders, woman may also experience various benign neoplasms of the reproductive tract, such as cervical polyps, uterine leiomyomas (fibroids), ovarian cysts, genital fistulas, and Bartholin's cysts. This chapter provides an overview of various pelvic floor disorders and benign neoplasms, discussing the assessment, treatment, and prevention strategies for each. It also addresses female genital cutting in the context of it being a harmful practice that affects girls' and women's health.

PELVIC FLOOR DISORDERS

Pelvic floor disorders such as pelvic organ prolapse or genital prolapse and urinary and fecal incontinence are common in aging women. Researchers funded by the National Institutes of Health (NIH, 2015a) reported that more than one-third of women in the United States have a pelvic floor disorder, and nearly one-quarter of women in the United States have one or more pelvic floor disorders that cause symptoms. The study reported that the frequency of pelvic floor disorders increases with age, affecting more than 40% of women from 60 to 79 years of age, and about 50% of women 80 years and older. The NIH analysis is the first to document in a nationally representative sample the extent of pelvic floor disorders, a cluster of health problems that causes physical discomfort and limits activity.

Pelvic floor disorders cause significant physical and psychological morbidity and can diminish women's social interactions, emotional well-being, and overall quality of life. Because these disorders increase with age, the problem will grow worse as our population ages. The term "pelvic floor" refers to the group of muscles that form a sling or hammock across the pelvis. Together with their surrounding tissues, these muscles hold the pelvic organs (uterus, bladder, and bowel), in place so that they can function correctly. These disorders occur as a result of weakness of the connective tissue and muscular support of pelvic organs due to a number of factors: Pregnancy, vaginal childbirth, obesity, lifting, chronic cough from smoking, straining at defecation secondary to constipation, radiation to the pelvis for cancer, and estrogen deficiency (American College of Obstetricians and Gynecologists (ACOG, 2015a). The female anatomy is susceptible to the development of pelvic floor disorders because of its vertical structures placement. The bony pelvis has an exaggerated lumbar spinal curve and downward tilt to it. The bladder rests on the symphysis and the posterior organs rest on the sacrum and coccyx. The pelvis holds the organs, but a woman's erect posture causes a funneling effect and constant downward pressure.

Pelvic Organ Prolapse

Pelvic organ prolapse (POP) (from the Latin *prolapsus*, "a slipping forth") refers to the abnormal descent or herniation of the pelvic organs from their original attachment sites or their normal position in the pelvis. POP occurs when structures of the pelvis shift and protrude into or outside of the vaginal canal. This disorder affects a woman's micturition, defecation, and sexual activity. The Egyptians were the first to describe prolapse of the genital organs. Hippocrates in 400 BC made reference to placing a pomegranate half into the vagina to treat organ prolapse. A disorder exclusive to women, POP rarely results in severe morbidity or mortality but can affect a woman's daily activities and quality of life (Brown, 2015). It is difficult to determine the incidence of POP, because the disorder is often asymptomatic and many women do not seek treatment. It has been estimated, however, that up to 75% of all women who have had a vaginal birth have POP (ACOG, 2015a). Each year, over 250,000 women undergo surgery to repair the prolapse at a cost of over $1 billion for hospitalization and physician fees alone (Maher & Haya, 2015). As the older adult population is expected to double in number by 2030, POP and its associated symptoms will become more prevalent (Mukwege et al., 2015).

Obesity is associated with a high prevalence of pelvic floor disorders. Obesity can also aggravate symptoms of pelvic organ prolapse, fecal incontinence, sexual dysfunction, stress urinary incontinence, and increase the risk of endometrial polyps and symptomatic fibroids. Weight reduction enhances reproductive outcomes, diminishes symptoms of urinary incontinence, improves sexual dysfunction, and reduces morbidity following gynecologic surgery. Sustained and substantial weight loss, however, is difficult to achieve for many women with their current lifestyle and dietary choices (Ramalingam & Monga, 2015).

The treatment and diagnosis of POP is challenging and problematic.

Types of Pelvic Organ Prolapse

The four most common types of pelvic or genital prolapse are cystocele, rectocele, enterocele, and uterine prolapse (Fig. 7.1):

- **Cystocele** occurs when the posterior bladder wall protrudes downward through the anterior vaginal wall.
- **Rectocele** occurs when the rectum sags and pushes against or into the posterior vaginal wall.
- **Enterocele** occurs when the small intestine bulges through the posterior vaginal wall (especially common when straining).

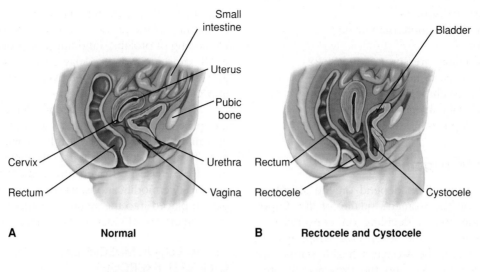

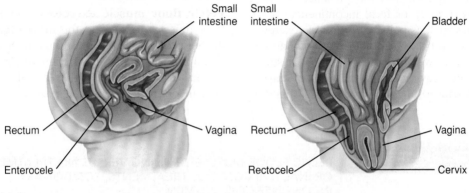

FIGURE 7.1 Types of pelvic prolapses. (**A**) Normal. (**B**) Rectocele and cystocele. (**C**) Enterocele. (**D**) Uterine prolapse.

- **Uterine prolapse** occurs when the uterus descends through the pelvic floor and into the vaginal canal. Multiparous women are at particular risk for uterine prolapse. The extent of uterine prolapse is classified in terms of stages:
  - *Stage 0:* No descent of pelvic structure during straining.
  - *Stage I:* The prolapsed descending organ is >1 cm above the hymenal ring.
  - *Stage II:* The prolapsed organ extends ~1 cm below the hymenal ring.
  - *Stage III:* The prolapsed organ extends 2 to 3 cm below the hymenal ring.
  - *Stage IV:* The vagina is completely everted or the prolapsed organ is >3 cm below the hymenal ring (Riss & Koch, 2015).

Etiology

Anatomic support of the pelvic organs is mainly provided by the levator ani muscle complex and the connective tissue attachments of the pelvic organ fascia. Dysfunction of one or both of these components can lead to loss of support and eventually POP. Weakened pelvic floor muscles also prevent complete closure of the urethra, resulting in urine leakage during physical stress. This problem is not limited to older women: Urinary incontinence has been documented in women of varying ages, including young (<25 years old) women (Walters, 2015).

Many risk factors for POP have been suggested, but the true cause is likely to be multifactorial. Causes might include:

- Constant downward gravity because of erect human posture
- Atrophy of supporting tissues with aging and decline of estrogen levels
- Weakening of pelvic support related to childbirth trauma
- Reproductive surgery, including hysterectomy
- Instrumental childbirth
- Multiparity
- Uncontrolled rapid birth
- Family history of POP
- Young age at first birth

- Connective tissue disorders
- Infant birth weight of more than 4,500 g
- Pelvic radiation
- Increased abdominal pressure secondary to:
  - Lifting of children or heavy objects
  - Straining due to chronic constipation
  - Respiratory problems or chronic coughing
  - Obesity (Rodriguez-Mias et al., 2015).

Therapeutic Management

Treatment options for POP depend on the symptoms and their effect on the woman's quality of life. Important considerations when deciding on nonsurgical or surgical options include the severity of symptoms, the woman's preferences, the woman's health status, age, and suitability for surgery, and the presence of other pelvic conditions (urinary or fecal incontinence). Conservative measures such as pelvic floor muscle exercises (PFME) or Kegel exercises supplemented by lifestyle interventions such as weight loss, avoidance of straining (reducing lifting heavy weights, treatment of chronic cough and constipation) are recommended as first-line management. PFME is aimed to increase the strength and endurance of the pelvic floor supports, prevent or delay worsening of prolapse, and improve prolapse symptoms. PFME can help women delay or avert the need for surgery and pre and postoperatively have been found to improve outcomes after surgery.

When surgery is being considered, the nature of the procedure and the likely outcome must be fully explained and discussed with the woman and her partner. Treatment options for POP include pelvic floor muscle exercises, estrogen replacement therapy, dietary and lifestyle modifications, use of a pessary (a removable device placed into the vagina to support pelvic organs), and surgery (see Evidence-Based Practice 7.1).

PELVIC FLOOR MUSCLE EXERCISES OR KEGEL EXERCISES

Pelvic floor muscle exercises strengthen the pelvic floor muscles to support the inner organs and prevent further prolapse. Pelvic floor muscle exercises are generally accepted as first-line treatment for stress and urge urinary incontinence and they are also widely used for anal incontinence. Over the past 30 years a wealth of

---

EVIDENCE-BASED PRACTICE 7.1	PELVIC FLOOR MUSCLE TRAINING VERSUS NO TREATMENT, OR INACTIVE CONTROL TREATMENTS, FOR URINARY INCONTINENCE IN WOMEN

STUDY

Involuntary leakage of urine (urinary incontinence) affects women of all ages, particularly older women who live in residential care such as nursing homes. Some women leak urine during exercise or when they cough or sneeze (stress urinary incontinence) and this may occur as a result of weakness of the pelvic floor muscles such as damage during childbirth. Other women leak urine before going to the toilet when there is a sudden and compelling need to pass urine (urgency urinary incontinence). This may be caused by involuntary contraction of the bladder muscle. Mixed urinary incontinence is the combination of both stress and urgency urinary incontinence. Pelvic floor muscle training is a supervised physical therapy treatment and it involves muscle-clenching exercises to strengthen the pelvic floor muscles. It is a common treatment used by women to stop urine leakage. Other treatments are also available which can either be used alone or in combination with pelvic floor muscle training (PFMT).

PFMT is a conservative treatment for urinary incontinence in women. This systematic review evaluated the effects of PFMT when compared to no treatment, placebo, or other inactive control treatments for urinary incontinence in women.

This study was done to compare the effects PFMT to no treatment, placebo, or other inactive control treatments in the management of women with urinary incontinence.

Findings

Randomized or quasi-randomized trials were used. Twenty-one trials (1,281 women) met the eligibility criteria for inclusion, comprising women with stress urinary incontinence, urgency urinary incontinence or mixed urinary incontinence, and they compared PFMT added to no treatment, placebo or other inactive control treatments.

This systematic review found support for the widespread recommendation that PFMT should be included in first-line conservative management programs for women with stress and any type of urinary incontinence. In women with stress incontinence, there was high quality evidence that PFMT is associated with improvement or cure.

Nursing Implications

Overall, according to this study, there is sufficient evidence to support the widespread recommendation that PFMT should be included in a first-line conservative management program for women with stress, urge, or mixed urinary incontinence. Previous studies have validated that pelvic floor exercises do help in bringing tone to the muscles that control micturition. Nurses can continue to instruct women with urinary incontinence to perform PFMT daily to improve their urinary control and their quality of life.

Adapted from Dumoulin, C., Hay-Smith, E. J., Mac Habee-Sequin, G. M., & Mercier, J. (2015). Pelvic floor muscle training verses no treatment, or inactive control treatments, for urinary incontinence in women. *Neurourology & Urodynamics, 34*(4), 300–308.

research has proven the benefits of pelvic floor muscle exercises in treating both urinary incontinence and pelvic organ prolapse (McClurg, Gerrard, & Hove, 2015). The purpose of pelvic floor exercises is to increase the muscle volume, which will result in a stronger muscular contraction. Pelvic floor muscle exercises might limit the progression of mild prolapse and alleviate mild prolapse symptoms, including low back pain and pelvic pressure. They will not, however, help severe uterine prolapse.

HORMONE REPLACEMENT THERAPY

Hormone replacement therapy, or HRT (orally, transdermally, low-dose vaginal ring or vaginal cream) may improve the tone, natural thickness, and vascularity of the supporting tissue in perimenopausal and menopausal women by increasing blood perfusion and the elasticity of the vaginal wall. HRT has many benefits, as well as risks. It is essential that the benefits are weighed out against the risks before this therapy is initiated.

Take Note!

Before hormone therapy is considered, a thorough medical history must be taken to assess a woman's risk for complications (e.g., endometrial cancer, myocardial infarction, stroke, breast cancer, pulmonary emboli, and deep vein thrombosis). Because of these risks, estrogens, with or without progestins, should be given at the lowest effective dose and for the shortest duration consistent with the treatment goals and risks for the individual woman (ACOG, 2015a).

DIETARY AND LIFESTYLE MODIFICATIONS

Dietary and lifestyle modifications may help prevent pelvic relaxation and chronic problems later in life. Specific lifestyle changes would include avoiding constipation, bladder irritants, heavy lifting, high impact exercise, weight loss, and smoking cessation. Dietary habits can exacerbate the prolapse by causing constipation and consequently chronic straining. The stools of a constipated woman are hard and dry, and typically she must strain while bearing down to defecate. This straining to pass a hard stool increases intra-abdominal pressure, which over time causes the pelvic organs to prolapse. Dietary modifications can help to establish regular bowel movements without discomfort and eliminate flatus and bloating. A weight loss regimen might also need to be instituted if the woman is overweight.

PESSARIES

Vaginal **pessaries** are synthetic devices inserted in the vagina to provide support to the bladder and other pelvic organs as a corrective measure for urinary incontinence and/or pelvic organ prolapse (Fig. 7.2). Today almost all pessaries are made of medical-grade silicone, which provides many advantages. Silicone pessaries are

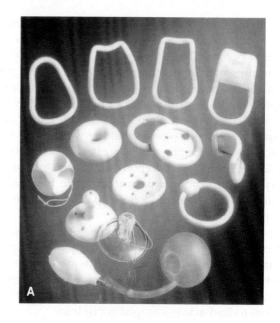

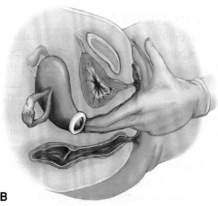

FIGURE 7.2 Examples of pessaries. **A.** Various shapes and sizes of pessaries available. **B.** Insertion of one type of pessary. A link to a web site for a picture of Colpexin Sphere is located on.

pliable and have a long shelf life; lack odor and secretion absorption; are biologically inert, nonallergenic, and noncarcinogenic; and they can be boiled or autoclaved for sterilization. Because most pessaries are made of silicone, pessary style and size are the main considerations when selecting a pessary (Colyar, 2015). Although many types and shapes are available, the most commonly used pessary is a firm ring that presses against the wall of the vagina and urethra to help decrease leakage and support a prolapsed vagina or uterus. Pessaries are a low risk treatment option with the advantage of being cost effective and minimally invasive, and provide immediate relief of symptoms.

Indications for pessary use include uterine prolapse or cystocele, especially among elderly clients for whom surgery is contraindicated; younger women with prolapse who plan to have additional children; and women with marked prolapse who prefer to use a pessary rather than undergo surgery (Ralph & Tamussino, 2015). Many women use pessaries for only a short period of time and become free of symptoms. Long-term use can lead to pressure necrosis and the development of fistulas in some women; in this situation other methods of support should be explored. Pessaries are fitted by trial and error; the woman often needs to try several sizes or styles. The largest pessary that the woman can wear comfortably is generally the most effective. The woman should be instructed to report any discomfort or difficulty with urination or defecation while wearing the pessary and also to attend follow-up care appointments to check positioning.

Nurses need to be aware of the personal isolation and embarrassment and social and cultural implications that urinary incontinence may cause as well as the subjective experiences of using a pessary. With appropriate support, vaginal pessaries can provide women with the freedom to lead active, engaged social lives.

SURGICAL INTERVENTIONS

Surgical interventions for pelvic or genital organ prolapse are designed to correct specific defects, with the goals being to restore normal anatomy and to preserve function. Approximately 260,000 stress incontinence surgical procedures are performed annually in the United States (Kirby, Tan-Kim, & Nager, 2015). Surgery is not an option for all women. Women who are at high risk of suffering recurrent prolapse after a surgical repair or who have morbid obesity, chronic obstructive pulmonary disease, or medical conditions in which general anesthesia would be risky are not good candidates for surgical repair (Alexander et al., 2015), and noninvasive treatment strategies should be discussed with them.

Surgical interventions might include anterior or posterior colporrhaphy (to repair a cystocele or rectocele) and vaginal hysterectomy (for uterine prolapse). This can be done laparoscopically whereby the uterus is removed through the vagina. An anterior and posterior colporrhaphy may be effective for a first-degree prolapse. This surgical procedure tightens the anterior and posterior vaginal wall, thus repairing a cystocele or rectocele. The pubocervical fascia (supportive tissue between the vagina and bladder) is folded and sutured to bring the bladder and urethra in proper position (Nilsson, 2015).

A vaginal hysterectomy is the treatment of choice for uterine prolapse because it removes the prolapsed organ that is bringing down the bladder and rectum with it. It can be combined with an anterior and posterior repair if a cystocele or rectocele is present.

Nursing Assessment

Nursing assessment for women with POP includes a thorough health history, a physical examination, and several laboratory and diagnostic tests.

HEALTH HISTORY AND CLINICAL MANIFESTATIONS

A history and general assessment of the client is important to exclude pathology and evaluate various factors that may influence choice and success of management. Evaluation of systems such as bowel, urinary and sexual function, coexistent morbidities, medical and surgical history, any physical or mental impairment, and lifestyle are noticeably very important, particularly in older women. The client's social circumstances and support systems, desire for treatment, and expectations will have implications on the management options.

The cause of prolapse is multifactorial, with vaginal childbirth, advancing age, heavy work, poor nutrition, vaginal surgery, and increasing body mass index being the most consistent risk factors (Rodriguez-Mias et al., 2015). Assessment of risk factors (chronic straining, hysterectomy, normal aging, and abnormalities of connective tissue) in the woman's history will assist the health care provider in the diagnosis and treatment of POP. The history should include questions about:

- The woman's obstetrical history (number of pregnancies, weight of newborns, pregnancy spacing)
- Chronic respiratory condition (chronic coughing)
- Menopausal status
- Weight history (loss or gain)
- Constipation (frequency and chronicity)
- Age
- Work history (e.g., physical labor or light office work)
- Nutritional assessment
- Family history (family member with POP)
- Urinary incontinence
- Previous pelvic surgeries

Assess for clinical manifestations of POP. POP is often asymptomatic, but when symptoms do occur, they are often related to the site and type of prolapse. Symptoms common to all types of prolapses are a feeling of dragging, a lump in the vagina, or something "coming down." Women with POP can present either with one symptom, such as vaginal bulging or pelvic pressure, or with several complaints, including many bladder, bowel, and pelvic symptoms. Symptoms associated with POP are summarized in Box 7.1.

Women present with varying degrees of uterine descent. Uterine prolapse is the most troubling type of pelvic relaxation because it is often associated with concomitant defects of the vagina in the anterior, posterior, and lateral compartments (Lazarou & Grigorescu, 2015).

PHYSICAL EXAMINATION

The pelvic examination performed by the health care provider includes an external genital inspection to visualize any obvious protrusion of the uterus, bladder, urethra, or vaginal wall occurring at the vaginal opening. Usually the woman is asked to perform the Valsalva maneuver (bearing

SYMPTOMS ASSOCIATED WITH PELVIC ORGAN PROLAPSE

- Urinary symptoms
- Stress incontinence
- Frequency (diurnal and nocturnal)
- Urgency and urge incontinence
- Hesitancy
- Poor or prolonged stream
- Feeling of incomplete emptying
- Bowel symptoms
- Difficulty with defecation
- Incontinence of flatus or liquid or solid stool
- Urgency of defecation
- Feeling of incomplete evacuation
- Rectal protrusion or prolapse after defecation
- Sexual symptoms
- Inability to have frequent intercourse
- Dyspareunia
- Lack of satisfaction or orgasm
- Incontinence during sexual activity
- Other local symptoms
- Pressure or heaviness in the vagina
- Pain in the vagina or perineum
- Low back pain after long periods of standing
- Palpable bulge in the vaginal vault
- Difficulty in walking due to a protrusion from the vagina
- Difficulty inserting or keeping a tampon in place
- Vaginal–cervical mucosa hypertrophy, excoriation, ulceration, and bleeding
- Abdominal pressure or pain

Adapted from American College of Obstetricians and Gynecologists [ACOG]. (2015a) Pelvic support problems. *ACOG Educational Pamphlet.* Retrieved from http://www.acog.org/~/media/For%20Patients/faq012.pdf?dmc=1&ts=20140128T1159591406; and Lazarou, G., & Grigorescu, B. A. (2015). Pelvic organ prolapse. *eMedicine.* Retrieved from http://emedicine.medscape.com/article/276259-overview

down) while the examiner notes which organ prolapses first and the degree to which it occurs. Any urine leakage during the examination is important to note. The woman is asked to contract the pubococcygeal muscles (pelvic floor muscle exercise); the health care provider inserts two fingers into the vagina to assess the strength and symmetry of the contraction. Because pelvic or genital organ prolapse can cause urinary symptoms such as incontinence, bladder function should be assessed by determining postvoid residual with a catheter. If the woman has more than 100 mL of retained urine, she should be referred for further urodynamic evaluation and testing.

LABORATORY AND DIAGNOSTIC TESTS

Common laboratory tests that may be ordered to determine the cause of POP include a urinalysis to rule out a bacterial infection, urine culture to identify the specific organism if present, visualization of urine loss during the pelvic examination, and measurement of postvoid urine volume.

Nursing Management

Help the woman understand the nature of the condition, the treatment options, and the likely outcomes. Nursing considerations might include the following:

- Describe normal anatomy and causes of pelvic prolapse.
- Assess how this condition has affected the woman's life.
- Outline the options, with the advantages and disadvantages of each.
- Allow the client to make the decision that is right for her.
- Provide education.
- Schedule preoperative activities needed for surgery.
- Reassure the client that there is a solution for her symptoms.
- Provide community education about genital prolapse.

Nursing Care Plan 7.1 provides an overview of care for a woman with POP.

PROMOTE PREVENTION STRATEGIES

Limited data are available on ways to prevent POP, but a nurse needs first to understand its incidence, risk factors, prevalence, clinical implications, and treatment options to be an effective caretaker of the woman. The nurse's understanding will not only improve his or her ability to treat this growing client population, but will also help in developing preventive strategies to address a woman's suffering from this condition.

Approaches include lifestyle changes that reduce modifiable risk factors, such as losing weight, avoiding heavy lifting, and relieving constipation. Explore with the woman what factors in her lifestyle might be modified to reduce her risk of developing POP (primary prevention) or to improve her quality of life after receiving treatment (secondary prevention).

ENCOURAGE PELVIC FLOOR MUSCLE TRAINING

Encourage the woman to perform pelvic floor muscle exercises daily (Teaching Guidelines 7.1). Discuss current research findings and educate the woman about estrogen therapy, allowing the woman to make her own decision on whether to use hormones. Controversy still exists regarding the benefits versus the risks of taking hormones, so the woman must weigh this option carefully (ACOG, 2015a).

Teaching Guidelines 7.1
PERFORMING PELVIC FLOOR EXERCISES

- Squeeze the muscles in your rectum as if you are trying to prevent passing flatus.
- Stop and start urinary flow to help identify the pubococcygeus muscle.

Overview of a Woman with Pelvic Organ Prolapse

Katherine, a 62-year-old multiparous woman, came to her gynecologist with complaints of a chronic dragging or heavy painful feeling in her pelvis, lower backache, constipation, and urine leakage. Her symptoms increase when she stands for long periods. She has not had menstrual cycles for at least a decade. She tells you, "I'm not taking any of those menopausal hormones." She also states that she is very self-conscious and embarrassed about her urine leakage and restricts her outside activities.

NURSING DIAGNOSIS: Body image changes related to relaxation of pelvic support and elimination difficulties.

Outcome Identification and Evaluation

The client will report an improved body image after management of pelvic organ prolapse and improved urinary control.

Interventions: *Providing Pain Management*

- Obtain a thorough history, including ongoing embarrassing experiences, methods of urine control used, what worked, what didn't, any changes in sexual practices related to this, and the effect of this condition on her activities of daily living *to provide a baseline and enable a systematic approach to address it.*
- Assess the frequency, severity, precipitating factors, and aggravating/alleviating factors *to identify characteristics of the client's abnormal urinary patterns to plan appropriate interventions.*
- Educate client about any medications prescribed (correct dosage, route, side effects, and

precautions) *to increase the client's understanding of the therapy and promote compliance.*
- Assess problematic elimination patterns *to identify underlying factors from which to plan appropriate prevention strategies.*
- Encourage client to increase fluids and fiber in diet and increase physical activity daily *to promote peristalsis.*
- Assist client with establishing regular toileting patterns by setting aside time daily for bowel elimination *to promote regular bowel function and evacuation.*
- Urge client to avoid the routine use of laxatives *to reduce risk of compounding constipation.*

NURSING DIAGNOSIS: Deficient knowledge related to causes of structural disorders and treatment options.

Outcome Identification and Evaluation

The client will demonstrate an understanding of current condition and treatments as evidenced by identifying treatment options, making health-promoting lifestyle choices, verbalizing appropriate health care practices, and adhering to treatment plan.

Interventions: *Providing Client Education*

- Assess client's understanding of pelvic organ prolapse and its treatment options *to provide a baseline for teaching.*
- Review information provided about surgical procedures and recommendations for healthy lifestyle, obtaining feedback frequently, *to validate client's understanding of instructions.*
- Discuss association between uterine, bladder, and rectal prolapse and symptoms *to help client understand the etiology of her symptoms and pain.*
- Have client verbalize and discuss information related to diagnosis, surgical procedure, preoperative routine, and postoperative regimen *to ensure adequate understanding and provide time for correcting or clarifying any misinformation or misconceptions.*

NURSING CARE PLAN 7.1

Overview of a Woman with Pelvic Organ Prolapse (continued)

- Provide written material with pictures *to promote learning and help client visualize what has occurred to her body secondary to aging, weight gain, childbirth, and gravity.*
- Discuss pros and cons of hormone replacement therapy, osteoporosis prevention, and cardiovascular events common in postmenopausal women *to promote informed decision making by the client about available menopausal therapies.*
- Inform client about the availability of community resources and make appropriate referrals as needed *to provide additional education and support.*
- Document details of teaching and learning *to allow for continuity of care and further education, if needed.*

- Tighten the pubococcygeus muscle for a count of three, and then relax it.
- Contract and relax the pubococcygeus muscle rapidly 10 times.
- Try to bring up the entire pelvic floor and bear down 10 times.
- Repeat pelvic floor muscle exercises at least five times daily.

ENCOURAGE DIETARY AND LIFESTYLE MODIFICATIONS

Instruct clients to increase dietary fiber and fluids to prevent constipation. A high-fiber diet with an increase in fluid intake alleviates constipation by increasing stool bulk and stimulating peristalsis. It is accomplished by replacing refined, low-fiber foods with high-fiber foods. The recommended daily intake of fiber for women is 25 g (Meyer, 2015). In addition to increasing the amount of fiber in her diet, also encourage the woman to drink eight 8-oz glasses of fluid daily and to engage in regular low-impact aerobic exercise, which promotes muscle tone and stimulates peristalsis.

Educate the client about other lifestyle changes that will assist with prolapse, such as:

- Achieve ideal weight to reduce intra-abdominal pressure and strain on pelvic organs, including pressure on the bladder.
- Wear a girdle or abdominal support to support the muscles surrounding the pelvic organs.
- Avoid lifting heavy objects to reduce the risk of increasing intra-abdominal pressure, which can push the pelvic organs downward.
- Avoid high-impact aerobics, jogging, or jumping repeatedly to minimize the risk of increasing intra-abdominal pressure, which places downward pressure on the organs.
- Give up smoking to minimize the risk for a chronic "smoker's cough," which increases intra-abdominal pressure and forces the pelvic organs downward.

PROVIDE TEACHING FOR PESSARY USE

Educate the woman about pessary use. Discuss complications as part of the instruction. Although the pessary is a safe device, it is still a foreign body in the vagina. Because of this, the most common side effects of the pessary are increased vaginal discharge, urinary tract infections, vaginitis, and odor. Odors can be reduced by douching with dilute vinegar or hydrogen peroxide. Postmenopausal women with thin vaginal mucosa are susceptible to vaginal ulceration with the use of a pessary. Advise the woman to use estrogen cream to make the vaginal mucosa more resistant to erosion and to strengthen the vaginal walls.

The woman must be capable of managing use of the pessary, either alone or with the help of a caretaker. The most common recommendations for pessary care include removing the pessary twice weekly and cleaning it with soap and water; using a lubricant for insertion; and having regular follow-up examinations every 6 to 12 months after an initial period of adjustment.

Besides cleaning, clients must properly reinsert the device into their vaginal cavity, and the woman must also be willing to participate in all aspects of care of the pessary for this treatment option to be successful. All women choosing this option must be instructed in the care of her pessary so that she feels comfortable with all aspects of it before leaving the health care facility. Health care visits should allow adequate time for women to share their concerns, anxieties, and fears surrounding the transition to life with a pessary.

PROVIDE PERIOPERATIVE CARE

Prepare the woman for surgery by reinforcing the risks and benefits of surgery and describing the postoperative course. Explain that a Foley catheter will be in place for up to one week, and that she might not be able to urinate due to the swelling after the catheter has been removed. Provide home care instructions for the Foley catheter. She should cleanse the perineal area daily with mild soap and water, especially around where the catheter enters the urinary meatus. If the woman is provided with a leg bag to be worn during waking hours, instruct her to empty it frequently and keep it below the level of the bladder to prevent backflow. The same principles are applied to the primary Foley bag when emptying it.

During the recovery period, instruct the client to avoid for several weeks activities that cause an increase in abdominal pressure, such as straining, sneezing, and coughing. In addition, advise her to avoid lifting anything heavy or straining to push anything. Explain to the woman that stool softeners and gentle laxatives might be prescribed to prevent constipation and straining with bowel movements. Avoiding vaginal intercourse will be recommended until the operative area is healed in six weeks.

Urinary Incontinence

Urinary incontinence (UI) is defined by the International Continence Society (2015) as the involuntary loss of urine that represents a hygienic or social problem to the individual. This disorder affects over 15 million women in the United States (Walters, 2015), but is underreported. It has been estimated that 50% of all women experience UT at some time in their life, varying in severity from mild to severe (Files, Mayer, & Chutka, 2015). The psychosocial costs and morbidities are even more difficult to quantify. Embarrassment and depression are common. The affected individual may experience a decrease in social interactions, excursions out of the home, and sexual activity (Su, Sun, & Jiann, 2015). It is more common than diabetes and Alzheimer's disease, both of which receive a great deal of press attention. Despite the considerable impact of incontinence on quality of life, many women are unlikely to bring up the subject of their lack of bladder control and very few women seek help or treatment for incontinence concerns. The following are several possible explanations for why clients do not talk about their bladder control issues. The client may:

- Feel that UI is inevitable and not amenable to treatment.
- Feel that UI is a "normal" part of aging.
- Believe that UI is part of being "female." Women tend to accept urinary symptoms such as UI more so than men.
- Feel embarrassment and try to deny that it is a real problem.
- Think that the only treatment option is surgical.
- The client may consider a UI a hygiene problem and not a medical condition.

Take Note!

Incontinence is preventable, treatable, and often curable. However, many women believe that loss of bladder function is a normal and expected part of aging.

Incontinence can have far-reaching effects. Some women experience anxiety, depression, social isolation, embarrassment, insomnia, fear, feelings of uncleanliness, worry, vulnerability, shame, limit her ability to travel far from home or have social engagements and disruptions in their self-esteem and dignity. UI can cause the woman to stop working, traveling, socializing, and enjoying sexual relationships. In addition, incontinence can create a tremendous burden for caretakers and is a common reason for admission to a long-term care facility. Depression and high levels of stress are typical in these women (Kwak, Kwon, & Kim, 2015).

Women often try to cope with UI through lifestyle modifications such as wearing protective pads, avoiding certain activities, emptying the bladder frequently, and modifying diet/fluid intake. Women who experience UI are generally most distressed by the social implications and many go to great efforts to hide their symptoms. In some cultures, UI is abhorred to the point where women are shunned by their communities. A sense of control, normality, and self-esteem are central issues in living with UI. Generally with time and a worsening of symptoms, women pursue medical evaluation and treatment (Waetjen et al., 2015).

The types of urinary incontinence are defined based on their presenting symptoms and signs. The three most common types of incontinence are urgency urinary incontinence (overactive bladder caused by detrusor muscle contractions), stress incontinence (inadequate urinary sphincter function), and mixed incontinence (involves both stress and urge incontinence) (King et al., 2015). Comparison Chart 7.1 details these types of UI.

Pathophysiology and Etiology

Urinary continence requires several factors, including effective functioning of the bladder, adequate pelvic floor muscles, neural control from the brain, and integrity of the neural connections that facilitate voluntary control. The bladder neck and proximal urethra function as a sphincter. During urination the sphincter relaxes and the bladder empties. The ability to control urination requires the integrated function of numerous components of the lower urinary tract, which must be structurally sound and functioning normally.

Incontinence can develop if the bladder muscles become overactive due to weakened sphincter muscles, if the bladder muscles become too weak to contract properly, or if signals from the nervous system to the urinary structures are interrupted. A major factor in women that contributes to urinary continence is the estrogen level, because this hormone helps maintain bladder sphincter tone. In perimenopausal or menopausal women, incontinence can be a problem as estrogen levels begin to decline and genitourinary changes occur. In simple terms, the bladder is the reservoir, the urethra

COMPARISON CHART 7.1	URGE INCONTINENCE VS. STRESS INCONTINENCE	
	Urge Incontinence	**Stress Incontinence**
Description	Precipitous loss of urine, preceded by a strong urge to void, with increased bladder pressure and detrusor contraction	Accidental leakage of urine that occurs with increased pressure on the bladder from coughing, sneezing, laughing, or physical exertion
Etiology	Causes might be neurologic, idiopathic, or infectious	Develops commonly in women in their 40s and 50s, usually as the result of weakened muscles and ligaments in the pelvis following childbirth
Signs and Symptoms	Urgency, frequency, nocturia, and a large amount of urine loss	Involuntary loss of a small amount of urine in response to physical activity that raises intra-abdominal pressure

is the seal, and the levator ani muscle is the gate that holds pressure against the outflow of urine by supporting the urethra and bladder from below. When any of these three structures is not functioning normally, incontinence occurs.

Contributing factors in urinary incontinence include:

* Fluid intake, especially alcohol, carbonated drinks, and caffeinated beverages
* Constipation: alters the position of the pelvic organs and puts pressure on the bladder
* Habitual "preventive" emptying: may result in training the bladder to hold only small amounts of urine
* Menopause and depletion of estrogen
* Chronic disease such as stroke, multiple sclerosis or diabetes
* Smoking: nicotine increases detrusor muscle contractions
* Advancing age: age-related anatomic changes provide less pelvic support
* Pregnancy and childbirth: damage to pelvic structures during childbirth
* Obesity: increases abdominal pressure (Schuiling & Likis, 2016).

Therapeutic Management

Treatment options depend on the type of UI. In general, the least invasive procedure with the fewest risks is the first choice for treatment. Surgery is used only if other methods have failed. There is a widespread belief that UI is an inevitable problem of getting older and that little or nothing can be done to relieve symptoms or reverse it. Nothing is further from the truth, and attitudes must change so that women will feel comfortable seeking help for this embarrassing condition.

For many women with urge incontinence, simple reassurance and lifestyle interventions might help. The promotion of a healthy weight can help to reduce incontinence related to obesity. However, if more than simple lifestyle measures are needed, effective treatments might include:

* Bladder training to establish normal voiding intervals (every 3 to 5 hours)
* Pelvic floor muscle exercises to strengthen the pelvic floor musculature
* Pessary ring to support pelvic structures that have weakened
* Pharmacotherapy to reduce the urge to void. Anticholinergic agents such as oxybutynin (Ditropan) or tolterodine (Detrol) or oxybutynin (Oxytrol) might be prescribed. The most common side effects of anticholinergic agents are dry mouth, blurred vision, constipation, nausea, dizziness, and headaches (King et al., 2015).

For women with stress incontinence, treatment is not always a cure, but it can minimize the impact of this condition on the woman's quality of life. Some treatment options for stress incontinence might include:

* Weight loss if needed
* Avoidance of constipation
* Smoking cessation
* Pelvic floor muscle exercises to strengthen the pelvic floor
* Pessaries
* Weighted vaginal cones to improve the tone of pelvic floor muscles
* Periurethral injection (injecting a bulking agent [collagen] to form a bulge that brings the urethral walls closer together to achieve a better closure)
* Medications such as duloxetine (Cymbalta, Yentreve) to increase urethral sphincter contractions during the storage phase of the urination cycle
* Estrogen replacement therapy to improve bladder sphincter tone
* Surgery to correct genital prolapse and improve urethral and bladder tone.

Consider This

Life can be complicated and embarrassing at times when we least expect it. I met a man in church who seemed interested in me, and he asked me out for coffee after Sunday services. I have been alone for 10 years and this prospect seemed exciting to me. We talked for hours over coffee and seemed to have a great deal in common, especially since both of us had lost our spouses to cancer. He asked me to go square dancing with him, since that was an activity we both had enjoyed in the past with our spouses. I hadn't been out or physically active for ages and didn't realize how my body had changed with age.

It was during the first dance that I noticed a wet sensation between my legs, which I was unable to control. I managed to continue on and pretend that all was fine, but then realized what many of my friends were talking about—stress incontinence. Not being able to control one's urine is very embarrassing and it complicates your life, but I made up my mind that it wasn't going to control me!

Thoughts: *Gravity and childbirth take a toll on women's reproductive organs by pushing them downward. This woman is not going to let stress incontinence curtail her outside activity, which demonstrates a good attitude. What can be done about her embarrassing accidents? Were there any preventive strategies she could have used at an earlier age?*

Nursing Assessment

The assessment of the woman experiencing UI includes a history, physical examination, laboratory tests, and possibly urodynamic testing. The onset, frequency, severity, and pattern of incontinence should be determined, as well as any associated symptoms such as frequency, dysuria, urgency, and nocturia. Incontinence may be quantified by asking the woman if she wears a pad and how often the pad is changed. A review of the woman's current medications, including over-the-counter medications, should be included in the history.

A complete physical examination should be carried out by the health care provider; it should include a neurologic assessment and pelvic and rectal examinations. The presence of associated POP should be noted because it can contribute to the woman's voiding problems and may have an impact on diagnosis and treatment. A rectal examination is done to evaluate sphincter tone and perineal sensation. A "cough stress test' can be performed by asking the woman to cough with a full bladder and subsequently observing for leakage of urine from the urethra can also help in assessing the client's ability to control voiding.

A urinalysis is performed to look for hematuria, pyuria, glucosuria, or proteinuria. A urine culture is done if there is pyuria or bacteriuria. Postvoid residual should be measured either with pelvic ultrasound or directly with a catheter. If the residual exceeds the limit set, urodynamic testing is then used to diagnose the incontinence.

Nursing Management

Incontinence can be devastating and can cause psychosocial concerns and isolation. Nurses can encourage women with troublesome symptoms to seek help. Discuss the treatment options with the client, including benefits and potential outcomes, and encourage her to select the continence treatment best for her lifestyle. Provide education about good bladder habits and strategies to reduce the incidence or severity of incontinence (Teaching Guidelines 7.2). Provide support and encouragement to ensure adherence to the guidelines. Remember that aging can increase the risk of incontinence, but incontinence is not an inevitable part of aging. Review the anatomy and physiology of the urinary system and offer simple explanations to help the woman cope with urinary alterations. Therapeutic listening is important. Be aware of the courage it takes for a woman to disclose an embarrassing condition.

Teaching Guidelines 7.2
MANAGING URINARY INCONTINENCE

- Avoid drinking too much fluid (i.e., 1.5 L total daily limit), but do not decrease your intake of fluids.
- Reduce intake of fluids and foods that are bladder irritants and precipitate urgency, such as chocolate, caffeine, sodas, alcohol, artificial sweetener, hot spicy foods, orange juice, tomatoes, and watermelon.
- Increase fiber and fluids in your diet to reduce constipation.
- Control blood glucose levels to prevent polyuria.
- Treat chronic cough.
- Remove any barriers that delay you from reaching the toilet.
- Practice good perineal hygiene by using mild soap and water. Wipe from front to back to prevent urinary tract infections.
- Become aware of adverse drug effects.
- Take your medications as prescribed.
- Continue to do pelvic floor muscle exercises.

Adapted from Files, J. A., Mayer, A. P., & Chutka, D. S. (2015). Urinary incontinence: Not just a mid-laugh crisis. *Journal of Women's Health*, *24*(1), 107–108; McClurg, D., Gerrard, J., & Hove, R. T. (2015). Reducing the incidence of incontinence. *British Journal of Midwifery*, *23*(1), 17–20; and Vasavada, S. P., Carmel, M. E., & Rackley, R. (2015). Urinary incontinence. *eMedicine*. Retrieved from http://emedicine.medscape.com/article/452289-overview

Take Note!

Simple diet and lifestyle alterations, combined with a proper pelvic floor muscle strengthening program, can often produce significant improvements for women of all ages.

BENIGN GROWTHS

The most common benign growths of the reproductive tract include cervical, endocervical, and endometrial polyps; uterine fibroids (leiomyomas); genital fistulas; Bartholin's cysts; and ovarian cysts.

Polyps

Polyps are small, usually benign growths. The incidence of malignancy in cervical polyps is 1 in 1,000. Malignancy is more common in perimenopausal or postmenopausal women (Nelson, Papa, & Ritchie, 2015). The cause of polyp growth is not well understood, but they are frequently the result of infection. Polyps might be associated with chronic inflammation, an abnormal local response to increased levels of estrogen, or local congestion of the cervical vasculature (Stewart, 2016). Single or multiple polyps might occur. They are most common in multiparous women. Polyps can appear anywhere but are most common on the cervix and in the uterus (Fig. 7.3).

Cervical polyps often appear after menarche. They occur in 2% to 5% of women, and approximately 2% of these polyps have cancerous changes (Schuiling & Likis, 2016). Endocervical polyps are commonly found in multiparous women ages 40 to 60. Endocervical polyps are more common than cervical polyps, with a stalk of varied width and length. Endometrial polyps are benign tumors or localized overgrowths of the endometrium. Most endometrial polyps are solitary, and they rarely occur in women younger than 20 years of age. The incidence of these polyps rises steadily with increasing age, peaks in the fifth decade of life, and gradually declines after menopause. They are present in up to 25% of women being seen for abnormal bleeding (Lieng, 2015).

Therapeutic Management

Treatment of polyps usually consists of simple removal with small forceps done on an outpatient basis, removal during hysteroscopy, or dilation and curettage. The polyp base can be removed by laser vaporization. Because many polyps are infected, an antibiotic may be ordered after removal as a preventive measure or to treat early signs of infection.

Although polyps are rarely cancerous, a specimen should be sent after surgery to a pathology laboratory to exclude malignancy. A cervical biopsy typically reveals mildly atypical cells and signs of infection. Polyps rarely return after they are removed. Regularly scheduled Pap smears are suggested for women with cervical polyps to detect any future abnormal growths that may be malignant.

Nursing Assessment

Nursing assessment for a woman with polyps includes assisting with the physical examination and preparing the collected specimen to be sent to the cytologist.

CLINICAL MANIFESTATIONS

Assess for clinical manifestations of polyps. Most endocervical polyps are cherry red, whereas most cervical polyps are grayish-white (Heller, 2015). Cervical and endocervical polyps are often asymptomatic, but they can produce mild symptoms such as abnormal vaginal bleeding (after intercourse or douching, between menses) or discharge. The most common clinical manifestation of endometrial polyps is metrorrhagia (irregular, acyclic uterine bleeding).

PHYSICAL EXAMINATION AND LABORATORY AND DIAGNOSTIC STUDIES

Typically, cervical polyps are diagnosed when the cervix is visualized through a speculum during the woman's annual gynecologic examination (Nelson, Papa, & Ritchie, 2015). Endometrial polyps are not detected on physical examination, but rather with ultrasound or hysteroscopy (introduction of a small camera through the cervix to visualize the uterine cavity).

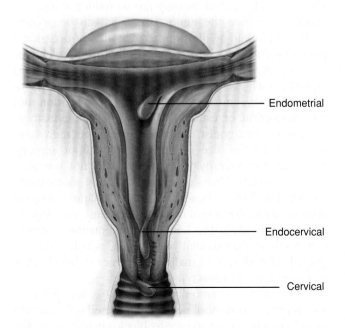

Endometrial

Endocervical

Cervical

FIGURE 7.3 Cervical, endocervical, and endometrial polyps.

Nursing Management

Nursing management of polyps involves explaining the condition and the rationale for removal and giving follow-up care instructions. The nurse also assists the health care provider with the removal procedure.

Uterine Fibroids

Uterine fibroids, also known as myomas or leiomyomas, are benign tumors composed of smooth muscle and fibrous connective tissue in the uterus. Unlike cancerous tumors, fibroids usually grow slower responding to present estrogen levels and their cells do not break away and invade other parts of the body. Fibroids are classified according to their position in the uterus and on the uterine layer most involved (Fig. 7.4):

- *Subserosol fibroids:* lie underneath the outermost peritoneal layer of the uterus and grow outside the uterus. They are attached to the uterus by a stalk or peduncle.
- *Intramural fibroids:* grow within the wall of the uterus and are the most common type
- *Submucosal fibroids:* grow from immediately below the inner uterine surface (endometrium) into the uterine cavity (King et al., 2015).

Fibroids are estrogen-dependent and thus grow rapidly during the childbearing years, when estrogen

is plentiful, but they shrink during menopause, when estrogen levels decline. It is believed that these benign tumors develop in up to 70% of all women over 30 years of age, but up to 50% are asymptomatic (Stewart, 2015). It is difficult to be precise because fibroids may cause no symptoms, and thus many women do not know they have them.

Fibroids are the most common indication for hysterectomy in the United States. The peak incidence occurs around age 45, and they are three times more prevalent in African American women than White women (Stewart, 2015).

Etiology

Although the cause of fibroids is unknown, several predisposing factors have been identified, including:

- Age (late reproductive years)
- Genetic predisposition
- African-American ethnicity
- Hypertension
- Nulliparity
- Obesity (Alexander et al., 2014).

Therapeutic Management

Treatment depends on the size of the fibroids and the woman's symptoms, which can include heavy or painful menses, feeling "full" in the lower pelvis, urinating frequently, pain during sexual relations, lower back pain, and infertility (NIH, 2015b). Several treatment options exist, ranging from watchful waiting to surgery.

MEDICAL MANAGEMENT

The goals of medical therapy are to reduce symptoms and/or to reduce the tumor size. This can be accomplished with pain medications to treat mild or occasional pain from fibroids; birth control pills to control heavy menses; or gonadotropin-releasing hormone (GnRH) agonists such as leuprolide (Lupron), nafarelin (Synarel), or goserelin (Zoladex), which stop ovulation and the production of estrogen, or low-dose mifepristone, a progestin antagonist. Both have produced regression and reduced the size of the tumors without surgery, but long-term therapy is expensive and not tolerated by most women. The side effects of GnRH medications include hot flashes, headaches, mood changes, vaginal dryness, musculoskeletal malaise, bone loss, and depression (King et al., 2015). Long-term mifepristone therapy can result in endometrial hyperplasia, which increases the risk of endometrial malignancy. Once either therapy is stopped, the fibroids typically recur.

Uterine artery embolization (UAE) is an option in which polyvinyl alcohol pellets are injected into selected blood vessels via a catheter to block circulation to the fibroid, causing it to shrink and producing symptom

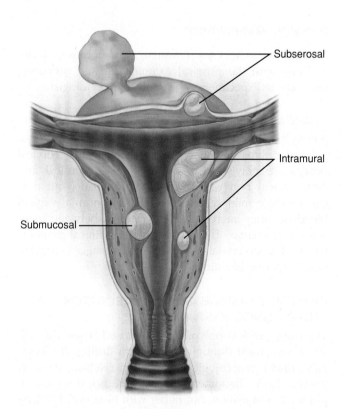

FIGURE 7.4 Submucosal, intramural, and subserosal fibroids.

Subserosal

Intramural

Submucosal

resolution. The procedure is carried out by an interventional radiologist who makes a tiny incision in the groin, introduces a fine catheter into the main artery leading to the uterus, and injects tiny particles of plastic or gelatin sponge into the artery that supplies blood to the fibroid. These particles stop the flow of blood, causing the fibroid to shrink or disappear completely over time. UAE has short-term advantages over surgery. Over the mid and long term, the benefits were similar, except for a higher re-intervention rate after UAE (Hehenkamp, Huirne, & Brolmann, 2015). There remains a need for a treatment that is noninvasive and that preserves fertility.

SURGICAL MANAGEMENT

For women with large fibroids or severe menorrhagia, surgery is preferred over medical treatment. Surgical management might involve myomectomy, laser surgery, or hysterectomy.

Myomectomy. Myomectomy involves removing the fibroid alone. A myomectomy is performed via laparoscopy, through an abdominal incision or through a vaginal approach. The advantage is that only the fibroid is removed; fertility is not jeopardized because this procedure leaves the uterine muscle walls intact. Myomectomy relieves symptoms but does not affect the underlying process; thus, fibroids grow back and further treatment will be needed in the future.

Laser Surgery. Laser surgery (or electrocauterization) involves destroying small fibroids with lasers. Laser therapy can be done using a vaginal approach or laparoscopically. The laser treatment preserves the uterus, but the process may cause scarring and adhesions, thus impairing fertility (Shigetomi et al., 2015). Fibroids can return after this procedure. Controversy remains as to whether laser treatment weakens the uterine wall and thus may contribute to uterine rupture in the future.

Hysterectomy. A hysterectomy is the surgical removal of the uterus. It is the most effective treatment for symptomatic fibroids with no recurrence. After cesarean section, it is the second most frequently performed surgical procedure for women in the United States. Approximately 600,000 hysterectomies are performed annually in the United States (Centers for Disease Control and Prevention [CDC], 2015). The top three conditions associated with hysterectomies are fibroids, endometriosis, and uterine prolapse (CDC, 2015). A hysterectomy to remove fibroids eliminates both the symptoms and the risk of recurrence, but it also terminates the woman's ability to bear children. Three types of hysterectomy surgeries are available: vaginal hysterectomy, laparoscopically assisted vaginal hysterectomy, and abdominal hysterectomy.

In a vaginal hysterectomy, the uterus is removed through an incision in the posterior vagina. Advantages include a shorter hospital stay and recovery time and no abdominal scars. Disadvantages include a limited operating space and poor visualization of other pelvic organs.

In a laparoscopically assisted vaginal hysterectomy, the uterus is removed through a laparoscope, through which structures within the abdomen and pelvis are visualized. Small incisions are made in the abdominal wall to permit the laparoscope to enter the surgical site. Advantages include a better surgical field, less pain, lower cost, and a shorter recovery time. Disadvantages include potential injury to the bladder and the inability to remove enlarged uteruses and scar tissue.

In an abdominal hysterectomy, the uterus and other pelvic organs are removed through an incision in the abdomen. This procedure allows the surgeon to visualize all pelvic organs and is typically used when a malignancy is suspected or a very large uterus is present. Disadvantages include the need for general anesthesia, a longer hospital stay and recovery period, more pain, higher cost, and a visible scar on the abdomen.

Complications of hysterectomy vary based on route of surgery and technique. The most common complications include infection, venous thromboembolic, genitourinary and gastrointestinal injuries, and hemorrhage (Goldman et al., 2015). With astute nursing observations and assessments, these complications can be reduced or minimized. A summary of treatment options for uterine fibroids is presented in Table 7.1.

Nursing Assessment

Nursing assessment for the woman with uterine fibroids includes a thorough health history, physical examination, and laboratory and diagnostic studies.

HEALTH HISTORY AND CLINICAL MANIFESTATIONS

The history should include questions about the woman's menstrual cycle, including alterations in the menstrual pattern (e.g., pain or pressure, aggravating and alleviating factors), history of infertility, and any history of spontaneous abortion, which might indicate a space-occupying uterine lesion. Ask if any female relatives have had fibroids, because there is a familial predisposition. Assess for clinical manifestations of uterine fibroids. Symptoms of fibroids depend on their size and location and may include:

- Chronic pelvic pain
- Low back pain
- Iron-deficiency anemia secondary to bleeding
- Bloating
- Constipation
- Infertility (with large tumors)
- Dysmenorrhea
- Miscarriage
- Sciatica

TABLE 7.1	SUMMARY OF TREATMENT OPTIONS FOR UTERINE FIBROIDS	
Method	**Advantages**	**Disadvantages**
Hormones	Noninvasive Reduces size of fibroids Symptom improvement	Serious side effects with long-term use Fibroids regrow when meds stopped
Uterine artery embolization	Minimally invasive Dramatic decrease in symptoms Future fertility possible	Procedure frequently painful Requires radiation and contrast dye Permanently implanted material Possible negative fertility impact
Myomectomy	Performed as minor surgery Uterus is preserved	Requires general anesthesia New growth of fibroids occurs
Hysterectomy	Complete removal of fibroids Immediate symptom relief	Requires general anesthesia Major surgery with associated risks Fertility not preserved
Laser surgery	Can be done as an outpatient procedure to destroy small fibroids.	Vaporization process can cause scarring and adhesions, affecting future fertility.

- Dyspareunia
- Urinary frequency, urgency, incontinence
- Irregular vaginal bleeding (menorrhagia)
- Feeling of heaviness in the pelvic region

PHYSICAL EXAMINATION AND LABORATORY AND DIAGNOSTIC STUDIES

The bimanual examination performed by the health care provider typically shows an enlarged, irregular uterus. The uterus may be palpable abdominally if the fibroid is very large. Ultrasound may be used to confirm the diagnosis.

Nursing Management

The level of support that nurses can provide women with fibroids depends on the type of treatment offered and her choice of them. Nurses should be able to explain any current treatment options and the implications of a diagnosis of fibroids. Many women have not heard of fibroids previously and need reassurance that they are both common and benign. If medication is prescribed, it is essential to explain the possible side effects and why medication can only be taken for a limited duration. If surgery is selected, verbal and written information about it and the aftercare should be addressed (Box 7.2).

A woman undergoing a hysterectomy for the treatment of fibroids often needs special care and can benefit from presurgical and postsurgical support provided by nurses. Personalized nursing, tailored to the individual woman's needs, enhances the client's coping strategies and alleviates different adverse psychological sequelae following gynecologic surgery. Women must cope with a variety of psychological adjustment difficulties, related to the changes in self-image, self-esteem, loss of femininity

or identity, and sexual dysfunction. The incidence of post-surgical problems can be reduced greatly with proper client-centered perioperative nursing care.

Genital Fistulas

Genital fistulas are an underestimated problem worldwide and have devastating consequences for women. Genital fistulas are abnormal openings between a genital tract organ and another organ, such as the urinary tract or the gastrointestinal tract. A fistula can result from a congenital anomaly, surgical complications, Bartholin's gland abscesses, radiation, or malignancy, but the majority of fistulas that occur worldwide are related to obstetric trauma and female genital cutting (Spurlock, 2015). During normal labor, the bladder is displaced upward into the abdomen, and the anterior vaginal wall, the base of the bladder, and the urethra are compressed between the fetal head and the posterior pubis. When labor is obstructed or prolonged, this unrelieved compression causes ischemia, which causes pressure necrosis and subsequent fistula formation.

Common types of fistulas include:
- *Vesicovaginal:* communication between the bladder and genital tract
- *Urethrovaginal:* communication between the urethra and the vagina
- *Rectovaginal:* communication between the rectum or sigmoid colon and the vagina

The direct consequences of this damage include urinary incontinence and fecal incontinence if the rectum is involved. This tragic condition has plagued women since the beginning of history (Taylor & Rakinic, 2015). Another

---

BOX 7.2

NURSING INTERVENTIONS FOR A WOMAN UNDERGOING A HYSTERECTOMY

Preoperative Care
- Instruct the client and her family about the procedure and aftercare.
- Provide interventions to reduce anxiety (due to perceived threats to the woman's self-concept and role functioning) and fear of alteration in body image, complications, and pain. Prepare the woman so that she knows what to expect throughout her perioperative experience. Explain postoperative pain management procedures that will be used. Identify the high-risk woman early to reduce her stress.
- Teach turning, deep breathing, and coughing before surgery to prevent postoperative atelectasis and respiratory complications such as pneumonia.
- Encourage the woman to discuss her feelings. Some women equate their femaleness with their reproductive capability, and loss of the uterus could evoke grieving.
- Complete all preoperative orders in a timely manner to allow for rest.

Postoperative Care
- Provide comfort measures.
- Administer analgesics promptly or use a patient-controlled anesthesia pump.
- Administer antiemetics to control nausea and vomiting per order.
- Change the client's linens and gown frequently to promote hygiene.
- Change the client's position frequently and use pillows for support to promote comfort and pain management.
- Assess the incision, the dressing, and vaginal bleeding and report if bleeding is excessive (soaking perineal pad within an hour).

- Monitor elimination and provide increased fluids and fiber to prevent constipation and straining.
- Encourage ambulation and active range-of-motion exercises when in bed to prevent thrombophlebitis and venous stasis.
- Monitor vital signs to detect early complications.
- Be comfortable discussing sexual concerns with the client.

Discharge Planning
- Advise the client to reduce her activity level to avoid fatigue, which might inhibit healing.
- Advise the client to rest when she is tired and to increase her activity level slowly.
- Educate the client on the need for pelvic rest (nothing in the vagina) for 6 weeks.
- Instruct the client to avoid heavy lifting or straining for about 6 weeks to prevent an increase in intra-abdominal pressure, which could weaken her sutures.
- Teach the client the signs and symptoms of infection.
- Advise the woman to take showers instead of tub baths to reduce the risk for infection.
- Encourage the client to eat a healthy diet with increased intake of fluids to prevent dehydration and fluid and electrolyte imbalance.
- Instruct the client to change her perineal pad frequently to prevent infection.
- Explain and schedule follow-up care appointments as needed.
- Provide information about community resources for support/help.

---

major cause of genital trauma leading to the development of genital fistulas is female genital cutting. This cultural practice, primarily carried out in Africa and Asia, is receiving worldwide attention as part of the international public health agenda to move toward reducing its incidence. Reasons for continuing this practice include rite of passage, preserving chastity, ensuring marriageability, religion, hygiene, improving fertility, and enhancing sexual pleasure for men (Nour, 2015). Because of migration, health care providers are increasingly confronted with the range of negative urogynecological effects that result from this practice. Nurses need to have a deeper understanding of the history, cultural beliefs, medical complications, and methods of surgical reconstruction to provide culturally competent care to this unique group of women. This cultural practice will be addressed in detail in Chapter 9.

Therapeutic Management

Many small fistulas will heal without treatment, but large fistulas often require surgical repair; surgery may

be postponed until the edema or inflammation in the surrounding tissues has dissipated. Surgical repair of fistulas is associated with a high success rate if it is done in a timely manner, but larger fistulas and those of long duration have a poorer prognosis (Jellison & Raz, 2015).

Nursing Assessment

The history should include questions about any changes in the woman's urinary and bowel patterns. Assess for common signs and symptoms of fistulas, which are related to the type of fistula. If the opening involves the rectum, feces and flatus will leak through the vagina. If it involves the bladder, urine will leak from the vagina. Depending on the location and size of the fistula, the woman may or may not experience discomfort. The health care provider can detect these abnormal openings through inspection and palpation during the pelvic examination. Diagnostic or laboratory tests are generally not ordered once this condition is found.

Nursing Management

Provide guidance and support. Offer information to help the woman learn about her condition and, with appropriate intervention, to improve her quality of life. Begin by making sure the woman understands her anatomy and why she is having such symptoms. Provide a thorough explanation of the treatment options so that she can make an informed decision. Be sensitive to the woman's feeling of shame and fear about her incontinence; these feelings may be why she delayed seeking treatment. Address all of the woman's needs, both physical and emotional.

Bartholin's Cysts

A Bartholin's cyst is a swollen, fluid-filled, sac-like structure that results when one of the ducts of the Bartholin's gland becomes blocked. The cyst may become infected and an abscess may develop in the gland. The Bartholin's glands are two mucus-secreting glandular structures with duct openings bilaterally at the base of the labia minora near the opening of the vagina that provide lubrication during sexual arousal. Normally these glands cannot be felt or seen unless they are infected. Bartholin's cysts are the most common cystic growths in the vulva, affecting approximately 2% of women at some time in their life (Reif et al., 2015).

Therapeutic Management

Treatment can be conservative or surgical depending on the symptoms, the size of the cyst, and whether it is infected or not. Small asymptomatic cysts do not require treatment. Sitz baths along with analgesics are used to reduce discomfort. Antibiotics are prescribed if the gland is infected. The aim of treatment for a cyst or abscess is to create a fistulous tract from the dilated duct to the outside vulva by incision and drainage. However, cysts or abscesses tend to return if this option is used.

Other treatment options beyond incision and drainage include placement of a Word catheter or a small loop of plastic tubing secured in place to prevent closure and to allow drainage. The use of a carbon dioxide laser to remove the cyst is also possible. After the Word catheter is inserted, the balloon tip is inflated and it is left in place for 4 to 6 weeks. The follow-up of the plastic tubing for removal is in approximately 3 weeks. Both procedures are safe and effective alternatives to surgery (Prabhu & Gardella, 2015). Treatment for a pregnant woman with a Bartholin's cyst depends on the severity of the symptoms and whether an infection is present. Surgery may be delayed until after the woman gives birth if there are no symptoms.

Nursing Assessment

Nursing assessment for the woman with a Bartholin's cyst includes a thorough health history, physical examination, and laboratory and diagnostic tests.

HEALTH HISTORY

The history should include questions about the woman's sexual practices and protective measures used. Assess for common signs and symptoms of Bartholin's cysts. The woman may be asymptomatic if the cyst is small (less than 5 cm) and not infected. If infection is present, symptoms include varying degrees of pain, especially when walking or sitting; unilateral edema; redness around the gland; and dyspareunia. Extensive inflammation may cause systemic symptoms. Abscess formation occurs when the cystic fluid becomes infected. An abscess usually develops rapidly over a 2- to 3-day period and may spontaneously rupture. A history of sudden relief of pain following profuse discharge is highly suggestive of spontaneous rupture (Schuiling & Likis, 2016).

PHYSICAL EXAMINATION AND LABORATORY AND DIAGNOSTIC STUDIES

The diagnosis of Bartholin's cysts or abscesses is primarily made during a physical examination when a protruding tender labial mass is located. In women over the age of 40, there is an increased risk of malignancy, typically sarcomas which account for 2% of all invasive vulvar malignancies. They are characterized by rapid growth, high metastatic potential, frequent recurrences, aggressive behavior, and high mortality rate (Chokoeva et al., 2015). Cultures of the purulent abscess fluid and of the cervix should be obtained for *Neisseria gonorrhoeae* and *Chlamydia trachomatis* to rule out a sexually transmitted infection.

Nursing Management

Nurses must be aware of and knowledgeable about vulvar cysts and treatment options. The woman may be aware of a vulvar cyst secondary to the pain or may be unaware of it if it is asymptomatic. A Bartholin's cyst may be an incidental finding during a routine pelvic examination. Explain the cause of the cyst and assist with cultures if needed. Provide reassurance and support.

Ovarian Cysts

An **ovarian cyst** is a fluid-filled sac that forms on the ovary (Fig. 7.5). These very common growths are benign 90% of the time and are asymptomatic in many women. The cysts are discovered incidentally during an ultrasound or routine pelvic exam. Ovarian cysts occur in 30% of women with regular menses, 50% of women with irregular menses, and 7% of postmenopausal women (Templeman,

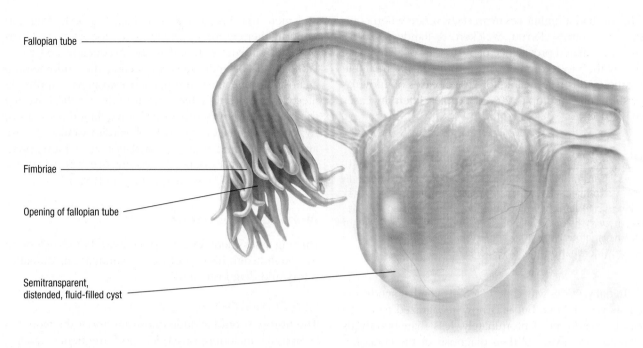

Fallopian tube

Fimbriae

Opening of fallopian tube

Semitransparent,
distended, fluid-filled cyst

FIGURE 7.5 Ovarian cyst. (Asset provided by Anatomical Chart Co.)

2015). When the cysts grow large and exert pressure on surrounding structures, women often seek medical help.

Types of Ovarian Cysts

The most common benign ovarian cysts are follicular cysts, corpus luteum (lutein) cysts, theca-lutein cysts, and polycystic ovarian syndrome (PCOS).

FOLLICULAR CYSTS

Small follicular cysts are commonly found in the ovaries of prepubertal girls and women of reproductive age, and in most cases, they are of no clinical significance. They are usually self-limiting and resolve spontaneously. Follicular cysts are caused by the failure of the ovarian follicle to rupture at the time of ovulation. Follicular cysts seldom grow larger than 5 cm in diameter; most regress and require no treatment. They can occur at any age and are rare after menopause. They are detected by vaginal ultrasound.

CORPUS LUTEUM (LUTEIN) CYSTS

A corpus luteum cyst forms when the corpus luteum becomes cystic or hemorrhagic and fails to degenerate after 14 days. These cysts might cause pain and delay the next menstrual period. A pelvic ultrasound helps to make this diagnosis. Typically these cysts appear after ovulation and resolve without intervention.

THECA-LUTEIN CYSTS

Prolonged abnormally high levels of human chorionic gonadotropin (hCG) stimulate the development of theca-lutein cysts. Although rare, these cysts are associated with hydatidiform mole, choriocarcinoma, polycystic ovary syndrome, and Clomid therapy.

POLYCYSTIC OVARY SYNDROME

Polycystic ovary syndrome is the most common endocrine condition in women of reproductive age. It is a heterogeneous condition that involves the presence of multiple inactive follicle cysts within the ovary that interfere with ovarian function. It is a multifaceted disorder, and central to its pathogenesis are hyperandrogenemia and hyperinsulinemia, which are targets for treatment (King et al., 2015). It is associated with obesity, hyperinsulinemia, elevated luteinizing hormone levels (linked to ovulation), elevated androgen levels (virilization), hirsutism (male-pattern hair growth), obstructive sleep apnea, follicular atresia (ovarian growth failure), ovarian growth and cyst formation, anovulation (failure to ovulate), infertility, type 2 diabetes, sleep apnea, amenorrhea (absence of menstruation or irregular periods), metabolic syndrome, which is characterized by abdominal obesity (waist circumference >35 in), dyslipidemia (triglyceride level >150 mg/dL, high-density lipoprotein cholesterol level <50 mg/dL), elevated blood pressure, a proinflammatory state characterized by an elevated C-reactive protein level, and a prothrombotic state characterized by elevated PAI-1 and fibrinogen levels. Recent studies also indicate that PCOS is associated with an increase in the risk of uterine fibroids, depression, adverse pregnancy outcomes and neonatal complications. A recent meta-analysis found that women with PCOS demonstrated a significantly higher risk of developing gestational diabetes, gestational hypertension, preeclampsia, preterm birth, and had a higher cesarean section rate when compared to controls (Kyrou, Weickert, & Randeva, 2015). With an estimated prevalence of 5% to 10% of all females, PCOS is the most common cause of medically treatable infertility and is responsible for 70% of cases of anovulatory subfertility and up to 20% of couples' infertility cases (NIH, 2015c).

Take Note!

Careful attention should be given to this condition because affected women are at increased risk for long-term health problems such as cardiovascular disease, hypertension, dyslipidemia, type 2 diabetes (half of all women), infertility, and cancer (endometrial, breast, and ovarian) (Moran, Norman, & Teede, 2015).

Initially PCOS was called Stein–Leventhal syndrome after its researchers, but it is now recognized to be an anabolic syndrome. Unfortunately, less than two-thirds of women are aware of their diagnosis or the concomitant high risk for developing type 2 diabetes mellitus and cardiovascular disease related to metabolic syndrome. Its etiology is not clearly understood, but studies suggest a genetic (autosomal-dominant) component. Women with PCOS have abnormalities in the metabolism of androgens and estrogen and in the control of androgen production. In addition, they have peripheral insulin resistance and hyperinsulinemia and obesity (Trikudanathan, 2015). All of these clinical manifestations must be addressed throughout the lifespan with an emphasis on prevention of cardiometabolic risks in the treatment plan.

Therapeutic Management

Treatment is centered on the clinical manifestations and should be initiated early to prevent/limit long-term complications such as metabolic syndrome, diabetes, endometrial carcinoma, and infertility (Ganie, Chakraborty, & Rehman, 2015). Oral contraceptives, antidiabetic agents, and statins are some of the common therapies used to address the symptoms of this complex hormonal condition. Weight loss and surgery may also be beneficial as non-drug options.

Treatment of ovarian cysts focuses on differentiating a benign cyst from a solid ovarian malignancy. Transvaginal ultrasound is useful in distinguishing fluid-filled cysts from solid masses. Laparoscopy may be needed to remove the cyst if it is large and pressing on surrounding structures. For smaller cysts, monitoring with repeat ultrasounds every 3 to 6 months might be in order (Lucidi, 2015). Oral contraceptives are often prescribed to suppress gonadotropin levels, which may help resolve the cysts. Pain medication is also prescribed if needed.

Medical management of PCOS is aimed at the treatment of metabolic derangements, anovulation, hirsutism, and menstrual irregularity. This includes both drug and nondrug therapy, along with lifestyle modifications. Goals of therapy focus on reducing the production and circulating levels of androgens, protecting the endometrium against the effects of unopposed estrogens, supporting lifestyle changes to achieve ideal body weight, lowering the risk of cardiovascular disease, avoiding the effects of hyperinsulinemia on the risk of cardiovascular disease and diabetes, and inducing ovulation to achieve pregnancy if desired (Evidence-Based Practice 7.2). Treatment modalities for PCOS are highlighted in Box 7.3.

Nursing Assessment

Nursing assessment for the woman with PCOS includes a thorough health history, physical examination, and laboratory and diagnostic tests.

HEALTH HISTORY

The history should include questions about the woman's symptoms, including onset, location, frequency, quality, intensity, and aggravating and alleviating factors of her discomfort. Note the last menstrual period and whether or not her cycles are regular. Ask about her overall general health and any changes recently noticed, such as a change in abdominal girth without a concomitant weight gain. Assess for common signs and symptoms of ovarian cysts. Findings might include:

- Hirsutism (face and chin, upper lip, areola, lower abdomen, and perineum)
- Alopecia (frontal region and crown of head)
- Virilization (clitoral hypertrophy, deepening of voice, increased muscle mass, breast atrophy, male-pattern baldness)
- Menstrual irregularity and infertility (menorrhagia, anovulation)
- Polycystic ovaries (12 or more follicles on ovaries)
- Obesity (occurs in more than 50% of women with PCOS; occurs in abdominal region, with an increase in the waist–hip ratio)
- Insulin resistance (chronic hyperinsulinemia leads to type 2 diabetes)
- Metabolic syndrome (elevated cholesterol, triglycerides, low-density lipoprotein; risk of cardiovascular disease)
- Increased risk for endometrial cancer, ovarian cancer, breast cancer
- Psychological impact (depression, frustration, anxiety, eating disorders)
- Acne (face and shoulders) (Lucidi, 2015).

PHYSICAL EXAMINATION AND LABORATORY AND DIAGNOSTIC STUDIES

The physical examination includes inspection, auscultation, and palpation of the abdomen because large ovarian masses may cause visible changes in the abdomen. A complete pelvic examination is performed to assess the

EVIDENCE-BASED PRACTICE 7.2 **IT'S NOT JUST PHYSICAL: THE ADVERSE PSYCHOSOCIAL EFFECTS OF POLYCYSTIC OVARY SYNDROME IN ADOLESCENTS**

STUDY

The prevalence of depression and other psychological disorders in women with PCOS is high and varies in numerous studies. In particular, women with PCOS have been found to be at an increased risk of social phobia and suicide attempts. The reasons for a higher prevalence of psychological disorders in women with PCOS are likely to be complex. Some investigators suggest that physical symptoms experienced by women with PCOS are the likely cause of psychological distress. However, evidence is inconsistent. While acne, hirsutism and obesity have been linked to increased psychological distress in some studies, no link is demonstrated in others. It is likely that multiple factors contribute to the high prevalence of psychosocial disorders in women with PCOS.

This study sheds light on the fact that this gynecologic disorder of endocrine origin can be associated with a great number of psychological symptoms (e.g., depression, anxiety, body image dissatisfaction, eating and sexual disorders, and poor quality of life). The goal of the study was to address the prevalence of psychological disorders and determinants of well-being.

Findings

An overwhelming majority of scientific literature on PCOS has focused on the medical approach to analyze the disorder and only a few studies have investigated its predisposing psychological factors. The literature review revealed several psychological disorders that accompany this syndrome with limited attention given to them to help women cope. The symptoms typically associated with PCOS, including amenorrhea, oligomenorrhea, hirsutism, obesity, infertility, anovulation, and acne, can lead to symptoms of depression, withdrawal from society, emotional distress, embarrassment, lower self-esteem, anxiety, body image disturbances, eating disorders, marital and social maladjustment, and impaired sexual functioning.

Nursing Implications

PCOS is closely associated with psychological disorders with important implications that necessitate identification and treatment of the disorders. The high prevalence rate of these psychological disorders in this population suggests that initial evaluation of all women with PCOS should also include an assessment of their mental health. Psychological support by nurses should take on an important role in the management of the affected women with PCOS. This should not suggest that medical treatment of PCOS is not required, but a thorough cooperation between medical treatment and psychological support would improve the situation of PCOS affected women. The physical and psychosocial aspects of management of PCOS go hand in hand. Meeting physical management goals (e.g. weight loss, reduction in hyperandrogenism manifestations) can lessen some of the distressing psychosocial effects, and enhance self-esteem.

Adapted from Lee, J. S. (2015). It's not just physical: The adverse psychosocial effects of polycystic ovary syndrome in adolescents. *Women's Healthcare, 3*(1), 20–28.

BOX 7.3

TREATMENT MODALITIES FOR PCOS

- Oral contraceptives to treat menstrual irregularities and acne
- Mechanical hair removal (shaving, waxing, plucking, or electrolysis) to treat hirsutism
- Glucophage (metformin), which improves insulin uptake by fat and muscle cells, to treat hyperinsulinemia; thiazolinediones (Actos, Avandia) to decrease insulin resistance
- Ovulation induction agents (Clomid) to treat infertility
- Lifestyle changes (e.g., weight loss, exercise, balanced low-fat diet)
- Referral to support groups to help improve emotional state and build self-esteem

Adapted from King, T. L., Brucker, M. C., Kriebs, J. M., Fahey, J. O., Gegor, C. L., & Varney, H. (2015). *Varney's Midwifery* (5th ed.), Burlington, MA: Jones & Bartlett Learning; Kyrou, I., Weickert, M. O., & Randeva, H. S. (2015). Diagnosis and management of polycystic ovary syndrome (PCOS). In *Endocrinology and Diabetes* (pp. 99–113). London, England: Springer Publishers; and Lucidi, R. S. (2015). Polycystic ovarian syndrome. *EMedicine.* Retrieved from at http://emedicine.medscape.com/article/256806-overview

location, size, shape, texture, mobility, and tenderness of any palpable mass.

Diagnostic tests include a pregnancy test to rule out ectopic pregnancy. Gonorrhea and chlamydia testing is warranted if an ovarian abscess is suspected. An ultrasound may be ordered to differentiate between functional or simple ovarian cysts and a solid tumor. Additional tests may be performed depending on the findings.

Remember Liz, the client with irregular menses, facial hair, and acne? Her glucose level is elevated, multiple cysts were felt on her ovaries during the pelvic examination, and laboratory tests found elevated lipid and lipoprotein levels. What education should the nurse provide Liz regarding her PCOS diagnosis? What medications might be prescribed to address her abnormal laboratory values?

Nursing Management

Nursing care should include education about the condition, treatment options, diagnostic test arrangements, and referral for surgery if needed. Provide support and reassurance during the diagnostic period to allay anxiety in the client and her family. Reassure the woman that the majority of ovarian cysts are benign, but regardless stress the importance of follow-up care. Listen to the woman's concerns about her appearance, infertility, and facial hair growth. Offer suggestions to help the woman feel better about herself and her health.

Nurses can have a positive impact on women with PCOS through counseling and education. Provide support for women dealing with negative self-image secondary to the physical manifestations of PCOS. Through education, help the woman understand the syndrome and its associated risk factors to prevent long-term health problems. Encourage the woman to make positive lifestyle changes. Make community referrals to local support groups to help the woman build her coping skills.

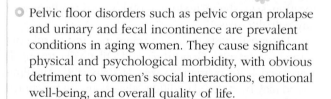

Liz returns to the clinic a month later for reevaluation of her PCOS. She has been taking metformin to reduce her insulin resistance and has followed her exercise regimen and reduced her caloric intake to lose weight, but she still complains about her facial hair and acne. What interventions might be helpful to address this problem? What medication might also be prescribed to regularize her menses and relieve the hirsutism?

KEY CONCEPTS

○ Pelvic floor disorders such as pelvic organ prolapse and urinary and fecal incontinence are prevalent conditions in aging women. They cause significant physical and psychological morbidity, with obvious detriment to women's social interactions, emotional well-being, and overall quality of life.

○ The four most common types of genital prolapse are cystocele, rectocele, enterocele, and uterine prolapse.

○ The purpose of pelvic floor muscle exercises is to increase the muscle volume, which will result in a stronger muscular contraction. These exercises might limit the progression of mild prolapse and alleviate mild prolapse symptoms, including low back pain and pelvic pressure.

○ UI is the involuntary loss of urine sufficient enough to be a social or hygiene problem. It affects approximately 15 million women in the United States.

○ The three most common types of incontinence are urge incontinence (overactive bladder caused by detrusor muscle contractions), stress incontinence

(inadequate urinary sphincter function), and mixed incontinence (involves both stress and urge incontinence).

○ The most common benign growths of the reproductive tract include cervical, endocervical, and endometrial polyps; uterine fibroids (leiomyomas); genital fistulas; Bartholin's cysts; and ovarian cysts.

○ PCOS involves the presence of multiple inactive follicle cysts within the ovary that interfere with ovarian function. Hyperandrogenism, insulin resistance, and chronic anovulation characterize PCOS. Careful attention should be given to this condition because women with it are at increased risk for long-term health problems such as cardiovascular disease, hypertension, dyslipidemia, infertility, type 2 diabetes, and cancer (endometrial, breast, and ovarian).

References and Recommended Readings

Alexander, L. L., LaRosa, J. H., Bader, H., & Garfield, S. (2014). *New dimensions in women's health* (6th ed.). Sudbury, MA: Jones & Bartlett.

Alexander, L., Shakespeare, K., Barradell, V., & Orme, S. (2015). Management of urinary incontinence in frail elderly women. *Obstetrics, Gynecology & Reproductive Medicine, 25*(3), 75–82.

American College of Obstetricians and Gynecologists [ACOG]. (2015a) Pelvic support problems. *ACOG Educational Pamphlet*. Retrieved from http://www.acog.org/~/media/For%20Patients/faq012.pdf?dmc=1&ts=20140128T1159591406

Brown, D. N. (2015). Pelvic organ prolapse: a consequence of nature or nurture?. *Menopause, 22*(5), 477–479.

Centers for Disease Control and Prevention [CDC]. (2015). *Women's reproductive health: Hysterectomy*. Retrieved from http://www.cdc.gov/reproductivehealth/WomensRH/Hysterectomy.htm

Chokoeva, A. A., Tchernev, G., Cardoso, J. C., Patterson, J. W., Dechev, I., Valkanov, S., et al. (2015). Vulvar sarcomas: Short guideline for histopathological recognition and clinical management. Part 1. *International Journal of Immunopathology and Pharmacology, 28*(2), 168–177.

Colyar, M. R. (2015). *Advanced practice nursing procedures*. Philadelphia, PA: F.A. Davis Company.

Dumoulin, C., Hay-Smith, E. J., Mac Habee-Sequin, G. M., & Mercier, J. (2015). Pelvic floor muscle training verses no treatment, or inactive control treatments, for urinary incontinence in women. *Neurourology & Urodynamics, 34*(4), 300–308.

Files, J. A., Mayer, A. P., & Chutka, D. S. (2015). Urinary incontinence: Not just a mid-laugh crisis. *Journal of Women's Health, 24*(1), 107–108.

Ganie, M. A., Chakraborty, S., & Rehman, H. (2015). Treatment of polycystic ovary syndrome: recent trial results. *Clinical Investigation, 5*(3), 337–350.

Goldman, N. A., Lynch, K., Jones, H., Rutledge, J., & Burke, W. M. (2015). Comparison of complications in patients undergoing robotic-assisted hysterectomy for large leiomyomas [107]. *Obstetrics & Gynecology, 125*, 40S.

Hehenkamp, W. J., Huirne, J. A., & Brölmann, H. A. (2015). Uterine artery embolization and new ablation techniques. In A. Tinelli & A. Malvasi (Eds.), *Uterine myoma, myomectomy and minimally invasive treatments* (pp. 153–168). Switzerland: Springer International Publishing.

Heller, D. S. (2015). Diseases of the cervix. In *OB-GYN pathology for the clinician* (pp. 91–106). Switzerland: Springer International Publishing.

International Continence Society. (2015). *Urinary Incontinence*, Retrieved from http://www.icsoffice.org/Home.aspx

Jellison, F. C., & Raz, S. (2015). Vaginal fistula repairs. In *Female pelvic surgery* (pp. 145–163). New York, NY: Springer Publishers.

King, T. L., Brucker, M. C., Kriebs, J. M., Fahey, J. O., Gegor, C. L., & Varney, H. (2015). *Varney's midwifery* (5th ed.). Burlington, MA: Jones & Bartlett Learning

Kirby, A. C., Tan-Kim, J., & Nager, C. W. (2015). Dynamic maximum urethral closure pressures measured by high-resolution manometry increase markedly after sling surgery. *International Urogynecology Journal*, 1–5.

Kwak, Y., Kwon, H., & Kim, Y. (2015). Health-related quality of life and mental health in older women with urinary incontinence. *Aging & Mental Health*, 1–8.

Kyrou, I., Weickert, M. O., & Randeva, H. S. (2015). Diagnosis and management of polycystic ovary syndrome (PCOS). In *Endocrinology and diabetes* (pp. 99–113). London, England: Springer Publishers.

Lazarou, G., & Grigorescu, B. A. (2015). Pelvic organ prolapse. *eMedicine*, Retrieved from http://emedicine.medscape.com/article/276259-overview

Lee, J. S. (2015). It's not just physical: The adverse psychosocial effects of polycystic ovary syndrome in adolescents. *Women's Healthcare*, 3(1), 20–28.

Lieng, M. (2015). Endometrial polyps. In *Minimally invasive gynecological surgery* (pp. 61–73). Berlin, Heidelberg, Germany: Springer Publishers.

Lucidi, R. S. (2015). Polycystic ovarian syndrome. *EMedicine*. Retrieved from http://emedicine.medscape.com/article/256806-overview

Maher, C., & Haya, N. (2015). Changing trends in pelvic organ prolapse surgery. *Obstetrics, Gynecology & Reproductive Medicine*, 25(6), 147–151.

McClurg, D., Gerrard, J., & Hove, R. T. (2015). Reducing the incidence of incontinence. *British Journal of Midwifery*, 23(1), 17–20.

Meyer, D. (2015). Health benefits of prebiotic fibers. *Advances in Food and Nutrition Research*, 74, 47–91.

Moran, L. J., Norman, R. J., & Teede, H. J. (2015). Metabolic risk in PCOS: Phenotype and adiposity impact. *Trends in Endocrinology & Metabolism*, 26(3), 136–143.

Mukwege, A. A., El-Nashar, S. A., Rhodes, D., Dowdy, S. C., & Trabuco, E. C. (2015). Are demographic and clinical characteristics of women presenting with advanced pelvic organ prolapse different compared with women presenting in earlier stages?[374]. *Obstetrics & Gynecology*, 125, 116S–117S.

National Institutes of Health [NIH]. (2015a) *Pelvic floor disorders*. Retrieved from https://www.nichd.nih.gov/health/topics/pelvicfloor/Pages/default.aspx

National Institutes of Health [NIH] (2015b) *Uterine fibroids*. Retrieved from http://www.nichd.nih.gov/health/topics/uterine/condition-info/Pages/default.aspx

National Institutes of Health [NIH] (2015c) *Polycystic ovarian syndrome*. Retrieved from http://www.nichd.nih.gov/health/topics/PCOS/Pages/default.aspx

Nelson, A. L., Papa, R. R., & Ritchie, J. J. (2015). Asymptomatic cervical polyps: can we just let them be?. *Women's Health*, 11(2), 121–126.

Nilsson, C. G. (2015). Creating a gold standard surgical procedure: the development and implementation of TVT. *International Urogynecology Journal*, 1–3.

Nour, N. M. (2015, January). Female genital cutting: Impact on women's health. *In Seminars in Reproductive Medicine*. 33(1), 41–46.

Prabhu, A., & Gardella, C. (2015). Common vaginal and vulvar Disorders. *Medical Clinics of North America*, 99(3), 553–574.

Ralph, G., & Tamussino, K. (2015). Conservative management of pelvic organ prolapse. In A. Tamilselvi & Ajay Rane (Eds.), *Principles and practice of urogynecology* (pp. 115–122). New Delhi, India: Springer Publishers.

Ramalingam, K., & Monga, A. (2015). Obesity and pelvic floor dysfunction. *Best Practice & Research Clinical Obstetrics & Gynecology*, 29(4), 541–547. DOI: http://dx.doi.org/10.1016/j.bpobgyn.2015.02.002

Reif, P., Ulrich, D., Bjelic-Radisic, V., Häusler, M., Schnedl-Lamprecht, E., & Tamussino, K. (2015). Management of Bartholin's cyst and abscess using the Word catheter–implementation, recurrence rates and costs. *European Journal of Obstetrics & Gynecology and Reproductive Biology*, 190, 81–84.

Riss, P., & Koch, M. (2015). Evaluation of pelvic organ prolapse. In *Principles and practice of urogynecology* (pp. 107–114). New Delhi, India: Springer Publishers.

Rodríguez-Mias, N. L., Martínez-Franco, E., Aguado, J., Sánchez, E., & Amat-Tardiu, L. (2015). Pelvic organ prolapse and stress urinary incontinence, do they share the same risk factors?. *European Journal of Obstetrics & Gynecology and Reproductive Biology*, 190: 52-57.

Schuiling, K. D., & Likis, F. E. (2016). *Women's gynecologic health* (3rd ed.). Sudbury, MA: Jones & Bartlett.

Shigetomi, H., Oka, K., Seki, T., & Kobayashi, H. (2015). Design and preclinical validation of the composite-type optical fiberscope for minimally invasive procedure of intrauterine disease. *Journal of Minimally Invasive Gynecology*, 22(6), 985–991.

Spurlock, J. (2015). Vesicovaginal fistula. *eMedicine*. Retrieved from: http://emedicine.medscape.com/article/267943-overview#a0102

Stewart, E. A. (2015). Uterine fibroids. *New England Journal of Medicine*, 372(17), 1646–1655.

Stewart, E. A. (2016). Endometrial polyps. *UpToDate*, Retrieved from http://www.uptodate.com/contents/endometrial-polyps

Su, C. C., Sun, B. Y., & Jiann, B. P. (2015). Association of urinary incontinence and sexual function in women. *International Journal of Urology*, 22(1), 109–113.

Taylor, D., & Rakinic, J. (2015). Rectovaginal fistula. *eMedicine*. Retrieved from: http://emedicine.medscape.com/article/193277-overview

Templeman, C. (2015). Ovarian cysts. *Journal of Pediatric and Adolescent Gynecology*, 17, 297–298.

Trikudanathan, S. (2015). Polycystic ovarian syndrome. *Medical Clinics of North America*, 99(1), 221–235.

Vasavada, S. P., Carmel, M. E., & Rackley, R. (2015). Urinary incontinence. *eMedicine*. Retrieved from http://emedicine.medscape.com/article/452289-overview

Waetjen, L. E., Xing, G., Johnson, W. O., Melnikow, J., & Gold, E. B., Study of Women's Health Across the Nation (SWAN). (2015). Factors associated with seeking treatment for urinary incontinence during the menopausal transition. *Obstetrics & Gynecology*, 125(5), 1071–1079.

Walters, M. (2015), Urinary incontinence in women comes and goes, and reasons remain elusive. *BJOG: An International Journal of Obstetrics & Gynecology*, 122, 824.

CHAPTER WORKSHEET

MULTIPLE CHOICE QUESTIONS

1. When you are interviewing a client with uterine fibroids, what subjective data would you expect to find in her history?
   a. Cyclic migraine headaches
   b. Urinary tract infections
   c. Chronic pelvic pain
   d. Chronic constipation

2. Conservative treatment options available for women with pelvic organ prolapse are:
   a. Pessaries and PFM exercises
   b. External pelvic fixation devices
   c. Weight gain and yoga
   d. Firm panty-and-girdle garments

3. Which of the following dietary and lifestyle modifications might the nurse recommend to help prevent pelvic relaxation as women age?
   a. Eat a high-fiber diet to avoid constipation and straining.
   b. Avoid sitting for long periods; get up and walk around frequently.
   c. Limit the amount of exercise to prevent overdeveloping muscles.
   d. Space children a year apart to reduce wear and tear on the uterus.

4. Women with PCOS are at increased risk for developing which of the following long-term health problems?
   a. Osteoporosis
   b. Lupus
   c. Type 2 diabetes
   d. Migraine headaches

5. Side effects experienced by women taking GnRH agonists for the treatment of fibroids closely resemble those of:
   a. Anorexia nervosa
   b. Osteoarthritis
   c. Depression
   d. Menopause

6. In securing a health history of a 65-year-old woman, which clinical manifestation described by the client would the nurse suspect is related to pelvic organ prolapse?
   a. Chronic abdominal pain
   b. Heavy feeling or dragging in vagina
   c. Uterine cramping and backache
   d. Weight gain and edema of ankles

CRITICAL THINKING EXERCISE

1. Faith, a 42-year-old multiparous woman, presents to the women's health clinic complaining of pelvic pain, menorrhagia, and vaginal discharge. She says she has been having these problems for several months. On examination, her uterus is enlarged and irregular in shape. Her blood studies reveal anemia.
   a. What condition might Faith have, based on her symptoms?
   b. What treatment options are available to address this condition?
   c. What educational interventions should the nurse discuss with Faith?

STUDY ACTIVITIES

1. Prepare an educational session to teach women how to do Pelvic floor muscle exercises to prevent stress incontinence and pelvic floor relaxation.

2. In a small group, discuss the personal, social, and sexual issues that might affect a woman with pelvic organ prolapse. How might these issues affect her socialization? How might a support group help?

3. List the symptoms that a woman with uterine fibroids might have. Discuss how these symptoms might mimic a more frightening condition and why the woman might delay seeking treatment.

4. A bladder that herniates into the vagina is a _____.

5. A rectum that herniates into the vagina is a _____.

BRINGING IT ALL TOGETHER: CASE STUDY

Elizabeth, a 52-year-old woman presents to the gynecologic clinic to discuss a 'horrible personal problem' that is ruining her life. She appears very distressed and only wants to talk to the nurse in private about it. A few months ago when she was out walking her dog, she experienced a sudden rectal urgency that she thought was gas, but she expelled feces instead. Over the past few months, her fecal incontinence has increased in severity and frequency causing her extreme stress. To avoid embarrassment, she has had to cover and excuse herself from work situations and turn down social invitations. She now has to wear a protective pad and disposable pants.

ASSESSMENT

Elizabeth is otherwise healthy and takes no prescription medications presently. She has had five vaginal births with three episiotomies. She has a body mass index of 27, mild stress urinary incontinence, and a low-grade rectocele with slightly decreased anal sphincter tone. Her pelvic exam demonstrated pelvic organ prolapse. The digital rectal exam ruled out fecal impaction and any rectal mass. A detailed history of her incontinence episodes was also taken.

Go to thePoint **to find questions to consider about this case.**

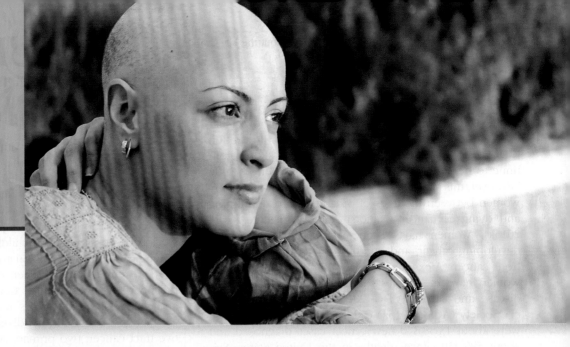

8

Cancers of the Female Reproductive Tract

Learning Objectives

Upon completion of the chapter, you will be able to:

1. Evaluate the major modifiable risk factors for reproductive tract cancers.

2. Analyze the screening methods and treatment modalities for cancers of the female reproductive tract.

3. Outline the nursing management needed for the most common malignant reproductive tract cancers in women.

4. Examine lifestyle changes and health screenings that can reduce the risk of or prevent reproductive tract cancers.

5. Assess at least three web site resources available for a woman diagnosed with cancer of the reproductive tract.

6. Appraise the psychological distress felt by women diagnosed with cancer, and outline information that can help them to cope.

Carmella is an obese, 55-year-old woman who presents to her woman's health care provider with vaginal bleeding. She has been through menopause and wonders why she is having a period again. Her history includes infertility and hypertension. Three years ago she had a mastectomy for breast cancer, and she has been taking tamoxifen (Nolvadex) to prevent recurrent breast cancer since her surgery. What risk factors in Carmella's history might predispose her to a reproductive tract cancer? What additional information is needed to make a diagnosis?

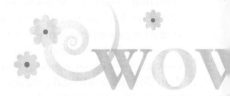

Words of Wisdom
The word "cancer" can strike fear into anyone who hears it. But when it involves a reproductive organ, this fear is often magnified.

INTRODUCTION

Cancer is the second leading cause of death for women in the United States, surpassed only by cardiovascular disease (Centers for Disease Control and Prevention [CDC], 2015a). Cardiovascular disease is, and should continue to be, a major focus of efforts in women's health. However, this should not overshadow the fact that many women between the ages of 35 and 74 are developing and dying of cancer (National Cancer Institute [NCI], 2015a). Women have a one-in-three lifetime risk of developing cancer, and one out of every four deaths is from cancer (Alexander et al., 2014). African American women have the highest death rates from both heart disease and cancer (CDC, 2015a). The American Cancer Society (ACS) (2015a) estimated that, in 2015, there were about 1,658,370 new cancer cases diagnosed and about 589,430 cancer deaths in the United States. Scientific evidence suggested that about one third of these cancer deaths expected to occur in 2015 were related to obesity, physical inactivity, and poor nutrition, and thus could have been prevented. Certain cancers are related to infectious agents, such as hepatitis B virus (HBV), human papillomavirus (HPV), human immunodeficiency virus (HIV), and *Helicobacter pylori* (*H. pylori*), and can be prevented through behavioral changes, vaccines, or antibiotics (Herrington, Coates, & Duprex, 2015). In addition, many of the more than 2 million skin cancers that are diagnosed annually could be prevented by protecting the skin from the sun's rays and avoiding indoor tanning. Sunburns, especially if they occur repetitively in childhood, may lead to melanoma. Most melanomas are treated successfully if discovered early, but metastatic melanoma has no good treatment (Balk, 2015).

It has been estimated that in the United States, half of all premature deaths, one third of acute disabilities, and one half of chronic disabilities are preventable, including some cancers (NCI, 2015b). Nurses need to focus their energies on screening, education, and early detection to reduce these numbers. Because cancer risk is strongly associated with lifestyle and behavior, screening programs are of particular importance for early detection. There is evidence that prevention and early detection have reduced cancer mortality rates and prevented reproductive cancers (CDC, 2015b).

This chapter begins with a nursing process overview of the care of women with reproductive cancer. It then describes selected cancers of the reproductive system: ovarian, endometrial, cervical, vaginal, and vulvar cancer. The chapter discusses the nurse's role through diagnosis, intervention, and follow-up care. Cancer management requires a multidisciplinary approach, including specialists in surgical, medical, and radiation oncology. The nurse can provide guidance and support to the client as she finds her way through the health care maze.

NURSING PROCESS OVERVIEW FOR WOMEN WITH CANCER OF THE REPRODUCTIVE TRACT

The word *cancer* is laden with fear and dread. These feelings may worsen when the cancer involves a woman's reproductive tract. The diagnosis of a reproductive tract cancer can have a profound impact on a woman's sexuality because it affects the very core of her identity as a female. The loss of the reproductive body part as well as the possible loss of childbearing ability can have a significant effect on women and their partners. Nurses need to remember this when counseling women and their partners about cancer treatment and side effects and changes in gender roles and sexuality.

When a woman is first diagnosed with a reproductive tract cancer, two primary needs arise: information and emotional support. When the diagnosis is made, the woman typically has many questions, such as "What is going to happen to me?" "How will this change my life?" and "Will I survive?" Nurses can play a major role in helping women find the answers to their questions and directing them to the resources they need. Two reliable sources of general cancer information are the NCI and the American Cancer Society. They can be reached via the Internet or by phone.

The nurse also plays a key role in offering emotional support, determining appropriate sources of support, and helping the woman use effective coping strategies. A recent research study found that social support from the woman's family, friends, and coworkers is one of the strongest predictors of how well she will cope (Garner et al., 2015). Implications for nurses working with women following a cancer diagnosis include assessing women's definitions and availability of support; respecting varied needs for informational support; providing a supportive clinical environment; educating clinicians, family, and friends regarding unsupportive responses within the cultural context; and validating women's control and balancing of support needs. Nurses are well positioned to provide women with anticipatory guidance from diagnosis to the end of treatment (Shirvani & Alhani, 2015). Women without a social support network may need a social work referral or may need to be guided toward support groups to receive the emotional support they need.

In addition, cancer clients have a strong need for hope. Strategies for inspiring hope may include active listening, touch, presence, and helping clients overcome communication barriers. Often it is not what nurses say or do but just their presence that counts.

Assessment

Assessment of a woman with cancer of the reproductive tract involves a thorough history and physical examination. In addition, various laboratory and diagnostic tests may be done to evaluate for a malignancy.

Health History and Physical Examination

Interview the woman carefully to determine any current or past factors that might increase her risk of cancer, such as early menarche, late menopause, sexually transmitted infections (STIs), use of hormonal agents, or infertility. Find out if the woman has a family history of cancer. Be thorough in obtaining the woman's past medical history, especially her reproductive, obstetric, and gynecologic history. Ask about her lifestyle and behaviors, including risky behaviors such as engaging in unprotected sexual intercourse or sexual intercourse with multiple partners. Find out if she has had routine or recommended screening procedures.

Ask if the woman has had any symptoms, such as abnormal vaginal bleeding or discharge or vaginal discomfort. Often the symptoms of cancer are vague and nonspecific and the woman may attribute them to another problem, such as aging, stress, or improper diet.

Perform a complete physical examination, including a review of body systems and a pelvic examination. Observe for lesions or masses in the perineal area. Note any masses when palpating the abdomen or when performing the pelvic examination.

Laboratory and Diagnostic Testing

Some of the laboratory and diagnostic tests used to help diagnose cancer of the reproductive tract are discussed in Common Laboratory and Diagnostic Tests 8.1.

COMMON LABORATORY AND DIAGNOSTIC TESTS 8.1

Test	Explanation	Indications	Nursing Implications
Clinical breast examination	Assessment of the breast for abnormal findings; client may discover lump herself; high-risk history for breast cancer	Identifies palpable mass, skin change, inverted nipple, or unresolved rash	• Educate client to perform breast self-examination and report any abnormalities of high risk. • Reinforce the need for frequent clinical breast examinations if risk factors are present.
Mammography	Screening modality for breast cancer or any distortion in breast tissue architecture	Detects calcifications, densities, and nonpalpable cancer lesions	Stress the importance of annual mammograms for all women after the age of 40 or 50, depending on their risk history.
Pap smear	Cervical cytology screening to diagnose cervical cancers	Aids in detecting abnormal cells of the cervix (from squamocolumnar junction of the cervix; most cervical cancers arise here)	Encourage all sexually active women to receive a pelvic examination, including a Pap smear if they have a high risk profile, to promote early detection of cervical cancer.
Transvaginal ultrasound	Screening for pelvic pathology to assist in diagnosing endometrial cancers	Allows measurement of endometrial thickness to determine if endometrial biopsy is needed for postmenopausal bleeding	• Review the risk factors for the development of endometrial cancer and reason for this screening test. • Assist in preparing the client for this examination.
CA-125	Nonspecific blood test used as a tumor marker	Elevation of marker suggests malignancy but is not specific to ovarian cancer.	• Review risk factors for ovarian cancer and explain that a series of diagnostic tests may be performed (transvaginal ultrasound, CT scan, CA-125) to assist in the diagnosis and treatment plan. • Elevated marker levels are not specific to ovarian cancer; they can be elevated in other types of cancer.

Adapted from American Cancer Society [ACS]. (2015b). *American Cancer Society guidelines for the early detection of cancer.* Retrieved from http://www.cancer.org/Healthy/FindCancerEarly/CancerScreeningGuidelines/american-cancer-society-guidelines-for-the-early-detection-of-cancer; Centers for Disease Control and Prevention [CDC]. (2015b). *Cancer prevention and control.* Retrieved from http://www.cdc.gov/cancer/dcpc/prevention/other.htm; and National Cancer Institute [NCI]. (2015c). *General cancer prevention.* Retrieved from http://www.cancer.gov/cancertopics/prevention#General+Cancer+Prevention+Information.

Nursing Diagnoses and Related Interventions

Upon completion of a thorough assessment, the nurse might identify several nursing diagnoses, including:

- Deficient knowledge
- Disturbed body image
- Anxiety
- Fear
- Pain

Nursing goals, interventions, and evaluation for women with a reproductive cancer are based on the nursing diagnoses. Nursing Care Plan 8.1 may be used as a guide in planning nursing care for women with a reproductive cancer. It should be individualized based on the woman's symptoms and needs.

Nurses have traditionally served as advocates in the health care arena and should continue to be on the forefront of health education and diagnosis, acting as leaders in the fight against cancer. Over half a

---

NURSING CARE PLAN 8.1

Overview of a Woman with a Reproductive Tract Cancer

Molly, a thin 28-year-old woman, comes to the free health clinic complaining of a thin, watery vaginal discharge and spotting after sex. Molly says she has had multiple sex partners since the age of 15. She had an abnormal Pap smear "a while back" but didn't return to the clinic for follow-up. Cervical cancer is suspected.

NURSING DIAGNOSIS: Anxiety related to uncertainty of diagnosis, possible diagnosis of cancer, and eventual outcome as evidenced by client's report of signs and symptoms and statements of being worried and not knowing what she would do

Outcome Identification and Evaluation

The client will demonstrate measures to cope with anxiety *as evidenced by statements acknowledging anxiety, use of positive coping strategies, and verbalization that anxiety has decreased.*

Interventions: *Reducing Anxiety*

- Encourage client to express her feelings and concerns *to reduce her anxiety and to determine appropriate interventions.*
- Assess the meaning of the diagnosis to the client, clarify misconceptions, and provide reliable, realistic information *to enhance her understanding of her condition, subsequently reducing her anxiety.*
- Assess client's psychological status *to determine the degree of emotional distress related to diagnosis and treatment options.*

- Identify and address verbalized concerns, providing information about what to expect *to decrease uncertainty about the unknown.*
- Assess the client's use of coping mechanisms in the past and their effectiveness *to foster use of positive strategies.*
- Teach client about early signs of anxiety and help her recognize them (e.g., fast heartbeat, sweating, or feeling flushed) *to minimize escalation of anxiety.*
- Provide positive reinforcement that the client's condition can be managed *to relieve her anxiety.*

NURSING DIAGNOSIS: Deficient knowledge related to diagnosis, prevention strategies, disease course, and treatment as evidenced by client's statements about hoping nothing bad is wrong, lack of follow-up for previous abnormal Pap test, and high-risk behaviors

Outcome Identification and Evaluation

The client will demonstrate an understanding of diagnosis, *as evidenced by making health-promoting lifestyle choices, verbalizing appropriate health care practices, describing condition once diagnosed, and adhering to measures to comply with therapy.*

NURSING CARE PLAN 8.1

Overview of a Woman with a Reproductive Tract Cancer (continued)

Interventions: *Providing Client Teaching*

- Assess client's current knowledge about her diagnosis and proposed therapeutic regimen *to establish a baseline from which to develop a teaching plan.*
- Review contributing factors associated with development of reproductive tract cancer, including lifestyle behaviors, *to foster an understanding of the etiology of cervical cancer.*
- Review information about treatments and procedures and recommendations for healthy lifestyle, obtaining feedback frequently *to validate adequate understanding of instructions.*
- Discuss strategies, including using condoms and limiting the number of sexual partners, *to reduce the risk of transmission of STIs*, including HPV, which is associated with cervical cancer.
- Encourage client to obtain prompt treatment of any vaginal or cervical infections *to minimize the risk for cervical cancer.*
- Urge the client to have an annual Pap smear and/or HPV test *to allow screening and early detection.*
- Describe the treatment measures used *to provide client with knowledge of what may be necessary.*
- Provide written material with pictures *to allow for client review and to help her visualize what is occurring in her body.*
- Inform client about available community resources and make appropriate referrals as needed *to provide additional education and support.*
- Document details of teaching and learning *to allow for continuity of care and further education, if needed.*

NURSING DIAGNOSIS: Disturbed body image related to suspected reproductive tract cancer and impact on client's sexuality and sense of self as evidenced by statement of being worried about not being the same

Outcome Identification and Evaluation

The client will verbalize or demonstrate a positive self-esteem in relation to body image as evidenced by positive statements about self, sexuality, and participation in activities with others.

Interventions: *Promoting Healthy Body Image*

- Assess client's use of self-criticism to determine client's current state of coping and adjustment.
- Determine if the client's change in body image has contributed to social isolation to provide a direction for care.
- Provide opportunities for client to explore her feelings related to issues of sexuality, including past behaviors that may have placed her at risk, to minimize feelings of guilt about her condition.
- Acknowledge the client's feelings about possible changes in her body and sexuality and her illness to foster trust and allow client to ventilate feelings and concerns.
- Facilitate contact with other clients with the same type of cancer to promote sharing of feelings and decrease feelings of isolation.
- Initiate referrals for counseling and community support groups as necessary to assist client in gaining a positive image of herself.

million women in the United States will be diagnosed with cancer this year alone and more than half will die of it (Siegel, Miller, & Jemal, 2015). The public needs to know that not only are these deaths preventable, but many of the cancers themselves are preventable. Nurses need to work to improve the availability and quality of cancer-screening services, making them accessible to underserved and socioeconomically disadvantaged clients. Through a unified effort by health care providers, health policy experts, government agencies, health insurance companies, the media, educational institutions, and women themselves, along with consistency and continuity, nurses can offer quality care to all women with cancer.

Educating to Prevent Cancer

Globally, there are nearly 13 million new cases of cancer and 8 million deaths from cancer each year. The most important cause of cancer is tobacco, which causes 30% of cancer deaths. Dietary factors, including obesity, are estimated to cause around 25% of cancer deaths, and alcohol about 6% of cancer deaths. All of these factors associated with cancer are preventable (Key, 2015). Nurses need to provide clients with information to help prevent disease and enhance quality of life. Educate women about the importance of consistent and timely screenings to identify cancer early. Emphasize the importance of having an annual pelvic examination. Also, stress the need for follow-up screenings as recommended. Provide clients with information if further diagnostic testing is required. Nurses also play a key role in promoting cancer awareness, prevention, and control. Advocate improving the availability of cancer-screening services and work to provide public education about risk factors for cancer.

Nurses can be instrumental in helping women to identify and change behaviors that put them at risk for various reproductive tract cancers (Teaching Guidelines 8.1). Do not limit your interventions to providing preventive education only: inform women about the consequences of doing nothing about their conditions and what the long-range outcomes might be without treatment. For example, stress the importance of visiting a health care provider if certain signs and symptoms appear:

- Blood in a bowel movement is considered abnormal
- Unusual vaginal discharge or chronic vulvar itching
- Persistent abdominal bloating or constipation
- Irregular vaginal bleeding
- Persistent low backache not related to standing
- Elevated or discolored vulvar lesions
- Bleeding after menopause
- Pain or bleeding after sexual intercourse

Teaching Guidelines 8.1
REDUCING YOUR RISK FOR CANCER

- Do not smoke; smoking is linked to lung cancer development.
- Drink alcohol only in moderation (no more than one drink daily).
- Be physically active daily.
- Eat a healthy diet.
- Stay current with immunizations.
- Use a condom with every sexual encounter.
- Reach and maintain a healthy weight.
- Take preventive medicines if needed.
- Get recommended screening tests:
  - Body mass index (BMI) to identify obesity
  - Mammogram every 1 to 2 years starting at age 40
  - Pap smear every 1 to 3 years if sexually active, between the ages of 21 and 65
  - Cholesterol checked annually starting at age 45
  - Blood pressure checked at least every 2 years
  - Diabetes test if hypertensive or hypercholesterolemia
  - Check for STIs if sexually active

Adapted from Agency for Healthcare Research and Quality. (2014). *Cancer screening and treatment in women: Recent findings.* Retrieved from http://www.ahrq.gov/research/findings/factsheets/women/cancerwom/; American Cancer Society [ACS]. (2015b). *American Cancer Society guidelines for the early detection of cancer.* Retrieved from http://www.cancer.org/Healthy/FindCancerEarly/CancerScreeningGuidelines/american-cancer-society-guidelines-for-the-early-detection-of-cancer; Mayo Clinic. (2015). *Cancer prevention: 7 steps to reduce your risk.* Retrieved from http://www.mayoclinic.org/cancer-prevention/art-20044816; National Cancer Institute [NCI]. (2015c). *General cancer prevention.* Retrieved from http://www.cancer.gov/cancertopics/prevention#General+Cancer+Prevention+Information; and World Health Organization. (2015). Cancer prevention and control. Retrieved from http://www.who.int/nmh/a5816/en/.

Teaching the Client About Her Diagnosis

Provide information about tests that may be required to confirm or rule out the diagnosis. Review with the woman what she has been told about her diagnosis and her understanding of her condition. It is not unusual for the woman to hear the diagnosis and then become overwhelmed by the thought of cancer, blocking out whatever is said after that. Answer any questions she may have. Go slowly and repeat the information as necessary. Use written materials to explain and reinforce the teaching. Provide information about her condition and recommended therapies. For example, if a client is undergoing surgery, discuss postoperative issues such as incision care, pain, and activity level. Instruct the client on health maintenance activities after treatment, and inform her and her family about available support resources.

Providing Emotional Support

Once the diagnosis is made, provide the woman and her family with emotional support. Validate the client's feelings and provide realistic hope, using a nonjudgmental approach and therapeutic communication skills during all interactions. Nurses can be invaluable when assisting women who are coping with the uncertainty of their future by providing positive communication and support. Nurses need to focus on the physical, psychosocial, and economic concerns, from diagnosis through treatment and, if applicable, until the end of life, for all of the women for whom they care. Individualize the care based on the client's cultural traditions and beliefs, as explained in the following section.

ENSURING CULTURALLY COMPETENT CANCER CARE

Cultural diversity in America is increasing, and as diverse cultures interact, conflicts inevitably ensue. These conflicts can affect health care outcomes. Providing culturally competent cancer care can improve outcomes and decrease disparities in care. If nurses are to meet the needs of ethnically diverse populations, they must be culturally sensitive, appreciative of differing health beliefs and practices, and very flexible in the way they approach health care. It is we who must adapt, expand, and learn.

Nurses have the opportunity to learn about diverse cultures, religions, and faith traditions that support clients and families during their cancer journey and while facing a serious life-limiting illness. Nursing care practices should embrace all clients with whom they come in contact and, by having a better understanding of diverse groups, nurses can build trust in clients seeking oncology care needs that range from detection to diagnosis to treatment possibly through palliative and end-of-life care also.

Be aware of the client's cultural background, religion, migration history, degree of acculturation, living conditions, educational level, and legal status, because each of these factors can affect the client's understanding of her diagnosis and the eventual outcome. A woman's reaction to a cancer diagnosis and her decisions about treatment are influenced by an individual's cultural values and how the community views cancer. A diagnosis of cancer carries deep physical, psychosocial, and cultural implications. Sensitive cross-cultural communication and cultural competence are vital for all nurses to deliver equal care to all cancer clients. Nurses need to understand the disparities and the influence of those disparities on health outcomes. Women with cancer reflect the demographic changes occurring in the United States and represent increasing differences in culture, religion, socioeconomic status, race, and lifestyle. Through embracing and learning from these differences, nurses become stronger care providers (Surbone, 2015).

In some cultures, sharing news of a serious illness like cancer is considered disrespectful and impolite. For example, some Europeans view such sharing as inhumane; the Asian culture views a cancer diagnosis as unnecessarily cruel. The Chinese, out of respect for aging family members, withhold discussions of serious illness to avoid causing unnecessary anxieties (Lofters, 2015). Integrate this knowledge in your care to ensure a culturally competent approach.

Take Note!

When a diagnosis of cancer is made, assessing an individual's strengths and weaknesses from a cultural perspective will help the nurse to provide culturally competent care.

As life becomes increasingly multilingual, multicultural, and multi-religious, learning about clients' values and cultural beliefs becomes challenging. Be willing to learn about client preferences; doing so promotes caring and nurturing.

SUPPORTING THE PREGNANT WOMAN WITH CANCER

Pregnancy complicated by cancer is relatively rare, occurring in one out of every 1,000 pregnancies (CancerNet, 2015a). The incidence is increasing because women in Western societies are tending to delay childbearing to the third and fourth decade of life; this phenomenon is going to be encountered more often in the future by nurses. The most frequent malignancies diagnosed during pregnancy are breast cancer, cervical cancer, hematologic malignancies (lymphomas and acute leukemia), and melanoma. Breast cancer is the most common cancer diagnosed in pregnant women which affects approximately one in 3,000 pregnancies. Less common tumors during pregnancy are gastrointestinal, ovarian, urologic, and lung cancers (Amant et al., 2015).

Theoretically, changes in the mother's immune system during pregnancy can increase the risk of malignancy because cell-mediated immunity, which is suppressed in pregnant women, normally protects against cancerous tumors (Kim & Chu, 2015). Some research has hinted at an increased rate of progression and decreased survival times in women who develop breast and cervical cancer and then become pregnant, but this generally has not been validated by research studies. With the cooperation of multidisciplinary teams, treatment of cancer during pregnancy with normal fetal outcome is feasible (Andersson et al., 2015).

Ovarian cancer during pregnancy is rare because the disease typically occurs in older women. Because most pregnant women receive frequent medical care, including pelvic examinations, most ovarian cancers in pregnant women are found at early stages; this carries a good prognosis for both the mother and the newborn. The presence of ascites indicates advanced disease (de Haan, Verheecke, & Amant, 2015).

Endometrial cancer is the most common neoplasia of the female reproductive system, with the highest incidence among uterine malignancies. It is rarely associated with pregnancy. Adenocarcinoma associated with pregnancy is typically endometrioid, focal, well-differentiated, and minimally invasive. Active treatment of endometrial cancer is incompatible with the continuation of the pregnancy. Since routine screening for endometrial cancer is currently not recommended in the general population, few cases would be detected in the relatively young pregnant population (*Cancer in Pregnancy*, 2015a). Cervical cancer is more common in the pregnant population than other reproductive malignancies, and it can affect the woman's health status and the pregnancy. Approximately 30% of women diagnosed with cervical cancer are in their reproductive years, whereas 3% of cervical cancers are diagnosed during pregnancy (*Cancer in Pregnancy*, 2015b). Management of cervical cancer during pregnancy depends on the following factors:

- Stage of the disease (and the tumor size)
- Nodal status
- Histologic subtype of the tumor
- Term of the pregnancy
- Whether the client wishes to continue her pregnancy
- Woman's desire for future fertility

In women with early-stage disease and absence of nodal involvement who are diagnosed during the first two trimesters of pregnancy, there is an increasing tendency to preserve the pregnancy while awaiting fetal maturity. The birth (when the fetal maturity is attained) should be performed using a cesarean section (ACS, 2015c). Treatment decisions are influenced by the stage of the cancer, the histologic type, the stage of the pregnancy, and the client's wishes. Both maternal and fetal safety and well-being have to be taken into account. Termination of pregnancy is not indicated in all cases. Pregnancy preservation in tumors diagnosed during early gestation is feasible in carefully selected cases. Discussion with the client and her family is essential and treatment has to be individualized (ACS, 2015c).

Nurses caring for young clients with cervical cancer must be aware of the surgical fertility preservation options, which clients are candidates for these surgeries, and the options for future assisted reproductive technology. Nurses need to be able to coordinate care for these clients with gynecologic oncologists and reproductive endocrinologists in order to facilitate optimal outcomes.

Women diagnosed with any malignancy during pregnancy must confront the reality of the disease and its impact on their future fertility and live with the risk of recurrence. The prognosis for a pregnant woman with cancer is often the same as other women of the same age with the same type of cancer (Cancer.Net, 2015a). The wishes of the pregnant woman and her family are of paramount importance when making decisions about continuing the pregnancy and undergoing cancer treatment. Some women will decide to terminate the pregnancy for the sake of their own health; others will undergo treatment during the pregnancy to preserve the life of the unborn child. Regardless of the woman's decision, provide support, hope, and education during treatment, birth, and beyond.

OVARIAN CANCER

Ovarian cancer is a malignant neoplastic growth of the ovary (Fig. 8.1). It is the ninth most common cancer among women and the fifth most common cause of cancer deaths for women in the United States. It accounts for more deaths than any other cancer of the reproductive system (ACS, 2015d). A woman's risk of getting invasive ovarian cancer in her lifetime is about 1 in 75. Her lifetime chance of dying from invasive ovarian cancer is about 1 in 100 (ACS, 2015d). This cancer mainly develops in older women. About half of the women who are diagnosed with ovarian cancer are 63 years or older. It is more common in White women than in African American women (ACS, 2015d).

The most important variable influencing the prognosis is the extent of the disease. Survival depends on the stage of the tumor, grade of differentiation, gross findings at surgery, amount of residual tumor after surgery, and effectiveness of any adjunct treatment postoperatively. Many women with ovarian cancer will experience recurrence despite best efforts to eradicate the cancer through surgery, radiation, or chemotherapy to eliminate residual tumor cells. The likelihood of long-term survival in the event of recurrence is dismal (Matsumoto, Onada, & Yaegashi, 2015). The 5-year survival rates (the percentage of women who live at least 5 years after their diagnosis) are shown in Table 8.1 according to stage.

Pathophysiology

Ovarian cancer, the cause of which is unknown, can originate from different cell types. Most ovarian cancers are thought to originate in the ovarian epithelium. New insights now propose a pivotal role for the fallopian tube during ovarian cancer pathogenesis. Increasing evidence suggests

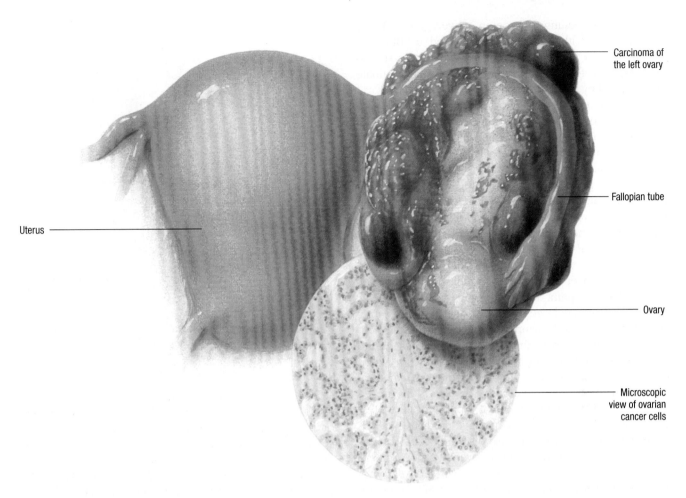

FIGURE 8.1 Ovarian cancer. (Asset provided by Anatomical Chart Co.)

that serous ovarian cancer originates from the fimbriated distal end of the fallopian tube, whereas the ovary gets only involved at a later stage. These represent 50% to 60% of all epithelial ovarian cancers. Based on this finding, a post-reproductive salpingectomy deserves consideration as a prophylactic intervention that may confer protection against an often deadly disease (Poole et al., 2015).

TABLE 8.1	FIVE-YEAR SURVIVAL RATES FOR OVARIAN CANCER
Stage	Five-Year Relative Survival Rates
I	80%–94%
II	57%–76%
III	34%–45%
IV	18%

Adapted from American Cancer Society [ACS]. (2015o). *Survival rates for ovarian cancer by stage.* Retrieved from http://www.cancer.org/cancer/ovariancancer/detailedguide/ovarian-cancer-survival-rates.

Tumors usually present as solid masses that have spread beyond the ovary and seeded into the peritoneum prior to diagnosis. A thorough understanding of the true pathogenesis of this cancer's origin could lead to the development of new and more effective therapies as well as novel biomarkers in early detection.

Screening and Diagnosis

Women with ovarian cancer are typically diagnosed at a late stage, when the cancer has spread into the peritoneal cavity and complete surgical removal is challenging. Seventy-five percent of ovarian cancers are not diagnosed until the cancer has advanced to stage III or IV, primarily because there is still no adequate screening test. The five-year survival time for women diagnosed at this stage is 30%, in contrast with a five-year survival of 90% for women diagnosed at an early stage (Wright et al., 2015). The United States Preventive Services Task Force (USPSTF) (2015), along with the American College of Obstetricians and Gynecologists (ACOG) and the American Medical Association (AMA), recently reviewed the evidence for ovarian cancer screening and did not recommend screening for women at average risk. However, women with increased risk related to BRCA ½ mutations or a family history of ovarian cancer should be considered for genetic counseling to further evaluate their risk (Cliby et al., 2015).

Two genes, BRCA1 and BRCA2, are linked with hereditary breast and ovarian cancers. Blood tests can be performed to assess DNA in white blood cells to detect mutations in the BRCA genes. These genetic markers do not predict whether the person will develop cancer. Rather, they provide information regarding the risk of developing cancer: a woman who is BRCA positive may have up to an 80% chance of developing breast cancer and a 40% chance of developing ovarian cancer (Liede, Sun, & Narod, 2015).

To assist in screening, researchers have developed an ovarian cancer symptom index that includes pelvic and abdominal pain, urinary frequency and urgency, increased abdominal size (bloating), and difficulty eating (feeling full). But this symptom index is not much help in detecting the disease early, as these symptoms tend to go unrecognized, leading to delays in diagnosis. When the presentation of such symptoms triggers a medical evaluation for ovarian cancer, the disease is diagnosed in only 1 in 100 women. The NCI reports that the present symptom index has a "low positive predictive value," especially for early-stage disease discovery (2015d).

Specific clinical guidelines for ovarian cancer screening have not been developed, so the disease is often not diagnosed until it has metastasized. The USPSTF recommends against routine screening for ovarian cancer with serum CA-125 or transvaginal ultrasound because earlier detection would have a small effect, at best, on mortality. CA-125 is a biologic tumor marker associated with ovarian cancer. Although its levels are elevated in many women with ovarian cancer, CA-125 is not specific for this cancer, and the levels may be elevated with other malignancies too (pancreatic, liver, colon, breast, and lung cancers). Despite the discovery that CA-125 and other serum markers increase before the clinical onset of ovarian cancer, it has proven surprisingly difficult to devise a successful screening program for asymptomatic women with ovarian cancer. Currently, it is not sensitive enough to serve as a screening tool alone (Ebell et al., 2015). The USPSTF (2015) reports that there is no supporting evidence that any screening test, including CA-125, ultrasound, or pelvic exam, reduces mortality from ovarian cancer. Thus, they recommend against routine screening for ovarian cancer.

Therapeutic Management

Treatment options for ovarian cancer vary depending on the stage and severity of the disease. Usually, a laparoscopy (abdominal exploration with an endoscope) is performed for diagnosis and staging, as well

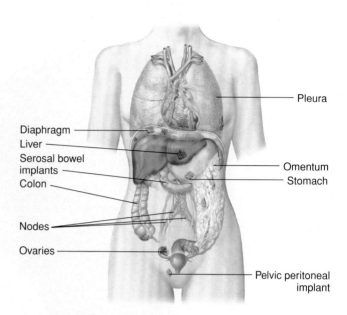

FIGURE 8.2 Common metastatic sites for ovarian cancer. (Asset provided by Anatomical Chart Co.)

as evaluation for therapy. In stage I, the cancer is limited to the ovaries. In stage II, the growth involves one or both ovaries, with pelvic extension. Stage III cancer has spread to the lymph nodes and other organs or structures inside the abdominal cavity. In stage IV, the cancer has metastasized to distant sites (Alexander et al., 2014). Figure 8.2 shows the likely metastatic sites for ovarian cancer.

Surgical intervention remains the mainstay of management of ovarian cancer. Surgery generally includes a total abdominal hysterectomy, bilateral salpingo-oophorectomy, peritoneal biopsies, omentectomy (excision of all or part of the omentum, which is a sheet of fat covered by the peritoneum that protects the abdominal structures), and pelvic para-aortic lymph node sampling to evaluate cancer extension (Nick et al., 2015). Because most women are diagnosed with advanced-stage ovarian cancer, aggressive management involving debulking or cytoreductive surgery is commonly performed. This surgery involves resecting all visible tumors from the peritoneum, taking peritoneal biopsies, sampling lymph nodes, and removing all reproductive organs and the omentum. This aggressive surgery has been shown to improve long-term survival rates.

Additional therapy with radiation may be warranted. Chemotherapy is recommended for all stages of ovarian cancer. Intraperitoneal chemotherapy, combined with surgery, has produced encouraging results for overall survivals at acceptable morbidity and mortality rates. Despite all of these therapies, virtually, the only agreement about treatment for advanced disease is that surgery and chemotherapy play a role, and that current treatment is effective in far too many women (Helm, 2015a).

Nursing Assessment

Ovarian cancers are considered the worst of all the gynecologic malignancies, primarily because they develop slowly and remain silent without symptoms until the cancer is far advanced. It has been described as the "overlooked disease" or "silent killer" because women and health care providers often ignore or rationalize early symptoms. For example, women may attribute gastrointestinal problems to stress and midlife changes. However, these vague complaints may precede more obvious symptoms by months. The most common early symptoms include abdominal bloating, early satiety, fatigue, vague abdominal pain, urinary frequency, diarrhea or constipation, malaise, and unexplained weight loss or gain. The later symptoms include anorexia, dyspepsia, ascites, a palpable abdominal mass, pelvic pain, and back pain (Goldstein et al., 2015).

Obtain a thorough history of the woman's symptoms, including their onset, duration, and frequency. Review the woman's history for risk factors such as:

- Nulliparity
- Early menarche (before 12 years old)
- Late menopause (after 55 years old)
- Increasing age after menopause
- High-fat diet
- Obesity
- Persistent ovulation over time
- First-degree relative with ovarian cancer
- Genetics—women of Ashkenazi Jewish decent
- Use of perineal talcum powder or hygiene sprays
- Older than 30 years at first pregnancy
- Positive BRCA1 and BRCA2 mutations
- Personal history of breast, bladder, or colon cancer
- Hormone replacement therapy (HRT) for more than 10 years
- Infertility (CDC, 2015c)

Perform a complete physical examination. Inspect the abdomen, noting any distention or bloating. Palpate the abdomen. Be alert for a mass or pain on palpation. Anticipate further testing to confirm the diagnosis.

Nursing Management

The complexities of ovarian cancer make a multidisciplinary approach necessary for optimal management. With the subtle nature and high risk of recurrence and mortality of this condition, most women find it an emotionally exhausting and devastating experience. The presence of hope is essential for women at the time of the diagnosis; they want to believe in being cured and able to continue their life as usual with loved ones, friends, and relatives. Still, the newly received cancer diagnosis makes women oscillate between hope and hopelessness, between positive expectations of getting cured and frightening feelings of the disease taking command. Nurses are invaluable resources in inspiring clients to find hope in life when diagnosed with cancer. Nursing management needs to focus on measures to promote early detection, educate the woman about the disease and its treatments, and provide emotional support. Nurses should show a positive attitude that communicates understanding and reassurance.

Promoting Early Detection

Nurses need to ensure that women are aware of the risk factors for ovarian cancer. Urge women not to dismiss seemingly innocuous symptoms as "just a part of aging." Encourage women to describe such nonspecific complaints at health visits.

Assess the woman's family and personal history for risk factors and encourage genetic testing for women with affected family members. Outline screening guidelines for women with hereditary cancer syndrome and inform women at high risk about the appropriate screening strategies.

Urge women to have yearly bimanual pelvic examinations and a transvaginal ultrasound to allow identification of ovarian masses in their early stages. After menopause, a mass on an ovary is not a cyst: physiologic cysts can arise only from a follicle that has not ruptured or from the cystic degeneration of the corpus luteum. Ovarian cancer is not always silent, and may manifest with several vague gastrointestinal symptoms. Although screening the general population is not recommended, nurses need to know what factors place women at high risk and really listen to women's complaints to detect this type of cancer before it becomes advanced.

Take Note!

A small ovarian "cyst" found on ultrasound in an asymptomatic postmenopausal woman should arouse suspicion. Any mass or ovary palpated in a postmenopausal woman should be considered cancerous until proven otherwise (Helm, 2015b).

Educating the Client

Education is a major focus of nursing care. This teaching involves risk reduction and health promotion. Teach the woman about risk reduction strategies; for instance, pregnancy, use of oral contraceptives, and breast-feeding reduce the risk of ovarian cancer. Instruct women to avoid using talc and hygiene sprays on their genitals. Review the lifetime risks related to *BRCA1* and *BRCA2* genes and options available should the woman test positive for these genes. Help to promote community awareness of ovarian cancer by educating the public about risk-reducing behaviors. See research on reproductive cancer risk factor (Evidence-Based Practice 8.1).

EVIDENCE-BASED PRACTICE 8.1   **DOES OVARIAN STIMULATION FOR IVF INCREASE GYNECOLOGICAL CANCER RISK? A SYSTEMATIC REVIEW AND META-ANALYSIS**

STUDY

Drugs to stimulate ovulation have been widely used for various types of subfertility since the early 1960s, and their use has increased in recent years. The use of assisted reproductive techniques is increasing, but the possible link between fertility drugs and reproductive cancer remains controversial. Subfertile women are commonly exposed to these agents, which may be administered at high doses for long periods of time during treatment for subfertility. There is uncertainty about the safety of these drugs and the potential risk of causing cancers associated with their use. The objective of this study was to evaluate the risk of reproductive cancer in women previously treated with ovulation-stimulating drugs for infertility.

Findings

A systematic review and meta-analysis was conducted. Clinical trials that examined the association between ovarian stimulation for IVF and gynecologic cancers were included. Twelve cohort studies with 178,396 women exposed to IVF were included. The meta-analysis found no significant association between ovarian stimulation for IVF and increased ovarian, endometrial, cervical, and breast cancer risk. Ovarian stimulation for IVF, therefore, does not increase the gynecologic risk, whether hormone-dependent endometrial and breast cancer risk, or non–hormone-dependent ovarian and cervical cancer. This study found no convincing evidence of an increased risk of reproductive cancer with fertility drug treatment.

Nursing Implications

Nurses can use the information from this study to reassure women that having experienced infertility and undergone in vitro fertilization treatments in the past are not increasing their risk of having reproductive cancer later in life. When women are trying to decide to undergo fertility treatment using drug therapy, it can be very anxiety producing for them as well as their partners. Knowing that in vitro fertilization treatment will not increase their risk of reproductive cancer as they age based on earlier exposure to ovulation-stimulating drug therapy can reduce their anxiety regarding their decision.

Adapted from Li, Y., Zhao, J., Zhang, Q., & Wang, Y. (2015). Does ovarian stimulation for IVF increase gynecological cancer risk? A systematic review and meta-analysis. *Reproductive BioMedicine Online*. doi: 10.1016/j.rbmo.2015.03.008.

Instruct the woman about the importance of healthy lifestyles. Stress the importance of maintaining a healthy weight to reduce risk. Encourage women to eat a low-fat diet. Factors associated with a reduced risk of ovarian cancer include the use of oral contraceptives for 3 years or longer, pregnancy and breastfeeding before the age of 30, bilateral tubal ligation, and removal of the ovaries (Memorial Sloan Kettering Cancer Center, 2015).

For the woman who is diagnosed with ovarian cancer, describe in simple terms the tests, treatment modalities, and follow-up needed. For example, if the woman will be having surgery, the nurse needs to provide thorough teaching about what to expect before, during, and after surgery. Outline the treatment options and the implications of choices. Assist the woman and her family to decipher the myriad of information related to staging, tests, and treatments. Teach the woman about additional treatment measures, such as radiation therapy or chemotherapy, including how to handle the common adverse effects of treatment.

Supporting the Client and Family

The diagnosis of ovarian cancer, like any cancer, can be overwhelming. In addition, the treatments and their effects can be highly stressful, both physically and emotionally. Provide one-to-one support for women facing treatment for ovarian cancer. Ovarian cancer involves the reproductive system, which has a direct impact on the

Consider This

I felt I was a lucky woman because I had been in remission from breast cancer for 12 years, and I had been given the gift of life to share with my beloved family. Recently I became ill with stomach problems: pain, indigestion, bloating, and nausea. My doctor treated me for gastric reflux disease, but the symptoms persisted. I then was referred to a gastroenterologist, a urologist, and then a gynecologist, who did an ultrasound, which was negative. I received reassurance from all three that there was nothing wrong with me. As time went by, I experienced more pain, more symptoms, and increased frustration. Six months after seeing all three specialists, a repeat ultrasound revealed I had ovarian cancer, and I needed surgery as soon as possible. I underwent a complete hysterectomy and my surgeon found I was in stage III. Since then, I have undergone chemotherapy and participated in a clinical cancer study that wasn't successful for me, and now I am facing the fact that I am going to die soon.

Thoughts: This woman has tried everything to save her life, but, alas, time has run out for her with advanced ovarian cancer. Women diagnosed with breast cancer are at a significant risk for developing ovarian cancer later in life. Of the string of doctors she saw, one has to ponder why none ordered more extensive testing, given her history of breast cancer. We are haunted with the question: If they had, would she be in stage III now? We will never know.

woman's view of herself. Encourage open discussion of sexuality and the impact of cancer. Listen and support the woman and her family as they try to cope with this disease. By being aware of women's individual needs and different coping strategies, nurses can improve support to women in this vulnerable situation. Encourage the use of appropriate coping strategies to allow for the best quality of life. Try to restore hope to women with ovarian cancer, and stress treatment compliance. Nurses should not forget about the family caregivers who need help with managing emotions about prognosis, balancing their own and the client's needs, work, and decision-making when there is uncertainty. If appropriate, encourage participation in clinical trials to offer hope for all women. Continue to offer support to the woman and her family members as they experience sadness and grief.

ENDOMETRIAL CANCER

Endometrial cancer (also known as uterine cancer) is a malignant neoplastic growth of the uterine lining. It is the fourth most common gynecologic malignancy and accounts for 6% of all cancers in women in the United States or 1 in 37 women. The NCI (2015e) estimates that about 54,870 new cases will be diagnosed in women in 2015 and that approximately 10,170 of these women will die. Endometrial cancer is responsible for over 75,000 deaths annually among women worldwide (Siegel et al., 2015). It is uncommon before the age of 55, but as women age, their risk of endometrial cancer increases. Approximately 80% of these malignancies are carcinomas of the endometrium. Because endometrial cancer is usually diagnosed in the early stages, it has a better prognosis than cervical or ovarian cancer (ACS, 2015e).

The increasing incidence and prevalence of endometrial cancer can be explained by the increase in life expectancy, increased caloric intake, increased obesity rates, infertility, null parity (never bearing children), older age of first pregnancy, and long-term use of unopposed estrogens for HRT. Protection against endometrial cancer includes increased parity, daily physical activity, use of combined oral contraceptives, and increased age of women at last childbirth (Schmid et al., 2015).

Pathophysiology

Two mechanisms are believed to be involved in the development of endometrial cancer. A history of exposure to unopposed estrogen is the cause in approximately 80% of women. Those that are spontaneous and are unrelated to estrogen or endometrial hyperplasia represent the other 25% of endometrial cancers. There has been an increase in the incidence of women using estrogen replacement therapy (without progestin) and in obesity rates (adipose fat converts androstenedione to estrone,

thereby increasing circulating estrogen levels) that may contribute to endometrial cancer (Temple, 2015).

Endometrial cancer may originate in a polyp or in a diffuse multifocal pattern. The pattern of spread partially depends on the degree of cellular differentiation. Well-differentiated tumors tend to limit their spread to the surface of the endometrium. Metastatic spread occurs in a characteristic pattern and most commonly involves the lungs, inguinal and supraclavicular nodes, liver, bones, brain, and vagina (NCI, 2015f). Early tumor growth is characterized by friable and spontaneous bleeding. Later tumor growth is characterized by myometrial invasion and growth toward the cervix (Fig. 8.3).

Adenocarcinoma of the endometrium is typically preceded by hyperplasia. Carcinoma in situ is found only on the endometrial surface. Type I carcinomas, the most common, begin as endometrial hyperplasia and progress to carcinomas. Giving estrogen preparations without progestin for HRT leads to an increased risk for endometrial cancer. Type I is generally found at an earlier stage and treatment results are more favorable.

Unlike type I endometrial carcinoma, type II carcinomas appear spontaneously, are associated with a poorly differentiated cell type, and have a poor prognosis. They account for less than 10% of all endometrial cancers but contribute to the majority of all endometrial deaths. This type is unrelated to estrogen or endometrial hyperplasia (ACS, 2015f).

Remember Carmella, the woman with postmenopausal bleeding? In postmenopausal women, any bleeding is abnormal and warrants further assessment. What testing would the nurse anticipate as being ordered to confirm the diagnosis? What would be the nurse's role during this testing?

Screening and Diagnosis

There is no specific screening test currently available to detect endometrial cancer. Screening for endometrial cancer is not routinely done because it is not practical or cost effective. The ACS (2015f) recommends that women be informed about the risks and symptoms of endometrial cancer at the onset of menopause and strongly encouraged to report any unexpected bleeding or spotting to their health care provider. A pelvic examination is frequently normal in the early stages of the disease. Changes in the size, shape, or consistency of the uterus or its surrounding support structures may exist when the disease is more advanced.

During the past two decades, the role of ultrasound in the evaluation of postmenopausal bleeding has changed markedly, from little or no role to a major role today. In the intervening years, numerous studies have

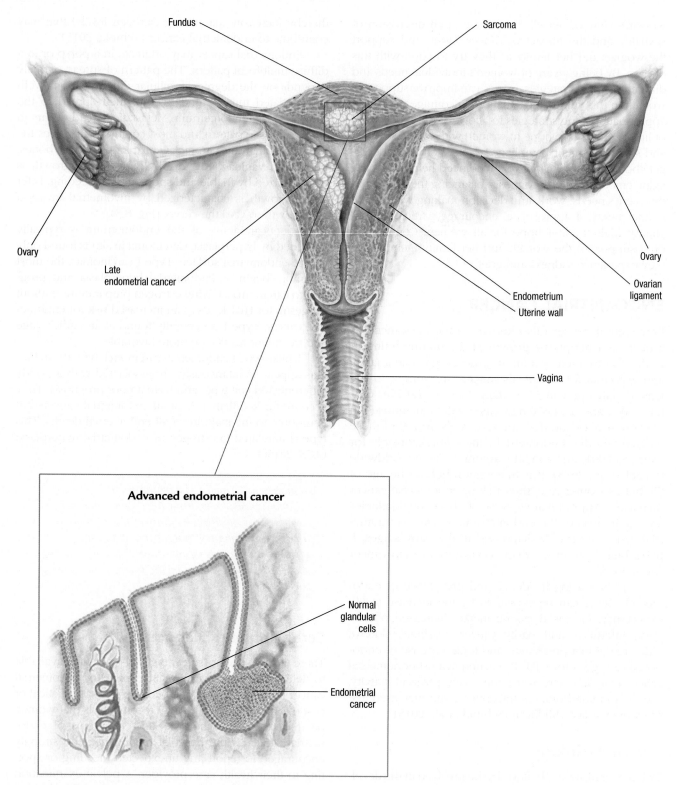

FIGURE 8.3 Progression of endometrial cancer. (Image 1 provided by Anatomical Chart Co.)

shown that ultrasound is at least as sensitive as endometrial biopsy for endometrial cancer and that ultrasound can reliably exclude cancer without the need for biopsy in some women with postmenopausal bleeding. The depth of myometrium is an important diagnostic factor.

In particular, numerous studies have shown that women with an endometrial thickness of 4 mm or less have an extremely low likelihood of endometrial cancer and thus do not need to undergo endometrial biopsy. Ultrasound can also help in the selection of an appropriate biopsy technique. In a woman with postmenopausal bleeding and a thick endometrium, a sonohysterogram can determine whether the endometrium is diffusely thick or has focal areas of thickening. With diffuse thickening, an endometrial biopsy is appropriate. When one or more focal areas of thickening are present, hysteroscopic biopsy is likely to be the better choice. Typically, the noninvasive ultrasound is done first before an invasive endometrial biopsy is attempted (Dueholm et al., 2015).

Transvaginal ultrasound can be used to evaluate the endometrial cavity and measure the thickness of the endometrial lining. It can be used to detect endometrial hyperplasia. If the endometrium measures less than 4 mm, then the client is at low risk for malignancy. Large prospective studies have shown that an endometrial thickness of ≤4 mm on transvaginal ultrasound in postmenopausal women with bleeding has a low risk of malignancy. Thus, in postmenopausal clients with bleeding, biopsy is not indicted when endometrial thickness is ≤4 mm, thereby avoiding invasive diagnostics (Wong et al., 2015).

Endometrial biopsy is an office procedure that is also one of the first steps in the diagnosis of endometrial cancer in a woman with postmenopausal bleeding. The biopsy is obtained through an endometrial suction catheter that is inserted through the cervix into the uterine cavity and a tissue sample is taken. The sensitivity and specificity of the biopsy procedure tend to be in the range of 95% for detection of endometrial cancer or other pathologies (King et al., 2015).

As indicated earlier, staging is the process of looking at all of the information the doctors have learned about the tumor to determine how much the cancer may have spread. The stage of an endometrial cancer is the most important factor in choosing a treatment plan. It can spread *locally* to other parts of the uterus or *regionally* to nearby lymph nodes. The regional lymph nodes are found in the pelvis and farther away along the aorta. Finally, the cancer can spread (*metastasize*) to distant lymph nodes or organs such as lung, liver, bone, brain, and others

In stage I, the tumor is confined to the corpus uteri. In stage II, it has spread to the cervix, but not outside the uterus. In stage III, it has spread locally and regionally. In stage IV, it has invaded the bladder mucosa and bowel mucosa, with distant metastases to the lungs, liver, and bone (International Federation of Gynecology and Obstetrics, 2015).

Therapeutic Management

Typically, the stage of the disease directs treatment. It usually involves surgery with adjunct therapy based on pathologic findings. Surgery most often involves removal of the uterus (hysterectomy) and the fallopian tubes and ovaries (salpingo-oophorectomy). Removal of the fallopian

tubes and ovaries is recommended because tumor cells spread early to the ovaries, and any dormant cancer cells could be stimulated to grow by ovarian estrogen. In more advanced cancers, radiation and chemotherapy are used as adjuncts to surgery. Routine surveillance intervals for follow-up care are typically every 3 to 4 months for the first 2 years, since 85% of recurrences occur in the first 3 years after diagnosis (Brennan et al., 2015).

Nursing Assessment

Obtain a thorough history from the woman, ascertaining her primary complaint. Most commonly, the major initial symptom of endometrial cancer is abnormal and painless vaginal bleeding. Obtain a menstrual history and inquire if the woman is taking any hormones. Also ascertain if she has a personal or family history of breast, ovarian, or colon cancer. These key pieces of information will assist in identifying the woman at high risk for endometrial cancer.

Take Note!

Any episode of bright-red bleeding that occurs after menopause should be investigated. Abnormal uterine bleeding is rarely the result of uterine malignancy in a young woman, but in the postmenopausal woman it should be regarded with suspicion.

Also review the woman's history for any risk factors, including:
- Nulliparity
- Obesity (more than 50 lb overweight)
- Liver disease
- Infertility
- Diabetes mellitus
- Hypertension
- History of pelvic radiation
- Polycystic ovary syndrome
- Early menarche (before 12 years old)
- High-fat diet
- Use of prolonged exogenous unopposed estrogen with an intact uterus
- Endometrial hyperplasia
- Family history of endometrial cancer
- Personal history of hereditary nonpolyposis colon cancer
- Personal history of breast, colon, or ovarian cancer
- History of uterine fibroids
- Late onset of menopause (after age 52 years)
- Tamoxifen use
- Chronic anovulation (Moses, 2015)

Assess the woman for additional manifestations, such as dyspareunia, low back pain, purulent genital discharge, dysuria, pelvic pain, weight loss, and a change in bladder and bowel habits. These may suggest advanced disease.

Perform a physical examination or assist with, as appropriate, a pelvic examination. Observe for vaginal discharge. Note any changes in the size, shape, or consistency of the uterus or surrounding structures or client reports of pain during examination. Anticipate the need for transvaginal ultrasound to identify endometrial hyperplasia (usually greater than 4 mm) and endometrial biopsy to identify malignant cells.

Nursing Management

Ensure that the woman understands all of the treatment options. Address any concerns the woman expresses, including questions about sexuality. Ensure that follow-up appointments are scheduled appropriately. Refer the client to a support group. Offer the woman and family explanations and emotional support throughout.

Educate the client about preventive measures or follow-up care if she has been treated for cancer. Education may be the most important tool currently available for the early detection of endometrial cancer. Many risk factors for endometrial cancer are modifiable or treatable, including obesity, hypertension, and diabetes. Educating women about risk factors and ways to decrease the risks is essential so that women can learn about their own risk profile and can become partners in the fight against this gynecologic cancer (Teaching Guidelines 8.2).

Teaching Guidelines 8.2
PREVENTIVE AND FOLLOW-UP MEASURES FOR ENDOMETRIAL CANCER

- Schedule regular pelvic examinations after the age of 21.
- Visit health care practitioner for early evaluation of any abnormal bleeding after menopause.
- Maintain a low-fat diet throughout life.
- Exercise daily.
- Manage weight to discourage hyperestrogenic states, which predispose to endometrial hyperplasia.
- Pregnancy serves as a protective factor by reducing estrogen.
- Ask your doctor about the use of combination estrogen and progestin pills.
- When combination oral contraceptives are taken to facilitate the regular shedding of the uterine lining, take risk reduction measures.
- Be aware of risk factors for endometrial cancer and make modifications as needed.
- Report any of the following symptoms immediately:
  - Bleeding or spotting after sexual intercourse
  - Bleeding that lasts longer than a week
  - Reappearance of bleeding after 6 months or more of no menses

- After cancer therapy, schedule follow-up appointments for the next few years.
- After cancer therapy, frequently communicate with your health care provider concerning your status.
- After surgery, maintain a healthy weight.

Carmella's endometrial biopsy indicates endometrial adenocarcinoma. Her health care provider recommends surgery and adjuvant radiation therapy. How long will Carmella need to follow up after surgery? What lifestyle changes will the nurse need to stress with Carmella?

CERVICAL CANCER

Cervical cancer is a malignancy located in the uterine cervix. It is the third most common genital malignancy in women in the United States, after cancers of the endometrium and the ovary. The ACS (2015g) estimates that over 13,000 cases of invasive cervical cancer will be diagnosed in the United States in women in 2015 and that approximately 4,100 of these women will die. Some researchers estimate that noninvasive cervical cancer (carcinoma in situ) is about four times more common than invasive cervical cancer. The 5-year survival rate for all stages of cervical cancer is 72% (ACS, 2015g). Cervical cancer is five to eight times more common in women affected with HIV or AIDS than those who are not. Hispanic women are most likely to get cervical cancer, followed by African Americans, Asians and Pacific Islanders, and Whites. Cervical cancer remains a disease of socioeconomic disparity. The high mortality rates of minorities are indicative of barriers to health care among those living in poverty. Hispanic women also have the highest rates of poverty, poor access to health care, and language and cultural barriers. Barriers to screening and prevention of cervical cancer include procrastination, fear of finding out that they have cancer, and embarrassment about having a Papanicolaou (Pap) test. In addition, most have little to no knowledge about HPV and its link with cancer (Strohl et al., 2015).

The incidence and mortality rates of cervical cancer have decreased noticeably in the past several decades, with most of the reduction attributed to the Pap test, which detects cervical cancer and some precancerous lesions. The Pap test (also known as a Pap smear) is a procedure used to obtain cells from the cervix for cytology screening. Cervical cancer is one of the most treatable cancers when detected at an early stage (ACS, 2015g). *Healthy People 2020* identifies several goals that address cervical cancer (*Healthy People 2020* 8.1; U.S. Department of Health & Human Services, 2015). Cervical cancer tends to occur in midlife. Most cases are found

Objectives	Nursing Significance
C-3 Reduce the female breast cancer death rate **C-4** Reduce the death rate from cancer of the uterine cervix **C-10** Reduce invasive uterine cervical cancer **C-11** Reduce late-stage female breast cancer **C-15** Increase the proportion of women who receive a cervical cancer screening based on the most recent guidelines **C-17** Increase the proportion of women who receive a breast cancer screening based on the most recent guidelines **C-18** Increase the proportion of women who were counseled about mammograms and Pap smear cancer screening consistent with current guidelines **C-20** Increase the proportion of persons who participate in behaviors that reduce their exposure to harmful ultraviolet (UV) irradiation and avoid sunburn	• Will help improve mortality rates and quality of life for women, and reduce health care costs related to treatment of malignancies. • Will help to promote screening and early detection. The National Institutes of Health (2015) reported that half of women diagnosed with invasive cervical cancer have never had a Pap smear and 10% have not had Pap smears during the past 5 years. • Will raise awareness of cancer screening and prevention on a local and national level to improve and promote the health of all women. • Will reduce the number of new cancer cases, as well as the illness, disability, and death caused by cancer. • Will reflect the importance of promoting evidence-based screening for cervical and breast cancer by lower mortality rates.

Note: *All cancer objectives project a 10% improvement from the baseline by 2020.*
Healthy People objectives based on data from http://www.healthypeople.gov.

in women younger than age 50. It rarely develops in women younger than age 20. Many older women do not realize that the risk of developing cervical cancer is still present as they age. The probability of a woman in the United States developing cervical cancer is approximately 1 in 120, but this statistic is age dependent; the highest incidence is in women 40 to 49 years of age (Sawaya et al., 2015).

Pathophysiology

Cervical cancer starts with abnormal changes in the cellular lining or surface of the cervix. Typically, these changes occur in the squamous–columnar junction of the cervix. Here, cylindrical secretory epithelial cells (columnar) meet the protective flat epithelial cells (squamous) from the outer cervix and vagina in what is termed the transformation zone. The continuous replacement of columnar epithelial cells by squamous epithelial cells in this area makes these cells vulnerable to taking up foreign or abnormal genetic material (ACS, 2015h). Figure 8.4 shows the pathophysiology of cervical cancer.

HPV infection must be present for cervical cancer to occur. HPV infections occur in a high percentage of sexually active women, but a successful immune response results in viral control or clearance of HPV. Most people

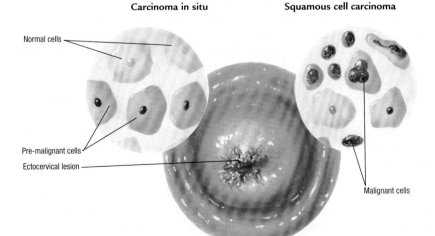
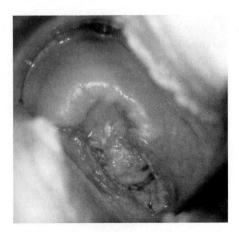

FIGURE 8.4 Cervical cancer. (Illustration is from The Anatomical Chart Company. [2009]. *Atlas of pathophysiology* [3rd ed.]. Philadelphia, PA: Lippincott Williams & Wilkins.)

who have HPV are asymptomatic and, therefore, do not realize they have the virus. More than 90% of squamous cervical cancers contain HPV DNA, and the virus is now accepted as a major causative factor in the development of cervical cancer and its precursor, cervical dysplasia (disordered growth of abnormal cells). Since only a small proportion of HPV infections progress to cancer, other factors must be involved in the process of carcinogenesis.

Screening and Diagnosis

Screening for cervical cancer is very effective because the presence of a precursor lesion, cervical intraepithelial neoplasia, helps determine whether further tests are needed. Lesions start as *dysplasia* and progress in a predictable fashion over a long period, allowing ample opportunity for intervention at a precancerous stage. Progression from low-grade to high-grade dysplasia takes an average of 9 years, and progression from high-grade dysplasia to invasive cancer takes up to 2 years. Three main factors have been postulated to influence the progression of low-grade dysplasia to high-grade dysplasia. These include the type and duration of viral infection, with high-risk HPV type and persistent infection predicting a higher risk for progression; host conditions that compromise immunity, such as multiparity or poor nutritional status; and environmental factors such as smoking, oral contraceptive use, or vitamin deficiencies. In addition, various gynecologic factors, including age of menarche, age of first intercourse, and number of sexual partners, significantly increase the risk for cervical cancer (Broadman & Matthews, 2015).

Widespread use of the Pap test is credited with saving tens of thousands of women's lives and decreasing deaths from cervical cancer. Routine Pap smear testing for all sexually active women has been one of the primary screening methods for early detection of cervical irregularities related to HPV and is crucial for the prevention of cervical cancer.

Despite its outstanding record of success as a screening tool for cervical cancer (it detects approximately 90% of early cancer changes), the conventional Pap smear has a 20% false-negative rate. High-grade abnormalities missed by human screening are frequently detected by computerized instruments (NCI, 2015g). Thus, many technologies have been developed to improve the sensitivity and specificity of Pap testing, including:

- *Thin-Prep:* In this liquid-based technique, the cervical specimen is placed into a vial of preservative solution rather than on a glass slide.
- *Computer-assisted automated Pap test rescreening (Autopap):* An algorithm-based decision-making technology identifies slides that should be rescreened by cytopathologists by selecting samples that exceed a certain threshold for the likelihood of abnormal cells.

- *HPV-DNA typing (Hybrid Capture):* This system uses the association between certain types of HPV (16, 18, 31, 33, 35, 45, 51, 52, and 56) and the development of cervical cancer. This system can identify high-risk HPV types and improves detection and management.
- *Computer-assisted technology (Cytyc CDS-1000, Auto-Cyte, AcCell):* These computerized instruments can detect abnormal cells that are sometimes missed by technologists (CDC, 2015d).

The high rate of false-negative results may also be due to other factors, including errors in sampling the cervix, in preparing the slide, and in client preparation. Although cytology-based nationwide cervical screening has been helpful in identifying abnormal cervical cells, the sensitivity of cytology for the detection of high-grade precursor lesions is limited. Additionally, adenocarcinoma and its precursors are often missed by cytology. The current insight that infection with HPV is the causative agent of cervical cancer and its precursors has led to the development of molecular tests for the detection of HPV. Strong evidence now supports the use of HPV testing in the prevention of cervical cancer. It is evident that HPV can be detected in urine-based testing which might eventually become a helpful tool in cervical cancer screening and HPV surveillance efforts. Nurses need to keep up to date on the latest research developments as well as the strengths and weaknesses of various screening methods (Fontenot, 2015).

Although professional medical organizations disagree as to the recommended frequency of screening for cervical cancer, ACOG (2015) recommends that cervical cancer screening should begin at age 21 years (regardless of sexual history), since women younger than age 21 are at very low risk of cancer. In addition, ACOG advises Pap smears every 3 years for women between ages 21 and 29 years and every 3 years for women between ages 30 and 65 years. A HPV co-test should be done every 5 years for this older age group. Cervical cancer screening can be stopped for women >65 years old with an adequate screening history. Women who have had a hysterectomy should stop screening. Women who have received the HPV vaccine should be screened according to the same guidelines as women who have not been vaccinated. In addition, women must have a clear understanding of the results of Pap smear testing and follow-up guidelines. High-risk women should continue to have annual Pap smears throughout their life (Table 8.2).

Pap smear results are classified using the Bethesda System (Box 8.1), which provides a uniform diagnostic terminology that allows clear communication between the laboratory and the health care provider. The information provided by the laboratory is divided into three categories: specimen adequacy, general categorization

TABLE 8.2	PAP SMEAR GUIDELINES
First Pap	Cervical cancer screening should begin at age 21. Women under age 21 should not be tested.
Ages 21–30 years	Should have a Pap smear every 3 years. HPV testing should not be used in this age group unless it is needed after an abnormal pap test result.
Ages 30–65 years	Should have a Pap smear plus an HPV test every 5 years. This is the preferred approach, but having a Pap smear alone every 3 years is okay also.
Ages >65 years	Women whom have had regular cervical testing with normal results should not be tested for cervical cancer. Women with a history of serious cervical pre-cancer lesions should continue testing for at least 20 years after that diagnosis, even if it continues after age 65.
HPV vaccination	Women whom have received the HPV vaccine should follow the screening recommendations for her age group.

Adapted from American Cancer Society [ACS]. (2015b). *American Cancer Society guidelines for the early detection of cancer.* Retrieved from http://www.cancer.org/healthy/findcancerearly/cancerscreeningguidelines/american-cancer-society-guidelines-for-the-early-detection-of-cancer

---

BOX 8.1

THE BETHESDA SYSTEM FOR CLASSIFYING PAP SMEARS

Specimen Type: Conventional Pap smear vs. liquid-based
Specimen Adequacy: Satisfactory or unsatisfactory for evaluation
General Categorization: (optional)
• Negative for intraepithelial lesion or malignancy
• Epithelial cell abnormality. See interpretation/result
Automated Review: If case was examined by automated device or not
Ancillary Testing: Provides a brief description of the test methods and report results so that the health care provider understands
Interpretation/Result:
• Negative for intraepithelial lesion or malignancy
• Organisms: *Trichomonas vaginalis*; fungus; bacterial vaginosis; herpes simplex
• Other non-neoplastic findings: Reactive cellular changes associated with inflammation, radiation, intrauterine devices, atrophy
• Other: Endometrial cells in a woman >40 years of age
• Epithelial cell abnormalities:
• *Squamous cell*
  • Atypical squamous cells
    • Of undetermined significance (ASC-US)
    • Cannot exclude HSIL (ASC-H)
  • Low-grade squamous intraepithelial lesion (LSIL)
    • Encompassing HPV/mild dysplasia/CIN-1
  • High-grade squamous intraepithelial lesion (HSIL)
  • Encompassing moderate and severe dysplasia CIS/CIN-2 and CIN-3
  • With features suspicious for invasion
  • Squamous cell carcinoma
• *Glandular cell*: Atypical
  • Endocervical, endometrial, or glandular cells
    • Endocervical cells—favor neoplastic
    • Glandular cells—favor neoplastic
    • Endocervical adenocarcinoma in situ
  • Adenocarcinoma
    • Endocervical, endometrial, extrauterine
• Other malignant neoplasms (specify)

Educational Notes and Suggestions: (optional)

Adapted from American Society of Cytopathology. (2015). *The Bethesda System for reporting cervical cytology: Definitions, criteria and explanatory notes.* Retrieved from http://www.cytopathology.org/the-bethesda-system-for-reporting-cervical-cytology-definitions-criteria-and-explanatory-notes-3rd-edition/; National Cancer Institute [NCI]. (2015k). *Cervical cancer prevention.* Retrieved from http://www.cancer.gov/cancertopics/pdq/prevention/cervical/Patient/page3; and Schuiling, K. D., & Likis, F. E. (2016). *Women's gynecologic health* (3rd ed.). Sudbury, MA: Jones & Bartlett.

---

of cytologic findings, and interpretation/result (ACS, 2015h).

Therapeutic Management

Treatment for abnormal Pap smears depends on the severity of the results and the health history of the woman. Therapeutic choices all involve destroying as many affected cells as possible. With the introduction of multimodality therapy for cervical cancer, many women will be long-term survivors in need of comprehensive surveillance care. Obesity and smoking are significant comorbidities that may complicate care in cervical cancer survivors. Nurses can focus their interventions at modifying these risk factors to increase the quality of life for cervical cancer survivors. Box 8.2 describes treatment options.

Using the Bethesda System, the following management guidelines for abnormal Pap results were developed by the NCI to provide direction to health care providers and clients:
• *ASC-US:* Repeat the Pap smear in 4 to 6 months or refer for colposcopy.
• *ASC-H:* Refer for colposcopy with HPV testing.

• *Atypical glandular cells (AGC) and adenocarcinoma in situ (AIS):* Immediate colposcopy; follow-up is based on the findings.

Colposcopy is a microscopic examination of the lower genital tract using a magnifying instrument called a colposcope. Specific patterns of cells that correlate well with certain histologic findings can be visualized.

BOX 8.2

TREATMENT OPTIONS FOR CERVICAL CANCER

- **Cryotherapy**—destroys abnormal cervical tissue by freezing with liquid nitrogen, Freon, or nitrous oxide. Studies show a 90% cure rate (NCI, 2015g). Healing takes up to 6 weeks, and the client may experience a profuse, watery vaginal discharge for 3 to 4 weeks.
- **Cone biopsy or conization**—removes a cone-shaped section of cervical tissue. The base of the cone is formed by the ectocervix (outer part of the cervix) and the point or apex of the cone is from the endocervical canal. The transformation zone is contained within the cone sample. The cone biopsy is also a treatment and can be used to completely remove any precancers and very early cancers. Two methods are commonly used for cone biopsies:
- **LEEP (loop electrosurgical excision procedure) or LLETZ (large loop excision of the transformation zone)**—the abnormal cervical tissue is removed with a wire that is heated by an electrical current. For this procedure, a local anesthetic is used. It is performed in the health care provider's office in approximately 10 minutes. Mild cramping and bleeding may persist for several weeks after the procedure.
- **Cold knife cone biopsy**—a surgical scalpel or a laser is used instead of a heated wire to remove tissue. This procedure requires general anesthesia and is done in a hospital setting. After the procedure, cramping and bleeding may persist for a few weeks.
- **Laser therapy**—destroys diseased cervical tissue by using a focused beam of high-energy light to vaporize it (burn it off). After the procedure, the woman may experience a watery brown discharge for a few weeks. Very effective in destroying precancers and preventing them from developing into cancers.
- **Hysterectomy**—removes the uterus and cervix surgically
- **Radiation therapy**—delivered by internal radium applications to the cervix or external radiation therapy that includes lymphatics of the pelvis
- **Chemoradiation**—weekly cisplatin therapy concurrent with radiation. Investigation of this therapy is ongoing (ACS, 2015h).

Nursing Assessment

Obtain a thorough history and physical examination of the woman. Investigate her history for risk factors such as:

- Early age at first intercourse (within 1 year of menarche)
- Lower socioeconomic status
- Promiscuous male partners
- Unprotected sexual intercourse
- Family history of cervical cancer (mother or sisters)
- Sexual intercourse with uncircumcised men
- Female offspring of mothers who took diethylstilbestrol (DES)
- Infections with genital herpes or chronic chlamydia
- Multiple sex partners
- Cigarette smoking
- Immunocompromised state
- HIV infection
- Oral contraceptive use
- Moderate dysplasia on Pap smear within past 5 years
- HPV infection (CDC, 2015e)

Question the woman about any signs and symptoms. Clinically, the first sign is abnormal vaginal bleeding, usually after sexual intercourse. Also be alert for reports of vaginal discomfort, malodorous discharge, and dysuria. In some cases, the woman is asymptomatic, with detection occurring at an annual gynecologic examination and Pap test.

Perform a physical examination. Inspect the perineal area for vaginal discharge or genital warts. Perform or assist with a pelvic examination, including the collection of a Pap smear as indicated (Nursing Procedure 8.1).

Take Note!

Suspect advanced cervical cancer in women with pelvic, back, or leg pain, weight loss, anorexia, weakness and fatigue, and fractures.

Prepare the woman for further diagnostic testing if indicated, such as a colposcopy. In a colposcopy, the woman is placed in the lithotomy position and her cervix is cleansed with acetic acid solution. Acetic acid makes abnormal cells appear white, which is referred to as *acetowhite*. These white areas are then biopsied and sent to the pathologist for assessment. Although this test is not painful, it has minor side effects (minor bleeding, cramping, and a risk of an infection developing after the biopsy), and can be performed safely in the clinic or office setting, and women may be apprehensive or anxious about it because it is done to identify and confirm potential abnormal cell growth. Some health care providers request that the woman pre-medicate with a mild analgesic such as ibuprofen prior to undergoing the procedure.

Nursing Management

The nurse's role involves primary prevention by educating women about risk factors and ways to prevent cervical dysplasia. Cervical cancer rates have decreased in the United States because of the widespread use of Pap testing, which can detect precancerous lesions of the cervix before they develop into cancer.

 Concept Mastery Alert

Cervical Cancer Prevention

The key points to remember in cervical cancer prevention are smoking cessation, limiting alcohol consumption, and encouraging teens to refrain from early sexual activity.

NURSING PROCEDURE 8.1

Assisting with Collection of a PAP Smear

Purpose: To Obtain Cells From the Cervix for Cervical Cytology Screening

1. Explain procedure to the client (Fig. A).
2. Instruct client to empty her bladder.
3. Wash hands thoroughly.
4. Assemble equipment, maintaining sterility of equipment (Fig. B).
5. Position client on stirrups or foot pedals so that her knees fall outward.
6. Drape client with a sheet for privacy, covering the abdomen but leaving the perineal area exposed.

7. Open packages as needed.
8. Encourage client to relax.
9. Provide support to client as the practitioner obtains a sample by spreading the labia; inserting the speculum; inserting the cytobrush and swabbing the endocervix; and inserting the plastic spatula and swabbing the cervix (Figs. C–H).

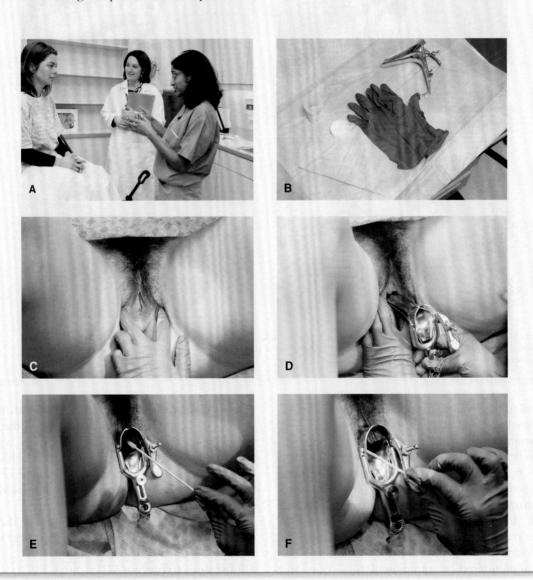

(continued)

NURSING PROCEDURE 8.1

Assisting with Collection of a PAP Smear (continued)

10. Transfer specimen to a container (Fig. I) or a slide. If a slide is used, spray the fixative on the slide holding the spray container about 12 inches away from the slide

11. Place sterile lubricant on the practitioner's fingertip when indicated for the bimanual examination.

12. Wash hands thoroughly.

13. Label specimen according to facility policy.

14. Rinse reusable instruments and dispose of waste appropriately (Fig. J).

15. Wash hands thoroughly.

16. Assist the client up after the exam is completed.

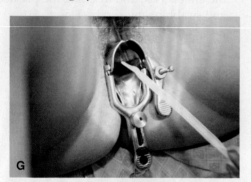

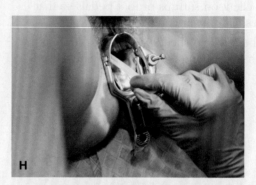

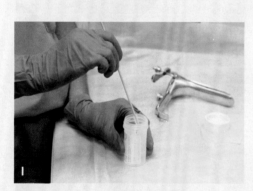

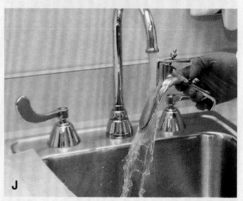

Adapted from King, T. L., Brucker, M. C., Kriebs, J. M., Fahey, J. O., Gegor, C. L., & Varney, H. (2015). *Varney's midwifery* (5th ed.). Burlington, MA: Jones & Bartlett Learning; and Schuiling, K. D., & Likis, F. E. (2016). *Women's gynecologic health* (3rd ed.). Burlington, MA: Jones & Bartlett Learning.

Gardasil and Cervarix are vaccines approved by the United States Food and Drug Administration to protect girls and women from HPV and thus prevent cervical cancer. The vaccines prevent infection from four HPV types: HPV 6, 11, 16, and 18. These types are responsible for 70% of cervical cancers and 90% of genital warts (NCI, 2015h). Clinical trials indicate that the vaccine has high efficacy in preventing persistent HPV infection, cervical cancer precursor lesions, vaginal and vulvar cancer precursor lesions, and genital warts (NCI, 2015h). The vaccine is administered by intramuscular injection, and the recommended schedule is a three-dose series with the second and third doses administered 2 and 6 months after the first dose. The recommended age for vaccination of females is 9 to 26 years (Castle & Schmeler, 2015).

The vaccines protect against infection with these types of HPV for 6 to 8 years. It is not known if the protection lasts longer. The vaccines do not protect women who are already infected with HPV (NCI, 2015h). However, the vaccine is not a substitute for routine cervical cancer screening, and vaccinated women should have Pap smears as recommended.

Focus primary prevention education on the following:
- Identify high-risk behaviors in clients and teach them how to reduce such behaviors
- Take steps to prevent STIs.
- Avoid early sexual activity.
- Faithfully use barrier methods of contraception.
- Avoid smoking and drinking.
- Receive the HPV vaccine.

• Instruct women on the importance of screening for cervical cancer by having annual Pap smears. Outline the proper preparation before having a Pap smear (Teaching Guidelines 8.3). Reinforce specific guidelines for screening.

• Interferes with visual evaluation of the sample (Schuiling & Likis, 2016).

Teaching Guidelines 8.3
STRATEGIES TO OPTIMIZE PAP SMEAR RESULTS

• Schedule your Pap smear appointment about 2 weeks (10 to 18 days) after the first day of your last menses to increase the chance of getting the best sample of cervical cells without menses.

• Refrain from intercourse for 48 hours before the test because additional matter such as sperm can obscure the specimen.

• Do not douche within 48 hours before the test to prevent washing away cervical cells that might be abnormal.

• Do not use tampons, birth control foams, jellies, vaginal creams, or vaginal medications for 72 hours before the test, because they could cover up or obscure the cervical cell sample.

• Cancel your Pap appointment if vaginal bleeding occurs, because the presence of blood cells interferes with visual evaluation of the sample.

Nurses also can advocate for clients by making sure that the Pap smear is sent to an accredited laboratory for interpretation. Doing so reduces the risk of false-negative results. The identification and treatment of early precancerous lesions is critical to prevention of cervical cancer. Prevention measures should include educating women that the risk of infection can be reduced by delaying the onset of sexual activity, decreasing the number of sexual partners, using condoms consistently, and never start smoking.

Secondary prevention focuses on reducing or limiting the area of cervical dysplasia. Tertiary prevention focuses on minimizing disability or the spread of cervical cancer. Explain in detail all procedures that might be needed. Encourage the client who has undergone any cervical treatment to allow the pelvic area to rest for approximately 1 month. Discuss this rest period with the client and her partner to gain his cooperation. Outline alternatives to vaginal intercourse, such as cuddling, holding hands, and kissing. Remind the woman about any follow-up procedures that are needed and assist her with scheduling if necessary.

Tertiary prevention of cervical cancer involves the diagnosis and treatment of confirmed cases of cancer. Treatment is typically through surgery, radiotherapy, and, frequently, chemotherapy. Palliative care is provided to women when the disease has already reached an incurable stage. Knowing that the woman and her family have been told about her prognosis, the nurse is in a position to support them when the impact of the diagnosis is realized.

Throughout the process, provide emotional support to the woman and her family. During the decision-making process, the woman may be overwhelmed by the diagnosis and all the information being presented. Refer the woman and her family to appropriate community resources and support groups as indicated. It is crucial for all women to be given correct information regarding safe sexual practices, informed about the preventive role of the HPV vaccination, and become educated about the role of the Pap test as a secondary screening measure for cervical cancer. The emotional needs of the woman diagnosed with cancer can best be met by a warm, friendly personality, an attitude of empathy rather than sympathy, and skilled communication. Nurses across all settings are in a powerful position to be advocates for safe health care practices of women through education at personal, community, and national levels.

VAGINAL CANCER

Vaginal cancer is a rare malignant tissue growth arising in the vagina. Only about 1 of every 1,100 women will develop vaginal cancer in her lifetime. In 2015, the ACS (2015i) estimate that more than 4,000 new cases will be diagnosed in women and that over 900 of those women will die from this cancer. The peak incidence of vaginal cancer occurs at 60 to 65 years of age. The prognosis of vaginal cancer depends largely on the stage of disease and the type of tumor. The overall 5-year survival rate for squamous cell carcinoma is about 42%; that for adenocarcinoma is about 78% (NCI, 2015i). Vaginal cancer can be effectively treated, and when found early it is often curable.

Pathophysiology

The etiology of vaginal cancer has not been identified. Malignant diseases of the vagina are either primary vaginal cancers or metastatic forms from adjacent or distant organs. About 80% of vaginal cancers are metastatic, primarily from the cervix and endometrium. These cancers invade the vagina directly. Cancers from distant sites that metastasize to the vagina through the blood or lymphatic system are typically from the colon, kidneys, skin (melanoma), or breast. Tumors in the vagina commonly occur on the posterior wall and spread to the cervix or vulva (NCI, 2015i).

Squamous cell carcinomas that begin in the epithelial lining of the vagina account for about 85% of vaginal cancers. This type of cancer usually occurs in women over age 50. The SCCs develop slowly over a period of years, commonly in the upper third of the vagina. They tend to spread early by directly invading the bladder and rectal walls. They also metastasize through blood and lymphatics. The remaining 15% are adenocarcinomas, which differ from SCC by an increase in pulmonary metastases and supraclavicular and pelvic node involvement (ACS, 2015j).

Therapeutic Management

Treatment of vaginal cancer depends on the type of cells involved and the stage of the disease. If the cancer is localized, radiation, laser surgery, or both may be used. If the cancer has spread, radical surgery might be needed, such as a hysterectomy, or removal of the upper vagina with dissection of the pelvic nodes in addition to radiation therapy.

Nursing Assessment

Begin the history and physical examination by reviewing for risk factors. Although direct risk factors for the initial development of vaginal cancer have not been identified, associated risk factors include advancing age (over 60 years old), previous pelvic radiation, exposure to DES in utero, vaginal trauma, history of genital warts (HPV infection), HIV infection, cervical cancer, chronic vaginal discharge, smoking, and low socioeconomic level (ACS, 2015k).

Question the woman about any symptoms. Most women with vaginal cancer are asymptomatic. Those with symptoms have painless vaginal bleeding (often after sexual intercourse), abnormal vaginal discharge, dyspareunia, dysuria, constipation, and pelvic pain (NCI, 2015i). During the physical examination, observe for any obvious vaginal discharge or genital warts or changes in the appearance of the vaginal mucosa. Anticipate colposcopy with biopsy of suspicious lesions to confirm the diagnosis.

Nursing Management

Nursing management for this cancer is similar to that for other reproductive cancers, with emphasis on sexuality counseling and referral to local support groups. Women undergoing radical surgery need intensive counseling about the nature of the surgery, risks, potential complications, changes in physical appearance and physiologic function, and sexuality alterations. Nurses should focus their care on client education, client pain and symptom management, communication with the woman and her family, and coordination of care across of all settings.

VULVAR CANCER

Vulvar cancer is an abnormal neoplastic growth on the external female genitalia including the clitoris, vaginal lips, and opening to the vagina (Fig. 8.5). Vulvar cancer

accounts for approximately 5% of all female genital malignancies. In the United States, women have a 1 in 333 chance of developing vulvar cancer at some point in their lifetime. It is the fourth most common gynecologic cancer, after endometrial, ovarian, and cervical cancers (NCI, 2015j). The ACS (2015h) estimates that, in 2015, over 5,000 cancers of the vulva will be diagnosed in the United States and over 1,000 women will die of this cancer. When detected early, it is highly curable. Typically, vulvar cancer can be advanced at diagnosis, though it is a visible cancer that can be seen by the woman as an abnormal lesion/growth in her genital region.

Vulvar cancer is found most commonly in older women in their mid-60s to mid-70s, but the incidence in women younger than 35 years old has increased during the past few decades. The overall 5-year survival rate when lymph nodes are not involved is 90%, but it drops to 50% to 70% when the lymph nodes have been invaded (ACS, 2015m).

Pathophysiology

Vulvar cancer can be classified into two groups according to predisposing factors: the first type correlates with a HPV infection and occurs mostly in younger women. The second group is not HPV associated and occurs in elderly women without cancerous disorders. Approximately 80% of vulvar tumors are squamous cell carcinomas. This type of cancer forms slowly over several years and is usually preceded by precancerous changes. These precancerous changes are termed vulvar intraepithelial neoplasia (VIN). The two major types of VIN are classic (undifferentiated) and simplex (differentiated). Classic VIN, the more common one, is associated with HPV infection (genital warts due to types 16, 18, 31, 33, 35, 45, and 54) and smoking (Alkatout et al., 2015). It typically occurs in women between 30 and 40 years old. In contrast to classic VIN, simplex VIN usually occurs in postmenopausal women and is not associated with HPV but chronic irritation over time (Cancer.Net, 2015b).

Screening and Diagnosis

Annual vulvar examination is the most effective way to prevent vulvar cancer. Careful inspection of the vulva during routine annual gynecologic examinations remains the most productive diagnostic technique. Liberal use of biopsies of any suspicious vulvar lesion is usually necessary to make the diagnosis and to guide treatment. However, many women do not seek health care evaluation for months or years after noticing an abnormal lump or lesion. Leading presenting complaints of women with vulvar cancer include dyspareunia, long history of pruritus, ulcers on the "outside" genitalia, vulvar swelling, vulvar bleeding, and urinary problems (Alkatout

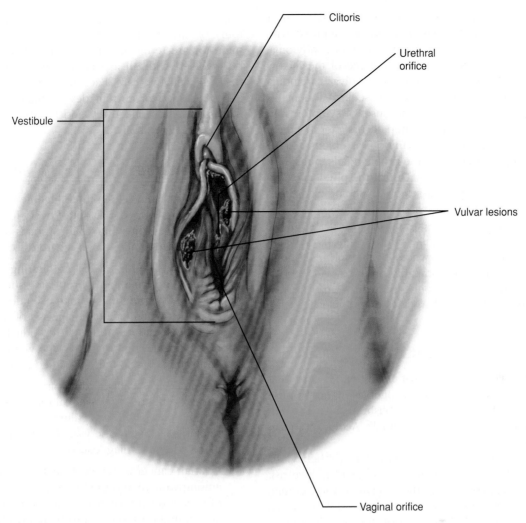

Clitoris

Urethral orifice

Vestibule

Vulvar lesions

Vaginal orifice

FIGURE 8.5 Vulvar cancer. (The Anatomical Chart Company. [2009]. *Atlas of pathophysiology* [3rd ed.]. Philadelphia, PA: Lippincott Williams & Wilkins.)

et al., 2015). The diagnosis of vulvar cancer is made by a biopsy of the suspicious lesion, which is usually found on the labia majora.

Take Note!

Vulvar pruritus or a lump is present in the majority of women with vulvar cancer. Lumps should be biopsied even if the woman is asymptomatic.

Therapeutic Management

Treatment varies depending on the extent of the disease. Laser surgery, cryosurgery, or electrosurgical incision may be used. Larger lesions may need more extensive surgery and skin grafting. The traditional treatment for vulvar cancer has been radical vulvectomy, but more conservative techniques are being used to improve psychosexual outcomes and less morbidity, without compromising survival (Forner, Dakhil, & Lampe, 2015).

Nursing Assessment

Typically, no single specific clinical symptom heralds this disease, so diagnosis is often delayed significantly. Therefore, it is important to review the woman's history for risk factors such as:

- Exposure to HPV type 16
- Age over 50 years
- HIV infection
- VIN
- Lichen sclerosus (a patchy skin disorder)
- Melanoma or atypical moles
- Exposure to HSV type 2
- Multiple sex partners
- Smoking
- Herpes simplex
- History of breast cancer
- Immune suppression
- Hypertension
- Diabetes mellitus
- Obesity (ACS, 2015n).

In most cases, the woman reports persistent vulvar itching, burning, and edema that do not improve with the use of creams or ointments. A history of condyloma, gonorrhea, and herpes simplex are some of the factors for greater risk for VIN. Diagnosis of vulvar carcinoma is often delayed. Women neglect to seek treatment for an average of 6 months from the onset of symptoms. In addition, a delay in diagnosis often occurs after the client presents to her physician. In many cases, a biopsy of the lesion is not performed until the problem fails to respond to numerous topical therapies. During the physical examination, observe for any masses or thickening of the vulvar area. A vulvar lump or mass is most often noted. The vulvar lesion is usually raised and may be fleshy, ulcerated, leukoplakic (looking like white patches), or warty. The cancer can appear anywhere on the vulva, although about three fourths arise primarily on the labia (Vargo & Beriwal, 2015). Less commonly, the woman may present with vulvar bleeding, discharge, dysuria, and pain.

Nursing Management

Women with vulvar cancer must clearly understand their disease, treatment options, and prognosis. To accomplish this, provide information and establish effective communication with the client and her family. Act as an educator and advocate.

Teach the woman about healthy lifestyle behaviors, such as smoking cessation and measures to reduce risk factors. For example, instruct the woman how to examine her genital area, urging her to do so monthly between menstrual periods. Tell her to look for any changes in appearance (e.g., whitened or reddened patches of skin); changes in feel (e.g., areas of the vulva becoming itchy or painful); or the development of lumps, moles (e.g., changes in size, shape, or color), freckles, cuts, or sores on the vulva. Urge the woman to report these changes to the health care provider (ACS, 2015m).

Teach the woman about preventive measures such as not wearing tight undergarments and not using perfumes and dyes in the vulvar region. Also educate her about the use of barrier methods of birth control (e.g., condoms) to reduce the risk of contracting HIV, HSV, and HPV. Other prevention measures include delaying first sexual intercourse, avoiding sexual intercourse with multiple partners, not starting smoking or quitting if a smoker already, and getting the HPV vaccine available for all boys and girls and women between 9 and 26 years old.

For the woman diagnosed with vulvar cancer, provide information and support. Discuss potential changes in sexuality if radical surgery is performed. Encourage her to communicate openly with her partner. Refer her to appropriate community resources and support groups. All nurses should come in contact with women in their clinical practices who have the potential to become cancer clients, already have suspicious signs or symptoms of cancer, are already undergoing cancer treatment, or are terminal cancer clients. The nurse should be involved with all aspects of cancer, from diagnosis through palliative care. Each nurse has an obligation to keep informed of current developments in the cancer field to function effectively and be able to educate the woman and her family.

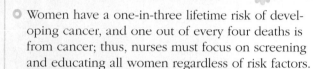

KEY CONCEPTS

- Women have a one-in-three lifetime risk of developing cancer, and one out of every four deaths is from cancer; thus, nurses must focus on screening and educating all women regardless of risk factors.

- The nurse plays a key role in offering emotional support, determining appropriate sources of support, and helping the woman use effective coping strategies when facing a diagnosis of cancer of the reproductive tract. Although reproductive tract cancer is rare during pregnancy, the woman's vigilance and routine screenings should continue throughout.

- A woman's sexuality and culture are inextricably interwoven, and it is essential that nurses working with women of various cultures recognize this and remain sensitive to the vast changes that will take place when the diagnosis of cancer is made.

- Ovarian cancer is the eighth most common cancer among women and the fourth most common cause of cancer deaths for women in the United States, accounting for more deaths than any other cancer of the reproductive system.

- Ovarian cancer has been described as the "overlooked disease" or "silent killer" because women and health care practitioners often ignore or rationalize early symptoms. It is typically diagnosed in advanced stages.

- Unopposed endogenous and exogenous estrogens, obesity, nulliparity, menopause after the age of 52 years, and diabetes are the major etiologic risk factors associated with the development of endometrial cancer.

- The American Cancer Society recommends that women should be informed about risks and symptoms of endometrial cancer at the onset of menopause and strongly encouraged to report any unexpected bleeding or spotting to their health care providers.

- Malignant diseases of the vagina are either primary vaginal cancers or metastatic forms from adjacent or distant organs. Vaginal cancer tumors can be effectively treated and, when found early, are often curable.

- Cervical cancer incidence and mortality rates have decreased noticeably in the past several decades, with most of the reduction attributed to the Pap test, which detects cervical cancer and precancerous lesions.

- The nurse's role involves primary prevention of cervical cancer through education of women regarding risk factors and preventive vaccines to avoid cervical dysplasia.

- About 80% of the diagnosed vaginal cancers are metastatic, primarily from the cervix and endometrium. These cancers invade the vagina directly. Vulvar cancer is often delayed significantly because there is no single specific clinical symptom that heralds it. The most common presentation is persistent vulvar itching that does not improve with the application of creams or ointments.

References and Recommended Readings

Agency for Healthcare Research and Quality. (2014). *Cancer screening and treatment in women: Recent findings*. Retrieved from http://www.ahrq.gov/research/findings/factsheets/women/cancerwom/

Alexander, L. L., LaRosa, J. H., Bader, H., & Garfield, S. (2014). *New dimensions in women's health* (6th ed.). Sudbury, MA: Jones & Bartlett.

Alkatout, I., Schubert, M., Garbrecht, N., Weigel, M. T., Jonat, W., Mundhenke, C., et al. (2015). Vulvar cancer: Epidemiology, clinical presentation, and management options. *International Journal of Women's Health, 7*, 305–313.

Amant, F., Han, S. N., Gziri, M. M., Vandenbroucke, T., Verheecke, M., & Van Calsteren, K. (2015). Management of cancer in pregnancy. *Best Practice & Research Clinical Obstetrics & Gynecology, 29*(5), 741–753.

American Cancer Society [ACS]. (2015a). *Key statistics about lung cancer*. Retrieved from http://www.cancer.org/cancer/lungcancer-non-smallcell/detailedguide/non-small-cell-lung-cancer-key-statistics

American Cancer Society [ACS]. (2015b). *ACS guidelines for the early detection of cancer*. Retrieved from http://www.cancer.org/healthy/findcancerearly/cancerscreeningguidelines/american-cancer-society-guidelines-for-the-early-detection-of-cancer

American Cancer Society [ACS]. (2015c). *Cervical cancer and pregnancy*. Retrieved from http://www.cancer.org/cancer/cervical-cancer/overviewguide/cervical-cancer-overview-treating-pregnancy

American Cancer Society [ACS]. (2015d). *What are the key statistics about ovarian cancer?* Retrieved from http://www.cancer.org/cancer/ovariancancer/detailedguide/ovarian-cancer-key-statistics

American Cancer Society [ACS]. (2015e). *What are the key statistics about endometrial cancer?* Retrieved from http://www.cancer.org/cancer/endometrialcancer/detailedguide/endometrial-uterine-cancer-key-statistics

American Cancer Society [ACS]. (2015f). *Endometrial (uterine) cancer*. Retrieved from http://www.cancer.org/acs/groups/cid/documents/webcontent/003097-pdf.pdf

American Cancer Society [ACS]. (2015g). *What are the key statistics about cervical cancer?* Retrieved from http://www.cancer.org/cancer/cervicalcancer/detailedguide/cervical-cancer-key-statistics

American Cancer Society [ACS]. (2015h). *Cervical cancer*. Retrieved from http://www.cancer.org/acs/groups/cid/documents/webcontent/003094-pdf.pdf

American Cancer Society [ACS]. (2015i). *What are the key statistics about vaginal cancer?* Retrieved from http://www.cancer.org/cancer/vaginalcancer/detailedguide/vaginal-cancer-key-statistics

American Cancer Society [ACS]. (2015j). *Vaginal cancer*. Retrieved from http://www.cancer.org/cancer/vaginalcancer/detailedguide/

American Cancer Society [ACS]. (2015k). *What are risk factors for vaginal cancer?* Retrieved from http://www.cancer.org/cancer/vaginalcancer/detailedguide/vaginal-cancer-risk-factors

American Cancer Society [ACS]. (2015l). *What are the key statistics about vulvar cancer?* Retrieved from http://www.cancer.org/cancer/vulvarcancer/detailedguide/vulvar-cancer-key-statistics

American Cancer Society [ACS]. (2015m). *What is vulvar cancer?* Retrieved from http://www.cancer.org/cancer/vulvarcancer/detailedguide/vulvar-cancer-what-is-vulvar-cancer

American Cancer Society [ACS]. (2015n). *What are the risk factors for vulvar cancer?* Retrieved from http://www.cancer.org/cancer/vulvarcancer/detailedguide/vulvar-cancer-risk-factors

American Cancer Society [ACS]. (2015o). *Survival rates for ovarian cancer by stage*. Retrieved from http://www.cancer.org/cancer/ovariancancer/detailedguide/ovarian-cancer-survival-rates

American College of Obstetricians and Gynecologists [ACOG]. (2015). *The ACOG cervical cancer screening guidelines: Key changes*. Retrieved from https://www.hpv16and18.com/hcp/cervical-cancer-screening-guidelines/acog-guidelines.html

American Society of Cytopathology. (2015). *The Bethesda System for reporting cervical cytology: Definitions, criteria and explanatory notes*. Retrieved from http://www.cytopathology.org/the-bethesda-system-for-reporting-cervical-cytology-definitions-criteria-and-explanatory-notes-3rd-edition/

Andersson, T. M., Johansson, A. L., Fredriksson, I., & Lambe, M. (2015). Cancer during pregnancy and the postpartum period: A population-based study. *Cancer, 121*(12), 2072–2077.

Balk, S. J. (2015). Pediatricians can play role in reducing skin cancer epidemic. *AAP News, 36*(1), 8.

Brennan, D. J., Hackethal, A., Mann, K. P., Mutz-Dehbalaie, I., Fiegl, H., Marth, C., et al. (2015). Serum HE4 detects recurrent endometrial cancer in patients undergoing routine clinical surveillance. *BMC Cancer, 15*(1), 33–36.

Broadman, C. H., & Matthews, K. J. (2015). Cervical cancer. *eMedicine*. Retrieved from http://emedicine.medscape.com/article/253513-overview

Cancer in Pregnancy. (2015a). *Endometrial cancer*. Retrieved from http://www.cancerinpregnancy.org/node/103

Cancer in Pregnancy. (2015b). *Cervical cancer*. Retrieved from http://www.cancerinpregnancy.org/node/52

Cancer.Net. (2015a). *Cancer during pregnancy*. Retrieved from http://www.cancer.net/coping/emotional-and-physical-matters/sexual-and-reproductive-health/cancer-during-pregnancy

Cancer.Net. (2015b). *Vulvar cancer*. Retrieved from http://www.cancer.net/cancer-types/vulvar-cancer/risk-factors-and-prevention

Castle, P. E., & Schmeler, K. M. (2015). HPV vaccination: For women of all ages? *The Lancet, 384*(9961), 2178–2180.

Centers for Disease Control and Prevention [CDC]. (2015a). *Cancer among women*. Retrieved from http://www.cdc.gov/cancer/dcpc/data/women.htm

Centers for Disease Control and Prevention [CDC]. (2015b). Cancer prevention and control. Retrieved from http://www.cdc.gov/cancer/dcpc/prevention/other.htm

Centers for Disease Control and Prevention [CDC]. (2015c). *Ovarian cancer risk factors*. Retrieved from http://www.cdc.gov/cancer/ovarian/basic_info/risk_factors.htm

Centers for Disease Control and Prevention [CDC]. (2015d). *Cervical cancer screening*. Retrieved from http://www.cdc.gov/cancer/cervical/basic_info/screening.htm

Centers for Disease Control and Prevention [CDC]. (2015e). *Cervical cancer risk factors*. Retrieved from http://www.cdc.gov/cancer/cervical/basic_info/risk_factors.htm

Cliby, W. A., Powell, M. A., Al-Hammadi, N., Chen, L., Miller, J. P., Roland, P. Y., et al. (2015). Ovarian cancer in the United States: Contemporary patterns of care associated with improved survival. *Gynecologic Oncology, 136*(1), 11–17.

de Haan, J., Verheecke, M., & Amant, F. (2015). Management of ovarian cysts and cancer in pregnancy. *Facts, Views & Vision in ObGyn, 7*(1), 25–31.

Dueholm, M., Marinovskij, E., Hansen, E. S., Møller, C., & Ørtoft, G. (2015). Diagnostic methods for fast-track identification of endometrial cancer in women with postmenopausal bleeding and endometrial thickness greater than 5 mm. *Menopause, 22*(6), 616–626.

Ebell, M. H., Culp, M., Lastinger, K., & Dasigi, T. (2015). A systematic review of the bimanual examination as a test for ovarian cancer. *American Journal of Preventive Medicine, 48*(3), 350–356.

Fontenot, H. B. (2015). Urine-based HPV testing as a method to screen for cervical cancer. *Nursing for Women's Health, 19*, 59–65.

Forner, D. M., Dakhil, R., & Lampe, B. (2015). Quality of life and sexual function after surgery in early stage vulvar cancer. *European Journal of Surgical Oncology (EJSO), 41*(1), 40–45.

Garner, M. J., McGregor, B. A., Murphy, K. M., Koenig, A. L., Dolan, E. D., & Albano, D. (2015). Optimism and depression: A new look at social support as a mediator among women at risk for breast cancer. *Psycho-Oncology, 24*(12), 1708–1713.

Goldstein, C. L., Susman, E., Lockwood, S., Medlin, E. E., & Behbakht, K. (2015). Awareness of symptoms and risk factors of ovarian cancer in a population of women and healthcare providers. *Clinical Journal of Oncology Nursing, 19*(2), 206–212.

Helm, C. W. (2015a). Hyperthermic intraperitoneal chemotherapy for ovarian cancer: Is there a role? *Journal of Gynecologic Oncology, 26*(1), 1–2.

Helm, C. W. (2015b). Ovarian cysts. *eMedicine.* Retrieved from http://emedicine.medscape.com/article/255865-overview

Herrington, C., Coates, P., & Duprex, W. (2015). Viruses and disease: Emerging concepts for prevention, diagnosis and treatment. *Journal of Pathology, 235*, 149–152.

International Federation of Gynecology & Obstetrics. (2015). *Endometrial carcinoma staging.* Retrieved from http://www.figo.org/search/node/endometrial+cancer+staging

Key, T. (2015). Cancer prevention and treatment. In *Nutrition for the primary care provider* (Vol. 111, pp. 123–129). Oxford, UK: Karger Publishers.

Kim, R. H., & Chu, Q. D. (2015). Breast cancer during pregnancy. In *Surgical oncology* (pp. 163–168). New York, NY: Springer Publishers.

King, T. L, Brucker, M. C., Kriebs, J. M., Fahey, J. O., Gegor, C. L., & Varney, H. (2015). *Varney's midwifery* (5th ed.). Burlington, MA: Jones & Bartlett Learning.

Li, Y., Zhao, J., Zhang, Q., & Wang, Y. (2015). Does ovarian stimulation for IVF increase gynecological cancer risk? A systematic review and meta-analysis. *Reproductive BioMedicine Online, 31*(1), 20–29.

Liede, A., Sun, P., & Narod, S. (2015). Effect of breast cancer after ovarian cancer on mortality for BRCA mutation carriers. *JAMA Surgery, 150*(5), 490–491.

Lofters, A. K. (2015). Ethnicity and breast cancer stage at diagnosis: An issue of health equity. *Current Oncology, 22*(2), 80–81.

Matsumoto, K., Onda, T., & Yaegashi, N. (2015). Pharmacotherapy for recurrent ovarian cancer: Current status and future perspectives. *Japanese Journal of Clinical Oncology, 45*(5), 408–410.

Mayo Clinic. (2015). *Cancer prevention: 7 steps to reduce your risk.* Retrieved from http://www.mayoclinic.org/cancer-prevention/art-20044816</bib>

Memorial Sloan Kettering Cancer Center. (2015). *Ovarian cancer risk factors.* Retrieved from http://www.mskcc.org/cancer-care/adult/ovarian/risk-factors

Moses, S. (2015). Endometrial cancer risk factors. *Family Practice Notebook.* Retrieved from http://www.fpnotebook.com/Gyn/HemeOnc/EndmtrlCncrRskFctr.htm

National Cancer Institute [NCI]. (2015a). *SEER cancer statistics review.* Retrieved from http://seer.cancer.gov/csr/1975_2010/

National Cancer Institute [NCI]. (2015b). *The burden of cancer.* Retrieved from http://www.cancer.gov/cancertopics/pdq/prevention/overview/HealthProfessional

National Cancer Institute [NCI]. (2015c). *General cancer prevention.* Retrieved from http://www.cancer.gov/cancertopics/prevention#General+Cancer+Prevention+Information

National Cancer Institute [NCI]. (2015d). *General information about ovarian epithelial cancer.* Retrieved from http://www.cancer.gov/cancertopics/pdq/treatment/ovarianepithelial/healthprofessional

National Cancer Institute [NCI]. (2015e). *Stat fact sheets: Endometrial cancer.* Retrieved from http://seer.cancer.gov/statfacts/html/corp.html

National Cancer Institute [NCI]. (2015f). *Endometrial cancer.* Retrieved from http://www.cancer.gov/cancertopics/types/endometrial

National Cancer Institute [NCI]. (2015g). *Screening and testing to detect cervical cancer.* Retrieved from http://www.cancer.gov/cancertopics/screening/cervical

National Cancer Institute [NCI]. (2015h). *Human papillomavirus (HPV) vaccines.* Retrieved from http://www.cancer.gov/cancertopics/factsheet/prevention/HPV-vaccine

National Cancer Institute [NCI]. (2015i). *General information about vaginal cancer.* Retrieved from http://www.cancer.gov/cancertopics/pdq/treatment/vaginal/Patient/page1

National Cancer Institute [NCI]. (2015j). *General information about vulvar cancer.* Retrieved from http://www.cancer.gov/cancertopics/pdq/treatment/vulvar/HealthProfessional/page1

National Cancer Institute [NCI]. (2015k). *Cervical cancer prevention.* Retrieved from http://www.cancer.gov/cancertopics/pdq/prevention/cervical/Patient/page3

National Institutes of Health [NIH]. (2015). *Cervical cancer.* Retrieved from http://report.nih.gov/nihfactsheets/viewfactsheet.aspx?csid=76

Nick, A. M., Coleman, R. L., Ramirez, P. T., & Sood, A. K. (2015). A framework for a personalized surgical approach to ovarian cancer. *Nature Reviews Clinical Oncology, 12*(4), 239–245.

Poole, E. M., Rice, M. S., Crum, C. P., & Tworoger, S. S. (2015). Salpingectomy as a potential ovarian cancer risk-reducing procedure. *Journal of the National Cancer Institute.* doi: 10.1093/jnci/dju490

Sawaya, G. F., Kulasingam, S., Denberg, T., Qaseem, A, & Clinical Guidelines Committee of American College of Physicians. (2015). Cervical cancer screening in average-risk women: Best practice advice from the clinical guidelines committee of the American college of physicians. *Annals of Internal Medicine, 162*(12), 851–859.

Schmid, D., Behrens, G., Keimling, M., Jochem, C., Ricci, C., & Leitzmann, M. (2015). A systematic review and meta-analysis of physical activity and endometrial cancer risk. *European Journal of Epidemiology, 30*(5), 397–412.

Schuiling, K. D., & Likis, F. E. (2016). *Women's gynecologic health* (3rd ed.). Sudbury, MA: Jones & Bartlett.

Shirvani, H., & Alhani, F. (2015). Challenges nursing role on improving quality of life in women with breast cancer undergoing chemotherapy. *Journal of Clinical Nursing and Midwifery, 3*(4), 1–12.

Siegel, R. L., Miller, K. D., & Jemal, A. (2015). Cancer statistics, 2015. *CA: A Cancer Journal for Clinicians, 65*, 5–29.

Strohl, A. E., Mendoza, G., Ghant, M. S., Cameron, K. A., Simon, M. A., Schink, J. C., et al. (2015). Barriers to prevention: Knowledge of HPV, cervical cancer, and HPV vaccinations among African American women. *American Journal of Obstetrics and Gynecology, 212*(1), 65–70.

Surbone, A. (2015). A review of cultural attitudes about cancer. In K. D. Miller & M. Simon (Eds.),*Global perspectives on cancer: Incidence, care, and experience* (2 vols., pp. 19–37). Santa Barbara, CA: ABC-CLIO Publisher.

Temple, S. V. (2015). Cancers of the reproductive system. In J. K. Itano, J. K. Brant, F. A. Conde, & M. G. Saria (Eds.), *Core curriculum for oncology nursing* (5th ed., pp. 103–116). St. Louis, MO: Elsevier.

U.S. Department of Health and Human Services. (2015). *Healthy people 2020.* Retrieved from http://www.healthypeople.gov/2020/topicsobjectives2020

U.S. Preventive Services Task Force [USPSTF]. (2015). *Screening for ovarian cancer. U.S. Preventive Services Task Force summary of recommendations.* Retrieved from http://www.ahrq.gov/clinic/pocketgd1011/gcp10s2.htm

Vargo, J. A., & Beriwal, S. (2015). Vulvar cancer. In *Target volume delineation for conformal and intensity-modulated radiation therapy* (pp. 349–358). Switzerland: Springer International Publishing.

Wong A. S., Lao T. T., Cheung C. W., Yeung S. W., Fan H. L., Ng P. S., et al. (2015). Reappraisal of endometrial thickness for the detection of endometrial cancer in postmenopausal bleeding: A retrospective cohort study. *British Journal of Obstetrics and Gynaecology, 123*(3), 439–446.

World Health Organization. (2015). *Cancer prevention and control.* Retrieved from http://www.who.int/nmh/a5816/en/

Wright, J. D., Chen, L., Tergas, A. I., Patankar, S., Burke, W. M., Hou, J. Y., et al. (2015). Trends in relative survival for ovarian cancer from 1975 to 2011. *Obstetrics & Gynecology, 125*(6), 1345–1352.

MULTIPLE CHOICE QUESTIONS

1. When describing ovarian cancer to a local women's group, the nurse states that ovarian cancer often is not diagnosed early because:
   a. The disease progresses very slowly.
   b. The early stages produce very vague symptoms.
   c. The disease usually is diagnosed only at autopsy.
   d. Clients do not follow up on acute pelvic pain.

2. A postmenopausal woman reports that she has started spotting again. Which of the following would the nurse do?
   a. Instruct the client to keep a menstrual diary for the next few months.
   b. Tell her not to worry, since this a common but not serious event.
   c. Have her start warm-water douches to promote healing.
   d. Anticipate that the doctor will assess her endometrium thickness.

3. Which of the following would the nurse identify as the priority psychosocial need for a women diagnosed with reproductive cancer?
   a. Research findings
   b. Hand-holding
   c. Cheerfulness
   d. Offering of hope

4. When teaching a group of women about screening and early detection of cervical cancer, the nurse would include which of the following as most effective?
   a. Fecal occult blood test
   b. CA-125 blood test
   c. Pap smear and HPV test
   d. Sigmoidoscopy

5. After teaching a group of students about reproductive tract cancers, the nursing instructor determines that the teaching was successful when the students identify which of the following as the deadliest type of female reproductive cancer?
   a. Vulvar
   b. Ovarian
   c. Endometrial
   d. Cervical

6. The nurse is attempting to reassure her obese female client about the discovery of an ovarian cyst after her pelvic exam. Which of the following statements is true concerning ovarian cysts? They are:
   a. Frequently seen in polycystic kidney disease
   b. Always painful and need to be removed surgically
   c. A precursor to ovarian carcinoma
   d. Part of a syndrome that includes hypertension and diabetes

7. Which of the following is considered a risk factor for vulvar cancer?
   a. Vitamin B_{12} deficiency
   b. Epstein–Barr virus
   c. Human papillomavirus
   d. Adenovirus

CRITICAL THINKING EXERCISES

1. A 27-year-old sexually active White woman visits the Health Department family planning clinic and requests information about the various available methods of contraception. In taking her history, the nurse learns that she started having sex at age 15 and has had multiple sex partners since then. She smokes two packs of cigarettes daily. Because she has been unemployed for a few months, her health insurance policy has lapsed. She has never previously obtained any gynecologic care.
   a. Based on her history, which risk factors for cervical cancer are present?
   b. What recommendations would you make for her and why?
   c. What are this client's educational needs concerning health maintenance?

2. A 60-year-old nulliparous woman presents to the gynecologic oncology clinic after her health care provider palpated an adnexal mass on her right ovary. In taking her history, the nurse learns that she has experienced mild abdominal bloating and weight loss for the past several months but felt fine otherwise. She was diagnosed with breast cancer 15 years ago and was treated with a lumpectomy and radiation. She has occasionally used talcum powder in her perineal area over the past 20 years.

A transvaginal ultrasound reveals a complex mass in the right adnexa. She undergoes a total abdominal hysterectomy and bilateral salpingo-oophorectomy and lymph node biopsy. Pathology confirms a diagnosis of stage III ovarian cancer with abdominal metastasis and positive lymph nodes.
   a. Is this client's profile typical for a woman with this diagnosis?
   b. What in her history might have increased her risk for ovarian cancer?
   c. What can the nurse do to increase awareness of this cancer for all women?

STUDY ACTIVITIES

1. During your surgical clinical rotation, interview a female client undergoing surgery for cancer of her reproductive organs. Ask her to recall the symptoms that brought her to the health care provider. Ask her

what thoughts, feelings, and emotions went through her mind before and after her diagnosis. Finally, ask her how this experience will change her life in the future.

2. Visit an oncology and radiology treatment center to find out about the various treatment modalities available for reproductive cancers. Contrast the various treatment methods and report your findings to your class.

3. Visit one of the web sites listed in the extensive list of websites provided on to explore a topic of interest concerning reproductive cancers. How correct and current is the content? What is its level? Share your assessment with your classmates.

4. Taking oral contraceptives provides protection against _____ cancer.

5. Two genes, *BRCA1* and *BRCA2*, are linked with hereditary _____ and _____ cancers.

BRINGING IT ALL TOGETHER: CASE STUDY

Jill, a 38-year old obese female with a history of infertility and irregular bleeding, returns to her OB/GYN doctor as a follow-up appointment. She had a D&C the week before to stop a profuse bleeding episode. She is informed by the doctor that her pathology report came back from the D&C showing endometrial adenocarcinoma. She is in shock over the diagnosis at her young age.

ASSESSMENT

The nurse takes Jill's history, which includes irregular menstrual cycles since her menarche. She has a BMI of 32. She takes medication to manage her diabetes and hypertension. She had been previously diagnosed with Polycystic ovary syndrome (PCOS) when she was a teenager. Her pelvic exam demonstrates an enlarged uterus. She had been to see her doctor several times because of her irregular bleeding, but she had been treated with medications until a D&C was done after months of unsuccessful drug therapy.

Go to thePoint **to find questions to consider about this case.**

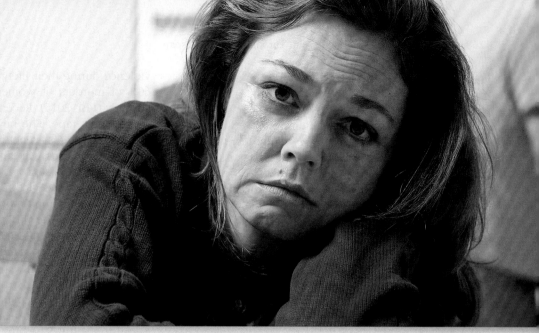

9

Violence and Abuse

Learning Objectives

Upon completion of the chapter, you will be able to:

1. Examine the incidence of violence in women.
2. Characterize the cycle of violence and appropriate interventions.
3. Evaluate the various myths and facts about violence.
4. Analyze the dynamics of rape and sexual abuse.
5. Select the resources available to women experiencing abuse.
6. Outline the role of the nurse who cares for abused women.

Dorothy came to the prenatal clinic with a complaint of recurring headaches. She had been in twice this week already, but insisted she be seen today and started to cry. When the nurse called her into the examination room, Dorothy's cell phone rang. She hurried to answer it and told the person on the other end that she was at the store. When the nurse asked if she was afraid at home, Dorothy answered "at times." What cues did the nurse pick up on to ask that question? How frequent is this problem in women?

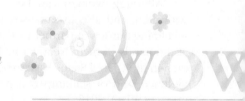

Words of Wisdom
After being traumatized, women can decide to stay in the shallow end of the pool or they can find support and swim in the ocean.

INTRODUCTION

Imagine if you were subjected to assault, rape, sexual slavery, torture, verbal abuse, mutilation, even murder—all because of your gender. It seems rarely acknowledged that violence against women and girls exists on the scale it does. Many of these females are brutalized from cradle to grave simply because of their gender. This abuse is the most pervasive human rights violation in the world today, and yet remains silent to many ears around the globe.

Gender-based violence is a major global public health and human rights problem and one that often goes unrecognized and unreported. It is a common source of physical, psychological, and emotional morbidity. It occurs in all countries, irrespective of social, economic, religious, or cultural group. It affects women across race, ethnicity, age, socioeconomic status, religion, sexual orientation, and geographic boundaries. No segments of society are immune from the vestiges of this problem. Due to the unequal power relations between men and women, women are violated either in the family, in the community, or in the country in which they live. The causes are multidimensional and are social, economic, cultural, political, and religious. Pregnancy is a time of unique vulnerability to intimate partner violence (IPV) victimization because of changes in women's physical, social, emotional, and economic needs during pregnancy. Although the true prevalence of violence during pregnancy is unclear, research suggests it is substantial and often continues into the postpartum period. Gender-based violence is one of the most rigorous challenges of women's health and well-being; it is a harrowing worldwide public health concern with serious consequences for individuals, families, and societies (Berthold, 2015).

Female-perpetrated violence against male partners receives little attention. Although women are victims of violence more frequently than men, the prevalence of violence among men nonetheless represents a significant public health concern. One out of every four men has experienced rape, physical violence, and/or stalking by an intimate partner in their lifetime (National Coalition Against Domestic Violence, 2015).

Although women can be violent in relationships with men, and also in same-sex partnerships, the overwhelming burden of partner violence is borne by women at the hands of men. Nearly 4 in 10 women and 1 in 10 men in the United States have experienced rape, physical violence, and/or stalking by a partner with IPV-related impact (WHO, 2015a).

For all the strides American women have made in the past 100 years, obliterating violence against themselves is not one of them. Violence against women is a growing problem and in many countries is still accepted as part of normal behavior. According to the Federal Bureau of Investigation (FBI) (2015), up to half of all women in the United States will experience some form of physical violence during their lifetime. In North America, 40% to 60% of murders of women are committed by intimate partners (FBI, 2015). Recently, the FBI has broadened its definition of rape. The new definition, as it appears on the FBI website, is "Penetration, no matter how slight, of the vagina or anus with any body part or object, or oral penetration by a sex organ of another person, without the consent of the victim." This broader definition will have a dramatic impact on the way rape is tracked and reported nationwide (FBI, 2015).

Federal funding for the problem is trickling down to local programs, but it is not reaching victims fast enough. For example, the United States has three times more shelters for animals than for battered women (Bouchet & Braswell, 2015). In many cases, a victim escapes her abuser only to be turned away from a local shelter because it is full. The number of abused women is staggering: one woman is being battered every 12 seconds in the United States (CDC, 2015a).

Nurses play a major role in assessing women who have suffered some type of violence. Nurses have a central ethic of caring and an agenda of early intervention and health promotion for their clients to improve their health status and well-being. Often, after a woman is victimized, she will complain about physical ailments that will give her the opportunity to visit a health care setting. A visit to a health care agency is an ideal time for women to be assessed for violence. Because nurses are viewed as trustworthy and sensitive about very personal subjects, women often feel comfortable confiding in them and discussing these issues with them. As a professional nurse, the act of screening women seen in every health care setting is often the first step for a victim to start thinking about a better future. Remember, your words carry weight with your client who looks to you for help, support, and encouragement.

Take Note!

Nurses will come in contact with violence and sexual abuse no matter what health care setting they work in. Nurses must be ready to ask the right questions and to act on the answers, because such action could be lifesaving.

This chapter addresses several types of gender-based violence: IPV, female genital cutting (FGC), human trafficking, and sexual abuse. All of these types of violence against women have devastating and costly consequences for all of society.

INTIMATE PARTNER VIOLENCE

IPV is actual or threatened physical or sexual violence or psychological/emotional abuse. Research suggests that physical violence in intimate relationships is often accompanied by psychological abuse and in one third to over one half of cases by sexual abuse (CDC, 2015b). Intimate partners include individuals who are currently

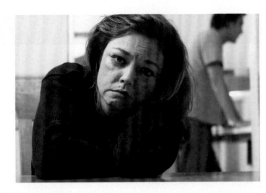

FIGURE 9.1 Intimate partner violence has significant physical, psychological, social, and economic consequences. An important role of the health care provider is to identify abusive or potentially abusive situations as soon as possible and provide support for the victim.

in dating, cohabiting, or marital relationships, or those who have been in such relationships in the past. Some of the common terms used to describe IPV are domestic abuse, spouse abuse, domestic violence, gender-based violence, battering, and rape. IPV affects a distressingly high percentage of the population and has physical, psychological, social, and economic consequences (Fig. 9.1).

Because a nurse may be the first health care provider to assess and identify the signs of IPV, a nurse can have a profound impact on a woman's decision to seek help. Thus, it is important for nurses to be able to identify abuse and aid the victim. IPV can leave significant psychological scars, and a well-trained nurse can have a positive impact on the victim's mental and emotional health.

Incidence

Overall, lifetime, and 1-year estimates for sexual violence, stalking, and IPV are alarmingly high for adult Americans, with IPV alone affecting more than 12 million people each year. On average, 20 persons per minute are victims of rape, physical violence, or stalking by an intimate partner in the United States. Women are disproportionately affected. The estimated cost of violence in the United States exceeds $70 billion each year. Each year, IPV results in an estimated 2,500 deaths and 3 million injuries among women (CDC, 2015c).

Women are at risk for violence at nearly every stage of their lives. Old, young, beautiful, unattractive, married, single—no woman is completely safe from the risk of IPV. Current or former husbands or lovers kill over half of the murdered women in the United States. IPV against women causes more serious injuries and deaths than automobile accidents, rapes, and muggings combined. IPV is expensive. The medical cost of IPV approaches $4.4 trillion each year globally to pay for medical and surgical care, counseling, child care, burden on the justice system, incarceration, attorney fees, and loss of work productivity (Lomborg, 2015).

IPV is pervasive and crosses all boundaries of sexual orientation, race, and class. The intimidation of another person through abusive acts and words is not a gender issue. Violence within these relationships may go unreported for fear of harassment or ridicule. The medical community's efforts to address IPV have often neglected members of the lesbian, gay, bisexual, and transgender (LGBT) population. Heterosexual women are primarily targeted for IPV screening and intervention despite the similar prevalence of IPV in LGBT individuals and its detrimental health effects (Cannon & Buttell, 2015). Perhaps because of the multiple barriers that confront LGBT abuse victims and the invisibility of the problem in the context of IPV services, the role of the nurse as their advocate is all the more critical.

Little is known about the national prevalence of IPV, sexual violence, and stalking among the LGBT community in the United States. Research documents that rates of IPV among LGBT individuals are equal to or greater than rates observed among heterosexual individuals. Risk factors are also similar to those documented among heterosexual individuals, in addition to help-seeking leaving, and recovery process (Edwards, Sylaska, & Neal, 2015). Current findings seem to also indicate some disparities in perceptions of what constitutes abuse among same and opposite sex couples (Russell & Chapleau, 2015). The *Violence against Women Act* has recently been renewed. It now includes coverage of same-sex partners—a big sign that attitudes are changing and improving for gays seeking shelters and help. As individuals and society come to realize same-sex partner violence as an existing problem, there is hope.

Background

Until the mid-1970s, our society tended to legitimize a man's power and control over a woman. The United States legal and judicial systems considered intervention into family disputes wrong and a violation of the family's right to privacy. IPV was often tolerated and even socially acceptable. Fortunately, attitudes and laws have changed to protect women and punish abusers. In *Healthy People 2020*, there are 13 measurable violence prevention objectives displayed in the *Healthy People 2020* table that follows. In addition to the 13 objectives listed, there are seven developmental objectives that focus on preventing sexual violence across the lifespan and preventing the different forms of partner violence including physical and sexual violence, emotional abuse, and stalking by a current or former partner.

Characteristics of Intimate Partner Violence

Although more research is needed in this area, studies have found certain risk factors for IPV in men. These

HEALTHY PEOPLE 2020 • 9.1

Violence Prevention Objectives

Objectives	Baseline (Year)	Target (2020)
IVP-29 Reduce homicides per 100,000 population	6.1 (2007)	5.5
IVP-30 Reduce firearm-related deaths per 100,000 population	10.3 (2007)	9.3
IVP-31 Reduce nonfatal firearm-related injuries per 100,000 population	20.7 (2007)	18.6
IVP-32 Reduce nonfatal physical assault injuries per 100,000 population	512.5 (2008)	461.2
IVP-33 Reduce physical assaults per 1,000 population (12+ years)	21.2 (2008)	19.2
IVP-34 Reduce physical fighting among adolescents in grades 9–12	31.5 (2009)	28.4
IVP-35 Reduce bullying among adolescents in grades 9–12	19.9 (2009)	17.9
IVP-36 Reduce weapon carrying by adolescents on school property	5.6 (2009)	4.6
IVP-37Reduce child maltreatment deaths per 100,000 population	2.3 (2008)	2.1
IVP-38 Reduce nonfatal child maltreatment per 100,000 population	9.4 (2008)	8.5
IVP-41 Reduce nonfatal intentional self-harm injuries per 100,000	124.9 (2008)	112.4
IVP-42 Reduce children's exposure to violence <18 years old	58.8 (2008)	52.9
IVP-43 Increase the number of states that link data on violent deaths	16 states	50 states

Nursing Significance

- Will increase men and women's quality and years of healthy life
- Eliminate health disparities for survivors of violence
- Goal is to have improved adherence to screening for IPV by health care providers
- Meeting these objectives will reflect the importance of early detection, intervention, and evaluation
- Eliminating LGBT health disparities and enhancing efforts to improve LGBT health are necessary to ensure that LGBT individuals can lead long, healthy lives

Healthy People objectives based on data from http://www.healthypeople.gov.

Adapted from U.S. Department of Health and Human Services [(USDHHS], (2015b). *Healthy People.gov.* Retrieved from www.healthypeople.gov/2020/default.aspx

risk factors can be divided into four different categories: individual factors, relationship factors, community factors, and societal factors. Specific risk factors within each category are listed in Table 9.1.

Generation-to-Generation Continuum of Violence

Violence is a learned behavior that, without intervention, is self-perpetuating. It is a cyclical health problem. The long-term effects of violence on victims and children can be profound. Children who witness one parent abuse another are more likely to become delinquents or batterers themselves because they see abuse as an integral part of a close relationship. Thus, an abusive relationship between father and mother can perpetuate future abusive relationships. Violence in childhood and adolescence is linked to the child's perception of the family as a hostile environment and of violence against

women as a corrective measure, and insults, swearing, and humiliation by their partner is acceptable (Song et al., 2015). If one considers violence against children and spouses, the psychological consequences are huge, stemming from the paradox of the victim being abused by a member of the family with whom he or she expects to have a supportive, loving, and respectful relationship. Research has found that children who witness IPV are at risk for developing psychiatric disorders, post-traumatic stress disorder (PTSD), developmental problems, school failure, violence against others, and low self-esteem (Cater et al., 2015).

Childhood maltreatment is a major health problem that is associated with a wide range of physical conditions and leads to high rates of psychiatric morbidity and social problems in adulthood. Consequences of violence extend far beyond the physical and mental suffering of victims and their families and have an impact on schools, neighborhoods, businesses, and the legal and health care

TABLE 9.1	COMMON MYTHS AND FACTS ABOUT VIOLENCE
Myths	**Facts**
Battering of women occurs only in lower socioeconomic classes	Violence occurs in all socioeconomic classes
Substance abuse causes the violence	Violence is a learned behavior and can be changed. The presence of drugs and alcohol can make a bad problem worse
Men have the right to discipline their partners. Battering is not a crime	In the past, our patriarchal legal system afforded men the right to physically chastise their wives and children; we no longer live under that system. Women and children are no longer considered the property of men, and violence against them is a crime in every state
Violence occurs to only a small percentage of women	One in four women will be victims of violence
Intimate partner violence (IPV) is typically a one time, isolated occurrence	Battering is a pattern of coercion and control that one person exerts over another. It is repeated using a number of tactics, including intimidation, threats, physical injury, economic deprivation, isolation, and sexual abuse. The various forms of abuse utilized by batterers help maintain power and control over their victims
Women can easily choose to leave an abusive relationship	Women stay in the abusive relationship because they feel they have no options
Only men with mental health problems commit violence against women	Abusers often seem normal and do not appear to suffer from personality disorders or other forms of mental illness
Pregnant women are protected from abuse by their partners	One in five women is physically abused during pregnancy. The effects of violence on infant outcomes can include preterm delivery, fetal distress, low birth weight, and child abuse
Women provoke their partners to abuse them	Women may be willing to blame themselves for someone else's bad behavior, but nobody deserves to be beaten
Violent tendencies have gone on for generations and are accepted	The police, justice system, and society are beginning to make IPV socially unacceptable
IPV is only a heterosexual issue	There is as much IPV in the lesbian/gay/bisexual/transgender population as in heterosexual relationships with the added psychological abuse of "outing" (when one partner threatens to disclose the others sexual preference in an effort to maintain power and control)

Adapted from Domestic Violence Organization.(2015a). *Common myths and why they are wrong.* Retrieved from http://www.domesticviolence.org/common-myths/; Tahoe Safe Alliance. (2015). *Myths about intimate partner violence in the LGBTQUA community.* Retrieved from http://tahoesafealliance.org/for-lgbqtia/lgbtqiamyths/; and Medicine Net. (2015b). *Domestic violence.* Retrieved from http://www.medicinenet.com/domestic_violence/page4.htm#what_are_the_causes_or_risk_factors_for_intimate_partner_violence

systems. Women who were physically or sexually abused as children have an increased risk of victimization and fear of crime, poor general health, and in addition experience adverse mental health conditions such as depression, anxiety, and low self-esteem as adults (Barrios et al., 2015).

In many cases when a parent is abused, the children are abused as well. Approximately one in eight children is abused annually in the United States. The lifetime economic cost to society of childhood maltreatment is estimated to be $124 billion dollars (Jackson & Deye, 2015). Young children who live with family violence represent a disempowered group. Developmentally, young children have relatively limited verbal skills and emotional literacy. In addition, the environment becomes one of secrecy and intimidation, as well as reduced emotional availability from the child's main caretaker. Taken together, these factors severely restrict these young children's capacity and opportunity to make their voices and needs heard (Jackson & Deye, 2015). Exposure to violence has a negative impact on children's physical, emotional, and cognitive well-being. The cycle continues into another generation through learned responses and violent acting out. Although there are always exceptions, most children deprived of their basic physical, psychological, and spiritual needs do not develop healthy personalities. They grow up with feelings of fear, behavioral problems, substance abuse, relationship difficulties, inadequacy, anxiety, anger, hostility, guilt, and rage. They often lack coping skills, blame others, demonstrate poor impulse control, have early delinquent behavior, and generally struggle with authority (Huang et al., 2015). Unless this cycle is broken, more than half become abusers themselves (CDC, 2015e).

The Cycle of Violence

In an abusive relationship, the cycle of violence comprises three distinct phases: the tension-building phase, the acute battering phase, and the honeymoon phase (Lawrence, 2015). The cyclical behavior begins with a time of tension-building arguments, progresses to violence, and settles into a making-up or calm period. This cycle of violence increases in frequency and severity as it is repeated over and over again. The cycle can cover a long or short period of time. The honeymoon phase gradually shortens and eventually disappears altogether. Abuse in relationships typically becomes accelerated and thus more dangerous over time. The abuser no longer feels the need to apologize and indulge in a honeymoon phase as the woman becomes increasingly disempowered in the relationship.

PHASE 1: TENSION BUILDING

During the first—and usually the longest—phase of the cycle, tension escalates between the couple. Excessive drinking, jealousy, or other factors might lead to name-calling, hostility, and friction. The woman might sense that her partner is reacting to her more negatively, that he is on edge and reacts heatedly to any trivial frustration. A woman often will accept her partner's building anger as legitimately directed toward her. She internalizes what she perceives as her responsibility to keep the situation from exploding. In her mind, if she does her job well, he remains calm. But if she fails, the resulting violence is her fault.

PHASE 2: ACUTE BATTERING

The second phase of the cycle is the explosion of violence. The batterer loses control both physically and emotionally. This is when the victim may be assaulted or murdered. After a battering episode, most victims consider themselves lucky that the abuse was not worse, no matter how severe their injuries. They often deny the seriousness of their injuries and refuse to seek medical treatment.

PHASE 3: HONEYMOON

The third phase of the cycle is a period of calm, loving, and contrite behavior on the part of the batterer. He may

---

<table>
<tr><td>

BOX 9.1

CYCLE OF VIOLENCE (FEMALE VICTIM AND MALE ABUSER)

- *Phase 1—Tension building:* Verbal or minor battery occurs. Almost any subject, such as housekeeping or money, may trigger the buildup of tension. There is a breakdown of communication. The victim attempts to calm the abuser. Victim feels like "walking on egg shells" around the abuser.
- *Phase 2—Acute battering:* Characterized by uncontrollable discharge of tension. Violence is rarely triggered by the victim's behavior: she is battered no matter what her response. The start of the battering episode is unpredictable and beyond the victim's control.
- *Phase 3—Reconciliation (honeymoon)/calm phase:* First, the abuser is ashamed of his behavior. The batterer tries to minimize the abuse and blame it on the partner. The batterer becomes loving, kind, and apologetic and expresses guilt. Then the abuser works on making the victim feel responsible. This loving behavior strengthens the bond between partners and will probably convince the victim, once again, that leaving the relationship is not necessary.

Adapted from Domestic Violence Organization.(2015b) *Cycle of violence.* Retrieved from http://www.domesticviolence.org/cycle-of-violence/; Domestic Violence Roundtable.(2015). *The cycle of domestic violence.* Retrieved from http://www.domesticviolenceroundtable.org/domestic-violence-cycle.html; and National Stress Clinic.(2015). *Domestic abuse: Understanding and breaking the cycle of violence.* Retrieved from http://www.nationalstressclinic.com/domestic-abuse-understanding-and-breaking-the-cycle-of-violence/

</td></tr>
</table>

be genuinely sorry for the pain he caused his partner. He attempts to make up for his brutal behavior and believes he can control himself and never hurt the woman he loves. The victim wants to believe that her partner really can change. She feels responsible, at least in part, for causing the incident, and she feels responsible for her partner's well-being (Box 9.1).

Types of Abuse

Abusers may use whatever it takes to control a situation—from emotional abuse and humiliation to physical assault. Victims often tolerate emotional, physical, financial, and sexual abuse. Many remain in abusive relationships because they believe they deserve the abuse.

Emotional Abuse

Emotional abuse includes:
- Promising, swearing, or threatening to hit the victim
- Forcing the victim to perform degrading or humiliating acts

- Threatening to harm children, pets, or close friends
- Humiliating the woman by name-calling and insults
- Threatening to leave her and the children
- Isolation from family and friends
- Destroying valued possessions
- Controlling the victim's every move

Physical Abuse

Physical abuse includes:
- Hitting or grabbing the victim so hard that it leaves marks
- Throwing things at the victim
- Slapping, spitting at, biting, burning, pushing, choking, or shoving the victim
- Kicking or punching the victim, or slamming her against things
- Attacking the victim with a knife, gun, rope, or electrical cord
- Controlling access to health care for injury

Financial Abuse

Financial abuse includes:
- Preventing the woman from getting a job
- Sabotaging a current job
- Controlling how all money is spent
- Failing to contribute financially

Sexual Abuse

Sexual abuse includes:
- Forcing the woman to have vaginal, oral, or anal intercourse against her will
- Biting the victim's breasts or genitals
- Shoving objects into the victim's vagina or anus
- Forcing the woman to do something sexual that she finds degrading or humiliating
- Forcing the victim to perform sexual acts on other people or animals

Myths and Facts About Intimate Partner Violence

Table 9.2 lists many of the myths about IPV. Health care providers should take steps to dispel these myths.

Abuse Profiles

Victims

Ironically, victims rarely describe themselves as abused. In battered woman syndrome, the woman has experienced deliberate and repeated physical or sexual assault by an intimate partner. She is terrified and feels trapped, helpless, and alone. She reacts to any expression of anger or threat by avoidance and withdrawal behavior. Some women believe that the abuse is caused by a personality flaw or inadequacy in themselves (e.g., inability to keep the man happy). These feelings of failure are reinforced and exploited by their partners. After being told repeatedly that they are "bad," some women begin to believe it. Many victims were abused as children and may have poor self-esteem, poor health, PTSD, depression, insomnia, low education achievement, or a history of suicide attempts, injury, or drug and alcohol abuse (Barrios et al., 2015).

Abusers

Abusers come from all walks of life and often feel insecure, powerless, and helpless; feelings that are not in line with the macho image they would like to project. The abuser expresses his feelings of inadequacy through violence or aggression toward others (Lawson, 2015).

Violence typically occurs at home and is usually directed toward the man's intimate partner or the children who live there. Abusers refuse to share power and choose violence to control their victims. They often exhibit childlike aggression or antisocial behaviors. They may fail to accept responsibility or blame others for their own problems. They might also have a history of substance abuse problems, trouble with the justice system, few close relationships, being sensitive to criticism, having a tendency to hold grudges, involved in power struggles, emotionally dysregulated, lacking in insight, prone to feeling misunderstood, mistreated, or victimized, mental illness, arrests, troubled relationships, obsessive jealousy, controlling behaviors, generally violent behavior, erratic employment history, and financial problems (Lawson, 2015).

Violence Against Pregnant Women

Many think of pregnancy as a time of celebration and planning for the unborn child's future, but in a troubled relationship it can be a time of escalating violence. The strongest predictor of abuse during pregnancy is prior abuse. Violence against pregnant women seems to be more prevalent than diseases routinely investigated during prenatal care, such as preeclampsia and diabetes (Lévesque & Chamberland, 2015). For women who have been abused before, beatings and violence during pregnancy are "business as usual" for them.

Women are at a higher risk for violence during pregnancy. Recent research findings indicate that having children does not protect women from IPV. On the contrary, the IPV appears to last longer if women have children, and this also seems to be the case even after the partnership has come to an end (Mauri et al., 2015). Pregnant women are vulnerable during this time, and abusers can take advantage of it. An estimated 325, 000 pregnant

TABLE 9.2   COMMON MYTHS AND FACTS ABOUT RAPE

Myths	Facts
Women who are raped get over it quickly	It can take several years to recover emotionally and physically from rape
Most rape victims tell someone about it	The majority of women never tell anyone about it. In fact, almost two thirds of victims never report it to the police
Once the rape is over, a survivor can again feel safe in her life	The victim feels vulnerable, betrayed, and insecure afterward
If a woman does not want to be raped, it cannot happen	A woman can be forced and overpowered by most men
Women who feel guilty after having sex then say they were raped	Few women falsely cry "rape." It is very traumatizing to be a victim
Victims should report the violence to the police and judicial system	Only 1% of rapists are arrested and convicted. Factoring unreported rapes together with the odds of being arrested and getting a felony conviction, only 6% of rapists will ever spend a day in jail. In other words, 15 of 16 rapists walk free
Women blame themselves for the rape, believing they did something to provoke the rape	Women should never blame themselves for being the victim of someone else's violence
When it comes to sex, men can be provoked to "a point of no return"	Men are physically able to stop at any point during sexual activity. Rape is not an act of impulsive, uncontrolled passion; it is a premeditated act of violence
Women who wear tight, short clothes are "asking for it"	No victim invites sexual assault, and what she wears is irrelevant
Women have rape fantasies and want to be raped	Reality and fantasy are different. Dreams have nothing to do with the brutal violation of rape
Only attractive women are raped	Anyone can be raped. Children, the elderly, and people with physical and mental disabilities are easy targets of rape because of their vulnerability
Medication can help women forget about the rape	Initially medication can help, but counseling is needed

Adapted from Centers for Disease Control and Prevention [CDC]. (2015f). *Understanding sexual violence*. Retrieved from http://www.cdc.gov/violenceprevention/pdf/svfactsheet2013-a.pdf; Rape Crisis. (2015). *Common myths about rape*. Retrieved from http://www.rapecrisis.org.uk/commonmyths2.php; Women Against Violence Against Women [WAVAW]. (2015). *Rape myths*. Retrieved from http://www.wavaw.ca/mythbusting/rape-myths/; and WELLWVU The Student's Center of Health. (2015). *Rape myths and facts*. Retrieved from: https://well.wvu.edu/articles/rape_myths_and_facts

women are abused by their partners each year (CDC, 2015a). Abuse during pregnancy poses special risks and dynamics. Various factors may lead to battering during pregnancy, including:

- Inability of the couple to cope with the stressors of pregnancy
- Young age at time of pregnancy
- Having less than a high school education for both partners
- Unemployment for either or both in partnership
- Violence in the family of origin
- Cohabitation and single marital status
- Sexual proprietariness on the part of the male partner
- Heavy drinking by partner
- Resentment toward the interference of the growing fetus and change in the woman's shape
- Doubts about paternity or the expectant mother's fidelity during pregnancy
- Perception that the baby will be a competitor
- Outside attention the pregnancy brings to the woman
- Unwanted pregnancy
- The woman's new interest in herself and her unborn baby
- Insecurity and jealousy about the pregnancy and the responsibilities it brings
- Financial burden related to expense of pregnancy and loss of income

- Stress of role transition from adult man to becoming the father of a child
- Physical and emotional changes of pregnancy that make the woman vulnerable
- Previous isolation from family and friends that limit the couple's support system

Abuse during pregnancy threatens the well-being of the mother and fetus. Physical violence may involve injuries to the head, face, neck, thorax, breasts, and abdomen. The mental health consequences are also significant. Several studies have confirmed the relationship between abuse and poor mental health, especially depression and PTSD; poor quality of life; increased distress, fearfulness, anxiousness, and stressfulness; and increased use of tobacco, alcohol, and/or illicit drugs (Lawson, 2015). For the pregnant woman, many of these conditions most often manifest during the postpartum period.

Take Note!

Frequently the fear of harm to her unborn child will motivate a woman to escape an abusive relationship.

Women assaulted during pregnancy are at risk for:
- Injuries to themselves and the fetus
- Depression
- Panic disorder
- Fetal and maternal deaths
- Chronic anxiety
- Miscarriage
- Stillbirth

- Poor nutrition
- Insomnia
- Placental abruption
- Uterine rupture
- Excessive weight gain or loss
- Smoking and substance abuse
- Delayed or no prenatal care
- Preterm labor
- Higher rate of surgical births
- Chorioamnionitis
- Vaginitis
- Sexually transmitted infections (STIs)
- Urinary tract infections
- Premature and low-birth-weight infants (AWHONN, 2015)

Signs of abuse can emerge during pregnancy and may include poor attendance at prenatal visits, unrealistic fears, weight fluctuations, difficulty with pelvic examinations, and nonadherence to treatment. See Evidence-Based Practice 9.1 for an intervention utilized for pregnant women experiencing IPV.

Uncovering abuse in pregnant women requires a consistent and direct approach to every client by the nurse. Multiple assessments may enhance reporting by enabling the nurse to establish trust and rapport with the woman and identify changes in her behavior. Once abuse is discovered in a pregnant woman, interventions should include safety assessment, emotional support, counseling, referral to community services, and ongoing prenatal care to avoid adverse health outcomes (Hewitt, 2015).

| EVIDENCE-BASED PRACTICE 9.1 | EFFECTIVENESS OF HOME VISITING IN REDUCING PARTNER VIOLENCE FOR FAMILIES EXPERIENCING ABUSE: A SYSTEMATIC REVIEW |

STUDY

IPV against women is a major, global societal problem with tremendous health consequences both for mother and child. Home visiting interventions by nurses for families at risk of abuse seem promising in decreasing IVP. In this systematic review, the effectiveness of home visiting was assessed as an intervention to reduce IPV experienced by mothers.

Findings

A systematic review was conducted of 1,258 articles; nineteen of them met the inclusion criteria and were examined in detail. Sixteen reported lower rates of physical assault with home visits by nurses and three studies showed no significant reduction of IPV. This systematic review found that home visiting interventions that support abused women during their pregnancy and beyond to

stop IPV seem to be effective in reducing the incidence of IPV. However, it is not known whether these results are effective in long-term.

Nursing Implications

By nurses making home visits, a trusting relationship can be established between the client and nurse. By addressing factors that may increase the risk of IPV in general, such as stress as well as other contributing factors, IPV can be reduced and the cycle of violence can be broken. A major benefit of home-visiting interventions is that they succeed in reaching high-risk young pregnant women, who are notoriously hard to reach for regular prenatal services during a vulnerable stage in their lives. Nurses can see the home environment and can detect risk factors and plan interventions to address them.

Adapted from Prosman, G. J., Wong, S. H., van der Wouden, J. C., & Lagro-Janssen, A. L. (2015). Effectiveness of home visiting in reducing partner violence for families experiencing abuse: A systematic review. *Family Practice*, 32(3), 247–256. (Online: 5/6/15).

Violence Against Older Women

IPV affects women of all ages, but often the literature focuses on women in the childbearing years, ignoring the problems of aging women who experience abuse. Elder mistreatment (i.e., abuse and neglect) is defined as intentional actions that cause harm or create a serious risk of harm to a vulnerable elder by a caregiver or other person who stands in a trust relationship to the elder. All 50 states have laws requiring health care providers to report elder or vulnerable person abuse. Estimates suggest that 500,000 to 2 million cases of elder abuse and neglect occur annually in the United States. It is estimated that one in ten older adults experience abuse, but only one in five to as little as one in twenty-four are reported. Research suggests that female elders are abused at a higher rate than males and that the older one is, the more likely one is to be abused. Elder abuse is expected to increase as the population ages (Wang et al., 2015). Types of abuse experienced by the older woman may include physical abuse, neglect, emotional abuse, sexual abuse, and financial/exploitation abuse (National Center on Elder Abuse, 2015).

Although an injury may bring the older woman into the health care system, the physical and emotional sequelae of IPV may be more subtle and may include depression, insomnia, chronic pain, difficulty trusting others, low self-esteem, thoughts of suicide, substance abuse, anger issues, atypical chest pain, or other kinds of somatic symptoms. Research suggests that older women usually have endured long-term abuse, have developed unhealthy strategies to cope (substance abuse, keeping the family together at all cost, and physical/mental health consequences), and shoulder blame from their adult children, yet have developed empowerment from within to be able to cope with the abuse (Policastro & Finn, 2015).

Accurate detection and assessment of abuse in older women are essential duties of all nurses. Nurses have frequent contact with older victims of abuse, providing them the opportunity to play a significant role in detecting, reporting, and intervening in such cases. As part of a thorough screening, nurses should determine what the client has done to attempt to resolve the abuse and the effectiveness of those strategies. Actions taken by the client, prior to revealing her abuse issue to the nurse, might have included passive acceptance, calling law enforcement, counseling, or other measures. In addition, taking time to establish rapport with older women builds a sense of trust, safety, and openness. Nurses must listen carefully and nonjudgmentally. Judging or criticizing the victim for her decisions might lead to the impression that she deserves the abuse or that she is to blame. Finally, nurses should attempt to stay current in their knowledge of referral resources to assist the older woman experiencing abuse. Some of these resources may be housing, transportation, medical services, employment, social services, and local support groups. A coordinated and comprehensive response to IPV is essential to reduce its sequelae.

Nursing Management of Intimate Partner Violence Victims

Nurses encounter thousands of abuse victims each year in their practice settings, but many victims slip through the cracks. As universal violence assessment has increased in recent years, nurses need to be aware of not only how to screen for violence, but how to respond in a way that is helpful, sincere, nonjudgmental, and legally adequate. This will require nurses to move beyond a description of violence toward a response that is action-oriented and evidence-based, which includes safety planning and referrals. There are many things that nurses can do to help victims. Early recognition and intervention can significantly reduce the morbidity and mortality associated with IPV. To stop the cycle of violence, nurses need to know how to assess for and identify IPV and implement appropriate actions.

Assessment

Routine screening for IPV is the first way to detect abuse. The nurse should build rapport by listening, showing an interest in the concerns of the woman, and creating an atmosphere of openness. Communicating support through a nonjudgmental attitude and telling the woman that no one deserves to be abused are first steps toward establishing trust and rapport. Rather than overlooking abused women as "chronic complainers," astute nurses need to be vigilant for subtle clues of abuse. Learning how to assess for abuse is critical. Some basic assessment guidelines follow.

SCREEN FOR ABUSE DURING EVERY HEALTH CARE VISIT

Screening for violence takes only a few minutes and can have an enormously positive effect on the outcome for the abused woman. Any woman could be a victim; no single sign marks a woman as an abuse victim, but the following clues may be helpful:

- *Injuries*—Bruises on their chest and abdomen, scars from blunt trauma, minor lacerations, or weapon wounds on the face, head, and neck
- *Injury sequelae*—Headaches, hearing loss from ruptured ear drums, joint pain, sinus infections, teeth marks, clumps of hair missing, dental trauma, pelvic pain, and breast or genital injuries
- Reported history of injury that is not consistent with the actual presenting problem
- *Mental health problems*—Depression, anxiety, substance abuse, eating disorders, suicidal ideation or suicide attempts, anger toward health care provider, and PTSD
- Frequent tranquilizer or sedative use
- Delay in seeking medical attention and patterns of repeated injury
- Bruises to the upper arm, neck and face, abdomen, or breasts

- Comments about emotional or physical abuse of "a friend"
- STIs or pelvic inflammatory disease
- Appears nervous, ashamed, or evasive when asked questions
- Frequent health care visits for chronic, stress-related disorders such as chest pain, headaches, back or pelvic pain, insomnia, injuries, anxiety, and gastrointestinal disturbances.
- Partner's behavior at the health care visit: appears overly solicitous or overprotective, is unwilling to leave her alone with the health care provider, answers questions for her, and attempts to control the situation (Ghandour, Campbell, & Lloyd, 2015).

Dorothy, who you met at the beginning of the chapter, has been frequenting the clinic with vague somatic complaints in recent weeks and admits she is sometimes afraid at home. She tells the nurse her partner doesn't want her to work, although he is only sporadically employed at low-paying jobs. What cues in her assessment might indicate abuse? What physical signs might the nurse observe?

ISOLATE CLIENT IMMEDIATELY FROM FAMILY

If abuse is detected, immediately isolate the woman to provide privacy and to prevent potential retaliation from the abuser. Asking about abuse in front of the perpetrator may trigger an abusive episode during the interview or at home. Ways to ensure the woman's safety would be to take the victim to an area away from the abuser to ask questions. The assessment can take place anywhere that is private and away from the abuser, for example, x-ray area, ultrasound room, elevator, ladies' room, or laboratory.

If abuse is detected, the nurse can do the following to enhance the nurse–client relationship:
- Educate the woman about the connection between the violence and her symptoms.
- Help the woman acknowledge what has happened to her and begin to deal with the situation.
- Offer her referrals so she can get the help that will allow her to begin to heal.

Dorothy returns to the prenatal clinic a month later with anemia, inadequate weight gain, bruises on her face and neck, and second-trimester bleeding. This time she is accompanied by her partner, who stays close to Dorothy. What questions should the nurse ask to assess the situation? Where is the appropriate location to ask these questions? What legal responsibilities does the nurse have concerning her observations?

ASK DIRECT OR INDIRECT QUESTIONS ABOUT ABUSE

Violence against women is often unseen, unknown, and hidden in families. Questions to screen for abuse should be routine and handled just like any other question. Many nurses feel uncomfortable asking questions of this nature, but broaching the subject is important even if the answer comes later. Opening up the possibility for women to express themselves about their experience of abuse to a nurse sends out a clear message that violence should never be tolerated and not kept hidden; it also conveys the message that nurses care about women's experiences and want to offer a best practice initial response. Just knowing that someone else knows about the abuse offers a victim some relief and may help her disclose it.

Ask difficult questions in an empathetic and non-threatening manner and remain nonjudgmental in all responses and interactions. Choose the type of question that makes you most comfortable. Direct and indirect questions produce the same results. "Does your partner hit you?" or "Have you ever been or are you now in an abusive relationship?" are direct questions. If that approach feels uncomfortable, try indirect questions: "We see many women with injuries or complaints like yours and often they are being abused. Is that what is happening to you?" or "Many women in our community experience abuse from their partners. Is anything like that happening in your life?" With either approach, nurses need to maintain a nonjudgmental acceptance of whatever answers the woman offers. The SAVE Model is a screening protocol that nurses can use when assessing women for violence (Box 9.2).

ASSESS IMMEDIATE SAFETY

It is essential to assist the woman by assessing her safety and the safety of her children. To do this, speak to the woman alone and ask her:
- Does she feel safe going home after her meeting with you?
- Does she need an immediate place of safety for herself or her children?
- Does she have a plan of escape if she becomes at risk for her safety?
- Does she need to consider an alternative exit from this building?
- Who are the people she could contact for help or support?

The Danger Assessment Tool (Box 9.3) helps women and health care providers assess the potential for homicidal behavior in an ongoing abusive relationship. It is based on research that showed several risk factors for abuse-related murders:
- Increased frequency or severity of abuse
- Presence of firearms
- Sexual abuse

BOX 9.2

SAVE MODEL

SCREEN all of your clients for violence by asking:
- Within the last year, have you been physically hurt by someone?
- Do you feel you are in control of your life?
- Within the last year, has anyone forced you to engage in sexual activities?
- Can you talk about your abuse with me now?
- In general, how would you describe your present relationship?

ASK direct questions in a nonjudgmental way:
- Begin by normalizing the topic to the woman.
- Make continuous eye contact with the woman.
- Stay calm; avoid emotional reactions to what she tells you.
- Never blame the woman, even if she blames herself.
- Do not dismiss or minimize what she tells you, even if she does.
- Wait for each answer patiently. Do not rush to the next question.
- Do not use formal, technical, or medical language.
- Avoid using leading questions; be direct and to the point.
- Use a nonthreatening, accepting approach.

VALIDATE the client by telling her:
- You believe her story.
- You do not blame her for what happened.
- It is brave of her to tell you this.
- Help is available for her.
- Talking with you is a hopeful sign and a first big step.

EVALUATE, educate, and refer this client by asking her:
- What type of violence was it?
- Is she now in any danger?
- How is she feeling now?
- Does she know that there are consequences to violence?
- Is she aware of community resources available to help her?

Adapted from USDHHS. (2015c). Screening for domestic violence in health care settings. *Office of the Assistant Secretary for Planning and Evaluation.* Retrieved from http://aspe.hhs.gov/hsp/13/dv/pb_screeningdomestic.cfm; Association of Women's Health, Obstetric and Neonatal Nurses [AWHONN]. (2015). Intimate partner violence. *Journal of Obstetric, Gynecologic & Neonatal Nursing, 44*(3), 405–408.; and Canadian Domestic Homicide Prevention Initiative. (2015). *Risk assessment, risk management and safety planning.* Retrieved from http://www.learningtoendabuse.ca/cdhpi/risk-assessment-risk-management-and-safety-planning

- Substance abuse
- Precipitated by arguments and conflicts
- Generally violent behavior outside of the home
- Control issues (e.g., daily chores, friends, job, money)
- Physical abuse during pregnancy
- Suicide threats or attempts (victim or abuser)
- Child abuse (Sugg, 2015).

DOCUMENT AND REPORT YOUR FINDINGS

If the interview reveals a history of abuse, accurate documentation is critical because this evidence may support the woman's case in court. Documentation must include details about the frequency and severity of abuse; the location, extent, and outcome of injuries; and any treatments or interventions. When documenting, use direct quotes and be very specific: "He choked me." Describe any visible injuries, and use a body map (outline of a woman's body) to show where the injuries are. Obtain photos (with informed consent) or document her refusal if the woman declines photos. Pictures or diagrams can be worth a thousand words. Figure 9.2 shows a sample documentation form for IPV.

Laws in many states require health care providers to alert the police to any injuries that involve knives, firearms, or other deadly weapons or that present life-threatening emergencies. If assessment reveals suspicion or actual indication of abuse, nurses can explain to the woman that they are required by law to report it.

Nursing Diagnosis

When violence is suspected or validated, the nurse needs to formulate nursing diagnoses based on the completed assessment. Possible nursing diagnoses related to violence against women might include the following:
- Deficient knowledge related to understanding the cycle of violence and availability of resources
- Anxiety related to threat to self-concept, situational crisis of abuse
- Situational low self-esteem related to negative family interactions
- Powerlessness related to lifestyle of helplessness
- Compromised individual and family coping related to abusive patterns

Interventions

The response of nurses to battered women can have a profound effect on their willingness to open up or seek help. Some responses to assist successful communication in these circumstances could include:
- *Listening*—"I hear and understand what you are saying." Being listened to can be an empowering experience for a woman who has been abused.
- *Communicating belief*—"That must have been very frightening for you."
- *Validating the decision to disclose*—"It must have been difficult for you to talk about this today."
- *Emphasizing the unacceptability of this violence*—"You don't deserve to be treated this way."

If abuse is identified, nurses can undertake interventions that can increase the woman's safety and improve her health. The goal of intervention is to enable the victim to gain control of her life. Provide sensitive, predictable

---

BOX 9.3

DANGER ASSESSMENT TOOL

Several risk factors have been associated with increased risk of homicides (murders) of women and men in violent relationships. No one can predict what will happen in your case, but we would like you to be aware of the danger of homicide in situations of abuse and for you to see how many of the risk factors apply to your situation. ("He" refers to your husband, partner, ex-husband, ex-partner, or whoever is currently physically hurting you).

_____1. Has the physical violence increased in severity or frequency over the past year?

_____2. Does he own a gun?

_____3. Have you left him after living together during the past year?

_____4. Is he unemployed?

_____5. Has he ever used a weapon against you or threatened you with a lethal weapon?

_____6. Does he threaten to kill you?

_____7. Has he avoided being arrested for domestic violence?

_____8. Do you have a child who is not his?

_____9. Has he ever forced you to have sex when you did not wish to do so?

_____10. Does he ever try to choke you?

_____11. Does he use illegal drugs? By drugs, I mean "uppers" or amphetamines, "meth," speed, angel dust, cocaine, "crack," street drugs, or mixtures.

_____12. Is he an alcoholic or problem drinker?

_____13. Does he control most or all of your daily activities? For instance: does he tell you who you can be friends with, when you can see your family, how much money you can use, or when you can take the car?

_____14. Is he violently and constantly jealous of you? (For instance, does he say "If I can't have you, no one can").

_____15. Have you ever been beaten by him while you were pregnant?

_____16. Has he ever threatened or tried to commit suicide?

_____17. Does he threaten to harm your children?

_____18. Do you believe he is capable of killing you?

_____19. Does he follow or spy on you, leave threatening notes or messages on answering machine, destroy your property, or call you when you don't want him to?

_____20. Have you ever threatened or tried to commit suicide?

_____ Total "Yes" Answers

Thank you. Please talk to your nurse, advocate, or counselor about what the Danger Assessment means in terms of your situation.

Source: March of Dimes Danger Assessment questionnaire. From Campbell, J. (1986). Nursing assessment for risk of homicide with battered women. *Advances in Nursing Science, 8*(4), 36–51.

---

care in an accepting setting. Offer step-by-step explanations of procedures. Provide educational materials about violence. Allow the victim to actively participate in her care and have control over all health care decisions. Pace your nursing interventions and allow the woman to take the lead. Communicate support through a nonjudgmental attitude. Carefully document all of your assessment findings and nursing interventions.

 Concept Mastery Alert

Priorities in Intimate Partner Violence Interventions

Although it is certainly important that the woman in an abusive situation is safe, it is most important for a woman to regain a sense of control in her life. A lack of control is what prevents a woman from escaping an abusive situation.

A public health approach to violence prevention requires input from and coordination across sectors, including health, education, social services, justice, and policy. The goal of public health is to improve the health of the entire community or society. Depending on when in the cycle of violence the nurse encounters the abused woman, goals may fall into three groups:

- *Primary prevention*—aimed at breaking the abuse cycle through community educational initiatives by nurses, physicians, law enforcement, teachers, and clergy.
- *Secondary prevention*—focuses on screening high-risk individuals and dealing with victims and abusers in early stages, with the goal of preventing progression of abuse.
- *Tertiary prevention*—activities are geared toward helping severely abused women and children

Domestic Violence Screening/Documentation Form

| DV Screen
☐ DV + (Positive)
☐ DV? (Suspected) | Date _____ Patient ID# _____
Patient Name _____
Provider Name _____
Patient Pregnant? ☐ Yes   ☐ No |

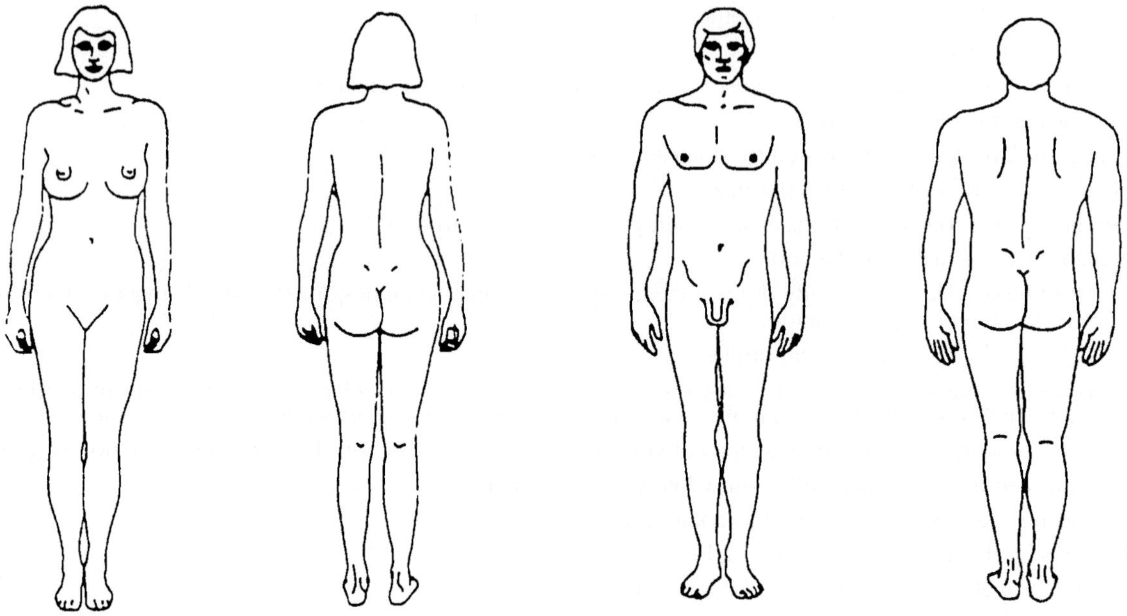

Assess Patient Safety

☐ Yes ☐ No   Is abuser here now?

☐ Yes ☐ No   Is patient afraid of their partner?

☐ Yes ☐ No   Is patient afraid to go home?

☐ Yes ☐ No   Has physical violence increased in severity?

☐ Yes ☐ No   Has partner physically abused children?

☐ Yes ☐ No   Have children witnessed violence in the home?

☐ Yes ☐ No   Threats of homicide?

By whom? _____

☐ Yes ☐ No   Threats of suicide?

By whom? _____

☐ Yes ☐ No   Is there a gun in the home?

☐ Yes ☐ No   Alcohol or substance abuse?

☐ Yes ☐ No   Was safety plan discussed?

Referrals

☐ Hotline number given

☐ Legal referral made

☐ Shelter number given

☐ In-house referral made

Describe: _____

☐ Other referral made

Describe: _____

Reporting

☐ Law enforcement report made

☐ Child Protective Services report made

☐ Adult Protective Services report made

Photographs

☐ Yes ☐ No   Consent to be photographed?

☐ Yes ☐ No   Photographs taken?

Attach photographs and consent form

FIGURE 9.2 Intimate partner violence documentation form. (Reprinted from Home Healthcare Nurse, 17, Cassidy K, How to assess *and intervene in domestic violence situations, 644–72, Copyright 1999, with permission from Lippincott Williams & Wilkins.*)

recover and become productive members of society and rehabilitating abusers to stop the cycle of violence. These activities are typically long term and expensive.

A modified tool developed by Holtz and Furniss (1993)—the ABCDES—provides a framework for providing sensitive nursing interventions to abused women (Box 9.4). Specific nursing interventions for the abused woman include educating her about community services, providing emotional support, and offering a safety plan.

BOX 9.4

THE ABCDES OF CARING FOR ABUSED WOMEN

- **A** is reassuring the woman that she is not alone. The isolation by her abuser keeps her from knowing that others are in the same situation and that health care providers can help her.
- **B** is expressing the belief that violence against women is not acceptable in any situation and that it is not her fault. Demonstrate by your actions and words that you believe her disclosure.
- **C** is confidentiality, since the woman might believe that if the abuse is reported, the abuser will retaliate. Interview her in private, without her partner or family members being present. Assure her that you will not release her information without her permission.
- **D** is documentation, which includes the following:
  - A clear quoted statement about the abuse in the woman's own words
  - Accurate descriptions of injuries and the history of them
  - Information on the first, the worst, and the most recent abusive incident
  - Photos of the injuries (with the woman's consent)
- **E** is education about the cycle of violence and that it will escalate:
  - Educate about abuse and its health effects.
  - Help her understand that she is not alone.
  - Offer appropriate community support and referrals.
  - Display posters and brochures to foster awareness of this public health problem.
- **S** is safety, the most important aspect of the intervention, to ensure that the woman has resources and a plan of action to carry out when she decides to leave.

Adapted from Centers for Disease Control & Prevention [CDC]. (2015a). *Understanding intimate partner violence: Fact sheet.* Retrieved from http://www.cdc.gov/violenceprevention/pub/ipv_factsheet.html; Human Rights Watch. (2015). *Abused and expelled.* Retrieved from http://www.hrw.org/sites/default/files/reports/morocco0214_ForUpload.pdf; and Ghandour, R. M., Campbell, J. C., & Lloyd, J. (2015). Screening and counseling for intimate partner violence: A vision for the future. *Journal of Women's Health, 24*(1), 57–61.

EDUCATE THE WOMAN ABOUT COMMUNITY SERVICES

A wide range of support services are available to meet the needs of victims of violence. Nurses should be prepared to help the woman take advantage of these opportunities. Services will vary by community but might include psychological counseling, legal advice, social services, crisis services, support groups, hotlines, housing, vocational training, and other community-based referrals.

Give the woman information about shelters or services even if she initially rejects it. Give the woman the National Domestic Violence hotline number: (800) 799-7233. The Joint Commission on the Accreditation of Hospitals and Health care Organizations (JCAHO), American Medical Association (AMA), American College of Obstetrician Gynecologists (ACOG), and the United States Preventive Services Task Force (USPSTF) all recommend routine IVP screening, counseling, and referrals in all health care agencies (USDHHS, 2015c).

PROVIDE EMOTIONAL SUPPORT

Providing reassurance and support to a victim of abuse is essential if the violence is to end. The physical, psychological, and emotional effects of IPV on women and their children can be severe and long-lasting. Nurses in all clinical settings can help victims to feel a sense of personal power and provide them with a safe and supportive environment. Appropriate action can help victims to express their thoughts and feelings in constructive ways, manage stress, and move on with their lives. Appropriate interventions are:

- Strengthen the woman's sense of control over her life by:
  - Teaching coping strategies to manage her stress
  - Assisting with activities of daily living to improve her lifestyle
  - Allowing her to make as many decisions as she can
  - Educating her about the symptoms of PTSD and their basis
- Encourage the woman to establish realistic goals for herself by:
  - Teaching problem-solving skills
  - Encouraging social activities to connect with other people
  - Providing support and allow the woman to grieve for her losses by:
    - Listening to and clarifying her reactions to the traumatic event
    - Discussing shock, disbelief, anger, depression, and acceptance
- Explain to the woman that:
  - Abuse is never OK. She didn't ask for it and she doesn't deserve it
  - She is not alone and help is available
  - Abuse is a crime and she is a victim
  - Alcohol, drugs, money problems, depression, or jealousy does not cause violence, but these things

can give the abuser an excuse for losing control and abusing her
- The actions of the abuser are not her fault
- Her history of abuse is believed
- Making a decision to leave an abusive relationship can be very hard and takes time

OFFER A SAFETY PLAN

The choice to leave must rest with the victim. Nurses cannot choose a life for the victim; they can only offer choices. Leaving is a process, not an event. Victims may try to leave their abusers as many as seven or eight times before succeeding. Frequently, the final attempt to leave may result in the death of the victim. Women planning to leave an abusive relationship should have a safety plan, if possible (Teaching Guidelines 9.1).

Teaching Guidelines 9.1

SAFETY PLAN FOR LEAVING AN ABUSIVE RELATIONSHIP

- When leaving an abusive relationship, take the following items:
  - Driver's license or photo ID
  - Social Security number or green card/work permit
  - Birth certificates for you and your children
  - Phone numbers for social services or women's shelter
  - The deed or lease to your home or apartment
  - Any court papers or orders
  - A change of clothing for you and your children
  - Pay stubs, checkbook, credit cards, and cash
  - Health insurance cards
- If you need to leave a domestic violence situation immediately, turn to authorities for assistance in gathering this material.
- Develop a "game plan" for leaving and rehearse it.
- Don't use phone cards—they leave a trail to follow.

Adapted from Burnett, L. B., & Adler, J. (2015). Domestic violence. *eMedicine*. Retrieved from http://emedicine.medscape.com/article/805546-overview; Murray, C. E., Horton, G. E., Johnson, C. H., Notestine, L., Garr, B., Pow, A. M., et al. (2015). Domestic violence service providers' perceptions of safety planning: A focus group study. *Journal of Family Violence*, 30(3), 381–392; and Chang, J. C. (2015). Domestic violence: Epidemiology and risk factors. *Clinical Gynecology* (2nd ed., pp. 94–101). Cambridge, UK: Cambridge University Press.

Nurses need to remember that their role is that of a guide, not a savior. A woman will make the best decision she sees fit at that moment in time. A nurse may be her most effective resource in her stress-filled environment. Just allowing the woman to talk may be the most valuable intervention. The impact of the nurse's presence and support will stay with the woman, no matter what decision she makes.

SEXUAL VIOLENCE

Sexual violence is both a public health problem and a human rights violation. Sexual violence includes IPV, human trafficking, incest, FGC, forced prostitution, bondage, exploitation, neglect, infanticide, and sexual assault. It occurs worldwide and affects up to one third of women over a lifetime (Bagwell-Gray, Messing, & Baldwin-White, 2015). Once every 2 minutes, 30 times an hour, 1,871 times a day, girls and women in America are raped. One in five women and 1 in 71 men will be sexually assaulted during their lifetime (Rape, Abuse, & Incest National Network [RAINN], 2015a). Rape has been reported against females from age 6 months to 93 years, but it still remains one of the most underreported violent crimes in the United States. Once every 2 minutes, a woman is sexually assaulted in the United States (RAINN, 2015a). The National Center for Prevention and Control of Sexual Assault estimates that two thirds of sexual assaults will not be reported (CDC, 2015f). Over the course of their lives, women may experience more than one type of violence.

Sexual violence can have a variety of devastating short- and long-term effects. Women can experience psychological, physical, and cognitive symptoms that affect them daily. They can include chronic pelvic pain, headaches, backache, STIs, pregnancy, anxiety, denial, fear, withdrawal, sleep disturbances, guilt, nervousness, phobias, substance abuse, depression, sexual dysfunction, and PTSD. Many contemplate suicide (CDC, 2015f). A traumatic experience not only damages a woman's sense of safety in the world, but it can also reduce her self-esteem and her ability to continue her education, to earn money and be productive, to have children and, if she has children, to nurture and protect them. Overall, sexually assaulted women exhibit lower functioning as adults afterward (MacGregor et al., 2015).

Take Note!

Sexual violence has been called a "tragedy of youth." More than half of all rapes (54%) of women occur before age 18 (Medicine Net, 2015a).

Characteristics of Assailants

Assailants, like their victims, come from all walks of life and all ethnic backgrounds; there is no typical profile. More than half are under age 25, and the majority are married and leading "normal" sex lives. Why do men rape? No theory provides a satisfactory explanation. So few assailants are caught and convicted that a clear profile remains elusive. What is known is that many assailants have trouble dealing with the stresses of daily life. Such men become angry and experience feelings of powerlessness. They become jealous easily; do not view women as equals; frequently are hot tempered; have a need to be reassured of their manhood; and do not handle stress in their lives well. They commit a sexual assault as an expression of power and control (Kilmartin, 2015).

Sexual Abuse

Sexual abuse occurs when a woman is forced to have sexual contact of any kind (vaginal, oral, or anal) without her consent. Current estimates indicate that one of five girls is sexually abused, and the peak ages of such abuse are from 8 to 12 years of age. At every age in the life span, females are more likely to be sexually abused by father, brother, family member, neighbor, boyfriend, husband, partner, or ex-partner than by a stranger or anonymous assailant. Sexual abuse knows no economic or cultural barriers (de Jong et al., 2015). Marriage does not constitute a tacit agreement for a spouse to inflict one's demands on the other without permission.

Childhood sexual abuse is any type of sexual exploitation that involves a child younger than 18 years old. It might include disrobing, nudity, masturbation, fondling, digital penetration, forced performance of sexual acts on the perpetrator, and intercourse (Dutton, 2015). Childhood sexual abuse has a lifelong impact on its survivors.

There is strong evidence that sexual assault in childhood or adolescence is a serious risk factor for mental illness (Brooker & Durmaz, 2015). Women who were sexually abused during childhood are at a heightened risk for repeat abuse. This is because the early abuse lowers their self-esteem and their ability to protect themselves and set firm boundaries. Childhood sexual abuse is a trauma that influences the way victims form relationships, deal with adversity, cope with daily problems, relate to their children and peers, protect their health, and live. See Evidence-Based Practice 9.2 for study regarding childhood sexual abuse. Studies have shown that the more victimization a woman experiences, the more likely it is she will be revictimized (Brenner & Ben-Amitay, 2015).

Interventions for sexually abused children or women should include referral for mental health counseling. Follow up for any medical problems (e.g., genitourinary complaints) should be arranged with the child's or woman's primary care physician. If the community has an abuse referral center, refer the victim there for follow-up care according to local protocol.

The medical consequences of sexual abuse require the prophylaxis and treatment of STIs, emergency contraception, and treatment of any injuries that resulted from

---

EVIDENCE-BASED PRACTICE 9.2

SIBLING SEXUAL ABUSE: AN EXPLORATORY STUDY OF LONG-TERM CONSEQUENCES FOR SELF-ESTEEM AND COUNSELING CONSIDERATIONS

Today, health care providers recognize childhood sexual abuse within the family as a significant and widespread problem with consequences lasting long into adulthood. Despite this progression, the research related to interfamilial incest conducted by researchers has focused primarily on father to daughter incest, largely ignoring the experience of sibling sexual assault, although it is more common than parental incest. Clearly, sibling incest is a pandemic problem that requires more attention from health care providers.

STUDY

This study addresses experiencing sibling sexual abuse as a child and how it inversely affects the level of self-esteem in adulthood. One hundred college students were used as the sample size; 67% were female and 33% were male with a diverse cultural representation. The age of the students ranged from 20 to 59 years old. A survey with two sections was used. The first section addressed recollection of the prevalence and severity of sibling abuse; the second section of the survey addressed self-esteem using the Rosenberg Self-Esteem Scale. Reliability and validity of this tool reflected a Cronbach's alpha coefficient of 0.82.

Findings

This study supported the likelihood that sibling sexual abuse could be the most common form of child sexual

abuse in the United States. In spite of the apparent prevalence of this, it is disturbing how little has been done to address the complexity surrounding this form of abuse. Both survivors and offenders of sibling sexual abuse experience the lasting impact of the abuse as they become adults in their social interactions, school, work, and family life. In addition to a low self-esteem, other mental health issues experienced include symptoms of PTSD, anxiety disorders, depression, eating disorders, angry outbursts, self-injury, somatic complaints, and suicidal ideation. Many engage in at-risk behaviors such as unprotected sex, self-medication with drugs and alcohol, and dating violence. Clearly, ignoring the problem of sibling sexual abuse has a negative effect on a sense of well-being as these children become adults.

Nursing Implications

One of the most important aspects is to establish trust with these clients and create a safe environment. An important role for nurses is in primary prevention of sibling sexual abuse through educating parents. When parents understand how to promote positive parent–child relationships and sibling interactions, the risk of abuse in the entire family tends to be reduced. Nurses can take a lead role through promotion of structured parent education programs within their communities and referrals to national networks such as Family Support America.

Adopted from Morrill, M. (2014). Sibling sexual abuse: An exploratory study of long term consequences for self-esteem and counseling considerations. *Journal of Family Violence, 29*(2), 205–213.

the abuse. Victims with post-assault bleeding require an emergent evaluation and may need emergency treatment by a gynecologist for repair of genital injury. The psychosocial aspects of sexual abuse must also be addressed because appropriate therapeutic follow-up is essential to the victim's future emotional well-being.

Incest

Incest is defined as sexual activity between persons so closely related that marriage between them is legally or culturally prohibited (Dorland's Medical Dictionary, 2015). The exact incidence of child sexual victimization is unknown. Such sexual abuse is not only a crime but also a symptom of acute and irreversible family dysfunction. Childhood incest abuse involves any kind of sexual exploitation between a child and another person that violates the social taboos of family roles; children cannot yet understand these activities and cannot give informed consent. Adult women with a history of incest exhibit a clinical syndrome that includes low self-esteem, difficulty with intimate relationships, sexual dysfunction, flashbacks and nightmares, repeated victimization, as well as suicidality, depressive symptomatology, eating disorders, and substance abuse (Harkins, 2015). Survivors of incest are often tricked, coerced, or manipulated. All adults appear to be powerful to children. Perpetrators might threaten victims so that they are afraid to disclose the abuse or might tell them the abuse is their fault. Often these threats serve to silence victims.

Incestuous relationships in the home endanger not only the child's intellectual and moral development, but also the health of the child. Many children do not ask for help because they do not want to expose their "secret." For this reason, just the tip of the iceberg is statistically visible: serious injuries, internal damage, STIs, or pregnancy. Incest can have serious long-term effects on its victims, which may include eating disorders, sexual problems in adult life, difficulty in interpersonal relationships, anxiety, PTSD, intense guilt and shame, low self-esteem, depression, and self-destructive behavior (National Center for Victims of Crime [NCVC], 2015a).

Whether an incest victim endured an isolated incident of abuse or ongoing assaults over an extended period, recovery can be painful and difficult. The recovery process begins with admission of abuse and the recognition that help and services are needed. Resources for incest victims include books, self-help groups, workshops, therapy programs, and possibly legal remedies. In addition to listening to and believing incest victims, nurses need to search for ways to prevent future generations from enduring such abuse and from continuing the cycle of abuse in their own family and relationships. Nurses have the ability and the responsibility to function within an interdisciplinary system responsible for the assessment and ongoing treatment of incestuous families. Nurses can fulfill their roles as advocates for children, while at the same time adding necessary referrals to social services and legal authorities. Forming this partnership with the social service and judicial communities will help protect the child from future abuse and ensure the child a safe environment in which to grow and develop.

Take Note!

Childhood sexual abuse is a trauma that can affect every aspect of the victim's life.

Rape

Rape is an expression of violence, not a sexual act. Rape distorts one of the most intimate forms of human interaction. It is not an act of lust or an overzealous release of passion: it is a violent, aggressive assault on the victim's body and integrity. Those who rape do so for a number of reasons, but they basically involve the motives of anger, power, eroticized cruelty, and opportunistic mating (Keygnaert, Vettenburg, & Temmerman, 2015). Rape is a legal rather than a medical term. It denotes penile penetration of the vagina, mouth, or rectum of the female or male without consent. It may or may not include the use of a weapon. Statutory rape is sexual activity between an adult and a person under the age of 18 and is considered to have occurred even if the underage person was willing (RAINN, 2015b). Nine out of every 10 rape victims are female (Alexander et al., 2014). Enforcement of laws, education, and

Consider This

At 53 years old, I stood and looked at myself in the mirror. The image staring back at me was one of a frightened, middle-aged, cowardly woman hiding her past. I had been sexually abused by my father for many years as a child and never told anyone. My mother knew of the abuse but felt helpless to make it stop. I married right out of high school to escape and felt I lived a "happy normal life" with my husband and three children. My children have left home and live away, and my husband recently died of a sudden heart attack. I am now experiencing dreams and thoughts about my past abuse and feeling afraid again.

Thoughts: This woman suppressed her abusive past for most of her life and now her painful experience has surfaced. What can be done to reach out to her at this point? Did her health care providers miss the "red flags" that are common to women with a history of childhood sexual abuse all those years?

TABLE 9.3   FOUR PHASES OF RAPE RECOVERY

Phase	Survivor's Response
Acute phase (disorganization)	Shock, fear, disbelief, anger, shame, guilt, feelings of uncleanliness; insomnia, nightmares, and sobbing
Outward adjustment phase (denial)	Appears outwardly composed and returns to work or school; refuses to discuss the assault and denies need for counseling
Reorganization	Denial and suppression do not work, and the survivor attempts to make life adjustments by moving or changing jobs and uses emotional distancing to cope
Integration and recovery	Survivor begins to feel safe and starts to trust others. She may become an advocate for other rape victims

Adapted from National Center for Victims of Crime [NCVC]. (2015b). *The trauma of victimization*. Retrieved from http://victimsofcrime. org/help-for-crime-victims/get-help-bulletins-for-crime-victims/trauma-of-victimization#ptsd; Rape, Abuse, and Incest National Network [RAINN]. (2015d). *Recovery from sexual assault*. Retrieved from http://www.rainn.org/get-information/sexual-assault-recovery; and The Advocacy Center (2015). *The path toward recovery for survivors of sexual violence*. Retrieved from http://advocacycenter.syr.edu/students/path-of-recovery/

community empowerment are all needed to prevent rape.

Many people believe that rape usually occurs on a dark night when a stranger assaults a provocatively dressed, promiscuous woman. They believe that rapists are sex-starved people seeking sexual gratification. Rape myths are destructive beliefs about sexual aggression (i.e., its scope, causes, context, and consequences) that serve to deny, downplay, or justify sexually aggressive behavior that men commit against women. A rape victim's recovery is frequently complicated by the public's failure to believe the victim and restore justice (Klaus, Buczkowski, & Wiktorska, 2015). Rape myths serve to blame victims and exonerate perpetrators. Such myths and the facts are presented in Table 9.3.

Acquaintance Rape

In acquaintance rape, someone is forced to have sex by a person he or she knows. Rape by a coworker, a teacher, a husband's friend, or a boss is considered acquaintance rape. Date rape, an assault that occurs within a dating relationship or marriage without consent of one of the

participants, is a form of acquaintance rape. Acquaintance and date rapes commonly occur on college campuses. One in four college women has been raped—that is, has been forced, physically or verbally, actively or implicitly, to engage in sexual activity (Wilson & Miller, 2015).

These forms of rape are physically and emotionally devastating for the victims. Research has indicated that the survivors of acquaintance rape report similar levels of depression, anxiety, complications in subsequent relationships, and difficulty attaining prerape levels of sexual satisfaction to those reported by survivors of stranger rape. Acquaintance rape remains a controversial topic because there is lack of agreement on the definition of consent. Despite the violation and reality of physical and emotional trauma, victims of acquaintance assault often do not identify their experience as sexual assault. Instead of focusing on the violation of the sexual assault, victims of acquaintance rape often blame themselves for the assault (RAINN, 2015c).

Although acquaintance rape and date rape do not always involve drugs, a rapist might use alcohol or other drugs to sedate his victim. In 1996, the federal government passed a law making it a felony to give an unsuspecting person a "date rape drug" with the intent of raping him or her. Even with penalties of large fines and up to 20 years in prison, the use of date rape drugs is growing (USDHHS, 2015a). Date rape drugs are also known as "club drugs" because they are often used at dance clubs, fraternity parties, and all-night raves. The most common is rohypnol (also known as "roofies," "forget pills," "mind erasers," or the "drop drug"). It comes in the form of a liquid or pill that quickly dissolves in liquid with no odor, taste, or color. This drug is 10 times as strong as diazepam (Valium). The effects can be felt within 30 minutes and produces memory loss for up to 8 hours. Gamma hydroxybutyrate (GHB; called "liquid ecstasy" or "easy lay") produces euphoria, an out-of-body high, sleepiness, increased sex drive, and memory loss. GHB takes effects in about 15 minutes and can last 3 to 4 hours. It comes in a white powder or liquid and may cause unconsciousness, depression, and coma. The third date rape drug, ketamine (known as "Special K," "vitamin K," or "super acid"), and acts on the central nervous system very quickly to separate perception and sensation. Combining ketamine with other drugs can be fatal. Date rape drugs can be very dangerous, and women can protect themselves against them in a variety of ways (Teaching Guidelines 9.2).

Teaching Guidelines 9.2
PROTECTING YOURSELF AGAINST DATE RAPE DRUGS

- Avoid parties where alcohol is being served.
- Never leave a drink of any kind unattended.

- Don't accept a drink from someone else.
- Accept drinks from a bartender or in a closed container only.
- If a drink is left unattended, pour it out, don't drink it.
- Don't drink anything that tastes or smells strange.
- Don't drink from a punch bowl or a keg.
- If you think someone drugged you, call 911.

Rape Recovery

Rape survivors take a long time to heal from their traumatic experience. Some women never heal and never get professional counseling, but most can cope. Rape is viewed as a situational crisis that the survivor is unprepared to handle because it is an unforeseen event. Survivors typically go through four phases of recovery following rape (Table 9.4).

A significant proportion of women who are raped also experience symptoms of PTSD. PTSD develops when an event outside the range of normal human experience occurs that produces marked distress in the person. Symptoms of PTSD are divided into three groups:

1. Intrusion (reexperiencing the trauma, including nightmares, flashbacks, recurrent thoughts)
2. Avoidance (avoiding trauma-related stimuli, social withdrawal, emotional numbing)
3. Hyperarousal (increased emotional arousal, exaggerated startle response, irritability)

Not every traumatized female develops full-blown or even minor PTSD. Symptoms usually begin within 3 months of the incident, but occasionally may only emerge years later. They must last more than a month to be considered PTSD. The condition varies from person to person. Some women recover within months, while others have symptoms for much longer. In some people, the condition becomes chronic (Darnell et al., 2015; Friedman, 2015).

Nursing Management of Rape Victims

Health care providers, along with sexual assault nurse examiners (SANE), can make a difference in the lives of survivors by understanding the facts, the effects this violence can have on mental and physical health, where to find information for themselves and their clients, and how to properly care for a survivor. A SANE is a registered nurse specially trained to conduct sexual assault evidentiary examinations for rape victims. In addition to the collection of forensic evidence, they also provide access to

TABLE 9.4	RISK FACTORS FOR INTIMATE PARTNER VIOLENCE IN MEN		
Individual Factors	**Relationship Factors**	**Community Factors**	**Societal Factors**
Young age	Martial conflict	Weak sanctions against IPV	Traditional gender norms
Heavy drinking	Economic stress	Poverty	Social norms supportive of violence
Personality disorders	Dysfunctional family	Low social capital	
Depression	Marital instability		
Low academic achievement	Male dominance in family		
Witnessing violence as a child	Cohabitation		
Low income and/or unemployment	Having outside sexual partners		
Experiencing violence as a child			
Desire for power and control in all relationships			
Anger and hostility	Taking aggression out on others while growing up		

Adapted from CDC. (2015d). *Intimate partner violence: Risk and protective factors*. Retrieved from http://www.cdc.gov/violenceprevention/intimatepartnerviolence/riskprotectivefactors.html; The Christian Broadcasting Network [CBN]. (2015). *12 traits of an abuser*. Retrieved from http://www.cbn.com/family/marriage/petherbridge_abusertraits.aspx; and Ghandour, R. M., Campbell, J. C., & Lloyd, J. (2015). Screening and counseling for intimate partner violence: A vision for the future. *Journal of Women's Health, 24*(1), 57–61.

crisis intervention, STI testing, and emergency contraception (International Association of Forensic Nurses, 2015).

Research has found that rape survivors undergo a profound and complex trauma. Exposure therapy has been used to help victims confront their trauma-related memories, feelings, and stimuli that evoke fear and anxiety (Nacasch, Rachamim, & Foa, 2015). The survivor should be provided with a safe and comfortable environment for a forensic examination. Nursing care of the rape survivor should focus on providing supportive care, collecting and documenting evidence, assessing for STIs, preventing pregnancy, and assessing for PTSD. Once initial treatment and evidence collection have been completed, follow-up care should include counseling, medical treatment, and crisis intervention. There is mounting evidence that early intervention and immediate counseling speed a rape survivor's recovery. By early intervention, it means interventions that implemented in the initials hours, days, or weeks after the traumatic event (Bryant, 2015). Nursing Care Plan 9.1 highlights a sample plan of care for a victim of rape.

NURSING CARE PLAN 9.1

Overview of the Woman Who is a Victim of Rape

Lucia, a 20-year-old college junior, was admitted to the emergency room after police found her when a passerby called 911 to report an assault. She stated, "I was raped a few hours ago while I was walking home through the park." Assessment reveals the following: numerous cuts and bruises of varying sizes on her face, arms, and legs; lip swollen and cut; right eye swollen and bruised; jacket and shirt ripped and bloodied; hair matted with grass and debris; vital signs within acceptable parameters; client tearful, clutching her clothing, and trembling; perineal bruising and tearing.

NURSING DIAGNOSIS: Rape-trauma syndrome related to report of recent sexual assault

Outcome Identification and Evaluation

Client will demonstrate adequate coping skills related to effects of rape as evidenced by her ability to discuss the event, verbalize her feelings and fears, and exhibit appropriate actions to return to her precrisis level of functioning.

Interventions: *Promoting Adequate Coping Skills*

- Stay with the client to promote feelings of safety.
- Explain the procedures to be completed based on facility's policy to help alleviate client's fear of the unknown.
- Assist with physical examination for specimen collection to obtain evidence for legal proceedings.
- Administer prophylactic medication as ordered to prevent pregnancy and STIs.
- Provide care to wounds as ordered to prevent infection.
- Assist client with hygiene measures as necessary to promote self-esteem.
- Allow client to describe the events as much as possible to encourage ventilation of feelings about the incident; engage in active listening and offer nonjudgmental support to facilitate coping and demonstrate understanding of the client's situation and feelings.
- Help the client identify positive coping skills and personal strengths used in the past to aid in effective decision making.
- Assist client in developing additional coping strategies and teach client relaxation techniques to help deal with the current crisis and anxiety.
- Contact the rape counselor in the facility to help the client deal with the crisis.
- Arrange for follow-up visit with rape counselor to provide continued care and to promote continuity of care.
- Encourage the client to contact a close friend, partner, or family member to accompany her home to provide support.
- Provide the client with the telephone number of a counseling service or community support groups to help her cope and obtain ongoing support.
- Provide written instructions related to follow-up appointments, care, and testing to ensure adequate understanding.

Take Note!

Many rape survivors seek treatment in the hospital emergency department if no rape crisis center is available. Unfortunately, many emergency department doctors and nurses have little training in how to treat rape survivors or in collecting evidence. To make matters worse, if they have to wait for hours in public waiting rooms, survivors may leave the hospital, never to receive treatment or supply the evidence needed to arrest and convict their assailants.

PROVIDING SUPPORTIVE CARE

Establishing a therapeutic and trusting relationship will help the survivor describe her experience. Take the woman to a secure, isolated area away from family, friends, and other clients and staff so she can be open and honest when asked about the assault. Provide a change of clothes, access to a shower and toiletries, and a private waiting area for family and friends.

COLLECTING AND DOCUMENTING EVIDENCE

The victim should be instructed to bring all clothing, especially undergarments, worn at the time of the assault to the medical facility. The victim should not shower or bathe before presenting for care. Typically a specially trained nurse will collect the evidence from the victim.

ASSESSING FOR SEXUALLY TRANSMITTED INFECTIONS

As part of the assessment, a pelvic examination will be done to collect vaginal secretions to rule out any STIs. This examination is very emotionally stressful for most women and should be carried out very gently and sensitively.

PREVENTING PREGNANCY

An essential element in the care of rape survivors involves offering them pregnancy prevention. After unprotected intercourse, including rape, pregnancy can be prevented by using an emergency contraceptive pill, sometimes called postcoital contraception. Emergency contraceptive pills involve high doses of the same oral contraceptives that millions of women take every day. The emergency regimen consists of one dose taken within 72 to 120 hours of the unprotected intercourse. Emergency contraception works by preventing ovulation, fertilization, or implantation. It does not disrupt an established pregnancy and should not be confused with mifepristone (RU-486), a drug approved by the Food and Drug Administration for abortion in the first 49 days of gestation. Emergency contraception is most effective if it is taken within 12 hours of the rape; it

becomes less effective with every 12 hours of delay thereafter.

ASSESSING FOR POSTTRAUMATIC STRESS DISORDER

Nurses can begin to assess the extent to which a survivor is suffering from PTSD by asking the following questions:
- To assess the presence of intrusive thoughts:
  - Do upsetting thoughts and nightmares of the trauma bother you?
  - Do you feel as though you are actually reliving the trauma?
  - Does it upset you to be exposed to anything that reminds you of that event?
- To assess the presence of avoidance reactions:
  - Do you find yourself trying to avoid thinking about the trauma?
  - Do you stay away from situations that remind you of the event?
  - Do you have trouble recalling exactly what happened?
  - Do you feel numb emotionally?
- To assess the presence of physical symptoms:
  - Are you having trouble sleeping?
  - Have you felt irritable or experienced outbursts of anger?
  - Do you have heart palpitations and sweating?
  - Do you have muscle aches and pains all over? (NCVC, 2015b).

With a growing body of knowledge about rape-related PTSD, help is available through most rape crisis and trauma centers. Support groups have been established where survivors can meet regularly to share experiences to help relieve the symptoms of PTSD. For some survivors, medication prescribed along with therapy is the best combination to relieve the pain. Just as in the treatment of any other illness, at the first opportunity, the woman should be encouraged to talk about the traumatic experience. This ventilating provides a chance to receive needed support and comfort, as well as an opportunity to begin making sense of the experience. To diminish symptoms of PTSD, survivors must work on two fronts: coming to terms with the past and alleviating stress in the present (Bryant, 2015).

In order to have a better understanding of the aftermath of criminal victimization such as sexual assault, nurses must begin to accept the reality that crime is random, senseless, and can happen to anyone regardless of the precautions that are taken to prevent it. Nurses must also understand that a victim's life is turned upside down when he or she becomes a victim of crime. In order to help victims to trust society again and regain a sense of balance and self-worth, nurses must educate all those who come in contact with victims and survivors to be sensitive to their needs.

Female Genital Cutting

FGC, also referred to as female genital mutilation (FGM) or female circumcision, is defined as a procedure involving any injury of the external female genitalia for cultural or nontherapeutic reasons. It confers severe health consequences for girls and women. The international community views this practice as a human rights violation (Gayle & Rymer, 2015). It is the surgical removal of a portion or portions of the genitalia of female infants, girls, and women, including the clitoris (type I), clitoris and labia minora (type II), and clitoris, labia minora, labia majora, and then suturing of the remaining tissue, known as fibulation, to leave only a small opening for urination, menstruation, intercourse, and childbirth (type III). There is a type IV, which encompasses all other mutilations of the female genital area such as pricking, piercing, cutting, cauterizing, and scraping of the vaginal tissue, incisions to the clitoris and vagina, and burning, scarring, or cauterizing of tissue with the aim of tightening or narrowing the vagina (Nour, 2015).

FGC is a worldwide practice that affects millions of women and girls. According to the World Health Organization (WHO) (2015b) and UNICEF, 140 million women are victims of FGC with about 130 million girls between infancy and age 15 undergoing FGC every year. Countries where this is practiced include 30 African countries and parts of the Middle East and Asia. Prevalence in countries such as Sudan and Egypt has been estimated as high as 99% (Johnsdotter, 2015). The exact origins of FGC are not known. Although FGC may be interwoven into the culture, it is not mandated by any religion. This practice predates both Islam and Christianity (Gruenbaum & Wirtz, 2015). In some cultures, it is associated with feminine beauty and often signifies a rite of passage from childhood to adulthood. Female cutting is performed to decrease a woman's sexual desires and to ensure her chastity until marriage and receipt of a dowry from the prospective groom (Farage et al., 2015). Ultimately, the reality of being ostracized by the community and the possibility of being ineligible to marry create enormous social pressure to have FGC carried out, pressure that outweighs the known physical and emotional damage of this practice (Nour, 2015).

Complications vary, depending on the type of cutting and the way it was performed. It is frequently performed without anesthesia under nonsterile conditions. Cutting tools can be anything from razors blades to knives to pieces of glass or tin can lids. Complications can include infertility, dysmenorrhea, dyspareunia, sexual dysfunction, infection, hemorrhage after the procedure, vaginal stenosis, chronic vaginitis, pelvic inflammatory disease, chronic urinary tract infections, incontinence, genital fistulas, recurrent abscesses, transmission of HIV and hepatitis during the procedure, severe pain and shock after the procedure, difficulty walking or using stairs due to severe scarring, urinary retention, inability to experience orgasm, and difficulty in giving birth. Long-term complications related to FGC include chronic pain, dyspareunia, and difficult childbirth. The most common long-term complication is the formation of inclusion clitoral dermoid cysts and labial fusion. These become large as a grapefruit and can lead to difficulty in walking, sitting and can cause psychological distress from the deformity. The psychological effects range from eating disorders, insomnia, depression, PTSD, and negative effects on the women's self-esteem and identity (Creighton, 2015).

As immigration to the United States increases, nurses are increasingly likely to encounter women affected by FGC and its complications. The psychological pressure and trauma of being torn between two cultures and feeling different may lie heavily on the women in a new setting where FGC is foreign and banned. Nurses need updated education regarding women with FGC so that appropriate care for this population can be provided for this very sensitive health care problem. Well-informed nurses are the best tool for providing culturally sensitive care to this population. Nurses are in a unique position to contact and educate women who have been cut or are at risk for mutilation. To advocate for these women, a thorough understanding of the practice of FGC, its cultural overtones, religious implications, and psychosocial effects is needed.

Take Note!

From a Western perspective, FGC is hard to comprehend. Because it is not talked about openly in communities that practice it, women who have undergone it accept it without question and assume it is done to all girls (Gruenbaum & Wirtz, 2015).

Background

Reasons for performing the ritual reflect the ideology and cultural values of each community that practices it. Some consider it a rite of passage into womanhood; others use it as a means of preserving virginity until marriage. In cultures where it is practiced, it is an important part of culturally defined gender identity. In any case, all the reasons are cultural and traditional and are not rooted

FOUR MAJOR TYPES OF FEMALE GENITAL MUTILATION PROCEDURES

Type I: Excision of the prepuce with excision of part or the entire clitoris

Type II: Excision of the clitoris and part or all of the labia minora

Type III (Infibulation): Excision of all or part of the external genitalia and stitching/narrowing of the vaginal opening

Type IV: Pricking, piercing, or incision of the clitoris or labia

- Stretching of the clitoris and/or labia
- Cauterizing by burning the clitoris and surrounding tissues
- Scraping or cutting the vaginal orifice
- Introduction of a corrosive substance into the vagina
- Placing herbs into the vagina to narrow it

Adapted from World Health Organization [WHO]. (2015b). *Female genital mutilation*. Retrieved from http://www.who.int/mediacentre/factsheets/fs241/en/print.html; Nour, N. M. (2015). Female genital cutting: Impact on women's health. *Seminars in Reproductive Medicine, 33*(1), 41–46; and Research Action and Information Network for the Bodily Integrity of Women [RAINBO]. (2015). *Caring for women with circumcision: Fact sheet for physicians.* Retrieved from http://www.rainbo.org/factsheet.html.

in any religious texts (Research Action and Information Network for the Bodily Integrity of Women [RAINBO], 2015). Since FGC has no health benefits and often leaves women with lifelong physical and emotional trauma, there is a human rights justification to end the practice. International pressure to end FGC has been mounting since 1997, when the WHO, UNICEF, and UNFPA issued a joint statement to call on governments to ban the practice (Borsand et al., 2015). Box 9.5 lists types of FGC procedures.

Nursing Management of Female Genital Cutting Client

Because of increasing migration, nurses throughout the world are increasingly exposed to women who have experienced these procedures and thus need to know about its impact on women's reproductive health. Helping women who have had an FGC procedure requires good communication skills and often an interpreter, since many may not speak English. As nurses, we are educated to provide comprehensive, culturally sensitive care regardless of our client's circumstances. Nurses must keep in mind that FGC is considered normal in many cultures and to not have it done would be unthinkable. Nurses have the opportunity to educate clients by

providing accurate information and positive health care experiences. Make sure that you are comfortable with your own feelings about this practice before dealing with clients. Some guidelines are as follows:

- Let the client know you are concerned and interested and want to help.
- Speak clearly and slowly, using simple, accurate terms.
- Use the term or name for this practice that the recipient uses, not "female genital cutting."
- Use pictures and diagrams to help the woman understand what you are saying.
- Be patient in allowing the client to answer questions.
- Include men in any education, as they are influential in this practice.
- Repeat back your understanding of the client's statements.
- Always look and talk directly to the client, not the interpreter.
- Place no judgment on the cultural practice.
- Maintain respect for older women who have experienced FGC.
- Encourage the client to express herself freely.
- Maintain strict confidentiality.
- Provide culturally attuned care to all women.

In short, FGC is a form of violence against women, and it is only through education and empowerment of women that real changes in this practice can be made. Because this practice often defines a woman and becomes a part of her identity, nurses must understand this to be able to assist women who have had this done to them. Only through intense education will the next generation of girls be saved from this practice.

Human Trafficking

The United Nations defines human trafficking as the recruitment, transportation, transfer, harboring or receipt of persons, by means of the threat or use of force, of abduction, of fraud, or deception to achieve the consent of a person having control over another person, for the purpose of exploitation (United Nations Office on Drugs and Crime, 2015).

A girl who was just 14 years old was held captive in a tiny trailer room, where she was forced to have sex with as many as 30 men a day. On her nightstand was a teddy bear that reminded her of her childhood in Mexico from where she was abducted and forced into sexual slavery.

This scenario describes human trafficking, the enslavement of immigrants for profit in America. Within our borders, thousands of foreign nationals and US citizens, many of them children, are forced or coerced into sex work or various forms of labor every year (Weitzer,

2015). Human trafficking is both a global problem and a domestic problem. The United States is a major receiver of trafficked persons. Human trafficking is a modern form of slavery that affects nearly 1 million people worldwide and approximately 20,000 persons in the United States annually (U.S. Department of State, 2015). Women and children are the primary victims of human trafficking, many in the sex trade as described above and others through forced-labor domestic servitude. Poverty and lack of economic opportunity make women and children potential victims of traffickers associated with international criminal organizations. They are vulnerable to false promises of job opportunities in other countries. Many of those who accept these offers from what appear to be legitimate sources find themselves in situations where their documents are destroyed, they or their families threatened with harm, or they are bonded by a debt that they have no chance of repaying.

Trafficking persons is hugely profitable: one estimate places global profits at approximately $35 billion annually. Among illegal enterprises, trafficking is second only to drug dealing and is tied with the illegal arms industry in its ability to generate dollars (Aronowitz & Koning, 2015).

The United States is a profitable destination country for traffickers, and these profits contribute to the development of organized criminal enterprises worldwide. According to findings of the Victims of Trafficking and Violence Protection Act of 2000:

- Victims are primarily women and children who lack education, employment, and economic opportunities in their own countries.
- Traffickers promise victims employment as nannies, maids, dancers, factory workers, sales clerks, or models in the United States.
- Traffickers transport the victims from their counties to unfamiliar destinations away from their support systems.
- Once they are here, traffickers coerce them, using rape, torture, starvation, imprisonment, threats, or physical force, into prostitution, pornography, the sex trade, forced labor, or involuntary servitude.

These victims are exposed to serious and numerous health risks such as rape; physical injury such as cigarette burns, fractures, bruises; torture; HIV/AIDS; STIs; cervical cancer; violence; hazardous work environments; poor nutrition; and drug and alcohol addiction (Greenbaum et al., 2015). Health care is one of the most pressing needs of these victims, but no comprehensive care is available to undocumented immigrants. Nurses and other health care providers who encounter victims of trafficking often do not realize it, and opportunities to intervene are lost. Although no one sign can demonstrate with certainty

---

> **BOX 9.6**
>
> ### IDENTIFYING VICTIMS OF HUMAN TRAFFICKING
>
> Look beneath the surface and ask yourself: Is this person...
> - A female or a child in poor health?
> - Foreign-born and doesn't speak English?
> - Lacking immigration documents?
> - Giving an inconsistent explanation of injury?
> - Reluctant to give any information about self, injury, home, or work?
> - Fearful of authority figure or "sponsor" if present? ("Sponsor" might not leave victim alone with health care provider).
> - Living with the employer?
>
> Sample questions to ask the potential victim of human trafficking:
> - Can you leave your job or situation if you wish?
> - Can you come and go as you please?
> - Have you been threatened if you try to leave?
> - Has anyone threatened your family with harm if you leave?
> - What are your working and living conditions?
> - Do you have to ask permission to go to the bathroom, eat, or sleep?
> - Is there a lock on your door so you cannot get out?
> - What brought you to the United States? Are your plans the same now?
> - Are you free to leave your current work or home situation?
> - Who has your immigration papers? Why don't you have them?
> - Are you paid for the work you do?
> - Are there times you feel afraid?
> - How can your situation be changed?
>
> Adapted from United Nations Office on Drugs and Crime [UNODC]. (2015). *Human trafficking.* Retrieved from http://www.unodc.org/unodc/en/human-trafficking/what-is-human-trafficking.html; Sanchez, R., & Stark, S. (2014). The hard truth about human trafficking. *Nursing Management, 45*(1), 18–23; and Weitzer, R. (2015). Human trafficking and contemporary slavery. *Annual Review of Sociology, 41*(1). Retrieved from http://www.annualreviews.org/doi/abs/10.1146/annurev-soc-073014-112506

when someone is being trafficked, clinicians should be aware of several indicators. It is important to be alert for trafficking victims in any setting and to recognize cues (Box 9.6).

Nursing interventions in the case of trafficking victims would include the following:
- Building trust is the number-one priority
- Take the time to listen and develop rapport
- Screen in a private place to ensure confidentiality and safety
- Reassure the potential victim
- One-on-one interactions are ideal
- Specifically ask about the client's safety

- Offer reworded stories
- Stay calm and on an even keel
- Understand the risk these victims are taking by disclosing their plight
- Always document your suspicion in your notes, at the very least
- Call the human trafficking hotline for guidance: 1-866-US-TIPLINE

Human trafficking is a violation of human rights. Few crimes are more repugnant than the sex trafficking of helpless and innocent victims. Nurses are one of the few groups of professionals likely to interact with trafficked victims while they are still in captivity. They have the opportunity to screen, identify, intervene, and rescue these victims. If you suspect a trafficking situation, notify local law enforcement and a regional social service organization that has experience in dealing with trafficking victims. It is imperative to reach out to these victims and stop the cycle of abuse by following through on your suspicions. Nurses can also reach out within their communities to bring about awareness through community education to human trafficking to uncover the hard truth about it to our nation's blind eyes.

SUMMARY

The causes of violence against women are complex. Previously, violence against women was largely invisible, natural, and trivial. Many laughed at the notion that intimate or community violence against women should be seen as a human rights violation. Raising awareness and developing evidence-based programs, practices, and policies to prevent IPV and sexual assault are essential in stopping violent behavior before it starts. Many women will experience some type of violence in their lives, and it can have a debilitating effect on their health and future relationships. Nurses have the skills, professional experience, and perspective to be an important part of comprehensive violence prevention efforts in communities. Violence is a preventable public health problem if multiple sectors understand patterns of violence and implement prevention strategies to reduce it (Copelon, 2015).

Violence frequently leaves a "legacy of pain" to future generations. Nurses can empower women and encourage them to move forward and take control of their lives. When women live in peace and security, free from violence, they have an enormous potential to contribute to their own communities and to the national and global society. Nurses can play an important role

in working toward the creation of a violence-free community, but they must first become informed. Nurses must insist that health care agencies that employ them accept this responsibility and work together to reach out to those being abused. The time is ripe for nurses to act and ensure serious inroads are made in improving the health and well-being of all women across the globe.

Violence against women is not normal, legal, or acceptable and it should never be tolerated or justified. It can and must be stopped by the entire world community. Early education and prevention provide the best hope for creating healthy futures and fostering a global society without violence.

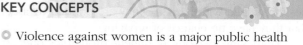

KEY CONCEPTS

- Violence against women is a major public health and social problem because it violates a woman's very being and causes numerous mental and physical health sequelae.
- Every woman has the potential to become a victim of violence.
- Several *Healthy People 2020* objectives focus on reducing the rate of physical assaults and the number of rapes and attempted rapes.
- Abuse may be mental, physical, or sexual in nature or a combination of all of these.
- The cycle of violence includes three phases: tension building, acute battering, and honeymoon.
- Many women experience PTSD after being sexually assaulted. PTSD can inhibit a survivor from adapting or coping in a healthy manner.
- Pregnancy can precipitate violence toward the woman or escalate it.
- FGC is practiced worldwide and nurses in the United States need to become knowledgeable about it and place no judgment on this cultural practice.
- Human trafficking is a violation against human rights, and nurses who suspect it should report it to stop the cycle of abuse against young children and women.
- The nurse's role in dealing with survivors of violence is to establish rapport; open up lines of communication; apply the nursing process to assess and screen all clients in all settings; and implement and intervene as appropriate.

References and Recommended Readings

Alexander, L. L., LaRosa, J. H., Bader, H., & Garfield, S. (2014). *New dimensions in women's health* (6th ed.). Sudbury, MA: Jones & Bartlett.

Aronowitz, A. A., & Koning, A. (2015). Understanding human trafficking as a market system: addressing the demand side of trafficking for sexual exploitation. *Revue International de droit Pénal, 85*(3), 669–696.

Association of Women's Health, Obstetric and Neonatal Nurses [AWHONN]. (2015). Intimate partner violence. *JOGNN, 44*(3), 405–408.

Bagwell-Gray, M. E., Messing, J. T., & Baldwin-White, A. (2015). Intimate partner sexual violence: A review of terms, definitions, and prevalence. *Trauma, Violence, & Abuse, 16*(3), 316–335.

Barrios, Y. V., Gelaye, B., Zhong, Q., Nicolaidis, C., Rondon, M. B., Garcia, P. J., et al . (2015). Association of childhood physical and sexual abuse with intimate partner violence, poor general health and depressive symptoms among pregnant women. *PLoS One, 10*(1), e0116609.

Berthold, S. M. (2015). Intimate partner violence and a rights-based approach to healing. *Human rights-based approaches to clinical social work* (pp. 85–113). Springer International Publishing.

Borsand, M., Friedman, B., Mirzayan, N., & Borsand, A. (2015). Female genital cutting: An ancient practice embedded in an ever-evolving world. *American Journal of Cosmetic Surgery, 32*(1), 31–36.

Bouchet, S., & Braswell, K. (2015). *Beyond silence and violence.* Dunwoody, GA: Fathers Incorporated. www.fathersincorporated.com

Brenner, I., & Ben-Amitay, G. (2015). Sexual revictimization: The impact of attachment anxiety, accumulated trauma, and response to childhood sexual abuse disclosure. *Violence and Victims, 30*(1), 49–65.

Brooker, C., & Durmaz, E. (2015). Mental health, sexual violence and the work of Sexual Assault Referral centres (SARCs) in England. *Journal of Forensic and Legal Medicine, 31,* 47–51.

Bryant, R. A. (2015). Early intervention after trauma. *Evidence based treatments for trauma-related psychological disorders* (pp. 125–142). Springer International Publishing.

Burnett, L. B., & Adler, J. (2015). Domestic violence. *eMedicine.* Retrieved from http://emedicine.medscape.com/article/805546-overview

Canadian Domestic Homicide Prevention Initiative. (2015). *Risk assessment, risk management and safety planning.* Retrieved from http://www.learningtoendabuse.ca/cdhpi/risk-assessment-risk-management-and-safety-planning

Cannon, C., & Buttell, F. (2015). Illusion of inclusion: The failure of the gender paradigm to account for intimate partner violence in LGBT relationships. *Partner Abuse, 6*(1), 65–70.

Cater, Å. K., Miller, L. E., Howell, K. H., & Graham-Bermann, S. A. (2015). Childhood exposure to intimate partner violence and adult mental health problems: Relationships with gender and age of exposure. *Journal of Family Violence, 1–12.* doi: 10.1007/s10896-015-9703-0

Centers for Disease Control & Prevention [CDC]. (2015a). *Understanding intimate partner violence: Fact sheet.* Retrieved from http://www.cdc.gov/violenceprevention/pub/ipv_factsheet.html

Centers for Disease Control and Prevention [CDC]. (2015b). *Intimate partner violence: definitions.* Retrieved from http://www.cdc.gov/violenceprevention/intimatepartnerviolence/definitions.html

Centers for Disease Control and Prevention [CDC]. (2015c). *CDC grand rounds: A public health approach to prevention of intimate partner violence.* Retrieved from http://www.cdc.gov/violenceprevention/intimatepartnerviolence/definitions.html

Centers for Disease Control & Prevention [CDC]. (2015d). *Intimate partner violence: Risk and protective factors.* Retrieved from http://www.cdc.gov/violenceprevention/intimatepartnerviolence/riskprotectivefactors.html

Centers for Disease Control and Prevention [CDC]. (2015e). *Understanding child mistreatment.* Retrieved from http://www.cdc.gov/violenceprevention/pdf/cm-factsheet–2013.pdf

Centers for Disease Control and Prevention [CDC]. (2015f). *Understanding sexual violence.* Retrieved from http://www.cdc.gov/violenceprevention/pdf/svfactsheet2013-a.pdf

Chang, J. C. (2015). Domestic violence: epidemiology and risk factors. *Clinical gynecology* (2nd ed., pp. 94–101). Cambridge, UK: Cambridge University Press.

Copelon, R. (2015). Violence against women: The potential and challenge of a human rights perspective. *Women's Health Journal,* (2-3), 62–67.

Creighton, S. M. (2015). Female genital mutilation (FGM) and the lower urinary tract. *International Journal of Urological Nursing, 1*(5), 208–211.

Darnell, D., Peterson, R., Berliner, L., Stewart, T., Russo, J., Whiteside, L., et al. (2015). Factors associated with follow-up attendance among rape victims seen in acute medical care. *Psychiatry, 78*(1), 89–101.

de Jong, R., Alink, L., Bijleveld, C., Finkenauer, C., & Hendriks, J. (2015). Transition to adulthood of child sexual abuse victims. *Aggression and Violent Behavior, 24,* 175–187.

Domestic Violence Organization. (2015a). *Common myths and why they are wrong.* Retrieved from http://www.domesticviolence.org/common-myths/

Domestic Violence Organization. (2015b). *Cycle of violence.* Retrieved from http://www.domesticviolence.org/cycle-of-violence/

Domestic Violence Roundtable. (2015). *The cycle of domestic violence.* Retrieved from http://www.domesticviolenceroundtable.org/domestic-violence-cycle.html

Dorland, W.A. N. (2015). *Dorland's dictionary of medical acronyms & abbreviations* (7th ed.). Philadelphia, PA: Elsevier Health Sciences.

Dutton, M.A. (2015). Mindfulness-based stress reduction for underserved trauma populations. *Mindfulness-oriented interventions for trauma: Integrating contemplative practices.* New York, NY: The Guilford Press.

Edwards, K. M., Sylaska, K. M., & Neal, A. M. (2015). Intimate partner violence among sexual minority populations: A critical review of the literature and agenda for future research. *Psychology of Violence, 5*(2), 112–121.

Farage, M. A., Miller, K. W., Tzeghai, G. E., Azuka, C. E., Sobel, J. D., & Ledger, W. J. (2015). Female genital cutting: Confronting cultural challenges and health complications across the lifespan. *Women's Health, 11*(1), 79–94.

Federal Bureau of Investigation [FBI]. (2015). *Intimate partner violence.* Retrieved from http://www.ojp.usdoj.gov/bjs/pub/ascii/ipv.txt.

Friedman, M. J. (2015). Overview of posttraumatic stress disorder (PTSD). *Posttraumatic and acute stress disorders* (pp. 1–8). Springer International Publishing.

Gayle, C. M., & Rymer, J. M. (2015). Female genital mutilation. *Clinical gynecology* (2nd ed., pp. 102–111). Cambridge, UK: Cambridge University Press.

Ghandour, R. M., Campbell, J. C., & Lloyd, J. (2015). Screening and counseling for intimate partner violence: A vision for the future. *Journal of Women's Health, 24*(1), 57–61.

Greenbaum, J., Crawford-Jakubiak, J. E., Christian, C. W., Flaherty, E. G., Leventhal, J. M., Lukefahr, J. L., et al. (2015). Child sex trafficking and commercial sexual exploitation: Health care needs of victims. *Pediatrics, 135*(3), 566–574.

Gruenbaum, E., & Wirtz, E. (2015). Female genital cutting debates. *The International Encyclopedia of Human Sexuality,* (Online 4/20/15), doi: 10.1002/9781118896877.wbiehs147

Harkins, G. (2015). Incest. *The International Encyclopedia of Human Sexuality.* 583–625. doi: 10.1002/9781118896877.wbiehs231

Hewitt, L. N. (2015). Intimate partner violence: The role of nurses in protection of patients. *Critical Care Nursing Clinics of North America, 27*(2), 271–275.

Huang, C. C., Vikse, J. H., Lu, S., & Yi, S. (2015). Children's exposure to intimate partner violence and early delinquency. *Journal of Family Violence, 1–13.* doi: 10.1007/s10896-015-9727-5

Human Rights Watch. (2015). *Abused and expelled.* Retrieved from http://www.hrw.org/sites/default/files/reports/morocco0214_ForUpload.pdf

Holtz, H., & Furniss, K. K. (1993). The health care provider's role in domestic violence. *Trends in Health Care Law and Ethics, 15,* 519–522.

International Association of Forensic Nurses. (2015). *Sexual assault nurse examiners.* Retrieved from http://www.forensicnurses.org/?page=aboutsane

Jackson, A. M., & Deye, K. (2015). Aspects of abuse: consequences of childhood victimization. *Current Problems in Pediatric and Adolescent Health Care, 45*(3), 86–93.

Joint Commission. (2015). *The Joint Commission accreditation manual for hospitals.* Chicago: Author.

Johnsdotter, S. (2015). Genital cutting, female. *The International Encyclopedia of Human Sexuality,* (Online 4/20/15), *121*(5), 800.

Keygnaert, I., Vettenburg, N., & Temmerman, M. (2015). Hidden violence is silent rape. *Culture, Health and Sexuality: An Introduction,* 189–206.

Kilmartin, C. (2015). Men's violence against women: An overview. *Religion and men's violence against women* (pp. 15–25). New York, NY: Springer Publishers.

Klaus, W., Buczkowski, K., & Wiktorska, P. (2015). Empowering the victims of crime: A real goal of the criminal justice system or no more than a pipe dream?. *Trust and legitimacy in criminal justice* (pp. 65–91). Springer International Publishing.

Lawrence, D. (2015). Breaking the cycle of violence. *Nursing Standard (1987), 29,* 18–21.

Lawson, D. M. (2015). *Family violence: Explanations and evidence-based clinical practice.* Hoboken, NJ: John Wiley & Sons.

Lévesque, S., & Chamberland, C. (2015). Intimate partner violence among pregnant young women: A qualitative inquiry. *Journal of Interpersonal Violence,* pii: 0886260515584349.

Lomborg, B. (2015). Why domestic violence costs more than war. *World Economic Forum.* Retrieved from https://agenda.weforum.org/2015/09/domestic-violence-cost-war-development-goals/

MacGregor, K. E., Villalta, L., Clarke, V., Viner, R. M., Kramer, T., & Khadr, S. N. (2015). G146 A systematic review of mental health outcomes in young people following sexual assault. *Archives of Disease in Childhood, 100*(Suppl 3), A63.

Mauri, E. M., Nespoli, A., Persico, G., & Zobbi, V. F. (2015). Domestic violence during pregnancy: Midwives experiences. *Midwifery, 31*(5), 498–504.

Medicine Net. (2015a). *Sexual assault.* Retrieved from http://www.medicinenet.com/rape_sexual_assault/article.htm#rape_sexual_assault_facts

Medicine Net. (2015b). *Domestic violence.* Retrieved from http://www.medicinenet.com/domestic_violence/page4.htm#what_are_the_causes_or_risk_factors_for_intimate_partner_violence

Morrill, M. (2014). Sibling sexual abuse: An exploratory study of long term consequences for self-esteem and counseling considerations. *Journal of Family Violence, 29*(2), 205–213.

Murray, C. E., Horton, G. E., Johnson, C. H., Notestine, L., Garr, B., Pow, A. M., et al. (2015). Domestic violence service providers' perceptions of safety planning: A focus group study. *Journal of Family Violence, 30*(3), 381–392.

Nacasch, N., Rachamim, L., & Foa, E. B. (2015). Prolonged exposure treatment. *Future directions in post-traumatic stress disorder* (pp. 245–251). Philadelphia, PA: Springer Publishers.

National Center for Victims of Crime [NCVC]. (2015a). *Incest.* Retrieved from http://www.victimsofcrime.org/

National Center for Victims of Crime [NCVC]. (2015b). *The trauma of victimization.* Retrieved from http://victimsofcrime.org/help-for-crime-victims/get-help-bulletins-for-crime-victims/trauma-of-victimization#ptsd

National Center on Elder Abuse. (2015). *Statistics/Data: Elder abuse: The size of the problem.* Retrieved from http://www.ncea.aoa.gov/Library/Data/

National Coalition Against Domestic Violence. (2015). *Fact sheet: National statistics.* Retrieved from http://www.ncadv.org/learn/statistics

National Stress Clinic. (2015). *Domestic abuse: Understanding and breaking the cycle of violence.* Retrieved from http://www.national-stressclinic.com/domestic-abuse-understanding-and-breaking-the-cycle-of-violence/

Nour, N. M. (2015). Female genital cutting: Impact on women's health. *Seminars in Reproductive Medicine, 33*(1), 41–46.

Policastro, C., & Finn, M. A. (2015). Coercive control and physical violence in older adults analysis using data from the National Elder Mistreatment Study. *Journal of Interpersonal Violence,* pii: 0886260515585545.

Prosman, G. J., Wong, S. H., van der Wouden, J. C., & Lagro-Janssen, A. L. (2015). Effectiveness of home visiting in reducing partner violence for families experiencing abuse: a systematic review. *Family Practice, 32*(3), 247–256.

Rape, Abuse, and Incest National Network [RAINN]. (2015a). *Statistics.* Retrieved from https://www.rainn.org/statistics

Rape, Abuse, and Incest National Network [RAINN]. (2015b). *Who are the victims?* Retrieved from http://rainn.org/get-information/statistics/sexual-assault-victims

Rape, Abuse, and Incest National Network [RAINN]. (2015c). *Acquaintance rape.* Retrieved from https://www.rainn.org/get-information/types-of-sexual-assault/acquaintance-rape

Rape, Abuse, and Incest National Network [RAINN]. (2015d). *Recovery from sexual assault.* Retrieved from http://www.rainn.org/get-information/sexual-assault-recovery

Research Action and Information Network for the Bodily Integrity of Women [RAINBO]. (2015). *Caring for women with circumcision: Fact sheet for physicians.* Retrieved from http://www.rainbo.org/factsheet.html.

Russell, B., & Chapleau, K. (2015). When is it abuse? How assailant gender, sexual orientation, and protection orders influence perceptions of intimate partner abuse. *Partner Abuse, 6*(1), 47–64.

Sanchez, R., & Stark, S. (2014). The hard truth about human trafficking. *Nursing Management, 45*(1), 18–23.

Song, A., Wenzel, S. L., Kim, J. Y., & Nam, B. (2015). Experience of domestic violence during childhood, intimate partner violence, and the deterrent effect of awareness of legal consequences. *Journal of Interpersonal Violence,* pii: 0886260515586359..

Sugg, N. (2015). Intimate partner violence: prevalence, health consequences, and intervention. *Medical Clinics of North America, 99*(3), 629–649.

TahoeSafe Alliance. (2015). *Myths about intimate partner violence in the LGBTQUA community.* Retrieved from http://tahoesafealliance.org/for-lgbqtia/lgbtqiamyths/

The Advocacy Center. (2015). *The path toward recovery for survivors of sexual violence.* Retrieved from http://advocacycenter.syr.edu/students/path-of-recovery/

The Christian Broadcasting Network [CBN]. (2015). *12 traits of an abuser.* Retrieved from http://www.cbn.com/family/marriage/petherbridge_abusertraits.aspx

United Nations Office on Drugs and Crime [UNODC]. (2015). *Human trafficking.* Retrieved from http://www.unodc.org/unodc/en/human-trafficking/what-is-human-trafficking.html

U.S. Department of Health and Human Services [USDHHS]. (2015a). *Date rape drugs fact sheet.* National Women's Health Information Center. Retrieved from http://www.womenshealth.gov/publications/our-publications/fact-sheet/date-rape-drugs.html

U.S. Department of Health and Human Services [USDHHS]. (2015b). *Healthy People 2020.* Retrieved from http://www.healthypeople.gov/document/HTML/Volume2/15Injury.htm#_Toc490549392

USDHHS. (2015c). Screening for domestic violence in health care settings. *Office of the Assistant Secretary for Planning and Evaluation.* Retrieved from http://aspe.hhs.gov/hsp/13/dv/pb_screeningdomestic.cfm

U.S. Department of State. (2015). *What is modern slavery?* Retrieved from http://www.state.gov/j/tip/what/index.htm

Victims of Trafficking and Violence Protection Act of 2000, Pub. Law No. 106–386 [H.R. 3244]. (2000). Retrieved from http://ojp.gov/vawo/laws/vawo2000/stitle_a.htm.

Wang, X. M., Brisbin, S., Loo, T., & Straus, S. (2015). Elder abuse: An approach to identification, assessment and intervention. *CMAJ: Canadian Medical Association Journal, 187*(8), 575–581.

Weitzer, R. (2015). Human trafficking and contemporary slavery. *Annual Review of Sociology, 41*(1). Retrieved from http://www.annualreviews.org/doi/abs/10.1146/annurev-soc-073014-112506

WELLWVU The Student's Center of Health. (2015). *Rape myths and facts.* Retrieved from https://well.wvu.edu/articles/rape_myths_and_facts

Wilson, L. C., & Miller, K. E. (2015). Meta-analysis of the prevalence of unacknowledged rape. *Trauma, Violence, & Abuse*, pii: 1524838015576391..

Women Against Violence Against Women [WAVAW]. (2015). *Rape myths*. Retrieved from http://www.wavaw.ca/mythbusting/rape-myths/

World Health Organization [WHO]. (2015a). *Violence against women fact sheet*. Retrieved from http://www.who.int/mediacentre/fact-sheets/fs239/en/

World Health Organization [WHO]. (2015b). *Female genital mutilation*. Retrieved from http://www.who.int/mediacentre/factsheets/fs241/en/print.html

CHAPTER WORKSHEET

MULTIPLE-CHOICE QUESTIONS

1. The primary goal of intervention in working with abused women is to:
   a. Set up an appointment with a mental health counselor for the victim
   b. Convince them to set up a safety plan to use when they leave
   c. Help them develop courage and financial support to leave the abuser
   d. Empower them and improve their self-esteem to regain control of their lives

2. The first phase of the abuse cycle is characterized by:
   a. The woman provoking the abuser to bring about battering
   b. Tension building and verbal or minor battery
   c. A honeymoon period that lulls the victim into forgetting
   d. An acute episode of physical battering

3. Women recovering from abusive relationships need to learn ways to improve their:
   a. Educational level by getting a college degree
   b. Earning power so they can move to a better neighborhood
   c. Self-esteem and communication skills to increase assertiveness
   d. Relationship skills so they will be better prepared to deal with their partners

4. Which of the following statements might empower abuse victims to take action?
   a. "You deserve better than this."
   b. "Your children deserve to grow up in a two-parent family."
   c. "Try to figure out what you do to trigger his abuse and stop it."
   d. "Give your partner more time to come to his senses about this."

5. If a woman thinks she is being stalked when driving, a good safety measure is to:
   a. Drive to a local police or fire department
   b. Take short cuts through back streets to lose them
   c. Wave a handgun to intimidate them
   d. Roll down her window and confront them

6. Nurses play an important role in screening and assessment of any client abuse/violence. Which of the following statements is correct?
   a. Most clients are extremely reluctant to come forth with private matters
   b. Any intimate partner violence questions should be asked in the presence of both partners
   c. To invite disclosure, assure the woman that you won't document her statements
   d. The best statement to make to the abused victim is: "You don't deserve this."

7. What should the nurse do if a victim of intimate partner violence chooses not to disclose information about her abusive relationship during your interview?
   a. Confront the victim with the physical evidence and telltale signs of abuse
   b. Contact family members to tell you about their abusive relationship
   c. Call the local police department to inquire about domestic disturbance calls
   d. Respect the client's right of self-determination and provide her with resources

CRITICAL THINKING EXERCISE

1. Mrs. Boggs has three children under the age of 5 and is 6 months pregnant with her fourth child. She has made repeated unscheduled visits to your clinic with vague somatic complaints regarding the children as well as herself, but has missed several scheduled prenatal appointments. On occasion she has worn sunglasses to cover bruises around her eyes. As a nurse you sense there is something else bothering her, but she doesn't seem to want to discuss it with you. She appears sad and the children cling to her.
   a. Outline your conversation when you broach the subject of abuse with Mrs. Boggs.
   b. What is your role as a nurse in caring for a family in which you suspect abuse is occurring?
   c. What ethical/legal considerations are important in planning care for this family?

STUDY ACTIVITIES

1. Visit the BellaOnline Domestic Violence website for victims of violence. Discuss what you discovered on this site and your reactions to it.

2. Research the statistics about violence against women in your state. Are law enforcement and community interventions reducing the incidence of sexual assault and intimate partner violence?

3. Attend a dorm orientation at a local college to hear about measures in place to protect women's safety on campus. Find out the number of sexual assaults reported and what strategies the college uses to reduce this number.

4. Volunteer to spend a weekend evening at the local sheriff's department 911 hotline desk to observe the number and nature of calls received reporting domestic violence. Interview the dispatch operator about the frequency and trends of these calls.

5. Identify three community resources that could be useful to a victim of violence. Identify their sources of funding and the services they provide.

BRINGING IT ALL TOGETHER: CASE STUDY

A 23-year-old pregnant female presents to the public health maternity clinic for the third time in a month with many vague complaints including insomnia, diffuse body aches and pains, poor appetite, fatigue, and constipation. This is her first pregnancy, and it was unplanned. Her recent OB examination findings and laboratory survey are within normal limits. Her past medical history is remarkable for anxiety and depression. According to the client, she does not drink or smoke. She does not work outside of the home.

ASSESSMENT

On physical examination, the nurse notes a well-dressed, pleasant, but anxious young female. Her husband of a year usually accompanies her to the office visits, but is absent today. She tends to avoid eye contact with the nurse when asked questions about her symptoms. Her vital signs and fetal heart rate are all within the normal range. On further examination, the nurse notices several bruises on her upper arms and thighs. When questioned about these marks, the client looks away.

Go to thePoint **to find questions to consider about this case.**

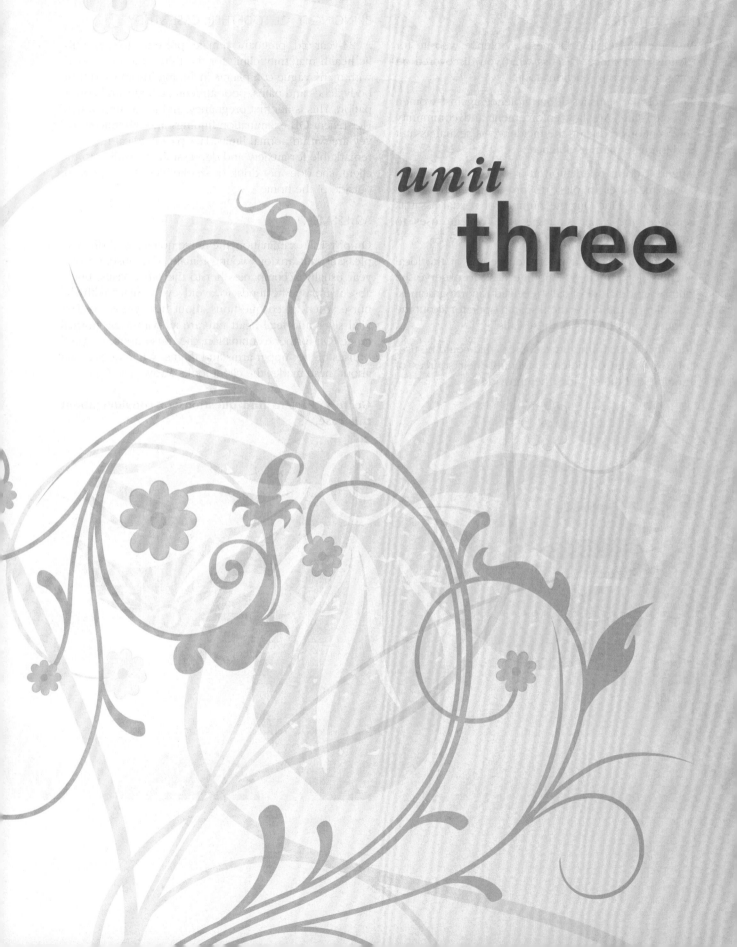

unit
three

Pregnancy

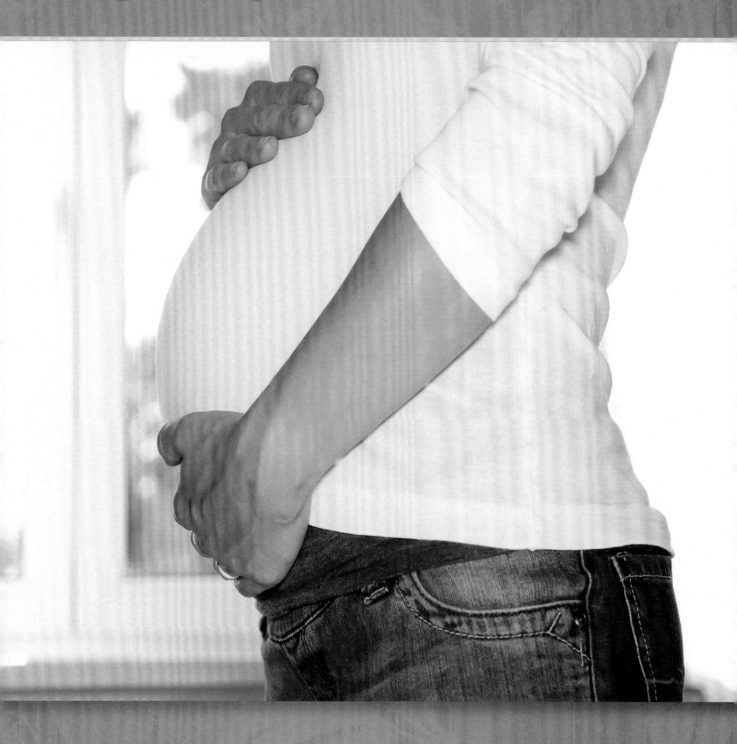

10

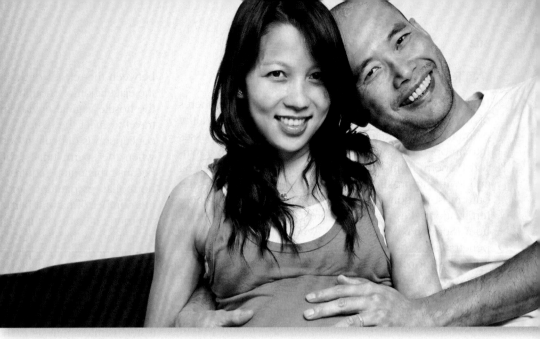

Fetal Development and Genetics

Learning Objectives

Upon completion of the chapter, you will be able to:

1. Characterize the process of fertilization, implantation, and cell differentiation.
2. Examine the functions of the placenta, umbilical cord, and amniotic fluid.
3. Outline normal fetal development from conception through birth.
4. Compare the various inheritance patterns, including nontraditional patterns of inheritance.
5. Analyze examples of ethical and legal issues surrounding genetic testing.
6. Research the role of the nurse in genetic counseling and genetic-related activities.

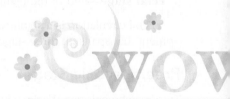

Words of Wisdom
Being a nurse without awe
is like food without spice.
Nurses only have to witness
the miracle of life to find
their lost awe.

*__Robert__ and __Kate Shafer__ have just received the good news that Kate's
pregnancy test was positive. It had been a long and anxious 3 years of trying
to start a family. Although both are elated about the prospect of becoming
parents, they are also concerned about the possibility of a genetic problem
because Kate is 41 years old. What might be their first step in looking into
their genetic concern? As a nurse, what might raise concerns for you?*

INTRODUCTION

Human reproduction is one of the most intimate spheres of an individual's life. Conception occurs when a healthy ovum from the woman is released from the ovary, passes into an open Fallopian tube, and starts its journey downward. Sperm from the male is deposited into the vagina and swims approximately 7 in to meet the ovum at the outermost portion of the Fallopian tube, the area where fertilization takes place. This process occurs in about an hour (Sermon & Viville, 2014). When one spermatozoon penetrates the ovum's thick outer membrane, a new living cell is formed that is unlike the cells of either parent. Soon, the two nuclei will fuse, bringing together about 25,000 genes to guide human development.

Nurses caring for the childbearing family need to have a basic understanding of conception and prenatal development so they can identify problems or variations and can initiate appropriate interventions should any problems occur. This chapter presents an overview of fetal development, beginning with conception. It also discusses hereditary influences on fetal development and the nurse's role in genetic counseling.

FETAL DEVELOPMENT

Fetal development during pregnancy is measured in number of weeks after fertilization. An average human pregnancy lasts for about 280 days or 40 weeks from the date of the last menstrual period (LMP). Traditionally, it has been calculated as 10 lunar months, or, in terms of the modern calendar, 9 months. Fertilization of the egg by the sperm, however, usually occurs (considering an average menstrual cycle of 28 days) 14 days after the last period. Thus, the average actual duration of a human pregnancy (gestation period) is 280 days − 14 days = 266 days.

The three stages of fetal development during pregnancy are the:
1. **Preembryonic stage**—fertilization through the second week
2. **Embryonic stage**—end of the second week through the eighth week
3. **Fetal stage**—end of the eighth week until birth

Fetal circulation is a significant aspect of fetal development that spans all three stages.

Preembryonic Stage

The preembryonic stage begins with **fertilization**, also called *conception*. Fertilization is the union of ovum and sperm, which is the starting point of pregnancy. Development during this stage takes place in an organized fashion that is cephalocaudal, proximal to distal, and general to specific. Fertilization typically occurs around 2 weeks after the last normal menstrual period in a 28-day cycle (Mader & Windelspecht, 2015). Fertilization requires a timely interaction between the release of the mature ovum at ovulation and the ejaculation of enough healthy, mobile sperm to survive the hostile vaginal environment through which they must travel to meet the ovum. All things considered, the act of conception is difficult at best. To say merely that it occurs when the sperm unites with the ovum is overly simple because this union requires an intricate interplay between hormonal preparation and overcoming an overwhelming number of natural barriers. A human being is truly an amazing outcome of this elaborate process.

Prior to fertilization, the ovum and the spermatozoon undergo the process of meiosis. The primary oocyte completes its first meiotic division before ovulation. The secondary oocyte begins its second meiotic division just before ovulation. Primary and secondary spermatocytes undergo meiotic division while still in the testes. Gametogenesis is the process by which gametes (ovum or sperm cells) are produced to initiate the development of a new individual. The gametes must have a haploid number of chromosomes (a single set, i.e., 23) so when they come together to form the zygote, the normal human diploid number of chromosomes (combination of two sets, i.e., 46) is established (Fig. 10.1). This smaller number of chromosome number found in eggs and sperm is vital because these gametes combine to form a new individual with 46 chromosomes.

Although each milliliter of ejaculated semen contains more than 200 million sperm, only one is able to enter the ovum to fertilize it. All others are blocked by the clear protein layer called the **zona pellucida**. The zona pellucida disappears in about 5 days. Once the sperm reaches the plasma membrane, the ovum resumes meiosis and forms a nucleus with half the number of chromosomes (23). When the nucleus from the ovum and the nucleus of the sperm make contact, they lose their respective nuclear membranes and combine their maternal and paternal chromosomes. Because each nucleus contains a haploid number of chromosomes (23), this union restores the diploid number (46). The resulting **zygote** begins the process of a new life.

The genetic information from both ovum and sperm establishes the unique physical characteristics of the individual. Sex determination is also determined at fertilization and depends on whether the ovum is fertilized by a Y-bearing sperm or an X-bearing sperm. Approximately 50% of sperms carry the XX chromosome while the other 50% carry XY. An XX zygote will become a female and an XY zygote will become a male (Fig. 10.2). That is why it is scientifically correct to say that the sex of the infant is determined by the father and not by the mother.

Fertilization takes place in the outer third of the ampulla of the Fallopian tube. When the ovum is fertilized by the sperm (now called a zygote), a great deal of activity immediately takes place. Mitosis, or *cleavage*, occurs as the zygote is slowly transported into the uterine cavity by tubal muscular movements (Fig. 10.3). After

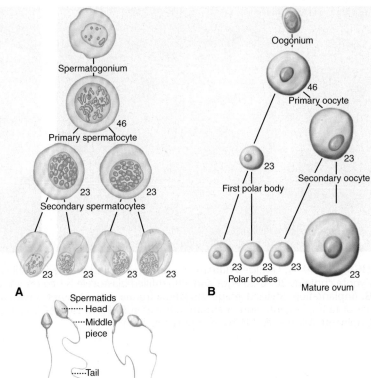

A

B

FIGURE 10.1 The formation of gametes by the process of meiosis is known as gametogenesis. **A.** Spermatogenesis. One spermatogonium gives rise to four spermatozoa. **B.** Oogenesis. From each oogonium, one mature ovum and three abortive cells are produced. The chromosomes are reduced to one half the number characteristic for the general body cells of the species. In humans, the number in the body cells is 46, and that in the mature spermatozoon and secondary oocyte is 23.

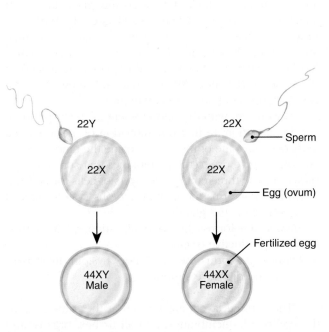

FIGURE 10.2 Inheritance of gender. Each ovum contains 22 autosomes and an X chromosome. Each spermatozoon (sperm) contains 22 autosomes and either an X chromosome or a Y chromosome. The gender of the zygote is determined at the time of fertilization by the combination of the sex chromosomes of the sperm (either X or Y) and the ovum (X).

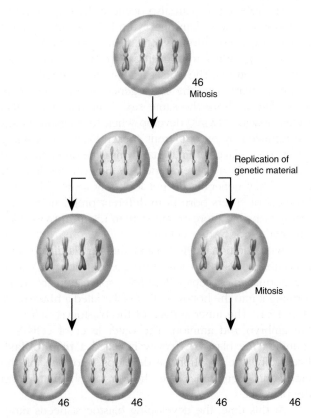

FIGURE 10.3 Mitosis of the stoma cells.

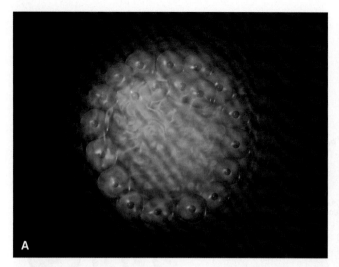
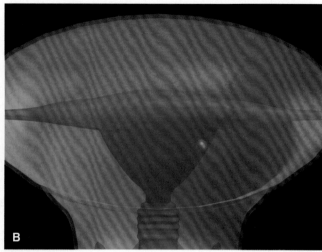

FIGURE 10.4 A. Fertilized human egg (zygote) having reached the blastocyst stage. Zygote contains 20 to 30 eggs and a fluid-filled blastocele is beginning to form. **B.** Implantation. Stylized image showing a frontal view of a uterus with a blastocyst about to implant into endometrium of the uterus. (From LifeART image copyright © 2011 Lippincott Williams & Wilkins. All rights reserved).

a series of four cleavages, the 16 cells appear as a solid ball of cells or **morula**, meaning "little mulberry." The morula continues to divide and transforms into a blastocyst as it moves further into the uterus. The morula reaches the uterine cavity about 72 hours after fertilization (Mueller, Hassel, & Grealy, 2015).

Multiple fetuses can also occur at the time of fertilization when more than one ovum is fertilized. Identical twins (also called monozygotic twins) occur when one fertilized egg splits and develops into two (or occasionally more) fetuses. The fetuses usually share one placenta. Identical twins have the same genes, so they generally look alike and are the same sex. Fraternal twins (also called dizygotic twins) develop when two separate eggs are fertilized by two different sperm. Each twin usually has its own placenta. Fraternal twins (like other siblings) share about 50% of their genes, so they can be different sexes. They generally do not look any more alike than brothers or sisters born from different pregnancies. Fraternal twins are more common than identical twins (see Chapter 19 for further details).

With additional cell division, the morula divides into specialized cells that will later form fetal structures. Within the morula, an off-center, fluid-filled space appears, transforming it into the hollow ball of cells called a **blastocyst** (Fig. 10.4). The inner surface of the blastocyst will form the embryo and amnion. The outer layer of cells surrounding the blastocyst cavity is called a **trophoblast**. Eventually, the trophoblast develops into one of the embryonic membranes, the chorion, and helps to form the placenta.

At this time, the developing blastocyst needs more food and oxygen to keep growing. The trophoblast

attaches itself to the surface of the endometrium for further nourishment. Normally, implantation occurs in the upper uterus (fundus), where a rich blood supply is available. This area also contains strong muscular fibers, which clamp down on blood vessels after the placenta separates from the inner wall of the uterus. Additionally, the lining is thickest here so the placenta cannot attach so strongly that it remains attached after birth. The process of attachment and placental formation is termed implantation. From a medical perspective, a pregnancy has not occurred until successful implantation has taken place (Jones & Lopez, 2014). Figure 10.5 shows the process of fertilization and implantation.

Concurrent with the development of the trophoblast and implantation, further differentiation of the inner cell mass occurs. Some of the cells become the embryo itself, and others give rise to the membranes that surround and protect it. The three embryonic layers of cells formed are:
1. *Ectoderm*—forms the central nervous system, special senses, skin, and glands.
2. *Mesoderm*—forms the skeletal, urinary, circulatory, and reproductive organs.
3. *Endoderm*—forms the respiratory system, liver, pancreas, and digestive system.

These three layers are formed at the same time as the embryonic membranes, and all tissues, organs, and organ systems develop from these three primary germ cell layers (El-Mazny, 2014). Box 10.1 summarizes pre-embryonic development.

Despite the intense and dramatic activities going on internally to create a human life, many women are unaware that pregnancy has begun. Several weeks will

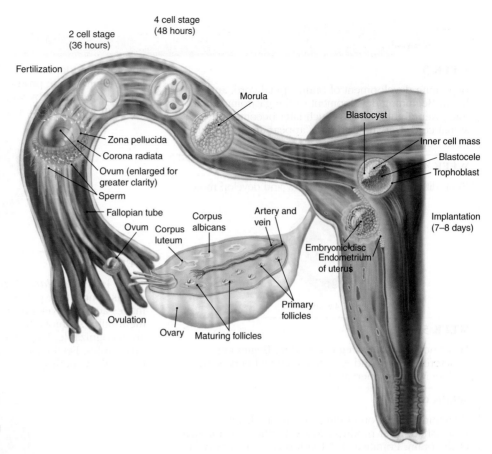

FIGURE 10.5 Fertilization and tubal transport of the zygote. From fertilization to implantation, the zygote travels through the fallopian tube, experiencing rapid mitotic division (cleavage). During the journey toward the uterus, the zygote evolves through several stages, including morula and blastocyst.

pass before even one of the presumptive signs of pregnancy—missing the first menstrual period—will take place.

Embryonic Stage

The embryonic stage of development begins at day 15 after conception and continues through week 8. Basic

---

BOX 10.1

SUMMARY OF PREEMBRYONIC DEVELOPMENT

- Fertilization takes place in ampulla of the Fallopian tube.
- Union of sperm and ovum forms a *zygote* (46 chromosomes).
- Cleavage cell division continues to form a morula (mass of 16 cells).
- The inner cell mass is called a *blastocyst*, which forms the embryo and amnion.
- The outer cell mass is called a *trophoblast*, which forms the placenta and chorion.
- Implantation occurs 7 to 10 days after conception in the endometrium.

---

structures of all major body organs and the main external features are completed during this time period, including internal organs. Table 10.1 and Figure 10.6 summarize embryonic development.

The embryonic membranes (Fig. 10.7) begin to form around the time of implantation. The chorion consists of trophoblast cells and a mesodermal lining. The chorion has finger-like projections called *chorionic villi* on its surface. The amnion originates from the ectoderm germ layer during the early stages of embryonic development. It is a thin protective membrane that contains amniotic fluid. Alongside of the amnion, a yolk sac develops as a second cavity about day 8 or 9 after conception. The yolk sac aids in transferring maternal nutrients and oxygen to the embryo during the second and third weeks of gestation when development of the uteroplacental circulation is under way. As the pregnancy progresses, the yolk sac atrophies and is incorporated into the umbilical cord. As the embryo grows, the amnion expands until it touches the chorion. These two fetal membranes form the fluid-filled amniotic sac, or bag of waters, that protects the floating embryo (Jordan et al., 2014).

Amniotic fluid surrounds the embryo and increases in volume as the pregnancy progresses, reaching approximately a liter at term. Amniotic fluid is derived from two sources: fluid transported from the maternal blood

TABLE 10.1 EMBRYONIC AND FETAL DEVELOPMENT

WEEK 3

Beginning development of brain, spinal cord, and heart; Beginning development of the gastrointestinal tract; Neural tube forms, which later becomes the spinal cord; Leg and arm buds appear and grow out from body

WEEK 4

Brain differentiates; Limb buds grow and develop more

4 weeks

WEEK 5

Heart now beats at a regular rhythm; Beginning structures of eyes and ears; Some cranial nerves are visible; Muscles innervated

WEEK 6

Beginning formation of lungs; Fetal circulation established; Liver produces RBCs; Further development of the brain; Primitive skeleton forms; Central nervous system forms; Brain waves detectable

WEEK 7

Straightening of trunk; Nipples and hair follicles form; Elbows and toes visible; Legs move; Diaphragm formed; Mouth with lips and early tooth buds

WEEK 8

Rotation of intestines. Facial features continue to develop; Heart development completes; Resembles a human being; Placenta is working; Eyelids form and grow, but are sealed shut

8 weeks

WEEKS 9–12

Sexual differentiation continues; Buds for all 20 temporary teeth laid down; Digestive system shows activity; Head makes up nearly half the fetus size. Face and neck are well formed; Urogenital tract completes

development; Red blood cells are produced in the liver; Urine begins to be produced and excreted; Fetal gender can be determined by week 12; Limbs are long and thin; digits are well formed; Fetus moves, kicks and swallows

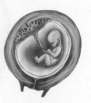

12 weeks

WEEKS 13–16

A fine hair called *lanugo* develops on the head; Fetal skin is almost transparent; Bones become harder; Fetus makes active movement; Sucking motions are made with the mouth; Amniotic fluid is swallowed; External genitalia are recognizable; Fingernails and toenails present; Weight quadruples; Fetal movement (also known as *quickening*) detected by mother

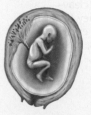

16 weeks

WEEKS 17–20

Rapid brain growth occurs; Fetal heart tones can be heard with stethoscope; Kidneys continue to secrete urine into amniotic fluid; Vernix caseosa, a white greasy film, covers the fetus; Eyebrows and head hair appear; Brown fat deposited to help maintain temperature; Nails are present on both fingers and toes; Muscles are well developed

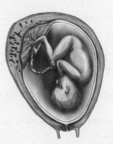

20 weeks

TABLE 10.1	EMBRYONIC AND FETAL DEVELOPMENT (continued)

WEEKS 21–24

Eyebrows and eyelashes are well formed; Fetus has a hand grasp and startle reflex; Alveoli forming in lungs; Skin is translucent and red; Eyelids remain sealed; Lungs begin to produce *surfactant*

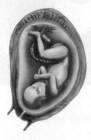

25 weeks

WEEKS 25–28

Fetus reaches a length of 15 in; Rapid brain development; Eyelids open and close; Nervous system controls some functions; Fingerprints are set; Subcutaneous fat is visible under the skin; Blood formation shifts from spleen to bone marrow; Fetus usually assumes head-down position; Fetus responds to light and sound; Fetus can open and shut eyes and suck thumb

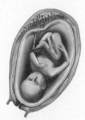

28 weeks

WEEKS 29–32

Rapid increase in the amount of body fat; Increased central nervous system control over body functions; Rhythmic breathing movements occur; Lungs are not fully mature; Pupillary light reflex is present; Fetus stores iron, calcium, and phosphorus

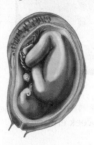

32 weeks

WEEKS 33–38

Testes are in scrotum of male fetus; Lanugo begins to disappear; Has strong hand grasp reflex; Increase in body fat; Earlobes formed and firm; Fingernails reach the end of fingertips; Small breast buds are present on both sexes; Mother supplies fetus with antibodies against disease; Fetus is considered full term at 38 weeks; Fetus fills uterus and moves to a head-down position

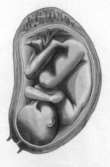

37 weeks

Adapted from March of Dimes. (2015c). *How your baby grows*. Retrieved from http://www.marchofdimes.com/pregnancy/yourbody_babygrowth.html; Jones, R. E., & Lopez, K. H. (2014). *Human reproductive biology* (4th ed.). Waltham, MA: Elsevier; Jordan, R. G., Engstrom, J., Marfell, J., & Farley, C. L. (2014). *Prenatal and postnatal care: A woman-centered approach*. Ames, Iowa: Wiley Blackwell.

across the amnion and fetal urine. Its volume changes constantly as the fetus swallows and voids. Sufficient amounts of amniotic fluid help maintain a constant body temperature for the fetus, permit symmetric growth and development, cushion the fetus from trauma, allow the **umbilical cord** to be relatively free from compression, and promote fetal movement to enhance musculoskeletal development. Amniotic fluid is composed of 98% water and 2% organic matter. It is slightly alkaline and contains albumin, urea, uric acid, creatinine, bilirubin, lecithin, sphingomyelin, epithelial cells, vernix, and fine hair called lanugo that floats in it. Amniotic fluid is essential for fetal growth and development, especially fetal lung development. It is dynamic, constantly changing as the fluid moves back and forth across the placental membrane (Zhang & Ducsay, 2014).

The volume of amniotic fluid is important in determining fetal well-being. It gradually fluctuates throughout the pregnancy. The rate of change of amniotic fluid volume depends on the gestational age. During the fetal

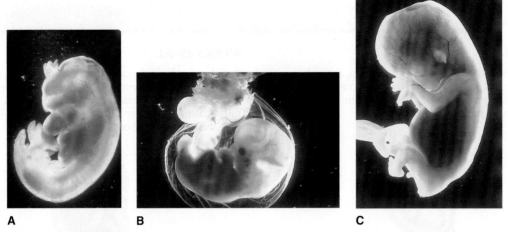

FIGURE 10.6 Embryonic development. **A.** Four-week embryo. **B.** Five-week embryo. **C.** Six-week embryo.

stage, the increase is 10 mL/week, and it increases to 50 to 60 mL/week at 19 to 25 weeks' gestation. The volume is at a maximum at 34 weeks' gestation before it undergoes a gradual decrease by term. Alterations in amniotic fluid volume can be associated with problems in the fetus. Too little amniotic fluid (<500 mL at term),

termed *oligohydramnios,* is associated with uteroplacental insufficiency, fetal renal abnormalities, and higher risk of surgical births and low-birth-weight infants. Too much amniotic fluid (>2,000 mL at term), termed *hydramnios,* is associated with maternal diabetes, neural tube defects, chromosomal deviations, and malformations of

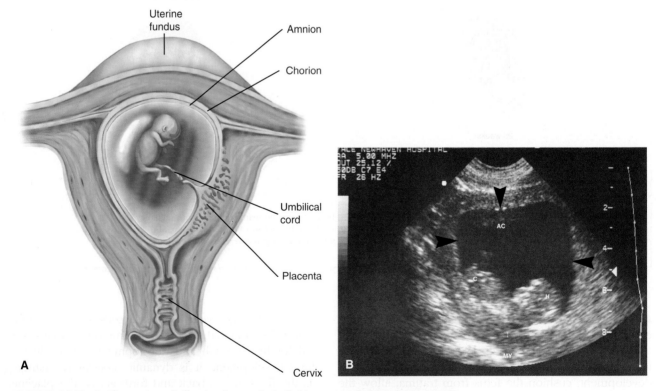

FIGURE 10.7   A. The embryo is floating in amniotic fluid, surrounded by the protective fetal membranes (amnion and chorion). **B.** Longitudinal sonogram of a pregnant uterus at 11 weeks showing the intrauterine gestational sac (*black arrowheads*) and the amniotic cavity (AC) filled with amniotic fluid; the fetus is seen in longitudinal section with the head (H) and coccyx (C) well displayed. The myometrium (MY) of the uterus can be identified. (Figure B is courtesy of L Scoutt).

the central nervous system and/or gastrointestinal tract that prevent normal swallowing of amniotic fluid by the fetus (Moore, 2015).

While the placenta is developing (end of the second week), the umbilical cord is also formed from the amnion. It is the lifeline from the mother to the growing embryo. It contains one large vein and two small arteries. Wharton's jelly (a specialized connective tissue) surrounds these three blood vessels in the umbilical cord to prevent compression, which would cut off fetal blood and nutrient supply. At term, the average umbilical cord is 22-in long and about an inch wide (King et al., 2015).

The precursor cells of the placenta—the trophoblasts—first appear 4 days after fertilization as the outer layer of cells of the blastocyst. These early blastocyst trophoblasts differentiate into all of the cells that form the **placenta**. When fully developed, the placenta serves as the interface between the mother and the developing fetus. Most commonly, the placenta develops at the uterine fundus. As early as 3 days after conception, the trophoblasts make human chorionic gonadotropin (hCG), a hormone that ensures that the endometrium will be receptive to the implanting embryo. During the next few weeks, the placenta begins to make hormones that control the basic physiology of the mother in such a way that the fetus is supplied with the nutrients and oxygen needed for growth. The placenta is the least understood human organ and arguably one of the most important. The placenta also protects the fetus from immune attack by the mother, removes waste products from the fetus, induces the mother to bring more food to the placenta and, near the time of delivery, produces hormones that ready fetal organs for life outside the uterus. The placenta allows the developing fetus to rely on the maternal circulation to fulfill its bioenergetics needs while growing undisturbed in the protected environment of the uterus (Fisher, 2015).

Theoretically, at no time during pregnancy does the mother's blood mix with fetal blood because there is no direct contact between their bloods; layers of fetal tissue always separate the maternal blood and the fetal blood. These fetal tissues are called the *placental barrier.* Materials can be interchanged only through diffusion. The maternal uterine arteries deliver the nutrients to the placenta, which in turn provides nutrients to the developing fetus; the mother's uterine veins carry fetal waste products away. The structure of the placenta is usually completed by week 12. During its transient existence, it performs actions that are later taken on by diverse separate organs, including the lungs, liver, gut, kidneys and endocrine glands.

The placenta is not only a transfer organ but a hormone factory as well. Placental hormones have profound effects on maternal metabolism, initially building up her energy reserves and then releasing these to support fetal growth in later pregnancy and lactation postnatally.

Several hormones are produced that are necessary for normal pregnancy:
- *hCG:* preserves the corpus luteum and its progesterone production so that the endometrial lining of the uterus is maintained; this is the basis for pregnancy tests.
- *Human placental lactogen (hPL) or human chorionic somatomammotropin (hCS):* modulates fetal and maternal metabolism, participates in the development of maternal breasts for lactation, and decreases maternal glucose utilization, which increases glucose availability to the fetus.
- *Estrogen (estriol):* causes enlargement of a woman's breasts, uterus, and external genitalia; stimulates myometrial contractility.
- *Progesterone (progestin):* maintains the endometrium, decreases the contractility of the uterus, stimulates maternal metabolism and breast development, provides nourishment for the early conceptus (the products of conception after fertilization in the early stages of growth and differentiation).
- *Relaxin:*acts synergistically with progesterone to maintain pregnancy, causes relaxation of the pelvic ligaments, and softens the cervix in preparation for birth (Freemark, 2015).

The placenta acts as a pass-through between the mother and fetus, not a barrier. Almost everything the mother ingests (food, alcohol, and drugs) passes through to the developing conceptus. This is why it is so important to advise pregnant women not to use unprescribed drugs, alcohol, and tobacco, because they can be harmful to the conceptus. Although prescription drug use is common during pregnancy, the human teratogenic risks are undetermined for more than 90% of drug treatments approved in the United States during the past decades (Dutta, 2015).

During the embryonic stage, the conceptus grows rapidly as all organs and structures are forming. During this critical period of differentiation the growing embryo is most susceptible to damage from external sources, including teratogens (substances that cause birth defects, such as alcohol and drugs), infections (such as rubella or cytomegalovirus), radiation, and nutritional deficiencies.

Teratogens

A **teratogen** is any substance, organism, physical agent, or deficiency state present during gestation that is capable of inducing abnormal postnatal structure or function by interfering with normal embryonic and fetal development (March of Dimes, 2015a). Teratogens are substances that may produce physical or functional defects in the human embryo or fetus after the pregnant woman has been exposed to that substance. Teratogens affect the fetus or embryo in a number of ways, causing physical deformities, problems in the behavioral or emotional development of the child, and decreased intellectual quotient (IQ) in the child. Additionally, teratogens may also affect pregnancies and cause complications such as preterm labors and spontaneous abortions. Susceptibility to teratogenic agents is dependent on the timing of the exposure and the developmental stage of the embryo or fetus. Teratogens are classified into four types: physical agents, metabolic conditions, infection, and drugs/chemical agents.

Selected harmful teratogens to newborns include:

- *Ionizing radiation*—leads to abnormal brain development, mental retardation, and leukemia in children.
- *Organic mercury*—leads to damage of neural system, mental retardation, behavioral and cognitive problems, and blindness in an infant.
- *Lead exposure*—can cause spontaneous abortions, delayed fetal development, increased risk of fetal death, or abnormal mental or physical development of a child.
- *Toxoplasma*—leads to spontaneous abortion, or stillbirth, underdeveloped fetal brain, blindness, and seizures.
- *Syphilis bacteria*—cause fetal death, spontaneous abortion, liver and spleen enlargement, and congenital syphilis.
- *Rubella virus*—leads to abnormal brain development in the fetus.
- *Cytomegalovirus*—leads to underdevelopment of the fetal brain, blindness, deafness, jaundice, liver and spleen dysfunction.
- *Varicella zoster*—leads to underdeveloped limbs, brain or eye malformations.
- *Herpes virus*—causes fetal death, microcephaly, herpetic pneumonia, and meningoencephalitis.
- *Maternal conditions*—obesity, diabetes, hypothyroidism, hyperthyroidism, and phenylketonuria (PKU).
- *Drugs*—thalidomide (limb malformations), alcohol (fetal alcohol syndrome), angiotensin-converting enzyme (ACE) inhibitors (antihypertensive agents) (prematurity, intrauterine growth restriction [IUGR]); cocaine (abruptio placenta, prematurity, microcephaly); and tetracycline (yellow-brown teeth discoloration); (Dutta, 2015).

Fetal Stage

The average pregnancy lasts 280 days from the first day of the LMP. The fetal stage is the time from the end of the eighth week until birth. It is the longest period of prenatal development. During this stage, the embryo is mature enough to be called a fetus. Although all major systems are present in their basic form, dramatic growth and refinement of all organ systems take place during the fetal period (Table 10.1). Figure 10.8 depicts a 12- to 15-week-old fetus.

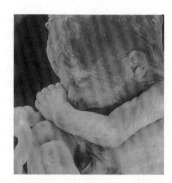

FIGURE 10.8 Fetal development: 12- to 15-week fetus.

Fetal Circulation

Fetal circulation differs from adult circulation due to the presence of certain vessels and shunts. These shunts will close after birth and most of these vessels will be seen as remnants in the adult circulation. The function of these shunts is to direct oxygen-rich venous blood to the systemic circulation and to ensure that oxygen-depleted venous blood bypasses the underdeveloped pulmonary circulation. The lungs finish their development after birth. Prior to this, the lung's function is taken over by the placenta, which therefore becomes the oxygen-transfer organ during fetal life (Finnemore & Groves, 2015).

The circulation through the fetus during uterine life differs from that of a child or an adult. In the extrauterine world, oxygenation occurs in the lungs and oxygenated blood returns via the pulmonary veins to the left side of the heart to be ejected by the left ventricle into the systemic circulation. In contrast, fetal circulation oxygenation occurs in the placenta, and the fetal lungs are nonfunctional as far as the transfer of oxygen and carbon dioxide is concerned. For oxygenated blood derived from the placenta to reach the fetus' systemic circulation, it has to travel through a series of shunts to accomplish this.

Thus, fetal circulation involves the circulation of blood from the placenta to and through the fetus, and back to the placenta. A properly functioning fetal circulation system is essential to sustain the fetus. Before it develops, nutrients and oxygen diffuse through the extraembryonic coelom and the yolk sac from the placenta. As the embryo grows, its nutrient needs increase and the amount of tissue easily reached by diffusion increases. Thus, the circulation must develop quickly and accurately (Jones & Lopez, 2014).

Three shunts also are present during fetal life:

1. *Ductus venosus*—connects the umbilical vein to the inferior vena cava.
2. *Ductus arteriosus*—connects the main pulmonary artery to the aorta.
3. *Foramen ovale*—anatomic opening between the right and left atrium.

Take Note!

Fetal circulation functions to carry highly oxygenated blood to vital areas (e.g., heart, brain) while first shunting it away from less important ones (e.g., lungs, liver). The placenta essentially takes over the functions of the lungs and liver during fetal life. As a result, large volumes of oxygenated blood are not needed.

The blood with the highest oxygen content is delivered to the fetal heart, head, neck, and upper limbs, while the blood with the lowest oxygen content is shunted toward the placenta.

The oxygenated blood is carried from the placenta to the fetus via the umbilical vein. About half of this blood passes through the hepatic capillaries and the rest flows through the ductus venosus into the inferior vena cava. Blood from the vena cava is mostly deflected through the foramen ovale into the left atrium, then to the left ventricle, into the ascending aorta, and on to the head and upper body. This allows the fetal coronary circulation and the brain to receive the blood with the highest level of oxygenation.

Deoxygenated blood from the superior vena cava flows into the right atrium, the right ventricle, and then the pulmonary artery. Because of high pulmonary vascular resistance, only a small percentage (5% to 10%) of the blood in the pulmonary artery flows to the lungs; the majority is shunted through the patent ductus arteriosus, and then to the descending aorta (American Heart Association [AHA], 2015). The fetal lungs are essentially nonfunctional because they are filled with fluid, making them resistant to incoming blood flow. They receive only enough blood for proper nourishment. Finally, two umbilical arteries carry the unoxygenated blood from the descending aorta back to the placenta.

At birth, a dramatic change in the fetal circulatory pattern occurs. The foramen ovale, ductus arteriosus, ductus venosus, and umbilical vessels are no longer needed. With the newborn's first breath, the lungs inflate, which leads to an increase in blood flow to the lungs from the right ventricle. This increase raises the pressure in the left atrium, causing a one-way flap on the left side of the foramen ovale, called the septum primum, to press against the opening, creating a functional separation between the two atria. Blood flow to the lungs increases because blood entering the right atrium can no longer bypass the right ventricle. As a result, the right ventricle pumps blood into the pulmonary artery and on to the lungs. Typically the foramen ovale is functionally closed within 1 to 2 hours after birth. It is physiologically closed by 1 month by deposits of fibrin that seal the shunt. Permanent closure occurs by the sixth month of life.

The ductus venosus, which links the inferior vena cava with the umbilical vein, usually closes with the clamping of the umbilical cord and inhibition of blood flow through the umbilical vein. This fetal structure closes by the end of the first week. The ductus arteriosus constricts partly in response to the higher arterial oxygen levels that occur after the first few breaths. This closure prevents blood from the aorta from entering the pulmonary artery. Functional closure of the ductus arteriosus in a term infant usually occurs within the first 72 hours after birth. Permanent closure occurs at 3 to 4 weeks of age (Yudkowitz, 2015). Frequently a functional or innocent murmur is auscultated by the nursery nurse when there are delayed fetal shunt closures, but they usually are not associated with a heart lesion. Successful transition from fetal to postnatal circulation requires increased pulmonary blood flow, removal of the placement and closure of the intracardiac (foramen ovale) and the extracardiac shunts (ductus venous and ductus arteriosus. All of these changes at birth leave the newborn with the typical adult pattern of circulation with right ventricle output equaling that of the left. Figure 10.9 shows fetal circulation. Also, view the following video of fetal circulation at this YouTube URL: https://www.youtube.com/watch?v=IRkisEtzskhttp://ndl.iitkgp.ac.in:8080/xmlui/handle/123456789/56006

GENETICS

Genetics is the study of individual genes and their role in heritance (Snustad, 2015). **Genomics**, a relatively new science, is the study of all genes and includes interactions among genes as well as interactions between genes and the environment. Genomics plays a role in complex conditions such as heart disease and diabetes. Another emerging area of research is that of pharmacogenomics, the study of genetic and genomic influences on pharmacodynamics and pharmacotherapeutics. While pharmacogenetics describes genetic variations between individuals and their influence on the efficacy and side effects of drugs, pharmacogenomics examines interactions of drugs with the entire genome. The main goal of both fields is the individual prediction of desirable and undesirable drug effects. An individual's genetics influences wellness and health issues throughout that individual's life cycle. The challenge for health care providers is to find the link between the client's genetic makeup and diseases (Brazeau, 2015).

According to the Centers for Disease Control and Prevention (2015a), birth defects and genetic disorders occur in 1 in 33 infants born in the United States and cause 1 in 5 infant deaths. Every 5 minutes an infant is born with a birth defect in the United States with nearly 120,000 infants affected annually. Traditionally, genetics has been associated with making decisions about childbearing and caring for children with genetic disorders. Currently, genetic and technological advances are expanding our understanding of how genetic changes affect human diseases such as diabetes, cancer,

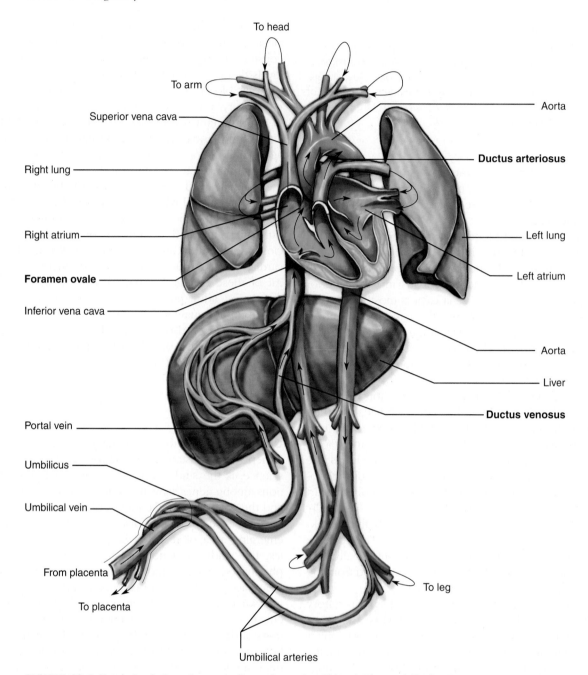

To head

To arm

Superior vena cava

Right lung

Right atrium

Foramen ovale

Inferior vena cava

Portal vein

Umbilicus

Umbilical vein

From placenta

To placenta

Aorta

Ductus arteriosus

Left lung

Left atrium

Aorta

Liver

Ductus venosus

To leg

Umbilical arteries

FIGURE 10.9 Fetal circulation. *Arrows* indicate the path of blood. The umbilical vein carries oxygen-rich blood from the placenta to the liver and through the ductus venosus. From there it is carried to the inferior vena cava to the right atrium of the heart. Some of the blood is shunted through the foramen ovale to the left side of the heart, where it is routed to the brain and upper extremities. The rest of the blood travels down to the right ventricle and through the pulmonary artery. A small portion of the blood travels to the nonfunctioning lungs, while the remaining blood is shunted through the ductus arteriosus into the aorta to supply the rest of the body.

Alzheimer's disease, and other multifactorial diseases that are prevalent in adults. Today's genetic technologies are not yet a crystal ball for seeing a child's future, but scientists are closer to routinely glimpsing the genetic blueprints of a fetus just months after sperm meets egg. The genomic reconstruction would reveal future disease risk and genetic traits in the first trimester of pregnancy. Recent research findings report that preimplantation with knowledge of the whole genome may facilitate the comprehensive diagnosis of diseases with a known genetic basis in embryos (Kumar et al., 2015). Newborn screening is perhaps the most widely used application of genetics in perinatal and neonatal care. Our ability to diagnose genetic conditions is more advanced than our ability to cure or treat the disorders. However, accurate diagnosis has led to improved treatment and outcomes for those affected with these disorders.

Take Note!

Genetic science has the potential to revolutionize health care with regard to national screening programs, predisposition testing, detection of genetic disorders, and pharmacogenetics.

Genetics has been a part of perinatal care for decades. Rapid development and implementation of advanced genetics technology in prenatal settings includes the ability to screen for and diagnose a broader range of diseases and conditions of the fetus in early gestational ages. Ultrasounds and maternal serum screening have become routine elements of prenatal care. Preconception carrier screening for conditions such as Tay–Sachs disease has been in place among high-risk populations such as Ashkenazi Jews. Amniocentesis and chorionic villus sampling are diagnostic tests that may confirm a genetic anomaly in a developing fetus, but they are all invasive techniques A fetal nuchal translucency test, seen on ultrasound, may suggest the presence of trisomy 21 or Down syndrome if increased nuchal thickness is found (Khalil & Coates, 2015).

Testing for genetic diseases before they cause symptoms, making a diagnosis in a person who has disease symptoms, and prescribing a type or dose of medication is early in its evolution. Genetic testing currently is rarely covered by health insurance companies, as the tests are still thought of as in research stages. This will change over the next several years as more associations between genomics and health are discovered.

Today, nurses are required to have basic skills and knowledge in genetics, genetic testing, and genetic counseling so they can assume new roles and provide information and support to women and their families. Roles for maternity nurses in genetic health care have expanded significantly as genetics education and counseling have become a standard of care. Today, nurses may provide preconception counseling for women at risk for the transmission of a genetic disorder. In addition, they may provide prenatal care for women with genetically linked disorders that require specialized care or may participate in screening infants for birth defects and genetic disorders. Nurses employed in prenatal care settings need to have accurate information they can provide to women so they understand the benefits and limitations of screening. Timely presentation of information and identification of available resources will help nurses minimize a couple's confusion and provide support for women as they proceed with pregnancy screening. Nurses at all levels should participate in risk assessments

for genetic conditions and disorders, explaining genetic risk and genetic testing, and supporting informed health decisions and opportunities for early intervention (Farrell, Nutter, & Agatisa, 2015). Nurses have a social and professional responsibility to ensure they provide current accurate information to clients and their families amid rapidly developing technology. This is especially true for nurses who value and support well-informed decision making that is woman-and-family-centered. For further information suitable for client education, nurses may want to access the following CDC web page on genomics: http://www.cdc.gov/genomics/public/index.htm/

It is very clear that genomics will have a profound effect on health and illness at all levels. Modern technology makes it possible to screen for and diagnose conditions prior to birth, such as open neural tube defects, chromosomal aneuploidies (i.e., trisomies 13, 18, and 21), congenital defects, and a myriad of single gene inheritable disorders (i.e., Tay–Sachs disease, cystic fibrosis, Huntington's disease, Duchenne muscular dystrophy, hemophilia). In the future, as the era of personalized health care moves forward, nurses will be responsible for ensuring that the scientific principles, ethical standards, and professional accountability of genetics and genomics practice are integrated into nursing practice. Nurses are increasingly doing this as they gain the necessary knowledge and skills. The strength of the nursing voice in genetics and genomic research will be the link to the bedside and the commitment to ensure that new knowledge is translated into competent, safe, effective, and evidence-based client care (Latendresse & Deneris, 2015).

Advances in Genetics and Genetic Technology

Human Genome Project

The publication of the first sequence of the human genome was regarded as one of the most ambitious and successful international research collaborations in modern biology. The Human Genome Project (HGP) was an international 13-year effort to produce a comprehensive sequence of the human genome. It was started in 1990 by the Department of Energy and the National Institutes of Health and was completed in May 2003. The goals of the HGP were to map, sequence, and determine the function of all human genes, which led to advances in the field of genetics and genetic testing (Kumar, Kingsley, & DiStefano, 2015). An individual's **genome** represents his or her genetic blueprint, which determines **genotype** (the gene pairs inherited from parents; the specific genetic makeup) and **phenotype** (observed outward characteristics of an individual). An individual's genetic profile can help guide decisions made regarding prevention, diagnosing, and treating disease. This is a profound shift in thinking from genetics that addressed rare disorders to the use of genetic information in all aspects of health care (Wilson & Nicholls, 2015).

A primary goal of the HGP was to translate the findings into new strategies for the prevention, diagnosis, and treatment of genetic diseases and disorders. Two key findings from the project were that all human beings are 99.9% identical at the deoxyribonucleic acid (DNA) level, and approximately 30,000 genes make up the human genome (International Human Genome Sequencing Consortium, 2015). Refer to thePoint for more information about the HGP.

Genetic Testing, Diagnosis, and Therapy

Recent advances in genetic knowledge and technology have affected all areas of health. These advances have increased the number of health interventions that can be undertaken with regard to genetic disorders. For example, genetic diagnosis is now possible very early in pregnancy (Evidence-Based Practice 10.1). Genetic testing can now identify presymptomatic conditions in children and adults. Gene therapy can be used to replace or repair defective or missing genes with normal ones.

Gene therapy has been used for a variety of disorders, including cystic fibrosis, melanoma, diabetes, HIV, and hepatitis. Gene therapy offers the possibility of accurately and specifically targeting particular genetic abnormalities through gene correction, addition, or replacement. This ability adds a new dimension of credible therapeutic choices (Cicalese & Aiuti, 2015). The potential exists for creation of increased intelligence and size through genetic intervention. Recent research using gene therapy shows promise for the generation of insulin-producing cells to cure diabetes; perhaps achieve long-term control of diabetes is on the horizon. Recent research is working toward beta cell replacement for diabetics to reliably and automatically maintain glucose levels within a tight range as the normal pancreas does (Johannesson et al., 2015). In the future, genetic agents may replace drugs, general surgery may be replaced by gene surgery, and genetic intervention may replace radiation. Recent successful trials on the treatment of ocular diseases and inherited immune deficiencies are particularly encouraging and have risen hopes that human gene therapy as a standard treatment option will finally become a reality. Continuous progress suggests that a wide range of

---

EVIDENCE-BASED PRACTICE 10.1

EFFECT OF ENHANCED INFORMATION, VALUES CLARIFICATION, AND REMOVAL OF FINANCIAL BARRIERS ON USE OF PRENATAL GENETIC TESTING: A RANDOMIZED CLINICAL TRIAL

Prenatal genetic testing guidelines have focused on identifying women at increased risk of giving birth to infants with chromosomal abnormalities. The use of prenatal genetic testing for clinical decision making is increasing exponentially. The current complexity of it brings concerns about the potential erosion of informed choice. It is difficult to ascertain if clients and their families truly understand what it is about and implications of the results. There currently are genetic tests for more than 2,500 diseases, with nearly 2,300 available for use in clinical decision making. The aim of this randomized study was to promote preference-based decision making and to assess the prenatal testing choices women make in the context of being fully informed about testing options.

STUDY

Of 1,932 women screened, 1,297 were eligible, and 744 enrolled in the study. They were then randomized into interventional and control groups. The women were diverse in ethnicity, language, education, and were at 20 weeks' gestation or less. Those in the intervention group had access to a computerized, interactive, prenatal testing support guide and were told that the study would pay for any tests for which they lacked health insurance coverage. Women in the control group received usual care, but no additional study intervention or financial support to cover prenatal testing. The goal was to determine

what choices women would make after being fully informed about the benefits and risks of prenatal testing.

Findings

After women received complete prenatal testing information and the opportunity to consider their values and preferences, they were less likely to undergo invasive testing and more likely to avoid testing for aneuploidy (i.e., trisomies 13, 18, and 21). Full implementation of prenatal testing guidelines may lead to more informed and preference-based prenatal decision making.

Nursing Implications

Based on this study's findings, nurses can utilize standard counseling in addition to computer-based interactive information to reinforce the information about genetic testing before decisions are made to proceed. The landscape for genetic testing is changing constantly and it is wise to have well-informed clients and their families making the right decisions for their situation. By utilizing computerized technology to assist in educating clients and their families about a vital decision affecting their future, nurses are providing evidence-based information to them. Nurses have a responsibility to be knowledgeable about available genetic tests so they can assist their clients to become informed consumers of genetic-based health care.

Adapted from Kuppermann, M., Pena, S., Bishop, J. T., Nakagawa, S., Gregorich, S. E., Sit, A., et al . (2015). Effect of enhanced information, values clarification, and removal of financial barriers on use of prenatal genetic testing: A randomized clinical trial. *Obstetrical & Gynecological Survey, 70*(1), 7–9.

diseases will be treated with gene therapy in the future (Lundstrom, 2015).

Current and potential applications of the HGP in health care include rapid and more specific diagnosis of disease, with hundreds of genetic tests available in research or clinical practice; earlier detection of genetic predisposition to disease; less emphasis on treating the symptoms of a disease and more emphasis on looking at the fundamental causes of the disease; new classes of drugs; avoidance of environmental conditions that may trigger disease; and augmentation or replacement of defective genes through gene therapy. This new genetic knowledge and technology, along with the commercialization of this knowledge, will change both professional and parental understanding of genetic disorders. Current reproductive applications, however, remain restricted to mostly the prevention of transmitting an at-risk gene or genes, but do not include treatment or cure. It is anticipated that this restriction might continue for years. As such, the scientific and ethical issues associated with reproductive applications will continue to affect decision making of at-risk individuals.

Ethical, Legal, and Social Issues of Genetic Technology

The potential benefits of these discoveries are vast, but so is the potential for misuse. These advances challenge all health care providers to consider the many ethical, legal, and social ramifications of genetics in human lives. In the near future, individual risk profiling based on an individual's unique genetic makeup will be used to tailor prevention, treatment, and ongoing management of health conditions. This profiling will raise issues associated with client privacy and confidentiality related to workplace discrimination and access to health insurance. Issues of autonomy are equally problematic as society considers how to address the injustices that will inevitably surface when disease risk can be determined years before the disease occurs. Nurses will play an important role in developing policies and providing direction and support in this arena, and to do so they will need a basic understanding of genetics, including inheritance and inheritance patterns. (For more information on the ethical, social, and legal issues surrounding human genetic research and advances, refer to thePoint).

Inheritance

DNA and Genetic Information

The nucleus within the cell is the controlling factor in all cellular activities because it contains chromosomes, long continuous strands of DNA that carry genetic information. Each chromosome is made up of **genes**. Genes are individual units of heredity of all traits and are organized into long segments of DNA that occupy a specific location on a chromosome and determine a particular characteristic in an organism.

DNA stores genetic information and encodes the instructions for synthesizing specific proteins needed to maintain life. DNA is double stranded and takes the form of a double helix. The side pieces of the double helix are made up of a sugar, deoxyribose, and a phosphate, occurring in alternating groups. The cross-connections or rungs of the ladder are attached to the sides and are made up of four nitrogenous bases: adenine, cytosine, thymine, and guanine. The sequence of the base pairs as they form each rung of the ladder is referred to as the genetic code (Travers & Muskhelishvili, 2015) (Fig. 10.10).

Each gene has a segment of DNA with a specific set of instructions for making proteins needed by body cells for proper functioning. Genes control the types of proteins made and the rate at which they are produced

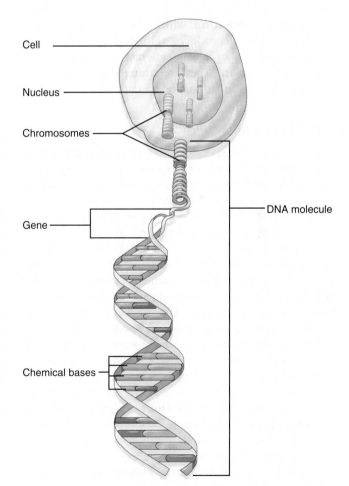

FIGURE 10.10 DNA is made up of four chemical bases. Tightly coiled strands of DNA are packaged in units called chromosomes, housed in the cell's nucleus. Working subunits of DNA are known as genes. (From the National Institutes of Health and National Cancer Institute. [1995]. Understanding gene testing [NIH Pub. No. 96-3905]. Washington, DC: U.S. Department of Human Services).

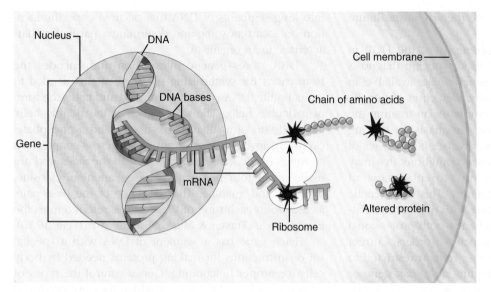

FIGURE 10.11 When a gene contains a mutation, the protein encoded by that gene will be abnormal. Some protein changes are insignificant, while others are disabling. (From the National Institutes of Health and National Cancer Institute. [1995]. Understanding gene testing [NIH Pub. No. 96-3905]. Washington, DC: U.S. Department of Human Services).

(Snustad, 2015). Any change in gene structure or location leads to a **mutation**, which may alter the type and amount of protein produced (Fig. 10.11). Genes never act in isolation; they always interact with other genes and the environment. They are arranged and lined up in a specific linear formation along a chromosome.

Genotypes and Alleles

The genotype—the specific genetic makeup of an individual, usually in the form of DNA—is the internally coded inheritable information. It refers to the particular **allele**, which is one of two or more alternative versions of a gene at a given position or locus on a chromosome that imparts the same characteristic of that gene. For instance, each human has a gene that controls height, but there are variations of these genes, called alleles, that code for a specific height. As another example, a gene that controls eye color may have an allele that can produce blue eyes or an allele that produces brown eyes. The genotype, together with environmental variation that influences the individual, determines the phenotype, or the observed, outward characteristics of an individual. A human inherits two genes, one from each parent. Therefore, one allele comes from the mother and one from the father. These alleles may be the same for the characteristic (**homozygous**) or different (**heterozygous**). For example, WW stands for homozygous dominant; ww stands for homozygous recessive. Heterozygous would be indicated as Ww. If the two alleles differ, such as Ww, the dominant one will usually be expressed in the phenotype of the individual.

Chromosomes

Human beings typically have 46 chromosomes. This includes 22 pairs of nonsex chromosomes or autosomes and 1 pair of sex chromosomes (two X chromosomes in females, and an X chromosome and a Y chromosome in males). Offspring receive one chromosome of each of the 23 pairs from each parent.

The pictorial analysis of the number, form, and size of an individual's chromosomes is termed the **karyotype**. This analysis commonly uses white blood cells and fetal cells in amniotic fluid. The chromosomes are numbered from the largest to the smallest, 1 to 22, and the sex chromosomes are designated by the letter X or Y. A female karyotype is designated as 46, XX and a male karyotype is designated as 46, XY. Figure 10.12 illustrates an example of a karyotyping pattern.

Genetic Mutations

Regulation and expression of the thousands of human genes are very complex processes and are the result of many intricate interactions within each cell. Alterations in gene structure, function, transcription, translation, and protein synthesis can influence an individual's health (Jones & Lopez, 2014). Gene mutations are a permanent change in the sequence of DNA.

Gene mutations can be inherited, spontaneous, or acquired. Inherited gene mutations are passed on from parent to child in the egg and sperm, and are passed on to all cells in that child's body when the body cells reproduce. Cystic fibrosis is an example of an inherited mutation. A spontaneous mutation can occur in individual eggs or sperm at the time of conception. A person who has the new spontaneous mutation has the risk of passing it on to his or her offspring. An example of a spontaneous mutation would be Marfan syndrome. Acquired mutations occur in body cells other than egg or sperm. They involve changes in DNA that take place after conception, during a person's lifetime. Acquired mutations are passed on when they reproduce to daughter cells. These changes can be caused by environmental factors such

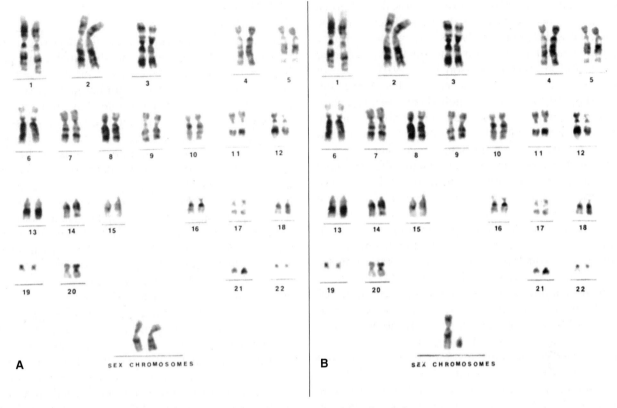

FIGURE 10.12 Karyotype pattern. **A.** Normal female karyotype. **B.** Normal male karyotype.

as ultraviolet radiation from the sun, or can occur if a mistake is made as DNA copies itself during cell division (National Institutes of Health [NIH], 2015a). Some mutations have no significant effect, whereas others can have a tremendous impact on the health of the individual. Several genetic disorders such as cancer, sickle cell disease, PKU, and hemophilia, can result from these mutations.

Patterns of Inheritance for Genetic Disorders

Patterns of inheritance demonstrate how a genetic disorder can be passed on to offspring. A genetic disorder is a disease caused by an abnormality in an individual's genetic material or genome. Diagnosis of a genetic disorder is usually based on clinical signs and symptoms or on laboratory confirmation of the presence of an altered gene associated with the disorder. Accurate diagnosis can be aided by recognition of the pattern of inheritance within a family. The pattern of inheritance is also vital to understand when teaching and counseling families about the risks in future pregnancies. Some genetic conditions are caused by mutations in a single gene. These conditions are typically inherited in one of several straightforward patterns, depending on the gene involved. Some genetic disorders occur in multiple family members, while others may occur in only a single family member.

A genetic disorder is caused by completely or partially altered genetic material, whereas a familial disorder is more common in relatives of the affected individual but may be caused by environmental influences and not genetic alterations.

Monogenic Disorders

The principles of genetic disease inheritance of single-gene disorders are the same principles that govern the inheritance of other traits, such as eye and hair color. These are known as Mendel's laws of inheritance, named for the genetic work of Gregor Mendel, an Austrian naturalist. These patterns occur due to a single gene being defective and are referred to as monogenic or sometimes Mendelian disorders. If the defect occurs on the autosome, the genetic disorder is termed *autosomal*; if the defect is on the X chromosome, the genetic disorder is termed *X linked*. The defect also can be classified as dominant or recessive. Monogenic disorders include autosomal dominant, autosomal recessive, X-linked dominant, and X-linked recessive patterns.

AUTOSOMAL DOMINANT INHERITANCE DISORDERS

Autosomal dominant inheritance disorders occur when a single gene in the heterozygous state is capable of producing the phenotype. In other words, the abnormal or mutant gene overshadows the normal gene and the individual will demonstrate signs and symptoms of the disorder. The affected person generally has one affected parent, and an affected person has a 50% chance of passing the abnormal gene to each of his or her children (Fig. 10.13). Affected individuals are present in every generation. Males and family members who are phenotypically normal (do not show signs or symptoms of the disorder) do not transmit the condition to their offspring. Females and males are equally affected and a male can pass the disorder on to his son. This male-to-male transmission is important in distinguishing autosomal dominant inheritance from X-linked inheritance. There are varying degrees of presentation among individuals in a family. Therefore, a parent with a mild form could have a child with a more severe form. Common types of genetic disorders that follow the autosomal dominant pattern of inheritance include neurofibromatosis (genetic disorders affecting the development and growth of neural cells and tissues); Huntington's disease (a genetic disorder affecting the nervous system characterized by abnormal involuntary movements and progressive dementia); achondroplasia (a genetic disorder resulting in disordered growth and abnormal body proportion); and polycystic kidney disease (a genetic disorder involving the growth of multiple, bilateral, grape-like clusters of fluid-filled cysts in the kidneys that eventually compress and replace functioning renal tissue).

AUTOSOMAL RECESSIVE INHERITANCE DISORDERS

Autosomal recessive inheritance disorders occur when two copies of the mutant or abnormal gene in the homozygous state are necessary to produce the phenotype. In other words, two abnormal genes are needed for the individual to demonstrate signs and symptoms of the disorder. These disorders are generally less common than autosomal dominant disorders (NIH, 2015a). Both parents of the affected person must be heterozygous carriers of the gene (clinically normal but carry the gene), and their offspring have a 25% chance of being homozygous (a 50% chance of getting the mutant gene from each parent and therefore a 25% chance of inheriting two mutant genes). If the child is clinically normal, there is a 50% chance that he or she is a carrier (Fig. 10.14). Affected individuals are usually present in only one generation of the family. Females and males are equally affected and a male can pass the disorder on to his son. The chance that any two parents will both be carriers of the mutant gene is increased if the couple is consanguineous (having a common ancestor). Common types of genetic disorders that follow the autosomal recessive inheritance pattern include cystic fibrosis (a genetic disorder involving generalized dysfunction of the exocrine glands); PKU (a disorder involving a deficiency in a liver enzyme that leads to the inability to process the essential amino acid phenylalanine); Tay–Sachs disease (a disorder due to insufficient activity of the enzyme hexosaminidase A, which is necessary for

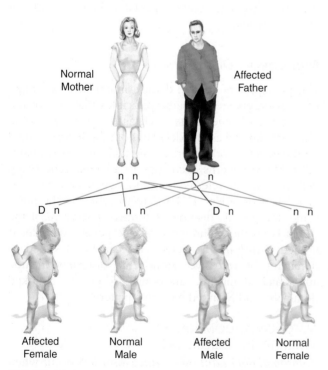

FIGURE 10.13 Autosomal dominant inheritance.

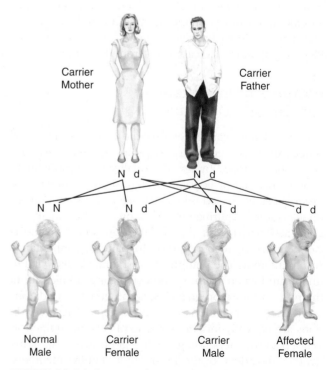

FIGURE 10.14 Autosomal recessive inheritance.

the breakdown of certain fatty substances in the brain and nerve cells); and sickle cell disease (a genetic disorder in which the red blood cells carry an ineffective type of hemoglobin instead of the normal adult hemoglobin).

X-LINKED INHERITANCE DISORDERS

X-linked inheritance disorders are those associated with altered genes present on the X chromosome. They differ from autosomal disorders. If a male inherits an X-linked altered gene, he will express the condition. Because a male has only one X chromosome, all the genes on his X chromosome will be expressed (the Y chromosome carries no normal allele to compensate for the altered gene). Because females inherit two X chromosomes, they can be either heterozygous or homozygous for any allele. Therefore, X-linked disorders in females are expressed similarly to autosomal disorders.

 Concept Mastery Alert

Male Children in Pattern of Inheritance of Duchenne Muscular Dystrophy

The gene for Duchenne muscular dystrophy is X-linked, which means that a male child who inherits this gene will be affected by, not a carrier of, the disease. A female child will not be affected by the disease.

Most X-linked disorders demonstrate a recessive pattern of inheritance. Males are more affected than females. A male has only one X chromosome and all the genes on his X chromosome will be expressed, whereas a female will usually need both X chromosomes to carry the disease. There is no male-to-male transmission (since no X chromosome from the male is transmitted to male offspring), but any man who is affected will have carrier daughters. If a woman is a carrier, there is a 50% chance that her sons will be affected and a 50% chance that her daughters will be carriers (Fig. 10.15). Common types of genetic disorders that follow X-linked recessive inheritance patterns include hemophilia (a genetic disorder involving a deficiency of one of the coagulation factors in the blood); color blindness; and Duchenne muscular dystrophy (a disorder involving progressive muscular weakness and wasting).

X-linked dominant inheritance is present if heterozygous female carriers demonstrate signs and symptoms of the disorder. All of the daughters and none of the sons of an affected male have the condition, while both male and female offspring of an affected woman have a 50% chance of inheriting and presenting with the condition (Fig. 10.16). X-linked dominant disorders are rare. The most common is hypophosphatemic (vitamin D–resistant) rickets (a disorder involving a softening or weakening of the bones). Fragile X syndrome is another X-linked dominant condition

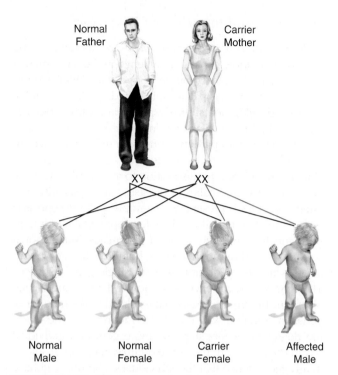

FIGURE 10.15 X-linked recessive inheritance.

that causes a range of developmental problems including learning disabilities and cognitive impairment. A characteristic of X-linked dominant is that fathers cannot pass X-linked traits to their sons (no male-to-male transmission).

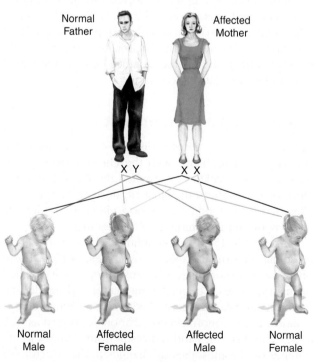

FIGURE 10.16 X-linked dominant inheritance.

Multifactorial Inheritance Disorders

Multifactorial inheritance disorders are thought to be caused by multiple genetic (polygenic) and environmental factors. Many of the common congenital malformations, such as cleft lip, cleft palate, spina bifida, pyloric stenosis, clubfoot, developmental hip dysplasia, and cardiac defects, are attributed to multifactorial inheritance. A combination of genes from both parents, along with unknown environmental factors, produces the trait or condition. An individual may inherit a predisposition to a particular anomaly or disease. The anomalies or diseases vary in severity, and often a sex bias is present. For example, pyloric stenosis is seen more often in males, while developmental hip dysplasia is much more likely to occur in females. Multifactorial conditions tend to run in families, but the pattern of inheritance is not as predictable as with single-gene disorders. The chance of recurrence is also lower than in single-gene disorders, but the degree of risk is related to the number of genes in common with the affected individual. The closer the degree of relationship, the more genes an individual has in common with the affected family member, resulting in a higher chance that the individual's offspring will have a similar defect. In multifactorial inheritance, the likelihood that both identical twins will be affected is not 100%, indicating that there are nongenetic factors involved.

Nontraditional Inheritance Patterns

Molecular studies have revealed that some genetic disorders are inherited in ways that do not follow the typical patterns of dominant, recessive, X-linked, or multifactorial inheritance. Examples of nontraditional inheritance patterns include mitochondrial inheritance and genomic imprinting. As the science of molecular genetics advances and more is learned about inheritance patterns, other nontraditional patterns of inheritance may be discovered or found to be relatively common.

Chromosomal Abnormalities

In some cases of genetic disorders, the abnormality occurs due to problems with the chromosomes. Chromosomal abnormalities arise when the normal complement of 46 chromosomes that produces a karyotype is altered, usually during cell division, either by an increase or decrease in the number of chromosomes.

About 1 in 150 live-born infants is born with a chromosomal abnormality (March of Dimes, 2015a). These often cause major defects because they involve added or missing genes. Congenital anomalies and intellectual disability are often associated with chromosomal abnormalities. These abnormalities occur on autosomal as well as sex chromosomes and can result from changes in the number of chromosomes or changes in the structure of the chromosomes.

Numerical Abnormalities

Chromosomal abnormalities of number often result from nondisjunction or failure of the chromosome pair to separate during cell division, meiosis, or mitosis. Few chromosomal numerical abnormalities are compatible with full-term development and most result in spontaneous abortion. One type of chromosomal number abnormality is **polyploidy**. Polyploidy causes an increase in the number of haploid sets (23) of chromosomes in a cell. Triploidy refers to three whole sets of chromosomes in a single cell (in humans, a total of 69 chromosomes per cell); tetraploidy refers to four whole sets of chromosomes in a single cell (in humans, a total of 92 chromosomes per cell). Polyploidy usually results in an early spontaneous abortion and is incompatible with life.

Some numerical abnormalities do support development to term because the chromosome on which the abnormality is present carries relatively few genes (such as chromosome 13, 18, 21, or X). Two common abnormalities of chromosome number are monosomies or trisomies. In **monosomies**, there is only one copy of a particular chromosome instead of the usual pair (an entire single chromosome is missing). In these cases, all fetuses spontaneously abort in early pregnancy. Survival is seen only in mosaic forms of these disorders. In **trisomies**, there are three of a particular chromosome instead of the usual two (an entire single chromosome is added). Trisomies may be present in every cell or may present in the mosaic form. The most common trisomies include trisomy 21 (Down syndrome), trisomy 18, and trisomy 13.

TRISOMY 21

Down syndrome is an example of a trisomy. The cause of Down syndrome is one of three types of abnormal cell division involving chromosome 21. All three abnormalities result in extra genetic material from chromosome 21, which is responsible for the characteristic features and developmental problems of Down syndrome. The three genetic variations that can cause Down syndrome include trisomy 21, where the infant has three copies of chromosome 21—instead of the usual two copies—in all of his or her cells; mosaic, where infants have some cells with an extra copy of chromosome 21; and translocation, where part of chromosome 21 becomes attached (translocated) to another chromosome, before or at conception. More than 90% of the cases of Down syndrome are caused by trisomy 21 (March of Dimes, 2015b) (Fig. 10.17).

Down syndrome affects 1 in 691 live-born babies. About 6,000 infants with Down syndrome are born in the United States annually. The risk of this and other trisomies increases with maternal age. The risk of having a baby with Down syndrome is about 1 in 1,250 for a woman at age 25, 1 in 1,000 at 30, 1 in 400 at 35, 1 in 100 at age 40, and 1 in 30 at age 45 (March of Dimes, 2015b). Children with Down syndrome have

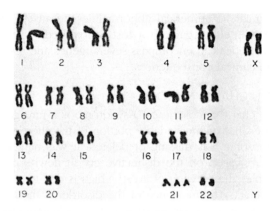

FIGURE 10.17 Karyotype of a child with Down syndrome.

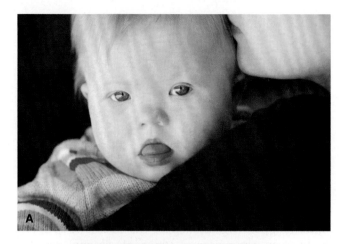

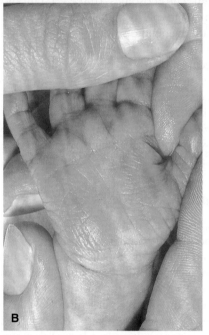

FIGURE 10.18 A. Typical facial features of an infant with Down syndrome. **B.** A simian line, a horizontal crease in the palm of children with Down syndrome.

characteristic features that are usually identified at birth (Fig. 10.18). These common characteristics include:
• Small, low-set ears that may fold over a little at the pinna
• Hyperflexibility
• Muscle hypotonia
• Small hands and feet
• A short neck
• Wide-spaced eyes that slant upward
• Ulnar loop on the second digit
• Deep crease across palm (termed a *simian crease*)
• Flat facial profile
• Short stature in childhood and adulthood
• Small white, crescent-shaped spots on irises
• Small mouth with protruding tongue
• Broad, short fingers (National Down Syndrome Society [NDSS], 2015a)

The outlook for children with Down syndrome is much brighter now than it was years ago. Most children with Down syndrome have an intellectual disability in the mild-to-moderate range. With early intervention and special education, many learn to read and write and participate in diverse childhood activities (Grieco et al., 2015). Life expectancy for individuals with Down syndrome has increased dramatically in recent years, with the average life span approaching that of peers without Down syndrome (NDSS, 2015b).

TRISOMY 18 AND TRISOMY 13

Two other common trisomies are trisomy 18 and trisomy 13. Trisomy 18 and trisomy 13 are, respectively, the second and third most commonly diagnosed autosomal trisomies in live-born infants. These conditions are associated with a high degree of infant mortality, with most dying before their first birthday (Trisomy 18 Foundation, 2015).

Trisomy 18, or Edward syndrome, occurs in 1 of every 2,500 pregnancies in the United States, about 1 in 6,000 live births (Trisomy 18 Foundation, 2015). Prenatally, several findings are apparent on ultrasound: IUGR, hydramnios or oligohydramnios, cardiac malformations,

a single umbilical artery, and decreased fetal movement. Additionally, trisomy 18 has been associated with a decrease in maternal serum levels of maternal serum alpha-fetoprotein (MSAFP) and hCG. Most affected newborns are female, with a 4:1 ratio to males. Affected newborns have 47 chromosomes (three at chromosome 18) and are characterized by severe intellectual disability, growth deficiency of the cranium (microcephaly), low-set ears, facial malformations, small-for-gestational-age size, seizures, drooping eyelids, webbing of fingers, kidney and congenital heart defects, rocker-bottom feet, and severe hypotonia (National Organization for Rare Disorders [NORD], 2015a). Infants with trisomy 18 have multiple anomalies that are severe, and life expectancy is greatly reduced beyond a few months.

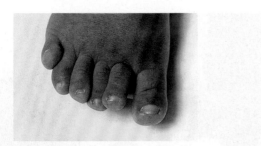

FIGURE 10.19 An infant with trisomy 13 has supernumerary digits (polydactyly).

Trisomy 13, or Patau syndrome, affects 1 of 10,000 live births (Support Organization for Trisomies [SOFT], 2015). Forty-seven chromosomes (three of chromosome 13) are present. Maternal age is also thought to be a causative factor in this genetic disorder. The common abnormalities associated with trisomy 13 are microcephaly, cardiac defects, small eyes, kidney malformations, central nervous system anomalies, rocker-bottom feet, neural tube defects, omphalocele, cleft lip and palate, cryptorchidism, polydactyly (Fig. 10.19), severe intellectual disability, severe hypotonia, and seizures. Life expectancy is only a few days for most infants with trisomy 13 (NORD, 2015b). Care for these infants is supportive.

Structural Abnormalities

Chromosomal abnormalities of structure usually occur when a portion of one or more chromosomes is broken or lost, and during the repair process the broken ends are rejoined incorrectly. Structural abnormalities usually lead to having too much or too little genetic material. Altered chromosome structure can take on several forms. Deletions occur when a portion of the chromosome is missing, resulting in a loss of that chromosomal material. Duplications are seen when a portion of the chromosome is duplicated and an extra chromosomal segment is present. Clinical findings vary depending on how much chromosomal material is involved. Inversions occur when a portion of the chromosome breaks off at two points and is turned upside down and reattached; therefore, the genetic material is inverted.

The most clinically significant structural abnormality is a translocation. This occurs when part of one chromosome is transferred to another chromosome and an abnormal rearrangement is present.

Structural abnormalities can be balanced or unbalanced. Balanced abnormalities involve the rearrangement of genetic material with neither an overall gain nor loss. Individuals who inherit a balanced structural abnormality are usually phenotypically normal but are at a higher risk for miscarriages and having chromosomally abnormal offspring. Examples of structural rearrangements that can be balanced include inversions, translocations, and ring chromosomes. Unbalanced structural abnormalities

are similar to numerical abnormalities because genetic material is either gained or lost. Unbalanced structural abnormalities can encompass several genes and result in severe clinical consequences.

CRI DU CHAT SYNDROME

Cri du chat ("cry of the cat") syndrome is a rare genetic disorder in which a variable portion of the short arm of chromosome 5 is missing or deleted. It was named "cri du chat" based on the distinctive cry in newborns that resembles the mewing of a cat, which is due to a laryngeal defect. The incidence of the disorder is thought to be approximately 1 in 50,000 live births (NORD, 2015d). In addition to the cat-like, high-pitched cry in infancy, it is also associated with intellectual and psychomotor disability, microcephaly, speech delay, low birth weight and slow growth, hypotonia, failure to thrive, wide-set eyes, small jaw, low-set ears, and various organ malformations. Symptoms vary greatly from case to case depending upon the exact size and location of the deleted genetic material.

No specific treatment is available for this syndrome. With contemporary interventions, the child may survive to adulthood: 75% of deaths occur during the first several months of life and almost 90% occur in the first year. Death occurs in 6% to 8% of the overall population affected with the syndrome. Pneumonia, aspiration pneumonia, congenital heart defects, and respiratory distress are the common causes of death (Chen, 2015a). Parents should be referred for genetic counseling.

FRAGILE X SYNDROME

Fragile X syndrome, also termed Martin–Bell syndrome, is a structural abnormality involving the X chromosome, which demonstrates breaks and gaps. It is a common form of intellectual disability and autism spectrum disorder. The syndrome is usually diagnosed by the age of 3 by molecular DNA studies. Conservative estimates report that fragile X syndrome affects approximately 1 in 5,000 males and 1 in 8,000 females (CDC, 2015c). Typically, a female becomes the carrier and will be mildly affected. The male who receives the X chromosome that has a fragile site will exhibit the full effects of the syndrome. Fragile X syndrome is characterized by intellectual disability, hyperactivity, large head, long face, short attention span, hand flapping, strabismus, hypotonia, speech delay, inflexible behavior, autistic-like behavior, poor eye contact, tactile defensiveness, double-jointedness, and perseverative speech (continued repetition of words or phrases). It is the most common form of male intellectual disability (NORD, 2015e).

Aside from the morbidity associated with intellectual disability and cognitive/behavioral/neuropsychological problems, the life span of an individual with fragile X syndrome is unaffected. This syndrome is currently not included in newborn screening panels in the United States, as it does not meet the standards for recommendation.

There is no cure for this disorder. Speech, occupational, and physical therapy services usually are needed, as well as special education and counseling.

Sex Chromosome Abnormalities

Chromosomal abnormalities can also involve sex chromosomes. These cases are usually less severe in their clinical effects than autosomal chromosomal abnormalities. Sex chromosome abnormalities are gender specific and involve a missing or extra sex chromosome. They affect sexual development and may cause infertility, growth abnormalities, and possibly behavioral and learning problems. Many affected individuals lead essentially normal lives. Examples are Turner syndrome (in females) and Klinefelter syndrome (in males).

TURNER SYNDROME

Turner syndrome is a common abnormality of the sex chromosome in which a portion or all of the X chromosome is missing. It affects about 1 in 2,000 live-born female infants worldwide (March of Dimes, 2015a). It is highly variable and can differ dramatically from one person to another. Most cases of Turner syndrome are not inherited. Clinical manifestations include a low posterior hairline and webbing of the neck, short stature, broad skeletal abnormalities, kidney abnormalities, osteoporosis, heart defects, a shield-like chest with widely spaced nipples, lymphedema, cataracts, scoliosis, puffy feet, underdeveloped secondary sex characteristics, heart defects, and infertility (NORD, 2015c). Only about a third of cases are diagnosed as newborns; the remaining two thirds are diagnosed in early adolescence when they experience primary amenorrhea. No cure exists for this syndrome. Growth hormone typically is given; hormone replacement therapy also may be used to induce puberty and stimulate continued growth. Most females with Turner syndrome are of normal intelligence and usually live essentially normal lives (NIH, 2015b).

KLINEFELTER SYNDROME

Klinefelter syndrome is a sex chromosomal abnormality that occurs only in males. About 1 in 500 to 1,000 males are born with Klinefelter syndrome (Chen, 2015b). With this syndrome an extra X chromosome (XXY) is present. The extra genetic material causes abnormal development of the testicles, resulting in decreased production of sperm and male sex hormones. Clinical manifestations may include:

- Mild intellectual disability
- Small testes that do not produce adequate testosterone
- Infertility
- Learning disabilities
- Delayed speech and language development
- Long arms and legs
- Enlarged breast tissue (gynecomastia)
- Scant facial and body hair
- Decreased sex drive (libido) (NORD, 2015f)

No treatment can correct this genetic abnormality, but testosterone replacement therapy can improve symptoms resulting from the deficiency. Surgery may be done to reduce gynecomastia. Most males with Klinefelter syndrome (XXY) are diagnosed in late puberty. Infertility is common and life expectancy is normal (Chen, 2015b).

Genetic Evaluation and Counseling

Genetic counseling is the process by which clients or relatives at risk for an inherited disorder are advised of the consequences and nature of the disorder, the probability of developing or transmitting it, and the options open to them in management and family planning in order to prevent, avoid, or ameliorate it. Nurses have long been on the forefront of genetic counseling for their clients. The knowledge derived from the HGP is transforming the health care model, with implications for nursing in genetic counseling, practice, and research (Lopes, de Omena Bomfim, & Flória-Santos, 2015). An individual should be referred for genetic counseling for any of a variety of reasons. Box 10.2 lists those who may benefit from genetic counseling. In many cases, geneticists and genetic counselors provide information to families regarding genetic diseases. However, an experienced family physician, pediatrician, or

Consider This

As I waited for the genetic counselor to come into the room, my mind was filled with numerous fears and questions. What does an inconclusive amniocentesis really mean? What if this pregnancy produced an abnormal baby? How would I cope with a special child in my life? If only I had gone to the midwife sooner when I thought I was pregnant, but still in denial. Why did I not stop drinking and smoking when I found out I was pregnant? If only I had started to take my folic acid pills when prescribed. Why didn't I research my family's history to know of any hidden genetic conditions? What about my sister with a Down syndrome child? What must I have been thinking? I guess I could play the "what-if" game forever and never come up with answers. Is it was too late to do anything about this? I am 37 years old and alone.... I started to pray silently when the counselor opened the door....

Thoughts: *This woman is reviewing the past few weeks, looking for answers to her greatest fears. Inconclusive screenings can introduce emotional torment for many women as they wait for validating results. Are these common thoughts and fears for many women facing potential genetic disorders? What supportive interventions might the nurse offer?*

THOSE WHO MAY BENEFIT FROM GENETIC COUNSELING

- Women who are pregnant or planning to be after age 35
- Paternal age 50 years or older
- Previous child, parents, or close relatives with an inherited disease, congenital anomalies, metabolic disorders, developmental disorders, or chromosomal abnormalities
- Consanguinity or incest
- Pregnancy screening abnormality, including alphafetoprotein, triple screen, amniocentesis, or ultrasound
- Stillborn with congenital anomalies
- Two or more pregnancy losses
- Exposure to drugs, medications, radiation, chemicals, or infections
- Concerns about genetic defects that occur frequently in their ethnic or racial group (for instance, those of African descent are most at risk for having a child with sickle cell anemia)
- Abnormal newborn screening
- Couples with a family history of X-linked disorders
- Carriers of autosomal recessive or dominant diseases
- Child born with one or more major malformations in a major organ system
- Child with abnormalities of growth
- Child with developmental delay, intellectual disability, blindness, or deafness

Adapted from March of Dimes. (2015d). *Genetic counseling*. Retrieved from http://www.marchofdimes.com/pregnancy/genetic-counseling.aspx; National Human Genome Research Institute. (2015). *What is genetic counseling and evaluation?* Retrieved from https://www.genome.gov/19016905; and Dayal, M. B., & Athanasiadis, I. (2015). Preimplantation genetic diagnosis. *eMedicine*. Retrieved from http://emedicine.medscape.com/article/273415-overview#aw2aab6b3.

nurse who has received special training in genetics may also provide the information.

A genetic consultation involves evaluation of an individual or a family. Its purposes are to confirm, diagnose, or rule out genetic conditions; to identify medical management issues; to calculate and communicate genetic risks to a family; to discuss ethical and legal issues; and to provide and arrange psychosocial support. Genetic counselors serve as educators and resource persons for other health care providers and the general public.

The ideal time for genetic counseling is before conception. Preconception counseling gives couples the chance to identify and reduce potential pregnancy risks, plan for known risks, and establish early prenatal care. Unfortunately, many women delay seeking prenatal care until their second or third trimester, after the crucial time of organogenesis. Therefore, it is important that preconception counseling be offered to all women as they seek health care throughout their childbearing years, especially if they are contemplating pregnancy.

This requires health care providers to take a proactive role.

Genetic screening and counseling can raise serious ethical and moral issues for a couple. The results of prenatal genetic testing can lead to the decision to terminate a pregnancy, even if the results are not conclusive but indicate a strong possibility that the child will have an abnormality. The severity of the abnormality may not be known, and some may find the decision to terminate unethical. Another difficult situation that provides an example of the ethical and moral issues surrounding genetic screening and counseling involves disorders that affect only one gender of offspring. A mother may find she is a carrier of a gene for a disorder for which there is no prenatal screening test available. In these cases, the couple may decide to terminate any pregnancy where the fetus is the affected sex, even though there is a 50% chance that the child will not inherit the disorder. In these situations, the choice is the couple's and information and support must be provided in a nondirective, nonjudgmental manner.

Genetic counseling is particularly important if a congenital anomaly or genetic disease has been diagnosed prenatally or if a child is born with a life-threatening congenital anomaly or genetic disease. In these cases, families need information urgently so they can make immediate decisions. If a diagnosis with genetic implications is made later in life, if a couple with a family history of a genetic disorder or a previous child with a genetic disorder is planning a family, or if there is suspected teratogen exposure, urgency of information is not such an issue. In these situations, the family needs time to ponder all their options. This may involve several meetings over a longer period of time.

Genetic counseling involves gathering information regarding birth history, past medical history, and current health status as well as a family history of congenital anomalies, intellectual disability, genetic diseases, reproductive history, general health, and causes of death. A detailed family history is imperative and in most cases will include the development of a pedigree, which is like a family tree (Fig. 10.20). Information is ideally gathered on three generations, but if the family history is complicated, information from more distant relatives may be needed. Families receiving genetic counseling may benefit from being told in advance that this information will be necessary; they may need to discuss these sensitive, private issues with family members to obtain the needed facts. When necessary, medical records may be requested for family members, especially those who have a genetic disorder, to help ensure accuracy of the information. Sometimes a pedigree may reveal confidential information not known by all family members, such as an adoption, a child conceived through in vitro fertilization, or a husband not being the father of a baby. Therefore, maintaining confidentiality is extremely important. After

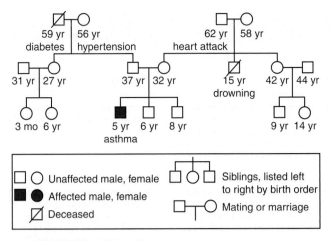

FIGURE 10.20 A pedigree is a diagram made using symbols that demonstrates the links between family members and focuses on medical and health information for each relative.

careful analysis of the data obtained, referral to a genetic counselor when indicated is appropriate.

Medical genetic knowledge has increased dramatically during the past few decades. Not only is it possible to detect specific diseases with genetic mutations, but it is also possible to test for a genetic predisposition to various diseases or conditions and certain physical characteristics. This leads to complex ethical, moral, and social issues. Maintaining client privacy and confidentiality and administering care in a nondiscriminatory manner are essential while maintaining sensitivity to cultural differences. It is essential to respect client autonomy and present information in a nondirective, nonjudgmental manner.

NURSING ROLES AND RESPONSIBILITIES

Nurses are at the forefront of client care, and will participate fully in genetic-based and genomic-based activities. Nurses will therefore have a critical role advocating for, educating, counseling, and supporting clients and families who are making gene-based health care decisions (Association of Genetic Nurses and Counselors [AGNC], 2015). The nurse is likely to interact with the client in a variety of ways related to genetics: taking a family history, scheduling genetic testing, explaining the purposes of all screening and diagnostic tests, answering questions, providing information and psychosocial support to individuals and families, and addressing concerns raised by family members. Nurses are often the first health care providers to encounter women with preconception and prenatal issues. Nurses play an important role in beginning the preconception counseling process and referring women and their partners for further genetic testing when indicated.

Nurses working with families involved with genetic counseling typically have certain responsibilities. These include:

- Using interviewing and active listening skills to identify genetic concerns
- Knowing basic genetic terminology and inheritance patterns
- Explaining basic concepts of probability and disorder susceptibility
- Safeguarding the privacy and confidentiality of clients' genetic information
- Providing complete informed consent to facilitate decisions about genetic testing
- Discussing costs of genetic services and the benefits and risks of using health insurance to pay for genetic services, including potential risks of discrimination
- Recognizing and defining ethical, legal, and social issues
- Providing accurate information about the risks and benefits of genetic testing
- Using culturally appropriate methods to convey genetic information
- Monitoring clients' emotional reactions after receiving genetic analysis
- Providing information on appropriate local support groups
- Knowing their own limitations and making appropriate referrals (Sermon & Viville, 2014)

An accurate and thorough family history is an essential part of preconception counseling. Nurses in any practice setting can obtain a client's history during the initial encounter. The purpose is to gather client and family information that may provide clues as to whether the client has a genetic trait, inherited condition, or inherited predisposition (International Society of Nurses in Genetics, 2015). At a basic level, all nurses should be able to take a family medical history to help identify those at risk for genetic conditions, and then initiate a referral when appropriate. Box 10.3 presents examples of focused assessment questions that can be used. Based on the information gathered during the history, the nurse must decide whether a referral to a genetic specialist is necessary or whether further evaluation is needed. Families identified with genetic issues need unique clinical care including management of acute illnesses, screening for long-term complications, discussion of the etiology of the condition, connections to social supports, and clarification of the recurrence risks and prenatal testing and treatment options. Prenatal testing to assess for genetic risks and defects might be used to identify genetic disorders. These tests are described in Common Laboratory and Diagnostic Tests 10.1.

Remember Robert and Kate Shafer? Based on the information gathered from their genetic history, they were referred to a genetic specialist. What prenatal tests might be ordered to assess their risk for genetic disorders? What would be the nurse's role related to genetic counseling?

COMMON LABORATORY AND DIAGNOSTIC TESTS 10.1

PRENATAL TESTS TO ASSESS RISK FOR GENETIC DISORDERS

Test	Description	Indication	Timing
Alpha-fetoprotein	A sample of the woman's blood is drawn to evaluate plasma protein that is produced by the fetal liver, yolk sac, and gastrointestinal tract, and crosses from the amniotic fluid into the maternal blood	Increased levels might indicate a neural tube defect, Turner syndrome, tetralogy of Fallot, multiple gestation, omphalocele, gastroschisis, or hydrocephaly. Decreased levels might indicate Down syndrome or trisomy 18	Typically performed between 15 and 18 weeks' gestation
Amniocentesis	Amniotic fluid aspirated from the amniotic sac; safety concerns include infection, pregnancy loss, and fetal needle injuries	To perform chromosome analysis, alpha-fetoprotein, DNA markers, viral studies, karyotyping, tests are done to identify cystic fibrosis, sickle cell trait or disease	Usually performed between 15 and 20 weeks' gestation to allow for adequate amniotic fluid volume to accumulate; results take 2 to 4 weeks
Chorionic villus sampling	Removal of small tissue specimen from the fetal portion of the placenta, which reflects the fetal genetic makeup; main complications include severe transverse limb defects and spontaneous pregnancy loss	To detect fetal karyotype, sickle-cell anemia, phenylketonuria, Down syndrome, sickle cell trait or disease, Duchenne muscular dystrophy, cystic fibrosis, and numerous other genetic disorders	Typically performed between 10 and 12 weeks' gestation, with results available in less than a week
Percutaneous umbilical blood sampling	Insertion of a needle directly into a fetal umbilical vessel under ultrasound guidance; two potential complications: fetal hemorrhage and risk of infection	Used for prenatal diagnosis of inherited blood disorders such as hemophilia A, karyotyping; detection of fetal infection; determination of acid–base status; and assessment and treatment of isoimmunization	Generally performed after 16 weeks' gestation
Fetal nuchal translucency (FNT)	An intravaginal ultrasound that measures fluid collection in the subcutaneous space between the skin and the cervical spine of the fetus	To identify fetal anomalies; abnormal fluid collection can be associated with genetic disorders (trisomies 13, 18, and 21), Turner syndrome, cardiac deformities, and/or physical anomalies. When the FNT is greater than 3 mm, the measurement is considered abnormal	Performed between 10 and 14 weeks' gestation
Level III ultrasound/fetal scan	Use of high-frequency sound waves to visualize the fetus	Enables early evaluation of structural changes	Typically performed after 18 weeks' gestation
Triple and quad screening tests	Triple screening includes alpha-fetoprotein, estriol, and beta-hCG; Quad screening includes alpha-fetoprotein, estriol, beta-hCG, and inhibin A	To identify risk for Down syndrome, neural tube defects, and other chromosomal disorders. Elevated hCG combined with lower-than-normal estriol and MSAFP levels indicate increased risk for Down syndrome or other trisomy condition	Performed between 15 and 18 weeks' gestation
Preimplantation genetic diagnosis	Genetic testing of embryos produced through in vitro fertilization (IVF)	Identifies embryos carrying specific genetic alterations that can cause disease. Only those without genetic alterations are later transferred into the woman's uterus to start a pregnancy. Prevents inheritable genetic disease before implantation	Usually on day 3 after egg retrieval and 2 days after fertilization, a single blastomere is removed from the developing embryo to be evaluated
Cell-free fetal DNA (cffDNA)	A noninvasive prenatal test using maternal plasma that holds a mixture of maternal and fetal DNA after 4 weeks' gestation	Determines fetal sex in pregnancies at risk for sex-linked conditions; RhD genotyping in pregnancies at risk of hemolytic disease of the newborn and fetal chromosomal abnormalities such as Down syndrome	A maternal blood sample is taken and next generation sequencing is used to analyze the cffDNA at approximately 10 weeks' gestation

Adapted from Latendresse, G. & Deneris, A. (2015). An update on current prenatal testing options: First trimester and noninvasive prenatal testing. *Journal of Midwifery & Women's Health, 60*(1), 24–36; Dayal, M. B. & Athanasiadis, I. (2015). Preimplantation genetic diagnosis. *eMedicine.* Retrieved from http://emedicine.medscape.com/article/273415-overview#aw2aab6b3; and Khalil, A. & Coates, A. (2015). Prenatal diagnosis of chromosomal abnormalities. *Arias' Practical Guide to High-Risk Pregnancy and Delivery: A South Asian Perspective*, (pp. 1–13, 4th ed.). Haryana, India: Elsevier.

BOX 10.3

FOCUSED HEALTH ASSESSMENT: GENETIC HISTORY

- What was the cause and age of death for deceased family members?
- Does any consanguinity exist between relatives?
- Do any serious illnesses or chronic conditions exist? If so, what was the age of onset?
- Do any female family members have a history of miscarriages, stillbirths, or diabetes?
- Do any female members have a history of alcohol or drug use during pregnancy?
- What were the ages of female members during childbearing, especially if older than 35 years?
- Do any family members have an intellectual disability or developmental delays?
- Do any family members have a known or suspected metabolic disorder such as PKU?
- What is the maternal age of both parents presently with this pregnancy?
- Do any family members have an affective disorder such as bipolar disorder?
- Have any close relatives been diagnosed with any type of cancer?
- What is your ethnic background (explore as related to certain disorders)?
- Do any family members have a known or suspected chromosomal disorder?
- Do any family members have a progressive neurologic disorder?

Adapted from Edelman, C. L., Kudzma, E. C., & Mandle, C. L. (2014). *Health promotion throughout the lifespan* (8th ed.). St. Louis, MO: Mosby Elsevier; Snustad, D.P. (2015). *Principles of genetics* (7th ed.). New York, NY: Wiley Publishers; Latendresse, G. & Deneris, A. (2015). An update on current prenatal testing options: First trimester and noninvasive prenatal testing. *Journal of Midwifery & Women's Health*, 60(1), 24–36; and Genetic Alliance. (2015). *Family health history*. Retrieved from http://geneticalliance.org/programs/genesinlife/fhh

---

Talking with family members who have recently been diagnosed with a genetic disorder or who have had a child born with congenital anomalies is very difficult. Many times the nurse may be the one who has first contact with these parents and will be the one to provide follow-up care. Genetic disorders are significant, life-changing, and possibly life-threatening situations. Genetic information is highly technical and the field is undergoing significant technological advances. Nurses need an understanding of who will benefit from genetic counseling and must be able to discuss the role of the genetic counselor with families. The goal is to ensure that families at risk are aware that genetic counseling is available before they attempt to have another baby.

Based on the results of their genetic tests, Robert and Kate are placed at moderate risk for having an infant with an autosomal recessive genetic disorder.

The couple asks the nurse what all of this means. What information should the nurse provide about concepts of probability and disorder susceptibility for this couple? How can the nurse help this couple to make knowledgeable decisions concerning their reproductive future?

Nurses play an essential role in providing emotional support to the family through this challenging time. Genetics permeates all aspects of health care. Today, everyone is embracing quality and evidence-based care. Nurses who have an understanding of genetics and genomics will possess the foundation to provide quality, evidence-based care especially with follow-up counseling after the couple or family has been to the genetic specialist.

Take Note!

Nurses need to be actively engaged with clients and their families and help them consider the facts, values, and context in which they are making decisions. Nurses need to be open and honest with families as they discuss these sensitive and emotional choices.

Nurses should provide ongoing support and education for clients and their families. This includes coping with the disease burden, helping clients and families adapt to a condition in the family, and ensuring adequate understanding of the genetic risks and the available prenatal diagnostic and reproductive choices. The nurse is in an ideal position to help families review what has been discussed during the genetic counseling sessions and to answer any additional questions they might have. Referral to appropriate agencies, support groups, and resources, such as a social worker, a chaplain, or an ethicist, is another key role when caring for families with suspected or diagnosed genetic disorders.

KEY CONCEPTS

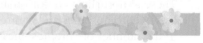

- Fertilization, which takes place in the outer third of the ampulla of the fallopian tube, leads to the formation of a zygote. The zygote undergoes cleavage, eventually implanting in the endometrium about 7 to 10 days after conception.

- Three embryonic layers of cells are formed: ectoderm, which forms the central nervous system, special senses, skin, and glands; mesoderm, which forms the skeletal, urinary, circulatory, and reproductive systems; and endoderm, which forms the respiratory system, liver, pancreas, and digestive system.

- Amniotic fluid surrounds the embryo and increases in volume as the pregnancy progresses, reaching approximately a liter by term.

- At no time during pregnancy is there any direct connection between the blood of the fetus and the blood of the mother, so there is no mixing of blood.

- The placenta protects the fetus from immune attack by the mother, removes waste products from the fetus, induces the mother to bring more food to the placenta, and, near the time of delivery, produces hormones that mature fetal organs in preparation for life outside the uterus.

- The purpose of fetal circulation is to carry highly oxygenated blood to vital areas (heart and brain) while first shunting it away from less vital ones (lungs and liver).

- Humans have 46 paired chromosomes that are found in all cells of the body, except the ovum and sperm cells, which have just 23 chromosomes. Each person has a unique genetic constitution, or genotype.

- Research from the HGP has provided a better understanding of the genetic contribution to disease.

- Genetic disorders can result from abnormalities in patterns of inheritance or chromosomal abnormalities involving chromosomal number or structure.

- Autosomal dominant inheritance occurs when a single gene in the heterozygous state is capable of producing the phenotype. Autosomal recessive inheritance occurs when two copies of the mutant or abnormal gene in the homozygous state are necessary to produce the phenotype. X-linked inheritance disorders are those associated with altered genes present on the X chromosome. They can be dominant or recessive.

- In some cases of genetic disorders, a chromosomal abnormality occurs. Chromosomal abnormalities do not follow straightforward patterns of inheritance. These abnormalities occur on autosomal as well as sex chromosomes and can result from changes in the number of chromosomes or changes in the structure of the chromosomes.

- Genetic counseling involves evaluation of an individual or a family. Its purpose is to confirm, diagnose, or rule out genetic conditions, identify medical management issues, calculate and communicate genetic risks to a family, discuss ethical and legal issues, and assist in providing and arranging psychosocial support.

- Legal, ethical, and social issues that can arise related to genetic testing include the privacy and confidentiality of genetic information, who should have access to personal genetic information, psychological impact and stigmatization due to individual genetic differences, use of genetic information in reproductive decision making and reproductive rights, and whether testing is to be performed if no cure is available.

- Preconception screening and counseling can raise serious ethical and moral issues for a couple. The results of prenatal genetic testing can lead to the decision to terminate a pregnancy.

- Nurses play an important role in beginning the preconception counseling process and referring women and their partners for further genetic information when indicated. Many times the nurse is the one who has first contact with these women and will be the one to provide follow-up care.

- Nurses need to have a solid understanding of who will benefit from genetic counseling and must be able to discuss the role of the genetic counselor with families, ensuring that families at risk are aware that genetic counseling is available before they attempt to have another baby.

- Nurses play an essential role in providing emotional support and referrals to appropriate agencies, support groups, and resources when caring for families with suspected or diagnosed genetic disorders. Nurses can assist clients with their decision making by referring them to a social worker, a chaplain, or an ethicist.

References and Recommended Readings

American Heart Association [AHA]. (2015). *Fetal circulation.* Retrieved from https://www.heart.org/HEARTORG/Conditions/Congenital-HeartDefects/SymptomsDiagnosisofCongenitalHeartDefects/Fetal-Circulation_UCM_315674_Article.jsp

Association of Genetic Nurses and Counselors [AGNC]. (2015). *Getting the message across.* Retrieved from http://www.agnc.org.uk/news-events/news/

Centers for Disease Control and Prevention [CDC]. (2015a). *Facts about birth defects.* Retrieved from http://www.cdc.gov/ncbddd/birthdefects/facts.html

Centers for Disease Control and Prevention [CDC]. (2015b). *Facts about Down syndrome.* Retrieved from http://www.cdc.gov/ncbddd/birthdefects/downsyndrome.html

Centers for Disease Control and Prevention [CDC]. (2015c). *Fragile X syndrome: Data & statistics.* Retrieved from http://www.cdc.gov/ncbddd/fxs/data.html

Chen, H. (2015a). Cri du chat syndrome. *eMedicine.* Retrieved from http://emedicine.medscape.com/article/942897-overview

Chen, H. (2015b). Klinefelter syndrome. *eMedicine.* Retrieved from http://emedicine.medscape.com/article/945649-overview

Cicalese, M. P., & Aiuti, A. (2015). Clinical applications of gene therapy for primary immunodeficiencies. *Human Gene Therapy, 26*(4), 210–219.

Dayal, M. B., & Athanasiadis, I. (2015). Preimplantation genetic diagnosis. *eMedicine.* Retrieved from http://emedicine.medscape.com/article/273415-overview#aw2aab6b3

Dutta, S. (2015). Human teratogens and their effects: A critical evaluation. *International Journal of Informative Research and Review*, *2*(3), 525–536.

Edelman, C. L., Kudzma, E.C., & Mandle, C. L. (2014). *Health promotion throughout the lifespan* (8th ed.). St. Louis, MO: Mosby Elsevier.

El-Mazny, A. (2014). *Human reproduction: Basic anatomy and physiology*. Charleston, SC: Amazon CreateSpace Publishers.

Farrell, R. M., Nutter, B., & Agatisa, P. K. (2015). Patient-centered prenatal counseling: Aligning obstetric healthcare professionals with needs of pregnant women. *Women & Health*, *55*(3), 280–296.

Fisher, S. (2015). Placenta: The forgotten organ. *Annual Review of Cell and Developmental Biology*, *31*(1), 523–552 Retrieved from http://www.annualreviews.org/doi/abs/10.1146/annurev-cellbio-100814-125620

Finnemore, A., & Groves, A. (2015). Physiology of the fetal and transitional circulation. *Seminars in Fetal and Neonatal Medicine*, *20*(4), 210–216 (Online 4/24/15).

Freemark, M. (2015). Placental hormones and the control of fetal growth. *International Journal of Pediatric Endocrinology*, *2015*(Suppl 1), O13. d

Genetic Alliance. (2015). *Family health history*. Retrieved from http://geneticalliance.org/programs/genesinlife/fhh

Grieco, J., Pulsifer, M., Seligsohn, K., Skotko, B., & Schwartz, A. (2015). Down syndrome: Cognitive and behavioral functioning across the lifespan. *American Journal of Medical Genetics Part C: Seminars in Medical Genetics*, 1–15.

International Human Genome Sequencing Consortium. (2015). *Celebrating a decade of discovery since the Human Genome project*. Retrieved from http://genome.wellcome.ac.uk/doc_WTX060109.html

International Society of Nurses in Genetics [ISONG]. (2015). *What can genetics nurses do for you?* Retrieved from http://www.isong.org/ISONG_genetic_nurse.php

Johannesson, B., Sui, L., Freytes, D. O., Creusot, R. J., & Egli, D. (2015). Toward beta cell replacement for diabetes. *The Excellence in the Life Sciences Journal (EMBO)*, *34*(7), 841–855.

Jones, R. E., & Lopez, K. H. (2014). *Human reproductive biology* (4th ed.). Waltham, MA: Elsevier.

Jordan, R. G., Engstrom, J., Marfell, J., & Farley, C. L. (2014). *Prenatal and postnatal care: A woman-centered approach*. Ames, Iowa: Wiley Blackwell

Khalil, A., & Coates, A. (2015). Prenatal diagnosis of chromosomal abnormalities. *Arias' practical guide to high-risk pregnancy and delivery: A South Asian perspective*, (4th ed., pp. 1–13). Haryana, India: Elsevier

King, T. L., Brucker, M. C., Kriebs, J. M., Fahey, J. O., Gegor, C. L., & Varney, H. (2015). *Varney's midwifery* (5th ed.). Burlington, MA: Jones & Bartlett Learning.

Kumar, A., Ryan, A., Kitzman, J. O., Wemmer, N., Snyder, M. W., Sigurjonsson, S., et al. (2015). Whole genome prediction for preimplantation genetic diagnosis. *Genome Medicine*, *7*(1), 35.

Kumar, S., Kingsley, C., & DiStefano, J. K. (2015). The Human Genome Project: Where are we now and where are we going?. *Genome mapping and genomics in human and non-human primates* (pp. 7–31). Berlin Heidelberg: Springer Publishers.

Kuppermann, M., Pena, S., Bishop, J. T., Nakagawa, S., Gregorich, S. E., Sit, A., et al . (2015). Effect of enhanced information, values clarification, and removal of financial barriers on use of prenatal genetic testing: A randomized clinical trial. *Obstetrical & Gynecological Survey*, *70*(1), 7–9.

Latendresse, G., & Deneris, A. (2015). An update on current prenatal testing options: First trimester and noninvasive prenatal testing. *Journal of Midwifery & Women's Health*, *60*(1), 24–36.

Lea, D. H., Cheek, D., Brazeau, D., & Brazeau, G. (2015). Pharmacogenomics/pharmacogenetics and interprofessional education and practice. *Mastering pharmacogenomics: A nurse's handbook for success* (pp. 191–204). Indianapolis, IN: Sigma Theta Tau International.

Lundstrom, K. (2015). New era in gene therapy. *Novel approaches and strategies for biologics, vaccines and cancer therapies*, (pp. 15–40). San Diego, CA: Elsevier.

Lopes, L. C., de Omena Bomfim, E., & Flória-Santos, M. (2015). Genomics-based health care: Implications for nursing. *International journal of Nursing Didactics*, *5*(02), 11–15.

Mader, S., & Windelspecht, M. (2015). *Human biology* (14th ed.). New York, NY: McGraw-Hill Higher Education

Maeda, K. (2015). Prenatal fetal life in the mother. *Journal of Health & Medical Informatics*, *6*, 177.

March of Dimes. (2015a). *Chromosomal abnormalities*. Retrieved from http://www.marchofdimes.com/hbhb_syndication/15530_1209.asp

March of Dimes. (2015b). *Down syndrome*. Retrieved from http://www.marchofdimes.com/baby/down-syndrome.aspx#

March of Dimes. (2015c). *How your baby grows*. Retrieved from http://www.marchofdimes.com/pregnancy/how-your-baby-grows.aspx#

March of Dimes. (2015d). *Genetic counseling*. Retrieved from http://www.marchofdimes.com/pregnancy/genetic-counseling.aspx

Moore, T. R. (2015). Abnormal amniotic fluid. *Protocols for high-risk pregnancies: An evidence-based approach*, (6th ed., pp. 315–328). Oxford, UK: John Wiley & Sons.

Mueller, W. A., Hassel, M., & Grealy, M. (2015). The human. *Development and reproduction in humans and animal model species* (pp. 169–213). Berlin Heidelberg: Springer Publishers.

National Down Syndrome Society [NDSS]. (2015a). *What is Down syndrome?* Retrieved from https://www.ndss.org/Down-Syndrome/What-Is-Down-Syndrome/

National Down Syndrome Society [NDSS]. (2015b). *Myths and truths about Down syndrome*. Retrieved from http://www.ndss.org/Down-Syndrome/Myths-Truths/

National Human Genome Research Institute. (2015). *What is genetic counseling and evaluation?* Retrieved from https://www.genome.gov/19016905

National Institutes of Health [NIH]. (2015a). *Mutations and health*. Retrieved from http://ghr.nlm.nih.gov/handbook/mutationsanddisorders

National Institutes of Health [NIH]. (2015b). *Turner syndrome*. Retrieved from http://ghr.nlm.nih.gov/condition/turner-syndrome

National Organization for Rare Disorders [NORD]. (2015a). *Trisomy 18 syndrome*. Retrieved from https://www.rarediseases.org/rare-disease-information/rare-diseases/byID/217/viewAbstract

National Organization for Rare Disorders [NORD]. (2015b). *Trisomy 13 syndrome*. Retrieved from https://www.rarediseases.org/rare-disease-information/rare-diseases/byID/218/viewAbstract

National Organization for Rare Disorders [NORD]. (2015c). Turner syndrome. Retrieved from https://www.rarediseases.org/rare-disease-information/rare-diseases/byID/112/viewAbstract

National Organization for Rare Disorders [NORD]. (2015d). Cri du chat syndrome. Retrieved from http://www.rarediseases.org/search/rdbdetail_abstract.html?disname=Cri%20du%20Chat%20Syndrome

National Organization for Rare Disorders [NORD]. (2015e). Fragile X syndrome. Retrieved from http://www.rarediseases.org/search/rdbdetail_abstract.html?disname=Fragile%20X%20Syndrome

National Organization for Rare Disorders [NORD]. (2015f). Klinefelter syndrome. Retrieved from http://www.rarediseases.org/search/rdbdetail_abstract.html?disname=Klinefelter%20Syndrome

Sermon, K., & Viville, S. (2014). *Textbook of human reproductive genetics*. New York, NY: Cambridge University Press.

Snustad, D. P. (2015). *Principles of genetics* (7th ed.). New York, NY: Wiley Publishers.

Support Organization for Trisomies [SOFT]. (2015). *Trisomy 13 facts*. Retrieved from http://trisomy.org/trisomy-13-facts-2/

Travers, A., & Muskhelishvili, G. (2015). DNA structure and function. *Federation of European Biochemical Societies (FEBS) Journal*, *282*(12), 2279–2295.

Trisomy 18 Foundation. (2015). *What is Trisomy 18?* Retrieved from http://www.trisomy18.org/site/PageServer?pagename=whatisT18_whatis

Wilson, B. J., & Nicholls, S. G. (2015). The Human Genome Project, and recent advances in personalized genomics. *Risk Management and Healthcare Policy*, *8*, 9–20.

Yudkowitz, F. S. (2015). Fetal-neonatal physiology and circulation. *Obstetric anesthesia* (pp. 17–23). New York, NY: McGraw-Hill Education.

Zhang, L., & Ducsay, C. A. (2014). *Advances in fetal and neonatal physiology*. New York, NY: Spring Publishers.

CHAPTER WORKSHEET

MULTIPLE-CHOICE QUESTIONS

1. After teaching a group of students about fertilization, the instructor determines that the teaching was successful when the group identifies which as the usual site of fertilization?
   a. Fundus of the uterus
   b. Endometrium of the uterus
   c. Upper portion of fallopian tube
   d. Follicular tissue of the ovary

2. Working in a reproductive health services clinic, the nurse is aware that the goal of the Human Genome project was to:
   a. Link specific abnormal genes to specific diseases for better treatment
   b. Map, sequence, and determine the function of all human genes
   c. Understand the underlying causes of diseases to transform health care
   d. Measure the impact of certain chromosomes on disease prevention

3. The nurse is counseling a couple, one of whom is affected by an autosomal dominant disorder. They express concerns about the risk of transmitting the disorder. What is the best response by the nurse regarding the risk that their baby may have the disease?
   a. "You have a one in four (25%) chance."
   b. "The risk is 12.5%, or a one in eight chance."
   c. "The chance is 100%."
   d. "Your risk is 50%, or a one in two chance."

4. What is the first step in determining a couple's risk for a genetic disorder?
   a. Observing the client and family over time
   b. Conducting extensive psychological testing
   c. Obtaining a thorough family health history
   d. Completing an extensive exclusionary list

5. A nurse is working in a women's health clinic. Genetic counseling would be most appropriate for the woman who:
   a. Just had her first miscarriage at 10 weeks
   b. Is 30 years old and planning to conceive
   c. Has a history with a close relative with Down syndrome
   d. Is 18 weeks pregnant with a normal triple screen result

6. Klinefelter syndrome is caused by a nondisjunction resulting in a genotype of:
   a. YYY
   b. XYY
   c. XXX
   d. XXY

7. Down syndrome results from the:
   a. Absence of one chromosome in position 21
   b. Presence of an extra chromosome in position 21
   c. Absence of both chromosomes in position 21
   d. Crossing over of the chromosomes in position 21

CRITICAL THINKING EXERCISE

1. Mr. and Mrs. Martin wish to start a family, but they can't agree on something important: Mr. Martin wants his wife to be tested for cystic fibrosis (CF) to see if she is a carrier. Mr. Martin had a brother with CF and watched his parents struggle with the hardship and the expense of caring for him for years, and he doesn't want to experience it in his own life. Mr. Martin has found out he is a CF carrier. Mrs. Martin doesn't want to have the test because she figures that once a baby is in their arms, they will be glad, no matter what.
   a. What information/education should this couple consider before deciding whether to have the test?
   b. How can you assist this couple in their decision-making process?
   c. What is your role in this situation if you don't agree with their decision?

STUDY ACTIVITIES

1. Obtain the video *Miracle of Life*, which shows conception and fetal development. What are your impressions? Is the title of this video realistic?

2. Select one of the websites from the extensive list of websites provided on thePoint to explore the topic of genetics. Critique the information presented. Was it understandable to a layperson? What specifically did you learn? Share your findings with your classmates during a discussion group.

3. Draw your own family pedigree, identifying inheritance patterns. Share it with your family to validate its accuracy. What did you discover about your family's past health?

4. Select one of the various prenatal screening tests (alpha-fetoprotein, amniocentesis, chorionic villus sampling, or fetal nuchal translucency) and research it in depth. Role-play with another nursing student how you would explain its purpose, the procedure, and potential findings to an expectant couple at risk for a fetal abnormality.

BRINGING IT ALL TOGETHER: CASE STUDY

A 27-year-old female of African-American descent presents to the preconception care clinic with her husband. They have been married for 2 years and are planning a pregnancy. They want to know about sickle cell anemia and other hemoglobin abnormalities. They ask if prenatal tests exist for this condition, and if they can be tested to determine their carrier status. They also want to understand the risks related to their future offspring if they are carriers. They have known several people with sickle cell anemia at their church and wonder if everyone with this disorder is affected the same way.

ASSESSMENT

A family history is taken by the nurse to determine if any of the couple's relatives have this disease or manifestations of it. They may not be aware of the various manifestations of it, but can describe behaviors and observations of their various family members. An explanation of the screening procedure to determine if they are carriers of the sickle cell trait is then offered.

Go to thePoint **to find questions to consider about this case.**

11

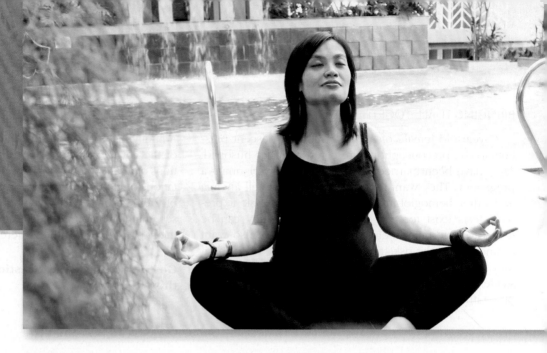

Maternal Adaptation During Pregnancy

Learning Objectives

Upon completion of the chapter, you will be able to:

1. Differentiate between subjective (presumptive), objective (probable), and diagnostic (positive) signs of pregnancy.

2. Describe maternal physiologic changes that occur during pregnancy.

3. Summarize the nutritional needs of the pregnant woman and her fetus.

4. Characterize the emotional and psychological changes that occur during pregnancy.

Marva, age 17, appeared at the health department clinic complaining that she had a stomach virus and needed to be seen right away. When the nurse asked her additional questions about her illness, Marva reported that she had been sick to her stomach and "beat tired" for days. She had stopped eating to avoid any more nausea and vomiting.

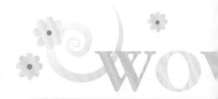

Words of Wisdom
When a woman discovers that she is pregnant, she must remember to protect and nourish the fetus by making wise choices.

INTRODUCTION

Pregnancy is a normal life event that involves considerable physical and psychological adjustments for the mother. A pregnancy is divided into three **trimesters** of 13 weeks each (Edelman, Kudzma, & Mandle, 2014). Within each trimester, numerous adaptations take place that facilitate the growth of the fetus. The most obvious are physical changes to accommodate the growing fetus, but pregnant women also undergo psychological changes as they prepare for parenthood. A thorough understanding of these numerous changes and adaptations is essential for all nurses caring for women during pregnancy.

SIGNS AND SYMPTOMS OF PREGNANCY

Traditionally, signs and symptoms of pregnancy have been grouped into the following categories: presumptive, probable, and positive (Box 11.1). The only signs that can determine a pregnancy with 100% accuracy are positive signs.

What additional information is necessary to complete the assessment of Marva, the 17-year-old with nausea and vomiting? What diagnostic tests might be done to confirm the nurse's suspicion that she is pregnant?

Subjective (Presumptive) Signs

Presumptive signs are those signs that the mother can perceive. The most obvious presumptive sign of pregnancy is the absence of menstruation. Skipping a period is not a reliable sign of pregnancy by itself, but if it is accompanied by consistent nausea, fatigue, breast tenderness, and urinary frequency, pregnancy would seem very likely.

Presumptive changes are the least reliable indicators of pregnancy because any one of them can be

Consider This

Jim and I decided to start our family, so I stopped taking the pill 3 months ago. One morning when I got out of bed to take the dog out, I felt queasy and light-headed. I sure hoped I was not coming down with the flu. By the end of the week, I was feeling really tired and started taking naps in the afternoon. In addition, I seemed to be going to the bathroom frequently, despite not drinking much fluid. When my breasts started to tingle and ache, I decided to make an appointment with my doctor to see what "illness" I had contracted.

After listening to my list of physical complaints, the office nurse asked me if I might be pregnant. My eyes opened wide: I had somehow missed the link between my symptoms and pregnancy. I started to think about when my last period was, and it had been 2 months ago. The office ran a pregnancy test and much to my surprise it was positive!

Thoughts: *Many women stop contraceptives in an attempt to achieve pregnancy but miss the early signs of pregnancy. This woman was experiencing several signs of early pregnancy—urinary frequency, fatigue, morning nausea, and breast tenderness. What advice can the nurse give this woman to ease these symptoms? What additional education related to her pregnancy would be appropriate at this time?*

BOX 11.1

SIGNS AND SYMPTOMS OF PREGNANCY

Presumptive (Time of Occurrence)	Probable (Time of Occurrence)	Positive (Time of Occurrence)
Fatigue (12 wks)	Braxton Hicks contractions (16–28 wks)	Ultrasound verification of embryo or fetus (4–6 wks)
Breast tenderness (3–4 wks)	Positive pregnancy test (4–12 wks)	Fetal movement felt by experienced clinician (20 wks)
Nausea and vomiting (4–14 wks)	Abdominal enlargement (14 wks)	Auscultation of fetal heart tones via Doppler (10–12 wks)
Amenorrhea (4 wks)	Ballottement (16–28 wks)	
Urinary frequency (6–12 wks)	Goodell's sign (5 wks)	
Hyperpigmentation of the skin (16 wks)	Chadwick's sign (6–8 wks)	
Fetal movements (**quickening**; 16–20 wks)	Hegar's sign (6–12 wks)	
Uterine enlargement (7–12 wks)		
Breast enlargement (6 wks)		

Adapted from Bope, E. T., & Kellerman, R. D. (2015). *Conn's current therapy 2015*. Philadelphia, PA: Saunders Elsevier; Shields, A. D. (2015). Pregnancy diagnosis. *eMedicine*. Retrieved from http://emedicine.medscape.com/article/262591-overview; and Jordan, R. G., Engstrom, J., Matrfell, J., & Farley, C. L. (2014). *Prenatal and postnatal care: A woman-centered approach*. Ames, Iowa: Wiley-Blackwell.

caused by conditions other than pregnancy (Shields, 2015). For example, amenorrhea can be caused by early menopause, endocrine dysfunction, malnutrition, anemia, diabetes mellitus, long-distance running, cancer, or stress. Nausea and vomiting can be caused by gastrointestinal disorders, food poisoning, acute infections, or eating disorders. Fatigue could be caused by anemia, stress, or viral infections. Breast tenderness may result from chronic cystic mastitis, premenstrual changes, or the use of oral contraceptives. Urinary frequency could have a variety of causes other than pregnancy, such as infection, cystocele, structural disorders, pelvic tumors, or emotional tension (Tharpe et al., 2016).

Objective (Probable) Signs

Physical Signs

Probable signs of pregnancy are those that can be detected on physical examination by a health care provider. Common probable signs of pregnancy include softening of the lower uterine segment or isthmus (Hegar's sign), softening of the cervix (Goodell's sign), and a bluish-purple coloration of the vaginal mucosa and cervix (Chadwick's sign). Other probable signs include changes in the shape and size of the uterus, abdominal enlargement, Braxton Hicks contractions, and **ballottement** (the examiner pushes against the woman's cervix during a pelvic examination and feels a rebound from the floating fetus).

Pregnancy Tests

Along with these physical signs, pregnancy tests are also considered a probable sign of pregnancy. In-home pregnancy testing became available in the United States in late 1977. In-home testing appealed to the general public because of convenience, cost, and confidentiality. Several pregnancy tests are available (Table 11.1). The tests vary in sensitivity, specificity, and accuracy and are influenced by the length of gestation, specimen concentration, presence of blood, and the presence of some drugs. Human chorionic gonadotropin (hCG) is detectable in the serum of approximately 5% of clients 8 days after conception and in more than 98% of clients by day 11 (Shields, 2015). At least 25 different home pregnancy tests are currently marketed in the United States. Most of these tests claim "99% accuracy" according to a U.S. Food and Drug Administration (FDA) guideline or make other similar statements on the packaging or product insert. The 99% accuracy statement in reference to the FDA guideline is misleading in that it has no bearing on the ability of the home pregnancy test to detect early pregnancy (Shields, 2015). The limitations of these tests must be understood so that pregnancy detection is not delayed significantly. Early pregnancy detection allows for the commencement of prenatal care, potential medication changes, and lifestyle changes to promote a healthy pregnancy.

hCG is a glycoprotein and the earliest biochemical marker for pregnancy. Many pregnancy tests are based on the recognition of hCG or a beta subunit of hCG. hCG levels in normal pregnancy usually double every 48 to 72 hours until they peak approximately 60 to 70 days after fertilization. At this point, they decrease to a plateau at 100 to 130 days of pregnancy. The hCG doubling time has been used as a marker by clinicians to differentiate normal from abnormal gestations. Low levels are associated with an ectopic pregnancy and

TABLE 11.1 SELECTED PREGNANCY TESTS

Type	Specimen	Example	Remarks
Agglutination inhibition tests	Urine	Pregnosticon, Gravindex	If hCG is present in urine, agglutination does not occur, which is positive for pregnancy; reliable 14–21 days after conception; 95% accurate in diagnosing pregnancy.
Immunoradiometric assay	Blood serum	Neocept, Pregnosis	Measures ability of blood sample to inhibit the binding of radiolabeled hCG to receptors; reliable 6–8 days after conception; 99% accurate in diagnosing pregnancy.
Enzyme-linked immunosorbent assay (ELISA)	Blood serum or urine	Over-the-counter home/office pregnancy tests; precise	Uses an enzyme to bond with hCG in the urine if present; reliable 4 days after implantation; 99% accurate if hCG specific.

Adapted from Jordan, R. G., Engstrom, J., Matrfell, J., & Farley, C. L. (2014). *Prenatal and postnatal care: A woman-centered approach.* Ames, Iowa: Wiley-Blackwell; King, T. L., Brucker, M. C., Kriebs, J. M., Fahey, J. O., Gegor, C. L., & Varney, H. (2015). *Varney's midwifery.* (5th ed.), Burlington, MA: Jones & Bartlett Learning; and Shields, A. D. (2015). Pregnancy diagnosis. *eMedicine.* Retrieved from http://emedicine.medscape.com/article/262591-overview.

higher-than-normal levels may indicate a molar pregnancy or multiple-gestational pregnancies (Zinaman, Johnson, & Marriott, 2015).

Take Note!

This elevation of hCG corresponds to the morning sickness period of approximately 6 to 12 weeks during early pregnancy.

Although probable signs suggest pregnancy and are more reliable than presumptive signs, they still are not 100% reliable in confirming a pregnancy. For example, uterine tumors, polyps, infection, and pelvic congestion can cause changes to uterine shape, size, and consistency. And although pregnancy tests are used to establish the diagnosis of pregnancy when the physical signs are still inconclusive, they are not completely reliable, because conditions other than pregnancy (e.g., ovarian cancer, choriocarcinoma, hydatidiform mole) can also elevate hCG levels.

Positive Signs

Usually within 2 weeks after a missed period, enough subjective symptoms are present so that a woman can be reasonably sure she is pregnant. However, an experienced health care provider can confirm her suspicions by identifying positive signs of pregnancy that can be directly attributed to the fetus. The positive signs of pregnancy confirm that a fetus is growing in the uterus. Visualizing the fetus by ultrasound, palpating for fetal movements, and hearing a fetal heartbeat are all signs that make the pregnancy a certainty.

If the pregnancy test is positive, the clinical visit should include an estimation of gestational age so that appropriate counseling can be provided. In addition, clients should receive information about the normal signs and symptoms of early pregnancy, and should be instructed to report any concerns to the health care provider for further evaluation. Once pregnancy has been confirmed, the health care provider will set up a schedule of prenatal visits to assess the woman and her fetus throughout the entire pregnancy. Assessment and education begins at the first visits and continues throughout the pregnancy (see Chapter 12).

Remember Marva, who thought she had a stomach virus? Her pregnancy test was positive. On questioning by the nurse, she acknowledged missing two menstrual periods and being sexually active with her boyfriend without using protection. What is the nurse's role at this point with Marva? What instructions might be given to her while she waits for her first prenatal visit?

PHYSIOLOGIC ADAPTATIONS DURING PREGNANCY

Every system of a woman's body changes during pregnancy to accommodate the needs of the growing fetus, and these changes occur with startling rapidity. The physical changes of pregnancy can be uncomfortable, although every woman reacts uniquely.

Reproductive System Adaptations

Significant changes occur throughout the woman's body during pregnancy to accommodate the growing human being within her. Many have a protective role for maternal homeostasis and are essential to meet the demands of both the mother and the fetus. Many adaptations are reversible after the woman gives birth, but some persist for life.

Uterus

The uterus grows at a steady and predictable rate during pregnancy. During the first few months of pregnancy, estrogen stimulates uterine growth, and the uterus undergoes a tremendous increase in size, weight, length, width, depth, volume, and overall capacity throughout pregnancy. The weight of the uterus increases from 70 g to about 1,100 to 1,200 g at term; its capacity increases from 10 to 5,000 mL or more at term (King et al., 2015). The uterine walls thin to 1.5 cm or less; the shape changes from pear shape to a solid globe in the first trimester, and then expands to become a hollow vessel.

Uterine growth occurs as a result of both hyperplasia and hypertrophy of the myometrial cells, which do not increase much in number but do increase in size. In early pregnancy, uterine growth is due to hyperplasia of uterine smooth muscle cells within the myometrium; however, the major component of myometrial growth occurs after mid-gestation due to smooth muscle cell hypertrophy caused by mechanical stretch of uterine tissue by the growing fetus (Osol & Moore, 2014). Blood vessels elongate, enlarge, dilate, and sprout new branches to support and nourish the growing muscle tissue, and the increase in uterine weight is accompanied by a large increase in uterine blood flow, which is necessary to perfuse the uterine muscle and accommodate the growing fetus. As pregnancy progresses, 80% to 90% of uterine blood flow goes to the placenta, with the remainder distributed between the endometrium and myometrium. During pregnancy, the diameter of the main uterine artery approximately doubles in size. This enlargement from a narrow to a larger-caliber vessel enhances the capacity of the uteroplacental vessels to accommodate the increased blood volume needed to supply the placenta (Osol & Moore, 2014).

Uterine contractility is enhanced as well. Spontaneous, irregular, and painless contractions, called **Braxton**

Hicks contractions, begin during the first trimester. These contractions continue throughout pregnancy, becoming especially noticeable during the last month, when they function to thin out or efface the cervix before birth (see Chapter 12 for more information).

The lower portion of the uterus (the isthmus) does not undergo hypertrophy and becomes increasingly thinner as pregnancy progresses, thereby forming the lower uterine segment. Changes in the lower uterus occurring during the first 6 to 8 weeks of gestation produce some of the typical findings, including a positive **Hegar's sign**. This softening and compressibility of the lower uterine segment results in exaggerated uterine anteflexion during the early months of pregnancy, which adds to urinary frequency (Heffner & Schust, 2014).

The uterus remains in the pelvic cavity for the first 3 months of pregnancy, after which it progressively ascends into the abdomen (Fig. 11.1). As the uterus grows, it presses on the urinary bladder and causes the increased frequency of urination experienced during early pregnancy. In addition, the heavy gravid uterus in the last trimester can fall back against the inferior vena cava in the supine position, resulting in vena cava compression, which reduces venous return and decreases cardiac output and blood pressure, with increasing orthostatic stress. This occurs when the woman changes

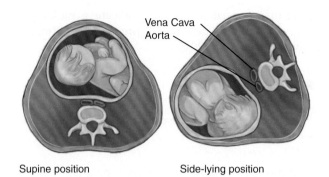

Supine position   Side-lying position

FIGURE 11.2 Supine hypotensive syndrome.

her position from recumbent to sitting to standing. This acute hemodynamic change, termed supine hypotensive syndrome, causes the woman to experience symptoms of weakness, light-headedness, nausea, dizziness, or syncope (Fig. 11.2). These changes are reversed when the woman is in the side-lying position, which displaces the uterus to the left and off the vena cava.

The uterus, which starts as a pear-shaped organ, becomes ovoid as length increases over width. By 20 weeks' gestation, the fundus, or top of the uterus, is at the level of the umbilicus and measures 20 cm. A monthly measurement of the height of the top of the uterus in centimeters, which corresponds to the number of gestational weeks, is commonly used to date the pregnancy.

Take Note!

Fundal height usually can be correlated with gestational weeks most accurately between 18 and 32 weeks. Obesity, hydramnios, and uterine fibroids interfere with the accuracy of this correlation.

The fundus reaches its highest level, at the xiphoid process, at approximately 36 weeks. Between 38 and 40 weeks, fundal height drops as the fetus begins to descend and engage into the pelvis. Because it pushes against the diaphragm, many women experience shortness of breath. By 40 weeks, the fetal head begins to descend and engage in the pelvis, which is termed *lightening*. For the woman who is pregnant for the first time, *lightening* usually occurs approximately 2 weeks before the onset of labor; for the woman who is experiencing her second or subsequent pregnancy, it usually occurs at the onset of labor. Although breathing becomes easier because of this descent, the pressure on the urinary bladder now increases and the woman now experiences urinary frequency again, as she did in the first trimester of pregnancy.

Cervix

Between weeks 6 and 8 of pregnancy, the cervix begins to soften (**Goodell's sign**) due to vasocongestion and the

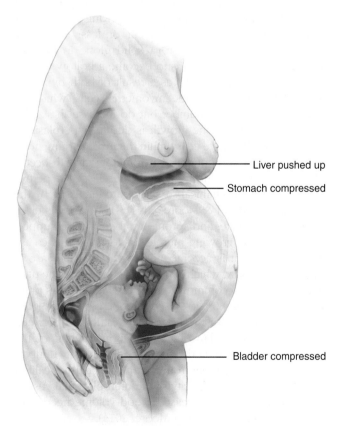

Liver pushed up

Stomach compressed

Bladder compressed

FIGURE 11.1 The growing uterus in the abdomen.

influence of estrogen. Along with the softening, the endocervical glands increase in size and number and produce more cervical mucus. Under the influence of progesterone, a thick mucus plug is formed that blocks the cervical os and protects the opening from bacterial invasion. At about the same time, increased vascularization of the cervix causes **Chadwick's sign**, a cyanosis or bluish purple discoloration Cervical ripening (softening, effacement, and increased distensibility) begins about 4 weeks before birth. The connective tissues of the cervix undergo biochemical modifications in preparation for labor that result in changes to its elasticity and strength. These changes are mediated through several factors, including inflammation, cervical stretch, pressure of the fetal presenting part, and release of hormones, including oxytocin, relaxin, nitric oxide, and prostaglandins (Myers et al., 2015).

Vagina

During pregnancy, vascularity increases because of the influences of estrogen, resulting in pelvic congestion and hypertrophy of the vagina in preparation for the distention needed for birth. The vaginal mucosa thickens, the connective tissue begins to loosen, the smooth muscle begins to hypertrophy, and the vaginal vault begins to lengthen (Bope & Kellerman, 2015). Vaginal secretions become more acidic, white, and thick. Most women experience an increase in a whitish vaginal discharge, called leukorrhea, during pregnancy. This is normal except when it is accompanied by itching and irritation, possibly suggesting *Candida albicans,* a monilial vaginitis, which is a very common occurrence in this glycogen-rich environment (King et al., 2015). Symptomatic vulvovaginal candidiasis affects 15% of pregnant women (Krapf, 2015). It is a benign fungal condition that is uncomfortable for the woman and can be transmitted from an infected mother to her newborn at birth. Neonates develop an oral infection known as thrush, which presents as white patches on the mucous membranes of their mouths. It is self-limiting and is treated with local antifungal agents.

Ovaries

The increased blood supply to the ovaries causes them to enlarge until approximately the 12th to 14th week of gestation. The ovaries are not palpable after that time because the uterus fills the pelvic cavity. Ovulation ceases during pregnancy because of the elevated levels of estrogen and progesterone, which block secretion of follicle-stimulating hormone (FSH) and luteinizing hormone (LH) from the anterior pituitary. The ovaries are very active in hormone production to support the pregnancy until about weeks 6 to 7, when the corpus luteum regresses and the placenta takes over the major production of progesterone.

Breasts

The breasts increase in fullness, become tender, and grow larger throughout pregnancy under the influence of estrogen and progesterone. The breasts become highly vascular and veins become visible under the skin. The nipples become larger and more erect. Both the nipples and the areola become deeply pigmented, and tubercles of Montgomery (sebaceous glands) become prominent. These sebaceous glands keep the nipples lubricated for breast-feeding.

Changes that occur in the connective tissue of the breasts, along with the tremendous growth, lead to striae (stretch marks) in approximately half of all pregnant women (Jordan et al., 2014). Initially they appear as pink to purple lines on the skin, but they eventually fade to a silver color. Although they become less conspicuous in time, they never completely disappear.

Creamy, yellowish breast fluid called colostrum can be expressed from the breast, if squeezed, by the third trimester. This fluid provides nourishment for the breast-feeding newborn during the first few days of life (see Chapters 15 and 16 for more information). Table 11.2 summarizes reproductive system adaptations.

General Body System Adaptations

In addition to changes in the reproductive system, the pregnant woman also experiences changes in virtually every other body system in response to the growing fetus.

Gastrointestinal System

The gastrointestinal system begins in the oral cavity and ends at the rectum. During pregnancy, the gums become hyperemic, swollen, and friable and tend to bleed easily. This change is influenced by estrogen and increased proliferation of blood vessels and circulation to the mouth. In addition, the saliva produced in the mouth becomes more acidic. Some women complain about excessive salivation, termed *ptyalism*, which may be caused by the decrease in unconscious swallowing by the woman when nauseated. Ptyalism typically resolves spontaneously, although in some women it endures throughout the pregnancy. Some women get temporary relief from gum chewing or sucking on hard candies (King et al., 2015). Dental plaque, calculus, and debris deposits increase during pregnancy and are all associated with gingivitis. An increased production of female hormones during pregnancy contributes to the development of gingivitis and periodontitis because vascular permeability and possible tissue edema are both increased. It is reported that as many as 50% to 70% of pregnant women will have some level of gingivitis during pregnancy as a result of hormonal changes that promote inflammation (Anil et al., 2015). Previous studies linked periodontal

TABLE 11.2	SUMMARY OF REPRODUCTIVE SYSTEM ADAPTATIONS
Reproductive Organ	**Adaptations**
Uterus	Size increases to 20 times that of nonpregnant size. Capacity increases by 2,000 times to accommodate the developing fetus. Weight increases from 2 oz to approximately 2 lb at term. Uterine growth occurs as a result of both hyperplasia and hypertrophy of the myometrial cells. Increased strength and elasticity allow uterus to contract and expel fetus during birth.
Cervix	Increases in mass, water content, and vascularization. Changes from a relatively rigid to a soft, distensible structure that allows the fetus to be expelled. Under the influence of progesterone, a thick mucus plug is formed, which blocks the cervical os and protects the developing fetus from bacterial invasion.
Vagina	Increased vascularity because of estrogen influences, resulting in pelvic congestion and hypertrophy. Increased thickness of mucosa, along with an increase in vaginal secretions to prevent bacterial infections.
Ovaries	Increased blood supply to the ovaries causes them to enlarge until approximately the 12th to 14th week of gestation. They actively produce hormones to support the pregnancy until weeks 6 to 7 when the placenta takes over the production of progesterone.
Breasts	Breast changes begin soon after conception; they increase in size and areolar pigmentation. The tubercles of Montgomery enlarge and become more prominent, and the nipples become more erect. The blood vessels become more prominent, and blood flow to the breast doubles.

disease with preterm birth; preeclampsia, and low-birth-weight risk, stillbirth and early-onset neonatal sepsis, but more recent research findings indicated no reduction in preterm births with the treatment of periodontal disease during pregnancy (Trivedi, Lal, & Singhal, 2015).

 Concept Mastery Alert

Gum Fragility in Pregnancy

Bleeding of gums during pregnancy, results from increased estrogen levels that cause blood vessel proliferation. This then leads to increased blood vessels in the gums and an increased chance of bleeding.

Smooth muscle relaxation and decreased peristalsis occur related to the influence of progesterone. Elevated progesterone levels cause smooth muscle relaxation, which results in delayed gastric emptying and decreased peristalsis. Transition time of food throughout the gastrointestinal tract may be so much slower that more water than normal is reabsorbed, leading to bloating and constipation. Constipation can also result from low-fiber food choices, reduced fluid intake, use of iron supplements, decreased activity level, and intestinal displacement secondary to a growing uterus. Constipation, increased venous pressure, and the pressure of the gravid uterus contribute to the formation of hemorrhoids.

The slowed gastric emptying combined with relaxation of the cardiac sphincter allows reflux, which causes heartburn. Acid indigestion or heartburn (pyrosis) seems to be a universal problem for pregnant women. It is caused by regurgitation of the stomach contents into the upper esophagus and may be associated with the generalized relaxation of the entire digestive system. Over-the-counter antacids will usually relieve the symptoms, but they should be taken with the health care provider's knowledge and only as directed.

The emptying time of the gallbladder is prolonged secondary to the smooth muscle relaxation from progesterone. Hypercholesterolemia can follow, increasing the risk of gallstone formation. Other risk factors for gallbladder disease include obesity, Hispanic ethnicity, and increasing maternal age (Heuman, Mihas, & Allen, 2015).

Nausea and vomiting, better known as morning sickness, plague about 80% of pregnant women. This condition is usually self-limiting, but the symptoms can be distressing and interfere with work, social activities, and interrupt sleep. Recently, the FDA approved doxylamine succinate 10 mg/pyridoxine hydrochloride 10 mg (Diclegis) as the first medication to specifically treat morning sickness in pregnancy (Pope, Maltepe, & Koren, 2015). Although it occurs most often in the morning, the nauseated feeling can last all day in some women. The highest incidence of morning sickness occurs between

6 and 12 weeks. The physiologic basis for morning sickness is still debatable. It has been linked to the high levels of hCG, high levels of circulating estrogens, prostaglandins, reduced stomach acidity, advancing maternal age, slowed peristalsis, genetic factors, and the lowered tone and motility of the digestive tract (King et al., 2015).

Cardiovascular System

Cardiovascular changes occur early during pregnancy to meet the demands of the enlarging uterus and the placenta for more blood and more oxygen. The changes include an increase in heart rate (25%); cardiac output increases by 30% to 50% and peaks at 25 to 30 weeks gestation; reduced total peripheral resistance; increased blood volume; increased plasma volume which leads to physiologic anemia. Perhaps the most striking cardiac alteration occurring during pregnancy is the increase in blood volume.

BLOOD VOLUME

Blood volume increases by approximately 1,500 mL, or up to 50% above nonpregnant levels, by the 32nd week of gestation, and remains more or less constant thereafter (Foo et al., 2015). The increase is made up of 1,000 mL plasma plus 450 mL red blood cells. It begins at weeks 10 to 12, peaks at weeks 32 to 34, and decreases slightly by week 40.

Take Note!

The rise in blood volume correlates directly with fetal weight, supporting the concept of the placenta as an arteriovenous shunt in the maternal vascular compartment.

This increase in blood volume is needed to provide adequate hydration of fetal and maternal tissues, to supply blood flow to perfuse the enlarging uterus, and to provide a reserve to compensate for blood loss at birth and during postpartum. The maternal blood volume expansion occurs at a larger proportion than the increase in red blood cell mass, which results in physiologic anemia and hemodilution. Criteria of physiologic anemia include hemoglobin 10 g or less; red blood cells 3.5 million/mm^3 and normal morphology with central pallor (Sabina et al., 2015). This increase is also necessary to meet the increased metabolic needs of the mother and to meet the need for increased perfusion of other organs, especially the woman's kidneys, because she is excreting waste products for herself and the fetus.

CARDIAC OUTPUT AND HEART RATE

Cardiac output, the product of stroke volume and heart rate, is a measure of the functional capacity of the heart. It increases from 30% to 50% over the nonpregnant rate by the 32nd week of pregnancy and declines to about a 20%

increase at 40 weeks' gestation. The increase in cardiac output is associated with an increase in venous return and greater right ventricular output, especially in the left lateral position (Bope & Kellerman, 2015). Heart rate increases by 10 to 15 bpm between 14 and 20 weeks of gestation, and this persists to term. There is slight hypertrophy or enlargement of the heart during pregnancy. This is probably to accommodate the increase in blood volume and cardiac output. The heart works harder and pumps more blood to supply the oxygen needs of the fetus as well as those of the mother. Both heart rate and venous return are increased in pregnancy, contributing to the increase in cardiac output seen throughout gestation. A woman with pre-existing heart disease may become symptomatic and begin to decompensate during the time the blood volume peaks. Close monitoring is warranted during 28 to 35 weeks' gestation.

BLOOD PRESSURE

Blood pressure, especially the diastolic pressure, declines slightly during pregnancy as a result of peripheral vasodilation caused by progesterone. It usually reaches a low point at midpregnancy and thereafter increases to prepregnancy levels until term. During the first trimester, blood pressure typically remains at the prepregnancy level. During the second trimester, the blood pressure decreases 5 to 10 mm Hg and thereafter returns to first-trimester levels (Gaillard & Jaddoe, 2015). Any significant rise in blood pressure during pregnancy should be investigated to rule out gestational hypertension. Gestational hypertension is a clinical diagnosis defined by the new onset of hypertension (systolic of 140 mm Hg or higher and/or diastolic of 90 mm Hg or higher) after 20 weeks gestation.

BLOOD COMPONENTS

The number of red blood cells also increases throughout pregnancy to a level which is 25% to 33% higher than nonpregnant values, depending on the amount of iron available. This increase is necessary to transport the additional oxygen required during pregnancy. Although there is an increase in red blood cells, there is a greater increase in the plasma volume as a result of hormonal factors and sodium and water retention. Because the plasma increase exceeds the increase of red blood cell production, normal hemoglobin and hematocrit values decrease. This state of hemodilution is referred to as **physiologic anemia of pregnancy**. Changes in red blood cell volume are due to increased circulating erythropoietin and accelerated red blood cell production. The rise in erythropoietin in the last two trimesters is stimulated by progesterone, prolactin, and human placental lactogen (Jones & Lopez, 2014).

Iron requirements during pregnancy increase because of the demands of the growing fetus and the increase in maternal blood volume. The fetal tissues prevail over the mother's tissues with respect to use of iron stores. With the accelerated production of red blood cells, iron is necessary for hemoglobin formation, the oxygen-carrying component of red blood cells.

> **Take Note!**
> Many women enter pregnancy with insufficient iron stores and thus need supplementation to meet the extra demands of pregnancy.

Both fibrin and plasma fibrinogen levels increase along with various blood-clotting factors. These factors make pregnancy a hypercoagulable state. These changes, coupled with venous stasis secondary to venous pooling, which occurs during late pregnancy after long periods of standing in the upright position with the pressure exerted by the uterus on the large pelvic veins, contribute to slowed venous return, pooling, and dependent edema. These factors also increase the woman's risk for venous thrombosis (DeLoughery, 2015).

Respiratory System

The growing uterus and the increased production of the hormone progesterone cause the lungs to function differently during pregnancy. Oxygen consumption reflects the uptick of maternal metabolism by increasing between 20% and 30% by the time full term is reached. During pregnancy, the amount of space available to house the lungs decreases as the uterus puts pressure on the diaphragm and causes it to shift upward by 4 cm above its usual position. The growing uterus does change the size and shape of the thoracic cavity, but diaphragmatic excursion increases, chest circumference increases by 2 to 3 in, and the transverse diameter increases by an inch, allowing a larger tidal volume, as evidenced by deeper breathing (Tidal volume, or the volume of air inhaled, increases by 30% to 40% (from 500 to 700 mL) as the pregnancy progresses. This increases results in maternal hyperventilation and hypocapnia. As a result of these changes, the woman's breathing becomes more diaphragmatic than abdominal. Concomitant with the increase in tidal volume is a 30% to 40% increase in maternal oxygen consumption due to the increased oxygen requirements of the developing fetus, placenta, and maternal organs.

Anatomic and physiologic changes of pregnancy predispose the mother to increased morbidity and mortality and increase the risks of a less than optimal outcome for the fetus. The frequency and significance of acute and chronic respiratory conditions in pregnant women have increased in recent years. Because of these various changes, pregnant women with asthma, pneumonia, or other respiratory pathology are more susceptible to early decompensation (Mehta et al., 2015).

A pregnant woman breathes faster and more deeply because she and the fetus need more oxygen. Oxygen consumption increases during pregnancy even as airway resistance and lung compliance remain unchanged. Changes in the structures of the respiratory system take place to prepare the body for the enlarging uterus and increased lung volume (Alexander et al., 2014). As muscles and cartilage in the thoracic region relax, the chest broadens, with a conversion from abdominal breathing to thoracic breathing. This leads to a 50% increase in air volume per minute. All of these structural alterations are temporary and revert back to their prepregnant state at the end of the pregnancy.

Increased vascularity of the respiratory tract is influenced by increased estrogen levels, leading to congestion. Rising levels of sex hormones and heightened sensitivity to allergens may influence the nasal mucosa, precipitating epistaxis (nosebleed) and rhinitis. This congestion gives rise to nasal and sinus stuffiness and changes in the tone and quality of the woman's voice (Jordan et al., 2014).

Renal/Urinary System

Hormonal changes during pregnancy allow for increased blood flow to the kidneys. The renal system must handle the effects of increased maternal intravascular and extracellular volume and metabolic waste products as well as excretion of fetal wastes. The predominant structural change in the renal system during pregnancy is dilation of the renal pelvis and uterus. Changes in renal structure occur as a result of the hormonal influences of estrogen and progesterone, pressure from an enlarging uterus, and an increase in maternal blood volume. Like the heart, the kidneys work harder throughout the pregnancy. Changes in kidney function occur to accommodate a heavier workload while maintaining a stable electrolyte balance and blood pressure. As more blood flows to the kidneys, the glomerular filtration rate (GFR) increases, leading to an increase in urine flow and volume, substances delivered to the kidneys, and filtration and excretion of urea, uric acid, creatinine, water and solutes (Cox & Reid, 2015).

Anatomically, the kidneys enlarge during pregnancy. Each kidney increases in length by approximately 1 to 1.5 cm and weight as a result of hormonal effects that cause increased tone and decreased motility of the smooth muscle. The renal pelvis becomes dilated. The ureters (especially the right ureter) elongate, widen, and become more curved above the pelvic rim as early as the 10th gestational week (Thadhani & Maynard, 2015). Progesterone is thought to cause both of these changes because of its relaxing influence on smooth muscle.

Blood flow to the kidneys increases by 50% to 80% as a result of the increase in cardiac output and relaxin which causes a decrease in both efferent and afferent resistance. This in turn leads to an increase in the GFR by as much as 40% to 60% starting during the second trimester, resulting in hyperfiltration. This elevation continues until birth. This change has important clinical implications for medication use because renally excreted drugs may require higher doses and more frequent administration for therapeutic blood levels during pregnancy (Larson, 2015).

The activity of the kidneys normally increases when a person lies down and decreases on standing. This difference is amplified during pregnancy, which is one reason a pregnant woman feels the need to urinate frequently while trying to sleep. Late in the pregnancy, the increase in kidney activity is even greater when the woman lies on her side rather than her back. Lying on either side relieves the pressure that the enlarged uterus puts on the vena cava carrying blood from the legs. Subsequently, venous return to the heart increases, leading to increased cardiac output. Increased cardiac output results in increased renal perfusion and glomerular filtration. As a rule, all the physiologic changes maximize by the end of the second trimester and then start to return to the prepregnant level. However, changes in the anatomy take up to 3 months postpartum to subside (King et al., 2015).

Musculoskeletal System

Changes in the musculoskeletal system are progressive, resulting from the influence of hormones, fetal growth, and maternal weight gain. Pregnancy is characterized by changes in posture and gait. By the 10th to 12th week of pregnancy, the ligaments that hold the sacroiliac joints and the pubis symphysis in place begin to soften and stretch, and the articulations between the joints widen and become more movable (Bope & Kellerman, 2015). The relaxation of the joints peaks by the beginning of the third trimester. The purpose of these changes is to increase the size of the pelvic cavity and to make delivery easier.

The postural changes of pregnancy—an increased swayback and an upper spine extension to compensate for the enlarging abdomen—coupled with the loosening of the sacroiliac joints may result in lower back pain. The woman's center of gravity shifts forward, requiring a realignment of the spinal curvatures. Factors thought to contribute to these postural changes include the alteration to the center of gravity that come with pregnancy, the influence of the pregnancy-related hormone relaxin on the pelvic joints, and the increasing weight and position of the growing fetus.

An increase in the normal lumbosacral curve (lordosis) occurs and a compensatory curvature in the cervicodorsal area develops to assist her in maintaining her balance (Fig. 11.3). In addition, relaxation and increased mobility of joints occur because of the hormones progesterone and relaxin, which lead to the characteristic "waddle" gait that pregnant women demonstrate toward term. Increased weight gain can add to this discomfort by accentuating the lumbar and dorsal curves (Kouhkan et al., 2015).

Integumentary System

There are a variety of skin changes that are associated with pregnancy. Increased activity of the maternal adrenal and pituitary glands, along with a contribution for the developing fetal endocrine glands, increasing cortisone

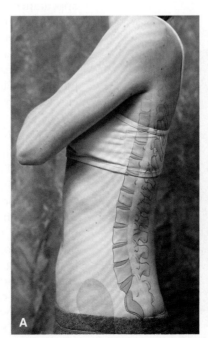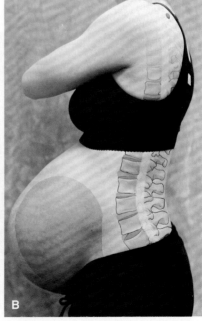

FIGURE 11.3 Postural changes during **(A)** the first trimester and **(B)** the third trimester.

levels, accelerated metabolism, and enhanced production of progesterone and estrogenic hormones are responsible for most skin changes in pregnancy (Tyler, 2015). Up to 90% of pregnant women will show signs of hyperpigmentation during pregnancy, and it is typically generalized and mild. The skin of pregnant women undergoes hyperpigmentation primarily as a result of estrogen, progesterone, and melanocyte-stimulating hormone levels. These changes are mainly seen on the nipples, areola, umbilicus, perineum, and axilla. Although many integumentary changes disappear after giving birth, some only fade. Many pregnant women express concern about stretch marks, skin color changes, and hair loss. Unfortunately, little is known about how to avoid these changes.

Complexion changes are not unusual. The increased pigmentation that occurs on the breasts and genitalia also develops on the face to form the "mask of pregnancy," which is also called facial melisma. It occurs in up to 70% of pregnant women. There is a genetic predisposition toward melasma, which is exacerbated by the sun, and it tends to recur in subsequent pregnancies. This blotchy, brownish pigment covers the forehead and cheeks in dark-haired women. Most facial pigmentation fades as the hormones subside at the end of the pregnancy, but some may linger. The skin in the middle of the abdomen may develop a pigmented line called **linea nigra**, which extends from the umbilicus to the pubic area (Fig. 11.4).

Striae gravidarum, or stretch marks, are irregular reddish streaks that appear on the abdomen, breasts, and buttocks in up to 90% of pregnant women. Striae are most prominent by 6 to 7 months. They result from genetics, reduced connective tissue strength resulting from the elevated adrenal steroid levels, and stretching of the structures secondary to growth (Tyler, 2015). They are more common in younger women, women with larger infants, and women with higher body mass indices. Nonwhites and women with a history of breast or thigh striae or a family history of striae gravidarum also are at higher risk. Several creams and lotions such as cocoa butter and olive oil have been touted as being able to prevent striae gravidarum, but research currently does not validate these claims. A study done by Tretti Clementoni and Lavagno (2015) did find that laser treatments did improve pigmentation, volume, and textural appearance of striae gravidarum in more than 50% of the women enrolled in the study.

VASCULAR-RELATED SKIN CHANGES

Vascular changes during pregnancy manifested in the integumentary system include varicosities of the legs, vulva, and perineum. Varicose veins commonly are the result of distention, instability, and poor circulation secondary to prolonged standing or sitting and the heavy gravid uterus placing pressure on the pelvic veins, preventing complete venous return. Interventions to reduce the risk of developing varicosities include:

- Elevating both legs when sitting or lying down
- Avoiding prolonged standing or sitting; changing position frequently
- Resting in the left lateral position
- Walking daily for exercise
- Avoiding tight clothing or knee-high hosiery
- Wearing support hose if varicosities are a pre-existing condition to pregnancy

Another skin manifestation, believed to be secondary to vascular changes and high estrogen levels, is the appearance of small blood vessels called vascular spiders. They may appear on the neck, thorax, face, and arms. They are especially obvious in white women and typically disappear after childbirth. Palmar erythema is a well-delineated pinkish area on the palmar surface of the hands. This integumentary change is also related to elevated estrogen levels (Trupin, 2015).

HAIR AND NAILS

Some women also notice a decline in hair growth during pregnancy. The hair follicles normally undergo a growing and resting phase. The resting phase is followed by a loss of hair; the hairs are then replaced by new ones. During pregnancy, fewer hair follicles go into the resting phase. After delivery, the body catches up with subsequent hair loss for several months. Nails typically grow faster during pregnancy. Pregnant women may experience increased brittleness, distal separation of the nail bed, whitish discoloration, and transverse grooves on the nails, but most of these conditions resolve in the postpartum period (King et al., 2015).

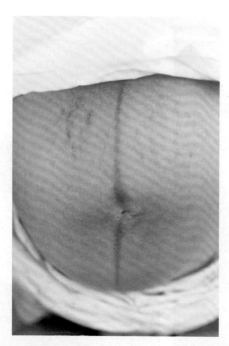

FIGURE 11.4 Linea nigra.

Endocrine System

The endocrine system undergoes many changes during pregnancy because hormonal changes are essential in meeting the needs of the growing fetus. Hormonal changes play a major role in controlling the supplies of maternal glucose, amino acids, and lipids to the fetus. Although estrogen and progesterone are the main hormones involved in pregnancy changes, other endocrine glands and hormones also change during pregnancy.

THYROID GLAND

The thyroid gland enlarges slightly and becomes more active during pregnancy as a result of increased vascularity and hyperplasia. Increased gland activity results in an increase in thyroid hormone secretion starting during the first trimester; levels taper off within a few weeks after birth and return to normal limits. Maternal thyroid hormone is transferred to the fetus beginning soon after conception and is critical for fetal brain development, neurogenesis, and organizational processes prior to 20 weeks when fetal thyroid production is low. However, even after the fetal thyroid is producing increasing amounts of hormone, much of the thyroxin (T_4) needed for development continues to be provided by the mother. Low maternal thyroid levels with thyroid insufficiency, hypothyroidism, or low or inadequate iodine intake may compromise fetal neurologic development (Pearce, 2015). With an increase in the secretion of thyroid hormones, the basal metabolic rate (the amount of oxygen consumed by the body over a unit of time in milliliters per minute) progressively increases by 25%, along with heart rate and cardiac output (Medici et al., 2015).

PITUITARY GLAND

During pregnancy, major endocrine and metabolic alterations occur due to the physiologic hormonal secretion from the placenta. The pituitary gland adapts to these changes and all secretory axes are affected. During pregnancy, the pituitary gland enlarges; it returns to normal size after birth.

The anterior lobe of the pituitary is glandular tissue and produces multiple hormones. The release of these hormones is regulated by releasing and inhibiting hormones produced by the hypothalamus. Some of these anterior pituitary hormones induce other glands to secrete their hormones. The increase in blood levels of the hormones produced by the final target glands (e.g., the ovary or thyroid) inhibits the release of anterior pituitary hormones. Changes in levels of pituitary hormones are discussed in the following paragraphs.

FSH and LH secretion are inhibited during pregnancy, probably as a result of hCG produced by the placenta and corpus luteum, and the increased secretion of prolactin by the anterior pituitary gland. Levels remain decreased until after delivery.

Thyroid-stimulating hormone (TSH) is reduced during the first trimester but usually returns to normal for the remainder of the pregnancy. Decreased TSH is thought to be one of the factors, along with elevated hCG levels, associated with morning sickness, nausea, and vomiting during the first trimester.

Growth hormone (GH) is an anabolic hormone that promotes protein synthesis. It stimulates most body cells to grow in size and divide, facilitating the use of fats for fuel and conserving glucose. During pregnancy, there is a decrease in the number of GH-producing cells and a corresponding decrease in GH blood levels. The action of human placental lactogen (hPL) is thought to decrease the need for and use of GH. During pregnancy, prolactin is secreted in pulses and increases 10-fold to promote breast development and the lactation process. High levels of progesterone secreted by the placenta inhibit the direct influence of prolactin on the breast during pregnancy, thus suppressing lactation. At birth, as soon as the placenta is expelled and there is a drop in progesterone, lactogenesis can begin. Prolactin, released from the anterior pituitary gland in response to suckling by the newborn is the major hormonal signal responsible for stimulation in the breasts (Crowley, 2015).

Melanocyte-stimulating hormone (MSH), another anterior pituitary hormone, increases during pregnancy. For many years, its increase was thought to be responsible for many of the skin changes of pregnancy, particularly changes in skin pigmentation (e.g., darkening of the areola, melasma, and linea nigra). However, currently it is thought that the skin changes are due to estrogen (and possibly progesterone) as well as the increase in MSH.

The two hormones oxytocin and antidiuretic hormone (ADH) released by the posterior pituitary are actually synthesized in the hypothalamus. They migrate along nerve fibers to the posterior pituitary and are stored until stimulated to be released into the general circulation. Oxytocin is released by the posterior pituitary gland, and its production gradually increases as the fetus matures (Kim, Bennett, & Terzidou, 2015). Oxytocin is responsible for uterine contractions, both before and after delivery. The muscle layers of the uterus (myometrium) become more sensitive to oxytocin near term. Toward the end of a term pregnancy, levels of progesterone decline and contractions that were previously suppressed by progesterone begin to occur more frequently and with stronger intensity. This change in the hormonal levels is believed to be one of the initiators of labor.

Oxytocin is responsible for stimulating the uterine contractions that bring about delivery. Contractions lead to cervical thinning and dilation. They also exert pressure, helping the fetus to descend in the pelvis for eventual delivery. After delivery, oxytocin secretion continues, causing the myometrium to contract and helping to constrict the uterine blood vessels, decreasing the amount of vaginal bleeding after delivery. Oxytocin is also responsible for milk ejection during breast-feeding. Stimulation of the breasts through sucking or touching stimulates the secretion of oxytocin from the posterior pituitary gland. Oxytocin causes contraction of the myoepithelial cells in the lactating mammary gland.

Women experience cramping pain and discomfort following childbirth as the uterus contracts and returns to its prepregnant size. These after pains are caused by involuntary contractions and usually last for a few days after childbirth. They are more evident in women who have previously had a baby. Breastfeeding signals the release of oxytocin, which stimulates the uterus to contract and increases the severity of after birth pains.

Vasopressin, also known as ADH functions to inhibit or prevent the formation of urine via vasoconstriction, which results in increased blood pressure. Vasopressin also exhibits an antidiuretic effect and plays an important role in the regulation of water balance (Cheng, 2015).

PANCREAS

The pancreas is an exocrine organ, supplying digestive enzymes and buffers, and an endocrine organ. The endocrine pancreas consists of the islets of Langerhans, which are groups of cells scattered throughout, each containing four cell types. One of the cell types is the beta cell, which produces insulin. Insulin lowers blood glucose by increasing the rate of glucose uptake and utilization by most body cells. The growing fetus needs significant amounts of glucose, amino acids, and lipids. Even during early pregnancy the fetus makes demands on the maternal glucose stores. Ideally, hormonal changes of pregnancy help meet fetal needs without putting the mother's metabolism out of balance.

A woman's insulin secretion works on a supply versus demand mode. As the demand to meet the needs of pregnancy increases, more insulin is secreted. Maternal insulin does not cross the placenta, so the fetus must produce his or her own supply to maintain glucose control. (Box 11.2 gives information about pregnancy, glucose, and insulin.)

Maternal glucose metabolism during pregnancy differs from the nongravid state to allow the mother to meet her own and the growing fetus's energy needs. During the first half of pregnancy, much of the maternal glucose is diverted to the growing fetus, and thus the mother's glucose levels are low. Human placental lactogen and other hormonal antagonists increase during the second half of pregnancy. Therefore, the mother must produce more insulin to overcome the resistance by these hormones. Insulin resistance (the inability of insulin to increase glucose uptake and utilization) in pregnancy is consequent to the physiologic adaptation necessary to provide glucose to the growing fetus. Disturbance in the maternal metabolism can induce structural and functional adaptations during fetal development (Nas, Breyer, & Tuu, 2015).

BOX 11.2

PREGNANCY, INSULIN, AND GLUCOSE

- During early pregnancy, maternal glucose levels decrease because of the heavy fetal demand for glucose. The fetus is also drawing amino acids and lipids from the mother, decreasing the mother's ability to synthesize glucose. Maternal glucose is diverted across the placenta to assist the growing embryo/fetus during early pregnancy, and thus levels decline in the mother. As a result, maternal glucose concentrations decline to a level that would be considered "hypoglycemic" in a nonpregnant woman.
- During early pregnancy there is also a decrease in maternal insulin production and insulin levels. The pancreas is responsible for the production of insulin, which facilitates entry of glucose into cells. Although glucose and other nutrients easily cross the placenta to the fetus, insulin does not. Therefore, the fetus must produce its own insulin to facilitate the entry of glucose into its own cells.
- After the first trimester, hPL from the placenta and steroids (cortisol) from the adrenal cortex act against insulin. hPL acts as an antagonist against maternal insulin, and thus more insulin must be secreted to counteract the increasing levels of hPL and cortisol during the last half of pregnancy.
- Prolactin, estrogen, and progesterone are also thought to oppose insulin. As a result, glucose is less likely to enter the mother's cells and is more likely to cross over the placenta to the fetus.

Adapted from Cunningham, F. G., Leveno, K. J., Bloom, S. L., Spong, C. Y., Dashe, J. S., Hoffman, B. L., et al. (2014). *William's Obstetrics* (24th ed.). New York, NY: McGraw Hill Education.

If the mother has normal beta cells of the islets of Langerhans, there is usually no problem meeting the demands for extra insulin. However, if the woman has inadequate numbers of beta cells, she may be unable to produce enough insulin and will develop glucose intolerance during pregnancy. If the woman has glucose intolerance, she is not able to meet the increasing demands and her blood glucose level increases.

ADRENAL GLANDS

Pregnancy does not cause much change in the size of the adrenal glands themselves, but there are changes in some secretions and activity. One of the key changes is the marked increase in cortisol secretion, which regulates carbohydrate and protein metabolism and is helpful in times of stress. Although pregnancy is considered a normal condition, it is a time of stress for a woman's body. The rate of secretion of cortisol by maternal adrenals is not increased in pregnancy, but the rate of clearance is decreased. Cortisol increases in response to increased estrogen levels throughout pregnancy and returns to normal levels within 6 weeks postpartum

(Banerjee & Williamson, 2015). During the stress of pregnancy, cortisol:

- Helps keep up the level of glucose in the plasma by breaking down noncarbohydrate sources, such as amino and fatty acids, to make glycogen. Glycogen, stored in the liver, is easily broken down to glucose when needed so that glucose is available in times of stress.
- Breaks down proteins to repair tissues and manufacture enzymes.
- Has anti-insulin, anti-inflammatory, and anti-allergic actions.
- Is needed to make the precursors of adrenaline, which the adrenal medulla produces and secretes (Jones & Lopez, 2014).

The amount of aldosterone, also secreted by the adrenal glands, is increased during pregnancy. It normally regulates absorption of sodium from the distal tubules of the kidney. During pregnancy, progesterone allows salt to be wasted (or lost) in the urine. Aldosterone is a key regulator of electrolyte and water homeostasis and plays a central role in blood pressure regulation. Hormonal changes during pregnancy, among them increased progesterone and aldosterone production, lead to the required plasma volume expansion of the maternal body as an accommodation mechanism for fetus growth. Aldosterone is produced in increased amounts by the adrenal glands as early as 15 weeks of pregnancy (Rossier, Baker, & Studer, 2015).

PROSTAGLANDIN SECRETION DURING PREGNANCY

Prostaglandins are not protein or steroid hormones; they are chemical mediators, or local hormones. Although hormones circulate in the blood to influence distant tissues, prostaglandins act locally on adjacent cells. The fetal membranes of the amniotic sac—the amnion and chorion—are both believed to be involved in the production of prostaglandins. Various maternal and fetal tissues, as well as the amniotic fluid itself, are considered to be sources of prostaglandins, but details about their composition and sources are limited. It is widely believed that prostaglandins play a part in softening the cervix and initiating and/or maintaining labor, but the exact mechanism is unclear. What is theorized is that when progesterone levels drop at term, an increased production of prostaglandins occurs, which facilitates uterine contractions and increases myometrial sensitivity to oxytocin that is needed for the labor process (King et al., 2015). Along with oxytocin, the influence of prostaglandins on the uterine myometrium predominates to promote uterine contractile activity.

PLACENTAL SECRETION

The placenta is an organ that serves to prevent the direct exchange between the blood of the fetus and the blood of the mother. The placenta is not only a transfer organ but a factory as well. It is capable of synthesizing enzymes and proteins, and manufactures fats and carbohydrates that serve as a source of stored energy. The placenta also functions as an endocrine gland, manufacturing and secreting hormones. The placenta has a feature possessed by no other endocrine organ—the ability to form protein and steroid hormones. Very early during pregnancy, the placenta begins to produce the following hormones:

- hCG
- hPL
- Relaxin
- Progesterone
- Estrogen

Table 11.3 summarizes the role of these hormones.

Immune System

The immune system is made up of organs and specialized cells whose primary purpose is to defend the body from foreign substances (antigens) that may cause tissue injury or disease. The mechanisms of innate and adaptive immunity work cooperatively to prevent, control, and eradicate foreign antigens in the body.

A general enhancement of innate immunity (inflammatory response and phagocytosis) and suppression of adaptive immunity (protective response to a specific foreign antigen) take place during pregnancy. These immunologic alterations help prevent the mother's immune system from rejecting the fetus (foreign body), increase her risk of developing certain infections such as urinary tract infections, and influence the course of chronic disorders such as autoimmune diseases. Some chronic conditions worsen (diabetes) while others seem to stabilize (asthma) during pregnancy, but this is individualized and not predictable. In general, immune function in pregnant women is similar to immune function in nonpregnant women. Table 11.4 summarizes the general body systems' adaptations to pregnancy.

Marva returns for her first prenatal appointment and tells the nurse that her whole body is "out of sorts." She is overwhelmed and feels poorly. Outline the bodily changes Marva can expect each trimester to help her understand the adaptations taking place. What guidance can the nurse give Marva to help her understand the changes of pregnancy?

CHANGING NUTRITIONAL NEEDS OF PREGNANCY

Maternal body weight and diet quality, even prepregnancy, can affect the uterine environment, birth weight, and the infant's subsequent health into adulthood.

TABLE 11.3	PLACENTAL HORMONES
Hormone	Description
Human chorionic gonadotropin (hCG)	• Responsible for maintaining the maternal corpus luteum, which secretes progesterone and estrogens, with synthesis occurring before implantation. • Production by fetal trophoblast cells until the placenta is developed sufficiently to take over that function. • Basis for early pregnancy tests because it appears in the maternal bloodstream soon after implantation. • Production peaks at 8 weeks and then gradually declines.
hPL (also known as human chorionic somatomammotropin [hCS])	• Preparation of mammary glands for lactation and involved in the process of making glucose available for fetal growth by altering maternal carbohydrate, fat, and protein metabolism. • Antagonist of insulin because it decreases tissue sensitivity or alters the ability to use insulin. • Increase in the amount of circulating free fatty acids for maternal metabolic needs and decrease in maternal metabolism of glucose to facilitate fetal growth.
Relaxin	• Secretion by the placenta as well as the corpus luteum during pregnancy. • Thought to act synergistically with progesterone to maintain pregnancy. • Increase in flexibility of the pubic symphysis, permitting the pelvis to expand during delivery. • Dilation of the cervix, making it easier for the fetus to enter the vaginal canal; thought to suppress the release of oxytocin by the hypothalamus, thus delaying the onset of labor contractions.
Progesterone	• Often called the "hormone of pregnancy" because of the critical role it plays in supporting the endometrium of the uterus. • Supports the endometrium to provide an environment conducive to fetal survival. • Produced by the corpus luteum during the first few weeks of pregnancy and then by the placenta until term. • Initially, causes thickening of the uterine lining in anticipation of implantation of the fertilized ovum. From then on, it maintains the endometrium, inhibits uterine contractility, and assists in the development of the breasts for lactation.
Estrogen	• Promotes enlargement of the genitals, uterus, and breasts, and increases vascularity, causing vasodilatation. • Relaxation of pelvic ligaments and joints. • Associated with hyperpigmentation, vascular changes in the skin, increased activity of the salivary glands, and hyperemia of the gums and nasal mucous membranes. • Aids in developing the ductal system of the breasts in preparation for lactation.

Adapted from Cunningham, F. G., Leveno, K. J., Bloom, S. L., Spong, C. Y., Dashe, J. S., Hoffman, B. L., et al. (2014). *William's Obstetrics* (24th ed.). New York, NY: McGraw Hill Education; Edelman, C. L., Kudzma, E.C., & Mandle, C. L. (2014). *Health promotion throughout the lifespan* (8th ed.). St. Louis, MO: Mosby Elsevier; and Shields, A. D. (2015). Pregnancy diagnosis. *eMedicine*. Retrieved from http://emedicine.medscape.com/article/262591-overview

Healthy eating during pregnancy enables optimal gestational weight gain and reduces complications, both of which are associated with positive birth outcomes. During pregnancy, maternal nutritional needs change to meet the demands of the pregnancy. Healthy eating can help ensure that adequate nutrients are available for both mother and fetus.

Nutritional intake during pregnancy has a direct effect on fetal well-being and birth outcome. Inadequate nutritional intake, for example, is associated with preterm birth, low birth weight, and congenital anomalies. Excessive nutritional intake is connected with fetal macrosomia (>4,000 g), leading to a difficult birth, neonatal hypoglycemia, and continued obesity in the mother and the potential for childhood obesity and the components of metabolic syndrome (Ojha et al., 2015).

Since the requirements for so many nutrients increase during pregnancy, pregnant women should take a vitamin and mineral supplement daily. Prenatal vitamins are prescribed routinely as a safeguard against a less-than-optimal diet. In particular, iron and folic acid need to be supplemented because their increased requirements during pregnancy are usually too great to be met through diet alone. With the exception of folic acid, there is little scientific evidence to support giving vitamin supplements to healthy pregnant women, but it seems to be the standard

TABLE 11.4	SUMMARY OF GENERAL BODY SYSTEM ADAPTATIONS
System	**Adaptation**
Gastrointestinal system	*Mouth and pharynx:* Gums become hyperemic, swollen, and friable and tend to bleed easily. Saliva production increases. *Esophagus:* Decreased lower esophageal sphincter pressure and tone, which increases the risk of developing heartburn. *Stomach:* Decreased tone and mobility with delayed gastric emptying time, which increases the risk of gastroesophageal reflux and vomiting. Decreased gastric acidity and histamine output, which improves symptoms of peptic ulcer disease. *Intestines:* Decreased intestinal tone motility with increased transit time, which increases risk of constipation and flatulence. *Gallbladder:* Decreased tone and motility, which may increase risk of gallstone formation.
Cardiovascular system	*Blood volume:* Marked increase in plasma (50%) and RBCs (25–33%) compared to nonpregnant values. Causes hemodilution, which is reflected in a lower hematocrit and hemoglobin. *Cardiac output and heart rate:* CO increases from 30% to 50% over the nonpregnant rate by the 32nd week of pregnancy. The increase in CO is associated with an increase in venous return and greater right ventricular output, especially in the left lateral position. Heart rate increases by 10–15 bpm between 14 and 20 weeks of gestation, and this increase will persist to term. *Blood pressure:* Diastolic pressure decreases typically 10–15 mm Hg to reach its lowest point by mid-pregnancy; it then gradually returns to nonpregnant baseline values by term. *Blood components:* The number of RBCs increases throughout pregnancy to a level 25–33% higher than nonpregnant values. Both fibrin and plasma fibrinogen levels increase, along with various blood-clotting factors. These factors make pregnancy a hypercoagulable state.
Respiratory system	Enlargement of the uterus shifts the diaphragm up to 4 cm above its usual position. As muscles and cartilage in the thoracic region relax, the chest broadens, with conversion from abdominal breathing to thoracic breathing. This leads to a 50% increase in air volume per minute. Tidal volume, or the volume of air inhaled, increases gradually by 30–40% (from 500 to 700 mL) as the pregnancy progresses.
Renal/urinary system	The renal pelvis becomes dilated. The ureters (especially the right ureter) elongate, widen, and become more curved above the pelvic rim. Bladder tone decreases and bladder capacity doubles by term. GFR increases 40–60% during pregnancy. Blood flow to the kidneys increases by 50–80% as a result of the increase in cardiac output.
Musculoskeletal system	Distention of the abdomen with growth of the fetus tilts the pelvis forward, shifting the center of gravity. The woman compensates by developing an increased curvature (lordosis) of the spine. Relaxation and increased mobility of joints occur because of the hormones progesterone and relaxin, which lead to the characteristic "waddle gait" that pregnant women demonstrate toward term.
Integumentary system	Hyperpigmentation of the skin is the most common alteration during pregnancy. The most common areas include the areola, genital skin, axilla, inner aspects of the thighs, and linea nigra. Striae gravidarum, or stretch marks, are irregular reddish streaks that may appear on the abdomen, breasts, and buttocks in about half of pregnant women. The skin in the middle of the abdomen may develop a pigmented line called linea nigra, which extends from the umbilicus to the pubic area. Melasma ("mask of pregnancy") occurs in up to 70% of pregnant women. It is characterized by irregular, blotchy areas of pigmentation on the face, most commonly on the cheeks, chin, and nose.
Endocrine system	Controls the integrity and duration of gestation by maintaining the corpus luteum via hCG secretion; production of estrogen, progesterone, hPL, and other hormones and growth factors via the placenta; release of oxytocin (by the posterior pituitary gland), prolactin (by the anterior pituitary), and relaxin (by the ovary, uterus, and placenta).
Immune system	A general enhancement of innate immunity (inflammatory response and phagocytosis) and suppression of adaptive immunity (protective response to a specific foreign antigen) take place during pregnancy. These immunologic alterations help prevent the mother's immune system from rejecting the fetus (foreign body), increase her risk of developing certain infections, and influence the course of chronic disorders such as autoimmune diseases.

of care today. Prenatal vitamins are prescribed in the United States almost universally (Jordan et al., 2014). Iron and folic acid are needed to form new blood cells for the expanded maternal blood volume and to prevent anemia. Iron is essential for fetal growth and brain development and in the prevention of maternal anemia. An increase in folic acid is essential before pregnancy and in the early weeks of pregnancy to prevent neural tube defects in the fetus. For most pregnant women, supplements of 27 mg of ferrous iron and 400 to 800 mcg of folic acid per day are recommended by the **dietary reference intakes (DRIs)** (American College of OB/GYN [ACOG], 2015a); (Hankey, 2015); and (U.S. Preventive Services Task Force [USPSTF], 2015). Women with a previous history of a fetus with a neural tube defect are often prescribed a higher dose of folic acid.

There is an abundance of conflicting advice about nutrition during pregnancy and what is good or bad to eat. Overall, the following guidelines are helpful:
- Increase consumption of fruits and vegetables.
- Replace saturated fats with unsaturated ones.
- Make half the plate fruits and vegetables.
- Choose whole grains in place of refined grains.
- Choose foods with a lot of fiber to prevent constipation.
- Avoid hydrogenated or partially hydrogenated fats.
- Do not consume any alcoholic beverages.
- Use reduced-fat spreads and dairy products instead of full-fat ones.
- Eat at least two servings of fish weekly, with one of them being an oily fish.
- Consume at least 2 quarts of water daily (USDA, 2015).

In the months before conception, food choices are key. The foods and vitamins consumed can ensure that the woman and her fetus will have the nutrients that are essential for the very start of pregnancy.

While most women recognize the importance of healthy eating during pregnancy, some find it challenging to achieve. Many women say they have little time and energy to devote to meal planning and preparation. Another barrier to healthy eating is conflicting messages from various sources, resulting in a lack of clear, reliable, and relevant information. Moreover, many women are eating less in an effort to control their weight, putting them at greater risk of inadequate nutrient intake.

Nutritional Requirements During Pregnancy

Pregnancy is one of the most nutritionally demanding periods of a woman's life. Gestation involves rapid cell division and organ development, and an adequate supply of nutrients is essential to support this tremendous fetal growth. Optimal maternal health via good nutritional practices during pregnancy reduces the risk of suboptimal fetal development.

Most women are usually motivated to eat properly during pregnancy for the sake of the fetus. The Food and Nutrition Board of the National Research Council has made recommendations for nutrient intakes for people living in the United States. The DRIs are more comprehensive than previous nutrient guidelines issued by the Board. They have replaced previous recommendations because they are not limited to preventing deficiency diseases. Rather, the DRIs incorporate current concepts about the role of nutrients and food components in reducing the risk of chronic disease, developmental disorders, and other related problems. The DRIs can be used to plan and assess diets for healthy people (Kruger & Butte, 2015).

These dietary recommendations also include information for women who are pregnant or lactating, because growing fetal and maternal tissues require increased quantities of essential dietary components. For example, the current DRIs suggest an increase in the pregnant woman's intake of protein from 60 to 80 g/day, iron from 18 to 27 g/day, and folic acid from 400 to 800 mcg/day, along with an increase of 300 calories/day over the recommended intake of 1,800 to 2,200 calories/day for nonpregnant women (Storck, 2015; Walsh & McAuliffe, 2015) (Table 11.5).

Gluten-free Diet During Pregnancy

In recent years, gluten-free foods have become popular, fueling a growing market for the Food Industry. Pregnant women may be missing out on important nutrients if they adopt gluten-free diets as many are also joining the ever-expanding "G-free" bandwagon. Many people feel that these products are healthier than their conventional counterparts. But is it really a health-promotion diet or just another trend during pregnancy? Gluten may have gotten its bad rap because it is frequently found in many processed and unhealthy foods. Several gluten-free foods contain more fat, including saturated, and sodium, but fewer minerals and vitamins than their equivalents with gluten (Pellegrini & Agostoni, 2015). Skipping processed foods altogether and focusing on fruits, vegetables, lean protein, and whole grains would provide a well-balanced healthy diet.

Eating a gluten-free diet can make it hard to get the recommended amount of folate, vitamin B, iron, calcium, fiber, and grain-servings that all pregnant women need. That is why, unless there is medical reason in which gluten must be eliminated from the diet due to celiac disease or a gluten allergy, there is no scientific reason to cut out wholesome, nutrient-dense grains from the diet (Neifeld, 2015).

USDA and MyPlate

For a pregnant woman to meet recommended DRIs, she should eat according to the U.S. Department of Agriculture (USDA) Food Guide *MyPlate* (Fig. 11.5). The

TABLE 11.5 DIETARY RECOMMENDATIONS FOR THE PREGNANT AND LACTATING WOMAN

Nutrient	Nonpregnant Women	Pregnant Woman	Lactating Woman
Calories	2,200	2,500	2,700
Protein	60 g	80 g	80 g
Water/fluids	6–8 glasses daily	8 glasses daily	8 glasses daily
Vitamin A	700 mcg	770 mcg	1,300 mcg
Vitamin C	75 mg	85 mg	120 mg
Vitamin D	5 mcg	5 mcg	5 mcg
Folate	400 mcg	600 mcg	500 mcg
Calcium	1,000 mg	1,000 mg	1,000 mg
Iodine			
Iron	18 mg	27 mg	9 mg

Adapted from American Pregnancy Association (2015). *Pregnancy nutrition.* Retrieved from http://americanpregnancy.org/pregnancyhealth/pregnancynutrition.html; Ural, S. H. (2015). Prenatal nutrition. *eMedicine.* Retrieved from http://emedicine.medscape.com/article/259059-overview; and Lutz, C. A., Mazur, E., & Litch, N. (2014). *Nutrition and diet therapy* (6th ed.). Philadelphia, PA: F.A. Davis.

USDA Food Guide *MyPlate* replaced the Food Guide Pyramid in 2011 as the government's primary food group symbol. *MyPlate* is an easy-to-understand visual cue to help consumers adopt healthy eating habits by encouraging them to build a healthy plate, consistent with the *Dietary Guidelines for Americans, 2015* (USDA & USDHHS, 2015), which are the basis for federal nutrition policy (USDA and U.S. Department of Health and Human Services [USDHHS], 2015). This new tool will serve as a basis for dietary instruction and it can be tailored to meet each woman's individual needs.

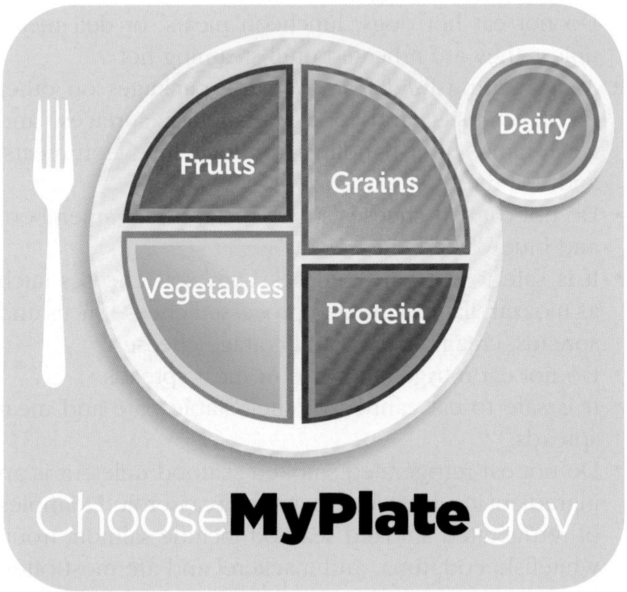

MyPlate provides guidance to help implement the dietary guidelines. The USDA has designed an interactive online diet-planning program called the Daily Food Plan for Moms that helps pregnant women personalize their dietary intake throughout their pregnancy. (Refer to thePoint for additional information about this food plan.) A summary of the new guidelines is as follows:

- Eat a variety of food from all food groups using portion control.
- Increase intake of vitamins, minerals, and dietary fiber.
- Lower intake of saturated fats, trans fats, and cholesterol.
- Consume adequate synthetic folic acid from supplements or from fortified foods.
- Increase intake of fruits, vegetables, and whole grains.
- Balance calorie intake with exercise to maintain ideal healthy weight (USDA, 2015).

An eating plan that follows *MyPlate* should provide sufficient nutrients for a healthy pregnancy. Except for iron, folic acid, and calcium, most of the nutrients a woman needs during pregnancy can be obtained by making healthy food choices. However, a vitamin and mineral supplement is generally prescribed.

Take Note!

Good food sources of folic acid include dark green vegetables, such as broccoli, romaine lettuce, and spinach; baked beans, black-eyed peas, citrus fruits, peanuts, and liver.

FIGURE 11.5 Food Guide *MyPlate* for pregnancy.

Food Concerns During Pregnancy

ARTIFICIAL SWEETENERS

Artificial sweeteners or intense sweeteners are sugar substitutes that are used as an alternative to table sugar. They are many times sweeter than natural sugar and contain no calories. Extensive scientific research has demonstrated the safety of the six low-calorie sweeteners currently approved for use in foods in the United States and Europe (stevia, acesulfame-K, aspartame, neotame, saccharin, and sucralose), if taken in acceptable quantities daily. But there is an ongoing debate over whether artificial sweeteners pose a health threat (Qurrat-ul-Ain & Khan, 2015).

The safety of artificial sweeteners consumed during pregnancy remains controversial also. Some health care providers advise their pregnant clients to avoid all nonnutritive sweeteners during pregnancy, while others suggest they can be used in moderation (Hankley, 2015). The debate continues on this matter until additional research can be completed.

FISH, SHELLFISH, AND LEVELS OF MERCURY

Fish and shellfish are an important part of a healthy diet because they contain high-quality protein, are low in saturated fat, and contain omega-3 fatty acids. However, nearly all fish and shellfish contain traces of mercury and some contain higher levels of mercury that may harm a developing fetus if ingested by pregnant women in large amounts. Human exposure to mercury occurs primarily through the consumption of fish contaminated through atmospheric mercury releases. The U.S. Environmental Protection Agency (EPA) and the United Nations Environment Program have identified coal-fired power plants as the source of 50% to 75% of the atmospheric mercury pollution in the United States and worldwide. Once airborne, rainfall transfers mercury particles into waterways where it is converted to the neurotoxic methylmercury form through a microbial process. Plankton absorbs the methylmercury and as the smaller fish eat the plankton and the larger predatory fish consume the smaller fish, the methylmercury bioaccumulates up the food chain to humans. Mercury exposure in pregnancy has been associated with both pregnancy complications and developmental problems in infants. Apart from the environmental exposure, mercury is likely to arise from predatory fish consumption. It would be prudent to advise all pregnant women to avoid these potential problems and minimize any risk.

All fish contain methylmercury regardless of the size or the geographic location of the waters from which the fish is caught, although size and type of fish as well as the geographic location of waters can influence lower or higher amounts of methylmercury. In addition, because methylmercury resides in the tissue of the fish, no method of cleaning or cooking will reduce the amount of mercury in a meal of contaminated fish (Nelson, 2015).

With this in mind, the FDA and the EPA are advising women who may become pregnant, pregnant women, and nursing mothers to do the following:

- Avoid consumption of fish with moderate-to-high mercury levels (e.g., for 6 to 12 months prior to conception and throughout pregnancy).
- Avoid eating shark, swordfish, king mackerel, orange roughy, ahi tuna, and tilefish because they are high in mercury levels.
- Eat up to 12 oz (two average meals) weekly of low-mercury-level fish such as shrimp, canned light tuna, salmon, pollock, and catfish.
- Check local advisories about the safety of fish caught by family and friends in local lakes, rivers, and coastal areas (FDA, 2015).

LISTERIOSIS AND PREGNANCY

Another food issue concern for pregnant women is consumption of food contaminated with the gram-positive bacillus *Listeria*. *Listeria* is a type of bacteria found in soil, water, and sometimes on plants. *Listeria* is commonly found in processed and prepared foods and in raw or unpasteurized milk. Listeriosis is associated with high morbidity and mortality. Though *Listeria* is all around our environment, most *Listeria* infections in people result from eating contaminated foods. Listeriosis during pregnancy usually presents as an unremarkable febrile illness in the mother, but can be fatal for the fetus and newborn. Reliable laboratory testing for early diagnosis is lacking. Listeriosis can be passed to an unborn baby through the placenta even if the mother is not showing signs of illness. This can lead to preterm births, miscarriages, stillbirths, and high neonatal mortality rates (Allerberger & Huhulescu, 2015). The Food Safety and Inspection Service and the FDA (2015) provide the following advice for pregnant women:

- Do not eat hot dogs, luncheon meats, or deli meats unless they are reheated until steaming hot.
- Avoid getting fluid from hot dog packages on other foods, utensils, and food preparation surfaces, and wash hands after handling hot dogs, luncheon meats, and deli meats.
- Do not eat soft cheeses such as feta, Brie, Camembert, and blue-veined cheeses.
- It is safe to eat hard cheeses, semi-soft cheeses such as mozzarella, pasteurized processed cheese slices and spreads, cream cheese, and cottage cheese.
- Do not eat refrigerated pâté or meat spreads.
- It is safe to eat canned or shelf-stable pâté and meat spreads.
- Do not eat refrigerated smoked seafood unless it is an ingredient in a cooked dish such as a casserole. Examples of refrigerated smoked seafood include salmon, trout, whitefish, cod, tuna, and mackerel and are most often labeled as "nova-style," "lox," "kippered," "smoked," or "jerky." These refrigerated smoked fish are found in the

refrigerated section or sold at deli counters of grocery stores and delicatessens.

- It is safe to eat canned fish such as salmon and tuna or shelf-stable smoked seafood.
- Do not drink raw (unpasteurized) milk or eat foods that contain unpasteurized milk.
- Use all refrigerated perishable items that are pre-cooked or ready-to-eat as soon as possible.
- Use a refrigerator thermometer to make sure that the refrigerator always stays at 40° F (about 5° C) or below.
- Do not eat salads made in the store such as ham salad, chicken salad, egg salad, tuna salad, or seafood salad.
- Clean your refrigerator regularly.

Maternal Weight Gain

The amount of weight that a woman gains during pregnancy is not as important as what she eats. A woman can lose extra weight after a pregnancy, but she can never make up for a poor nutritional status during the pregnancy. Earlier guidelines recommended weight gain that would be optimal for the infant, but new guidelines take into account the well-being of the mother too (Table 11.6).

In 2009, the Health and Medicine Division revised the recommendations regarding maternal gestational weight gain. The revisions took into account that presently American women (1) have more multiple pregnancies; (2) are becoming pregnant at an older age; (3) are exceeding the ideal weight gain during pregnancy; and (4) tend to be more overweight and obese when becoming pregnant.

TABLE 11.6	NORMAL DISTRIBUTION OF WEIGHT GAIN DURING PREGNANCY
Component	**Weight (pounds)**
Infant birth weight	7.5
Blood volume increase	4
Uterus	2
Increase in breast tissue	2
Placenta	1.5
Maternal fluid volume	4
Maternal fat tissue	7
Amniotic fluid	2
Approximate total weight gain	30

Adapted from American College of Obstetricians and Gynecologists [ACOG]. (2015b). *Weight gain guidelines by ACOG for pregnancy.* Retrieved from http://www.womenshealthcaretopics.com/weight_gain_during_pregnancy.htm; and Lutz, C. A., Mazur, E., & Litch, N. (2014). *Nutrition and diet therapy* (6th ed.). Philadelphia, PA: F. A. Davis.

BOX 11.3

BODY MASS INDEX

Body mass index (BMI) provides an accurate estimate of total body fat and is considered a good method to assess overweight and obesity in people. BMI is a weight-to-height ratio calculation that can be determined by dividing a woman's weight in kilograms by her height in meters squared. BMI can also be calculated by weight in pounds divided by the height in inches squared, multiplied by 704.5.

The Centers for Disease Control and Prevention (CDC) (2015) categorizes BMI as follows:
- Underweight: <18.5
- Healthy weight: 18.5–24.9
- Overweight: 25–29.9
- Obese: 30 or higher

Use this example to calculate BMI:
Mary is 5 ft 5 in tall and weighs 150 lb.
1. Convert weight into kilograms: 150 ÷ 2.2 lb/kg = 68.18 kg.
2. Convert height into meters:
   a. 5 ft 5 in = 65 in ÷ 2.54 cm/in = 165.1 cm
   b. 165.1 cm ÷ 100 cm = 1.65 m
3. Then square the height in meters: 1.65 × 1.65 = 2.72
4. Calculate BMI: 68.18 kg ÷ 2.72 = 25.

Adapted from Centers for Disease Control and Prevention [CDC]. (2015). *BMI for adults: Body mass index calculator.* Retrieved from http://www.cdc.gov/nccdphp/dnpa/bmi/calc-bmi.htm

---

The new recommendations are based on the woman's pregnancy body mass index (BMI) as follows (Box 11.3):
- Underweight (BMI < 18.5) total weight gain range = 28–40 lb.
- Normal weight (BMI = 18.5–24.9) total weight gain range = 25–35 lb.
- Overweight (BMI = 25–29.9) total weight gain range = 15–25 lb.
- Obese (BMI = 30 or higher) total weight gain range = 11–20 lb.

A woman who is underweight before pregnancy or who has a low maternal weight gain pattern should be monitored carefully because she is at risk of giving birth to a low-birth-weight infant (<2,500 g or 5.5 lb). Frequently these women simply need advice on what to eat to add weight. Encourage the woman to eat snacks that are high in calories such as nuts, peanut butter, milkshakes, cheese, fruit, yogurt, and ice cream. Any woman who has a prepregnancy BMI of less than 18.5 is considered to be at high risk and should be referred to a nutritionist (Sharma et al., 2015).

Conversely, women who start a pregnancy while overweight (BMI > 25–29) run the risk of having a high-birth-weight infant, with resulting cephalopelvic disproportion and, potentially, a surgical birth. Two thirds of reproductive-age women in the United States are overweight or obese and at risk for numerous adverse pregnancy outcomes, in addition to a surgical birth. Some researchers have suggested that the uterine environment may influence the potential development of offspring obesity later in life. In a recent study, just a 10% weight loss before conception, was associated with at least a 10% lower risk of preeclampsia, gestational diabetes, preterm birth, macrosomia, and still birth (Schummers et al., 2015). Dieting during pregnancy is never recommended, even for women who are obese. Severe restriction of caloric intake is associated with a decrease in birth weight. Because of the expansion of maternal blood volume and the development of fetal and placental tissues, some weight gain is essential for a healthy pregnancy. Women who gain more than the recommended weight during pregnancy and who fail to lose this weight 6 months after giving birth are at much higher risk of being obese nearly a decade later (American College of Obstetricians and Gynecologists [ACOG], 2015a). Women who are overweight when beginning a pregnancy should gain no more than 15 to 25 lb during the pregnancy, depending on their nutritional status and degree of obesity (American College of Obstetricians and Gynecologists [ACOG], 2015a).

The best way to assess whether a pregnant woman is consuming enough calories is to follow her pattern of weight gain. All pregnant women should aim for a steady rate of weight gain throughout pregnancy. If she is gaining in a steady, gradual manner, then she is taking in enough calories. However, consuming an adequate amount of calories does not guarantee that her nutrients are sufficient. It is critical to evaluate both the quantity and the quality of the foods eaten.

During the first trimester, for women whose prepregnancy weight is within the normal weight range, weight gain should be about 3.5 to 5 lb. For underweight women, weight gain should be at least 5 lb. For overweight women, weight gain should be about 2 lb. Much of the weight gained during the first trimester is caused by growth of the uterus and expansion of the blood volume.

During the second and third trimesters, the following pattern is recommended: For women whose prepregnancy weight is within the normal weight range, weight gain should be about 1 pound per week. For underweight women, weight gain should be slightly more than 1 pound per week. For overweight women, weight gain should be about two thirds of a pound per week (Hankley, 2015).

Nutrition Promotion

Through education, nurses can play an important role in ensuring adequate nutrition for pregnant women. During the initial prenatal visit, health care providers conduct a thorough assessment of a woman's typical dietary practices and address any conditions that may cause inadequate nutrition, such as nausea and vomiting or lack of access to adequate food. Assess and reinforce dietary information at every prenatal visit to promote good nutrition. A normal pregnancy and a well-balanced diet generally provide most of the recommended nutrients except iron and folate, both of which must be supplemented in the form of prenatal vitamins. (See Teaching Guidelines 11.1.)

Teaching Guidelines 11.1

TEACHING TO PROMOTE OPTIMAL NUTRITION DURING PREGNANCY

- Follow the USDA Food Guide *MyPlate* and select a variety of foods from each group.
- Gain between 15 and 40 lb in a gradual and steady manner depending on prepregnancy weight as follows:
  - Underweight (BMI > 18.5) total weight gain range = 28–40 lb
  - Normal weight (BMI = 18.5–24.0) total weight gain range = 25–35 lb
  - Overweight (BMI = 25–29) total weight gain range = 15–25 lb
  - Obese (BMI = 30 or higher) total weight gain range = 11–20 lb (HMD, 2009).
- Take your prenatal vitamin/mineral supplementation daily.
- Avoid weight-reduction diets during pregnancy.
- Do not skip meals; eat three meals with one or two snacks daily.
- Limit the intake of sodas and caffeine-rich drinks.
- Avoid the use of diuretics during pregnancy.
- Do not restrict the use of salt unless instructed to do so by your health care provider.
- Engage in reasonable physical activity daily.

Special Nutritional Considerations

Many factors play an important role in shaping a person's food habits, and these factors must be taken into account if nutritional counseling is to be realistic and appropriate. Nurses need to be aware of these factors to ensure individualized teaching and care.

Cultural Variations and Restrictions

Food is important to every cultural group. It is often part of celebrations and rituals. When working with women from various cultures, the nurse needs to adapt American nutritional guidelines to meet their nutritional needs within their cultural framework. Food choices and variations for different cultures might include the following:
- Bread, cereal, rice, and pasta group:
  - Bolillo
  - Couscous
  - Flaxseed
  - Hau juan

- Vegetable group:
  - Agave
  - Bok choy
  - Jicama
  - Okra
  - Water chestnuts
- Protein group:
  - Bean paste
  - Blood sausage
  - Legumes
  - Shellfish
- Fruit group:
  - Catalpa
  - Kumquats
  - Plantain
  - Yucca fruit
  - Zapote
- Milk and dairy:
  - Buffalo milk
  - Buttermilk
  - Soybean milk (Academy of Nutrition and Dietetics [AND], 2015a)

Lactose Intolerance

The best source of calcium is milk and dairy products, but for women with lactose intolerance, adaptations are necessary. Women with lactose intolerance lack an enzyme (lactase) needed for the breakdown of lactose into its component simple sugars, glucose, and galactose. Without adequate lactase, lactose passes through the small intestine undigested and causes abdominal discomfort, gas, and diarrhea. Lactose intolerance is especially common among women of African, Asian, and Middle Eastern descent (Szilagyi, 2015).

Additional or substitute sources of calcium may be necessary. These may include peanuts, almonds, sunflower seeds, broccoli, salmon, kale, and molasses (McIndoo, 2015). In addition, encourage the woman to drink lactose-free dairy products or calcium-enriched orange juice or soy milk (Evidence-Based Practice 11.1).

Vegetarians

Vegetarian diets are becoming increasingly prevalent in the United States. People choose a vegetarian diet for

EVIDENCE-BASED PRACTICE 11.1 — INTERVENTIONS FOR NAUSEA AND VOMITING IN EARLY PREGNANCY

Nausea, retching or dry heaving, and vomiting in early pregnancy are very common and can be very distressing for women. Many treatments are available to women with 'morning sickness', including drugs and complementary and alternative therapies. Because of concerns that taking medications may adversely affect the development of the fetus, this review aimed to examine if these treatments have been found to be effective and safe.

STUDY

The purpose of this study was to assess the effectiveness and safety of all interventions for nausea and vomiting in early pregnancy, up to 20 weeks of gestation. Thirty-seven trials involving 5,049 women met the inclusion criteria. These trials covered many interventions, including acupressure, acustimulation, acupuncture, ginger, chamomile, lemon oil, mint oil, vitamin B6, and several antiemetic drugs.

Evidence regarding the effectiveness of P6 acupressure, auricular (ear) acupressure, and acustimulation of the P6 point was limited. Acupuncture (P6 or traditional) showed no significant benefit to women in pregnancy. The use of ginger products may be helpful to women, but the evidence of effectiveness was limited and not consistent, though two recent studies support ginger over placebo. There was only limited evidence from trials to support the use of pharmacological agents including vitamin B6, and anti-emetic drugs to relieve mild or moderate nausea and vomiting. There was little information on maternal and fetal adverse outcomes and on psychological, social, or economic outcomes. The methodological quality of the included studies was mixed.

Findings

This review found a lack of high-quality evidence to back up any advice on which interventions to use. Some of the studies showed a benefit in improving nausea and vomiting symptoms for women, but generally effects were inconsistent and limited. Studies were carried out in a way that meant they were at high risk of bias and, therefore, it was difficult to draw firm conclusions. Most studies had different ways of measuring the symptoms of nausea and vomiting and therefore, could not be looked at these findings together. Few studies reported maternal and fetal adverse outcomes and there was very little information on the effectiveness of treatments for improving women's quality of life.

Nursing Implications

Given the high prevalence of nausea and vomiting in early pregnancy, women and nurses caring for them need clear guidance about effective and safe interventions based on systematically reviewed evidence. Diclegis is the only FDA approved medicine for treatment of morning sickness presently, but causes drowsiness, so women should avoid engaging in activities requiring complete mental alertness, such as driving. There is a lack of high-quality evidence to support any particular intervention at this time. This is not the same as saying that the interventions studied are ineffective, but that there is insufficient strong evidence for any one intervention. Advice provided by nurses to pregnant clients experiencing morning sickness should remain general and individualized, based on the findings of this study.

Adapted from Matthews, A., Haas, D. M., O'Mathúna, D. P., Dowswell, T., & Doyle, M. (2014). Interventions for nausea and vomiting in early pregnancy. *Cochrane Database of Systematic Reviews*, (3), CD007575.

various reasons including environmental, animal rights, philosophical, religious, and health beliefs (Dunlevy, 2015). Vegetarians choose not to eat meat, poultry, and fish. Their diets consist mostly of plant-based foods, such as legumes, vegetables, whole grains, nuts, and seeds. Vegetarians fall into groups defined by the types of foods they eat. Lacto-ovo-vegetarians omit red meat, fish, and poultry, but eat eggs, milk, and dairy products in addition to plant-based foods. Lacto-vegetarians consume milk and dairy products along with plant-based foods; they omit eggs, meat, fish, and poultry. Vegans eliminate all foods from animals, including milk, eggs, and cheese, and eat only plant-based foods (Foster & Samman, 2015).

The concern with any form of vegetarianism, especially during pregnancy, is that the diet may be inadequate in nutrients. Other risks of vegetarian eating patterns during pregnancy may include low gestational weight gain, iron-deficiency anemia, compromised protein utilization, and decreased mineral absorption (Piccoli et al., 2015). A diet can become so restrictive that a woman is not gaining weight or is consistently not eating enough from one or more of the food groups. Generally, the more restrictive the diet is, the greater the chance of nutrient deficiencies.

Well-balanced vegetarian diets that include dairy products provide adequate caloric and nutrient intake and do not require special supplementation; however, vegan diets do not include any meat, eggs, or dairy products. Pregnant vegetarians must pay special attention to their intake of protein, iron, calcium, and vitamin B_{12}. Suggestions include:

- *For protein:* substitute soy foods, beans, lentils, nuts, grains, and seeds.
- *For iron:* eat a variety of meat alternatives, along with vitamin C-rich foods.
- *For calcium:* substitute soy, calcium-fortified orange juice, and tofu.
- *For vitamin B_{12}:* eat fortified soy foods and a B_{12} supplement.

The Academy of Nutrition and Dietetics (2015b), used an evidence-based review to show that well-planned vegetarian diets are appropriate for individuals during all stages of the life cycle, including pregnancy, lactation, infancy, childhood, and adolescence, and for athletes.

Pica

Pica is a term used to describe the intense craving for and eating of non-food items. Many women experience unusual food cravings during their pregnancy. Having cravings during pregnancy is perfectly normal. Sometimes, however, women crave substances that have no nutritional value and can even be dangerous to themselves and their fetus. Pica is the compulsive ingestion of nonfood substances. Pica is derived from the Latin term for magpie, a bird that is known to consume a variety of nonfood substances. Unlike the bird, however, pregnant women who develop a pica habit typically have one or two specific cravings.

The exact cause of pica is not known. Many theories have been advanced to explain it, but none has been proven scientifically. The incidence of pica is difficult to determine, since it is underreported. It is more common in the United States among African American women compared with other ethnicities, but the practice of pica is not limited to any one geographic area, race, creed, or culture. In the United States, pica is also common in women from rural areas and women with a family history of it. Common substances ingested include dirt, clay, and laundry starch. Other pica cravings are burnt matches, stones, charcoal, mothballs, ice, cornstarch, toothpaste, soap, sand, plaster, coffee grounds, paint chips, coffee grounds, baking soda, and cigarette ashes (Jyothi, 2015).

The three main substances consumed by women with pica are soil or clay (geophagia), ice (pagophagia), and laundry starch (amylophagia). Nutritional implications include:

- *Soil:* replaces nutritive sources and causes iron-deficiency anemia.
- *Clay:* produces constipation; can contain toxic substances and cause parasitic infection.
- *Ice:* can cause iron-deficiency anemia, tooth fractures, freezer burn injuries.
- *Laundry starch:* replaces iron-rich foods, leads to iron deficiencies, and replaces protein metabolism, thus depriving the fetus of amino acids needed for proper development (American Pregnancy Association, 2015).

Clinical manifestations of anemia often precede the identification of pica because the health care provider rarely addresses the behavior and the woman does not usually volunteer such information (King et al., 2015). Secrecy surrounding this habit makes research and diagnosis difficult because some women fail to view their behavior as anything unusual, harmful, or worth reporting. Because of the clinical implications, pica should be discussed with all pregnant women as a preventive measure. The topic can be part of a general discussion of cravings, and the nurse should stress the harmful effects outlined above.

Suspect pica when the woman exhibits anemia although her dietary intake is appropriate. Ask about her usual dietary intake, and include questions about the ingestion of nonfood substances. Consider the potential negative outcomes for the pregnant woman and her fetus, and take appropriate action.

PSYCHOSOCIAL ADAPTATIONS DURING PREGNANCY

Pregnancy is a unique time in a woman's life. It is a time of dramatic alterations in her body and her appearance, as well as a time of change in her social status.

All of these changes occur simultaneously. Concurrent with the physiologic changes within her body systems are psychosocial changes within the mother and family members as they face significant role and lifestyle changes.

Maternal Emotional Responses

Motherhood, perhaps more than any role in the society, has acquired a special significance for women. Women are taught they should find fulfillment and satisfaction in the role of the "ever-bountiful, ever-giving, self-sacrificing mother." Pregnancy and transitioning to motherhood are critical experiences in a woman's life, stirring a whole range of powerful emotions (Einstein, 2015). With such high expectations, many pregnant women experience various emotions throughout their pregnancy. The woman's approach to these emotions is influenced by her emotional makeup, her sociologic and cultural background, her acceptance or rejection of the pregnancy, whether the pregnancy was planned, if the father is known, and her support network (Alexander et al., 2014).

Despite the wide-ranging emotions associated with the pregnancy, many women experience similar responses. These responses commonly include ambivalence, introversion, acceptance, mood swings, and changes in body image.

Ambivalence

The realization of a pregnancy can lead to fluctuating responses, possibly at the opposite ends of the spectrum. For example, regardless of whether the pregnancy was planned, the woman may feel proud and excited by the news, while at the same time fearful and anxious of the implications. The reactions are influenced by several factors, including the way the woman was raised, her current family situation, the quality of the relationship with the expectant father, and her hopes for the future. Some women express concern over the timing of the pregnancy, wishing that goals and life objectives had been met before becoming pregnant. Other women may question how a newborn or infant will affect their career or their relationships with friends and family. These feelings can cause conflict and confusion about the pregnancy.

Ambivalence, or having conflicting feelings at the same time, is a universal feeling and is considered normal when preparing for a lifestyle change and new role. Pregnant women commonly experience ambivalence during the first trimester. Usually ambivalence evolves into acceptance by the second trimester, when fetal movement is felt. The woman's personality, her ability to adapt to changing circumstances, and the reactions of her partner will affect her adjustment to being pregnant and her acceptance of impending motherhood.

Introversion

Introversion, or focusing on oneself, is common during the early part of pregnancy. The woman may withdraw and become increasingly preoccupied with herself and her fetus. As a result, she may participate less with the outside world, and she may appear passive to her family and friends.

This introspective behavior is a normal psychological adaptation to motherhood for most women. Introversion seems to heighten during the first and third trimesters, when the woman's focus is on behaviors that will ensure a safe and health pregnancy outcome. Couples need to be aware of this behavior and should be informed about measures to maintain and support the focus on the family.

Acceptance

During the second trimester, the physical changes of the growing fetus, including an enlarging abdomen and fetal movement, bring reality and validity to the pregnancy. There are many tangible signs that someone separate from herself is present. The pregnant woman feels fetal movement and may hear the heartbeat. She may see the fetal image on an ultrasound screen and feel distinct parts, recognizing independent sleep and wake patterns. She becomes able to identify the fetus as a separate individual and accepts this.

Many women will verbalize positive feelings about the pregnancy and will conceptualize the fetus. The woman may accept her new body image and talk about the new life within. Generating a discussion about the woman's feelings and offering support and validation at prenatal visits are important.

Mood Swings

Emotional liability is characteristic throughout most pregnancies. One moment a woman can feel great joy, and within a short time she can feel shock and disbelief. Frequently, pregnant women will start to cry without any apparent cause. Some women feel as though they are riding an emotional "roller-coaster." These extremes in emotion can make it difficult for partners and family members to communicate with the pregnant woman without placing blame on themselves for their mood changes. Clear explanations about how common mood swings are during pregnancy are essential.

Change in Body Image

The way in which pregnancy affects a woman's body image varies greatly from person to person. Some women feel as if they have never been more beautiful, whereas others spend their pregnancy feeling overweight and uncomfortable. For some women pregnancy is a relief from worrying about weight, whereas for others it only exacerbates their fears of weight gain. Changes in body image are normal but can be very stressful for the pregnant woman. Offering a thorough explanation and initiating discussion of the expected bodily changes may help the family to cope with them.

Becoming a Mother

Reva Rubin (1984) identified maternal tasks that a woman must accomplish to incorporate the maternal role into her personality. Accomplishing these tasks helps the expectant mother to develop her self-concept as a mother and to form a mutually gratifying relationship with her infant. These tasks are listed in Box 11.4.

BOX 11.4

BECOMING A MOTHER

- Ensuring safe passage throughout pregnancy and birth
  - Primary focus of the woman's attention
  - First trimester: woman focuses on herself, not on the fetus
  - Second trimester: woman develops attachment of great value to her fetus
  - Third trimester: woman has concern for herself and her fetus as a unit
  - Participation in positive self-care activities related to diet, exercise, and overall well-being
- Seeking acceptance of infant by others
  - First trimester: acceptance of pregnancy by herself and others
  - Second trimester: family needs to relate to the fetus as member
  - Third trimester: unconditional acceptance without rejection
- Seeking acceptance of self in maternal role to infant ("binding in")
  - First trimester: mother accepts idea of pregnancy, but not of infant
  - Second trimester: with sensation of fetal movement (quickening), mother acknowledges fetus as a separate entity within her
  - Third trimester: mother longs to hold infant and becomes tired of being pregnant
- Learning to give of oneself
  - First trimester: identifies what must be given up to assume new role
  - Second trimester: identifies with infant, learns how to delay own desires
  - Third trimester: questions her ability to become a good mother to infant

Adapted from Rubin, R. (1984). *Maternal identity and the maternal experience.* New York, NY: Springer.

Pregnancy and Sexuality

Sexuality is an important part of health and well-being. Sexual behavior modifies as pregnancy progresses, influenced by biologic, psychological, and social factors. The way a pregnant woman feels and experiences her body during pregnancy can affect her sexuality. The woman's changing shape, emotional status, fetal activity, changes in breast size, pressure on the bladder, and other discomforts of pregnancy result in increased physical and emotional demands. These can produce stress on the sexual relationship between the pregnant woman and her partner. As the changes of pregnancy ensue, many partners become confused, anxious, and fearful of how the relationship may be affected.

The sexual desire of pregnant women may change throughout the pregnancy. During the first trimester, the woman may be less interested in sex because of fatigue, nausea, and fear of disturbing the early embryonic development. During the second trimester, her interest may increase because of the stability of the pregnancy. During the third trimester, her enlarging size may produce discomfort during sexual activity (Bope & Kellerman, 2015).

Potential complications of sex during pregnancy include preterm labor, pelvic inflammatory disease, antepartum hemorrhage in placenta previa, and venous air embolism. Generally, sexual relations are generally considered safe in pregnancy. Abstinence is usually only recommended for women who are at risk for preterm labor or for antepartum hemorrhage because of placenta previa (Boynton, 2015).

A woman's sexual health is intimately linked to her own self-image. Sexual positions to increase comfort as the pregnancy progresses as well as alternative noncoital modes of sexual expression, such as cuddling, caressing, and holding, should be discussed. Giving permission to talk about and then normalizing sexuality can help enhance the sexual experience during pregnancy and, ultimately, the couple's relationship. If avenues of communication are open regarding sexuality during pregnancy, any fears and myths the couple may have can be dispelled.

Pregnancy and the Partner

Nursing care related to childbirth has expanded from a narrow emphasis on the physical health needs of the mother and infant to a broader focus on family-related social and emotional needs. One prominent feature of this family-centered approach is the recent movement toward promoting the mother–infant bond. To achieve a truly family-centered practice, nursing must make a comparable commitment to understanding and meeting the needs of the partner in the emerging family. Recent studies suggest that the partner's potential contribution to the infant's overall development has been misperceived or devalued and that the partner's ability and willingness to assume a more active role in the infant's care may have been underestimated.

Reactions to pregnancy and to the psychological and physical changes by the woman's partner vary greatly. Some enjoy the role of being the nurturer, whereas others experience alienation and may seek comfort or companionship elsewhere. Some expectant fathers may view pregnancy as proof of their masculinity and assume the dominant role, whereas others see their role as minimal, leaving the pregnancy up to the woman entirely. Each expectant partner reacts uniquely.

Emotionally and psychologically, expectant partners may undergo fewer visible changes than women, but most of these changes remain unexpressed and unappreciated (Davies, 2015). Expectant partners also experience a multitude of adjustments and concerns. Physically, they may gain weight around the middle and experience nausea and other GI disturbances—a reaction termed *couvade syndrome* that is a sympathetic response to their partner's pregnancy. They also experience ambivalence during early pregnancy, with extremes of emotions (e.g., pride and joy versus an overwhelming sense of impending responsibility).

During the second trimester of pregnancy, partners go through acceptance of their role of breadwinner, caretaker, and support person. They come to accept the reality of the fetus when movement is felt, and they experience confusion when dealing with the woman's mood swings and introspection. During the third trimester, the expectant partner prepares for the reality of this new role and negotiates what the role will be during the labor and birthing process. Many express concern about being the primary support person during labor and birth and worry how they will react when faced with their loved one in pain. Expectant partners share many of the same anxieties as their pregnant partners. However, it is uncommon for them to reveal these anxieties to the pregnant partner or health care providers. Often, how the expectant partner responds during the third trimester depends on the state of the marriage or partnership. When the marriage or partnership is struggling, the impending increase in responsibility toward the end of pregnancy acts to drive the expectant partner further away. Often it manifests as working late, staying out late with friends, or beginning new or superficial relationships. In the stable marriage or partnership, the expectant partner who may have been struggling to find his or her place in the pregnancy now finds concrete tasks to do—for example, painting the nursery, assembling the car seat, or attending Lamaze classes.

Pregnancy and Siblings

A sibling's reaction to pregnancy is age dependent. Some children might express excitement and anticipation,

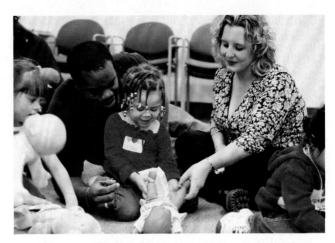

FIGURE 11.6 Parents preparing sibling for the birth of a new baby.

whereas others might have negative reactions. A young toddler might regress in toilet training or ask to drink from a bottle again. An older school-aged child may ignore the new addition to the family and engage in outside activities to avoid the new member. The introduction of an infant into the family is often the beginning of sibling rivalry, which results from the child's fear of change in the security of the relationship with his or her parents (Jordan et al., 2014). Preparation of the siblings for the anticipated birth is imperative and must be designed according to the age and life experiences of the sibling at home. Constant reinforcement of love and caring will help to reduce the older child's fear of change and worry about being replaced by the new family member.

If possible, parents should include siblings in preparation for the birth of the new baby to help them feel as if they have an important role to play (Fig. 11.6). Parents must also continue to focus on the older sibling after the birth to reduce regressive or aggressive behavior toward the newborn.

Pregnancy is an extremely busy time, not only in terms of the bodily changes taking place, but tasks that must be done such as choosing a provider to care for them, preparing for the new family member in a matter of months, and making lifestyle modifications to promote the best possible pregnancy outcome. We will explore this more in Chapter 12.

KEY CONCEPTS

○ Pregnancy is a normal life event that involves considerable physical, psychosocial, emotional, and relationship adjustments.

○ The signs and symptoms of pregnancy have been grouped into those that are subjective (presumptive) and experienced by the woman herself, those that are objective (probable) and observed by the health care provider, and those that are the positive, certain signs.

◎ Physiologically, almost every system of a woman's body changes during pregnancy with startling rapidity to accommodate the needs of the growing fetus. A majority of the changes are influenced by hormonal changes.

◎ The placenta is a unique kind of endocrine gland; it has a feature possessed by no other endocrine organ—the ability to form protein and steroid hormones.

◎ Occurring in conjunction with the physiologic changes in the woman's body systems are psychosocial changes occurring within the mother and family members as they face significant role and lifestyle changes.

◎ Commonly experienced emotional responses to pregnancy in the woman include ambivalence, introversion, acceptance, mood swings, and changes in body image.

◎ Reactions of expectant partners to pregnancy and to the physical and psychological changes in the woman vary greatly.

◎ A sibling's reaction to pregnancy is age dependent. The introduction of a new infant to the family is often the beginning of sibling rivalry, which results from the established child's fear of change in security of their relationships with their parents. Therefore, preparation of the siblings for the anticipated birth is imperative.

References and Recommended Readings

Academy of Nutrition and Dietetics [AND]. (2015a). *Eat right, your way, every day with foods from all ethnic traditions*. Retrieved from http://www.eatright.org/Media/content.aspx?id=6442474621#.U3DyestOXL8

Academy of Nutrition and Dietetics [AND]. (2015b). *Vegetarian pregnancy*. Retrieved from http://www.eatright.org/Public/content.aspx?id=6442478249&terms=vegetarian%20and%20pregnancy.

Alexander, L. L., LaRosa, J. H., Bader, H., & Garfield, S. (2014) *New dimensions in women's health* (6th edition). Sudbury, MA: Jones & Bartlett.

Allerberger, F., & Huhulescu, S. (2015). Pregnancy related listeriosis: Treatment and control. *Expert Review of Anti-infective Therapy, 13*(3), 395–403.

American College of Obstetricians and Gynecologists [ACOG]. (2015a). *Nutrition during pregnancy*. Retrieved from http://www.acog.org/~/media/For%20Patients/faq001.pdf?dmc=1&ts=20140510T1230032319

American College of Obstetricians and Gynecologists [ACOG]. (2015b). *Weight gain guidelines by ACOG for pregnancy*. Retrieved from http://www.womenshealthcaretopics.com/weight_gain_during_pregnancy.htm

American Pregnancy Association. (2015). Pregnancy and pica: Non-food cravings. Retrieved from http://www.americanpregnancy.org/pregnancyhealth/unusualcravingspica.html

Anil, S., Alrowis, R. M., Chalisserry, E. P., Chalissery, V. P., AlMoharib, H. S., & Al-Sulaimani, A. F. (2015). Oral health and adverse pregnancy outcomes. (pp. 631–662). Available at: http://dx.doi.org/10.5772/59517

Banerjee, A., & Williamson, C. (2015). Endocrine and metabolic emergencies in pregnancy. *Endocrine Reviews*, DOI: http://dx.doi.org/10.1210/EME.9781936704811.ch5

Bope, E. T., & Kellerman, R. D. (2015). *Conn's current therapy 2015*. Philadelphia, PA: Elsevier.

Boynton, P. M. (2015). Pregnancy: relationships advice. *The International Encyclopedia of Human Sexuality*. 861–1042.

Centers for Disease Control and Prevention. (2015). *BMI for adults: Body mass index calculator*. Retrieved from http://www.cdc.gov/nccdphp/dnpa/bmi/calc-bmi.htm

Cheng, H. M. (2015). Water balance. In *Physiology question-based learning* (pp. 127–135). Springer International Publishing. DOI: 10.1007/978-3-319-12790-3_14

Cox, S., & Reid, F. (2015). Urogynecological complications in pregnancy: an overview. *Obstetrics, Gynecology & Reproductive Medicine, 25*(5), 123–127.

Crowley, W. R. (2015). Neuroendocrine regulation of lactation and milk production. *Comprehensive Physiology. 5*(1), 255–291.

Cunningham, F. G., Leveno, K. J., Bloom, S. L., Spong, C. Y., Dashe, J. S., Hoffman, B. L., et al. (2014) *William's obstetrics* (24th ed.). New York, NY: McGraw Hill Education

Davies, J. (2015). Fatherhood Institute: Supporting fathers to play their part. *Community Practitioner, 88*(1), 13–14.

DeLoughery, T. G. (2015). Bleeding and thrombosis: Women's issues. In *Hemostasis and thrombosis* (pp. 151–155). Springer International Publishing.

Dunlevy, F. (2015). Nutritional assessment during pregnancy. *Topics in Clinical Nutrition, 30*(1), 71–79.

Edelman, C. L., Kudzma, E. C.,& Mandle, C. L. (2014). *Health promotion throughout the lifespan* (8th ed.). St. Louis, MO: Mosby Elsevier.

Einstein, A. (2015). Thinking about emotions.. *Thinking about Thinking: Cognition, science, and psychotherapy*, (pp. 68–85). New York, NY: Routledge.

Foo, L., Tay, J., Lees, C. C., McEniery, C. M., & Wilkinson, I. B. (2015). Hypertension in pregnancy: Natural history and treatment options. *Current Hypertension Reports, 17*(5), 1–18.

Foster, M. & Samman, S. (2015). Vegetarian diets across the lifecycle: impact on zinc intake and status. *Advances in Food and Nutrition Research, 74*,93--131.bib>

Food Safety and Inspection Service and Food and Drug Administration [FDA]. (2015). *Listeriosis and pregnancy*. Retrieved from http://www.fsis.usda.gov/Factsheets/Protect_Your_Baby/index.asp

Gaillard, R., & Jaddoe, V. W. (2015). Assessment of maternal blood pressure development during pregnancy. *Journal of Hypertension, 33*(1), 61–62.

Hankey, C. R. (2015). Importance of good health and nutrition before and during pregnancy. *Early years nutrition and healthy weight* (pp. 1–13). Somerset, NJ: John Wiley & Sons.

Health and Medicine Division (HMD). (2009). *Weight gain during pregnancy: Reexamining the guidelines*. Retrieved from http://www.iom.edu/Reports/2009/Weight-Gain-During-Pregnancy-Reexamining-the-Guidelines.aspx

Heffner, L. J., & Schust, D. J. (2014). *The reproductive system at a glance* (4th ed.) Sumerset, NJ: WileyBlackwell.

Heuman, D. M., Mihas, A. A., & Allen, J. (2015). Gallstones (Cholelithiasis). *eMedicine*. Available from: http://emedicine.medscape.com/article/175667-overview

Jones, R. E., & Lopez, K. H. (2014). *Human reproductive biology* (4th ed.). Waltham, MA: Elsevier.

Jordan, R. G., Engstrom, J., Matrfell, J., & Farley, C. L. (2014). *Prenatal and postnatal care: A woman-centered approach*. Ames, Iowa: Wiley-Blackwell.

Jyothi, N. (2015). Case study on post pregnancy related complication of pica. *International Journal of Nursing Care, 3*(1), 42–45.

Kim, S. H., Bennett, P. R., & Terzidou, V. (2015). Diverse roles of oxytocin. *Inflammation and Cell Signaling, 2*(1), 10–14.

King, T. L., Brucker, M. C., Kriebs, J. M., Fahey, J. O., Gegor, C. L., & Varney, H. (2015). *Varney's midwifery* (5th ed.). Burlington, MA: Jones & Bartlett Learning.

Kouhkan, S., Rahimi, A., Ghasemi, M., Naimi, S. S., & Baghban, A. A. (2015). Postural changes during first pregnancy. *British Journal of Medicine and Medical Research, 7*(9), 744–753.

Krapf, J. M. (2015). Vulvovaginitis. *eMedicine*. Available on: http://emedicine.medscape.com/article/2188931-overview

Kruger, H. S., & Butte, N. F. (2015). Nutrition in pregnancy and lactation. *Nutrition for the primary care provider*. *111*, 64–70.

Larson, L. (2015). Renal disease in pregnancy. In *Medical Management of the pregnant patient* (pp. 261–272). New York, NY: Springer Publishers.

Lutz, C. A., Mazur, E., & Litch, N. (2014). *Nutrition and diet therapy* (6th ed.). Philadelphia, PA: F.A. Davis

Matthews, A., Haas, D. M., O'Mathúna, D. P., Dowswell, T., & Doyle, M. (2014). Interventions for nausea and vomiting in early pregnancy. *Cochrane Database of Systematic Reviews*, (3). CD007575.

Mclndoo, H. (2015). The best plant-based milks. *Environmental Nutrition*, *38*(1), 5–6.

Medici, M., Korevaar, T. I., Visser, W. E., Visser, T. J., & Peeters, R. P. (2015). Thyroid function in pregnancy: What is normal?. *Clinical chemistry*, *61*(5), 704–713.

Mehta, N., Chen, K., Hardy, E., & Powrie, R. (2015). Respiratory disease in pregnancy. *Best Practice & Research Clinical Obstetrics & Gynecology*, *29*(5), 598–611.

Myers, K. M., Feltovich, H., Mazza, E., Vink, J., Bajka, M., Wapner, R. J., et al. (2015). The mechanical role of the cervix in pregnancy. *Journal of Biomechanics*. *48*(9), 1511–1523.

Nas, K., Breyer, H., & Tuu, L. (2015). The role of tailored treatment on conception and pregnancy at patients with insulin resistance. *Endocrine Abstracts*, *37*. DOI:10.1530/endoabs.37.EP189

Neifeld, R. (2015). Gluten free for the gluten tolerant during pregnancy. *BabyMed*. Retrieved from http://www.babymed.com/food-and-nutrition/gluten-free-gluten-tolerant-during-pregnancy

Nelson, R. (2015). To eat fish or not to eat fish. *American Journal of Nursing*, *115*(2), 18–19.

Ojha, S., Fainberg, H. P., Sebert, S., Budge, H., & Symonds, M. E. (2015). Maternal health and eating habits: metabolic consequences and impact on child health. *Trends in Molecular Medicine*, *21*(2), 126–133.

Osol G., & Moore L. G. (2014). Maternal uterine vascular remodeling during pregnancy. *Microcirculation*, *21*(1), 38–47.

Pearce, E. N. (2015). Thyroid disorders during pregnancy and post-partum. *Best Practice & Research Clinical Obstetrics & Gynecology*, *29*(5), 700–706.

Pellegrini, N., & Agostoni, C. (2015). Nutritional aspects of gluten-free products. *Journal of the Science of Food and Agriculture*, *95*(12), 2380–2385.

Piccoli, G., Clari, R., Vigotti, F., Leone, F., Attini, R., Cabiddu, G., et al. (2015). Vegan-vegetarian diets in pregnancy: danger or panacea? A systematic narrative review. *BJOG: An International Journal of Obstetrics & Gynecology*, *122*(5), 623–633.

Pope, E., Maltepe, C., & Koren, G. (2015). Comparing pyridoxine and doxylamine succinate-pyridoxine HCl for nausea and vomiting of pregnancy: A matched, controlled cohort study. *Journal of Clinical Pharmacology*, *57*(7), 809–814.

Qurrat-ul-Ain, & Khan, S. A. (2015). Artificial sweeteners: safe or unsafe? *JPMA. The Journal of the Pakistan Medical Association*, *65*(2), 225–227.

Rossier, B. C., Baker, M. E., & Studer, R. A. (2015). Epithelial sodium transport and its control by aldosterone: The story of our internal environment revisited. *Physiological Reviews*, *95*(1), 297–340.

Rubin, R. (1984). *Maternal identity and the maternal experience*. New York, NY: Springer.

Sabina, S., Iftequar, S., Zaheer, Z., Khan, M. M., & Khan, S. (2015) An overview of anemia in pregnancy. *Journal of Innovations in Pharmaceuticals and Biological Sciences*. *2*(2), 144–151.

Samra-Latif, O.M. (2015). Vulvovaginitis. *eMedicine*. Retrieved from http://emedicine.medscape.com/article/2188931-overview#a0101

Schummers, L., Hutcheon, J. A., Bodnar, L. M., Lieberman, E., & Himes, K. P. (2015). Risk of adverse pregnancy outcomes by pre-pregnancy body mass index: A population-based study to inform prepregnancy weight loss counseling. *Obstetrics & Gynecology*, *125*(1), 133–143.

Sharma, A. J., Vesco, K. K., Bulkley, J., Callaghan, W. M., Bruce, F. C., Staab, J., et al. (2015). Associations of gestational weight gain with preterm birth among underweight and normal weight women. *Maternal and Child Health Journal*, *19*(9), 2066–2073.

Shields, A. D. (2015). Pregnancy diagnosis. *eMedicine*. Retrieved from http://emedicine.medscape.com/article/262591-overview

Storck, S. (2015). Eating right during pregnancy. *MedlinePlus*. Retrieved from http://www.nlm.nih.gov/medlineplus/ency/patientinstructions/000584.htm

Szilagyi, A. (2015). Adult lactose digestion status and effects on disease. *Canadian Journal of Gastroenterology & Hepatology*, *29*(3), 149–156.

Thadhani, R. I., & Maynard, S. E. (2014). Renal and urinary physiology in normal pregnancy. *UpToDate*. Retrieved from http://www.uptodate.com/contents/renal-and-urinary-tract-physiology-in-normal-pregnancy

Thadhani, R.I., & Maynard, S.E. (2015). Renal and urinary tract physiology in normal pregnancy. *UpToDate*. Retrieved from http://www.uptodate.com/contents/renal-and-urinary-tract-physiology-in-normal-pregnancy

Tharpe, N. L., Farley, C. L., & Jordan, R. (2016). *Clinical practice guidelines for midwifery & women's health* (5th ed.). Sudbury, MA: Jones & Bartlett.

Tretti Clementoni, M., & Lavagno, R. (2015). A novel 1565 nm non-ablative fractional device for stretch marks: A preliminary report. *Journal of Cosmetic and Laser Therapy*, *17*(3), 148–155.

Trivedi, S., Lal, N., & Singhal, R. (2015). Periodontal diseases and pregnancy. *Journal of Orofacial Sciences*, *7*(1), 67–68.

Trupin, S. R. (2015). Common pregnancy complaints and questions. *eMedicine*. Retrieved from http://emedicine.medscape.com/article/259724-overview

Tyler, K. H. (2015). Physiological skin changes during pregnancy. *Clinical Obstetrics and Gynecology*, *58*(1), 119–124.

U.S. Department of Agriculture [USDA] (2015). *Health and nutrition information for pregnant and breastfeeding women*. Retrieved from http://www.choosemyplate.gov/pregnancy-breastfeeding/pregnancy-nutritional-needs.html

U.S. Food and Drug Administration [FDA] (2015). *What you need to know about mercury in fish and shellfish*. Retrieved from http://www.fda.gov/food/resourcesforyou/consumers/ucm110591.htm

U.S. Department of Agriculture [USDA] and U.S. Department of Health and Human Services [USDHHS]. *Dietary guidelines for Americans*, 2015 (8th ed.) Retrieved from http://www.health.gov/dietaryguidelines/2015.asp

U.S. Preventive Services Task Force [USPSTF]. (2015). Folic acid for the prevention of neural tube defects: U.S. Preventive Services Task Force recommendation statement. Retrieved from http://www.ahrq.gov/clinic/pocketgd1011/gcp10s2.htm

Walsh, J. M., & McAuliffe, F. M. (2015). Impact of maternal nutrition on pregnancy outcome–Does it matter what pregnant women eat?. *Best Practice & Research Clinical Obstetrics & Gynecology*, *29*(1), 63–78.

Zinaman, M. J., Johnson, S., & Marriott, L. (2015). Analysis of human chorionic gonadotropin levels in normal and failing pregnancies [40]. *Obstetrics & Gynecology*, *125*, 21S–22S.

CHAPTER WORKSHEET

MULTIPLE-CHOICE QUESTIONS

1. What factors would change during a pregnancy if the hormone progesterone were reduced or withdrawn?
   a. The woman's gums would become red and swollen and would bleed easily.
   b. The uterus would contract more and peristalsis would increase.
   c. Morning sickness would increase and would be prolonged.
   d. The secretion of prolactin by the pituitary gland would be inhibited.

2. Which of the following is a presumptive sign or symptom of pregnancy?
   a. Restlessness
   b. Elevated mood
   c. Urinary frequency
   d. Low backache

3. When obtaining a blood test for pregnancy, which hormone would the nurse expect the test to measure?
   a. Human chorionic gonadotropin (hCG)
   b. Human placental lactogen (hPL)
   c. Follicle-stimulating hormone (FSH)
   d. Luteinizing hormone (LH)

4. During pregnancy, which of the following should the expectant mother reduce or avoid?
   a. Raw meat or uncooked shellfish
   b. Fresh, washed fruits and vegetables
   c. Whole grains and cereals
   d. Protein and iron from meat sources

5. A feeling expressed by most women upon learning they are pregnant is:
   a. Acceptance
   b. Depression
   c. Jealousy
   d. Ambivalence

6. Reva Rubin identified four major tasks that the pregnant woman undertakes to form a mutually gratifying relationship with her infant. What is "binding in?"
   a. Ensuring safe passage through pregnancy, labor, and birth.
   b. Seeking acceptance of this infant by others.
   c. Seeking acceptance of self as mother to the infant.
   d. Learning to give of oneself on behalf of the infant.

7. A pregnant client close to term comes in the clinic for an exam. The woman complains about experiencing shortness of breath. The nurse knows that this complaint can be explained as the:
   a. Fetus needs more oxygen now that his/her size is larger.
   b. Fundus of the uterus is high and pushing the diaphragm upwards.
   c. Woman is experiencing an allergic reaction because of high histamine levels.
   d. Oxygen partial pressure concentration is lower in the third trimester.

8. Which of the following fish should be limited in a pregnant woman's diet because of the high mercury content?
   a. Salmon
   b. Cod
   c. Shrimp
   d. Sword fish

CRITICAL THINKING EXERCISES

1. When interviewing a woman at her first prenatal visit, the nurse asks about her feelings. The woman replies, "I'm frightened and confused. I don't know whether I want to be pregnant or not. Being pregnant means changing our whole life, and now having somebody to care for all the time. I'm not sure I would be a good mother. Plus I'm a bit afraid of all the changes that would happen to my body. Is this normal? Am I okay?"
   a. How should the nurse answer this question?
   b. What specific information is needed to support the client during this pregnancy?

2. Sally, age 23, is 9 weeks pregnant. At her clinic visit she says, "I'm so tired I can barely make it home from work. Then once I'm home, I don't have the energy to make dinner." She says she is so sick in the morning that she is frequently late to work and spends much of the day in the bathroom. Sally's current lab work is within normal limits.
   a. What explanation can the nurse offer Sally about her discomforts?
   b. What interventions can the nurse offer to Sally?

3. Bringing a new infant into the family affects the siblings. What strategies can a nurse discuss when a mother asks how to deal with this?

STUDY ACTIVITIES

1. Go to your local health department's maternity clinic and interview several women regarding their feelings and the bodily changes that have taken place since they became pregnant. Based on your findings, place them into appropriate trimesters of their pregnancy.

2. Search the Internet for information about the psychological changes that occur during pregnancy. Share information from the websites you found with your clinical group.

3. During pregnancy, the plasma volume increases by 50% but the RBC volume increases by only 25% to 33%. This disproportion is manifested as _____.

4. When a pregnant woman in her third trimester lies on her back and experiences dizziness and light-headedness, the underlying cause of this is _____.

BRINGING IT ALL TOGETHER: CASE STUDY

A 22-year-old pregnant client presents to the maternity clinic with a 4-day history of loss of appetite, constipation, and abdominal pain. She is in the first trimester of her first pregnancy and came to this country recently from India. Her mother accompanies her and answers most of the questions for her daughter. After much questioning, the mother reveals that her daughter frequently eats dirt, which is a common practice in her country.

ASSESSMENT

Examination reveals a tired-looking young woman, normal vital signs, moist pale mucous membranes, and a moderately distended abdomen. Bowel sounds are slow and faint. The fetal heart rate is within normal range.

Go to thePoint **to find questions to consider about this case.**

12

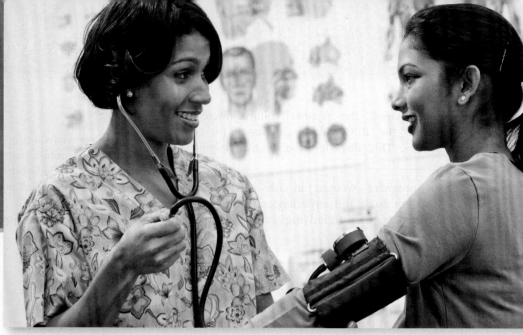

Nursing Management During Pregnancy

Learning Objectives

Upon completion of the chapter, you will be able to:

1. Relate the information typically collected at the initial prenatal visit.

2. Determine an appropriate reproductive life plan based on a couple's risk profile.

3. Select the assessments completed at follow-up prenatal visits.

4. Evaluate the tests used to assess maternal and fetal well-being, including nursing management for each.

5. Outline appropriate nursing management to promote maternal self-care and to minimize the common discomforts of pregnancy.

6. Examine the key components of perinatal education.

Linda and her husband, Rob, are eager to start a family within the next year. They are stable in their careers and financially secure. They decide to investigate a new nurse–midwife practice associated with the local hospital, and they go for a preconception appointment. They leave their appointment overwhelmed with all the information they were given about having a healthy pregnancy.

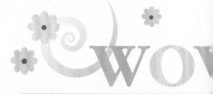

Words of Wisdom
The secret of human touch is simple: showing a sincere liking and interest in people. Nurses need to use touch often.

INTRODUCTION

Pregnancy is a time of many physiologic and psychological changes that can positively or negatively affect the woman, her fetus, and her family. Misconceptions, inadequate information, and unanswered questions about pregnancy, birth, and parenthood are common. The ultimate goal of any pregnancy is the birth of a healthy newborn, and nurses play a major role in helping the pregnant woman and her partner achieve this goal. Ongoing assessment and education are essential.

This chapter describes the nursing management required during pregnancy. It begins with a brief discussion of preconception care and then describes the assessment of the woman at the first prenatal visit and on follow-up visits. The chapter discusses tests commonly used to assess maternal and fetal well-being, including specific nursing management related to each test. The chapter also identifies important strategies to minimize the common discomforts of pregnancy and promote self-care. Finally, the chapter discusses perinatal education, including childbirth education, birthing options, health care provider options, preparation for breast-feeding or bottle-feeding, and final preparation for labor and birth.

PRECONCEPTION CARE

Ideally, couples thinking about having a child should schedule a visit with their health care provider for preconception counseling to ensure that they are in the best possible state of health before pregnancy. **Preconception care** is the promotion of the health and well-being of a woman and her partner before pregnancy. The goal of preconception care is to identify and modify biomedical, behavioral, and social risks to a woman's health or pregnancy outcome through prevention and management interventions (Centers for Disease Control and Prevention [CDC], 2015a).

Preconception care is advocated throughout the world as a tool for improving perinatal outcomes. Preconception care should occur any time a health care provider sees a woman of reproductive age. Primary care for all women of childbearing age by nurses should include a routine assessment of a woman's reproductive goals and planning. Women who could potentially become pregnant should be assessed for preconception risks and educated about the importance of maternal health in ensuring healthy pregnancies. Women may be motivated to address modified health risks by learning about the way their present health will affect a future pregnancy. For women not intending a pregnancy soon, preconception care should focus on contraception counseling (Callegari, Ma, & Schwartz, 2015). Personal and family history, physical examination, laboratory screening, reproductive plan, nutrition, supplements, weight, exercise, vaccinations, and injury prevention should be reviewed in all women.

Encourage folic acid 400 to 800 mcg per day depending on risk profile, as well as proper diet and exercise. Women should receive the influenza vaccine if planning pregnancy during flu season; the rubella and varicella vaccines if there is no evidence of immunity to these viruses; and tetanus/diphtheria/pertussis if lacking adult vaccination. Offer specific interventions to reduce morbidity and mortality for both the woman who has been identified with chronic diseases or exposed to teratogens or illicit substances and her baby. Several interventions have been proven to effectively improve pregnancy outcome when provided as preconception care. Recent research suggests that events that occur in the uterine decidua, even before a woman knows she is pregnant, may have a significant impact on fetal growth and the outcome of pregnancy. In addition, an intact immune system optimizes placental development and function and is essential for fetal survival (Regal, Gilbert, & Burwick, 2015). New insights reveal that the early embryo is extremely sensitive to signals from gametes, trophoblastic tissue, and periconception maternal lifestyles. Also, environmental factors prior to and after conception have an enormous impact on the developing embryo and cause long-term health problems. There is a growing body of evidence that environmental factors during embryonic development can cause irreversible alteration in epigenetic markers and induce various adult diseases, such as cardiovascular, neurologic, and metabolic disorders later in life (Keytash, Jones, & Frances, 2015). With this in mind, shifting the focus on the periconception period and the very early stages of pregnancy should offer significant benefits to the health of both the mother and her infant. The overall aim should be to effectively use every pregnancy as the health care opportunity of two lifetimes (Steeggers-Theunissen & Steegers, 2015).

The CDC (2015b) formulated 10 guidelines for preconception care (see Box 12.1).

Risk Factors for Adverse Pregnancy Outcomes

Preconception care is just as important as prenatal care to reduce adverse pregnancy outcomes such as maternal and infant mortality, preterm births, and low–birth-weight infants. Adverse pregnancy outcomes constitute a major public health challenge: 13% of infants are born premature; 8.3% are born with low birth weight; 1 in 33 live births have major birth defects; and 32% of women suffer pregnancy complications (CDC, 2015c). Risk factors for these adverse pregnancy outcomes are prevalent among women of reproductive age, as demonstrated by the following statistics:

- 10% of women smoke during pregnancy, contributing to fetal addiction to nicotine.
- 7.6% consume alcohol during pregnancy, leading to fetal alcohol spectrum disorder.

TEN GUIDELINES FOR PRECONCEPTION CARE

- **Recommendation 1.** Individual responsibility across the lifespan: Each woman, man, and couple should be encouraged to have a reproductive life plan.
- **Recommendation 2.** Consumer awareness: Increase public awareness of the importance of preconception health behaviors and preconception care services by using information and tools appropriate across various ages; literacy, including health literacy; and cultural/linguistic contexts.
- **Recommendation 3.** Preventive visits: As a part of primary care visits, provide risk assessment and educational and health promotion counseling to all women of childbearing age to reduce reproductive risks and improve pregnancy outcomes.
- **Recommendation 4.** Interventions for identified risks: Increase the proportion of women who receive interventions as follow-up to preconception risk screening, focusing on high-priority interventions (i.e., those with evidence of effectiveness and greatest potential impact).
- **Recommendation 5.** Interconception care: Use the interconception period to provide additional intensive interventions to women who have had a previous pregnancy that ended in an adverse outcome (i.e., infant death, fetal loss, birth defects, low birth weight, or preterm birth).
- **Recommendation 6.** Prepregnancy checkup: Offer, as a component of maternity care, one prepregnancy visit for couples and persons planning pregnancy.
- **Recommendation 7.** Health insurance coverage for women with low incomes: Increase public and private health insurance coverage for women with low incomes to improve access to preventive women's health and preconception and interconception care.
- **Recommendation 8.** Public health programs and strategies: Integrate components of preconception health into existing local public health and related programs, including emphasis on interconception interventions for women with previous adverse outcomes.
- **Recommendation 9.** Research: Increase the evidence base and promote the use of the evidence to improve preconception health.
- **Recommendation 10.** Monitoring improvements: Maximize public health surveillance and related research mechanisms to monitor preconception health.

Adapted from Centers for Disease Control and Prevention. (2015b). *Preconception care recommendations.* Retrieved from http://www.cdc.gov/preconception/hcp/recommendations.html

- 70% of women do not take folic acid supplements, increasing the risk of neural tube defects in the newborn. Taking folic acid reduces the incidence of neural tube defects by two thirds.

- 35% of women starting a pregnancy are obese, which may increase their risk of developing hypertension, diabetes, and thromboembolic disease and may increase the need for cesarean birth.
- 3% take prescription or over-the-counter drugs that are known teratogens (substances harmful to the developing fetus).
- 5% of women have preexisting medical conditions that can negatively affect pregnancy if unmanaged (CDC, 2015d).

All of the preceding factors pose risks to pregnancy and could be addressed with early interventions if the woman seeks preconception health care. Specific recognized risk factors for adverse pregnancy outcomes that fall into one or more of these categories are listed in Box 12.2.

The period of greatest environmental sensitivity and consequent risk for the developing embryo is between days 17 and 56 after conception. The first prenatal visit, which is usually a month or later after a missed menstrual period, may occur too late to affect reproductive outcomes associated with abnormal organogenesis secondary to poor lifestyle choices. In some cases, such as with unplanned pregnancies, women may delay seeking health care because they deny that they are pregnant. Thus, commonly used prevention practices may begin too late to avert the morbidity and mortality associated with congenital anomalies and low birth weight. A more global preventative strategy is needed to reduce the high rates of pregnancy complications in all populations. Securing international-level political priority for maternal and newborn care remains critical to accomplish the goal of better health for all families. All couples should take on the responsibility of developing their reproductive life plan and share it with their health care providers at office visits (Darmstadt, Shiffman, & Lawn, 2015).

What is the purpose of couples like Linda and Rob going for preconception counseling? What are the goals of preconception care for this couple? What psychological support can be offered by the nurse to this couple at this stage?

Nursing Management

In the United States, rates of maternal mortality, unintended pregnancies, low birth weight, and preterm infants continue to rise, making the need for preconception care a priority for all nurses. Traditionally, women have thought that preconception care is a single visit made before getting pregnant; however, the maximum benefits are obtained when the woman and her partner receive care throughout her reproductive years. The nurse's role is vital in identifying risk factors and encouraging healthier behaviors that potentially improve

BOX 12.2

RISK FACTORS FOR ADVERSE PREGNANCY OUTCOMES

- **Isotretinoins.** Use of isotretinoins (e.g., Accutane®) in pregnancy to treat acne can result in **alcohol misuse**. No time during pregnancy is safe to drink alcohol, and harm can occur early, before a woman has realized that she is or might be pregnant. Fetal alcohol syndrome and other alcohol-related birth defects can be prevented if women cease intake of alcohol before conception.
- **Antiepileptic drugs.** Certain antiepileptic drugs are known teratogens (e.g., valproic acid). Recommendations suggest that before conception, women who are on a regimen of these drugs and who are contemplating pregnancy should be prescribed a lower dosage of these drugs.
- **Diabetes (preconception).** The threefold increase in the prevalence of birth defects among infants of women with type 1 and type 2 diabetes is substantially reduced through proper management of diabetes.
- **Folic acid deficiency.** Daily use of vitamin supplements containing folic acid (400 mcg) has been demonstrated to reduce the occurrence of neural tube defects by two thirds.
- **Hepatitis B.** Vaccination is recommended for men and women who are at risk for acquiring hepatitis B virus (HBV) infection. Preventing HBV infection in women of childbearing age prevents transmission of infection to infants and eliminates risk to the woman of HBV infection and sequelae, including hepatic failure, liver carcinoma, cirrhosis, and death.
- **HIV/AIDS.** If HIV infection is identified before conception, timely antiretroviral treatment can be administered, and women (or couples) can be given additional information that can help prevent mother-to-child transmission.
- **Rubella seronegativity.** Rubella vaccination provides protective seropositivity and prevents congenital rubella syndrome.
- **Obesity.** Adverse perinatal outcomes associated with maternal obesity include neural tube defects, preterm delivery, diabetes, cesarean section, and hypertensive and thromboembolic disease. Appropriate weight loss and nutritional intake before pregnancy reduce these risks.
- **Sexually transmitted infections (STIs).** *Chlamydia trachomatis* and *Neisseria gonorrhoeae* have been strongly associated with ectopic pregnancy, infertility, and chronic pelvic pain. STIs during pregnancy might result in fetal death or substantial physical and developmental disabilities, including intellectual disability and blindness. Early screening and treatment prevent these adverse outcomes.
- **Smoking.** Preterm birth, low birth weight, and other adverse perinatal outcomes associated with maternal smoking in pregnancy can be prevented if women stop smoking before or during early pregnancy. Because only 20% of women successfully control tobacco dependency during pregnancy, cessation of smoking is recommended before pregnancy.

Adapted from Centers for Disease Control and Prevention. (2015a). *Preconception care and health care*. Retrieved from http://www.cdc.gov/preconception/hcp/; March of Dimes. (2015a). *Pregnancy complications*. Retrieved from http://www.marchofdimes.com/pregnancy/pregnancy-complications.aspx; National Institutes of Health. (2015). *Health problems in pregnancy*. Retrieved from http://www.nlm.nih.gov/medlineplus/healthproblemsinpregnancy.html; Senie, R. T. (2014). *Epidemiology of women's health*. Burlington, MA: Jones & Bartlett Learning.

maternal and perinatal outcomes. Preconception care involves obtaining a complete health history and physical examination of the woman and her partner. Key areas include:

- immunization status of the woman;
- underlying medical conditions, such as cardiovascular and respiratory problems or genetic disorders;
- reproductive health data, such as pelvic examinations, use of contraceptives, and STIs;
- sexuality and sexual practices, such as safer-sex practices and body image issues;
- nutrition history and present status;
- lifestyle practices, including occupation and recreational activities;
- psychosocial issues such as levels of stress and exposure to abuse and violence;
- medication and drug use, including use of tobacco, alcohol, over-the-counter and prescription medications, and illicit drugs;
- support system, including family, friends, and community.

Figure 12.1 gives a sample preconception screening tool.

This information provides a foundation for planning health promotion activities and education. For example, to have a positive impact on the pregnancy:

- ensure that the woman's immunizations are up to date;
- create a reproductive life plan to address and outline their reproductive needs;
- take a thorough history of both partners to identify any medical or genetic conditions that need treatment or a referral to specialists;
- identify history of STIs and high-risk sexual practices so they can be modified;
- complete a dietary history combined with nutritional counseling;
- gather information regarding exercise and lifestyle practices to encourage daily exercise for well-being and weight maintenance;
- stress the importance of taking folic acid to prevent neural tube defects;

PRECONCEPTION SCREENING AND COUNSELING CHECKLIST

NAME	BIRTHPLACE	AGE

DATE: /   /   ARE YOU PLANNING TO GET PREGNANT IN THE NEXT SIX MONTHS? ___ Y ___N

IF YOUR ANSWER TO A QUESTION IS YES, PUT A CHECK MARK ON THE LINE IN FRONT OF THE QUESTION. FILL IN OTHER INFORMATION THAT APPLIES TO YOU .

DIET AND EXERCISE

What do you consider a healthy weight for you?_____
___Do you eat three meals a day?
___Do you follow a special diet (vegetarian, diabetic, other)?
___Which do you drink (__ coffee __ tea __ cola __ milk __ water __ soda/pop
    other_____)?
___Do you eat raw or undercooked food (meat, other)?
___Do you take folic acid?
___Do you take other vitamins daily (__ multivitamin __ vitamin A __ other)?
___Do you take dietary supplements (__ black cohosh __ pennyroyal __ other)?
___Do you have current/past problems withh eating disorders?
___Do you exercise? Type/frequency:_____
Notes:

LIFESTYLE

___Do you smoke cigarettes or use other tobacco products?
    How many cigarettes/packs a day?_____
___Are you exposed to second-hand smoke?
___Do you drink alcohol?
    What kind?_____How often?_____How much?_____
___Do you use recreational drugs (cocaine, heroin, ecstasy, meth/ice, other?
    List:_____
___Do you see a dentist regularly?
    What kind of work do you do?_____
___Do you work or live near possible hazards (chemicals, x-ray or other radiation,
    lead)? List:_____
___Do you use saunas or hot tubs?
Notes:

MEDICATION /DRUGS

___Are you taking prescribed drugs (Accutane, valproic acid, blood thinners)? List
    them_____
___Are you taking non-prescribed drugs?
    List them:_____
___Are you using birth control pills?
___Do you get injectable contraceptives or shots for birth control?
___Do you use any herbal remedies or alternative medicine?
    List:_____
NOTES:

MEDICAL/FAMILY HISTORY

Do you have or have you ever had:
___Epilepsy?
___Diabetes?
___Asthma?
___High blood pressure?
___Heart disease?
___Anemia?
___Kidney or bladder disorders?
___Thyroid disease?
___Chickenpox?
___Hepatitis C?
___Digestive problems?
___Depression or other mental health problem?
___Surgeries?
___Lupus?
___Scleroderma?
___Other conditions?
Have you ever been vaccinated for:
___Measles, mumps, rubella?
___Hepatitis B?
___Chickenpox?
NOTES:

WOMEN'S HEALTH

___Do you have any problems with your menstrual cycle?
___How many times have you been pregnant?
    What was/ were the outcomes(s)?_____
___Did you have difficulty getting pregnant last time?
___Have you been treated for infertility?
    Have you had surgery on your uterus, cervix, ovaries, or tubes?
___Did you mother take the hormone DES during pregnancy?
    Have you ever had HPV, genital warts or chlamydia?
___Have you ever been treated for a sexually transmitted infection (genital herpes,
    gonorrhea, syphilis, HIV/AIDS, other)? List:_____
NOTES:

GENETICS

Does your family have a history of   Or   Your partner's family
___Hemophilia?   ___
___Other bleeding disorders?   ___
___Tay-Sachs disease?   ___
___Blood diseases (sickle cell, thalassemia, other)?   ___
___Muscular dystrophy?   ___
___Down syndrome/mental retardation?   ___
___Cystic fibrosis?   ___
___Birth defects (spine/heart/kidney)?   ___
Your ethnic background is:_____
Your partner's ethnic background is: _____
NOTES:

HOME ENVIRONMENT

___Do you feel emotionally supported at home?
___Do you have help from relatives or friends if needed?
___Do you feel you have serious money/financial worries?
___Are you in a stable relationship?
___Do you feel safe at home?
___Does anyone threaten or physically hurt you?
___Do you have pets (cats, rodents, exotic animals)? List:_____
___Do have any contact with soil, cat litter, or sandboxes?

Baby preparation (if planning pregnancy):
___Do you have a place for a baby to sleep?
___Do you need any baby items?
NOTES:

OTHER

IS THERE ANYTHING ELSE YOU'D LIKE ME TO KNOW?

ARE THERE ANY QUESTIONS YOU'D LIKE TO ASK ME?

FIGURE 12.1 Sample preconception screening tool. (Used with permission. Copyright March of Dimes.)

- urge the woman to achieve optimal weight before a pregnancy;
- identify work environment and any needed changes to promote health;
- address substance use issues, including smoking and drugs;
- identify victims of violence and assist them to get help;
- manage chronic conditions such as diabetes and asthma;
- educate the couple about environmental hazards, including metals and herbs;
- offer genetic counseling to identify carriers;
- suggest the availability of support systems, if needed (Hurst & Linton, 2015; Templeton, 2015).

Nurses can act as advocates and educators, creating healthy, supportive communities for women and their partners in the childbearing phases of their lives. It is important to enter into a collaborative partnership with the woman and her partner, enabling them to examine their own health and its influence on the health of their future baby. Provide information to allow the woman and her partner to make an informed decision about having a baby, but keep in mind that this decision rests solely with the couple.

Take Note!

Because all women of reproductive age, from menarche to menopause, benefit from preventive care, preconception care should be an integral part of that continuum (Boggess & Berggren, 2015).

Linda and Rob decide to change several aspects of their lifestyle and nutritional habits before conceiving a baby, based on advice from the nurse-midwife. They both want to lose weight, stop smoking, and increase their intake of fruits and vegetables. How will these lifestyle and dietary changes benefit Linda's future pregnancy? What other areas might need to be brought up to date to prepare for a future pregnancy?

THE FIRST PRENATAL VISIT

Once a pregnancy is suspected and, in some cases, tentatively confirmed by a home pregnancy test, the woman should seek prenatal care to promote a healthy outcome. Although the most opportune window (preconception) for improving pregnancy outcomes may be missed, appropriate nursing management starting at conception and continuing throughout the pregnancy can have a positive impact on the health of pregnant women and their unborn children.

The assessment process begins at this initial prenatal visit and continues throughout the pregnancy. The initial visit is an ideal time to screen for factors that might place the woman and her fetus at risk for problems such as preterm delivery. The initial visit also is an optimal time to begin educating the client about changes that will affect her life.

Prenatal care can be delivered in one of the two methods: individually or in a group format termed *centering*. The first method is the traditional model whereby a pregnant woman sees her health care provider at specified interims throughout her pregnancy and all visits occur on a one-to-one basis. The centering pregnancy model of group prenatal care involves groups of up to a dozen women in similar gestational ages meeting with their health care provider for 10 sessions of approximately 1.5 to 2 hours each. The centering group method has been theorized to produce better birth outcomes than traditional individually delivered prenatal care due to increased client–provider interaction, increased social support, and greater perceived empowerment (Tracy, 2014). See Evidence-Based Practice 12.1.

The International Association of Diabetes and Pregnancy Study Groups (IADPSG) recently issued recommendations on the diagnosis and classification of hyperglycemia in pregnancy. Specific recommendations for diagnosing hyperglycemic disorders in pregnancy include the following:

- At the *first prenatal visit*, measure fasting plasma glucose, HbA1c, or random plasma glucose of all women or all high-risk women based on her risk factors, weight status, and family history. Thresholds for diagnosis of overt diabetes during pregnancy are shown in Box 12.3.
- If glucose testing is not diagnostic of overt diabetes, the woman should be tested for gestational diabetes from 24 to 28 weeks of gestation with a 2-hour 75-g oral glucose tolerance test (American Diabetes Association [ADA], 2015).

Given our society's poor food choices, sedentary tendencies, obesity, increasing life stresses, and the increasing immigration of high-risk populations (Hispanic, African American, Southeast Asian, Arab, Afro-Caribbean, Mediterranean, and Native American), the incidence of gestational diabetes is growing. The American College of Obstetricians and Gynecologists (ACOG), the American

---

BOX 12.3

THRESHOLDS FOR DIAGNOSIS OF OVERT DIABETES DURING PREGNANCY

The thresholds for the diagnosis of overt diabetes during pregnancy are:
- Fasting plasma glucose: 126 mg/dL
- Hemoglobin A1c level: at least 6.5%
- Random plasma glucose: 200 mg/dL

EVIDENCE-BASED PRACTICE 12.1 THE EFFECTS OF CENTERING PREGNANCY GROUP PRENATAL CARE ON GESTATIONAL AGE, BIRTH WEIGHT, AND FETAL DEMISE

STUDY

Although rates of infant mortality in the United States have declined over the last several decades, rates of preterm births (<27 weeks gestation) and low birth weight (<2,500 g) have increased. Access to quality prenatal care has demonstrated improvement of maternal and child outcomes, and may help reduce infant mortality, preterm birth, and low-weight infants. The centering group prenatal care model has been theorized to produce better birth outcomes than traditional individually delivered prenatal care due to increased patient–provider interaction, increased social support, greater perceived empowerment, and increased exposure to useful skills and information about pregnancy, birthing, and childcare.

This study compared birth outcomes for women who received two different forms of prenatal care. The objective of this study was to examine the effects of centering prenatal care versus individually delivered prenatal care on gestational age, birth weight, and fetal demise. Samples of 6,155 women were divided into two groups—individual prenatal care and group prenatal care at five sites. The sample included women who received prenatal care at one of the five sites that offered both individual and group prenatal care.

Findings

Results indicated that women in the centering pregnancy group prenatal care, compared with women in traditional individually delivered prenatal care, had significantly longer gestational ages ($b = .35$, 95% CI [.29, .41]) and higher overall birth weights ($b = 28.6$, 95 % CI [4.8, 52.3]). Results also indicated that group-delivered prenatal care was associated with significantly and substantially lower odds of very low birth weight and fetal demise.

Nursing Implications

At present there is support to provide centering group prenatal care where possible according to guidelines. The results indicated largely beneficial effects of group prenatal care on women's birth outcomes. Health policy reforms aimed at reducing adverse birth outcomes may consider group prenatal care a promising alternative format for delivering prenatal care. Nurses should continue to encourage all women to obtain prenatal care (group or traditional) as part of their reproductive plan to enhance the outcomes of their pregnancy and all of their future children. Given the evidence of beneficial effects of centering group prenatal care and the cost implications of widespread implementation will be critical for informing state and local health policies aimed at improving maternal and perinatal health outcomes.

Adapted from Tanner-Smith, E., Steinka-Fry, K., & Lipsey, M. (2014). The effects of centering pregnancy group prenatal care on gestational age, birth weight, and fetal demise. *Maternal & Child Health Journal, 18*(4), 801–809.

Diabetes Association (ADA), and the World Health Organization (WHO) have all recommended screening at the first prenatal visit for women who are over 25 years old, overweight, have polycystic ovary syndrome, history of gestational diabetes, and a positive family history of diabetes (Satyan et al., 2015). Global guidelines for screening, diagnosis, and classification have been established, and offer the potential to stop the cycle of diabetes and obesity caused by hyperglycemia in pregnancy. Normoglycemia is the goal in all aspects of pregnancy and offers the benefits of decreased short-term and long-term complications of diabetes.

Counseling and education of the pregnant woman and her partner are critical to ensure healthy outcomes for mother and her infant. Pregnant women and their partners frequently have questions, misinformation, or misconceptions about what to eat, weight gain, physical discomforts, drug and alcohol use, sexuality, and the birthing process. The nurse needs to allow time to answer questions and provide anticipatory guidance during the pregnancy and to make appropriate community referrals to meet the needs of these clients. To address these issues and foster the overall well-being of pregnant women and their fetuses, specific national health goals have been established (see *Healthy People 2020*).

Comprehensive Health History

During the initial visit, a comprehensive health history is obtained, including age, menstrual history, prior obstetric history, past medical and surgical history, psychological screening, family history, genetic screening, dietary habits, lifestyle and health practices, medication or drug use, and history of exposure to STIs (Moses, 2015a). Often, use of a prenatal history form (Fig. 12.2) is the best way to document the data collected (see Evidence-Based Practice 12.2).

The initial health history typically includes questions about three major areas: the reason for seeking care; the client's past medical, surgical, and personal history, including that of the family and her partner; and the client's reproductive history. During the history-taking process, the nurse and client establish the foundation of a trusting relationship and jointly develop a plan of care for the pregnancy. They tailor this plan to the client's lifestyle as much as possible and focus primarily on education for overall wellness during the pregnancy. The ultimate goal for the first prenatal visit is to collect baseline data about the woman and her partner and to detect any risk factors that need to be addressed to facilitate a healthy pregnancy (King et al., 2015). See *Healthy People 2020 12.1*.

(text continues on page 372)

HEALTHY PEOPLE 2020 • *12.1*

Objective	Nursing Significance
MICH-10 Increase the proportion of pregnant women who receive early and adequate prenatal care by 10% over *HP 2010* goal.	Will contribute to reduced rates of perinatal illness, disability, and death by helping to identify possible risk factors and implementing measures to lessen these factors that contribute to poor outcomes
MICH-12 (Developmental) Increase the proportion of pregnant women who attend a series of prepared childbirth classes.	Will contribute to a positive birthing experience because women will be prepared for what they will face; will also help in reducing pain and anxiety
MICH-13 (Developmental) Increase the proportion of mothers who achieve a recommended weight gain during their pregnancies.	Will reduce the risks associated with weight for better perinatal outcomes for mother and infant
MICH-16 Increase the proportion of women delivering a live birth who received preconception care services and practiced key recommended preconception health behaviors: • Took multivitamins/folic acid prior to pregnancy • Did not smoke prior to pregnancy • Did not drink alcohol prior to pregnancy • (Developmental) Used contraception to plan pregnancy	The risk of maternal and infant mortality and pregnancy-related complications can be reduced by increasing access to quality preconception care. This will enhance healthy birth outcomes and early identification and treatment of health.

Adapted from U.S. Department of Health and Human Services. (2010). *Healthy People 2020*. Retrieved from http://www.healthypeople.gov/2020/topicsobjectives2020/objectiveslist.aspx?topicId=26

EVIDENCE-BASED PRACTICE 12.2 — ANTENATAL DIETARY EDUCATION AND SUPPLEMENTATION TO INCREASE ENERGY AND PROTEIN INTAKE

STUDY

Gestational weight gain is positively associated with fetal growth, and observational studies of food supplementation in pregnancy have reported increases in gestational weight gain and fetal growth. During pregnancy, the fetus develops based on the nutrition of the mother. Inadequate intake during pregnancy can lead to malnutrition and poor outcomes for the fetus. The objective of this study was to assess the effects of education during pregnancy to increase energy and protein intake, or of actual energy and protein supplementation, on energy and protein intake, and the effect on maternal and infant health outcomes.

Findings

The review included 17 randomized controlled trials, involving 9,030 women. Four main findings included (1) providing nutritional advice resulted in an increase in the mother's protein intake with resulting fewer preterm births and low birth weights; (2) giving mothers balanced energy and protein supplements was associated with fewer infants dying during labor and infants had an increase in birth weights; (3) high protein supplementation showed no benefit for women and potential harm for the infant with more becoming small for gestational age at birth; and (4) isocaloric protein supplementations showed no benefit for higher birth weight in the infant and weekly gestational gain for the mothers.

Nursing Implications

This review provides encouraging evidence that prenatal nutritional education with the aim of increasing energy and protein intake in the maternal population appears to be effective in reducing the risk of preterm birth, low birth weight, increasing head circumference at birth, increasing birth weight among undernourished women, and increasing protein intake. There remains question about high protein supplementation being beneficial. Nurses can continue to provide good sound evidence-based nutritional education to their pregnant clients to bring about healthy outcomes.

Adapted from Ota, E., Hori, H., Mori, R., Tobe-Gai, R., & Farrar, D. (2015). Antenatal dietary education and supplementation to increase energy and protein intake. *Cochrane Database of Systematic Reviews*, (6), CD000032. doi: 10.1002/14651858.CD000032. pub3.

Health History Summary
Maternal/Newborn Record System

Page 1 of 2

Patient's name _____

ID. No. _____

_____

_____

Demographic data

Date of birth _____ Age ____ Language □ _____ □ English □ N/A   □ None   Interpreter □ _____

Religion □ _____ Race/ethnicity _____

Marital status S M SEP D W   Name of baby's father _____

Allergy/sensitivity

□ None □ Latex

□ Other _____

Education	Occupation	Full	Part	Self	Unemp	Work Tel No	Home Tel No
Patient		□	□	□	□		
Father of baby		□	□	□	□		

Primary/referring physician

Menstrual history

Menarche yrs	Interval days	Length days	Abnormalities □ None

LMP ___/___/___   Certain □ Yes □ No   Normal □ Yes □ No   Positive pregnancy test ___/___/___   □ Blood □ Urine

EDD   By dates ___/___/___   By ultrasound ___/___/___   Date of ultrasound ___/___/___

Pregnancy history	Gravida	Full term	Premature	Spontaneous Ab	Induced Ab	Ectopic	Multiple births	Live

No	Month/ year	Infant sex	Weight at birth	Wks gest	Hours in labor	Type of delivery	Anesthesia	Comments/complications
1								
2								
3								
4								
5								
6								
7								

Medical history

Obstetric   Patient
1. Anemia _____ □
2. Fetal/neonatal death or anomaly _____ □
3. Gestational diabetes _____ □
4. Hemorrhage _____ □
5. Hyperemesis _____ □
6. Incompetent cervix _____ □
7. Intrauterine growth retardation _____ □
8. Isoimmunization _____ □
9. Polyhydramnios _____ □
10. Postpartum depression ____ □
11. Pregnancy-induced hypertension _____ □
12. Preterm labor or birth ____ □
13. PROM-chorioamnionitis ___ □
14. Rhogam given _____ □
15. RH neg _____ □

Gynecologic
16. Contraceptive use _____ □
17. Abnormal PAP _____ □
18. Fibroids _____ □
19. Gyn· surgery _____ □

Check and detail positive findings below. Use reference numbers.

Gynecologic (cont'd.)   Patient
20. Infertility _____ □
21. In utero exposure to DES ___ □
22. Uterine/cervical anomaly ____ □

Sexually transmitted diseases
23. Chlamydia _____ □
24. Gonorrhea _____ □
25. Herpes (HSV) _____ □
26. Syphilis _____ □

Vaginal/genital infections
27. Trichomonas _____ □
28. Condylomata _____ □
29. Candidiasis _____ □

Other infections
30. Toxoplasmosis _____ □
31. Group B streptococcus _____ □
32. Rubella or immunization _____ □
33. Varicella or immunization ____ □
34. Cytomegalovirus (CMV) _____ □
35. AIDS (HIV) _____ □
36. Hepatitis (type ____) _____ □
    or immunization (type ____)

FIGURE 12.2 Sample prenatal history form. (Used with permission. Copyright Briggs Corporation, 2001.)

Health History Summary
Maternal/newborn record system

Page 2 of 2

Patient's name _____

ID. No. _____

_____

_____

Check and detail positive findings below. Use reference numbers.

Cardiovascular

	Patient	Family
37. Myocardial infarction ___	☐	☐
38. Heart disease ___	☐	☐
39. Rheumatic fever ___	☐	
40. Valve disease ___	☐	
41. Chronic hypertension ___	☐	☐
42. Disease of the aorta ___	☐	☐
43. Varicosities Thrombophlebitis ___	☐	☐
44. Previous pulmonary embolism ___	☐	
45. Blood disorders ___	☐	☐
46. Anemia/ hemoglobinopathy ___	☐	☐
47. Blood transfusions ___	☐	
48. Other ___	☐	

Pulmonary

	Patient	Family
49. Asthma ___	☐	
50. Tuberculosis ___	☐	☐
51. Chronic obstructive pulmonary disease ___	☐	☐

Endocrine

	Patient	Family
52. Diabetes ___	☐	☐
53. Thyroid dysfunction ___	☐	☐
54. Maternal PKU ___	☐	
55. Endocrinopathy ___	☐	☐
56. Gastrointestinal ___	☐	
57. Liver disease ___	☐	

Renal disease

	Patient	Family
58. Cystitis ___	☐	
59. Pyelonephritis ___	☐	
60. Asymptomatic bacteriuria ___	☐	
61. Chronic renal disease ___	☐	☐
62. Autoimmune disease ___	☐	☐
63. Cancer ___	☐	☐

Neurologic disease

	Patient	Family
64. Cerebrovascular accident ___	☐	☐
65. Seizure disorder ___	☐	☐
66. Migraine headaches ___	☐	☐
67. Degenerative disease ___	☐	☐
68. Other ___	☐	

Psychological/surgical

	Patient	Family
69. Psychiatric disease Mental lillness ___	☐	☐
70. Physical abuse or neglect ___	☐	☐
71. Emotional abuse or neglect ___	☐	☐
72. Addiction (drug, alcohol, nicotine) ___	☐	☐
73. Major accidents ___	☐	
74. Surgery ___	☐	
75. Anesthetic complications ___	☐	
76. Non-surgical hospitalization ___	☐	
77. Other ___	☐	
78. **No known disease/problems** ___	☐	

Genetic history

	Patient	Father of baby	Family
79. Age 35 or older (female) 50 or older (male) ___	☐	☐	☐
80. Cerebral palsy ___	☐	☐	☐
81. Cleft lip/palate ___	☐	☐	☐
82. Congenital anomalies ___	☐	☐	☐
83. Congenital heart disease ___	☐	☐	☐
84. Consanguinity ___	☐	☐	☐
85. Cystic fibrosis ___	☐	☐	☐
86. Down's syndrome ___	☐	☐	☐
87. Hemophilia ___	☐	☐	☐
88. Huntington's chorea ___	☐	☐	☐
89. Mental retardation ___	☐	☐	☐
90. Muscular dystrophy ___	☐	☐	☐
91. Neural tube defect ___	☐	☐	☐
92. Sickle cell disease or trait ___	☐	☐	☐
93. Tay-sachs disease ___	☐	☐	☐
94. Test for fragile X ___	☐	☐	☐
95. Thalassemia A or B ___	☐	☐	☐
96. Other ___	☐	☐	☐
97. Other ___	☐	☐	☐
98. Other ___	☐	☐	☐

Historical risk status   ☐ No risk factors noted
☐ **At risk (identify)**

Signature

FIGURE 12.2 (continued)

Reason for Seeking Care

The woman commonly comes for prenatal care based on the suspicion that she is pregnant. She may report that she has missed her menstrual period or has had a positive result on a home pregnancy test. Ask the woman for the date of her last normal menstrual period (LMP). Also ask about any presumptive or probable signs of pregnancy that she might be experiencing. Typically a urine or blood test to check for evidence of human chorionic gonadotropin (hCG) is done to confirm the pregnancy.

Past History

Ask about the woman's past medical and surgical history. This information is important because conditions that the woman experienced in the past (e.g., urinary tract infections) may recur or be exacerbated during pregnancy. Also, chronic illnesses, such as diabetes or heart disease, can increase the risk for complications during pregnancy for the woman and her fetus. Ask about any history of allergies to medications, foods, or environmental substances. Ask about any mental health problems, such as depression or anxiety. Gather similar information about the woman's family and her partner.

The woman's personal history also is important. Ask about her occupation, possible exposure to teratogens, exercise and activity level, recreational patterns (including the use of substances such as alcohol, tobacco, and drugs), use of alternative and complementary therapies, sleep patterns, nutritional habits, and general lifestyle. Each of these may have an impact on the outcome of the pregnancy. For example, if the woman smokes during pregnancy, nicotine in the cigarettes causes vasoconstriction in the mother, leading to reduced placental perfusion. As a result, the newborn may be small for gestational age. The newborn will also go through nicotine withdrawal soon after birth. In addition, no safe level of alcohol ingestion in pregnancy has been determined. Many fetuses exposed to heavy alcohol levels during pregnancy develop fetal alcohol syndrome, a collection of deformities and disabilities.

Reproductive History

The woman's reproductive history includes a menstrual, obstetric, and gynecologic history. Typically, this history begins with a description of the woman's menstrual cycle, including her age at menarche, number of days in her cycle, typical flow characteristics, and any discomfort experienced. The use of contraception also is important, including when the woman last used any contraception.

Establishing an accurate due date is one of the most important assessments for a pregnant woman, one that has both social and medical significance. For women and their families, this estimated due date (EDD) represents

---

<table>
<tr><td colspan="2">**BOX 12.4**</td></tr>
<tr><td colspan="2">**NAGELE'S RULE FOR CALCULATING THE ESTIMATED DUE DATE (EDD)**</td></tr>
<tr><td>1. Use the first day of the last normal menstrual period</td><td>10/14/15</td></tr>
<tr><td>2. Subtract 3 from the number of months</td><td>7/14/15</td></tr>
<tr><td>3. Add 7 to the number of days</td><td>7/21/15</td></tr>
<tr><td>4. Adjust the year by adding 1 year</td><td>7/21/16</td></tr>
<tr><td colspan="2">5. Estimated due date (+ or − 2 weeks) = July 21, 2016</td></tr>
</table>

---

the long-awaited birthday of their child and is a time frame around which many economic and social activities are planned. This end point date provides guidance for the timing of specific maternal and fetal testing throughout pregnancy, gauges fetal growth parameters, and provides well-established timelines for specific interventions in the management of prenatal complications. In fact, critical decisions, such as preterm labor management, timing of postdate induction of labor, and identification of fetal growth restriction (FGR), are all based on the presumed gestational age of the fetus, which is calculated backwards from the EDD (Bond, 2015).

Ask the woman the date of her LMP to determine the estimated or EDD. Several methods may be used to estimate the date of birth. Nagele's rule can be used to establish the EDD (Box 12.4). Using this rule, subtract 3 months from the month of her LMP and then add 7 days to the first day of the LMP. Then correct the year by adding 1 to it where necessary. An alternative way is to add 7 days and then add 9 months = year where needed. This date has a margin of error of plus or minus 2 weeks. For instance, if a woman reports that her LMP was October 14, 2015, you would subtract 3 months (July) and add 7 days (21), then add 1 year (2016). The woman's EDD is July 21, 2016.

Because of the normal variations in women's menstrual cycles, differences in the normal length of gestation among ethnic groups, and errors in dating methods, there is no such thing as an exact due date. In general, a birth 2 weeks before or 2 weeks after the EDD is considered normal. Nagele's rule is less accurate if the woman's menstrual cycles are irregular, if the woman conceives while breast-feeding or before her regular menstrual cycle is established after childbirth, if she is ovulating although she is amenorrheic, or after she discontinues oral contraceptives (Schuiling & Likis, 2016).

A gestational or birth calculator or wheel can also be used to calculate the due date (Fig. 12.3). Some practitioners use ultrasound to more accurately determine the gestational age and date the pregnancy. Ultrasound is typically the most accurate method of dating a pregnancy.

Typically, an obstetric history provides information about the woman's past pregnancies, including any problems encountered during the pregnancy, labor, birth,

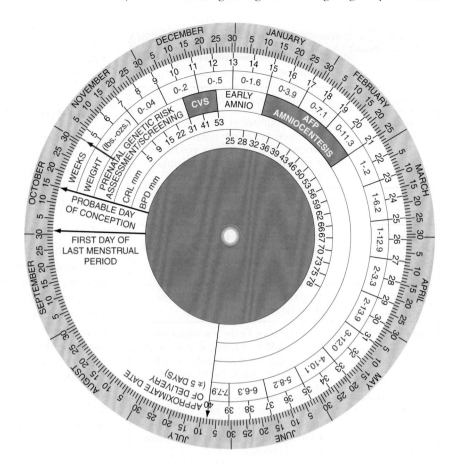

FIGURE 12.3 EDD using a birth wheel. The first day of the woman's last normal menstrual period was October 1. Using the birth wheel, her EDD would be approximately July 8 of the following year. (Used with permission. Copyright March of Dimes, 2015.)

and postpartum. Such information can provide clues to problems that might develop in the current pregnancy. Some common terms used to describe and document an obstetric history include gravid, **gravida**, gravida I (primigravida), gravida II (secundigravida), multigravida, and **para** (Table 12.1).

Other systems may be used to document a woman's obstetric history. These systems often break down the category of para more specifically (Box 12.5).

Information about the woman's gynecologic history is important. Ask about any reproductive tract surgeries the woman has undergone. For example, surgery on the uterus may affect its ability to contract effectively during labor. A history of tubal pregnancy increases the woman's risk for another tubal pregnancy. Also ask about safe-sex practices and any history of STIs.

Physical Examination

The next step in the assessment process is the physical examination, which detects any physical problems that may affect the pregnancy outcome. The initial physical examination provides the baseline for evaluating changes during future visits.

BOX 12.5

OBSTETRIC HISTORY TERMS: GTPAL OR TPAL

G, gravida; T, term births; P, preterm births; A, abortions; L, living children
- G—the current pregnancy to be included in count
- T—the number of term gestations delivering between 38 and 42 weeks
- P—the number of preterm pregnancies ending >20 weeks or viability but before completion of 37 weeks
- A—the number of pregnancies ending before 20 weeks or viability
- L—the number of children currently living

Consider this example:
Mary Johnson is pregnant for the fourth time. She had one abortion at 8 weeks gestation. She has a daughter who was born at 40 weeks gestation and a son born at 34 weeks. Mary's obstetric history would be documented as follows:
- Using the gravida/para method: gravida 4, para 2
- Using the TPAL method: 1112 (T = 1 [daughter born at 40 weeks]; P = 1 [son born at 34 weeks]; A = 1 [abortion at 8 weeks]; L = 2 [two living children])

TABLE 12.1	PREGNANCY TERMS
Term	**Definition**
Gravid	The state of being pregnant
Gravida/ Gravidity	The total number of times a woman has been pregnant, regardless of whether the pregnancy resulted in a termination or if multiple infants were born from a pregnancy.
Nulligravida	A woman who has never experienced pregnancy
Primigravida	A woman pregnant for the first time
Secundigravida	A woman pregnant for the second time
Multigravida	A woman pregnant for at least the third time
Para	The number of times a woman has given birth to a fetus of at least 20 gestational weeks (viable or not), counting multiple births as one birth event.
Parity	Refers to the number of pregnancies, not the number of fetuses, carried to the point of viability, regardless of the outcome
Nullipara (para 0)	A woman who has not produced a viable offspring.
Primipara	A woman who has given birth once after a pregnancy of at least 20 wks, commonly referred to as a "primip" in clinical practice.
Multipara	A woman who has had two or more pregnancies of at least 20 wks gestation resulting in viable offspring. Commonly referred to as a "multip."

Preparation

Instruct the client to undress and put on a gown. Also ask her to empty her bladder and, in doing so, to collect a urine specimen. Typically this specimen is a clean-catch urine specimen that is sent to the laboratory for a urinalysis to detect a possible urinary tract infection.

Begin the physical examination by obtaining vital signs, including blood pressure, respiratory rate, temperature, and pulse. Also measure the client's height and weight. Abnormalities such as an elevated blood pressure may suggest pregestational hypertension, requiring further evaluation. Abnormalities in pulse rate and respiration require further investigation for possible cardiac or respiratory disease. If the woman weighs less than 100 pounds or more than 200 pounds or there has been a sudden weight gain, report these findings to the primary care provider; medical treatment or nutritional counseling may be necessary.

Head-to-Toe Assessment

A complete head-to-toe assessment is usually performed by the health care provider. Every body system is assessed. Some of the major areas are discussed here. Throughout the assessment, be sure to drape the client appropriately to ensure privacy and prevent chilling.

HEAD AND NECK

Assess the head and neck area for any previous injuries and sequelae. Evaluate for any limitations in range of motion. Palpate for any enlarged lymph nodes or swelling. Note any edema of the nasal mucosa or hypertrophy of gingival tissue in the mouth; these are typical responses to increased estrogen levels in pregnancy. Palpate the thyroid gland for enlargement. Slight enlargement is normal, but marked enlargement may indicate hyperthyroidism, requiring further investigation.

CHEST

Auscultate heart sounds, noting any abnormalities. A soft systolic murmur caused by the increase in blood volume may be noted. Anticipate an increase in heart rate by 10 to 15 beats per minute (bpm) (starting between 14 and 20 weeks of pregnancy) secondary to increases in cardiac output and blood volume. The body adapts to the increase in blood volume with peripheral dilation to maintain blood pressure. Progesterone causes peripheral dilation.

Auscultate the chest for breath sounds, which should be clear. Also note symmetry of chest movement and thoracic breathing patterns. Estrogen promotes relaxation of the ligaments and joints of the ribs, with a resulting increase in the anteroposterior chest diameter. Expect a slight increase in respiratory rate to accommodate the increase in tidal volume and oxygen consumption.

Inspect and palpate the breasts and nipples for symmetry and color. Increases in estrogen and progesterone and blood supply make the breasts feel full and more nodular, with increased sensitivity to touch. Blood vessels become more visible and there is an increase in breast size. Striae gravidarum (stretch marks) may be visible in women with large breasts. Darker pigmentation of the nipple and areola is present, along with enlargement of Montgomery's glands. Colostrum (yellowish secretion that precedes mature breast milk) is excreted typically in the third trimester.

Take Note!

Use this opportunity to reinforce and teach breast self-examination if the woman has a high-risk history.

ABDOMEN

The appearance of the abdomen depends on the number of weeks of gestation. The abdomen enlarges progressively as the fetus grows. Inspect the abdomen for striae, scars, shape, and size. Inspection may reveal striae gravidarum (stretch marks) and **linea nigra**, a thin brownish black pigmented line running from the umbilicus to the symphysis pubis, depending on the duration of the pregnancy. Palpate the abdomen, which should be rounded and nontender. A decrease in muscle tone may be noted due to the influence of progesterone.

Typically, the height of the fundus is measured when the uterus arises out of the pelvis to evaluate fetal growth. At 12 weeks gestation the fundus can be palpated at the symphysis pubis. At 16 weeks gestation the fundus is midway between the symphysis and the umbilicus. At 20 weeks the fundus can be palpated at the umbilicus and measures approximately 20 cm from the symphysis pubis. By 36 weeks the fundus is just below the xiphoid process and measures approximately 36 cm. The uterus maintains a globular/ovoid shape throughout pregnancy (Bope & Kellerman, 2015).

EXTREMITIES

Inspect and palpate both legs for dependent edema, pulses, and varicose veins. If edema is present in early pregnancy, further evaluation may be needed to rule out gestational hypertension. During the third trimester, dependent edema is a normal finding. Ask the woman if she has any pain in her calf that increases when she ambulates. This might indicate a deep vein thrombosis (DVT). High levels of estrogen during pregnancy place women at higher risk for DVT.

Pelvic Examination

The pelvic examination provides information about the internal and external reproductive organs. In addition, it aids in assessing some of the presumptive and probable signs of pregnancy and allows for determination of pelvic adequacy. During the pelvic examination, remain in the examining room to assist the health care provider with any specimen collection, fixation, and labeling. Also provide comfort and emotional support for the woman, who might be anxious. Throughout the examination, explain what is happening and why, and answer any questions as necessary.

EXTERNAL GENITALIA

After the client is placed in the lithotomy position and draped appropriately, the external genitalia are inspected visually. They should be free from lesions, discharge, hematomas, varicosities, and inflammation upon inspection. A culture for STIs may be collected at this time.

INTERNAL GENITALIA

Next, the internal genitalia are examined via a speculum. The cervix should be smooth, long, thick, and closed. Because of increased pelvic congestion, the cervix will be softened (Goodell's sign), the uterine isthmus will be softened (Hegar's sign), and there will be a bluish coloration of the cervix and vaginal mucosa (Chadwick's sign).

The uterus typically is pear shaped and mobile, with a smooth surface. It will undergo cell hypertrophy and hyperplasia so that it enlarges throughout the pregnancy to accommodate the growing fetus.

During the pelvic examination, a Papanicolaou (Pap) smear may be obtained. Additional cultures, such as for gonorrhea and chlamydia screening, also may be obtained. Ensure that all specimens obtained are labeled correctly and sent to the laboratory for evaluation. A rectal examination is done last to assess for lesions, masses, prolapse, or hemorrhoids.

Once the examination of the internal genitalia is completed and the speculum is removed, a bimanual examination is performed to estimate the size of the uterus to confirm dates and to palpate the ovaries. The ovaries should be small and nontender, without masses. At the conclusion of the bimanual examination, the health care provider reinserts the index finger into the vagina and the middle finger into the rectum to assess the strength and regularity of the posterior vaginal wall.

PELVIC SIZE, SHAPE, AND MEASUREMENTS

The size and shape of the women's pelvis can affect her ability to deliver vaginally. Pelvic shape is typically classified as one of the four types: gynecoid, android, anthropoid, and platypelloid. Refer to Chapter 13 for an in-depth discussion of pelvic size and shape.

Taking internal pelvic measurements determines the actual diameters of the inlet and outlet through which the fetus will pass. This is extremely important if the woman has never given birth vaginally. Taking pelvic measurements is unnecessary for the woman who has given birth vaginally before (unless she has experienced some type of trauma to the area) because vaginal delivery demonstrates that the pelvis is adequate for the passage of the fetus.

Three measurements are assessed: diagonal conjugate, true conjugate, and ischial tuberosity (Fig. 12.4). The diagonal conjugate is the distance between the anterior surface of the sacral prominence and the anterior surface of the inferior margin of the symphysis pubis (Bope & Kellerman, 2015). This measurement, usually 12.5 cm or greater, represents the anteroposterior diameter of the pelvic inlet through which the fetal head passes first. The diagonal conjugate is the most useful measurement for estimating pelvic size because a misfit with the fetal head occurs if it is too small.

The true conjugate, also called the obstetric conjugate, is the measurement from the anterior surface

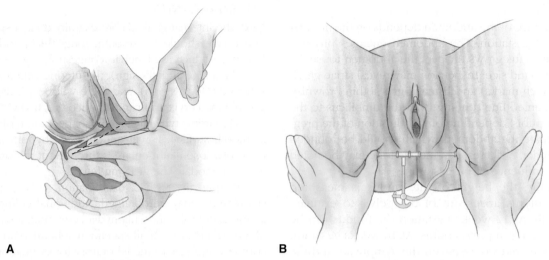

FIGURE 12.4 Pelvic measurements. **A.** Diagonal conjugate (*solid line*) and true conjugate (*dotted line*). **B.** Ischial tuberosity diameter.

of the sacral prominence to the posterior surface of the inferior margin of the symphysis pubis. This diameter cannot be measured directly; rather, it is estimated by subtracting 1 to 2 cm from the diagonal conjugate measurement. The average true conjugate diameter is at least 11.5 cm (Cunningham et al., 2014). This measurement is important because it is the smallest front-to-back diameter through which the fetal head must pass when moving through the pelvic inlet.

The ischial tuberosity diameter is the transverse diameter of the pelvic outlet. This measurement is made outside the pelvis at the lowest aspect of the ischial tuberosities. A diameter of 10.5 cm or more is considered adequate for passage of the fetal head (Tharpe, Farley, & Jordan, 2016).

Laboratory Tests

A series of tests is generally ordered during the initial visit so that baseline data can be obtained, allowing for early detection and prompt intervention if any problems occur. Tests that are generally conducted for all pregnant women include urinalysis and blood studies. The urine is analyzed for albumin, glucose, ketones, and bacteria casts. Blood studies usually include a complete blood count (CBC) (hemoglobin, hematocrit, red and white blood cell counts, and platelets), blood typing and Rh factor, glucose screening for high-risk women, a rubella titer, hepatitis B surface antibody antigen, HIV, venereal disease research laboratory (VDRL) or rapid plasma reagin (RPR) tests, and cervical smears to detect STIs (Common Laboratory and Diagnostic Tests 12.1). In addition, most offices and clinics have ultrasound equipment available to validate an intrauterine pregnancy and assess early fetal growth.

The need for additional laboratory studies is determined by a woman's history, physical examination findings, current health status, and risk factors identified in the initial interview. Additional tests can be offered (e.g., screening for genetic diseases, blood lead screening, rubeola, and so on), but ultimately the woman and her partner make the decision about undergoing them. Educate the client and her partner about the tests, including the rationale. In addition, support the client and her partner in their decision-making process, regardless of whether you agree with the couple's decision. The couple's decisions about their health care are based on the ethical principle of autonomy, which allows an individual the right to make decisions about his or her own body.

Remember Linda and Rob, the couple who want to start a family? Ten months after the preconception appointment, Linda calls to make a first prenatal appointment. What key areas will be addressed at this first prenatal visit? What interventions might be suggested for Linda to implement in order to ensure a healthy newborn? What emotional support might be needed by Linda at this time in her first trimester of pregnancy?

FOLLOW-UP VISITS

Continuous prenatal care is important for a successful pregnancy outcome. The recommended follow-up visit schedule for a healthy pregnant woman is as follows:
- Every 4 weeks up to 28 weeks (7 months)
- Every 2 weeks from 29 to 36 weeks
- Every week from 37 weeks to birth

At each subsequent prenatal visit, the following assessments are completed:
- Weight and blood pressure, which are compared with baseline values

COMMON LABORATORY AND DIAGNOSTIC TESTS 12.1

Test	Explanation
Complete blood cell count (CBC)	Evaluates hemoglobin (12–14 g) and hematocrit (42% ± 5%) levels and red blood cell count (4.2–5.4 million/mm^3) to detect the presence of anemia; identifies white blood cell level (5,000–10,000 mm^{-3}), which if elevated may indicate an infection; determines platelet count (150,000–450,000 mL^3) to assess clotting ability.
Blood typing	Determines woman's blood type and Rh status to rule out any blood incompatibility issues early; Rh-negative mother would likely receive RhoGAM (at 28 weeks gestation) and again within 72 hours after childbirth, if she is Rh sensitive.
Rubella titer	Detects antibodies for the virus that causes German measles; if titer is 1:8 or less, the woman is not immune; requires immunization after birth, and woman is advised to avoid people with undiagnosed rashes.
Hepatitis B	Determines if mother has hepatitis B by detecting presence of hepatitis antibody surface antigen (HbsAg) in her blood.
HIV testing	Detects HIV antibodies and if positive requires more specific testing, counseling, and treatment during pregnancy with antiretroviral medications to prevent transmission to fetus.
STI screening: VDRL or RPR serologic tests or by cervical smears, cultures, or visual identification of suspicious lesions	Detects STIs (such as syphilis, herpes, HPV, gonorrhea) so that treatment can be initiated early to prevent transmission to fetus.
Cervical smears	Detects abnormalities such as cervical cancer (Pap test) or infections such as gonorrhea, chlamydia, or group B streptococcus so that treatment can be initiated if positive.

Adapted from Fischbach, F., & Dunning, M. B. (2014). *A manual of laboratory and diagnostic tests* (9th ed.). Philadelphia, PA: Lippincott Williams & Wilkins; Ferri, F. F. (2014). *Ferri's best test: A practical guide to laboratory medicine and diagnostic imaging* (3rd ed.). Philadelphia, PA: Elsevier Health Sciences.

- Urine testing for protein, glucose, ketones, and nitrites
- Fundal height measurement to assess fetal growth
- Assessment for quickening/fetal movement to determine fetal well-being
- Assessment of fetal heart rate (should be 110 to 160 bpm)

At each follow-up visit answer questions, provide anticipatory guidance and education, review nutritional guidelines, and evaluate the client for adherence to prenatal vitamin therapy. Throughout the pregnancy, encourage the woman's partner to participate if possible.

Follow-Up Visit Intervals and Assessments

Up to 28 weeks gestation, follow-up visits involve assessment of the client's blood pressure and weight. The urine is tested for protein and glucose. Fundal height and fetal heart rate are assessed at every office visit.

The best procedure for screening and diagnosing gestational diabetes remains controversial. All strategies involve an oral glucose test, but there remains disagreement about how many grams of glucose (50, 75, or 100) the woman ingests and how long afterwards, her blood sample is drawn. A recent *Cochrane Review* concluded that there was insufficient evidence to permit assessment of which is the best method to use to identify women who have gestational diabetes (Farrar et al., 2015). Screening for gestational diabetes is best done between 24 and 28 weeks gestation, unless screening is warranted in the first trimester for high-risk reasons (obesity, >25 years old, family history of diabetes, history of gestational diabetes, or woman is of a certain ethnic group: Hispanic, Native Americans, Asian, or African American) (U.S. Preventive Services Task Force [USPSTF], 2015). Between weeks 24 and 28, a blood glucose level is obtained using an oral 50-g glucose load followed by a 1-hour plasma glucose determination. If the result is more than 130 (ADA) to140 (ACOG) mg/dL, further testing, such as a 3-hour 100-g glucose tolerance test, is warranted to determine whether gestational diabetes is present (Farrar et al., 2015). Because insulin resistance increases as pregnancy advances, testing at this gestational point yields a higher rate of abnormal test results.

During this time, review the common discomforts of pregnancy, evaluate any client complaints, and answer questions. Reinforce the importance of good nutrition and use of prenatal vitamins, along with daily exercise.

Between 29 and 36 weeks gestation, all the assessments of previous visits are completed, along with assessment for edema. Special attention is focused on the presence and location of edema during the last trimester. Pregnant women commonly experience dependent edema of the lower extremities from constriction of blood vessels secondary to the heavy gravid uterus. Periorbital edema around the eyes, edema of the hands, and pretibial edema (edema on the front, or shin part of the leg) are abnormal and could be signs of gestational hypertension. Inspecting and palpating both extremities, listening for complaints of tight rings on fingers, and observing for swelling around the eyes are important assessments. Abnormal findings in any of these areas need to be reported.

If the mother is Rh negative, her antibody titer is evaluated. RhoGAM is given if indicated. RhoGAM is used to prevent development of antibodies to Rh+ red cells whenever fetal cells are known or suspected of entering the maternal circulation such as after a spontaneous abortion or amniocentesis. It is also recommended for prophylaxis at 28 weeks gestation and following birth if the infant is Rh+ (King et al., 2015). The client also is evaluated for risk of preterm labor. At each visit, ask if she is experiencing any common signs or symptoms of preterm labor (e.g., uterine contractions, dull backache, feeling of pressure in the pelvic area or thighs, increased vaginal discharge, menstrual-like cramps, vaginal bleeding). If the woman has had a previous preterm birth, she is at risk for another and close monitoring is warranted. An initial preterm labor evaluation if the woman reports signs and symptoms of preterm labor includes: review of prenatal record for risk factors, evaluation of reported symptoms (uterine contractions, vital signs, fetal heart rate, pelvic exam for cervical dilation and effacement assessment, and status of fetal membranes), and a urine culture to diagnose asymptomatic bacteriuria (Jordan et al., 2014). If positive for preterm labor, the woman may be requested to rest and medications to stop contractions may be in order.

Counsel the woman about choosing a health care provider for the newborn, if she has not selected one yet. Along with completion of a breast assessment, the nurse should discuss and educate the client about the choice of breast-feeding versus bottle-feeding. The American Academy of Pediatrics (AAP) does encourage all mothers to breast-feed their offspring, but the decision to do so is the woman's ultimately. The nurse can refer the client to *Nursing Mothers* and *La Leche League* web sites for further information to assist her in making that decision. Reinforce the importance of daily fetal movement monitoring as an indicator of fetal well-being. Re-evaluate hemoglobin and hematocrit levels to assess for anemia.

Between 37 and 40 weeks gestation, the same assessments are done as for the previous weeks. In addition, screening for group B streptococcus, gonorrhea, and chlamydia is done. Fetal presentation and position (via Leopold's maneuvers) are assessed. Review the signs and symptoms of labor and forward a copy of the prenatal record to the hospital labor department for future reference. Review the client's desire for family planning after birth as well as her decision to breast-feed or bottle-feed. Remind the client that an infant car seat is required by law and must be used to drive the newborn home from the hospital or birthing center.

Fundal Height Measurement

Fundal height is the distance (in centimeters) measured with a tape measure from the top of the pubic bone to the top of the uterus (fundus) with the client lying on her back with her knees slightly flexed (Fig. 12.5). Measurement in this way is termed the McDonald's method. Fundal height typically increases as the pregnancy progresses; it reflects fetal growth and provides a gross estimate of the duration of the pregnancy.

Between 12 and 14 weeks gestation, the fundus can be palpated above the symphysis pubis. The fundus reaches the level of the umbilicus at approximately 20 weeks and measures 20 cm. Fundal measurement should approximately equal the number of weeks of gestation until week 36. For example, a fundal height of 24 cm suggests a fetus at 24 weeks gestation. After 36 weeks, the fundal height then drops due to lightening and may no longer correspond with the week of gestation.

It is expected that the fundal height will increase progressively throughout the pregnancy, reflecting fetal growth. However, if the growth curve flattens or stays stable, it may indicate the presence of FGR. If the fundal height measurement is greater than 4 cm from the estimated gestational age, further evaluation is warranted if

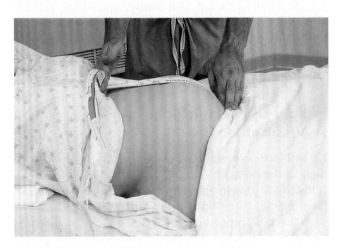

FIGURE 12.5 Fundal height measurement.

a multifetal gestation has not been diagnosed or hydramnios has not been ruled out (Weber & Kelley, 2014).

Fetal Movement Determination

Perception of fetal movement typically begins in the second trimester, and occurs earlier in multiparous women versus nulliparous women. The mother's first perception of fetal movement, termed "quickening," is commonly described as a gentle fluttering. This perceived fetal movement is most often related to trunk and limb motion and rollovers, or flips (Moses, 2015b). Maternal perception of fetal movement is an important screening method for fetal well-being, because decreased fetal movement is associated with a range of pregnancy pathologies and poor pregnancy outcomes. Decreased fetal movement may indicate asphyxia and FGR. If compromised, the fetus decreases its oxygen requirements by decreasing activity. Reduced fetal movement is thought to represent fetal compensation in a chronic hypoxic environment due to inadequacies in the placental supply of oxygen and nutrients (Fretts, 2014). A decrease in fetal movement may also be related to other factors as well, such as maternal use of central nervous system depressants, fetal sleep cycles, hydrocephalus, bilateral renal agenesis, stillbirth, placental dysfunction, and bilateral hip dislocation (Heazell, 2015).

Fetal movement counting is a method used by the mother to quantify her fetus's movement. However, the optimal number of movements and the ideal duration of counting them remain controversial. Many variations for determining fetal movement, also called fetal movement counts, have been developed, but the one most common method is described as follows. Determining fetal movement is a noninvasive method of screening and can be easily taught to all pregnant women. Any technique used requires client participation and cooperation.

Instruct the client about how to count fetal movements, the reasons for doing so, and the significance of decreased fetal movements. Urge the client to perform the counts in a relaxed environment and a comfortable position, such as semi-Fowler's or side-lying. Provide the client with detailed information concerning fetal movement counts and stress the need for consistency in monitoring (at approximately the same time each day) and the importance of informing the health care provider promptly of any reduced movements. Providing clients with "fetal kick count" charts to record movement helps promote adherence to your instructions. No values for fetal movement have been established that indicate fetal well-being, so the woman needs to be aware of a decrease in the number of movements when last assessed. The most common method used is "Count to 10," whereby a woman focuses her attention on her fetus's movement and records how long it takes to document 10 movements. If it takes longer than 2 hours, the woman should contact her health care provider for further evaluation. Fetal kick counting in current prenatal care appears to be underutilized and nurses need to educate women about this assessment in their pregnancy care.

Fetal Heart Rate Measurement

Fetal heart rate measurement is integral to fetal surveillance throughout the pregnancy. Auscultating the fetal heart rate with a handheld Doppler at each prenatal visit helps confirm that the intrauterine environment is still supportive to the growing fetus. The purpose of assessing fetal heart rate is to determine the rate and rhythm. The normal fetal heart rate range is 110 to 160 bpm. Nursing Procedure 12.1 lists the steps in measuring fetal heart rate.

NURSING PROCEDURE 12.1

Measuring Fetal Heart Rate

Purpose: To Assess Fetal Well-Being

1. Assist the woman onto the examining table and have her lie down.
2. Cover her with a sheet to ensure privacy, and then expose her abdomen.
3. Palpate the abdomen to determine the fetal lie, position, and presentation.
4. Locate the back of the fetus (the ideal position to hear the heart rate).
5. Apply lubricant gel to abdomen in the area where the back has been located.
6. Turn on the handheld Doppler device and place it on the spot over the fetal back.
7. Listen for the sound of the amplified heart rate, moving the device slightly from side to side as necessary to obtain the loudest sound. Assess the woman's pulse rate and compare it to the amplified sound. If the rates appear the same, reposition the Doppler device.
8. Once the fetal heart rate has been identified, count the number of beats in 1 minute and record the results.
9. Remove the Doppler device and wipe off any remaining gel from the woman's abdomen and the device.
10. Record the heart rate on the woman's medical record; normal range is 110 to 160 bpm.
11. Provide information to the woman regarding fetal well-being based on findings.

Teaching About the Danger Signs of Pregnancy

It is important to educate the client about danger signs during pregnancy that require further evaluation. Explain that she should contact her health care provider immediately if she experiences any of the following:

- *During the first trimester:* spotting or bleeding (miscarriage), painful urination (infection), severe persistent vomiting (hyperemesis gravidarum), fever >100 °F (37.7 °C; infection), and lower abdominal pain with dizziness and accompanied by shoulder pain (ruptured ectopic pregnancy)
- *During the second trimester:* regular uterine contractions (preterm labor); pain in calf, often increased with foot flexion (blood clot in deep vein); sudden gush or leakage of fluid from vagina (premature rupture of membranes); and absence of fetal movement for more than 12 hours (possible fetal distress or demise)
- *During the third trimester:* sudden weight gain; periorbital or facial edema, severe upper abdominal pain, or headache with visual changes (gestational hypertension and/or preeclampsia); and a decrease in fetal daily movement for more than 24 hours (possible demise). Any of the previous warning signs and symptoms can also be present in this last trimester (March of Dimes, 2015a).

Early Contractions

One of the warning signs that should be emphasized is early contractions, which can lead to preterm birth. The woman should not confuse these early preterm contractions with Braxton Hicks contractions, which are not true labor pains because they go away when walking around or resting. They often go away when the woman goes to sleep. Braxton Hicks contractions are usually felt in the abdomen versus in the lower back with true preterm labor contractions. Signs of preterm labor that a woman may experience include contractions every 10 minutes or more frequently, change in vaginal discharge, pelvic pressure, low, dull backache, pelvic cramps, and diarrhea (Nagtalon-Ramos, 2014).

All pregnant women need to be able to recognize early signs of contractions to prevent preterm labor, which is a major public health problem in the United States. Approximately 12% of all live births—or one out of nine infants —is born too soon. Our nation's rate of premature births has increased by 36% over the last 25 years. Worldwide, 15 million infants are born too soon each year (March of Dimes, 2015b). These preterm infants (born at less than 37 weeks gestation) can suffer lifelong health consequences such as intellectual disability, chronic lung disease, cerebral palsy, seizure disorders, and blindness (March of Dimes, 2015c). Preterm labor can happen to any pregnant women at any time.

In many cases it can be stopped with medications if it is recognized early, before significant cervical dilation has taken place. If the woman experiences menstrual-like cramps occurring every 10 minutes accompanied by a low, dull backache, she should stop what she is doing and lie down on her left side for 1 hour and drink two or three glasses of water. If the symptoms worsen or do not subside after 1 hour, she should contact her health care provider.

ASSESSMENT OF FETAL WELL-BEING

During the antepartum period, several tests are performed routinely to monitor fetal well-being and to detect possible problems. When a high-risk pregnancy is identified, additional antepartum testing can be initiated to promote positive maternal, fetal, and neonatal outcomes. **High-risk pregnancies** include those that are complicated by maternal or fetal conditions (coincidental with or unique to pregnancy) that jeopardize the health status of the mother and put the fetus at risk for uteroplacental insufficiency, hypoxia, and death (CDC, 2015d). However, additional antepartum fetal testing should take place only when the results obtained will guide future care, whether it is reassurance, more frequent testing, admission to the hospital, or the need for immediate delivery (Brown, 2015).

Ultrasonography

Since its introduction in the late 1950s, ultrasonography has become a very useful diagnostic tool in obstetrics. Real-time scanners can produce a continuous picture of the fetus on a monitor screen. A transducer that emits high-frequency sound waves is placed on the mother's abdomen and moved to visualize the fetus (Fig. 12.6). The fetal heartbeat and any malformations in the fetus can be assessed and measurements can be made accurately from the picture on the monitor screen.

Obstetric ultrasound is a standard component of prenatal care used to identify pregnancy complications and to establish an accurate gestational age in order to improve pregnancy outcomes. Because the ultrasound procedure is noninvasive, it is a safe, but not evidence-based practice for low-risk women, accurate, and cost-effective tool. It provides important information about fetal activity, growth, and gestational age; assesses fetal well-being; and determines the need for invasive intrauterine tests (Maeda, 2015).

There are no hard-and-fast rules as to the number of ultrasounds a woman should have during her pregnancy. A low-risk woman does not necessarily require any, but most practices do them as part of their prenatal care routine. A transvaginal ultrasound may be performed in the first trimester to confirm pregnancy, exclude ectopic (in which a fertilized egg implants somewhere other

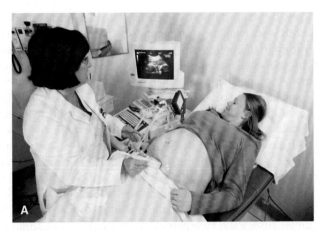
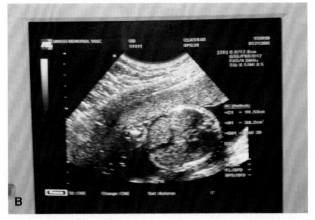

FIGURE 12.6 Ultrasound. **A.** Ultrasound device being applied to client's abdomen. **B.** View of monitor.

than the main cavity of the uterus) or molar (hydatidiform mole, a benign tumor that develops in the uterus) pregnancies, and confirm cardiac pulsation. A second abdominal scan may be performed at about 18 to 20 weeks to look for congenital malformations, exclude multifetal pregnancies, and verify dates and growth. A third abdominal scan may be done at around 34 weeks to evaluate fetal size, assess fetal growth, and verify placental position (Everett & Peebles, 2015). An ultrasound is used to confirm placental location during amniocentesis and to provide visualization during chorionic villus sampling (CVS). An ultrasound is also ordered whenever an abnormality is suspected.

During the past several years, ultrasound technology has advanced significantly. Now available for expecting parents is 3D/4D ultrasound imaging. Unlike traditional 2D imaging, which takes a look at the developing fetus from one angle (thus creating the "flat" image), 3D imaging takes a view of the fetus from three different angles. Software then takes these three images and merges them to produce a 3D image. Because the fourth dimension is time and movement, with 4D parents are able to watch the live movements of their fetus in 3D.

Nursing management during the ultrasound procedure focuses on educating the woman about the ultrasound test and reassuring her that she will not experience any sensation from the sound waves during the test. No special client preparation is needed before performing the ultrasound, although in early pregnancy the woman may need to have a full bladder. Inform her that she may experience some discomfort from the pressure on the full bladder during the scan, but it will last only a short time. Tell the client that the conducting gel used on the abdomen during the scan may feel cold initially.

Doppler Flow Studies

Comprehensive assessment of fetal well-being involves monitoring of fetal growth, placental function, central venous pressure, and cardiac function. Ultrasound evaluation of the fetus using 2D, color Doppler, and pulse-wave Doppler techniques forms the foundation of prenatal diagnosis of structural anomalies, rhythm abnormalities, and altered fetal circulation (Pruetz, Votava-Smith, & Miller, 2015). Doppler flow studies can be used to measure the velocity of blood flow via ultrasound. Doppler flow studies can detect fetal compromise in high-risk pregnancies. The test is noninvasive and has no contraindications. The color images produced help to identify abnormalities in diastolic flow within the umbilical vessels. The velocity of the fetal red blood cells can be determined by measuring the change in the frequency of the sound wave reflected off the cells. Thus, Doppler flow studies can detect the movement of red blood cells in vessels (Everett & Peebles, 2015). In pregnancies complicated by hypertension or FGRs, diastolic blood flow may be absent or even reversed (Alfirevic, Stampalija, & Medley, 2015). Doppler flow studies also can be used to evaluate the blood flow through other fetal blood vessels, such as the aorta and those in the brain. Research continues to determine the indications for Doppler flow studies to improve pregnancy outcomes. Nursing management of the woman undergoing Doppler flow studies is similar to that described for an ultrasound.

Alpha-Fetoprotein Analysis

Alpha-fetoprotein (AFP) is a glycoprotein produced initially by the yolk sac and fetal gut, and later predominantly by the fetal liver. In a fetus, the serum AFP level increases until approximately 14 to 15 weeks, and then falls progressively. In normal pregnancies, AFP from fetal serum enters the amniotic fluid (in microgram quantities) through fetal urination, fetal gastrointestinal secretions, and transudation across fetal membranes (amnion and placenta). About 30 years ago, elevated levels of maternal serum AFP or amniotic fluid AFP were first linked to the occurrence of fetal neural tube defects. This biomarker screening test is now recommended for all pregnant women along with other prenatal screening test depending on risk profile (ACOG, 2015b; Alexander et al., 2014).

AFP is present in amniotic fluid in low concentrations between 10 and 14 weeks of gestation and can be detected in maternal serum beginning at approximately 12 to 14 weeks of gestation (Callahan, 2016). If a developmental defect is present, such as failure of the neural tube to close, more AFP escapes into amniotic fluid from the fetus. AFP then enters the maternal circulation by crossing the placenta, and the level in maternal serum can be measured. The optimal time for AFP screening is 16 to 18 weeks of gestation. Currently, ACOG recommends offering screening and diagnostic tests to all pregnant women, regardless of age or risk factors present (2015b). Correct information about gestational dating, maternal weight, race, number of fetuses, and insulin dependency is necessary to ensure the accuracy of this screening test. If incorrect maternal information is submitted or the blood specimen is not drawn during the appropriate time frame, false-positive results may occur, increasing the woman's anxiety. Subsequently, further testing might be ordered based on an inaccurate interpretation, resulting in additional financial and emotional costs to the woman.

A variety of situations can lead to elevation of maternal serum AFP, including open neural tube defect, underestimation of gestational age, the presence of multiple fetuses, gastrointestinal defects, low birth weight, oligohydramnios, maternal age, diabetes, and decreased maternal weight (King et al., 2015). Lower-than-expected maternal serum AFP levels are seen when fetal gestational age is overestimated or in cases of fetal death, hydatidiform mole, increased maternal weight, maternal type 1 diabetes, and fetal trisomy 21 (Down syndrome) or trisomy 18 (Edward's syndrome) (Khalil & Coates, 2015).

Measurement of maternal serum AFP is minimally invasive, requiring only a venipuncture for a blood sample. AFP has now been combined with other biomarker screening tests to determine the risk of neural tube defects and Down syndrome.

Nursing management for AFP testing consists of preparing the woman for this screening test by gathering accurate information about the date of her LMP, weight, race, and gestational dating. Accurately determining the window of 16 to 18 weeks gestation will help to ensure that the test results are correct. Also explain that the test involves obtaining a blood specimen.

Marker Screening Tests

Using maternal serum is an effective, noninvasive method for identifying fetal risk for aneuploidy (trisomies 13, 18, and 21) and neural tube defects. Prenatal screening for Down syndrome in the early second trimester with multiple maternal serum markers has been available for more than 15 years. Abnormalities in maternal serum marker levels and fetal measurements obtained during the first trimester screening can be markers for not only certain chromosomal disorders and anomalies in the fetus, but also for specific pregnancy complications. Pregnancy-associated plasma protein A (PAPP-A) is a key regulator of insulin-like growth factor essential for normal fetal development. In maternal blood, this protein increases with gestational age. It is routinely used for Down syndrome screening in the first trimester. A low maternal serum PAPP-A, at 11 to 13 weeks of gestation, is associated with stillbirth, infant death, preterm birth, preeclampsia, and chromosomal abnormalities (Kalousová, Muravská, & Zima, 2014; Patil, Panchanadikar, & Wagh, 2014). Multiple blood screening tests may be used to determine the risk of open neural tube defects and Down syndrome: the triple-marker screen (AFP, hCG, and unconjugated estriol) or the quad screen, which includes the triple screening tests with the addition of a fourth marker, inhibin A (glycoprotein secreted by the placenta). The quad screen is used to enhance the accuracy of screening for Down syndrome in women younger than 35 years of age. Low inhibin A levels indicate the possibility of Down syndrome (ACOG, 2015b). These biomarkers are merely screening tests and identify women who need further definitive procedures (i.e., ultrasound, amniocentesis, and genetic counseling) to make a diagnosis of neural tube defects (anencephaly, spina bifida, and encephalocele) or Down syndrome in the fetus. Most screening tests are performed between 15 and 22 weeks of gestation (16 to 18 weeks is ideal), except for the cffDNA test which can be performed around 9 to 10 weeks gestation (Dempsey & Overton, 2015).

With these multiple screening tests, low maternal serum AFP (MSAFP), unconjugated estriol levels, and a high hCG level suggest the possibility of Down syndrome. Elevated levels of MSAFP are associated with open neural tube defects, ventral wall defects, some renal abnormalities, multiple gestation, certain skin disorders, fetal demise, and placental abnormality. The multiple marker combination with the highest screening performance currently available is AFP, unconjugated estriol (uE3), hCG, and inhibin A, together with maternal age (the so-called quad marker test). With this combination, a detection rate of 80% at a 5% false-positive rate is achieved (Hixson et al., 2015).

A number of factors influence the interpretation of an MSAFP value. The most important is the accuracy of the gestational age determination. A variation of 2 weeks can be misleading and lead to a wrong interpretation. Maternal weight (>250 pounds), ethnicity, maternal smoking habits, fetal gender, gravidity, para status, and women with insulin-dependent diabetes also may alter the levels of MSAFP and need to be taken into consideration when interpreting the results (Latendresse & Deneris, 2015). Recent research studies indicate prenatal testing with the use of cell free DNA (cfDNA) has significantly lower false positives and high positive predictive values for detection of trisomies than standard testing (Greeley, Kessler, & Vohra, 2015).

Nursing Management

Accurate test interpretation and risk determination are dependent on accurate pregnancy dating and reporting of relevant maternal characteristics. This is why it is so important for nurses, if an abnormal test result is reported, for them to confirm pregnancy dating and report any significant maternal factors relevant to test accuracy. In addition, nurses have a big role in providing education about the tests to the couples. Prenatal screening has become standard in prenatal care. However, for many couples it remains confusing, emotionally charged, and filled with uncertain risks. Offer a thorough explanation of the test, reinforcing the information given by the health care professional. Provide couples with a description of the risks and benefits of performing these screens, emphasizing that these tests are for screening purposes only. Remind the couple that a definitive diagnosis is not made without further tests such as an amniocentesis. Answer any questions about these prenatal screening tests and respect the couple's decision if they choose not to have them done. Many couples may choose not to know because they would not consider having an abortion regardless of the test results.

Nuchal Translucency Screening

Nuchal translucency screening (ultrasound) is also done in the first trimester between 11 and 14 weeks. This allows for early detection and diagnosis of some fetal chromosomal and structural abnormalities. Over the years, it has become clear that increased nuchal translucency is a marker for chromosomal abnormalities, and is also associated with a wide spectrum of structural anomalies, genetic syndromes, and high risk of abortion and fetal death (Rayburn, Jolley, & Simpson, 2015). Ultrasound is used to identify an increase in nuchal translucency, which is due to the subcutaneous accumulation of fluid behind the fetal neck. Increased nuchal translucency is associated with chromosomal abnormalities such as trisomies 21, 18, and 13. Infants with trisomies tend to have more collagen and elastic connective tissue, allowing for accumulation. In addition, diaphragmatic hernias, cardiac defects, and fetal skeletal and neurologic abnormalities have been associated with increased nuchal translucency measurements (Evans, Andriole, & Evans, 2015). See Chapter 10 for more information.

Amniocentesis

Amniocentesis involves a transabdominal puncture of the amniotic sac to obtain a sample of amniotic fluid for analysis. The fluid contains fetal cells that are examined to detect chromosomal abnormalities and several hereditary metabolic defects in the fetus before birth. In addition, amniocentesis is used to confirm a fetal abnormality when other screening tests detect a possible problem.

Amniocentesis is performed in the second trimester, usually between 15 and 18 weeks gestation. At this age, the amount of fluid is adequate (approximately 150 mL), and the ratio of viable to nonviable cells is the greatest (Hehir, Dalrymple, & Malone, 2015). More than 40 different chromosomal abnormalities, inborn errors of metabolism, and neural tube defects can be diagnosed with amniocentesis. It can replace a genetic probability with a diagnostic certainty, allowing the woman and her partner to make an informed decision about the option of therapeutic abortion.

Amniocentesis can be performed in any of the three trimesters of pregnancy. An early amniocentesis (performed between weeks 11 and 14) is done to detect genetic anomalies. However, early amniocentesis has been associated with a high risk of spontaneous miscarriage and postprocedural amniotic fluid leakage compared with transabdominal chorionic villus screening (King et al., 2015).

In the second trimester, the procedure is performed between 15 and 20 weeks to detect chromosomal abnormalities, evaluate the fetal condition when the woman is sensitized to the Rh-positive blood, diagnose intrauterine infections, and investigate amniotic fluid AFP when the MSAFP level is elevated (March of Dimes, 2015d).

In the third trimester, amniocentesis is most commonly indicated to determine fetal lung maturity after the 35th week of gestation via analysis of lecithin-to-sphingomyelin ratios and to evaluate the fetal condition with Rh isoimmunization. Table 12.2 lists amniotic fluid analysis findings and their implications.

Procedure

Amniocentesis is performed after an ultrasound examination identifies an adequate pocket of amniotic fluid free of fetal parts, the umbilical cord, or the placenta (Fig. 12.7). The health care provider inserts a long pudendal or spinal needle, a 22-gauge, 5-inch needle, into the amniotic cavity and aspirates amniotic fluid, which is placed in an amber or foil-covered test tube to protect it from light. When the desired amount of fluid has been withdrawn, the needle is removed and slight pressure is applied to the site. If there is no evidence of bleeding, a sterile bandage is applied to the needle site. The specimens are then sent to the laboratory immediately for the cytologist to evaluate.

Examining a sample of fetal cells directly produces a definitive diagnosis rather than a "best guess" diagnosis based on indirect screening tests. It is an invaluable diagnostic tool, but the risks include lower abdominal

TABLE 12.2	AMNIOTIC FLUID ANALYSIS AND IMPLICATIONS	
Test Component	**Normal Findings**	**Fetal Implications of Abnormal Findings**
Color	Clear with white flecks of vernix caseosa in a mature fetus	Blood of maternal origin is usually harmless. "Port wine" fluid may indicate abruptio placentae. Fetal blood may indicate damage to the fetal, placental, or umbilical cord vessels.
Bilirubin	Absent at term	High levels indicate hemolytic disease of the neonate in isoimmunized pregnancy.
Meconium	Absent (except in breech presentation)	Presence indicates fetal hypotension or distress.
Creatinine	More than 2 mg/dL in a mature fetus	Decrease may indicate immature fetus (less than 37 wks).
Lecithin-to-sphingomyelin ratio (L/S ratio)	More than 2 generally indicates fetal pulmonary maturity.	A ratio of less than 2 indicates pulmonary immaturity and subsequent respiratory distress syndrome.
Phosphatidylglycerol	Present	Absence indicates pulmonary immaturity.
Glucose	Less than 45 mg/dL	Excessive increases at term or near term indicate hypertrophied fetal pancreas and subsequent neonatal hypoglycemia.
Alpha-fetoprotein	Variable, depending on gestation age and laboratory technique; highest concentration (about 18.5 ng/mL) occurs at 13–14 wks	Inappropriate increases indicate neural tube defects such as spina bifida or anencephaly, impending fetal death, congenital nephrosis, or contamination of fetal blood.
Bacteria	Absent	Presence indicates chorioamnionitis.
Chromosomes	Normal karyotype	Abnormal karyotype may indicate fetal sex and chromosome disorders.
Acetylcholinesterase	Absent	Presence may indicate neural tube defects, exomphalos, or other serious malformations.

Adapted from Cunningham, F., Leveno, K., Bloom, S., Spong, K., Dashe, J. S., Hoffman, B. L., et al. (2014). *William's obstetrics* (24th ed.). New York, NY: McGraw-Hill Education; March of Dimes. (2015d). *Amniocentesis*. Retrieved from http://www.marchofdimes.com/pregnancy/amniocentesis.aspx; Springer, S. C. (2015). Prenatal diagnosis and fetal therapy. *eMedicine*. Retrieved from http://emedicine.medscape.com/article/936318-overview

discomfort and cramping that may last up to 48 hours after the procedure, spontaneous abortion (1 in 200), maternal or fetal infection, postamniocentesis chorioamnionitis that has an insidious onset, fetal–maternal hemorrhage, leakage of amniotic fluid in 2% to 3% of women after the procedure, and higher rates of fetal loss in earlier amniocentesis procedures (<15 weeks gestation) versus later ones (Akolekar et al., 2015). Obtaining the test results may take up to 3 weeks. Women today are choosing noninvasive prenatal testing rather than undergoing invasive testing such as amniocentesis or CVS despite those tests not being 100% correct. Women with reassuring noninvasive results and normal ultrasound findings seem satisfied over the risk of procedure-related pregnancy loss (Biswas & Choolani, 2015). The number of invasive procedures has declined since the availability of

noninvasive prenatal testing, and it is predicted that they will replace the more invasive procedures in the future.

Nursing Management

When preparing the woman for an amniocentesis, explain the procedure and its potential complications, and encourage her to empty her bladder just before the procedure to avoid the risk of bladder puncture. Inform her that a 20-minute electronic fetal monitoring strip usually is obtained to evaluate fetal well-being and obtain a baseline to compare after the procedure is completed. Obtain and record maternal vital signs.

After the procedure, assist the woman to a position of comfort and administer RhoGAM intramuscularly if the woman is Rh negative to prevent potential sensitization to

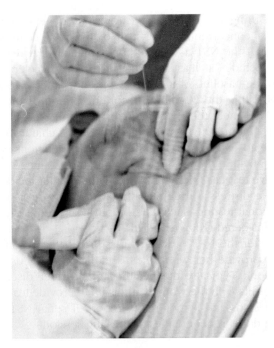

FIGURE 12.7 Technique for amniocentesis: Inserting needle.

fetal blood. Assess maternal vital signs and fetal heart rate every 15 minutes for an hour after the procedure. Observe the puncture site for bleeding or drainage. Instruct the client to rest after returning home and remind her to report fever, leaking amniotic fluid, vaginal bleeding, or uterine contractions or any changes in fetal activity (increased or decreased) to the health care provider.

When the test results come back, be available to offer support, especially if a fetal abnormality is found. Also prepare the woman and her partner for the need for genetic counseling. Trained genetic counselors can provide accurate medical information and help couples to interpret the results of the amniocentesis so they can make the decisions that are right for them as a family.

Chorionic Villus Sampling

Chorionic villus sampling (CVS) is an invasive procedure involving an 18-gauge needle stick through the abdomen or passage of a suction catheter through the cervix under ultrasound guidance. This test is used to obtain a sample of the chorionic villi from the placenta for prenatal evaluation of chromosomal disorders such as Down syndrome or cystic fibrosis, enzyme deficiencies, and fetal gender determination and to identify sex-linked disorders such as hemophilia, sickle cell anemia, and Tay–Sachs disease (Greeley et al., 2015). Chorionic villi are fingerlike projections that cover the embryo and anchor it to the uterine lining before the placenta is developed. Because they are of embryonic origin, sampling provides information about the developing fetus. CVS can be used to detect numerous genetic disorders, with the exception of neural tube defects (Latendresse & Deneris, 2015).

There has been an impetus to develop earlier prenatal diagnostic procedures so that couples can make an early decision to terminate the pregnancy if an anomaly is confirmed. Early prenatal diagnosis by CVS has been proposed as an alternative to routine amniocentesis, which carries fewer risks if done later in the pregnancy. In addition, results of CVS testing are available sooner than those of amniocentesis, usually within 48 hours.

Procedure

CVS is generally performed 10 to 13 weeks after the LMP. Earlier, chorionic villi may not be sufficiently developed for adequate tissue sampling and the risk of limb defects is increased (Khalil & Coates, 2015). First, an ultrasound is done to confirm gestational age and viability. Then, under continuous ultrasound guidance, CVS is performed using either a transcervical or transabdominal approach. With the transcervical approach, the woman is placed in the lithotomy position and a sterile catheter is introduced through the cervix and inserted in the placenta, where a sample of chorionic villi is aspirated. This approach requires the client to have a full bladder to push the uterus and placenta into a position that is more accessible to the catheter. A full bladder also helps in better visualization of the structures. With the transabdominal approach, an 18-gauge spinal needle is inserted through the abdominal wall into the placental tissue and a sample of chorionic villi is aspirated. Regardless of the approach used, the sample is sent to the cytogenetics laboratory for analysis.

Potential complications of CVS include postprocedure vaginal bleeding and cramping (most common), hematomas, spontaneous abortion, limb abnormalities, rupture of membranes, infection, chorioamnionitis, and fetal–maternal hemorrhage (March of Dimes, 2015e). The pregnancy loss rate or procedure-related miscarriage rate is approximately 0.5% to 1.0%, which is the same rate for amniocentesis. In addition, women who are Rh negative should receive immune globulin (RhoGAM) to avoid isoimmunization (Jordan et al., 2014).

Nursing Management

Explain to the woman that the procedure will last about 15 minutes. An ultrasound will be done first to locate the embryo, and a baseline set of vital signs will be taken before starting. Make sure she is informed of the risks related to the procedure, including their incidence. If a transabdominal CVS procedure is planned, advise her to fill her bladder by drinking increased amounts of water. Inform her that a needle will be inserted through her abdominal wall and samples will be collected. Once the samples are collected, the needle will be withdrawn and the samples will be sent to the genetics laboratory for evaluation.

For transcervical CVS, inform the women that a speculum will be placed into the vagina under ultrasound guidance. Then the vagina is cleaned and a small catheter is inserted through the cervix. The samples obtained through the catheter are then sent to a laboratory.

After either procedure, assist the woman to a position of comfort and clean any excess lubricant or secretions from the area. Instruct her about signs to watch for and report, such as fever, cramping, and vaginal bleeding. Urge her not to engage in any strenuous activity for the next 48 hours. Assess the fetal heart rate for changes and administer RhoGAM to an unsensitized Rh-negative woman after the procedure.

Nonstress Test

The nonstress test (NST) is the most common method of prenatal testing used in practice today. The NST provides an indirect measurement of uteroplacental function. Unlike the fetal movement counting done by the mother alone, this procedure requires specialized equipment and trained personnel. The basis for the NST is that the normal fetus produces characteristic fetal heart rate patterns in response to fetal movements. In the healthy fetus there is an acceleration of the fetal heart rate with fetal movement. Currently, an NST is recommended twice weekly (after 28 weeks of gestation) for clients with diabetes and other high-risk conditions, such as IUGR, preeclampsia, post-term pregnancy, renal disease, and multifetal pregnancies (Cunningham et al., 2014). NST is a noninvasive test that requires no initiation of contractions. It is quick to perform and there are no known side effects.

Procedure

Before the procedure, the client eats a meal to stimulate fetal activity. Then she is placed in the left lateral recumbent position to avoid supine hypotension syndrome. An external electronic fetal monitoring device is applied to her abdomen. The device consists of two belts, each with a sensor. One of the sensors records uterine activity, while the second sensor records fetal heart rate. The client is handed an "event marker" with a button that she pushes every time she perceives fetal movement. When the button is pushed, the fetal monitor strip is marked to identify that fetal movement has occurred. The procedure usually lasts 20 to 30 minutes.

Nursing Management

Prior to the NST, explain the testing procedure and have the woman empty her bladder. Position her in a semi-Fowler's position and apply the two external monitor belts. Document the date and time the test is started, client information, the reason for the test, and the maternal vital signs. Obtain a baseline fetal monitor strip over 15 to 30 minutes.

During the test, observe for signs of fetal activity with a concurrent acceleration of the fetal heart rate. Interpret the NST as reactive or nonreactive. A reactive NST includes at least two fetal heart rate accelerations from the baseline of at least 15 bpm for at least 15 seconds within the 20-minute recording period. If the test does not meet these criteria after 40 minutes, it is considered nonreactive. A nonreactive NST is characterized by the absence of two fetal heart rate accelerations using the 15-by-15 criterion in a 20-minute time frame. A nonreactive test has been correlated with a higher incidence of fetal distress during labor, fetal mortality, and IUGR. Additional testing, such as a biophysical profile, should be considered (King et al., 2015).

After the NST procedure, assist the woman off the table, provide her with fluids, and allow her to use the restroom. Typically the health care provider discusses the results with the woman at this time. Provide teaching about signs and symptoms to report. If serial NSTs are being done, schedule the next testing session.

Biophysical Profile

A **biophysical profile (BPP)** uses a real-time ultrasound and NST to allow assessment of various parameters of fetal well-being. A BPP includes ultrasound monitoring of fetal movements, fetal tone, and fetal breathing and ultrasound assessment of amniotic fluid volume with or without assessment of the fetal heart rate. A BPP is performed in an effort to identify infants who may be at risk of poor pregnancy outcome, so that additional assessments of well-being may be performed, or labor may be induced or a cesarean section performed to expedite birth. The primary objectives of the BPP are to reduce stillbirth and to detect hypoxia early enough to allow delivery in time to avoid permanent fetal damage resulting from fetal asphyxia. These parameters, together with the NST, constitute the biophysical profile. Each parameter is controlled by a different structure in the fetal brain: fetal tone by the cortex; fetal movements by the cortex and motor nuclei; fetal breathing movements by the centers close to the fourth ventricle; and the NST by the posterior hypothalamus and medulla. The amniotic fluid is the result of fetal urine volume. Some facilities do not perform an NST unless other parameters of the profile are abnormal (King et al., 2015). The BPP is based on the concept that a fetus that experiences hypoxia loses certain behavioral parameters in the reverse order in which they were acquired during fetal development (normal order of development: tone at 8 weeks; movement at 9 weeks; breathing at 20 weeks; and fetal heart rate reactivity at 24 weeks).

Scoring and Interpretation

The BPP is a scored test with five components, each worth two points if present. A total score of 10 is possible if the NST is used. Thirty minutes are allotted for testing, although less than 10 minutes is usually needed. The following criteria must be met to obtain a score of 2; anything less is scored as 0 (Moses, 2015c):

- *Body movements:* three or more discrete limb or trunk movements
- *Fetal tone:* one or more instances of full extension and flexion of a limb or trunk
- *Fetal breathing:* one or more fetal breathing movements of more than 30 seconds
- *Amniotic fluid volume:* one or more pockets of fluid measuring 2 cm
- *NST:* normal NST = 2 points; abnormal NST = 0 points

Interpretation of the BPP score can be complicated, depending on several fetal and maternal variables. Because it is indicated as a result of a nonreassuring finding from previous fetal surveillance tests, this test can be used to quantify the interpretation, and intervention can be initiated if appropriate. A maximum score of 10 can be achieved and the test is complete once all of the variables have been observed. For the test to be judged abnormal and a score of zero awarded for the absence of fetal movement, fetal tone, or fetal breathing movements, a period of not less than 30 minutes must have elapsed. Because of the excellent sensitivity of fetal NST for fetal acidemia, it has been proposed that this acute marker alone may be used for fetal assessment in combination with the amniotic fluid volume assessment, a chronic marker. This combination, also known as the modified BPP, has been shown to have excellent false-negative rates that compare with that of the complete BPP. In addition, a recent study reported that BPP scores correlates fairly closely with the APGAR scores obtained after birth (Nisa et al., 2015).

One of the important factors is the amniotic fluid volume, taken in conjunction with the results of the NST. Amniotic fluid is largely composed of fetal urine. As placental function decreases, perfusion of fetal organs, such as kidneys, decreases, and this can lead to a reduction of amniotic fluid. If oligohydramnios or decreased amniotic fluid is present, the potential exists for antepartum or intrapartum fetal compromise (Lakshmi & Jyothsna, 2015).

Overall, a score of 8 to 10 is considered normal if the amniotic fluid volume is adequate. A score of 6 or below is suspicious, possibly indicating a compromised fetus; further investigation of fetal well-being is needed.

Because the BPP is an ultrasonographic assessment of fetal behavior, it requires more extensive equipment and more highly trained personnel than other testing modalities. The cost is much greater than with less sophisticated tests. It permits conservative therapy and prevents premature or unnecessary intervention. There are fewer false-positive results than with the NST alone (Callahan, 2016).

Nursing Management

Nursing management focuses primarily on offering the client support and answering her questions. Expect to complete the NST before scheduling the biophysical profile, and explain why further testing might be needed. Tell the woman that the ultrasound will be done in the diagnostic imaging department.

NURSING MANAGEMENT FOR THE COMMON DISCOMFORTS OF PREGNANCY

Most women experience common discomforts during pregnancy and ask a nurse's advice about ways to minimize them. However, other women will not bring up their concerns unless asked. Therefore, the nurse needs to address the common discomforts that occur in each trimester at each prenatal visit and provide realistic measures to help the client deal with them (Teaching Guidelines 12.1). Nursing Care Plan 12.1 applies the nursing process to the care of a woman experiencing some discomforts of pregnancy.

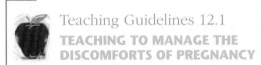

Teaching Guidelines 12.1
TEACHING TO MANAGE THE DISCOMFORTS OF PREGNANCY

Urinary Frequency or Incontinence
- Try pelvic floor exercises to increase control over leakage.
- Empty your bladder when you first feel a full sensation.
- Avoid caffeinated drinks, which stimulate voiding.
- Reduce your fluid intake after dinner to reduce night-time urination.

Fatigue
- Attempt to get a full night's sleep, without interruptions.
- Eat a healthy balanced diet.
- Schedule a nap in the early afternoon daily.
- When you are feeling tired, rest.

Nausea and Vomiting
- Avoid an empty stomach at all times.
- Eat dry crackers/toast in bed before arising.
- Eat several small meals throughout the day.
- Avoid brushing teeth immediately after eating to avoid gag reflex.
- Acupressure wristbands can be worn daily.
- Drink fluids between meals rather than with meals.
- Avoid greasy, fried foods or ones with a strong odor, such as cabbage or Brussels sprouts.

Backache
- Avoid standing or sitting in one position for long periods.

- Apply heating pad (low setting) to the small of your back.
- Support your lower back with pillows when sitting.
- Use proper body mechanics for lifting anything.
- Avoid excessive bending, lifting, or walking without rest periods.
- Wear supportive low-heeled shoes; avoid high heels.
- Stand with your shoulders back to maintain correct posture.

Leg Cramps
- Elevate legs above heart level frequently throughout the day.
- If you get a cramp, straighten both legs and flex your feet toward your body.
- Ask your health care provider about taking additional calcium supplements, which may reduce leg spasms.

Varicosities
- Walk daily to improve circulation to extremities.
- Elevate both legs above heart level while resting.
- Avoid standing in one position for long periods of time.
- Don't wear constrictive stockings and socks.
- Don't cross the legs when sitting for long periods.
- Wear support stockings to promote better circulation.

Hemorrhoids
- Establish a regular time for daily bowel elimination.
- Avoid constipation and straining during defecation.
- Prevent straining by drinking plenty of fluids and eating fiber-rich foods and exercising daily.
- Use warm sitz baths and cool witch hazel compresses for comfort.

Constipation
- Increase your intake of foods high in fiber and drink at least eight 8-ounce glasses of fluid daily.
- Ingest prunes or prune juice which are natural laxatives.
- Consume warm liquids (tea) on rising, to stimulate peristalsis.
- Exercise each day (brisk walking) to promote movement through the intestine.
- Reduce the amount of cheese consumed.

Heartburn/Indigestion
- Avoid spicy or greasy foods and eat small frequent meals.
- Sleep on several pillows so that your head is elevated 30 degrees.
- Stop smoking and avoid caffeinated drinks to reduce stimulation.
- Avoid lying down for at least 3 hours after meals.
- Try drinking sips of water to reduce burning sensation.
- Avoid foods that trigger symptoms—fried foods, citrus, soda, chocolate.
- Take antacids sparingly if burning sensation is severe.

Braxton Hicks Contractions
- Keep in mind that these contractions are a normal sensation. Try changing your position or engaging in mild exercise to help reduce the sensation.
- Drink more fluids if possible.

First-Trimester Discomforts

During the first 3 months of pregnancy, the woman's body is undergoing numerous changes. Some women experience many discomforts, but others have few. These discomforts are caused by the changes taking place within the body and they pass as the pregnancy progresses.

Urinary Frequency or Incontinence

Urinary frequency or incontinence is common in the first trimester because the growing uterus compresses the bladder. This also is a common complaint during the third trimester, especially when the fetal head settles into the pelvis. However, the discomfort tends to improve in the second trimester, when the uterus becomes an abdominal organ and moves away from the bladder region.

After infection and gestational diabetes have been ruled out as causative factors of increased urinary frequency, suggest that the woman decrease her fluid intake 2 to 3 hours before bedtime and limit her intake of caffeinated beverages. Increased voiding is normal, but encourage the client to report any pain or burning during urination. Also explain that increased urinary frequency may subside as she enters her second trimester, only to recur in the third trimester. Teach the client to perform pelvic floor muscle training exercises, formally termed Kegel exercises, to increase support of the uterus, bladder, small intestine, and rectum) throughout the day to help strengthen perineal muscle tone, thereby enhancing urinary control and decreasing the possibility of incontinence.

Fatigue

Fatigue plagues all pregnant women, primarily in the first and third trimesters (the highest energy levels typically occur during the second trimester), even if they get their normal amount of sleep at night. First-trimester fatigue most often is related to the many physical changes (e.g., increased oxygen consumption, increased levels of progesterone and relaxin, increased metabolic demands) and psychosocial changes (e.g., mood swings, multiple role demands) of pregnancy. Third-trimester fatigue can be caused by sleep disturbances from increased weight (many women cannot find a comfortable sleeping position due to the enlarging abdomen), physical discomforts such as heartburn, and insomnia due to mood swings, multiple role anxiety, and a decrease in exercise (Rigby, 2015).

NURSING CARE PLAN 12.1

Overview of the Woman Experiencing Common Discomforts of Pregnancy

Alicia, a 32-year-old, G1 P0, at 10 weeks gestation, comes to the clinic for a visit. During the interview she tells you, "I'm running to the bathroom to urinate it seems like all the time, and I'm so nauseous that I'm having trouble eating." She denies any burning or pain on urination. Vital signs are within acceptable limits.

NURSING DIAGNOSIS: Impaired urinary elimination related to frequency secondary to physiologic changes of pregnancy

Outcome Identification and Evaluation

The client will report a decrease in urinary complaints, as evidenced by a decrease in the number of times she uses the bathroom to void, reports that she feels her bladder is empty after voiding, and use of Kegel exercises.

Interventions: *Promoting Normal Urinary Elimination Patterns*

- Assess client's usual bladder elimination patterns to establish a baseline for comparison.
- Obtain a urine specimen for analysis to rule out infection or glucosuria.
- Review with client the physiologic basis for the increased frequency during pregnancy; inform client that frequency should abate during the second trimester and that it most likely will return during her third trimester. This will promote understanding of the problem.
- Encourage the client to empty her bladder when first feeling a sensation of fullness to minimize risk of urinary retention.
- Suggest client avoid caffeinated drinks, which can stimulate the need to void.
- Encourage client to drink adequate amounts of fluid throughout the day; however, have client reduce her fluid intake before bedtime to reduce nighttime urination.
- Urge client to keep perineal area clean and dry to prevent irritation and excoriation from any leakage.
- Instruct client in Kegel exercises to increase perineal muscle tone and control over leakage.
- Teach client about the signs and symptoms of urinary tract infection and urge her to report them should they occur to ensure early detection and prompt intervention.

NURSING DIAGNOSIS: Imbalanced nutrition, less than body requirements, related to nausea and vomiting

Outcome Identification and Evaluation

The client will ingest adequate amounts of nutrients for maternal and fetal well-being as evidenced by acceptable weight gain pattern and statements indicating an increase in food intake with a decrease in the number of episodes of nausea and vomiting.

Interventions: *Promoting Adequate Nutrition*

- Obtain weight and compare to baseline to determine effects of nausea and vomiting on nutritional intake.
- Review client's typical dietary intake over 24 hours to determine nutritional intake and patterns so that suggestions can be individualized.
- Encourage client to eat five or six small frequent meals throughout the day to prevent her stomach from becoming empty.
- Suggest that she munch on dry crackers, toast, cereal, or cheese, or drink a small amount of lemonade before arising to minimize nausea.

(continued)

NURSING CARE PLAN 12.1

Overview of the Woman Experiencing Common Discomforts of Pregnancy (continued)

- Encourage client to arise slowly from bed in the morning and avoid sudden movements to reduce stimulation of the vomiting center.
- Advise client to drink fluids between meals rather than with meals to avoid overdistention of the abdomen and subsequent increase in abdominal pressure.
- Encourage her to increase her intake of foods high in vitamin B_6 such as meat, poultry, bananas, fish, green leafy vegetables, peanuts, raisins, walnuts, and whole grains, as tolerated, to ensure adequate nutrient intake.
- Advise the client to avoid greasy, fried, or highly spiced foods and to avoid strong odors, including foods such as cabbage, to minimize gastrointestinal upset.
- Encourage the client to avoid wearing tight or restricting clothes to minimize pressure on the expanding abdomen.
- Arrange for consultation with nutritionist as necessary to assist with diet planning.

Once anemia, infection, and blood dyscrasias have been ruled out as contributing to the client's fatigue, advise her to arrange work, child care, and other demands in her life to permit additional rest periods. Work with the client to devise a realistic schedule for rest. Using pillows for support in the left-side-lying position relieves pressure on major blood vessels that supply oxygen and nutrients to the fetus when resting (Fig. 12.8). Also recommend the use of relaxation techniques, providing instructions as necessary, and suggest she increase her daily exercise level.

Nausea and Vomiting

It is estimated that somewhere between 70% and 80% of pregnant women experience nausea and vomiting. In the United States, this translates to approximately 4 million women. It is found more often in Western

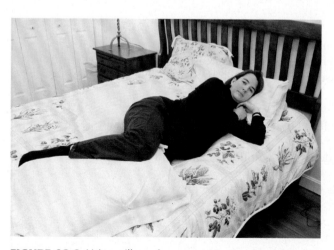

FIGURE 12.8 Using pillows for support in the side-lying position.

countries and urban populations, and is rare among Africans, Native Americans, Eskimos, and most Asian populations (Callahan, 2016). The problem is generally time limited, with the onset about the fifth week after the last menstrual period, a peak at 8 to 12 weeks, and resolution by 16 to 18 weeks. Despite popular use of the term *morning sickness*, nausea and vomiting of pregnancy persist throughout the day in the majority of affected women and has been found to be limited to the morning in less than 2% of women (Tyler & Nagtalon-Ramos, 2015). The physiologic changes that cause nausea and vomiting are unknown, but research suggests that unusually high levels of estrogen, progesterone, and hCG, and a vitamin B_6 deficiency may be contributing factors. Symptoms generally last until the second trimester and are generally associated with a positive pregnancy outcome, in terms of lower rates of miscarriages, congenital malformations, and preterm births (Cunningham et al., 2014). In summary, the etiology of nausea and vomiting in pregnancy is physiologic, thus assessment of the condition focuses on severity, and the management is largely supportive.

Nausea and vomiting of pregnancy can take a physical and psychological toll on the pregnant woman, and may have an adverse effect on her partner, family members, and even co-workers. The burden it places on the woman is usually minimized, as it is considered a normal part of pregnancy, thus it may not be worthy of evaluation, diagnosis, management, and emotional support. As a result, it may not be taken seriously because it is so common and time-limited; leading some women to feel frustrated and feel guilty that they are even complaining about their symptoms. Nurses need to pick up on this, address it, and provide support for her.

The goal of treatment is to improve symptoms while minimizing risks to mother and fetus. Treatment management ranges from simple dietary modifications to drug therapy. To help alleviate nausea and vomiting, advise the woman to eat small, frequent meals that are bland and low in fat (five or six times a day) to prevent her stomach from becoming completely empty. Other helpful suggestions include eating dry crackers, Cheerios, or cheese or drinking lemonade before getting out of bed in the morning and increasing her intake of foods high in vitamin B_6, such as meat, poultry, bananas, fish, green leafy vegetables, peanuts, raisins, walnuts, and whole grains, or making sure she is receiving enough vitamin B_6 by taking her prescribed prenatal vitamins.

Pharmacologic treatment of nausea and vomiting in pregnancy is limited. The Food and Drug Administration (FDA) recently approved doxylamine–pyridoxine therapy for use in pregnancy, which seems to work fairly well based on the current reviews (Slaughter et al., 2014). Other pharmacotherapies that might be considered may include diphenhydramine (e.g., Benadryl), dimenhydrinate (e.g., Dramamine), meclinine (e.g., Antivert), prochlorperazine (e.g., Compazine), promethazine (e.g., Phenergan), or ondansetron (e.g., Zofran).

Other helpful tips to deal with nausea and vomiting include the following:
• Get out of bed in the morning very slowly.
• Avoid sudden movements.
• Avoid triggers that stimulate or exacerbate nausea—strong food odors.
• Eat a high-protein snack before retiring at night to prevent an empty stomach.
• Take ginger (up to 1 g in divided doses daily; 250 mg capsules QID), which increases tone and peristalsis in the gastrointestinal tract.
• Open a window to remove odors of food being cooked.
• Eat more protein than carbohydrates and take in more liquids than solids.
• Limit intake of fluids or soups during meals (drink them between meals).
• Avoid fried foods and foods cooked with grease, oils, or fatty meats, because they tend to upset the stomach.
• Avoid highly seasoned foods such as those cooked with garlic, onions, peppers, and chili.
• Drink a small amount of caffeine-free carbonated beverage (ginger ale) if nauseated.
• Trying acupressure using a wristband has been FDA approved for nausea.
• Avoid wearing tight or restricting clothes, which might place increased pressure on the expanding abdomen.
• Avoid stress (Bope & Kellerman, 2015; Jordan et al., 2014; King et al., 2015).

Breast Tenderness

As a result of increased estrogen and progesterone levels, which cause the fat layer of breasts to thicken and the number of milk ducts and glands to increase during the first trimester, many women experience breast tenderness. Offering a thorough explanation to the woman about the reasons for the breast discomfort is important. Wearing a larger bra with good support can help alleviate this discomfort. Advise her to wear a supportive bra, even while sleeping. As her breasts increase in size, advise her to change her bra size to ensure adequate support.

Constipation

Constipation affects up to 38% of pregnancies (Verghese, Futaba, & Latthe, 2015). Increasing levels of progesterone during pregnancy lead to decreased contractility of the gastrointestinal tract, slowed movement of substances through the colon, and a resulting increase in water absorption. All of these factors lead to constipation. Lack of exercise or too little fiber or fluids in the diet can also promote constipation. In addition, the large bowel is mechanically compressed by the enlarging uterus, adding to this discomfort. The iron and calcium in prenatal vitamins can also contribute to constipation during the first and third trimesters.

Explain how pregnancy exacerbates the symptoms of constipation and offer the following suggestions:
• Eat fresh or dried fruit daily.
• Eat more raw fruits and vegetables, including their skins.
• Eat whole-grain cereals and breads such as raisin bran or bran flakes.
• Participate in physical activity every day.
• Engage in pelvis floor exercises, stretching exercises and yoga daily
• Eat meals at regular intervals.
• Establish a time of day to defecate, and elevate feet on a stool to avoid straining.
• Drink six to eight glasses of water daily.
• Decrease intake of refined carbohydrates.
• Drink warm fluids on arising to stimulate bowel motility.
• Decrease consumption of sugary sodas.
• Avoid eating large amounts of cheese.

If the suggestions above are ineffective, suggest that the woman use a bulk-forming laxative such as Metamucil®.

Nasal Stuffiness, Bleeding Gums, Epistaxis (Nosebleeds)

Increased levels of estrogen cause edema of the mucous membranes of the nasal and oral cavities. Advise the woman to drink extra water for hydration of the mucous membranes or to use a cool mist humidifier in her bedroom at night. If she needs to blow her nose to relieve nasal stuffiness, advise her to blow gently, one nostril at a time. Advise her to avoid the use of nasal decongestants and sprays.

If a nosebleed occurs, advise the woman to loosen the clothing around her neck, sit with her head tilted forward, pinch her nostrils with her thumb and forefinger for 10 to 15 minutes, and apply an ice pack to the bridge of her nose.

If the woman has bleeding gums, encourage her to practice good oral hygiene by using a soft toothbrush and flossing daily. Warm saline mouthwashes can relieve discomfort. If the gum problem persists, instruct her to see her dentist.

Cravings

Food craving refers to an intense desire to consume a specific food. Desires for certain foods and beverages are likely to begin during the first trimester but do not appear to reflect any physiologic need. Foods with a high sodium or sugar content often are the ones craved. At times, some women crave nonfood substances such as clay, cornstarch, laundry detergent, baking soda, soap, paint chips, dirt, ice, or wax. As explained in Chapter 11, this craving for nonfood substances, termed *pica*, may indicate a severe dietary deficiency of minerals or vitamins, or it may have cultural roots (Jyothi, 2015).

Leukorrhea

Increased vaginal discharge begins during the first trimester and continues throughout pregnancy. The physiologic changes behind leukorrhea arise from the high levels of estrogen, which cause increased vascularity and hypertrophy of cervical glands as well as vaginal cells (Cunningham et al., 2014). The result is progressively increasing vaginal secretions throughout pregnancy.

Advise the woman to keep the perineal area clean and dry, washing the area with mild soap and water during her daily shower. Also recommend that she avoid wearing pantyhose and other tight-fitting nylon clothes that prevent air from circulating to the genital area. Encourage the use of cotton underwear and suggest wearing a nightgown rather than pajamas to allow for increased airflow. Also instruct the woman to avoid douching and tampon use.

Second-Trimester Discomforts

A sense of well-being typically characterizes the second trimester for most women. By this time, the fatigue, nausea, and vomiting have subsided and the uncomfortable changes of the third trimester are a few months away. Not every woman experiences the same discomforts during this time, so nursing assessments and interventions must be individualized.

Backache

Musculoskeletal pain is a common occurrence in pregnancy and postpartum. Half of women report having back pain at some point during pregnancy. This can seriously impact the quality of life of women and have socioeconomic issues from loss days at work. The pain can be lumbar or sacroiliac. The pain may also be present only at night. Back pain is thought to be due to multiple factors, which include shifting of the center of gravity caused by the enlarging uterus, increased joint laxity due to an increase in relaxin, stretching of the ligaments (which are pain-sensitive structures), and pregnancy-related circulatory changes.

Treatment is heat and ice, acetaminophen, massage, proper posturing, good support shoes, and a good exercise program for strength and conditioning. Pregnant women may also relieve back pain by placing one foot on a stool when standing for long periods of time and placing a pillow between the legs when lying down (Plastaras & Appasamy, 2015). After exploring other reasons that might cause backache, such as uterine contractions, urinary tract infection, ulcers, or musculoskeletal back disorders, the following instructions may be helpful:

- Maintain correct posture, with head up and shoulders back.
- Wear low-heeled shoes with good arch support.
- When standing for long periods, place one foot on a stool or box.
- Use good body mechanics when lifting objects.
- When sitting, use foot supports and pillows behind the back.
- Try pelvic tilt or rocking exercises to strengthen the back (ACOG, 2015c).

The pelvic tilt or pelvic rock is used to alleviate pressure on the lower back during pregnancy by stretching the lower back muscles. It can be done sitting, standing, or on all fours. To do it on all fours, the hands are positioned directly under the shoulders and the knees under the hips. The back should be in a neutral position with the head and neck aligned with the straight back. The woman then presses up with the lower back and holds this position for a few seconds, then relaxes to a neutral position. This action of pressing upward is repeated frequently throughout the day to prevent a sore back (Rigby, 2015).

Leg Cramps

Many women experience leg cramps in pregnancy. They become more common as pregnancy progresses and are especially troublesome at night. They occur primarily in the second and third trimesters and could be related to the pressure of the gravid uterus on pelvic nerves and blood vessels. During pregnancy, up to 50% of women can be affected by leg cramps, and up to

25% can be affected by restless legs syndrome (King et al., 2015). Along with lack of exercise, diet can also be a contributing factor if the woman is not consuming enough of certain minerals, such as calcium and magnesium. The sudden stretching of leg muscles may also play a role in causing leg cramps (Kondhare & Khodgire, 2015).

Encourage the woman to gently stretch the muscle by dorsiflexing the foot up toward the body. Wrapping a warm, moist towel around the leg muscle can also help the muscle to relax. Advise the client to avoid stretching her legs, pointing her toes, and walking excessively. Stress the importance of wearing low-heeled shoes and support hose and arising slowly from a sitting position. If the leg cramps are due to deficiencies in minerals, the condition can be remedied by eating more foods rich in these nutrients. Also instruct the woman on calf-stretching exercises: have her stand 3 feet from the wall and lean toward it, resting her lower arms against it, while keeping her heels on the floor. This may help reduce cramping if it is done before going to bed.

Elevating the legs throughout the day will help relieve pressure and minimize strain. Wearing support hose and avoiding curling the toes may help to relieve leg discomfort. Also instruct the client to avoid standing in one spot for a prolonged period or crossing her legs. If she must stand for prolonged periods, suggest that she change her position at least every 2 hours by walking or sitting to reduce the risk of leg cramps. Encourage her to drink eight 8-ounce glasses of fluid throughout the day to ensure adequate hydration. Taking daily walks can also help reduce leg cramping because ambulation improves circulation to the muscles.

Varicosities of the Vulva and Legs

Varicosities of the vulva and legs are associated with the increased venous stasis caused by the pressure of the gravid uterus on pelvic vessels and the vasodilation resulting from increased progesterone levels. Progesterone relaxes the vein walls, making it difficult for blood to return to the heart from the extremities; pooling can result. Genetic predisposition, inactivity, obesity, and poor muscle tone are also contributing factors.

Encourage the client to wear support hose and teach her how to apply them properly. Advise her to elevate her legs above her heart while lying on her back for 10 minutes before she gets out of bed in the morning, thus promoting venous return before she applies the hose. Instruct the client to avoid crossing her legs and avoid wearing knee-high stockings. They cause constriction of leg vessels and muscles and contribute to venous stasis. Also encourage the client to elevate both legs above the level of the heart for 5 to 10 minutes at least twice a day (Fig. 12.9); to wear low-heeled shoes; and to avoid long periods of standing or sitting, frequently changing her

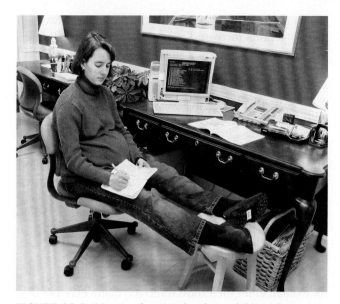

FIGURE 12.9 Woman elevating her legs while working.

position. If the client has vulvar varicosities, suggest she apply ice packs to the area when she is lying down.

Hemorrhoids

Hemorrhoids are varicosities of the rectum and may be external (outside the anal sphincter) or internal (above the sphincter) (ACOG, 2015d). They occur as a result of progesterone-induced vasodilation and from pressure of the enlarged uterus on the lower intestine and rectum. Hemorrhoids are more common in women with constipation, poor fluid intake or poor dietary habits, smokers, or those with a previous history of hemorrhoids (Zielinski, Searing, & Deibel, 2015).

Instruct the client in measures to prevent constipation, including increasing fiber intake and drinking at least 2 L of fluid per day. Recommend the use of topical anesthetics (e.g., Preparation H®, Anusol, witch hazel compresses such as Tucks®) to reduce pain, itching, and swelling, if permitted by the health care provider. Teach the client about local comfort measures such as warm sitz baths, witch hazel compresses, or cold compresses. To minimize her risk of straining while defecating, suggest that she elevates her feet on a stool. Also encourage her to avoid prolonged sitting or standing (ACOG, 2015d).

Flatulence With Bloating

Flatulence and gas pain are another result of decreased gastrointestinal motility. The physiologic changes that result in constipation (reduced gastrointestinal motility and dilation secondary to progesterone's influence) may also result in increased flatulence. As the enlarging uterus compresses the bowel, it delays the passage of food through the intestines, thus allowing more time for gas to be formed by bacteria in the colon. The woman usually reports increased passage of rectal gas, abdominal bloating, or belching. Instruct the woman to avoid gas-forming foods, such as beans, cabbage, and onions, as well as foods that have a high content of white sugar. Adding more fiber to the diet, increasing fluid intake, and increasing physical exercise are also helpful in reducing flatus. In addition, reducing the amount of swallowed air, if chewing gum, will reduce gas build-up. The knee–chest position may also help with discomfort from unexpelled gas. Reducing the intake of carbonated beverages and cheese and eating mints can also help reduce flatulence during pregnancy (Almansa, De Vault, & Houghton, 2015).

Third-Trimester Discomforts

As women enter their third trimester, many experience a return of the first-trimester discomforts of fatigue, urinary frequency, leukorrhea, and constipation. These discomforts are secondary to the ever-enlarging uterus compressing adjacent structures, increasing hormone levels, and the metabolic demands of the fetus. In addition to these discomforts, many women experience shortness of breath, heartburn and indigestion, swelling, and Braxton Hicks contractions.

Shortness of Breath and Dyspnea

Dyspnea is a common complaint in pregnant women. Physiologic and hemodynamic changes can result in a significant dyspnea in such cases. In some women, dyspnea in normal daily activities can be a sign of heart and lung disease and may be associated with poor perinatal and cardiac outcomes in which early detection can prevent adverse events. The increasing growth of the uterus prevents complete lung expansion late in pregnancy. As the uterus enlarges upward in the second and third trimesters, the expansion of the diaphragm is limited. Dyspnea can occur when the woman lies on her back and the pressure of the gravid uterus against the vena cava reduces venous return to the heart (Tara et al., 2015).

Explain to the woman that dyspnea is normal and will improve when the fetus drops into the pelvis (lightening). Instruct her to adjust her body position to allow for maximum expansion of the chest and to avoid large meals, which increase abdominal pressure. Raising the head of the bed on blocks or placing pillows behind her back is helpful too. Under normal circumstances, resting with the head elevated while taking slow, deep breaths reduces shortness of breath symptoms. In addition, stress to her that lying on her left side will displace the uterus off the vena cava and improve her breathing. Having the woman periodically stand up and stretch her arms above her head and take a deep breath is helpful to relieve dyspnea. Also, advise the woman to avoid exercise that precipitates dyspnea, to rest after exercise, and to avoid overheating in warm climates. If she still smokes, encourage her to stop.

Heartburn and Indigestion

Heartburn and indigestion result when high progesterone levels cause relaxation of the cardiac sphincter, allowing food and digestive juices to flow backward from the stomach into the esophagus. Irritation of the esophageal lining occurs, causing the burning sensation known as heartburn. It occurs in up to 70% of women at some point during pregnancy, with an increased frequency seen in the third trimester (King et al., 2015). The pain may radiate to the neck and throat. It worsens when the woman lies down, bends over after eating, or wears tight clothes. Indigestion (vague abdominal discomfort after meals) results from eating too much or too fast; from eating when tense, tired, or emotionally upset; from eating food that is too fatty or spicy; and from eating heavy food or food that has been badly cooked or processed (Nagtalon-Ramos, 2014). In addition, the stomach is displaced upward and compressed by the large uterus in the third trimester, thus limiting the stomach's capacity to empty quickly. Food sits, causing heartburn and indigestion.

Review the client's usual dietary intake and suggest that she limit or avoid gas-producing or fatty foods and large meals. Instruct the woman to pay attention to the timing of the discomfort. Usually it is heartburn when the pain occurs 30 to 45 minutes after a meal. Encourage the client to maintain proper posture and remain in the sitting position for 1 to 3 hours after eating to prevent reflux of gastric acids into the esophagus by gravity. Urge the client to consume small, frequent meals, to eat slowly, chewing her food thoroughly to prevent excessive swallowing of air, which can lead to increased gastric pressure. Instruct the client to avoid foods that act as triggers such as caffeinated drinks, greasy, gas-forming foods, citrus, spiced foods, chocolate, coffee, alcohol, and spearmint or peppermint. These items stimulate the release of gastric digestive acids, which may cause reflux into the esophagus. Avoid late-night or large meals and gum chewing. Avoid lying down within 3 hours after eating. Finally, elevate the head of the bed by 10 to 30 degrees.

Dependent Edema

Swelling is the result of increased capillary permeability caused by elevated hormone levels and increased blood volume. Sodium and water are retained and thirst increases. Edema occurs most often in dependent areas such as the legs and feet throughout the day due to gravity; it improves after a night's sleep. Warm weather or prolonged standing or sitting may increase edema. Generalized edema, appearing in the face, hands, and feet, can signal preeclampsia if accompanied by dizziness, blurred vision, headaches, upper quadrant pain, or nausea (Rigby, 2015). This edema should be reported to the health care provider. Appropriate suggestions to minimize dependent edema include the following:

- Elevate your feet and legs above the level of the heart periodically throughout the day.
- Wear support hose when standing or sitting for long periods.
- Change position frequently throughout the day.
- Walk at a sensible pace to help contract leg muscles to promote venous return.
- When taking a long car ride, stop to walk around every 2 hours.
- When standing, rock from the ball of the foot to the toes to stimulate circulation.
- Lie on your left side to keep the gravid uterus off the vena cava to return blood to the heart.
- Avoid foods high in sodium, such as lunch meats, potato chips, and bacon.
- Avoid wearing knee-high stockings.
- Drink six to eight glasses of water daily to replace fluids lost through perspiration.
- Avoid high intake of sugar and fats, because they cause water retention.

Braxton Hicks Contractions

Braxton Hicks contractions are irregular, painless contractions that occur without cervical dilation. Typically they intensify in the third trimester in preparation for labor. In reality, they have been present since early in the pregnancy but may have gone unnoticed. They are thought to increase the tone of uterine muscles for labor purposes (Grant, Strevens, & Thornton, 2015).

Reassure the client that these contractions are normal. Instruct the client in how to differentiate between Braxton Hicks and labor contractions. Explain that true labor contractions usually grow longer, stronger, and closer together and occur at regular intervals. Walking usually strengthens true labor contractions, whereas Braxton Hicks contractions tend to decrease in intensity and taper off. Advise the client to keep herself well hydrated and to rest in a left-side-lying position to help relieve the discomfort. Suggest that she use breathing techniques such as Lamaze techniques to ease the discomfort.

NURSING MANAGEMENT TO PROMOTE SELF-CARE

Pregnancy is considered a time of health, not illness. Health promotion and maintenance activities are essential to promoting an optimal outcome for the woman and her fetus. Pregnant women commonly have many questions about the changes occurring during pregnancy: how these changes affect their usual routine, such as working, traveling, exercising, or engaging in sexual activity; how the changes influence their typical self-care activities, such as bathing, perineal care, or dental care; and whether these changes are signs of a problem.

 Take Note!

Women may have heard stories about or been told by others what to do and what not to do during pregnancy, leading to many misconceptions and much misinformation.

Nurses can play a major role in providing anticipatory guidance and teaching to foster the woman's responsibility for self-care, helping to clarify misconceptions and correct any misinformation. Educating the client to identify threats to safety posed by her lifestyle or environment and proposing ways to modify them to avoid a negative outcome are important. Counseling should also include healthy ways to prepare food, advice to avoid medications unless they are prescribed for her, and advice on identifying teratogens within her environment or at work and how to reduce her risk from exposure. The pregnant client can better care for herself and the fetus if her concerns are anticipated and identified by the nurse and are incorporated into teaching sessions at each prenatal visit.

Personal Hygiene

Hygiene is a necessity for the maintenance of good health. Cleansing the skin removes dirt, bacteria, sweat,

Consider This

One has to wonder sometimes why women go through what they do. During my first pregnancy I was sick for the first 2 months. I would experience waves of nausea from the moment I got out of bed until midmorning. Needless to say, I wasn't the happiest camper around. After the third month, my life seemed to settle down and I was beginning to think that being pregnant wasn't too bad after all. For the moment, I was fooled. Then, during my last 2 months, another wave of discomfort struck—heartburn and constipation—a double whammy! I now feared eating anything that might trigger acid indigestion and also might remain in my body too long. I literally had to become the "fiber queen" to combat these two challenges. Needless to say, my "suffering" was well worth our bright-eyed baby girl in the end.

Thoughts: Despite the various discomforts associated with pregnancy, most women wouldn't change their end result. Do most women experience these discomforts? What suggestions could be made to reduce them?

dead skin cells, and body secretions. Counsel women to wash their hands and under their fingernails frequently throughout the day in order to lower the bacterial count on both. During pregnancy a woman's sebaceous (sweat) glands become more active under the influence of hormones, and sweating is more profuse. This increase may make it necessary to use a stronger deodorant and shower more frequently. The cervical and vaginal glands also produce more secretions during pregnancy. Frequent showering helps to keep the area dry and promotes better hygiene. Encourage the use of cotton underwear to allow greater air circulation. Taking a tub bath in early pregnancy is permitted, but closer to term, when the woman's center of gravity shifts, it is safer to shower to prevent the risk of slipping.

Hot Tubs and Saunas

Caution pregnant women to avoid using hot tubs, saunas, whirlpools, and tanning beds during pregnancy. The heat may cause fetal tachycardia as well as raise the maternal temperature. Exposure to bacteria in hot tubs that have not been cleaned sufficiently is another reason to avoid them during pregnancy.

Perineal Care

The glands in the cervical and vaginal areas become more active during pregnancy secondary to hormonal influences. This increase in activity will produce more vaginal secretions, especially in the last trimester. Advise pregnant women to shower frequently and wear all-cotton underwear to minimize the effects of these secretions. Caution pregnant women not to douche, because douching can increase the risk of infection, and not to wear panty liners, which block air circulation and promote moisture. Explain that they should also avoid perfumed soaps, lotions, perineal sprays, and harsh laundry detergents to help prevent irritation and potential infection.

Dental Care

Physiologic changes that occur in pregnant women can adversely affect oral health. Elevations in estrogen and progesterone enhance the inflammatory response and consequently alter gingival tissue. During pregnancy, the incidence of gingivitis and periodontitis increases (Anil et al., 2015). Pregnancy is a time when a woman can be very receptive to health messaging. Pregnancy is no longer a contraindication for dental treatment; it is also a time when nurses can help clients understand that good oral health is important to a healthy pregnancy and can decrease the risk of dental caries in their children. When women see oral health as a priority for themselves, they are more likely to place a high priority on their children's oral health.

Periodontal disease is a contributing factor to systemic conditions, such as heart disease, respiratory diseases, diabetes mellitus, adverse pregnancy outcomes (preterm births, low–birth-weight infants, and small-for-gestational-age infants), anemia, and stroke (Trivedi, Lal, & Singhal, 2015). Research has established that the elevated levels of estrogen and progesterone during pregnancy cause women to be more sensitive to the effects of bacterial dental plaque, which can cause gingivitis, an oral infection characterized by swollen and bleeding gums (ACOG, 2013). Brushing and flossing teeth twice daily will help reduce bacteria in the mouth. Advise the woman to visit her dentist early in the pregnancy to address any dental caries and have a thorough cleaning to prevent possible infection later in the pregnancy. Advise her to avoid exposure to x-rays by informing the hygienist of the pregnancy. If x-rays are necessary, the abdomen should be shielded with a lead apron.

Researchers have reported an association between prematurity and periodontitis, an oral infection that spreads beyond the gum tissues to invade the supporting structures of the teeth. Periodontitis is characterized by bleeding gums, loss of tooth attachment, loss of supporting bone, and bad breath due to pus formation. Unfortunately, because this infection is chronic and often painless, women frequently do not realize they have it and a preterm birth can result. During pregnancy, gingivitis occurs in 35% to 100% of women, depending upon the study (Trivedi et al., 2015). Nurses should assess all pregnant women's oral health status by taking an oral health history; checking their mouths for swollen or bleeding gums, untreated dental decay, mucosal lesions, and signs of infection; and document findings in the prenatal record.

Additional guidelines that the nurse should stress regarding maintaining dental health include the following:
- Seek professional dental care during the first trimester for assessment and care.
- Be reassured that oral health care is safe during pregnancy.
- Obtain treatment for dental pain and infection promptly during pregnancy.
- Brush twice daily for 2 minutes, especially before bed, with fluoridated toothpaste and rinse well. Use a soft-bristled toothbrush and be sure to brush at the gum line to remove food debris and plaque to keep gums healthy.
- Floss teeth daily with dental floss and rinse well afterward with plain water.
- Eat healthy foods, especially those high in vitamins A, C, and D, and calcium.
- Avoid sugary snacks.
- Chew sugar-free gum for 10 minutes after a meal if brushing is not possible.
- After vomiting, rinse your mouth immediately with baking soda (1/4 teaspoon) and warm water (1 cup)

to neutralize the acid (National Maternal and Child Oral Health Resource Center, 2015).

Breast Care

Because the breasts enlarge significantly and become heavier throughout pregnancy, stress the need to wear a firm, supportive bra with wide straps to balance the weight of the breasts. Instruct the woman to anticipate buying a larger-sized bra about halfway through her pregnancy because of the increasing size of the breasts. Advise her to avoid using soap on the nipple area because it can be very drying. Encourage her to rinse the nipple area with plain water while bathing to keep it clean. The Montgomery glands (located in the areolar part of the nipple) secrete a lubricating substance that keeps the nipples moist and discourages growth of bacteria, so there is no need to use alcohol or other antiseptics on the nipples.

If the mother has chosen to breast-feed, nipple preparation is unnecessary unless her nipples are inverted and do not become erect when stimulated. Breast shells can be worn during the last 2 months to address this issue (Alexander et al., 2014).

Around week 16 of pregnancy, colostrum secretion begins, which the woman may notice as moisture in her bra. Advise the woman to place breast pads or a cotton cloth in her bra and change them frequently to prevent buildup, which may lead to excoriation.

Clothing

Many contemporary clothes are loose fitting and layered, so the woman may not need to buy an entirely new wardrobe to accommodate her pregnancy. Some pregnant women may continue to wear tight clothes. Point out that loose clothing will be more comfortable for the client and her expanding waistline.

Advise pregnant women to avoid wearing constricting clothes and girdles that compress the growing abdomen. Urge the woman to avoid knee-high hose, which might impede lower-extremity circulation and increase the risk of developing DVT. Low-heeled shoes will minimize pelvic tilt and possible backache. Wearing layered clothing that can be removed as the temperatures fluctuate may be more comfortable, especially toward term, when the woman may feel overheated.

Exercise

A physically inactive lifestyle is associated with an increase in chronic diseases such as cardiovascular disease, type 2 diabetes, osteoporosis, and cancer. The proportion of pregnant women who are overweight or obese is increasing globally, thus exercise is essential to reduce these risks and promote a healthy pregnancy. Exercise is well tolerated by a healthy woman during pregnancy. It promotes a

feeling of well-being; improves circulation; helps reduce constipation, bloating, and swelling; may help prevent or treat gestational diabetes; promotes muscle tone, strength, and endurance; may improve the woman's ability to cope with labor; increases energy level; improves posture; helps sleep and promotes relaxation and rest; and relieves the lower back discomfort that often arises as the pregnancy progresses (Barakat, Lucia, & Ruiz, 2015). However, the duration and difficulty of exercise should be modified throughout pregnancy because of a decrease in performance efficiency with gestational age. Some women continue to push themselves to maintain their prior level of exercise, but most find that as their shape changes and their abdominal area enlarges, they must modify their exercise routines. Modification also helps to reduce the risk of injury caused by laxity of the joints and connective tissue due to the hormonal effects (Petrov, Glantz, & Fagevik Olsen, 2015).

Exercise during pregnancy is contraindicated in women with preterm labor, poor weight gain, anemia, facial and hand edema, pain, hypertension, threatened abortion, dizziness, shortness of breath, multiple gestation, decreased fetal activity, cardiac disease, and palpitations (Rigby, 2015).

Federal physical activity guidelines recommend at least 150 minutes of moderate-intensity exercise per week during pregnancy (Fig. 12.10) (Dietz, 2015). It is believed that pregnancy is a unique time for behavior modification and that healthy behaviors maintained or adopted during pregnancy may improve the woman's health for the rest of her life. The excess weight gained in pregnancy, which some women never lose, is a major public health problem (Truong et al., 2015). Exercise helps the woman avoid gaining excess weight during pregnancy.

Exercise during pregnancy helps return a woman's body to good health after the baby is born. The long-term benefits of exercise that begin in early pregnancy include improved posture, weight control, and improved muscle tone. Exercise also aids in the prevention of osteoporosis after menopause, reduces the risk of hypertension and diabetes, and assists in keeping the birth weight of the fetus within the normal range (Barakat et al., 2015). Teaching Guidelines 12.2 highlights recommendations for exercise during pregnancy.

Teaching Guidelines 12.2
TEACHING TO PROMOTE EXERCISE DURING PREGNANCY

- Consume liquids before, during, and after exercising.
- Ask your health care provider before you start a new exercise routine.
- Avoid exercising in hot, humid weather or when you have a fever.
- Stop exercising if you experience vaginal bleeding, dizziness, chest pain, headache, muscle weakness,

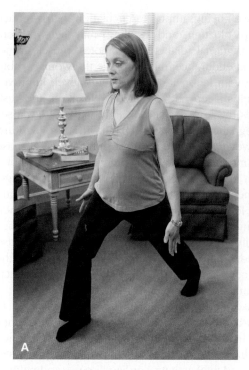

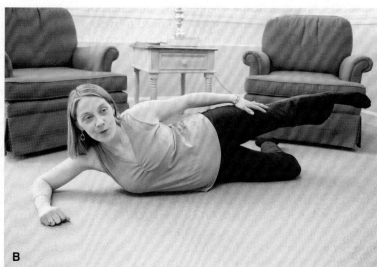

FIGURE 12.10 Exercising during pregnancy.

calf pain or swelling, uterine contractions, decreased fetal movement, or fluid leaking from the vagina.

* Exercise three or four times each week, not sporadically.
* Engage in brisk walking, swimming, biking, or low-impact aerobics; these are considered ideal activities.
* Avoid getting overheated during exercise.
* Wear comfortable exercise footwear that gives strong ankle and arch support.
* Contact sports should be avoided during pregnancy.
* Include relaxation and stretching before and after your exercise program.
* Reduce the intensity of workouts in late pregnancy.
* Avoid jerky, bouncy, or high-impact movements.
* Avoid lying flat (supine) after the fourth month because of hypotensive effect.
* Use pelvic tilt and pelvic rocking to relieve backache.
* Start with 5 to 10 minutes of stretching exercises.
* Rise slowly following an exercise session to avoid dizziness.
* Avoid activities such as skiing, surfing, scuba diving, and ice hockey.
* Never exercise to the point of exhaustion.

Adapted from Kader, M., & Naim-Shuchana, S. (2014). Physical activity and exercise during pregnancy. *European Journal of Physiotherapy*, *16*(1), 2–9; American College of Obstetricians & Gynecologists. (2015e). *Exercise during pregnancy*. Retrieved from https://www.acog.org/Search?Keyword=exercise+guidelines; American Pregnancy Association. (2014b). *Pregnancy exercise guidelines*. Retrieved from http://americanpregnancy.org/pregnancyhealth/exerciseguidelines.html

Sleep and Rest

Getting enough sleep helps a person feel better and promotes optimal performance levels during the day. The body releases its greatest concentration of growth hormone during sleep, helping the body to repair damaged tissue and grow. Also, with the increased metabolic demands during pregnancy, fatigue is a constant challenge to many pregnant women, especially during the first and third trimesters. The following tips can help promote adequate sleep:

* Stay on a regular schedule by going to bed and waking up at the same times.
* Eat regular meals at regular times to keep external body cues consistent.
* Take time to unwind and relax before bedtime.
* Establish a bedtime routine or pattern and follow it.
* Create a proper sleep environment by reducing the light and lowering the room temperature.
* Go to bed when you feel tired; if sleep does not occur, read a book until you are sleepy.
* Reduce caffeine intake later in the day.
* Limit fluid intake after dinner to minimize trips to the bathroom.
* Exercise daily to improve circulation and well-being.
* Use a modified Sims position to improve circulation in the lower extremities.
* Avoid lying on your back after the fourth month, which may compromise circulation to the uterus.
* Avoid sharply bending your knees, which promotes venous stasis below the knees.

• Keep anxieties and worries out of the bedroom. Set aside a specific area in the home or time of day for them.

Sexual Activity and Sexuality

Sexuality is an important part of health and well-being. Pregnancy is characterized by intense biologic, psychological, and social changes. These changes have direct and indirect, conscious and unconscious effects on a woman's sexuality. The woman experiences dramatic alterations in her physiology, her appearance, and her body, as well as her relationships. A woman's sexual responses during pregnancy vary widely. Common symptoms such as fatigue, nausea, vomiting, breast soreness, and urinary frequency may reduce her desire for sexual intimacy. However, many women report enhanced sexual desire due to increasing levels of estrogen. Usually sexual satisfaction does not change in pregnancy compared with the prepregnancy patterns despite a decline of sexual activity during the third trimester. A discussion of expected changes in sexuality should be routinely done in order to improve couples' perception of possible sexual modifications induced by pregnancy. It is clear that, despite some difficulties related to sexual activity during pregnancy, its need and importance are recognized for both participants.

Take Note!

Fluctuations in sexual desire are normal and a highly individualized response throughout pregnancy.

The physical and emotional adjustments of pregnancy can cause changes in body image, fatigue, mood swings, and sexual activity. The woman's changing shape, emotional status, fetal activity, changes in breast size, pressure on the bladder, and other common discomforts of pregnancy result in increased physical and emotional demands. These can produce stress on the sexual relationship of the pregnant woman and her partner. However, most women adjust well to the alterations and experience a satisfying sexual relationship. Research indicates that sexual intercourse is safe in the absence of ruptured membranes, bleeding, or placenta previa, but pregnant women engage in sex less often as the pregnancy progresses (ACOG, 2015f).

Often pregnant women ask whether sexual intercourse is allowed during pregnancy or whether there are specific times when they should refrain from having sex. This is a good opportunity to educate clients about sexual behavior during pregnancy and also to ask about their expectations and individual experience related to sexuality and possible changes. It is also a good time for nurses to address the impact of the changes associated with pregnancy on sexual desire and behavior. Couples may enjoy sexual activity more because there is no fear of pregnancy and no need to disrupt spontaneity by using birth control. An increase in pelvic congestion and lubrication secondary to estrogen influence may heighten orgasm for many women. Some women have a decrease in desire because of a negative body image, fear of harming the fetus by engaging in intercourse, and fatigue, nausea, and vomiting (Boynton, 2015). Condom use can be recommended to decrease the release of prostaglandins in the semen that may stimulate contractions. A couple may need assistance to adjust to the various changes brought about by pregnancy.

Reassure the women and her partner that sexual activity is permissible during pregnancy unless there is a history of any of the following:
• Vaginal bleeding
• Placenta previa
• Risk of preterm labor
• Cervical insufficiency
• Premature rupture of membranes
• Presence of infection (Rigby, 2015)

Inform the couple that the fetus will not be injured by intercourse. Suggest that alternative positions may be more comfortable (e.g., woman on top, side-lying), especially during the later stages of pregnancy. Some of the physical changes in pregnancy, which can affect a couple's relationship, for example, halitosis which can result from dehydration, but can be alleviated through extra fluids and better oral hygiene. Women can have breast tenderness and skin changes that can cause them feel unattractive to their partner during pregnancy. In addition, they can be worried about increases in vaginal discharge and need to know what is normal and what can be a sign of infection. Nurses should make women feel comfortable talking about their fears, encouraging them to take pride in their changing bodies.

Many women feel a particular need for closeness during pregnancy, and the woman should communicate this need to her partner (Halford, Petch, & Creedy, 2015). Emphasize to the couple that closeness and cuddling need not culminate in intercourse, and that other forms of sexual expression, such as mutual masturbation, foot massage, holding hands, kissing, and hugging can be very satisfying (Halford et al., 2015).

Sex in pregnancy is normal. Research suggests that prepregnancy sexuality plays an important role in maintaining sexuality during pregnancy and postpartum (Yildiz, 2015). There are very few proven contraindications and risks to intercourse in low-risk pregnancies, and therefore, these clients should be reassured. In pregnancies complicated by placenta previa or an increased risk of preterm labor, the evidence to support abstinence is lacking, but it is a reasonable benign recommendation given the theoretical catastrophic consequences (Yeniel & Petri, 2014).

Women will experience a myriad of symptoms, feelings, and physical sensations during their pregnancy. Having a satisfying sexual relationship during pregnancy is certainly possible, but it requires honest communication between partners to determine what works best for them and a good relationship with their health care provider to ensure safety (March of Dimes, 2015f).

Employment

Nearly three-quarters of pregnant women in the United States will continue to work outside the home until the last month of pregnancy (Jordan et al., 2014). For the most part, women can continue working until giving birth if they have no complications during their pregnancy and the workplace does not present any special hazards (Zolotor & Carlough, 2014). Hazardous occupations include health care workers, daycare providers, laboratory technicians, chemists, painters, hairstylists, veterinary workers, and carpenters (Guidotti, 2014). Jobs requiring strenuous work such as heavy lifting, climbing, carrying heavy objects, and standing for prolonged periods place a pregnant woman at risk if modifications are not instituted.

Assess for environmental and occupational factors that place a pregnant women and her fetus at risk for injury. Interview the woman about her employment environment. Ask about possible exposure to teratogens (substances with the potential to alter the fetus permanently in form or function) and the physical demands of employment: Is she exposed to temperature extremes? Does she need to stand for prolonged periods in a fixed position? A description of the work environment is important in providing anticipatory guidance to the woman. Stress the importance of taking rest periods throughout the day, because constant physically intensive workloads increase the likelihood of low birth weight and preterm labor and birth (Cunningham et al., 2014).

Because of the numerous physiologic and psychosocial changes that women experience during their pregnancies, the employer may need to make special accommodations to reduce the pregnant woman's risk of hazardous exposures and heavy workloads. The employer may need to provide adequate coverage so that the woman can take rest breaks; remove the woman from any areas where she might be exposed to toxic substances; and avoid work assignments that require heavy lifting, hard physical labor, continuous standing, or constant moving. Some recommendations for working while pregnant are given in Teaching Guidelines 12.3.

Teaching Guidelines 12.3
TEACHING FOR THE PREGNANT WORKING WOMAN
- Plan to take two 10- to 15-minute breaks within an 8-hour work day.
- Be sure there is a place available for you to rest, preferably in the side-lying position, with a restroom readily available.

- Avoid jobs that require strenuous workloads; if this is not possible, then request a modification of work duties (lighter tasks) to reduce your workload.
- Change your position from standing to sitting or vice versa at least every 2 hours.
- Ensure that you are allowed time off without penalty, if necessary, to ensure a healthy outcome for you and your fetus.
- Make sure the work environment is free of toxic substances.
- Ensure the work environment is smoke-free so passive smoking is not a concern.
- Minimize heavy lifting if associated with bending.

Travel

Pregnancy does not curtail a woman's ability to travel in a car or in a plane. However, women should follow a few safety guidelines to minimize risk to themselves and their fetuses. According to ACOG (2015g), pregnant women can travel safely throughout their pregnancy, although the second trimester is perhaps the best time to travel because there is the least chance of complications. Pregnant women considering international travel should evaluate the problems that could occur during the journey as well as the quality of medical care available at the destination.

A woman in the third trimester should be advised to defer overseas travel because of concerns about access to medical care in case of problems such as hypertension, phlebitis, or premature labor (CDC, 2015e). Pregnant women should be advised to consult with their health care providers before making any travel decisions.

Take Note!
Clinical manifestations that indicate the need for immediate medical attention while traveling are vaginal bleeding, passing tissue or clots, abdominal pain or cramps, contractions, ruptured membranes, excessive leg swelling or pain, headaches, or visual problems (Leggat & Zuckerman, 2015).

Advise pregnant women to be aware of the potential for injuries and traumas related to traveling, and teach women ways to prevent these from occurring. Teaching Guidelines 12.4 offers tips for safe travel on planes and to foreign areas.

Teaching Guidelines 12.4
TEACHING TO PROMOTE SAFE TRAVEL ON PLANES AND IN FOREIGN COUNTRIES
- Bring along a copy of the prenatal record if your travel will be prolonged in case there is a medical emergency away from home.

- When traveling abroad, carry a foreign dictionary that includes words or phrases for the most common pregnancy emergencies.
- Travel with at least one companion at all times for personal safety.
- Check with your health care provider before receiving any immunizations necessary for foreign travel; some may be harmful to the fetus.
- When in a foreign country, avoid fresh fruit, vegetables, and local water.
- Avoid any milk that is not pasteurized.
- Eat only meat that is well cooked to avoid exposure to toxoplasmosis.
- Request an aisle seat and walk about the airplane every 2 hours.
- While sitting on long flights, practice calf-tensing exercises to improve circulation to the lower extremities.
- Be aware of typical problems encountered by pregnant travelers, such as fatigue, heartburn, indigestion, constipation, vaginal discharge, leg cramps, urinary frequency, and hemorrhoids.
- Always wear support hose while flying to prevent the development of blood clots.
- Drink plenty of water to keep well hydrated throughout the flight.
- Postpone travel if risks outweigh benefits.

Adapted from American College of Obstetricians and Gynecologists. (2015e). *Travel during pregnancy: FAQ 055*. Retrieved from http://www.acog.org/~/media/for%20patients/faq055.ashx; Centers for Disease Control and Prevention. (2015e). *Pregnant travelers*. Retrieved from http://wwwnc.cdc.gov/travel/yellowbook/2014/chapter-8-advising-travelers-with-specific-needs/pregnant-travelers

When traveling by car, the major risk is a car accident. Motor vehicle accidents account for more than 50% of all traumas during pregnancy and 82% of fetal deaths occurring during these accidents (Eshaghabadi & Barati, 2015). The impact and momentum can lead to traumatic separation of the placenta from the wall of the uterus. Shock and massive hemorrhage might result. Tips that nurses can offer to promote safety during ground travel include the following:

- Always wear a three-point seat belt, no matter how short the trip, to prevent ejection or serious injury from collision.
- Apply a nonpadded shoulder strap properly; it should cross between the breasts and over the upper abdomen, above the uterus (Fig. 12.11).
- If no seat belts are available (buses or vans), ride in the back seat of the vehicle.
- Use a lap belt that crosses over the pelvis below the uterus.
- Deactivate the airbag if possible. If you cannot, move the seat as far back from the dashboard as possible to minimize impact on the abdomen.

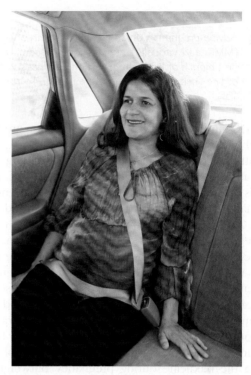

FIGURE 12.11 Proper application of a seat belt during pregnancy.

- Never use a cellular phone while driving to prevent distraction.
- Avoid driving when very fatigued in the first and third trimesters.
- Avoid late-night driving, when visibility might be compromised.
- Direct a tilting steering wheel away from the abdomen (CDC, 2015e).

Immunizations and Medications

Vaccines are among the greatest public health achievements of the twenty-first century, credited with significant reduction of morbidity and mortality from many diseases caused by bacteria and viruses (Senie, 2014). Ideally, clients should receive all childhood immunizations before conception to protect the fetus from any risk of congenital anomalies. If the client comes for a preconception visit, discuss immunizations such as measles, mumps, and rubella (MMR), hepatitis B, and diphtheria/tetanus (every 10 years); administer them at this time if needed.

The risk to a developing fetus from vaccination of the mother during pregnancy is primarily theoretical. Routine immunizations are not usually indicated during pregnancy. However, no evidence exists of risk from vaccinating pregnant women with inactivated virus or bacterial vaccines or toxoids. A number of other vaccines have not been adequately studied, and thus theoretical risks of vaccination must be weighed against the risks of the disease to mother and fetus (CDC, 2015f).

Take Note!

Advise pregnant women to avoid live virus vaccines (MMR and varicella) and to avoid becoming pregnant within 1 month of having received one of these vaccines because of the theoretical risk of transmission to the fetus (CDC, 2015f).

CDC guidelines for vaccine administration are highlighted in Box 12.6.

Little is known about the effects of taking most medications during pregnancy. Less than 10% of medications approved by the FDA since 1980 have enough information to determine their risk for birth defects (CDC, 2015g). Based on this lack of evidence, it is best for pregnant women not to take any medications during their pregnancy. At the very least, encourage them to discuss with the health care provider their current medications and any herbal remedies they take so that they can learn about any potential risks should they continue to take them during pregnancy. Generally, if the woman is taking medicine for seizures, high blood pressure, asthma, or depression, the benefits of continuing the medicine during pregnancy outweigh the risks to the fetus. The safety profile of some medications may change according to the gestational age of the fetus. Embryogenesis is completed by the end of the first trimester, when all fetal organs are complete. Thus, to cause a malformation, fetal drug exposure must occur in the first 12 weeks of gestation (Gadot & Koren, 2015).

The FDA has developed a system of ranking drugs that appears on drug labels and package inserts. These risk categories are summarized in Box 12.7. Always advise women to check with the health care provider for guidance.

A common concern of many pregnant women involves the use of over-the-counter medications and herbal agents. Many women consider these products benign simply because they are available without a prescription (King et al., 2015). Although herbal medications are commonly thought of as "natural" alternatives to other medicines, they can be just as potent as some prescription medications. A major concern about herbal medicine is the lack of consistent potency in the active ingredients in any given batch of product, making it difficult to know the exact strength by reading the label. Also, many herbs contain chemicals that cross the placenta and may cause harm to the fetus.

Nurses are often asked about the safety of over-the-counter medicines and herbal agents. Unfortunately, many drugs have not been evaluated in controlled studies, and it is difficult to make general recommendations for these products. Therefore, encourage pregnant women to check with their health care provider before taking anything. Questions about the use of over-the-counter and herbal products are part of the initial prenatal interview.

BOX 12.6

CDC GUIDELINES FOR VACCINE ADMINISTRATION DURING PREGNANCY

Vaccines That Should Be Considered if Otherwise Indicated
- Hepatitis B
- Influenza (inactivated) injection
- Tetanus/diphtheria (Tdap)
- Meningococcal
- Rabies

Vaccines Contraindicated During Pregnancy
- Influenza (live, attenuated vaccine) nasal spray
- Measles
- Mumps
- Rubella
- Varicella
- BCG (tuberculosis)
- Meningococcal
- Typhoid

Adapted from Centers for Disease Control and Prevention. (2015f). *Vaccines for pregnant women.* Retrieved from http://www.cdc.gov/vaccines/adults/rec-vac/pregnant.html; March of Dimes. (2015h). *Vaccinations during pregnancy.* Retrieved from http://www.marchofdimes.com/pregnancy/vaccinations-during-pregnancy.aspx

---

BOX 12.7

FDA PREGNANCY RISK CLASSIFICATION OF DRUGS

- The Pregnancy subsection will provide information relevant to the use of the drug in pregnant women, such as dosing and potential risks to the developing fetus, and will require information about whether there is a registry that collects and maintains data on how pregnant women are affected when they use the drug or biological product. Information in drug labeling about the existence of any pregnancy registries has been previously recommended but not required until now.
- The Lactation subsection will provide information about using the drug while breastfeeding, such as the amount of drug in breast milk and potential effects on the breastfed child.
- The Females and Males of Reproductive Potential subsection will include information about pregnancy testing, contraception and about infertility as it relates to the drug. This information has been included in labeling, but there was no consistent placement for it until now.

Retrieved from http://www.fda.gov/NewsEvents/Newsroom/PressAnnouncements/ucm425317.htm

NURSING MANAGEMENT TO PREPARE THE WOMAN AND HER PARTNER FOR LABOR, BIRTH, AND PARENTHOOD

Pregnancy and birth are unique to every woman. Women and families hold different expectations during childbearing based on their knowledge, experiences, belief systems, culture, and social and family backgrounds. These differences should be understood and respected by the nurse, and care to them adapted to meet the individual needs of the women and families. Knowing a woman's needs, values, cultural background, preferences, and expectations during childbirth helps nurses to provide high-quality care to them. Childbirth today is a very different experience from childbirth in previous generations. In the past, women were literally "put to sleep" with anesthetics, and they woke up with a baby. Most women never remembered the details and had a passive role in childbirth as the physician delivered the newborn. In the 1950s, consumers began to insist on taking a more active role in their health care, and couples desired to be together during the extraordinary event of childbirth. Beginning in the 1970s, the father or significant other support person remained with the mother throughout labor and birth. Fathers today want to be seen as individuals who are part of the laboring couple. If fathers are left out, they tend to feel helpless; this can result in a feeling of panic and can put their support for their partner at risk (Schytt & Bergstrom, 2014).

Health beliefs related to pregnancy and childbirth exist in various cultures globally. A woman's perception of her own status is critical to her decision-making process, because her personal behaviors can significantly alter her pregnancy-related risks. Pregnant women of diverse cultures hold a number of beliefs related to diet, behavior related to prenatal care, and the use of herbs during pregnancy and postnatally. Nurses need to be aware of these cultural beliefs so as to incorporate those into their practices, while those posing a health risk should be discouraged respectfully (M'soka, Mabuza, & Pretorius, 2015).

Childbirth education began because women demanded to become more involved in their birthing experience rather than simply turning control over to a health care provider. Nurses played a pivotal role in bringing about this change by providing information and supporting clients and their families, fostering a more active role in preparing for the upcoming birth.

Traditional childbirth education classes focused on developing and practicing techniques for use in managing pain and facilitating the progress of labor. Recently, the focus of this education has broadened: it now encompasses not only preparation for childbirth, but also preparation for breast-feeding, infant care, transition to new parenting roles, relationship skills, family health promotion, and sexuality (Varner, 2015). The term used to describe this broad range of topics is **perinatal education**. Subjects commonly addressed in perinatal education include the following:

- Anatomy and physiology of reproduction
- Fetal growth and development
- Prenatal maternal exercise
- Physiologic and emotional changes during pregnancy
- Sex during pregnancy
- Infant growth and development
- Nutrition and healthy eating habits during pregnancy
- Teratogens and their impact on the fetus
- Signs and symptoms of labor
- Preparation for labor and birth (for parents, siblings, and other family members)
- Options for birth
- Infant nutrition, including preparation for breast-feeding
- Infant care, including safety, CPR, and first aid
- Family planning (March of Dimes, 2015g)

Childbirth Education Classes

Childbirth education classes teach pregnant women and their support person about pregnancy, birth, and parenting. The classes are offered in local communities or online and are usually taught by certified childbirth educators. Most childbirth classes support the concept of **natural childbirth** (a birth without pain-relieving medications) so that the woman can be in control throughout the experience as much as possible. The classes differ in their approach to specific comfort techniques and breathing patterns. The three most common childbirth methods are the Lamaze (psychoprophylactic) method, the Bradley (partner-coached childbirth) method, and the Dick-Read (natural childbirth) method.

Lamaze Method

Lamaze is a psychoprophylactic ("mind prevention") method of preparing for labor and birth that promotes the use of specific breathing and relaxation techniques. Dr. Fernand Lamaze, a French obstetrician, popularized this method of childbirth preparation in the 1960s. Lamaze believed that conquering fear through knowledge and support was important. He also believed women needed to alter the perception of suffering during childbirth. This perception change would come about by learning conditioned reflexes that, instead of signaling pain, would signal the work of producing a child, and thus would carry the woman through labor awake, aware, and in control of her own body (Lamaze International, 2015). Lamaze felt strongly that all women have the right to deliver their babies with minimal or no medication while maintaining their dignity, minimizing their pain, maximizing their self-esteem, and enjoying the miracle of birth.

Lamaze classes include information on toning exercises, relaxation exercises and techniques, and breathing methods for labor. The breathing techniques are used in labor to enhance relaxation and to reduce the woman's perception of pain. The goal is for women to become aware of their own comfortable rate of breathing in order to maintain relaxation and adequate oxygenation of the fetus. The following breathing techniques are an effective attention-focusing strategy to reduce pain:

- *Paced breathing* involves breathing techniques used to decrease stress responses and therefore decrease pain. This type of breathing implies self-regulation by the woman. The woman starts off by taking a cleansing breath at the onset and end of each contraction. This cleansing breath symbolizes freeing her mind from worries and concerns. This breath enhances oxygenation and puts the woman in a relaxed state.
- *Slow-paced breathing* is associated with relaxation and should be half the normal breathing rate (6 to 9 breaths per minute). This type of breathing is the most relaxed pattern and is recommended throughout labor. Abdominal or chest breathing may be used. It is generally best to breathe in through the nose and breathe out either through the nose or mouth, whichever is more comfortable for the woman.
- *Modified-paced breathing* can be used for increased work or stress during labor to increase alertness or focus attention or when slow-paced breathing is no longer effective in keeping the woman relaxed. The woman's respiratory rate increases, but it does not exceed twice her normal rate. Modified-paced breathing is a quiet upper chest breath that is increased or decreased according to the intensity of the contraction. The inhalation and the exhalation are equal. This breathing technique should be practiced during pregnancy for optimal use during labor.
- *Patterned-paced breathing* is similar to modified-paced breathing but with a rhythmic pattern. It uses a variety of patterns, with an emphasis on the exhalation breath at regular intervals. Different patterns can be used, such as 4/1, 6/1, 4/1. A 4/1 rhythm is four upper chest breaths followed by an exhalation (a sighing out of air, like blowing out a candle). Random patterns can be chosen for use as long as the basic principles of rate and relaxation are met.

Couples practice these breathing patterns typically during the last few months of the pregnancy until they feel comfortable using them. Focal points (visual fixation

on a designated object), effleurage (light abdominal massage by woman or partner), massage, and imagery (journey of the mind to a relaxing place) are also added to aid in relaxation. From the nurse's perspective, encourage the woman to breathe at a level of comfort that allows her to cope. Always remain quiet during the woman's periods of imagery and focal point visualization to avoid breaking her concentration.

Bradley (Partner-Coached) Method

The Bradley method uses various exercises and slow, controlled abdominal breathing to accomplish relaxation. Dr. Robert Bradley, a Denver-based obstetrician, advocated a completely unmedicated labor and birth experience. The Bradley method emphasizes the pleasurable sensations of childbirth, teaching women to concentrate on these sensations while "turning on" to their own bodies (Bradley Method, 2014). In 1965, Bradley wrote *Husband-Coached Childbirth*, which advocated the active participation of the husband as labor coach.

A woman is conditioned to work in harmony with her body using breath control and deep abdominopelvic breathing to promote general body relaxation during labor. This method stresses that childbirth is a joyful, natural process and emphasizes the partner's involvement during pregnancy, labor, birth, and the early newborn period. Thus, the training techniques are directed toward the coach, not the mother. The coach is educated in massage/comfort techniques to use on the mother throughout the labor and birth process.

Dick-Read Method

In 1944, Grantly Dick-Read, a British obstetrician, wrote *Childbirth Without Fear*. He believed that the attitude of a woman toward her birthing process had a considerable influence on the ease of her labor, and he believed that fear is the primary pain-producing agent in an otherwise normal labor. He felt that fear builds a state of tension, creating an antagonistic effect on the laboring muscles of the uterus, which results in pain. A private, undisturbed, and dark environment, where women can feel safe, can promote the release of oxytocin, the hormone responsible for uterine contractions and though to promote the release of the pain-relieving hormones endorphins. When this is not achieved, women can experience fear–tension–pain syndrome, impeding labor progress and causing increased levels of pain (Westbury, 2015). Dick-Read sought to interrupt the circular pattern of fear, tension, and pain during the labor and birthing process. He promoted the belief that the degree of fear could be diminished with increased understanding of the normal physiologic response to labor (Alexander et al., 2014).

Dick-Read believed that prenatal instruction was essential for pain relief and that emotional factors during labor interfered with the normal labor progression. The woman achieves relaxation and reduces pain by arming herself with the knowledge of normal childbirth and using abdominal breathing during contractions.

Nursing Management and Childbirth Education

Childbirth education is less about methods than about mastery. The overall aim of any of the methods is to promote an internal locus of control that will enable each woman to yield her body to the process of birth. As the woman gains success and tangible benefits from the exercises she is taught, she begins to reframe her beliefs and gains practical knowledge, and the impetus will be there for her to engage in the conscious use of the techniques (Fig. 12.12). Nurses play a key role in supporting and encouraging each couple's use of the techniques taught in childbirth education classes.

Every woman's labor is unique, and it is important for nurses not to generalize or stereotype women. The most effective support a nurse can offer a couple using prepared childbirth methods is encouragement and presence. These nursing measures must be adapted to each individual throughout the labor process. Offering encouraging phrases such as "great job" or "you can do it" helps to reinforce their efforts and at the same time empowers them to continue. Using eye-to-eye contact to engage the woman's total attention is important if she appears overwhelmed or appears to lose control during the transition phase of labor.

Nurses play a significant role in enhancing the couple's relationship by respecting the involvement of the partner and demonstrating concern for his needs throughout labor. Offering to stay with the woman to give him a break periodically allows him to meet his needs while at the same time still actively participating. Offer anticipatory guidance to the couple and assist during critical times in labor. Demonstrate many of the coping techniques to the partner and praise their successful use, which increases self-esteem. Focus on their strengths and the positive elements of the labor experience. Congratulating the couple for a job well done is paramount.

Throughout the labor experience, demonstrate personal warmth and project a friendly attitude. Frequently, a nurse's touch may help to prevent a crisis by reassuring the mother that she is doing fine.

Options for Birth Settings and Care Providers

From the moment a woman discovers she is pregnant, numerous decisions await her—where the infant will be born, what birth setting is best, and who will assist with the birth. The majority of women are well and healthy and can consider the full range of birth settings—hospital, birth center, or home setting—and care providers. They should be given information about each to ensure the most informed decision.

Birth Settings

HOSPITALS

Hospitals are the most common site for birth in the United States. If the woman has a serious medical condition or is at high risk for developing one, she will probably need to plan to give birth in a hospital setting under the care of an obstetrician. Giving birth in a hospital is advantageous for several reasons. Hospitals are best equipped to diagnose and treat women and newborns with complications; trained personnel are available if necessary; and no transportation is needed if a complication should arise during labor or birth. Disadvantages include the high-tech atmosphere; strict policies and restrictions that might limit who can be with the woman; and the medical model of care.

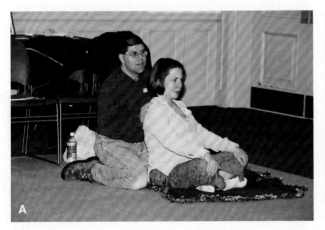
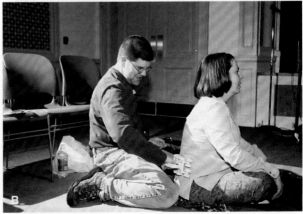

FIGURE 12.12 A couple practicing the techniques taught in a childbirth education class.

Within the hospital setting, however, choices do exist regarding birth environments. The conventional delivery room resembles an operating room, where the health care professional delivers the newborn from the woman, who is positioned in stirrups. The woman is then transferred to the recovery area on a stretcher and then again to the postpartum unit. The birthing suite is the other option within the hospital setting. In the birthing suite, the woman and her partner remain in one place for labor, birth, and recovery. The birthing suite is a private room decorated to look as homelike as possible. For example, the bed converts to allow for various birthing positions, and there may be a rocking chair or an easy chair for the woman's partner. Despite the homey atmosphere, the room is still equipped with emergency resuscitative obstetric equipment and electronic fetal monitors in case they are needed quickly (Fig. 12.13A). Such settings provide a more personal childbirth experience in a less formal and intimidating atmosphere compared to the traditional delivery room.

FREESTANDING BIRTH CENTER

A freestanding birth center offers women a comfortable setting where they can receive maternity care with appropriate levels of intervention. A freestanding birth center (Fig. 12.13B) can be a good choice for a woman who wants more personalized care than in a hospital but does not feel comfortable with a home birth. In contrast to the institutional environment in hospitals, most freestanding birth centers have a homelike atmosphere, and many are, in fact, located in converted homes. Some are located on hospital property and are affiliated with them. Birth centers are designed to provide maternity care to women judged to be at low risk for obstetric complications. Women are allowed and encouraged to give birth in the position most comfortable for them. Care in birth centers is often provided by midwives and is more relaxed, with no routine intravenous lines, fetal monitoring, and restrictive protocols. A disadvantage of

the birth center is the need to transport the woman to a hospital quickly if an emergency arises, because emergency equipment is not readily available. In a research study comparing homelike to conventional institutional settings, the author concluded that there appeared to be some benefits from homelike settings for childbirth, although increased support from caregivers may be more important (Alliman, Jolles, & Summers, 2015).

HOME BIRTHS

Rates of planned home births have been increasing since the 1970s, with 1 in 49 non-Hispanic White women giving birth outside the hospital setting now (Zielinski, Ackerson, & Low, 2015). Most women who choose a home birth believe that birth is a natural process that requires little medical intervention (Lewis, 2015). Research has shown that women believe that planned home births increase privacy, comfort, and convenience; are associated with reduced rates of medical interventions; and facilitate family involvement in a relaxed, peaceful atmosphere (Budin, 2015).

The safety of home births is an ongoing debate in the United States. The American College of Nurse Midwives (ACNM), the American Public Health Association (APHA), and WHO state that planned home birth is safe, as long as the woman falls under certain criteria, such as a low-risk pregnancy, singleton fetus, cephalic fetus at term, and the absence of pre-existing conditions (Declercq & Stotland, 2015). Home births can be safe if there are qualified, experienced attendants and an emergency transfer system in place in case of serious complications. Many women choose the home setting out of a strong desire to control their child's birth and to give birth surrounded by family members. Most home birth caregivers are midwives who have provided continuous care to the woman throughout the pregnancy. Disadvantages include the need to transport the woman to the hospital during or after labor if a problem arises, and the limited pain management available in the home setting.

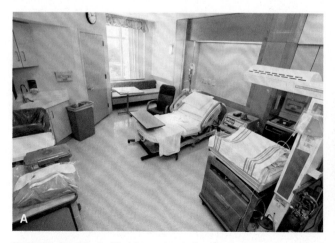 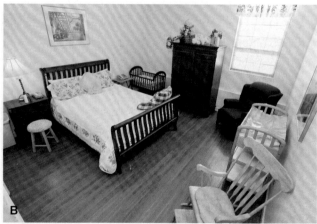

FIGURE 12.13 A. Birthing suite in hospital setting. **B.** Childbirth room in birthing center.

Care Providers

While most women in the United States still receive pregnancy care from an obstetrician, an increasing number are choosing a midwife for their care. The difference is a matter of degrees. Obstetricians must finish a 4-year residency in obstetrics and gynecology in addition to medical school. Certified nurse-midwives are registered nurses who have graduated from a nurse-midwifery education program accredited by the Accreditation Commission for Midwifery Education (ACME) and have passed a national certification examination to receive the professional designation of certified nurse-midwife. As of 2010, a graduate degree is required for entry into midwifery practice in the United States. Midwives usually care for low-risk women in a variety of settings. They are able to write prescriptions, provide prenatal care, childbirth care, postpartum care, newborn care, and well-women's care throughout the lifespan. Family practice doctors also provide maternity, woman's care, and well-baby care. Many deliver their clients' newborns in the hospital or birthing centers. Obstetricians can handle high-risk pregnancies and delivery emergencies; can administer or order pain-relief drugs; and are assisted by a support staff in the hospital setting. Midwives work in hospitals, birthing centers, and home settings to deliver care. They believe in the normalcy of birth and tolerate wide variations of what is considered normal during labor, which leads to fewer interventions applied during the childbirth process. Midwives attend approximately 8% of total United States births (American College of Nurse-Midwives, 2015). Midwives do handle high-risk and emergency births because many are not always predictable—they typically have an obstetrician as back up when they do occur to assist them.

In addition to the woman's primary health care provider, some women hire a doula to be with them during the childbearing process. *Doula* is a Greek word that means "woman's servant." A doula is a laywoman trained to provide women and their families with encouragement, emotional and physical support, and information through late pregnancy, labor, birth, and postpartum. Doulas provide the woman with continuous support throughout labor but do not perform any clinical procedures.

Preparation for Breast-Feeding or Bottle-Feeding

Pregnant women are faced with a decision about which method of feeding to choose. Educate the pregnant client about the advantages and disadvantages of each method, allowing the woman and her partner to make an informed decision about the best method for their situation. Providing the client and her partner with this information will increase the likelihood of a successful experience regardless of the method of feeding chosen.

As part of health promotion/evidence-based interventions, nurses should be encouraging and educating all women on breast-feeding.

Breast-Feeding

Substantial scientific evidence exists documenting the health benefits of breast-feeding for newborns. Current evidence cited by the AAP showed improved outcomes for breast-fed infants with regard to otitis media, lower respiratory infections, gastroenteritis, atopic dermatitis, childhood asthma, childhood obesity, type 1 and type 2 diabetes, childhood leukemia, sudden infant death syndrome, and cognitive development, and for their mothers with regard to breast cancer, ovarian cancer, and type 2 diabetes. The AAP recommends that infants be breast-fed exclusively until the age 6 months, and continue to be breast-fed for a year and for as long as it is mutually desired (2012). In addition, a lack of breast-feeding has a negative impact on the health care system by increasing the number of client visits, hospital admissions, rate of obesity, and health care costs. Most researchers agree that the duration of breast-feeding is inversely associated with overweight risk. Breast-feeding is a cost-effective, natural, and effective prevention strategy for reducing childhood obesity. A recent study estimates that $13 billion a year would be saved and 1,000 deaths prevented each year if 90% of infants in the United States were exclusively breast-fed until 6 months (Office on Women's Health, 2014).

Human milk provides an ideal balance of nutrients for newborns (ACOG, 2015h). Breast-feeding is advantageous for the following reasons:
- Human milk is digestible and economical and requires no preparation.
- Bonding between mother and child is promoted.
- Cost is less than purchasing formula.
- Ovulation is suppressed (however, this is not a reliable birth control method).
- The risk of ovarian cancer and the incidence of premenopausal breast cancer are reduced for the woman.
- Extra calories are used, which promotes weight loss gradually without dieting.
- Oxytocin is released to promote more rapid uterine involution with less bleeding.
- Sucking helps to develop the muscles in the infant's jaw.
- Absorption of lactose and minerals in the newborn is improved.
- The immunologic properties of breast milk help prevent infections in the baby.
- The composition of breast milk adapts to meet the infant's changing needs.
- Constipation in the baby is not a problem with adequate intake.
- Food allergies are less likely to develop in the breast-fed baby.

- The incidence of otitis media and upper respiratory infections in the infant is reduced.
- Breast-fed babies are less likely to be overfed, thus reducing the risk of adult obesity.
- Breast-fed newborns are less prone to vomiting (AAP 2015; ACOG, 2015h; American Academy of Family Physicians, 2015; Women, Infant & Children [WIC], 2015).

One could say that lactation and breast-feeding are so natural that they should just happen on their own accord, but this is not the case. Learning to breast-feed takes practice, requires support from the partner, and requires dedication and patience on the part of the mother; it may be necessary to work closely with a lactation consultant to be successful and comfortable when breast-feeding. (Figure 12.14 show the different positions that may be used for breast-feeding.) Nurses can encourage breast-feeding for all mothers except those that are HIV+, and are untreated, have active tuberculosis, use illicit drugs, or take prescribed cancer chemotherapeutic agents.

Breast-feeding also has some side effects. These include breast discomfort, sore nipples, mastitis, engorgement, milk stasis, vaginal dryness, and decreased libido (Alekseev, Vladimir, & Nadezhda, 2015). The most common cause of nipple pain is an improper latch and such discomfort is piercing, immediate, and short-lived, typically occurring as soon as the baby starts nursing and gradually subsiding during the feeding. Some mothers feel it is inconvenient or embarrassing, limits other activities, limits partner involvement, increases their dependency by being tied to the infant all the time, and restricts their use of alcohol or drugs. Nurses can help mothers to cope with their fear of dependency and feelings of obligation by emphasizing the positive aspects of breast-feeding and encouraging bonding experiences. Nurses can be instrumental in helping mothers prepare and continue to breastfeed after they return to work.

PREPARATION FOR BREAST-FEEDING

Nipple preparation is not necessary during the prenatal period unless the nipples are inverted and do not become erect when stimulated. Assess for this by placing the forefinger and thumb above and below the areola and compressing behind the nipple. If it flattens or inverts, advise the client to wear breast shields during the last 2 months of pregnancy. Breast shields exert a continuous pressure around the areola, pushing the nipple through a central opening in the inner shield (La Leche League International, 2014). The shields are worn inside the bra. Initially the shields are worn for 1 hour, and then the woman progressively increases the wearing time up to 8 hours daily. The client maintains this schedule until after childbirth, and then she wears the shield 24 hours a day until the infant latches on

easily (La Leche League International, 2014). In addition, suggest that the woman wear a supportive nursing bra 24 hours a day.

Encourage the woman to request a certified lactation specialist (CLS) at the hospital, if giving birth there. Lactation specialists are health care providers who specialize in the clinical management of breast-feeding. Some run their own breast-feeding support groups as well. In addition, suggest that the woman attends a breast-feeding support group (e.g., La Leche League), provide her with sources of information about infant feeding, and suggest that she reads a good reference book about lactation. All of these activities will help in her decision-making process and will be invaluable to her should she choose to breast-feed her newborn. Women returning to work can pump their breasts and store the milk in the freezer for future use.

Bottle-Feeding

Recent research indicates that infants who are fed formula within the first 6 months do have an increased incidence of otitis media, diabetes, asthma, atopic dermatitis, reflux, diarrhea, colic, constipation, and lower respiratory infections (Schram, 2014). It is important to inform mothers and their partners of this.

Bottle-feeding an infant is not just a matter of "open, pour, and feed." Parents need information on types of formulas, preparation and storage of formula, equipment, and feeding positions. It is recommended that normal full-term infants receive conventional cow's milk-based formula; the physician should direct this choice. If the infant has a reaction (diarrhea, vomiting, abdominal pain, excessive gas) to the first formula, another formula should be tried. Sometimes a soy-based formula is substituted. In terms of preparation of formula and its use, the following guidelines should be stressed:

- Obtain adequate equipment (six 4-ounce bottles, eight 8-ounce bottles, and nipples).
- Consistency is important. Stay with a nipple that is comfortable to the infant.
- Frequently assess nipples for any loose pieces of rubber at the opening.
- Correct formula preparation is critical to the health and development of the infant. Formula is available in three forms: ready-to-feed, concentrate, and powder.
- Read the formula label thoroughly before mixing.
- Correct formula dilution is important to avoid fluid imbalances. For ready-to-use formula, use as is without dilution. For concentrated formulas, dilute with equal parts of water. For powdered formulas, mix one scoop of powder with 2 ounces of water
- If the water supply is safe, sterilization is not necessary.
- Bottles and nipples should be washed in hot, sudsy water using a bottle brush.

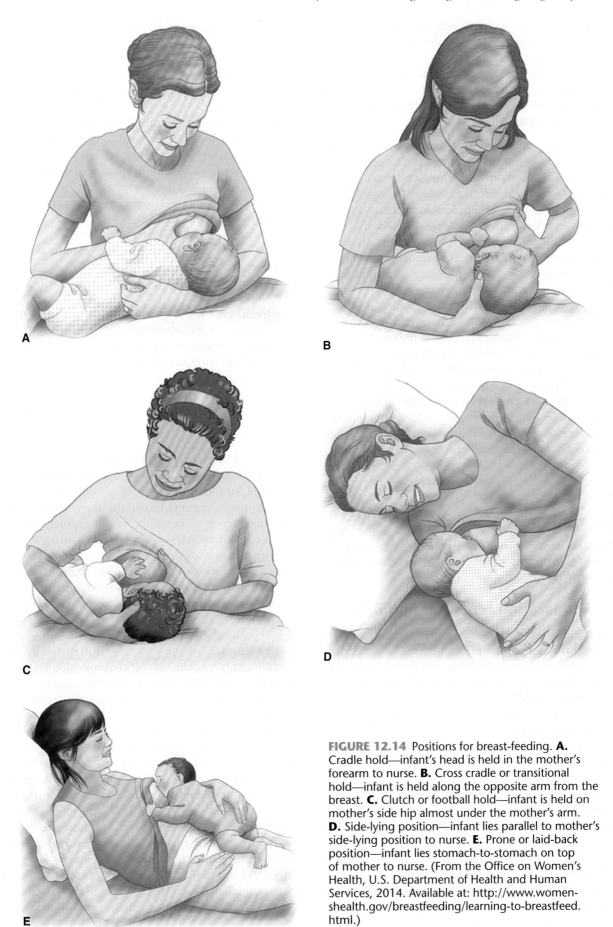

FIGURE 12.14 Positions for breast-feeding. **A.** Cradle hold—infant's head is held in the mother's forearm to nurse. **B.** Cross cradle or transitional hold—infant is held along the opposite arm from the breast. **C.** Clutch or football hold—infant is held on mother's side hip almost under the mother's arm. **D.** Side-lying position—infant lies parallel to mother's side-lying position to nurse. **E.** Prone or laid-back position—infant lies stomach-to-stomach on top of mother to nurse. (From the Office on Women's Health, U.S. Department of Health and Human Services, 2014. Available at: http://www.women-shealth.gov/breastfeeding/learning-to-breastfeed.html.)

- Formula should be served at room temperature.
- If the water supply is questionable, water should be boiled for 5 minutes before use.
- Formula should not be heated in a microwave oven, because it is heated unevenly.
- Formula can be prepared 24 hours ahead of time and stored in the refrigerator.

Teach the woman and other caretakers to feed the infant in a semi-upright position using the cradle hold in the arms. This position allows for face-to-face contact between the infant and caretaker. Advise the caretaker to hold the bottle so that the nipple is kept full of formula to prevent excessive air swallowing. Instruct the caretaker to feed the infant every 3 to 4 hours and adapt the feeding times to the infant's needs. Frequent burping of the infant (every ounce) helps prevent gas from building up in the stomach. Caution the caretaker not to prop the bottle; propping the bottle can cause choking.

Bottle-feeding should mirror breast-feeding as closely as possible. While nutrition is important, so are the emotional and interactive components of feeding. Encourage the caretaker to cuddle the infant closely and position the infant so that his or her head is in a comfortable position. Also encourage communication with the infant during feedings. Nurses should know the different types of formulas available to provide advice to mothers who have made the informed choice not to breastfeed or to stop breastfeeding.

Take Note!

Warn the caretaker about the danger of putting the infant to bed with a bottle. This can lead to "baby bottle tooth decay" (nursing caries) because sugars in the formula stay in contact with the infant's developing teeth for prolonged periods.

Final Preparation for Labor and Birth

The nurse has played a supportive/education role for the couple throughout the pregnancy and now needs to assist in preparing them for their "big event" by making sure they have made informed decisions and completed the following checklist:

- Attended childbirth preparation classes and practiced breathing techniques
- Selected a birth setting and made arrangements there
- Know what to expect during labor and birth
- Toured the birthing facility
- Packed a suitcase to take to the birthing facility when labor starts
- Made arrangements to have siblings and/or pets taken care of during labor
- Been instructed on signs and symptoms of labor and what to do
- Know what to do if membranes rupture prior to going into labor

- Know how to reach their health care provider when labor starts
- Communicated their needs and desires concerning pain management
- Discussed the possibility of a cesarean birth if complications occur
- Discussed possible names for the newborn
- Selected a feeding method (breast or bottle) with which they feel comfortable
- Made a decision regarding circumcision if they have a boy
- Purchased an infant safety car seat in which to bring their newborn home
- Decided on a pediatrician
- Have items needed to prepare for the newborn's homecoming:
  - Infant clothes in several sizes
  - Nursing bras
  - Infant crib with spaces between the slats that are 2 inches or less apart
  - Diapers (cloth or disposable)
  - Feeding supplies (bottles and nipples if bottle-feeding)
  - Infant thermometer
- Selected a family planning method to use after the birth

At each prenatal visit the nurse has had the opportunity to discuss and reinforce the importance of being prepared for the birth of the child with the parents. It is now up to the parents to use the nurse's guidance and put it into action to be ready for the upcoming birth.

A recent national survey entitled *Listening to Mothers III: Pregnancy and Birth* revealed concerns about overuse of maternity care practices and women's readiness to make informed decisions. Key findings point to the need for quality improvement, consumer engagement, and shared decision making (Declercq, Sakala, Corry, Applebaum, & Herrlick, 2014). These findings present a challenge for all nurses caring for maternity clients to thoroughly explain all procedures, along with their rationales, and truly listen to what the woman desires to make her childbirth experience outcome a positive one for her.

All nurses have the responsibility to impart their knowledge to all women and their families—and that starts with teaching themselves first. The evidence is clear that women have better outcomes when nurses intervene only when needed in the childbirth process. Nurses need to personalize their care to every woman based on her needs, her desires, and her state of health. Nurses must focus on teaching women and their families to understand the value of birth and its long-lasting effects on the family. In addition, nurses must provide birth settings that are safe, whether in the hospital, birth center, or at home. This includes, but is not limited to, providing continuous support in labor, allowing women the freedom to move and assume positions of choice, offering nourishment of the woman's body and spirit, using nonpharmacologic pain-relief modalities whenever possible, and ensuring seamless, collaborative teamwork. Continuous labor support is a nonpharmacologic, evidence-based strategy associated with reduced cesarean rates (Baum, Crawford, & Humphrey-Shelton, 2015).

KEY CONCEPTS

- Preconception care is the promotion of the health and well-being of a woman and her partner before pregnancy. The goal of preconception care is to identify any areas such as health problems, lifestyle habits, or social concerns that might unfavorably affect pregnancy.

- A thorough history and physical examination are performed on the initial prenatal visit.

- A primary aspect of nursing management during the antepartum period is counseling and educating the pregnant women and her partner to promote healthy outcomes for all involved.

- Nagele's rule can be used to establish the estimated date of birth. Using this rule, subtract 3 months from the month of their last LMP, add 7 days to the first day of the LMP, then correct the year by adding 1 to it. This date is within plus or minus 2 weeks (margin of error).

- Pelvic shape is typically classified as one of the four types: gynecoid, android, anthropoid, and platypelloid. The gynecoid type is the typical female pelvis and offers the best shape for a vaginal delivery.

- Continuous prenatal care is important for a successful outcome. The recommended schedule is every 4 weeks up to 28 weeks (7 months); every 2 weeks from 29 to 36 weeks; and every week from 37 weeks to birth.

- The height of the fundus is measured when the uterus arises out of the pelvis to evaluate fetal growth.

- The fundus reaches the level of the umbilicus at approximately 20 weeks and measures 20 cm. The fundal measurement should approximately equal to the number of weeks of gestation until week 36.

- At each visit the woman is asked whether she is having any common signs or symptoms of preterm labor, which might include uterine contractions, dull backache, pressure in the pelvic area or thighs, increased vaginal discharge, menstrual-like cramps, and vaginal bleeding.

- Prenatal screening has become standard in prenatal care to detect neural tube defects and genetic abnormalities.

- The nurse should address matter-of-factly common discomforts that occur in each trimester at all prenatal visits and should provide realistic measures to help the client deal with them effectively.

- The pregnant client can better care for herself and the fetus if her concerns are anticipated by the nurse and incorporated into guidance sessions at each prenatal visit.

- Iron and folic acid need to be supplemented because their increased requirements during pregnancy are usually too great to be met through diet alone.

- Throughout pregnancy, a well-balanced diet is critical for a healthy baby.

- Perinatal education has broadened its focus to include preparation for pregnancy and family adaptation to the new parenting roles. Childbirth education began because of increasing pressure from consumers who wanted to become more involved in their birthing experience.

- Three common childbirth education methods are Lamaze (psychoprophylactic), Bradley (partner-coached childbirth), and Dick-Read (natural childbirth).

- The great majorities of women in the United States are well and healthy and can consider the full range of birth settings: hospital, birth center, or home setting.

- All pregnant women need to be able to recognize early signs of contractions to prevent preterm labor.

References and Recommended Readings

Akolekar, R., Beta, J., Picciarelli, G., Ogilvie, C., & D'Antonio, F. (2015). Procedure-related risk of miscarriage following amniocentesis and chorionic villus sampling: a systematic review and meta-analysis. *Ultrasound in Obstetrics & Gynecology, 45*(1), 16–26.

Alekseev, N. P., Vladimir, I. I., & Nadezhda, T. E. (2015). Pathological postpartum breast engorgement: Prediction, prevention, and resolution. *Breastfeeding Medicine, 10*(4), 203–208.

Alexander, L. L., LaRosa, J. H., Bader, H., & Garfield, S. (2014). *New dimensions in women's health* (6th ed.). Sudbury, MA: Jones & Bartlett.

Alfirevic, Z., Stampalija, T., & Medley, N. (2015). Fetal and umbilical Doppler ultrasound in normal pregnancy. *Cochrane Database of Systematic Reviews 2015*, (4), CD001450. doi: 10.1002/14651858. CD001450.pub4

Alliman, J., Jolles, D., and Summers, L. (2015). The innovation imperative: Scaling freestanding birth centers, centering pregnancy, and midwifery-led maternity health homes. *Journal of Midwifery & Women's Health, 60*, 244–249.

Almansa, C., DeVault, K., & Houghton, L. A. (2015). Gas and bloating. In B. E. Lacy, M. D. Crowell, & J. K. DiBaise (Eds.), *Functional and motility disorders of the gastrointestinal tract* (pp. 113–123). New York, NY: Springer Publishers.

American Academy of Family Physicians. (2015). *Summary of recommendations for clinical preventive services*. Retrived from http://www.aafp.org/dam/AAFP/documents/patient_care/clinical_recommendations/cps-recommendations.pdf

American Academy of Pediatrics. (2012). Breastfeeding and the use of human milk. *Pediatrics, 129*(3), 827–841.

American Academy of Pediatrics. (2015). *Breastfeeding*. Retrieved from https://www2.aap.org/breastfeeding/index.html

American College of Nurse-Midwives. (2015). *About midwives*. Retrieved from http://www.midwife.org/About-Midwives

American College of Obstetricians & Gynecologists. (2013). *Oral health care during pregnancy and through the lifespan*. Retrieved from: http://www.acog.org/Resources-And-Publications/Committee-Opinions/Committee-on-Health-Care-for-Underserved-Women/Oral-Health-Care-During-Pregnancy-and-Through-the-Lifespan

American College of Obstetricians and Gynecologists. (2015a). *Routine tests in pregnancy FAQ 133*. Retrieved from http://www.acog.org/For_Patients/Search_FAQs?Topics=906bff1e-0656-4579-a7df-4a22f9bce483fb741a4b-41f7-4b37-8307-f4844738b26f

American College of Obstetricians and Gynecologists. (2015b). *Screening tests for birth defects*. Retrieved from http://www.acog.org/~/media/For%20Patients/faq165.pdf?dmc=1&ts=20140517T0925037578

American College of Obstetricians and Gynecologists. (2015c). *Easing back pain during pregnancy*. Retrieved from http://www.acog.org/~/media/For%20Patients/faq115.pdf?dmc=1&ts=201405 17T1536210126

American College of Obstetricians and Gynecologists. (2015d). *Problems of the digestive system*. Retrieved from http://www.acog.org/~/media/For%20Patients/faq120.pdf?dmc=1&ts=20140518T1321141397

American College of Obstetricians & Gynecologists. (2015e). *Exercise during pregnancy*. Retrieved from https://www.acog.org/Search?Keyword=exercise+guidelines

American College of Obstetricians & Gynecologists. (2015f). *Sexuality and sexual problems*. Retrieved from http://pause.acog.org/topics/sexuality-and-sexual-problems

American College of Obstetricians & Gynecologists. (2015g). *Travel during pregnancy*. Retrieved from http://www.acog.org/~/media/For%20Patients/faq055.pdf?dmc=1&ts=20140519T1526511729

American College of Obstetricians and Gynecologists. (2015h). *Breastfeeding your baby*. Retrieved from http://www.acog.org/~/media/For%20Patients/faq029.pdf?dmc=1&ts=20140520T0943394126

American Diabetes Association. (2015). Classification and diagnosis of diabetes. *Diabetes Care, 38*(suppl 1), S8–S16.

American Pregnancy Association. (2014a). *Maternal serum alpha-fetoprotein screening (MSAFP)*. Retrieved from http://americanpregnancy.org/prenataltesting/afp.html

American Pregnancy Association. (2014b). *Pregnancy exercise guidelines*. Retrieved from http://americanpregnancy.org/pregnancy-health/exerciseguidelines.html

Anil, S., Alrowis, R. M., Chalisserry, E. P., Chalissery, V. P., AlMoharib, H. S., & Al-Sulaimani, A. F. (2015). Oral health and adverse pregnancy outcomes. In S. V. Mandeep (Ed.), *Emerging trends in oral health sciences and dentistry* (pp. 631–662). http://dx.doi.org/10.5772/59517

Barakat, R., Lucía, A., & Ruiz, J. (2015). Exercise and pregnancy. In M. L. Mountjoy (Ed.), *Handbook of sports medicine and science: The female athlete* (pp. 110–119). Hoboken, NJ: John Wiley & Sons. doi: 10.1002/9781118862254.ch12

Baum, A., Crawford, P., & Humphrey-Shelton, M. (2015). Clinical inquiry: Does the presence of a trained support person during labor decrease C-section rates? *The Journal of Family Practice, 64*(3), 192–193.

Biswas, A., & Choolani, M. (2015). Prenatal diagnosis of chromosomal abnormalities—shifting paradigm. *Annals of the Academy of Medicine, Singapore, 44*(2), 40–42.

Boggess, K. A., & Berggren, E. K. (2015). Preconception care has the potential for a high return on investment. *American Journal of Obstetrics & Gynecology, 212*(1), A1–A20.

Bond, S. (2015). American College of Obstetricians and Gynecologists Releases Committee opinion on estimation of due date. *Journal of Midwifery & Women's Health, 60*(2), 220–224.

Bope, E. T., & Kellerman, R. D. (2015) *Conn's current therapy 2015*. Philadelphia, PA: Saunders Elsevier.

Boynton, P. M. 2015. Pregnancy: Relationships advice. *The International Encyclopedia of Human Sexuality*. 861–1042. doi: 10.1002/9781118896877.wbiehs372

Bradley Method. (2014). *Introduction to the Bradley method*. Retrieved from http://www.bradleybirth.com

Brown, H. L. (2015). ACOG guidelines at a glance: Antepartum fetal surveillance. *Contemporary OB/GYN*. Retrieved from http://contemporaryobgyn.modernmedicine.com/contemporary-obgyn/news/acog-guidelines-glance-antepartum-fetal-surveillance?page=full

Budin, W. C. (2015). Choosing wisely for birth. *The Journal of Perinatal Education, 24*(1), 3–5.

Callahan, T. L. (2016). *Tarascon Ob/Gyn pocketbook*. Burlington, MA: Jones & Bartlett Learning.

Callegari, L. S., Ma, E. W., & Schwarz, E. B. (2015). Preconception care and reproductive planning in primary care. *Medical Clinics of North America, 99*(3), 663–682.

Centers for Disease Control and Prevention. (2015a). *Preconception care and health care*. Retrieved from http://www.cdc.gov/preconception/hcp/

Centers for Disease Control and Prevention. (2015b). *Preconception care recommendations*. Retrieved from http://www.cdc.gov/preconception/hcp/recommendations.html

Centers for Disease Control and Prevention. (2015c). *Facts about birth defects*. Retrieved from http://www.cdc.gov/ncbddd/birthdefects/facts.html

Centers for Disease Control and Prevention. (2015d). *Pregnancy complications*. Retrieved from http://www.cdc.gov/reproductivehealth/MaternalInfantHealth/PregComplications.htm#n5

Centers for Disease Control and Prevention. (2015e). *Pregnant travelers*. Retrieved from http://wwwnc.cdc.gov/travel/yellowbook/2014/chapter-8-advising-travelers-with-specific-needs/pregnant-travelers

Centers for Disease Control and Prevention. (2015f). *Vaccines for pregnant women*. Retrieved from http://www.cdc.gov/vaccines/adults/rec-vac/pregnant.html

Centers for Disease Control and Prevention. (2015g). *Mediations and pregnancy*. Retrieved from http://www.cdc.gov/pregnancy/meds/

Cunningham, F., Leveno, K, Bloom, S., Spong, K., Dashe, J.S., Hoffman, B.L., et al. (2014) *William's obstetrics* (24th ed.). New York, NY: McGraw-Hill Education.

Darmstadt, G. L., Shiffman, J., & Lawn, J. E. (2015). Advancing the newborn and stillbirth global agenda: Priorities for the next decade. *Archives of Disease in Childhood, 100*(suppl 1), S13–S18.

Declercq, E. R., Sakala, C., Corry, M. P., Applebaum, S., & Herrlich, A. (2014). Major survey findings of listening to mothers (SM) III: New mothers speak out: Report of national surveys of women's childbearing experiences conducted October 2102 and January-April 2013. *Journal of Perinatal Education. Winter, 23(1),* 17–24. doi: 10.1891/1058-1243.23.1.17

Declercq, E, & Stotland, N. E. (2015). Planned home birth. *UpToDate*. Retrieved from http://0-www.uptodate.com.ksclib.keene.edu/contents/planned-homebirth?source=search_result&search=planned+home+birth&selectedTitle=1~150

Dempsey, Á. C., & Overton, T. G. (2015). Advances in fetal therapy. *Obstetrics, Gynecology & Reproductive Medicine*. (Online 5/8/15), doi:10.1016/j.ogrm.2015.04.003

Dietz, W. H. (2015). The response of the US Centers for Disease Control and Prevention to the obesity epidemic. *Annual Review of Public Health, 36*, 575–596.

Eshaghabadi, A., & Barati, P. (2015). P97: Motor vehicle accident during the pregnancy. *The Neuroscience Journal of Shefaye Khatam, 2*(4), 147–147.

Evans, M. I., Andriole, S., & Evans, S. M. (2015). Genetics: Update on prenatal screening and diagnosis. *Obstetrics and Gynecology Clinics of North America, 42*(2), 193–208.

Everett, T. R., & Peebles, D. M. (2015, April). Antenatal tests of fetal wellbeing. In *Seminars in Fetal and Neonatal Medicine*. WB Saunders.

Farrar, D., Duley, L., Medley, N., & Lawlor, D. A. (2015). Different strategies for diagnosing gestational diabetes to improve maternal and infant health. *Cochrane Database of Systematic Reviews, 2015*(1), CD007122. doi: 10.1002/14651858.CD007122.pub3

Ferri, F. F. (2014). *Ferri's best test: A practical guide to laboratory medicine and diagnostic imaging* (3rd ed.). Philadelphia, PA: Elsevier Health Sciences.

Fischbach, F., & Dunning, M. B. (2014). *A manual of laboratory and diagnostic tests* (9th ed.). Philadelphia, PA: Lippincott Williams & Wilkins.

Fretts, R. C. (2014). Evaluation of decreased fetal movements. *UpToDate*. Retrieved from http://www.uptodate.com/contents/evaluation-of-decreased-fetal-movements

Gadot, Y., & Koren, G. (2015). Medications in pregnancy: Can we treat the mother while protecting the unborn? In S. Macleod, S. Hill, G. Koren, & A. Rane (Eds.), *Optimizing treatment for children in the developing world* (pp. 65–70). Switzerland: Springer International Publishing.

Grant, N., Strevens, H., & Thornton, J. (2015). Physiology of labor. In G. Capogna (Ed.), *Epidural labor analgesia* (pp. 1–10). Switzerland: Springer International Publishing.

Greeley, E. T., Kessler, K. A., & Vohra, N. (2015). Clinical applications of noninvasive prenatal testing. *Journal of Fetal Medicine*, 1–7. doi: 10.1007/s40556-015-0035-1

Guidotti, T. L. (2014). Demystifying reproductive hazards in the workplace. *Archives of Environmental & Occupational Health*, 69(2), 125–126. doi:10.1080/19338244.2014.811996

Halford, W. K., Petch, J., & Creedy, D. (2015). Caring and sexuality. *Clinical Guide to Helping New Parents* (pp. 131–150). New York, NY: Springer Publishers.

Heazell, A. (2015). A kick in the right direction-reduced fetal movements and stillbirth prevention. *BMC Pregnancy and Childbirth*, 15(suppl 1), A7. doi:10.1186/1471-2393-15-S1-A7

Hehir, M. P., Dalrymple, J., & Malone, F. D. (2015). Decision-support guide and use of prenatal genetic testing. *JAMA*, 313(2), 199–199.

Hixson, L., Goel, S., Schuber, P., Faltas, V., Lee, J., Narayakkadan, A., et al. (2015). An overview on prenatal screening for chromosomal aberrations. *Journal of Laboratory Automation*. doi: 10.1177/2211068214564595.

Hurst, H. M., & Linton, D. M. (2015). Preconception care: Planning for the future. *The Journal for Nurse Practitioners*, 11(3), 335–340.

Jordan, R.G., Engstrom, J., Marfell, J., & Farley, C.L. (2014). *Prenatal and postnatal care: A women-centered approach*. Ames, IA: John Wiley & Sons.

Jyothi, M. N. (2015). A case report on pica: A rare pregnancy related complication. *Asian Journal of Nursing Education and Research*, 5(1), 137–139.

Kader, M., & Naim-Shuchana, S. (2014). Physical activity and exercise during pregnancy. *European Journal of Physiotherapy*, 16(1), 2–9.

Kalousová, M., Muravská, A., & Zima, T. (2014). Pregnancy-associated plasma protein A (PAPP-A) and preeclampsia. *Advances in Clinical Chemistry*, 63, 169–209.

Keytash, A., Jones, L., & Frances, A. (2015). Strong healthy behavioral change program for women. *Australian Nursing and Midwifery Journal*, 22(9), 45–46.

Khalil, A., & Coates, A. (2015). Prenatal diagnosis of chromosomal abnormalities. In F. Arias, A. G. Bhide, S. Arulkumaran, K. R. Damania, & S. N. Daftary (Eds.), *Arias' practical guide to high-risk pregnancy and delivery: A South Asian perspective* (4th ed., 1–13). New Delhi, India: Elsevier Health Sciences.

King, T. L., Brucker, M. C., Kriebs, J. M., Fahey, J. O., Gegor, C. L., & Varney, H. (2015). *Varney's midwifery* (5th ed.). Burlington, MA: Jones & Bartlett Learning

Kondhare, M. M., & Khodgire, U. (2015). Benefits of exercises on selected physiological common complaints during pregnancy. *Journal of Physical Education Research*, 1, 13–26.

Lakshmi, G. R., & Jyothsna, D. (2015). Influence of amniotic fluid index on fetal outcome. *Journal of Evidence Based Medicine and Healthcare*, 2(10), 1455–1463.

La LecheLeague International. (2014). *Breastfeeding help*. Retrieved from http://www.llli.org/resources/assistance.html?m=0,0

Lamaze International.(2015). *Healthy birth practices*. Retrieved from http://www.lamaze.org

Latendresse, G., & Deneris, A. (2015). An update on current prenatal testing options: First trimester and noninvasive prenatal testing. *Journal of Midwifery & Women's Health*, 60(1), 24–36.

Leggat, P. A., & Zuckerman, J. N. (2015). Pre-travel health risk assessment. In J. N. Zuckerman, G. Brunette, & P. Leggat (Eds.), *Essential travel medicine* (pp. 23–34). West Sussex: John Wiley & Sons.

Lewis, R. (2015). As home births increase, recent studies illuminate controversies and complexities. *JAMA*, 313(6), 553–555.

Maeda, K. (2015). Ultrasound diagnosis of the fetus in-utero. *Journal of Health Medical Informatics*, 6(174). doi:10.4172/2157-7420.1000174

March of Dimes. (2015a). *Pregnancy complications*. Retrieved from http://www.marchofdimes.com/pregnancy/pregnancy-complications.aspx

March of Dimes. (2015b). *The serious problem of premature birth*. Retrieved from http://www.marchofdimes.com/mission/prematurity-campaign.aspx

March of Dimes. (2015c). *Preterm labor*. Retrieved from http://www.marchofdimes.com/pregnancy/preterm-labor-and-birth.aspx

March of Dimes. (2015d). *Aminocentesis*. Retrieved from http://www.marchofdimes.com/pregnancy/amniocentesis.aspx

March of Dimes. (2015e). *Chorionic villus sampling*. Retrieved from http://www.marchofdimes.com/pregnancy/chorionic-villus-sampling.aspx

March of Dimes. (2015f). *Sex during pregnancy*. Retrieved from http://www.marchofdimes.com/pregnancy/physicalactivity_sex.html

March of Dimes. (2015g). *Childbirth education classes*. Retrieved from http://www.marchofdimes.com/pregnancy/childbirth-education-classes.aspx

March of Dimes. (2015h). *Vaccinations during pregnancy*. Retrieved from http://www.marchofdimes.com/pregnancy/vaccinations-during-pregnancy.aspx

Moses, S. (2015a). Routine obstetric visit. *Family PRACTICE NOTEBOOK*. Retrieved from: http://www.fpnotebook.com/ob/Exam/RtnObstrcVst.htm

Moses, S. (2015b). Fetal movement count. *Family practice notebook*. Retrieved from http://www.fpnotebook.com/ob/fetus/FtlMvmntCnt.htm

Moses, S. (2015c). Biophysical profile. *Family practice notebook*. Retrieved from http://www.fpnotebook.com/ob/fetus/BphysclPrfl.htm

M'soka, N. C., Mabuza, L. H., & Pretorius, D. (2015). Cultural and health beliefs of pregnant women in Zambia regarding pregnancy and child birth. *Curationis*, 38(1), 1–7.

Nagtalon-Ramos, J. (2014). *Best evidence-based practices in maternal-newborn care*. Philadelphia, PA: F. A. Davis Company.

National Institutes of Health. (2015). *Health problems in pregnancy*. Retrieved from http://www.nlm.nih.gov/medlineplus/healthproblemsinpregnancy.html

National Maternal and Child Health Resource Center. (2015). *Oral health care during pregnancy: A national consensus statement*. Retrieved from http://www.mchoralhealth.org/materials/consensus_statement.html

Nisa, M. U., Hamid, N., Nasreen, F., & Khanum, F. (2015). Co-relation of biophysical profile with APGAR score. *Cell*, 92. doi: 321–9001662.

Office on Women's Health. (2014). Why breastfeeding is important. *Womenshealth.gov*. Retrieved from http://www.womenshealth.gov/breastfeeding/why-breastfeeding-is-important/

Ota E, Hori H, Mori R, Tobe-Gai R, Farrar D. Antenatal dietary education and supplementation to increase energy and protein intake. (2015). *Cochrane Database of Systematic Reviews*, 2015(6), CD000032. doi: 10.1002/14651858.CD000032.pub3

Patil, M., Panchanadikar, T., & Wagh, G. (2014). Variation of PAPP-A level in the first trimester of pregnancy and its clinical outcome. *Journal of Obstetrics and Gynecology of India*, 64(2), 116–119.

Petrov Fieril, K., Glantz, A., & Fagevik Olsen, M. (2015). The efficacy of moderate-to-vigorous resistance exercise during pregnancy: A randomized controlled trial. *Acta Obstetricia et Gynecologica Scandinavica*, 94(1), 35–42.

Plastaras, C. T., & Appasamy, M. (2015). Interventional procedures for musculoskeletal pain in pregnancy and postpartum: Efficacy and safety. In C. Fitzgerald, & N. Segal (Eds.), *Musculoskeletal health in pregnancy and postpartum* (pp. 115–133). Switzerland: Springer International Publishing.

Pruetz, J. D., Votava-Smith, J., & Miller, D. A. (2015, March). Clinical relevance of fetal hemodynamic monitoring: Perinatal implications. *Seminars in fetal and neonatal medicine*, 20(4);217–224. doi:10.1016/j.siny.2015.03.007

Rayburn, W. F., Jolley, J. A., & Simpson, L. L. (2015). Advances in ultrasound imaging for congenital malformations during early gestation. *Birth Defects Research Part A: Clinical and Molecular Teratology*, 103, 260–268.

Regal, J. F., Gilbert, J. S., & Burwick, R. M. (2015). The complement system and adverse pregnancy outcomes. *Molecular Immunology*, 67(1), 56–70.

Rigby, F. B. (2015). Common pregnancy complaints and questions. *Emedicine*. Retrieved from http://emedicine.medscape.com/article/259724-overview

Satyan, M. T., Grothusen, J., Drummond, K., Kennedy, B., Weiner, C., & Lee, G. (2015). 200: A retrospective review of the impact of HAPO based screening guidelines for gestational diabetes. *American Journal of Obstetrics & Gynecology, 212*(1), S113–S114.

Schuiling, K. D., & Likis, F. E. (2016). *Women's gynecologic health* (3rd ed.). Burlington, MA: Jones & Bartlett Learning.

Schram, J. (2014). Food for thought. *World of Irish Nursing & Midwifery, 22*(3), 46–47.

Schytt, E., & Bergström, M. (2014). First-time fathers' expectations and experiences of childbirth in relation to age. *Midwifery, 30*(1), 82–88.

Senie, R.T. (2014). *Epidemiology of women's health*. Burlington, MA: Jones & Bartlett Learning.

Slaughter, S., Hearns-Stokes, R., van der Vlugt, T., & Joffe, H. (2014). FDA approval of doxylamine-pyridoxine therapy for use in pregnancy. *New England Journal of Medicine, 370*(12), 1081–1083.

Springer, S. C. (2015). Prenatal diagnosis and fetal therapy. *eMedicine*. Retrieved from http://emedicine.medscape.com/article/936318-overview#aw2aab6b5

Steegers-Theunissen, R. P., & Steegers, E. A. (2015). Embryonic health: New insights, health and personalized patient care. *Reproduction, Fertility and Development, 27*(4), 712–715.

Tanner-Smith, E., Steinka-Fry, K., & Lipsey, M. (2014). The effects of centering pregnancy group prenatal care on gestational age, birth weight, and fetal demise. *Maternal & Child Health Journal, 18*(4), 801–809.

Tara, F., Vakilian, F., Moosavi-Baigy, F., Salehi, M., & Moghiman, T. (2015). Prenatal and cardiovascular outcome in pregnant patients with dyspnea. *Research in Cardiovascular Medicine, 4*(2). doi: 10.5812/cardiovascmed.20950

Templeton, A. (2015). The public health importance of antenatal care. *Facts, Views & Vision in ObGyn, 7*(1), 5–6.

Tharpe, N. L., Farley, C. L., & Jordan, R. (2016). *Clinical practice guidelines for midwifery & women's health* (5th ed.). Sudbury, MA: Jones & Bartlett.

Tracy, M. (2014) Centering pregnancy: An alternative model of prenatal care. *The Citizen*. Retrieved from http://www.auburnhospital.org/news-events/articles/centering-pregnancy-an-alternate-model-of-prenatal-care

Trivedi, S., Lal, N., & Singhal, R. (2015). Periodontal diseases and pregnancy. *Journal of Orofacial Sciences, 7*(1), 67–68.

Truong, Y. N., Yee, L. M., Caughey, A. B., & Cheng, Y. W. (2015). Weight gain in pregnancy: Does the Institute of Medicine have it right? *American Journal of Obstetrics and Gynecology, 212*(3), 362–370.

Tyler, S., & Nagtalon-Ramos, J. (2015). Managing nausea and vomiting of pregnancy. *NP Women's Healthcare, 3*(2), 7–13.

U.S. Department of Health and Human Services. (2010). *Healthy People 2020*. Retrieved from http://www.healthypeople.gov/2020/topicsobjectives2020/objectiveslist.aspx?topicId = 26

U.S. Preventive Services Task Force. (2015). *Screening for gestational diabetes mellitus*. Retrieved from http://www.uspreventiveservices-taskforce.org/uspstf/uspsgdm.htm

Varner, C. A. (2015). Comparison of the Bradley method and HypnoBirthing childbirth education classes. *The Journal of Perinatal Education, 24*(2), 128–136.

Verghese, T. S., Futaba, K., & Latthe, P. (2015). Constipation in pregnancy. *The Obstetrician & Gynecologist, 17*(2), 111–115.

Weber, J., & Kelley, J. H. (2014). *Health assessment in nursing* (5th ed.). Philadelphia, PA: Lippincott Williams & Wilkins.

Westbury, B. (2015). The power of environment. *The Practicing Midwife, 18*(6), 24–26.

Women, Infants and Children. (2015). *Breastfeeding promotion and support in WIC*. Retrieved from http://www.fns.usda.gov/wic/breastfeeding-promotion-and-support-wic

Yeniel, A. A., & Petri, E. E. (2014). Pregnancy, childbirth, and sexual function: Perceptions and facts. *International Urogynecology Journal, 25*(1), 5–14.

Yıldız, H. (2015). The relation between prepregnancy sexuality and sexual function during pregnancy and the postpartum period: A prospective study. *Journal of Sex & Marital Therapy, 41*(1), 49–59.

Zielinski, R., Ackerson, K., & Low, L. K. (2015). Planned home birth: Benefits, risks, and opportunities. *International Journal of Women's Health, 7*, 361–377.

Zielinski, R., Searing, K., & Deibel, M. (2015). Gastrointestinal distress in pregnancy: Prevalence, assessment, and treatment of 5 common minor discomforts. *The Journal of Perinatal & Neonatal Nursing, 29*(1), 23–31.

Zolotor, A., & Carlough, M. (2014). Update on prenatal care. *American Family Physician, 89*(3), 199–208.

MULTIPLE CHOICE QUESTIONS

1. Which of the following biophysical profile findings indicate poor oxygenation to the fetus?
   a. Two pockets of amniotic fluid
   b. Well-flexed arms and legs
   c. Nonreactive fetal heart rate
   d. Fetal breathing movements noted

2. The nurse teaches the pregnant client how to perform Kegel exercises as a way to accomplish which of the following?
   a. Prevent perineal lacerations
   b. Stimulate labor contractions
   c. Increase pelvic muscle tone
   d. Lose pregnancy weight quickly

3. During a clinic visit, a pregnant client at 30 weeks gestation tells the nurse, "I've had some mild cramps that are pretty irregular. What does this mean?" The cramps are probably:
   a. The beginning of labor in the very early stages
   b. An ominous finding indicating that the client is about to have a miscarriage
   c. Related to over hydration of the woman
   d. Braxton Hicks contractions, which occur throughout pregnancy

4. The nurse is preparing her teaching plan for a woman who has just had her pregnancy confirmed. Which of the following should be included in it? Select all that apply.
   a. Prevent constipation by taking a daily laxative
   b. Balance your dietary intake by increasing your calories by 300 daily
   c. Continue your daily walking routine just as you did before this pregnancy
   d. Tetanus, measles, mumps, and rubella vaccines will be given to you now
   e. Avoid tub baths now that you are pregnant to prevent vaginal infections
   f. Sexual activity is permitted as long as your membranes are intact
   g. Increase your consumption of milk to meet your iron needs

5. A pregnant client's LMP was on August 10. Using Nagele's rule, the nurse calculates that her EDD will be which of the following?
   a. June 23
   b. July 10
   c. July 30
   d. May 17

6. Which of the following is not true about breast-feeding?
   a. Breast-fed infants experience more obesity and allergies
   b. Breast milk is perfectly suited to the infant's nutritional needs
   c. Breast milk contains maternal antibodies to stimulate infant's immunity
   d. Breast-feeding enhances maternal bonding and attachment

7. Practicing good oral hygiene is important for all women throughout their pregnancy. As a nurse providing anticipatory guidance for pregnant women, what condition can result from periodontal disease if good dental care isn't practiced?
   a. Postdates pregnancy
   b. Large for gestational age infant
   c. Advanced reproductive cancer
   d. Preterm or low–birth-weight infant

8. Anticipatory guidance regarding sexual activity during pregnancy includes: Select all that apply:
   a. Sexual activity is contraindicated throughout pregnancy
   b. Most women don't desire intimacy after the first trimester
   c. Sexual activity may continue up until the end of the second trimester
   d. Sexual intercourse is prohibited if a history of preterm labor exists
   e. Women's sexual desire may change throughout the pregnancy
   f. Couples can try a variety of positions of comfort during pregnancy

9. Which of the following would be considered risk factors for psychological well-being in pregnancy? Select all that apply:
   a. Limited support system and network of friends and family
   b. Introverted personality at any point in the pregnancy
   c. Ambivalence any time during the pregnancy
   d. High levels of stress due to family discord
   e. History of previous high-risk pregnancy with complications
   f. Depression prior to pregnancy and on medication

CRITICAL THINKING EXERCISES

1. Mary Jones comes to the Women's Health Center, where you work as a nurse. She is in her first trimester of pregnancy and tells you her main complaints are nausea and fatigue, to the point that she wants to sleep most of the time and eats one meal daily. She appears pale and tired. Her mucous membranes are pale. She reports that she gets 8 to 9 hours of sleep each night but still can't seem to stay awake and alert at work. She tells you she knows that she is not eating as she should, but she isn't hungry. Her hemoglobin and hematocrit are low.
   a. What subjective and objective data do you have to make your assessment?
   b. What is your impression of this woman?
   c. What nursing interventions would be appropriate for this client?
   d. How will you evaluate the effectiveness of your interventions?

2. Monica, a 16-year-old African-American high school student, is here for her first prenatal visit. Her LMP was 2 months ago, and she states she has been "sick ever since." She is 5 feet, 6 inches tall, and weighs 110 pounds. In completing her dietary assessment, the nurse asks about her intake of milk and dairy products. Monica reports that she doesn't like "that stuff" and doesn't want to put on too much weight because it "might ruin my figure."
   a. In addition to the routine obstetric assessments, which additional ones might be warranted for this teenager?
   b. What dietary instruction should be provided to this teenager based on her history?
   c. What follow-up monitoring should be included in subsequent prenatal visits?

3. Maria, a 27-year-old Hispanic woman in her last trimester of pregnancy (34 weeks), complains to the clinic nurse that she is constipated and feels miserable most of the time. She reports that she has started taking laxatives, but they don't help much. When questioned about her dietary habits, she replies that she eats beans and rice and drinks tea with most meals. She says she has tried to limit her fluid intake so she doesn't have to go to the bathroom so much because she doesn't want to miss any of her daytime soap operas on television.
   a. What additional information would the nurse need to assess her complaint?
   b. What interventions would be appropriate for Maria?
   c. What adaptations will Maria need to make to alleviate her constipation?

STUDY ACTIVITIES

1. Visit a freestanding birth center and compare it to a traditional hospital setting in terms of restrictions, type of pain management available, and costs.

2. Arrange to shadow a nurse-midwife for a day to see her role in working with the childbearing family.

3. Visit the student resources on and select two of the supplied websites that correspond to this chapter. Note their target audience, the validity of information offered, and their appeal to expectant couples. Present your findings.

4. Request permission to attend a childbirth education class in your local area and help a woman without a partner practice the paced breathing exercises. Present the information you learned and think about how you can apply it while taking care of a woman during labor.

5. A laywoman with a specialized education and experience in assisting women during labor is a _____.

BRINGING IT ALL TOGETHER: CASE STUDY

A 19-year-old female came to the public health clinic. This was her first prenatal visit, although she was 8 months pregnant. Her explanation as to why she had not been there before was: "It was summer and everything had been going good until my back starting hurting two days ago."

ASSESSMENT

Her vital signs were within in normal range. Weight was 175 pounds. On physical exam, the back area was normal without tenderness when palpated. Fundal height was 36 cm; fetal heart rate was 150 bpm; urinalysis was negative for blood, glucose, or leukocytes. The pelvic exam showed the cervix to be long, thick, and closed. Missed routine prenatal lab work was done since this was her first visit. When questioned further about when her back seemed to cause her the most discomfort, she stated that she was a waitress and when she finished her shift, she could barely walk home.

Go to thePoint **to find questions to consider about this case.**

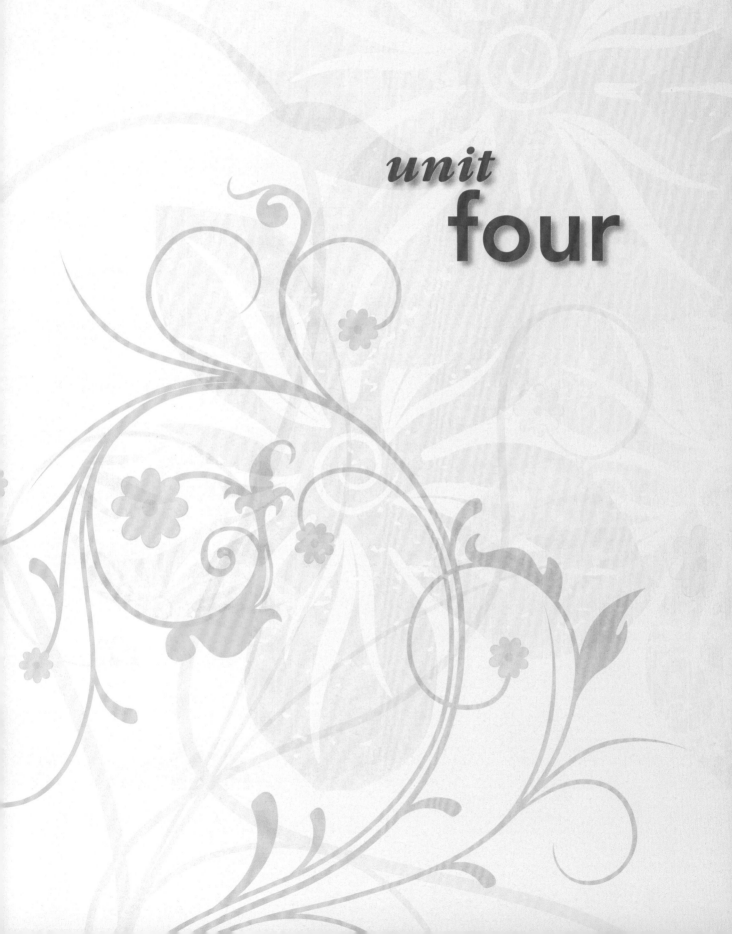

unit
four

Labor and Birth

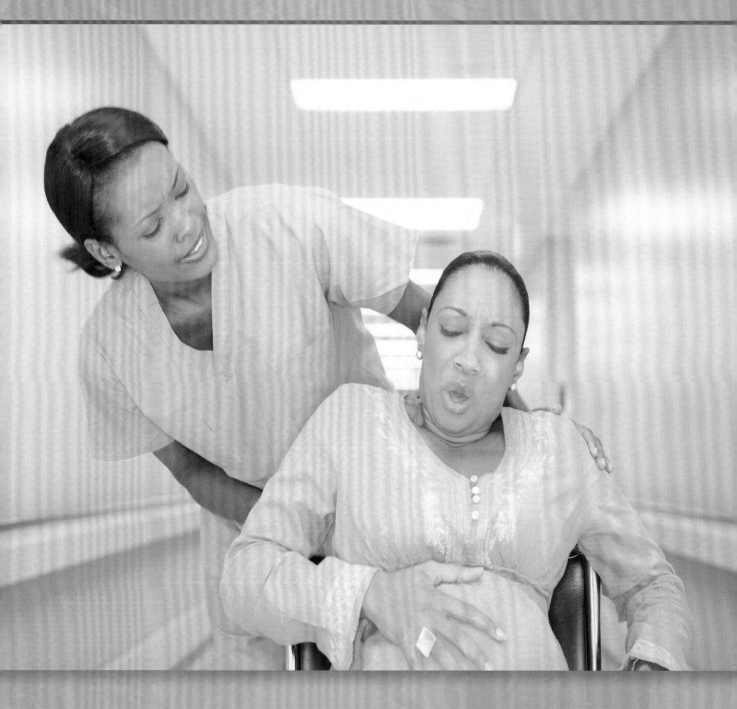

13

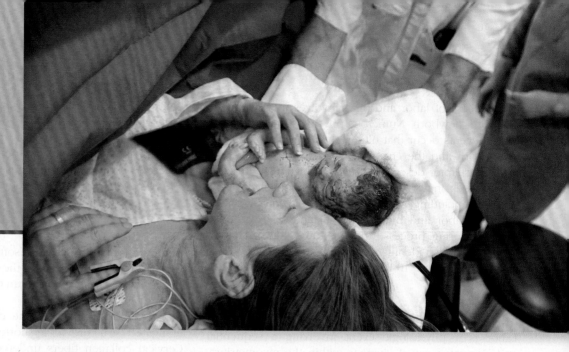

KEY TERMS

attitude
dilation
doula
duration
effacement
engagement
frequency
intensity
lie
lightening
molding
position
presentation
station

Labor and Birth Process

Learning Objectives

Upon completion of the chapter, you will be able to:

1. Relate premonitory signs of labor.

2. Compare and contrast true versus false labor.

3. Categorize the critical factors affecting labor and birth.

4. Analyze the cardinal movements of labor.

5. Evaluate the maternal and fetal responses to labor and birth.

6. Classify the stages of labor and the critical events in each stage.

7. Characterize the normal physiologic/psychological changes occurring during all four stages of labor.

8. Formulate the concept of pain as it relates to the woman in labor.

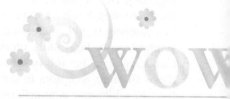

Kathy *and Chuck have been eagerly awaiting the birth of their first child for what seems to them an eternity. When Kathy finally feels contractions in her abdomen, she and Chuck rush to the birthing center. After the OB nurse finishes a complete history and physical assessment, she informs Kathy and her husband that she must have experienced "false labor" and that they should return home until she starts true labor.*

Words of Wisdom
Intense physical and emotional support promotes a positive and memorable birthing experience.

INTRODUCTION

The process of labor and birth involves more than the birth of a newborn. Numerous physiologic and psychological events occur that ultimately result in the birth of a newborn and the creation or expansion of the family. This chapter describes labor and birth as a process. It addresses initiation of labor, the premonitory signs of labor, including true and false labor, critical factors affecting labor and birth, maternal and fetal response to the laboring process, and the four stages of labor. The chapter also identifies critical factors related to each stage of labor: the "10 P's of labor."

INITIATION OF LABOR

Labor is a physiologic event involving a sequential and integrated set of changes within the myometrium, decidua, and cervix that occurs gradually over a period of days to weeks in order to expel the fetus from the uterus. It is difficult to determine exactly why labor begins and what initiates it. Although several theories have been proposed to explain the onset and maintenance of labor, none of these has been proved scientifically. It is widely believed that labor is influenced by a cascade of events, including uterine stretch from the fetus and amniotic fluid volume, progesterone withdrawal to estrogen dominance, increased oxytocin sensitivity, and increased release of prostaglandins.

One theory suggests that labor is initiated by a change in the estrogen-to-progesterone ratio. During the last trimester of pregnancy, estrogen levels increase and progesterone levels decrease. This change leads to an increase in the number of myometrium gap junctions. Gap junctions are proteins that connect cell membranes and facilitate coordination of uterine contractions and myometrial stretching (Norwitz, 2015).

Although physiologic evidence for the role of oxytocin in the initiation of labor is inconclusive, the number of oxytocin receptors in the uterus increases at the end of pregnancy. This creates an increased sensitivity to oxytocin. Estrogen, the levels of which are also rising, increases myometrial sensitivity to oxytocin. With the increasing levels of oxytocin in the maternal blood in conjunction with increasing fetal cortisol levels that synthesize prostaglandins, uterine contractions are initiated. Oxytocin also aids in stimulating prostaglandin synthesis through receptors in the decidua. Prostaglandins lead to additional contractions, cervical softening, gap junction induction, and myometrial sensitization, thereby leading to a progressive cervical **dilation** (the opening or enlargement of the external cervical os). Uterine contractions have two main functions: to dilate the cervix and to push the fetus through the birth canal (Funai & Norwitz, 2015).

PREMONITORY SIGNS OF LABOR

Before the onset of labor, a pregnant woman's body undergoes several changes in preparation for the birth of the newborn. The changes that occur often lead to characteristic signs and symptoms that suggest that labor is near. These premonitory signs and symptoms can vary, and not every woman experiences every one of them.

Cervical Changes

Before labor begins, cervical softening and possible cervical dilation with descent of the presenting part into the pelvis occur. These changes can occur 1 month to 1 hour before actual labor begins.

As labor approaches, the cervix changes from an elongated structure to a shortened, thinned segment. Cervical collagen fibers undergo enzymatic rearrangement into smaller, more flexible fibers that facilitate water absorption, leading to a softer, more stretchable cervix. These changes occur secondary to the effects of prostaglandins and pressure from Braxton Hicks contractions. The ripening and softening of the cervix are essential for effacement and dilation, which reflect the enhanced collagen breakdown that was previously inhibited by progesterone (Grant, Strevens, & Thornton, 2015).

Lightening

Lightening occurs when the fetal presenting part begins to descend into the true pelvis. The uterus lowers and moves into a more anterior position. The shape of the abdomen changes as a result of the change in the uterus. With this descent, the woman usually notes that her breathing is much easier and that there is a decrease in gastric reflux. However, she may complain of increased pelvic pressure, leg cramping, dependent edema in the lower legs, and low back discomfort. She may notice an increase in vaginal discharge and more frequent urination. In primiparas, lightening can occur 2 weeks or more before labor begins; among multiparas it may not occur until labor starts (Cheng & Caughey, 2015a).

Increased Energy Level

Some women report a sudden increase in energy before labor. This is sometimes referred to as nesting, because many women will focus this energy toward childbirth preparation by cleaning, cooking, preparing the nursery, and spending extra time with other children in the household. The increased energy level usually occurs 24 to 48 hours before the onset of labor. It is thought to be the result of an increase in epinephrine release caused by a decrease in progesterone (Jordan et al., 2014).

Bloody Show

At the onset of labor or before, the mucous plug that fills the cervical canal during pregnancy is expelled as a result of cervical softening and increased pressure of the presenting part. These ruptured cervical capillaries release a small amount of blood that mixes with mucus, resulting in the pink-tinged secretions known as bloody show.

Braxton Hicks Contractions

Braxton Hicks contractions, which the woman may have been experiencing throughout the pregnancy, may become stronger and more frequent. Braxton Hicks contractions are typically felt as a tightening or pulling sensation of the top of the uterus. They occur primarily in the abdomen and groin and gradually spread downward before relaxing. In contrast, true labor contractions are more commonly felt in the lower back. These contractions aid in moving the cervix from a posterior position to an anterior position. They also help in ripening and softening the cervix. However, the contractions are irregular and can be decreased by walking, voiding, eating, increasing fluid intake, or changing position.

Braxton Hicks contractions usually last about 30 seconds but can persist for as long as 2 minutes. As birth draws near and the uterus becomes more sensitive to oxytocin, the frequency and intensity of these contractions increase. However, if the contractions last longer than 30 seconds and occur more often than four to six times an hour, advise the woman to contact her health care provider so that she can be evaluated for possible preterm labor, especially if she is less than 38 weeks pregnant.

> **Take Note!**
>
> An infant born between 34 0/7 and 36 6/7 weeks of gestation is identified as "late preterm" and experiences many of the same health issues as other preterm birth infants (Horgan, 2015).

Spontaneous Rupture of Membranes

Rupture of membranes with loss of amniotic fluid prior to the onset of labor is termed prelabor rupture of membranes (PROM). It occurs in 8% to 10% of women with term pregnancies, the majority of whom will begin labor spontaneously within 24 hours (King et al., 2015). The rupture of membranes can result in either a sudden gush or a steady leakage of amniotic fluid. Although much of the amniotic fluid is lost when the rupture occurs, a continuous supply is produced to ensure protection of the fetus until birth.

After the amniotic sac has ruptured, the barrier to infection is gone and an ascending infection is possible.

In addition, there is a danger of cord prolapse if engagement has not occurred with the sudden release of fluid and pressure with rupture. Due to the possibility of these complications, advise women to notify their health care provider and go in for an evaluation.

Consider This

I always pictured myself a dignified woman and behaved in ways to demonstrate that, for that was the way I was raised. My mother and grandmother always stressed that you should look good, dress well, and do nothing to embarrass yourself in public. I did a fairly good job of living up to their expectations until an incident occurred at the end of my first pregnancy. I recall I was overdue according to my dates and was miserable in the summer heat. I decided to go to the store for some ice cream. As I waddled down the grocery aisles, all of a sudden my water broke and came pouring down my legs all over the floor. Not wanting to make a spectacle of myself and remembering what my mother always said about being dignified at all times in public, I quickly reached up onto the grocery shelf and "accidentally" knocked off a large jar of pickles right where my puddle was. As I walked hurriedly away from that mess without my ice cream, I heard on the store loudspeaker, "Clean-up on aisle 13!"

Thoughts: *We tend to live by what we are taught, and in this case, this woman needed to save face from her ruptured membranes. Many women experience ruptured membranes before the onset of labor, so it is not out of the ordinary for this to happen in public. What risks can occur when membranes do rupture? What action should this woman take now to minimize these risks? How will the nurse validate this woman's ruptured membranes?*

TRUE VERSUS FALSE LABOR

False labor is a condition occurring during the latter weeks of some pregnancies in which irregular uterine contractions are felt, but the cervix is not affected. In contrast, true labor is characterized by contractions occurring at regular intervals that increase in frequency, duration, and intensity. True labor contractions bring about progressive cervical dilation and effacement. Table 13.1 summarizes the differences between true and false labor. False labor, prodromal labor, and Braxton Hicks contractions are all names for contractions that do not contribute in a measurable way toward the goal of birth. Distinguishing between true and false labor is an essential nursing assessment skill and one that develops with experience.

TABLE 13.1	DIFFERENCES BETWEEN TRUE AND FALSE LABOR	
Parameters	True Labor	False Labor
Contraction timing	Regular, becoming closer together, usually 4–6 min apart, lasting 30–60 s	Irregular, not occurring close together
Contraction strength	Become stronger with time, vaginal pressure is usually felt	Frequently weak, not getting stronger with time or alternating (a strong one followed by weaker ones)
Contraction discomfort	Starts in the back and radiates around toward the front of the abdomen	Usually felt in the front of the abdomen
Any change in activity	Contractions continue no matter what positional change is made	Contractions may stop or slow down with walking or making a position change
Stay or go?	Stay home until contractions are 5 min apart, last 45–60 s, and are strong enough so that a conversation during one is not possible—then go to the hospital or birthing center.	Drink fluids and walk around to see if there is any change in the intensity of the contractions; if the contractions diminish in intensity after either or both—stay home.

Adapted from Cunningham, F. G., Leveno, K. J., Bloom, S. L., Spong, C. Y., Dashe, J. S., Hoffman, B. L., et al. (2014). *Williams' obstetrics* (24th ed.). New York, NY: McGraw-Hill Education; King, T. L., Brucker, M. C., Kriebs, J. M., Fahey, J. O., Gegor, C. L., & Varney, H. (2015). *Varney's midwifery* (5th ed.), Burlington, MA: Jones & Bartlett Learning.; and Tharpe, N. L., Farley, C. L., & Jordan, R. (2016). *Clinical practice guidelines for midwifery & women's health*(4th ed.). Sudbury, MA: Jones & Bartlett.

Many women fear being sent home from the hospital with false labor. All women feel anxious when they feel contractions, but they should be informed that labor could be a long process, especially if it is their first pregnancy. Encourage the woman to think of false labor or prelabor signs as positive, because they are part of the entire labor continuum. With first pregnancies, the cervix can take up to 20 hours to dilate completely (Cunningham et al., 2014).

Remember Kathy and Chuck, the anxious couple who came to the hospital too early? Kathy felt sure she was in labor and is now confused. What explanations and anticipatory guidance should be offered to this couple? What term would describe her earlier contractions?

FACTORS AFFECTING THE LABOR PROCESS

Traditionally, the critical factors that affect the process of labor and birth are outlined as the "five **P**s:"
1. **P**assageway (birth canal)
2. **P**assenger (fetus and placenta)
3. **P**owers (contractions)
4. **P**osition (maternal)
5. **P**sychological response

These critical factors are commonly accepted and discussed by health care providers. However, five additional "P's" can also affect the labor process:

1. **P**hilosophy (low tech, high touch)
2. **P**artners (support caregivers)
3. **P**atience (natural timing)
4. **P**atient (client) preparation (childbirth knowledge base)
5. **P**ain management (comfort measures)

These five additional **P**s are helpful in planning care for the laboring family. These client-focused factors are an attempt to foster labor that can be managed through the use of high touch, patience, support, knowledge, and pain management.

Passageway

The birth passageway is the route through which the fetus must travel to be born vaginally. Compared to other primates, childbirth is remarkably difficult in humans because the head of the neonate is large relative to the birth-relevant dimensions of the maternal pelvis. The passageway consists of the maternal pelvis and soft tissues. Of the two, however, the maternal bony pelvis is more important because it is relatively unyielding (except for the coccyx). Typically the pelvis is assessed and measured during the first trimester, often at the first visit to the health care provider, to identify any abnormalities that might hinder a successful vaginal birth. As the pregnancy progresses, the hormones relaxin and estrogen cause the connective tissues to become more relaxed and elastic and cause the joints to become more flexible to prepare the mother's pelvis for birth. Additionally, the soft tissues usually yield to the forces of labor.

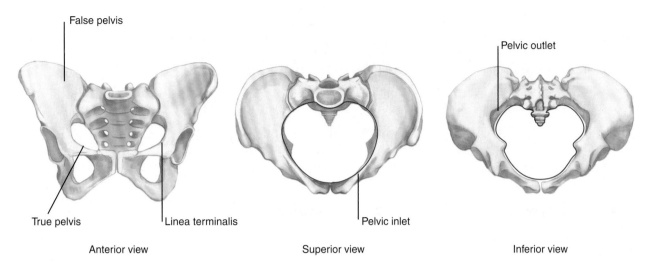

False pelvis

Pelvic outlet

True pelvis Linea terminalis

Pelvic inlet

Anterior view   Superior view   Inferior view

FIGURE 13.1 The bony pelvis.

Bony Pelvis

The maternal bony pelvis can be divided into the true and false portions. The false (or greater) pelvis is composed of the upper flared parts of the two iliac bones with their concavities and the wings of the base of the sacrum. The false pelvis is divided from the true pelvis by an imaginary line drawn from the sacral prominence at the back to the superior aspect of the symphysis pubis at the front of the pelvis. This imaginary line is called the linea terminalis. The false pelvis lies above this imaginary line; the true pelvis lies below it (Fig. 13.1). The true pelvis is the bony passageway through which the fetus must travel. It is made up of three planes: the inlet, the mid-pelvis (cavity), and the outlet.

PELVIC INLET

The pelvic inlet allows entrance to the true pelvis. It is bounded by the sacral prominence in the back, the ilium on the sides, and the superior aspect of the symphysis pubis in the front (Jones & Lopez, 2014). The pelvic inlet is wider in the transverse aspect (sideways) than it is from front to back.

MID-PELVIS

The mid-pelvis (cavity) occupies the space between the inlet and outlet. It is through this snug, curved space that the fetus must travel to reach the outside. As the fetus passes through this small area its chest is compressed, causing lung fluid and mucus to be expelled. This expulsion removes the space-occupying fluid so that air can enter the lungs with the newborn's first breath.

PELVIC OUTLET

The pelvic outlet is bound by the ischial tuberosities, the lower rim of the symphysis pubis, and the tip of the coccyx. In comparison with the pelvic inlet, the outlet is wider from front to back. For the fetus to pass through

the pelvis, the outlet must be large enough. To ensure the adequacy of the pelvic outlet for vaginal birth, the following pelvic measurements are assessed:

- Diagonal conjugate of the inlet (distance between the anterior surface of the sacral prominence and the anterior surface of the inferior margin of the symphysis pubis).
- Transverse or ischial tuberosity diameter of the outlet (distance at the medial and lowest aspect of the ischial tuberosities, at the level of the anus; a known hand span or clenched-fist measurement is generally used to obtain this measurement).
- True or obstetric conjugate (distance estimated from the measurement of the diagonal conjugate; 1.5 cm is subtracted from the diagonal conjugate measurement).

For more information about pelvic measurements, see Chapter 12.

If the diagonal conjugate measures at least 11.5 cm and the true or obstetric conjugate measures 10 cm or more (1.5 cm less than the diagonal conjugate, or about 10 cm), then the pelvis is large enough for a vaginal birth of what would be considered a normal-size newborn.

Pelvic Shape

In addition to size, the shape of a woman's pelvis is a determining factor for a vaginal birth. Each plane of the pelvis has a shape, which is defined by the anterior-posterior and transverse diameters. The pelvis is divided into four main shapes: gynecoid, anthropoid, android, and platypelloid (Fig. 13.2).

GYNECOID PELVIS

The gynecoid pelvis is considered the true female pelvis, occurring in about 40% of all women; it is less common in men (Fischer & Mitteroecker, 2015). Vaginal birth is most favorable with this type of pelvis because the inlet is round and the outlet is roomy. This shape offers the

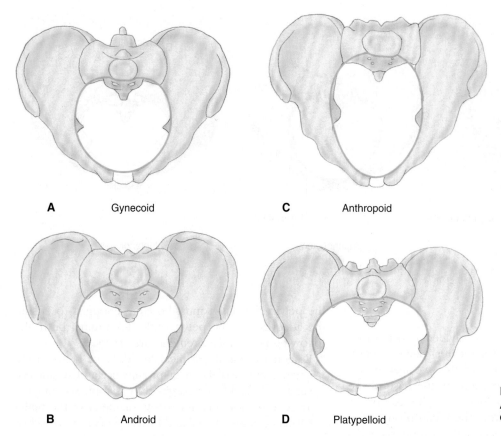

A   Gynecoid   **C**   Anthropoid

B   Android   **D**   Platypelloid

FIGURE 13.2 Pelvic shapes.
A. Gynecoid. **B.** Android.
C. Anthropoid. **D.** Platypelloid.

optimal diameters in all three planes of the pelvis. This type of pelvis allows early and complete fetal internal rotation during labor.

ANTHROPOID PELVIS

The anthropoid pelvis is common in men and is most common in the non-White women. It occurs in approximately 25% of women (Marani & Koch, 2014). The pelvic inlet is oval and the sacrum is long, producing a deep pelvis (wider front to back [anterior to posterior] than side to side [transverse]). Vaginal birth is more favorable with this pelvic shape compared with the android or platypelloid shape (Tharpe, Farley, & Jordan, 2016).

ANDROID PELVIS

The android pelvis is considered the male-shaped pelvis and is characterized by a funnel shape. It occurs in approximately 20% of women (Cunningham et al., 2014). The pelvic inlet is heart-shaped and the posterior segments are reduced in all pelvic planes. Descent of the fetal head into the pelvis is slow, and failure of the fetus to rotate is common. The prognosis for labor is poor, subsequently leading to cesarean birth.

PLATYPELLOID (FLAT) PELVIS

The platypelloid or flat pelvis is the least common type of pelvic structure among men and women, with an approximate incidence of 3% (King et al., 2015). The

pelvic cavity is shallow but widens at the pelvic outlet, making it difficult for the fetus to descend through the mid-pelvis. Labor prognosis is poor with arrest at the inlet occurring frequently. It is not favorable for a vaginal birth unless the fetal head can pass through the inlet. Women with this type of pelvis usually require cesarean birth.

An important principle is that most pelvises are not purely defined but occur in nature as mixed types. Many women have a combination of these four basic pelvis types, with no two pelves being exactly the same. Regardless of the shape, the newborn can be born vaginally if size and positioning remain compatible. The narrowest part of the fetus attempts to align itself with the narrowest pelvic dimension (e.g., biparietal to interspinous diameters, which means the fetus generally tends to rotate to the most ample portion of the pelvis).

Soft Tissues

The soft tissues of the passageway consist of the cervix, the pelvic floor muscles, and the vagina. Through **effacement**, the cervix effaces (thins) to allow the presenting fetal part to descend into the vagina.

Take Note!

The process of cervical effacement and dilation is similar to that of pulling a turtleneck sweater over your head.

The pelvic floor muscles help the fetus to rotate anteriorly as it passes through the birth canal. The soft tissues of the vagina expand to accommodate the fetus during birth.

Passenger

The fetus (with placenta) is the passenger. The fetal head (size and presence of molding), fetal attitude (degree of body flexion), fetal lie (relationship of body parts), fetal presentation (first body part), fetal position (relationship to maternal pelvis), fetal station, and fetal engagement are all important factors that have an impact on the ultimate outcome in the birthing process.

Fetal Head

The fetal head is the largest fetal structure, making it an important factor in relation to labor and birth. Considerable variation in the size and diameter of the fetal skull is often seen.

Compared with an adult's head, the fetal head is large in proportion to the rest of the body, usually about one quarter of the body surface area (Martin, Fanaroff, & Walsh, 2014). The bones that make up the face and cranial base are fused and essentially fixed. However, the five bones that make up the rest of the cranium (two frontal bones, two parietal bones, and the occipital bone) are not fused; rather, they are soft and pliable, with gaps between the plates of bone. These gaps, membranous spaces between the cranial bones, are called sutures, and the intersections of these sutures are called fontanelles. Sutures are important because they allow the cranial bones to overlap in order for the head to adjust in shape (elongate) when pressure is exerted on it by uterine contractions or the maternal bony pelvis. Some diameters shorten, whereas others lengthen as the head is molded during the labor and birthing process. This malleability of the fetal skull may decrease fetal skull dimensions by 0.5 to 1 cm (King et al., 2015). After birth, the sutures close as the bones grow and the brain reaches its full growth.

The changed (elongated) shape of the fetal skull at birth as a result of overlapping of the cranial bones is known as **molding**. Along with molding, fluid can also collect in the scalp (caput succedaneum) or blood can collect beneath the scalp (cephalohematoma), further distorting the shape and appearance of the fetal head. Caput succedaneum can be described as edema of the scalp at the presenting part. This swelling crosses suture lines and disappears within 3 to 4 days. Cephalohematoma is a collection of blood between the periosteum and the bone that occurs several hours after birth. It does not cross suture lines and is generally reabsorbed over the next 6 to 8 weeks (Collins & Reed, 2014).

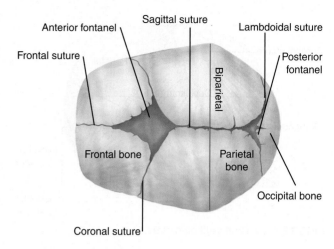

FIGURE 13.3 Fetal skull.

Take Note!

Parents may become concerned about the distortion of their newborn's head. However, reassurance that the oblong shape is only temporary is usually all that is needed to reduce their anxiety.

Sutures also play a role in helping to identify the position of the fetal head during a vaginal examination. Figure 13.3 shows a fetal skull. During a pelvic examination, palpation of these sutures by the examiner reveals the position of the fetal head and the degree of rotation that has occurred.

The anterior and posterior fontanelles are also useful in helping to identify the position of the fetal head. They allow for molding, and are important when evaluating the newborn. The anterior fontanelle is the famous "soft spot" of the newborn's head. It is a diamond-shaped space that measures from 1 to 4 cm. It remains open for 12 to 18 months after birth to allow for growth of the brain (Verklan & Walden, 2014). The posterior fontanelle corresponds to the anterior one but is located at the back of the fetal head; it is triangular. This one closes within 8 to 12 weeks after birth and measures, on average, 1 to 2 cm at its widest diameter (Weber & Kelley, 2014).

The diameter of the fetal skull is an important consideration during the labor and birth process. Fetal skull diameters are measured between the various landmarks of the skull. Diameters include occipitofrontal, occipitomental, suboccipitobregmatic, and biparietal (Fig. 13.4). The two most important diameters that can affect the birth process are the suboccipitobregmatic (approximately 9.5 cm at term) and the biparietal (approximately 9.25 cm at term) diameters. The suboccipitobregmatic diameter, measured from the base of the occiput to the center of the anterior fontanelle, identifies the smallest anteroposterior diameter of the fetal skull. The biparietal diameter measures the largest transverse diameter of the fetal skull: the distance between the two parietal bones.

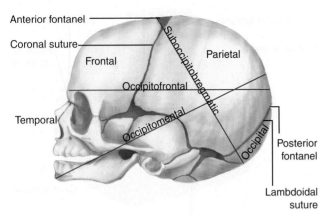

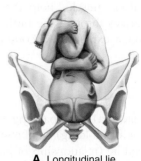

A. Longitudinal lie

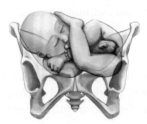

B. Transverse lie

FIGURE 13.4 Fetal skull diameters.

FIGURE 13.6 Fetal lie.

In a cephalic (head first) presentation, which occurs in 95% of all term births, if the fetus presents in a flexed position in which the chin is resting on the chest, the optimal or smallest fetal skull dimensions for a vaginal birth are demonstrated. If the fetal head is not fully flexed at birth, the anteroposterior diameter increases. This increase in dimension might prevent the fetal skull from entering the maternal pelvis.

Fetal Attitude

Fetal attitude is another important consideration related to the passenger. Fetal **attitude** refers to the posturing (flexion or extension) of the joints and the relationship of fetal parts to one another. The most common fetal attitude when labor begins is with all joints flexed—the fetal back is rounded, the chin is on the chest, the thighs are flexed on the abdomen, and the legs are flexed at the knees (Fig. 13.5). This normal fetal position is most favorable for vaginal birth, presenting the smallest fetal skull diameters to the pelvis.

When the fetus presents to the pelvis with abnormal attitudes (no flexion or extension), their nonflexed position can increase the diameter of the presenting part as it passes through the pelvis, increasing the difficulty of

birth. An attitude of extension tends to present larger fetal skull diameters, which may make birth difficult.

Fetal Lie

Fetal **lie** refers to the relationship of the long axis (spine) of the fetus to the long axis (spine) of the mother. There are three possible lies: longitudinal (which is the most common), transverse (Fig. 13.6), and oblique.

A longitudinal lie occurs when the long axis of the fetus is parallel to that of the mother (fetal spine to maternal spine side-by-side). A transverse lie occurs when the long axis of the fetus is perpendicular to the long axis of the mother (fetal spine lies across the maternal abdomen and crosses her spine). In an oblique lie, the fetal long axis is at an angle to the bony inlet, and no palpable fetal part is presenting. This lie is usually transitory and occurs during fetal conversion between other lies. A fetus in a transverse or oblique lie position cannot be delivered vaginally (Cunningham et al., 2014).

Fetal Presentation

Fetal **presentation** refers to the body part of the fetus that enters the pelvic inlet first (the "presenting part"). This is the fetal part that lies over the inlet of the pelvis or the cervical os. Knowing which fetal part is coming first at birth is critical for planning and initiating appropriate interventions.

The three main fetal presentations are cephalic (head first), breech (pelvis first), and shoulder (scapula

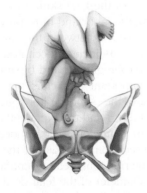

FIGURE 13.5 Fetal attitude: full flexion. Note that the smallest diameter presents to the pelvis.

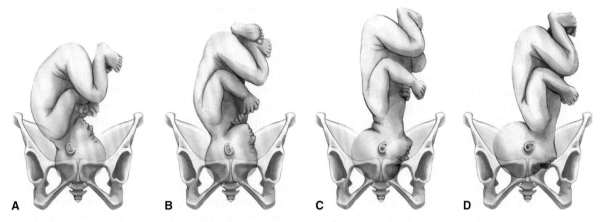

FIGURE 13.7 Fetal presentation: cephalic presentations. **A.** Vertex. **B.** Military. **C.** Brow. **D.** Face.

first). The majority of term newborns (95%) enter this world in a cephalic presentation; breech presentations account for 3% of term births, and shoulder presentations for approximately 2% (Tharpe et al., 2016).

In a cephalic presentation, the presenting part is usually the occipital portion of the fetal head (Fig. 13.7). This presentation is also referred to as a vertex presentation. Variations in a vertex presentation include the military, brow, and facial presentations.

BREECH PRESENTATION

By term, approximately 97% of infants actively turn to a cephalic presentation. It is determined by abdominal palpation (Hofmeyr, 2015). Breech presentation occurs when the fetal buttocks or feet enter the maternal pelvis first and the fetal skull enters last. This abnormal presentation poses several challenges at birth. Primarily, the largest part of the fetus (skull) is born last and may become "hung up" or stuck in the pelvis. In addition, the umbilical cord can become compressed between the

fetal skull and the maternal pelvis after the fetal chest is born because the head is the last to exit. Moreover, unlike the hard fetal skull, the buttocks are soft and are not as effective as a cervical dilator during labor compared with a cephalic presentation. Finally, there is the possibility of trauma to the head as a result of the lack of opportunity for molding.

The types of breech presentations are determined by the positioning of the fetal legs (Fig. 13.8). In a frank breech (50% to 70%), the buttocks present first with both legs extended up toward the face. In a full or complete breech (5% to 10%), the fetus sits crossed-legged above the cervix. In a footling or incomplete breech (10% to 30%), one or both legs are presenting. Breech presentations are associated with prematurity, placenta previa, multiparity, uterine abnormalities (fibroids), and some congenital anomalies such as hydrocephaly (Hofmeyr, 2015). A frank breech can result in a vaginal birth, but complete, footling, and incomplete breech presentations generally necessitate a cesarean birth.

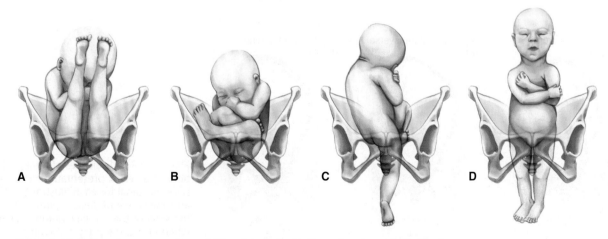

FIGURE 13.8 Breech presentations. **A.** Frank breech. **B.** Complete breech. **C.** Single footling breech. **D.** Double footling breech.

SHOULDER PRESENTATION

A shoulder presentation or shoulder dystocia occurs when the fetal shoulders present first, with the head tucked inside. Clinically, signs of shoulder dystocia appear while the woman is pushing as the neonate's head slowly extends and emerges over the perineum, but then retracts back into the vagina, commonly referred to as the "turtle sign." Odds of a shoulder presentation are 1 in 300 births (Cunningham et al., 2014). The fetus is in a transverse lie with the shoulder as the presenting part. Conditions associated with shoulder dystocia include placenta previa, prematurity, high parity, premature rupture of membranes, multiple gestation, or fetal anomalies. A cesarean birth is usually necessary if identified before labor begins, but will be evaluated based on the length of gestation, the size of the fetus, the position of the placenta, and whether the membranes have ruptured (Sharshiner & Silver, 2015).

Fetal Position

Fetal **position** describes the relationship of a given point on the presenting part of the fetus to a designated point of the maternal pelvis (King et al., 2015). The landmark fetal presenting parts include the occipital bone (O), which designates a vertex presentation; the chin (mentum [M]), which designates a face presentation; the buttocks (sacrum [S]), which designate a breech presentation; and the scapula (acromion process [A]), which designates a shoulder presentation.

In addition, the maternal pelvis is divided into four quadrants: right anterior, left anterior, right posterior, and left posterior. These quadrants designate whether the presenting part is directed toward the front, back, left, or right side of the pelvis. Fetal position is determined first by identifying the presenting part and then the maternal quadrant the presenting part is facing (Fig. 13.9). Position is indicated by a three-letter abbreviation as follows:

- The first letter defines whether the presenting part is tilted toward the left (L) or the right (R) side of the maternal pelvis.
- The second letter represents the particular presenting part of the fetus: O for occiput, S for sacrum (buttocks), M for mentum (chin), A for acromion process, and D for dorsal (refers to the fetal back) when denoting the fetal position in shoulder presentations (Cheng & Caughey, 2015a).

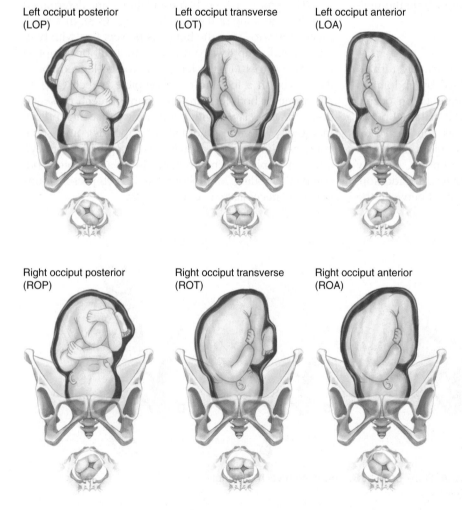

Left occiput posterior (LOP)

Left occiput transverse (LOT)

Left occiput anterior (LOA)

Right occiput posterior (ROP)

Right occiput transverse (ROT)

Right occiput anterior (ROA)

FIGURE 13.9 Examples of fetal positions in a vertex presentation. The lie is longitudinal for each illustration. The attitude is one of flexion. Notice that the view of the top illustration is seen when facing the pregnant woman. The bottom view is that seen with the woman in a dorsal recumbent position.

• The third letter defines the location of the presenting part in relation to the anterior (A) portion of the maternal pelvis or the posterior (P) portion of the maternal pelvis. If the presenting part is directed to the side of the maternal pelvis, the fetal presentation is designated as transverse (T).

For example, if the occiput is facing the left anterior quadrant of the pelvis, then the position is termed left occiput anterior and is recorded as LOA.

> ### Take Note!
> LOA is the most common (and most favorable) fetal position for birthing today, followed by right occiput anterior (ROA). The positioning of the fetus allows the fetal head to contour to the diameters of the maternal pelvis. LOA and ROA are optimal positions for a vaginal birth.

An occiput posterior position may lead to a long and difficult birth, and other positions may or may not be compatible with vaginal birth.

Fetal Station

Fetal **station** refers to the relationship of the presenting part to the level of the maternal pelvic ischial spines. Fetal station is measured in centimeters and is referred to as a minus or plus, depending on its location above or below the ischial spines. Typically, the ischial spines are the narrowest part of the pelvis and are the natural measuring point for the birth progress.

Zero (0) station is designated when the presenting part is at the level of the maternal ischial spines. When the presenting part is above the ischial spines, the distance is recorded as minus stations. When the presenting part is below the ischial spines, the distance is recorded as plus stations. For instance, if the presenting part is above the ischial spines by 1 cm, it is documented as being a −1 station; if the presenting part is below the ischial spines by 1 cm, it is documented as being a +1 station.

An easy way to understand this concept is to think in terms of meeting the goal, which is the birth. If the fetus is descending downward (past the ischial spines) and moving toward meeting the goal of birth, then the station is positive and the centimeter numbers grow bigger from +1 to +4. If the fetus is not descending past the ischial spines, then the station is negative and the centimeter numbers grow bigger from −1 to −4. The farther away the presenting part from the outside, the larger the negative number (−4 cm). The closer the presenting part of the fetus is to the outside, the larger the positive number (+4 cm). Figure 13.10 shows stations of the presenting part.

Fetal Engagement

Fetal **engagement** signifies the entrance of the largest diameter of the fetal presenting part (usually the fetal

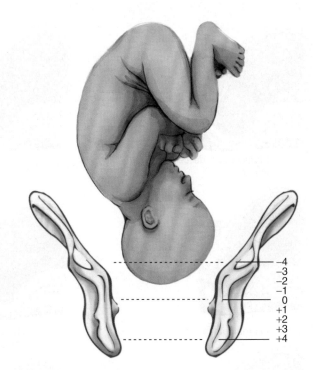

FIGURE 13.10 Fetal stations.

head) into the smallest diameter of the maternal pelvis (Alexander et al., 2014). The fetus is said to be engaged in the pelvis when the presenting part reaches 0 station. Engagement is determined by pelvic examination.

The largest diameter of the fetal head is the biparietal diameter. It extends from one parietal prominence to the other. It is an important factor in the navigation through the maternal pelvis. Engagement typically occurs in primigravidas 2 weeks before term, whereas multiparas may experience engagement several weeks before the onset of labor or not until labor begins.

> ### Take Note!
> The term *floating* is used when engagement has not occurred, because the presenting part is freely movable above the pelvic inlet.

Cardinal Movements of Labor

The fetus goes through many positional changes as it travels through the passageway. These positional changes are known as the cardinal movements of labor. They are deliberate, specific, and very precise movements that allow the smallest diameter of the fetal head to pass through a corresponding diameter of the mother's pelvic structure. Although cardinal movements are conceptualized as separate and sequential, the movements are typically concurrent (Fig. 13.11).

ENGAGEMENT

Engagement occurs when the greatest transverse diameter of the head in vertex (biparietal diameter) passes

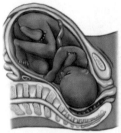
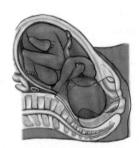

Engagement, descent, flexion

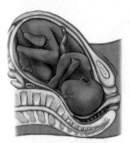
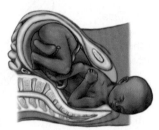

Internal rotation

External rotation (restitution)

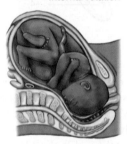
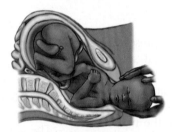

Extension beginning (rotation complete)

External rotation (shoulder rotation)

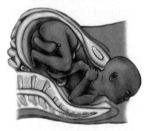
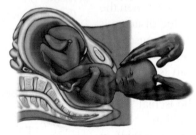

Extension complete

Expulsion

FIGURE 13.11 Cardinal movements of labor.

through the pelvic inlet (usually 0 station). The head usually enters the pelvis with the sagittal suture aligned in the transverse diameter.

DESCENT

Descent is the downward movement of the fetal head until it is within the pelvic inlet. Descent occurs intermittently with contractions and is brought about by one or more of the following forces:
- Pressure of the amniotic fluid
- Direct pressure of the fundus on the fetus's buttocks or head (depending on which part is located in the top of the uterus)

- Contractions of the abdominal muscles (second stage)
- Extension and straightening of the fetal body

Descent occurs throughout labor, ending with birth. During this time, the mother experiences discomfort, but she is unable to isolate this particular fetal movement from her overall discomfort.

FLEXION

Flexion occurs as the vertex meets resistance from the cervix, the walls of the pelvis, or the pelvic floor. As a result, the chin is brought into contact with the fetal thorax and the presenting diameter is changed from occipitofrontal to suboccipitobregmatic (9.5 cm), which achieves the smallest fetal skull diameter presenting to the maternal pelvic dimensions.

INTERNAL ROTATION

After engagement, as the head descends, the lower portion of the head (usually the occiput) meets resistance from one side of the pelvic floor. As a result, the head rotates about 45 degrees anteriorly to the midline under the symphysis. This movement is known as *internal rotation*. Internal rotation brings the anteroposterior diameter of the head in line with the anteroposterior diameter of the pelvic outlet. It aligns the long axis of the fetal head with the long axis of the maternal pelvis. The widest portion of the maternal pelvis is the anteroposterior diameter, and thus the fetus must rotate to accommodate the pelvis.

EXTENSION

With further descent and full flexion of the head, the nucha (the base of the occiput) becomes impinged under the symphysis. Resistance from the pelvic floor causes the fetal head to extend so that it can pass under the pubic arch. *Extension* occurs after internal rotation is complete. The head emerges through extension under the symphysis pubis along with the shoulders. The anterior fontanel, brow, nose, mouth, and chin are born successively.

EXTERNAL ROTATION (RESTITUTION)

After the head is born and is free of resistance, it untwists, causing the occiput to move about 45 degrees back to its original left or right position (restitution). The sagittal suture has now resumed its normal right-angle relationship to the transverse (bisacromial) diameter of the shoulders (i.e., the head realigns with the position of the back in the birth canal). *External rotation* of the fetal head allows the shoulders to rotate internally to fit the maternal pelvis.

EXPULSION

Expulsion of the rest of the body occurs more smoothly after the birth of the head and the anterior and posterior shoulders (Cheng & Caughey, 2015a). See Figure 13.3 for an image of a fetal skull.

Powers

The primary stimulus powering labor is uterine contraction. Contractions cause complete dilation and effacement of the cervix during the first stage of labor. The secondary powers in labor involve the use of intra-abdominal pressure (voluntary muscle contractions) exerted by the woman as she pushes and bears down during the second stage of labor.

Uterine Contractions

Uterine contractions are involuntary and therefore cannot be controlled by the woman experiencing them, regardless of whether they are spontaneous or induced. Uterine contractions are rhythmic and intermittent, with a period of relaxation between contractions. This pause allows the woman and the uterine muscles to rest. In addition, this pause restores blood flow to the uterus and placenta, which is temporarily reduced during each uterine contraction.

Uterine contractions are responsible for thinning and dilating the cervix, then thrusting the presenting part toward the lower uterine segment. The cervical canal reduces in length from 2 cm to a paper-thin entity and is described in terms of percentages from 0% to 100%. In primigravidas, effacement typically starts before the onset of labor and usually begins before dilation; in multiparas, however, neither effacement nor dilation may start until labor ensues (Fig. 13.12). On clinical examination the following may be assessed:

- Cervical canal 2 cm in length would be described as 0% effaced.
- Cervical canal 1 cm in length would be described as 50% effaced.
- Cervical canal 0 cm in length would be described as 100% effaced.

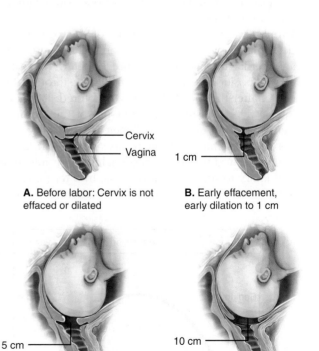

FIGURE 13.12 Cervical effacement and dilation. Cervical dilation is expressed in centimeters. **A.** Shows cervix not effaced or dilated. **B.** 50% effaced. **C.** 100% effaced. **D.** Fully dilated at 10 centimeters.

Dilation is dependent on the pressure of the presenting part and the contraction and retraction of the uterus. The diameter of the cervical os increases from less than 1 cm to approximately 10 cm to allow for birth. When the cervix is fully dilated, it is no longer palpable on vaginal examination. Descriptions may include the following:

• External cervical os closed: 0 cm dilated
• External cervical os half open: 5 cm dilated
• External cervical os fully open: 10 cm dilated

During early labor, uterine contractions are described as mild, they last about 30 seconds, and they occur about every 5 to 7 minutes. As labor progresses, contractions last longer (60 seconds), occur more frequently (2 to 3 minutes apart), and are described as being moderate to high in intensity. Each contraction has three phases: increment (buildup of the contraction), acme (peak or highest intensity), and decrement (descent or relaxation of the uterine muscle fibers; Fig. 13.13).

Uterine contractions are monitored and assessed according to three parameters: frequency, duration, and intensity.

1. **Frequency** refers to how often the contractions occur and is measured from the beginning of one contraction to the beginning of the next contraction.
2. **Duration** refers to how long a contraction lasts and is measured from the beginning of one contraction to the end of that same contraction.
3. **Intensity** refers to the strength of the contraction determined by manual palpation or measured by an internal intrauterine pressure catheter. The catheter is positioned in the uterine cavity through the cervix after the membranes have ruptured. It reports intensity by measuring the pressure of the amniotic fluid inside the uterus in millimeters of mercury. It is not recommended for routine use in low-risk laboring women due to the potential risk of infection and injury to the placenta or fetus. In a recent meta-analysis involving more than 2,000 laboring women,

the researchers found increase in surgical births and no advantages of using internal intrauterine pressure catheters over external monitoring during labor augmentation (Milton, Chelmow, & Ramus, 2015).

Intra-Abdominal Pressure

Increased intra-abdominal pressure (voluntary muscle contractions) compresses the uterus and adds to the power of the expulsion forces of the uterine contractions (Grant et al., 2015). Coordination of these forces in unison promotes birth of the fetus and expulsion of the fetal membranes and placenta from the uterus. Interference with these forces (such as when a woman is highly sedated or extremely anxious) can compromise the effectiveness of these powers.

Position (Maternal)

Positioning for normal labor and birth has evolved. Until about 250 years ago, women were depicted in art and described in essays as sitting upright with flexed hips, squatting, or less commonly standing or kneeling during the childbirth process. These positions maintain flexion at the hip joint and somewhat straighten the pelvis (Nieuwenhuijze et al., 2014). In the past 250 years, dorsal and dorsal lithotomy positions evolved for unclear reasons and have been ascribed to Western medicine. Childbirth medicalization has reduced laboring women's opportunity in a spontaneous position of choice to a recumbent one. Medical historians say the evolution was to facilitate forceps usage, to promote men's power over women and for convenience after administration of anesthesia (Marani & Koch, 2014).

Maternal positioning during labor has only recently been the subject of well-controlled research. Scientific evidence has shown that nonmoving, back-lying positions during labor are not healthy (Gizzo et al., 2014). However, despite this evidence to the contrary, many

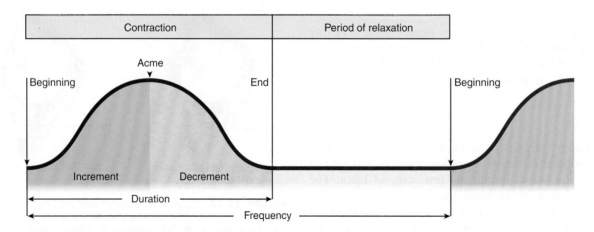

FIGURE 13.13 The three phases of a uterine contraction.

women continue to lie flat on their backs during labor. Some of the reasons why this practice continues include the beliefs that:

- laboring women need to conserve their energy and not tire themselves
- nurses cannot keep track of the whereabouts of ambulating women
- it is the preference of the health care provider
- the fetus can be monitored better in this position
- the supine position facilitates vaginal examinations and external belt adjustment
- a bed is "where one is supposed to be" in a hospital setting
- the position is more convenient for the delivering health care provider
- laboring women are "connected to things" that impede movement (Hanson & VandeVusse, 2014).

Although many labor and birthing facilities claim that all women are allowed to adopt any position of comfort during their laboring experience, many women spend their time on their backs during labor and birth. Women should be encouraged to assume any position of comfort for them. In a recently randomized, controlled study, the use of a peanut-shaped ball during labor decreased the length of labor and increased the rate of vaginal births. The peanut ball was associated with a significantly lower incidence of cesarean births. The peanut ball can be a potentially successful nursing intervention to help progress labor and support vaginal birth for women laboring under epidural analgesia (Tussey et al., 2015).

Take Note!

If the only furniture provided is a bed, this is what the woman will use. Furnishing rooms with comfortable chairs, beanbags, and other birth props allows a woman to choose from a variety of positions and to be free to move during labor.

Changing positions and moving around during labor and birth offer several benefits. Maternal position can influence pelvic size and contours. Changing position and walking affect the pelvis joints, which may facilitate fetal descent and rotation. Squatting enlarges the pelvic inlet and outlet diameters, whereas a kneeling position removes pressure on the maternal vena cava and helps to rotate the fetus from a posterior position to an anterior one to facilitate birth (Budin, 2015). The use of any upright or lateral position, compared with supine or lithotomy positions, may:

- reduce the length of the first stage of labor
- reduce the duration of the second stage of labor
- reduce the number of assisted deliveries (vacuum and forceps)
- reduce episiotomies and perineal tears
- contribute to fewer abnormal fetal heart rate patterns

- increase comfort/reduce requests for pain medication
- enhance a sense of control by the mother
- alter the shape and size of the pelvis, which assists in descent
- assist gravity to move the fetus downward (Cox & King, 2015)

Using the research available can bring better outcomes, heightened professionalism, and evidence-based practice to childbearing practices. The National Institute for Health and Care Excellence (NICE) guidelines recommend discouraging women from lying supine or semi-supine during labor and encourage them to adapt to any other position that they find comfortable since lying on their backs is associated with longer labors, increase in surgical births, increased pain, and a higher incidence of FHR abnormalities. The Cochrane collaboration supports the current NICE guidance of positions (Camorcia, 2015).

Psychological Response

Childbearing can be one of the most life-altering experiences for a woman. The experience of childbirth goes beyond the physiologic aspects: it influences a woman's self-confidence, self-esteem, and view of life, relationships, and children. Her state of mind (psyche) throughout the entire process is critical to bring about a positive outcome for her and her family. Factors promoting a positive birth experience include:

- clear information about procedures
- support; not being alone
- sense of mastery, self-confidence
- trust in staff caring for her
- positive reaction to the pregnancy
- personal control over breathing
- preparation for the childbirth experience

Having a strong sense of self and meaningful support from others can often help women manage labor well. Feeling safe and secure typically promotes a sense of control and ability to withstand the challenges of the childbearing experience. Anxiety and fear, however, decrease a woman's ability to cope with the discomfort of labor. Maternal catecholamines secreted in response to anxiety and fear can inhibit uterine blood flow and placental perfusion. In contrast, relaxation can augment the natural process of labor (Leonard, 2015). Preparing mentally for childbirth is important so that the woman can work with, rather than against, the natural forces of labor.

Philosophy

Not everyone views childbirth in the same way. A philosophical continuum exists that extends from viewing labor as a disease process to a normal process. One philosophy assumes that women cannot manage the birth experience adequately and therefore need constant expert monitoring and management. The other philosophy assumes that women are capable and reasoning individuals who can actively participate in their birth experience.

The health care system in the United States today appears to be leaning toward the former philosophy, applying technological interventions to most mothers who enter the hospital system. Giving birth in a hospital in the 21st century for many women has become "intervention intensive"—designed to start, continue, and end labor through medical management rather than allowing the normal process of birth to unfold. Advances in medical care have improved the safety for women with high-risk pregnancies. However, the routine use of intravenous therapy, electronic fetal monitoring, augmentation, and epidural anesthesia has not necessarily improved birth outcomes for all women (Leonard, 2015). Perhaps a middle-of-the-road philosophy for intervening when circumstances dictate, along with weighing the risks and benefits before doing so, may be appropriate.

During the 1970s, family-centered maternity care was developed in response to the consumer reaction to the depersonalization of birth. The hope was to shift the philosophy from "technologization" to personalization to humanize childbirth. The term *family-centered birthing* is more appropriate today to denote the low-tech, high-touch approach requested by many childbearing women, who view childbirth as a normal process.

Certified nurse midwives (CNMs) are champions of family-centered birthing, and their participation in the childbirth process is associated with fewer unnecessary interventions when compared with obstetricians. CNMs subscribe to a normal birth process where the woman uses her own instincts and bodily signs during labor. In short, midwives empower women within the birthing environment (Casey et al., 2015).

No matter what philosophy is held, it is ideal if everyone involved in the particular birth process—from the health care provider to the mother—shares the same philosophy toward the birth process.

Partners

Women desire support and attentive care during labor and birth. Caregivers can convey emotional support by offering their continued presence and words of encouragement. Throughout the world, few women are left to labor totally alone: emotional, physical, or spiritual support during labor is the norm for most cultures. According to the Childbirth Connection's ongoing *Listening to Mothers Initiative III survey*, almost all women (99%) reported having received some type of supportive care during labor (Edmonds, Cwiertniewicz, & Stoll, 2015). A caring partner can use massage, light touch, acupressure, hand-holding, stroking, and relaxation; can help

the woman communicate her wishes to the staff; and can provide a continuous, reassuring presence, all of which bring some degree of comfort to the laboring woman (Capogna, 2015). Although the presence of the mother's significant other at the birth provides special emotional support, a partner can be anyone who is present to support the woman throughout the experience. For many women, the essential ingredients for a safe and satisfying birth include a sense of empowerment and success in coping with or transcending the experience, in addition to having solid, positive encouragement from a support companion.

Worldwide, women usually support other women in childbirth. **Doula** is a Greek word meaning woman servant or caregiver. It now commonly refers to a woman who offers emotional and practical support to a mother or couple before, during, and after childbirth. A doula believes in "mothering the mother," but clinical support remains the job of the midwife or medical staff (Ahlemeyer & Mahon, 2015). The continuous presence of a trained female support person reduces the need for medication for pain relief, the use of vacuum or forceps delivery, and the need for cesarean births. Continuous support was also associated with a slight reduction in the length of labor. The doula, who is an experienced labor companion, provides the woman and her partner with emotional and physical support and information throughout the entire labor and birth experience.

A recent study in the United States found that nursing care decreases the likelihood of negative evaluations of the childbirth experience, feelings of tenseness during labor, and finding labor worse than expected. Also reported were less perineal trauma, reduced difficulty in mothering, and reduced likelihood of early cessation of breast-feeding. Continuous support by nurses included reassurance, encouragement, praise, and explanation (Iravani et al., 2015).

Given the many benefits of intrapartum support, laboring women should always have the option to receive partner support, whether from nurses, doulas, significant others, or family. Whoever the support partner is, he or she should provide the mother with continuous presence and hands-on comfort and encouragement. The overall objective of providing support for women during childbirth is to create a positive experience for her, while preserving her physical and psychological health.

Patience

The birth process takes time. If more time were allowed for women to labor naturally without intervention, the cesarean birth rate would most likely be reduced. In one study, continuous support provided by midwives during labor reduced the duration of labor and the number of cesarean births; this model of support should be available to all women (Cox & King, 2015). The literature suggests that delaying interventions can give a woman enough time to progress in labor and reduce the need for surgical intervention (American College of Obstetricians and Gynecologists [ACOG], 2014b; Society for Maternal-Fetal Medicine [SMFM], 2014).

Healthy People 2020 has two goals related to cesarean births in the United States:

1. Reduce the rate of cesarean births among low-risk (full-term, singleton, vertex presentation) women having their first child to 23.9% of live births, from a baseline of 26.5%.
2. Reduce the rate of cesarean births among women who have had a prior cesarean birth to 81.7% of live births, from a baseline of 90.8% (U.S. Department of Health and Human Services, 2010).

We are a long way from achieving these goals—the current cesarean birth rate in the United States, at 32.7%, approximately one in three births, is the highest since these data first became available from birth certificates in 1989. Cesarean birth rate is associated with increased morbidity and mortality for both mother and infant as well as increased inpatient length of stay and health care costs (Centers for Disease Control and Prevention [CDC], 2014a).

It is difficult to predict how a labor will progress and therefore equally difficult to determine how long a woman's labor will last. There is no way to estimate the likely strength and frequency of uterine contractions, the extent to which the cervix will soften and dilate, and how much the fetal head will mold to fit the birth canal. We cannot know beforehand whether the complex fetal rotations needed for an efficient labor will take place properly. All of these factors are unknown when a woman starts labor.

Induction of Labor

There is a trend in health care to attempt to manipulate the process of labor through medical means such as artificial rupture of membranes (amniotomy) and augmentation of labor with oxytocin (Kriebs, 2015). The labor induction rate has doubled in the United States since the 1990s (Moses, 2015).

Approximately one in four women are induced or have labor augmented with uterine-stimulating drugs or artificial rupture of membranes to accelerate her progress, and early term (in the 37th and 38th week) inductions have also increased. An amniotomy (artificial rupture of the fetal membranes) may be performed to augment or induce labor when the membranes have not ruptured spontaneously. Doing so allows the fetal head to have more direct contact with the cervix to dilate it. This procedure is performed with the fetal head at −2 station or lower, with the cervix dilated to at least 3 cm. Synthetic oxytocin (Pitocin) is also used to induce or augment labor by stimulating uterine contractions. It is

administered piggybacked into the primary intravenous line with an infusion pump titrated to uterine activity.

Elective induction of labor is at an all-time high in the United States despite known associated risks. It can lead to birth of an infant too early, a long labor, exposure to a high-alert medication with its potential side effects, unnecessary cesarean birth, and maternal and neonatal morbidity. Elective induction has a cascade of related interventions, such as an intravenous line, continuous electronic fetal monitoring, confinement to bed, amniotomy, pharmacologic labor-stimulating agents, parental pain medications, and regional anesthesia, each with its own set of potential complications and risks. These risks apply to all women having the procedure; however, for nulliparous women before 41 weeks of gestation with an unfavorable cervix, the main risk is cesarean birth after unsuccessful labor induction with the potential for maternal and neonatal morbidity and increased health care costs. When cesarean occurs, subsequent births are likely to be via cesarean as well (Caughey, 2014). Compelling evidence indicates that elective induction of labor may increase the risk of cesarean birth, especially for nulliparous women (Le Ray et al., 2015). Elective induction of labor in nulliparas is associated with increased rates of cesarean, postpartum hemorrhage, neonatal resuscitation, and longer hospitalizations without improvement in neonatal outcomes (Glavind & Uldbjerg, 2015). The belief is that many cesarean births could be avoided if women were allowed to labor longer and if the natural labor process were allowed to complete the job. The longer wait (using the intervention of patience) usually results in less intervention.

The ACOG attributes the dramatic increase in inductions in part to pressure from women, convenience for physicians, and liability concerns. Other reasons for the increase in inductions include the availability of better cervical ripening agents and a more relaxed attitude toward marginal indications for inductions. They recommend a cautious approach regarding elective induction until clinical trials can validate a more liberal use of labor inductions (ACOG, 2014b). Current medical indications for inducing labor include:

- spontaneous rupture of membranes and when labor does not start,
- large size fetus not expected to navigate the maternal pelvis,
- fetal growth restriction (FGR) where external intervention is needed,
- a pregnancy of more than 42 weeks' gestation,
- maternal hypertension, diabetes, or lung disease, and
- a uterine infection (March of Dimes, 2015).

When the laboring woman feels the urge to bear down, pushing begins. Most women respond extremely well to messages from their body without being directed by the nurse. A more natural, undirected approach allows the woman to wait and bear down when she feels the urge to push. Having patience and letting nature take its course will reduce the incidence of physiologic stress in the mother, resulting in less trauma to her perineal tissue.

Patient (Client) Preparation: Prenatal Education

Basic prenatal education can help women manage their labor process and feel in control of their birthing experience. The literature indicates that if a woman is prepared before the labor and birth experience, the labor is more likely to remain normal or natural (without the need for medical intervention) (Byrne et al., 2014). An increasing body of evidence also indicates that the well-prepared woman, with good labor support, is less likely to need analgesia or anesthesia and is unlikely to require cesarean birth (Hoang, 2014).

Prenatal education teaches the woman about the childbirth experience and increases her sense of control. She is then able to work as an active participant during the labor and birth experience (Jordan et al., 2014). The research also suggests that prenatal preparation may affect intrapartum and postpartum psychosocial outcomes (Budin, 2014). For example, prenatal education covering parenting communication classes had a significant effect on postpartum anxiety and postpartum adjustment. In a recent study of Hispanic women attending a community prenatal education program, they found that many women experienced anguish from unknowns during their pregnancy, leading to a yearning to learn and understand more, but with a desire to do so without sacrificing their cultural identity (Fitzgerald, Cronin, & Boccella, 2015). In another study involving Somali couples, most did not attend prenatal classes because their religion does not allow women and men to learn in the same room, and the men are not allowed to look at naked figures displayed in photos and videos (Wojnar, 2015). If the prenatal educational setting were more respectful of their beliefs, attendance would improve. These findings have important implications for nurses teaching prenatal classes to diverse cultures. Prenatal education should be viewed as an opportunity to strengthen families by providing anticipatory guidance and improving family members' life skills. In short, prenatal education helps to promote healthy families during the transition to parenthood and beyond (Woods & Chesser, 2015).

There is increasing evidence that women use herbs to induce labor and also during labor for pain relief. Desire to have control over their health has been cited as the strongest motive for women to use herbal medicine. A few of the herbs used include *Caulophyllum*, made from the herb blue cohosh to induce labor contractions; blue and black cohosh, raspberry leaves, castor oil, and evening primrose oil used for cervical ripening and induction of labor; and *Chanlibao* to shorten the

second stage of labor by strengthening the contractions (Ramasubramaniam et al., 2015). The use of herbs during labor have been found to benefit some women by easing the labor process without side effects, but clinical trials are lacking to prove the safety and effectiveness of them.

Take Note!

Learning about labor and birth allows women and couples to express their needs and preferences, enhance their confidence, and improve communication between themselves and the staff.

Pain Management

Labor and birth, although a normal physiologic process, can produce significant pain. Pain during labor is a nearly universal experience. Controlling the uterine discomfort without harm to the fetus or labor process is the major focus of pain management during childbirth. Pain is a subjective experience involving a complex interaction of physiologic, spiritual, psychosocial, cultural, and environmental influences (Van der Gucht & Lewis, 2015). Cultural values and learned behaviors influence perception and response to pain, as do anxiety and fear, both of which tend to heighten the sense of pain (Jones, 2015). The challenge for care providers is to find the right combination of pain/coping management methods to keep the discomfort manageable while minimizing the negative effect on the fetus, the normal physiology of labor, maternal–infant bonding, breast-feeding, and a woman's perception of the labor itself (King et al., 2015). Chapter 14 presents a full discussion of pain management during labor and birth.

PHYSIOLOGIC RESPONSES TO LABOR

Labor is the process by which the birth canal is prepared to allow the fetus to pass from the uterine cavity to the outside world. During pregnancy, progesterone secreted from the placenta suppresses the spontaneous contractions of a typical uterus, keeping the fetus within the uterus. In addition, the cervix remains firm and noncompliant. At term, however, changes occur in the cervix that make it softer. In addition, uterine contractions become more frequent and regular, signaling the onset of labor.

The labor process involves a series of rhythmic, involuntary, usually quite uncomfortable uterine muscle contractions. The contractions bring about a shortening that causes effacement and dilation of the cervix and a bursting of the fetal membranes. Uterine contractions of an intensity of 30 mm Hg or greater promote cervical dilation. Then, accompanied by both reflex and voluntary contractions of the abdominal muscles (pushing), the uterine contractions result in the birth of the baby (Grant et al., 2015). During labor, the mother and fetus make several physiologic adaptations.

Maternal Responses

As the woman progresses through childbirth, numerous physiologic responses occur that assist her to adapt to the labor process. The labor process stresses several of the woman's body systems, which react through numerous compensatory mechanisms. Maternal physiologic responses include:

- Heart rate increases by 10 to 20 bpm.
- Cardiac output increases by 12% to 31% during the first stage of labor and by 50% during the second stage of labor.
- Blood pressure increases by up to 35 mm Hg during uterine contractions in all labor stages.
- The white blood cell count increases to 25,000 to 30,000 cells/mm^3, perhaps as a result of tissue trauma.
- Respiratory rate increases and more oxygen is consumed related to the increase in metabolism.
- Gastric motility and food absorption decrease, which may increase the risk of nausea and vomiting during the transition stage of labor.
- Gastric emptying and gastric pH decrease, increasing the risk of vomiting with aspiration.
- Temperature rises slightly, possibly due to an increase in muscle activity.
- Muscular aches/cramps occur as a result of the stressed musculoskeletal system.
- Basal metabolic rate increases and blood glucose levels decrease because of the stress of labor (Cheng & Caughey, 2015a).

A woman's ability to adapt to the stress of labor is influenced by her psychological and physical state. Among the many factors that affect her coping ability are:

- Previous birth experiences and their outcomes (complications and previous birth outcomes)
- Current pregnancy experience (planned versus unplanned, discomforts experienced, age, risk status of pregnancy, chronic illness, weight gain)
- Cultural considerations (values and beliefs about health status)
- Support system (presence and support of a valued partner during labor)
- Childbirth preparation (attended childbirth classes and has practiced paced breathing techniques)
- Exercise during pregnancy (muscles toned; ability to assist with intra-abdominal pushing)
- Expectations of the birthing experience (viewed as a meaningful or stressful event)
- Anxiety level (excessive anxiety may interfere with labor progress)
- Fear of labor and loss of control (fear may enhance pain perception, augmenting fear)
- Fatigue and weariness (not up for the challenge/ duration of labor) (King et al., 2015)

Fetal Responses

Although the focus during labor may be on assessing the mother's adaptations, several physiologic adaptations occur in the fetus as well. The fetus is experiencing labor along with the mother. If the fetus is healthy, the stress of labor usually has no adverse effects. The nurse needs to be alert to any abnormalities in the fetus's adaptation to labor. Fetal responses to labor include:

- Periodic fetal heart rate accelerations and slight decelerations related to fetal movement, fundal pressure, and uterine contractions
- Decrease in circulation and perfusion to the fetus secondary to uterine contractions (a healthy fetus is able to compensate for this drop)
- Increase in arterial carbon dioxide pressure (PCO_2)
- Decrease in fetal breathing movements throughout labor
- Decrease in fetal oxygen pressure with a decrease in the partial pressure of oxygen (PO_2) (Verklan & Walden, 2014)

Take Note!

Respiratory changes during labor help to prepare the fetus for extrauterine respiration immediately after birth.

STAGES OF LABOR

Labor is typically divided into four stages: dilation, expulsive, placental, and restorative. Table 13.2 summarizes the major events of each stage.

The first stage is the longest: it begins with the first true contraction and ends with full dilation (opening) of the cervix. Because this stage lasts so long, it is divided into three phases, each corresponding to the progressive dilation of the cervix.

Stage two of labor, or the expulsive stage, begins when the cervix is completely dilated and ends with the birth of the newborn. The expulsive stage can last from minutes to hours. The contractions typically occur every 2 to 3 minutes, lasting 60 to 90 seconds and are strong by palpation. The woman is usually intent on the work of pushing during this stage.

The third stage, or placental expulsion, starts after the newborn is born and ends with the separation and birth of the placenta. Continued uterine contractions typically cause the placenta to be expelled within 5 to 30 minutes. If the newborn is stable, bonding of infant and mother takes place during this stage through touching, holding, and skin-to-skin contact.

The fourth stage, or the restorative stage or immediate postpartum period, lasts from 1 to 4 hours after birth. This period is when the mother's body begins to stabilize after the hard work of labor and the loss of the products of conception. The fourth stage is often not recognized

TABLE 13.2	STAGES AND PHASES OF LABOR			
	First Stage	**Second Stage**	**Third Stage**	**Fourth Stage**
Description	From 0–10 cm dilation; consists of three phases	From complete dilation (10 cm) to birth of the newborn; may last up to 3 h	Separation and delivery of the placenta; usually takes 5–10 min, but may take up to 30 min	1–4 h after the birth of the newborn; time of maternal physiologic adjustment
Phases	**Latent phase** (0–3 cm dilation) • Cervical dilation from 0 to 3 cm • Cervical effacement from 0% to 40% • Nullipara, lasts up to 9 h; multipara, lasts up to 5–6 h • Contraction frequency every 5–10 min • Contraction duration 30–45 s • Contraction intensity mild to palpation **Active phase** (4–7 cm dilation) • Cervical dilation from 4 to 7 cm • Cervical effacement from 40% to 80% • Nullipara, lasts up to 6 h; multipara, lasts up to 4 h • Contraction frequency every 2–5 min • Contraction duration 45–60 s • Contraction intensity moderate to palpation **Transition phase** (8–10 cm dilation) • Cervical dilation from 8 to 10 cm • Cervical effacement from 80% to 100% • Nullipara lasts up to 1 h; multipara, lasts up to 30 min • Contraction frequency every 1–2 min • Contraction duration 60–90 s • Contraction intensity strong by palpation	**Pelvic phase** (period of fetal descent) **Perineal phase** (period of active pushing) • Nullipara, lasts up to 1 h; multipara, lasts up to 30 min • Contraction frequency every 2–3 min or less • Contraction duration 60–90 s • Contraction intensity strong by palpation • Strong urge to push during the later perineal phase	**Placental separation:** detaching from uterine wall **Placental expulsion:** coming outside the vaginal opening	

Adapted from Cheng, Y. W., & Caughey, A. B. (2015a). Normal labor and delivery. *eMedicine.* Retrieved from http://emedicine. medscape.com/article/260036-overview; Cunningham, F. G., Leveno, K. J., Bloom, S. L., Spong, C. Y., Dashe, J. S., Hoffman, B. L., et al. (2014). *Williams' obstetrics* (24th ed.). New York, NY: McGraw-Hill Education; and King, T. L., Brucker, M. C., Kriebs, J. M., Fahey, J. O., Gegor, C. L., & Varney, H. (2015). *Varney's midwifery* (5th ed.). Burlington, MA: Jones & Bartlett Learning.

as a true stage of labor, but it is a critical period for maternal physiologic transition as well as new family attachment. Close monitoring of both the mother and her newborn are done during this stage (Green, 2015).

First Stage

During the first stage of labor, the fundamental change underlying the process is progressive dilation of the cervix. Cervical dilation is gauged subjectively by vaginal examination and is expressed in centimeters. The first stage ends when the cervix is dilated to 10 cm in diameter and is large enough to permit the passage of a fetal head of average size. The fetal membranes, or bag of waters, usually rupture during the first stage, but they may have burst earlier or may even remain intact until birth. For the primigravida, the first stage of labor lasts about 12 hours. However, this time can vary widely; for the multiparous woman, it is usually only half of that.

During the first stage of labor, women usually perceive the visceral pain of diffuse abdominal cramping and uterine contractions. Pain during the first stage of labor is primarily a result of the dilation of the cervix and lower uterine segment, and the distention (stretching) of these structures during contractions. The first stage is divided into three phases: latent or early phase, active phase, and transition phase.

Latent or Early Phase

The latent or early phase gives rise to the familiar signs and symptoms of labor. This phase begins with the start of regular contractions and ends when rapid cervical dilation begins. Cervical effacement occurs during this phase, and the cervix dilates from 0 to 3 cm.

Contractions usually occur every 5 to 10 minutes, last 30 to 45 seconds, and are described as mild by palpation by the nurse. Assessment of intensity is evaluated by pressing down on the fundus during a contraction to see if it can be dented with the nurse's fingers. The ability to indent the fundus at the peak of the contraction would typically indicate a mild contraction. Effacement of the cervix is from 0% to 40%. Most women are very talkative during this period, perceiving their contractions to be similar to menstrual cramps. Women may remain at home during this phase, contacting their health care provider about the onset of labor.

For the nulliparous woman, the latent phase typically lasts about 9 hours; in the multiparous woman, it lasts about 6 hours (Cheng & Caughey, 2015a). During this phase, women are apprehensive but excited about the start of their labor after their long gestational period.

Think back to the couple who were sent home from the hospital birthing center. Three days later Kathy awoke with a wet sensation and intense discomfort in her back, spreading around to her abdomen. She decided to go for a walk, but her contractions didn't diminish. Instead, her contractions continued to occur every few minutes and grew stronger in intensity. She and Chuck decided to go back to the hospital birthing center. Was there a difference in the location of Kathy's discomfort this time? What changes will the admission nurse find in Kathy if this is true labor?

Active Phase

The active phase of labor encompasses the time from an increase in the rate of cervical dilation (end of latent phase of labor) until completion of cervical dilation. Cervical dilation begins to occur more rapidly during the active phase. The cervix usually dilates from 4 to 7 cm, with 40% to 80% effacement taking place. This phase can last up to 6 hours for the nulliparous woman and 4.5 hours for the multiparous woman (Leap & Hunter, 2015). The fetus descends farther in the pelvis.

Contractions become more frequent (every 2 to 5 minutes) and increase in duration (45 to 60 seconds). The woman's discomfort intensifies (moderate to strong by palpation). She becomes more intense and inwardly focused, absorbed in the serious work of her labor. She limits interactions with those in the room. If she and her partner have attended childbirth education classes, she will begin to use the relaxation and paced breathing techniques that they learned to cope with the contractions. The typical dilation rate for the nulliparous woman is 1.2 cm/hr; for the multiparous woman, it is 1.5 cm/hr (Cunningham et al., 2014).

Transition Phase

The transition phase is the last phase of the first stage of labor. During this phase, dilation slows, progressing from 8 to 10 cm, with effacement from 80% to 100%. The transition phase is the most difficult and, fortunately, the shortest phase for the woman, lasting approximately 1 hour in the first birth and perhaps 15 to 30 minutes in successive births (Tharpe et al., 2016). During transition, the contractions are stronger (hard by palpation), more painful, more frequent (every 1 to 2 minutes), and they last longer (60 to 90 seconds). The average rate of fetal descent is 1 cm/hr in nulliparous women and 2 cm/hr in multiparous women. Pressure on the rectum is great, and there is a strong desire to contract the abdominal muscles and push.

Other maternal symptoms during the transitional phase include nausea and vomiting, trembling extremities, backache, increased apprehension and irritability, restless movement, increased bloody show from the vagina, inability to relax, diaphoresis, feelings of loss of control, and being overwhelmed (the woman may say, "I can't take it anymore") (Cunningham et al., 2014).

In assessing Kathy, the nurse finds she is 4 cm dilated and 50% effaced with ruptured membranes. In what stage and phase of labor would this assessment finding place Kathy?

Second Stage

The second stage of labor begins with complete cervical dilation (10 cm) and effacement and ends with the birth of the newborn. Although the previous stage of labor primarily involved the thinning and opening of the cervix, this stage involves moving the fetus through the birth canal and out of the body. The cardinal movements of labor occur during the early phase of passive descent in the second stage of labor.

Contractions occur every 2 to 3 minutes, last 60 to 90 seconds, and are described as strong by palpation. The average length of the second stage of labor in a nullipara is approximately 1 hour and less than half that time for the multipara. During this expulsive stage, the mother usually feels more in control and less irritable and agitated. She is focused on the work of pushing. The maternal urge to push is generally felt when there is direct contact of the fetus to the pelvic floor. Stretch receptors in the wall of the vagina, rectum, and perineum communicate the pressure of the fetus descending in the birth canal that, along with increased abdominal pressure, causes the overwhelming urge to push described by laboring women (Camorcia, 2015).

Pushing

The second stage of labor has two phases (pelvic and perineal) related to the existence and quality of the maternal urge to push and to obstetric conditions related to fetal descent. The early phase of the second stage is called the pelvic phase, because it is during this phase that the fetal head is negotiating the pelvis, rotating, and advancing in descent. The later phase is called the perineal phase, because at this point the fetal head is lower in the pelvis and is distending the perineum. The occurrence of a strong urge to push characterizes the later phase of the second stage and has also been called the phase of active pushing (Cheng & Caughey, 2015b).

The later perineal phase occurs when the mother feels a tremendous urge to push as the fetal head is lowered and is distending the perineum. The perineum bulges and there is an increase in bloody show. The fetal head becomes apparent at the vaginal opening but disappears between contractions. When the top of the head no longer regresses between contractions, it is said to have crowned. The fetus rotates as it maneuvers out. Evidence now shows that labor actually progresses slower than we thought in the past. Many women might need a little more time to labor and give birth vaginally instead of moving to a surgical birth (ACOG, 2014c). The second stage commonly lasts up to 3 hours in a first labor and up to an hour in subsequent ones (Fig. 13.14).

SPONTANEOUS PUSHING VERSUS DIRECTED PUSHING

There are two ways of conducting the second stage of labor: *spontaneous pushing* (following the mother's spontaneous urge) and *directed pushing* (pushing directed by the caregiver). Spontaneous pushing represents a natural way of managing the second stage of labor. However, lately, and as a result of epidural analgesia, health care providers frequently resort to directed pushing without taking into account the negative repercussions it has on the woman and her fetus.

Evidence is mounting that the management of the second stage, particularly pushing, is a modifiable risk factor in long-term perinatal outcomes (ACOG, 2014b).

Research supports spontaneous physiologic approaches to second stage labor care; however, many women in hospital settings continue to receive direction from nurses to use prolonged Valsalva (holding breath) bearing-down efforts as soon as the cervix is completely dilated. Traditionally, women have been taught to hold their breath to the count of 10, inhale again, push again, and repeat the process several times during a contraction. This sustained, strenuous style of pushing, i.e., Valsalva bearing-down and supine maternal positions, is linked to hemodynamic changes in the mother and interferes with oxygen exchange between the mother and the fetus. In addition, it is associated with pelvic floor damage: the longer the push, the more damage to the pelvic floor.

In clinical practice, health care providers sometimes resist delaying the onset of pushing after the second stage of labor has begun because of a belief that it will increase labor time. Delaying maternal bearing-down efforts during the second stage until the woman feels the urge to push (laboring down) allows for optimal use of maternal energy, has no detrimental maternal effects, and results in improved fetal oxygenation (Osborne & Hanson, 2014). Research shows that delaying pushing for up to 90 minutes after complete cervical dilation resulted in a significant decrease in the time mothers spend pushing without a significant increase in total time in second stage of labor (King et al., 2015). Because research does not support a policy of directed pushing, and some evidence suggests it may be harmful, the practice of directed pushing should be abandoned (Brodric, 2014). The newest protocol from the Association of Women's Health, Obstetric and Neonatal Nurses (AWHONN, 2014) recommends an open-glottis method in which air is released during pushing to prevent the buildup of intrathoracic pressure. Doing so also supports mother's involuntary bearing-down efforts (Holvey, 2014). The adoption of a physiologic, woman-directed approach to bearing down is advocated (King et al., 2015).

Behaviors demonstrated by laboring women during this time include pushing at the onset of the urge to bear down; using their own pattern and technique of bearing down in response to sensations they experience; using open-glottis bearing down with contractions; pushing with variations in strength and duration; pushing down with progressive intensity; and using multiple positions to increase progress and comfort. This approach is in stark contrast to management by arbitrary time limits and the directed bearing-down efforts seen in practice today. Labor nurses need to develop an evidence-based approach that acknowledges and reinforces women's innate ability to give birth and refrain from trying to direct women's pushing behaviors (Reed, 2015).

Laboring down (promotion of passive descent) is an alternative strategy for second-stage management in women with epidurals. Using this approach, the fetus descends and is born without coached maternal pushing.

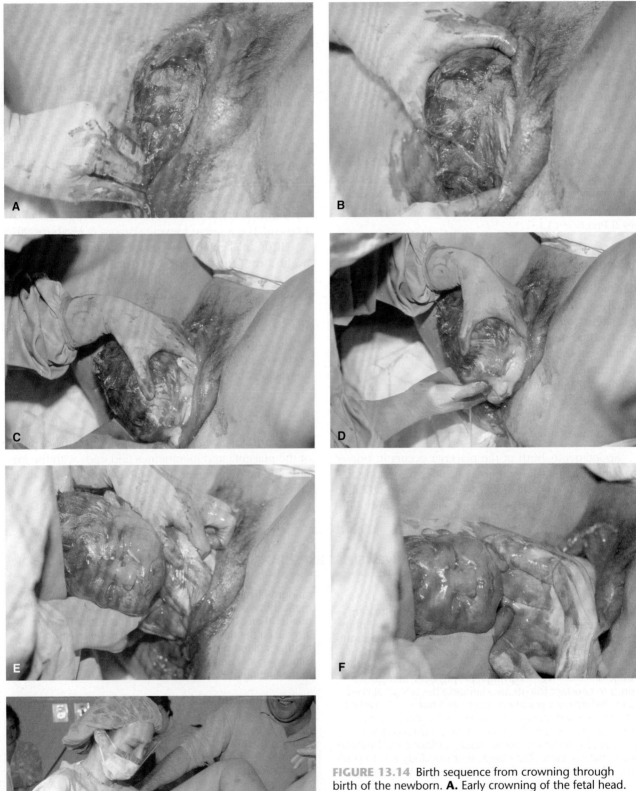

FIGURE 13.14 Birth sequence from crowning through birth of the newborn. **A.** Early crowning of the fetal head. Notice the bulging of the perineum. **B.** Late crowning. Notice that the fetal head is appearing face down. This is the normal OA position. **C.** As the head extends, you can see that the occiput is to the mother's right side–ROA position. **D.** The cardinal movement of extension. **E.** The shoulders are born. Notice how the head has turned to line up with the shoulders—the cardinal movement of external rotation. **F.** The body easily follows the shoulders. **G.** The newborn is held for the first time. (© B. Proud.)

Third Stage

The third stage of labor begins with the birth of the newborn and ends with the separation and birth of the placenta. It consists of two phases: placental separation and placental expulsion. Worldwide, approximately 800 women die each day from preventable causes related to childbirth. The single most common cause is severe bleeding, which can kill a woman within hours if care is delayed. Prompt and effective management is paramount to saving the lives of these women and prevention measures can be initiated in the third stage of labor. Controversy continues about active verses expectant management of the third stage of labor. See Evidence-Based Practice 13.1.

Placental Separation

After the infant is born, the uterus continues to contract strongly and can now retract, decreasing markedly in size. These contractions cause the placenta to pull away from the uterine wall. The following signs of separation indicate that the placenta is ready to deliver:

- The uterus rises upward.
- The umbilical cord lengthens.
- A sudden trickle of blood is released from the vaginal opening.
- The uterus changes its shape to globular.

Spontaneous birth of the placenta occurs in one of two ways: the fetal side (shiny gray side) presenting first (called Schultz's mechanism or more commonly called "shiny Schultz's") or the maternal side (red raw side) presenting first (termed Duncan's mechanism or "dirty Duncan").

Placental Expulsion

After separation of the placenta from the uterine wall, continued uterine contractions cause the placenta to be expelled within 2 to 30 minutes unless there is gentle external traction to assist. After the placenta is expelled, the uterus is massaged briefly by the attending physician or midwife until it is firm so that uterine blood vessels constrict, minimizing the possibility of hemorrhage. Normal blood loss is approximately 500 mL for a vaginal birth and 1,000 mL for a cesarean birth. Blood loss of over 1,000 mL is considered severe (Pavord & Maybury, 2015).

If the placenta does not spontaneously deliver, the health care provider assists with its removal by manual extraction. On expulsion, the placenta is inspected for its intactness by the health care provider and the nurse to make sure all sections are present. If any piece is still attached to the uterine wall, it places the woman at risk for postpartum hemorrhage because it becomes a space-occupying object that interferes with the ability of the uterus to contract fully and effectively.

Fourth Stage

The fourth stage begins with completion of the expulsion of the placenta and membranes and ends with the initial physiologic adjustment and stabilization of the mother (1 to 4 hours after birth). This stage initiates the postpartum period. The mother usually feels a sense of peace

---

EVIDENCE-BASED PRACTICE 13.1 | **ACTIVE VERSES EXPECTANT MANAGEMENT FOR WOMEN IN LABOR**

STUDY

Once birth has taken place, the uterus continues to contract, causing the placenta to separate from the wall of the uterus. The mother then delivers the placenta without outside intervention. This is termed expectant management of the third stage of labor. Active management of the third stage of labor involves giving a prophylactic uterotonic drug to contract the uterus, clamping the umbilical cord early before cord pulsations stops; and traction is applied to the cord with counter-pressure on the uterus to deliver the placenta. Active management was introduced to try to reduce postpartum hemorrhage, a major contributor to maternal mortality. The objective of this study was to compare the effectiveness of active verses expectant management of the third stage of labor.

Findings

Seven studies involving 8247 women were analyzed. Because of the clinical heterogeneity of the sample, random-effects were used in the analysis. Active management showed a significant decrease in primary blood loss greater than 500 mL and subsequent anemia. However it reduced the newborn's birthweight and increased the mother's blood pressure. Overall, the quality of the evidence was low and more data are needed to be confident in the findings.

Nursing Implications

Although there was lack of high-quality evidence in this review, active management of the third stage of labor reduced the risk of hemorrhage after childbirth, but adverse effects were identified. Women should be provided information on the benefits and harms of both methods to support informed choice. Given the concerns about early cord clamping and the potential adverse effects of uterotonic drugs, it is important to look at the individual components of third-stage management and work toward modifications to bring about the best outcomes.

Adapted from Begley, C. M., Gyte, G. M, Devane, D., McGuire, W., & Weeks, A. (2015). Active versus expectant management for women in the third stage of labor. *Cochrane Database of Systematic Reviews, 2015*, 3, CD007412.

and excitement, is wide awake, and is very talkative initially. The attachment process begins with her inspecting her newborn and desiring to cuddle and breast-feed him or her. The mother's fundus should be firm and well contracted. Typically it is located at the midline between the umbilicus and the symphysis, but it then slowly rises to the level of the umbilicus during the first hour after birth (Jordan et al., 2014). If the uterus becomes boggy, it is massaged to keep it firm. The lochia (vaginal discharge) is red, mixed with small clots, and of moderate flow. If the woman has had an episiotomy during the second stage of labor, it should be intact, with the edges approximated and clean and no redness or edema present.

The focus during this stage is to monitor the mother closely to prevent hemorrhage, bladder distention, and venous thrombosis. Usually the mother is thirsty and hungry during this time and may request food and drink. Her bladder is hypotonic and thus she has limited sensation to acknowledge a full bladder or to void. Vital signs, the amount and consistency of the vaginal discharge (lochia), and the uterine fundus are usually monitored every 15 minutes for at least 1 hour. The woman will be feeling cramp-like discomfort during this time due to the contracting uterus.

KEY CONCEPTS

- Labor is a complex, multifaceted interaction between the mother and fetus. Thus, it is difficult to determine exactly why labor begins and what initiates it.

- Before the onset of labor, a pregnant woman's body undergoes several changes in preparation for the birth of the newborn, often leading to characteristic signs and symptoms that suggest that labor is near. These changes include cervical changes, lightening, increased energy level, bloody show, Braxton Hicks contractions, and spontaneous rupture of membranes.

- False labor is a condition seen during the latter weeks of some pregnancies in which irregular uterine contractions are felt, but the cervix is not affected.

- The critical factors in labor and birth are designated as the 10 P's: passageway (birth canal), passenger (fetus and placenta), powers (contractions), position (maternal), psychological response, philosophy (low tech, high touch), partners (support caregivers), patience (natural timing), patient (client) preparation (childbirth knowledge base), and pain management (comfort measures).

- The size and shape of a woman's pelvis are determining factors for a vaginal birth. The female pelvis is classified according to four main shapes: gynecoid, anthropoid, android, and platypelloid.

- The labor process is comprised of a series of rhythmic, involuntary, usually quite uncomfortable uterine muscle contractions that bring about a shortening (effacement) and opening (dilation) of the cervix, and a bursting of the fetal membranes. Important parameters of uterine contractions are frequency, duration, and intensity.

- The diameters of the fetal skull vary considerably, with some diameters shortening and others lengthening as the head is molded during the labor and birth process.

- Pain during labor is a nearly universal experience for childbearing women. Having a strong sense of self and meaningful support from others can often help women manage labor well and reduce their sensation of pain.

- Preparing mentally for childbirth is important for women to enable them to work with the natural forces of labor and not against them.

- As the woman experiences and progresses through childbirth, numerous physiologic responses occur that assist her adaptation to the laboring process.

- Labor is typically divided into four stages that are unequal in length.

- During the first stage, the fundamental change underlying the process is progressive dilation of the cervix. It is further divided into three phases: latent phase, active phase, and transition.

- The second stage of labor is from complete cervical dilation (10 cm) and effacement through the birth of the infant.

- The third stage is that of separation and birth of the placenta. It consists of two phases: placental separation and placental expulsion.

- The fourth stage begins after the birth of the placenta and membranes and ends with the initial physiologic adjustment and stabilization of the mother (1 to 4 hours).

References and Recommended Readings

Ahlemeyer, J., & Mahon, S. (2015). Doulas for childbearing women. *MCN: The American Journal of Maternal/Child Nursing, 40*(2), 122–127.

Alexander, L. L., LaRosa, J. H., Bader, H., & Garfield, S. (2014). *New dimensions in women's health* (6th ed.). Sudbury, MA: Jones & Bartlett.

American College of Obstetricians and Gynecologists [ACOG]. (2014a). *Labor induction: FAQ 154.* Retrieved from http://www.acog.org/For_Patients/Search_FAQs

American College of Obstetricians & Gynecologists [ACOG] (2014b). *Nation's OB/GYNs take aim at preventing cesareans: New guidelines recommends allowing women to labor longer to help avoid cesarean*. Retrieved from http://www.acog.org/About_ACOG/News_Room/News_Releases/2014/Nations_Ob-Gyns_Take_Aim_at_Preventing_Cesareans

American College of Obstetricians & Gynecologists [ACOG] & Society for Maternal-Fetal Medicine [SMFM]. (2014c). Safe prevention of the primary cesarean delivery. *Obstetrics & Gynecology, 123*(3), 693–711.

Association of Women's Health, Obstetric and Neonatal Nurses [AWHONN]. (2014). *Nursing care and management of the 2nd stage of labor* (2nd ed.). Retrieved from https://www.awhonn.org/awhonn/content.do?name=08_Store/08_labormanagement.htm

Begley, C. M., Gyte, G. M., Devane, D., McGuire, W., & Weeks, A. (2015). Active versus expectant management for women in the third stage of labor. *Cochrane Database of Systematic Reviews 2015, 2*(3), CD007412.

Brodric, A. (2014). Too afraid to push: dealing with fear of childbirth. *Practicing Midwife, 17*(3), 15–17.

Budin, W. C. (2014). What to Teach? *Journal of Perinatal Education, 23*(2), 59–61.

Budin, W. C. (2015). Choosing wisely for birth. *The Journal of Perinatal Education, 24*(1), 3–5.

Byrne, J., Hauck, Y., Fisher, C., Bayes, S., & Schutze, R. (2014). Effectiveness of a mindfulness-based childbirth education pilot study on maternal self-efficacy and fear of childbirth. *Journal of Midwifery & Women's Health, 59*(2), 192–197.

Camorcia, M. (2015). The second and third stage of labor. In *Epidural labor analgesia* (pp. 103–119). Springer International Publishing. DOI: 10.1007/978-3-319-13890-9_9

Capogna, G. (2015). Humanization of childbirth and epidural analgesia. In *Epidural labor analgesia* (pp. 315–323). Springer International Publishing. DOI: 10.1007/978-3-319-13890-9_24

Casey M., Fealy G., Kennedy C., Hegarty J., Prizeman G., McNamara M., et al. (2015). Nurses', midwives' and key stakeholders' experiences and perceptions of a scope of nursing and midwifery practice framework. *Journal of Advanced Nursing, 71*(6), 1227–1237.

Caughey, A. (2014). Induction of labor: does it increase the risk of cesarean delivery? *BJOG: An International Journal of Obstetrics & Gynecology, 121*(6), 658–661.

Centers for Disease Control and Prevention [CDC]. (2014a). Primary cesarean delivery rates, by state: Results from the revised birth certificate, 2006–2012. *National vital statistics reports 63*(1), Hyattsville, MD: National Center for Health Statistics.

Cheng, Y. W., & Caughey, A. B. (2015a). Normal labor and delivery. *eMedicine*. Retrieved from http://emedicine.medscape.com/article/260036-overview

Cheng, Y. W., & Caughey, A. B. (2015b). Second stage of labor. *Clinical Obstetrics and Gynecology, 58*(2), 227–240.

Collins, K. A., & Reed, R. C. (2014). Birth trauma. *Forensic Pathology of Infancy and Childhood*, 139–168.

Cox, K. J., & King, T. L. (2015). Preventing primary cesarean births: Midwifery care. *Clinical Obstetrics and Gynecology, 58*(2), 282–293.

Cunningham, F. G., Leveno, K. J., Bloom, S. L., Spong, C. Y., Dashe, J. S., Hoffman, B. L., et al. (2014). *Williams' obstetrics* (24th ed.). New York, NY: McGraw-Hill Education.

Edmonds, J. K., Cwiertniewicz, T., & Stoll, K. (2015). Childbirth education prior to pregnancy? Survey findings of childbirth preferences and attitudes among young women. *The Journal of Perinatal Education, 24*(2), 93–101.

Fischer, B., & Mitteroecker, P. (2015). Covariation between human pelvis shape, stature, and head size alleviates the obstetric dilemma. *Proceedings of the National Academy of Sciences, 112*(18), 5655–5660.

Fitzgerald, E. M., Cronin, S. N., & Boccella, S. H. (2015). Anguish, yearning, and identity: Toward a better understanding of the pregnant Hispanic woman's prenatal care experience. *Journal of Transcultural Nursing*, pii: 1043659615578718.

Funai, E. F., & Norwitz, E. R. (2015). Mechanism of normal labor and delivery. *UpToDate*. Retrieved from http://www.uptodate.com/contents/mechanism-of-normal-labor-and-delivery

Gizzo, S., Di Gangi, S., Noventa, M., Bacile, V., Zambon, A., & Nardelli, G.B. (2014). Women's choice of positions during labor: Return to the past or a modern way to give birth? *BioMed Research International*. 2014, Article ID 638093.

Glavind, J., & Uldbjerg, N. (2015). Elective cesarean delivery at 38 and 39 weeks: Neonatal and maternal risks. *Current Opinion in Obstetrics and Gynecology, 27*(2), 121–127.

Grant, N., Strevens, H., & Thornton, J. (2015). Physiology of labor. In *Epidural labor analgesia* (pp. 1–10). Springer International Publishing.

Green, C. J. (2015). *Maternal newborn nursing care plans* (3rd ed.). Burlington, MA: Jones & Bartlett Learning.

Hanson, L., & VandeVusse, L. (2014). Supporting labor progress toward physiologic birth. *Journal of Perinatal & Neonatal Nursing, 28*(2), 101–107.

Hoang, S. (2014). Pregnancy and anxiety. *International Journal of Childbirth Education, 29*(1), 67–70.

Hofmeyr, G. J. (2015). Breech delivery. *Protocols for high-risk pregnancies: An evidence-based approach* (6th ed.). (pp. 423–427). West Sussex, UK: John Wiley & Sons.

Holvey, N. (2014). Supporting women in the second stage of labor. *British Journal of Midwifery, 22*(3), 182–186.

Horgan, M. J. (2015). Management of the late preterm infant: Not quite ready for prime time. *Pediatric Clinics of North America, 62*(2), 439–451.

Iravani, M., Zarean, E., Janghorbani, M., & Bahrami, M. (2015). Women's needs and expectations during normal labor and delivery. *Journal of Education and Health Promotion, 4*, 6.

Jones, L. V. (2015). Non-pharmacological approaches for pain relief during labor can improve maternal satisfaction with childbirth and reduce obstetric interventions. *Evidence Based Nursing, 18*(3), 70.

Jones, R. E., & Lopez, K. H. (2014). *Human reproductive biology* (4th ed.). Waltham, MA: Elsevier Health Sciences.

Jordan, R. G., Engstrom, J., Marfell, J., & Farley, C. L. (2014). *Prenatal and postnatal care: A women-centered approach*. Ames, Iowa: John Wiley & Sons

King, T. L., Brucker, M. C., Kriebs, J. M., Fahey, J. O., Gegor, C. L., & Varney, H. (2015). *Varney's midwifery* (5th ed.). Burlington, MA: Jones & Bartlett Learning.

Kriebs, J. M. (2015). Patient safety during induction of labor. *The Journal of Perinatal & Neonatal Nursing, 29*(2), 130–137.

Leap, N., & Hunter, B. (2015). *Supporting women for labor and birth: A companion*. Florence, KY: Routledge.

Leonard, P. (2015). Childbirth education: A handbook for nurses. *Nursing Spectrum*. Retrieved from http://ce.nurse.com/60057/Childbirth-Education-A-Handbook-for-Nurses

Le Ray C., Blondel B., Prunet C., Khireddine I., Deneux-Tharaux C., Goffinet F. (2015). Stabilizing the caesarean rate: Which target population? *BJOG, 122*(5), 690–699.

Marani, E., & Koch, W. (2014). *The pelvis: Structure, gender and society*. Philadelphia, PA: Springer Healthcare

March of Dimes. (2015). *Inducing labor: Medical reasons*. Retrieved from http://www.marchofdimes.org/videos/inducing-labor-medical-reasons.aspx

Martin, R. J., Fanaroff, A. A., & Walsh, M. C. (2014). *Neonatal-perinatal medicine* (10th ed.). St. Louis, MO: Elsevier Health Sciences.

Moses, S. (2015). Labor induction. *Family Practice Notebook*, Retrieved from http://www.fpnotebook.com/ob/ld/LbrIndctn.htm

Milton, S. K., Chelmow, D., & Ramus, R. M. (2015). Maternal and fetal outcomes with internal compared with external tocometry: A meta-analysis [218]. *Obstetrics & Gynecology, 125*, 71S.

Nieuwenhuijze, M., Low, L., Korstjens, I., & Lagro-Janssen, T. (2014). The role of maternity care providers in promoting shared decision making regarding birthing positions during the second stage of labor. *Journal of Midwifery & Women's Health, 59*(3), 277–285.

Norwitz, E. R. (2015). Physiology of parturition. *UpToDate*. Retrieved from http://www.uptodate.com/contents/physiology-of-parturition

Osborne, K., & Hanson, L. (2014). Labor down or bear down: A strategy to translate second-stage labor evidence to perinatal practice. *Journal of Perinatal & Neonatal Nursing, 28*(2), 117–126.

Pavord, S., & Maybury, H. (2015). How I treat postpartum hemorrhage. *Blood, 125*(18), 2759–2770.

Ramasubramaniam, S., Renganathan, L., Vijayalakshmi, G., & Mallo-Banatao, M. V. Use of herbal preparations among parturient women: Is there enough evidence-A review of literature. *International Journal of Herbal Medicine, 2*(5), 20–26.

Reed, R. (2015). Supporting women's instinctive pushing behavior during birth. *The Practicing Midwife, 18*(6), 13–15.

Sharshiner, R., & Silver, R. M. (2015). Management of fetal malpresentation. *Clinical Obstetrics and Gynecology, 58*(2), 246–255.

Tharpe, N. L., Farley, C. L., & Jordan, R. (2016). *Clinical practice guidelines for midwifery & women's health* (5th ed.). Sudbury, MA: Jones & Bartlett.

Tussey, C. M., Botsios, E., Gerkin, R. D., Kelly, L. A., Gamez, J., & Mensik, J. (2015). Reducing length of labor and cesarean surgery rate using a peanut ball for women laboring with an epidural. *The Journal of Perinatal Education, 24*(1), 16–24.

U.S. Department of Health and Human Services. (2010). *Healthy People 2020*. Retrieved from http://www.healthypeople.gov/2020/topicsobjectives2020

Van der Gucht, N., & Lewis, K. (2015). Women's experiences of coping with pain during childbirth: A critical review of qualitative research. *Midwifery, 31*(3), 349–358.

Verklan, T., & Walden, M. (2014). *Core curriculum for neonatal intensive care nursing* (4th ed.). St. Louis, MO: Saunders Elsevier

Weber, J., & Kelley, J. (2014). *Health assessment in nursing* (5th ed.). Philadelphia, PA: Lippincott Williams & Wilkins.

Wojnar, D. M. (2015). Perinatal experiences of Somali couples in the United States. *JOGNN: Journal of Obstetric, Gynecologic & Neonatal Nursing, 44*(3), 358–369.

Woods, N. K., & Chesser, A. (2015). Becoming a mom: Improving birth outcomes through a community collaborative prenatal education model. *Journal of Family Medicine & Disease Prevention, 1*(002), 1–4.

MULTIPLE-CHOICE QUESTIONS

1. When determining the frequency of contractions, the nurse would measure which of the following?
   a. Start of one contraction to the start of the next contraction
   b. Beginning of one contraction to the end of the same contraction
   c. Peak of one contraction to the peak of the next contraction
   d. End of one contraction to the beginning of the next contraction

2. Which fetal lie is most conducive to a spontaneous vaginal birth?
   a. Transverse
   b. Longitudinal
   c. Perpendicular
   d. Oblique

3. Which of the following observations would suggest that placental separation is occurring?
   a. Uterus stops contracting altogether.
   b. Umbilical cord pulsations stop.
   c. Uterine shape changes to globular.
   d. Maternal blood pressure drops.

4. As the nurse is explaining the difference between true versus false labor to her childbirth class, she states that the major difference between them is:
   a. Discomfort level is greater with false labor.
   b. Progressive cervical changes occur in true labor.
   c. There is a feeling of nausea with false labor.
   d. There is more fetal movement with true labor.

5. The shortest but most intense phase of labor is the:
   a. Latent phase
   b. Active phase
   c. Transition phase
   d. Placental expulsion phase

6. A laboring woman is admitted to the labor and birth suite at 6-cm dilation. She would be in which phase of the first stage of labor?
   a. Latent
   b. Active
   c. Transition
   d. Early

7. Which assessment would indicate that a woman is in true labor?
   a. Membranes are ruptured and fluid is clear.
   b. Presenting part is engaged and not floating.
   c. Cervix is 4 cm dilated, 90% effaced.
   d. Contractions last 30 seconds, every 5 to 10 minutes.

8. Interventions that are underutilized in promoting a normal birth. Select all that apply.
   a. Oral nutrition and fluids in labor
   b. Open glottis pushing in the second stage of labor
   c. Skin-to-skin contact after birth for infant bonding
   d. Routine artificial rupture of membranes (amniotomy)
   e. Labor induction with Pitocin given intravenously
   f. Routine episiotomy to shorten labor length

9. Physiologic preparation for labor would be demonstrated by:
   a. Decrease in Braxton Hicks contractions felt by mother
   b. Weight gain and an increase in appetite by mother
   c. Lightening, whereby the fetus drops into true pelvis
   d. Fetal heart rate accelerations and increased movements

CRITICAL THINKING EXERCISES

1. Cindy, a 20-year-old primipara, calls the birthing center where you work as a nurse and reports that she thinks she is in labor because she feels labor pains. Her due date is this week. The midwives have been giving her prenatal care throughout this pregnancy.
   a. What additional information do you need to respond appropriately?
   b. What suggestions/recommendations would you make to her?
   c. What instructions need to be given to guide her decision making?
   d. What other premonitory signs of labor might the nurse ask about?
   e. What manifestations would be found if Cindy is experiencing true labor?

2. You are assigned to lead a community education class for women in their third trimester of pregnancy to prepare them for their upcoming birth. Prepare an outline of topics that should be addressed.

STUDY ACTIVITIES

1. During clinical post conference, share with the other nursing students how the critical forces of labor influenced the length of labor and the birthing process for a laboring woman assigned to you.

2. The cardinal movements of labor include which of the following? Select all that apply.
   a. Extension and rotation
   b. Descent and engagement
   c. Presentation and position
   d. Attitude and lie
   e. Flexion and expulsion

3. Interview a woman on the mother–baby unit who has given birth within the past few hours. Ask her to describe her experience and examine psychological factors that may have influenced her laboring process.

4. On the following illustration, identify the parameters of uterine contractions by marking an "X" where the nurse would measure the duration of the contraction.

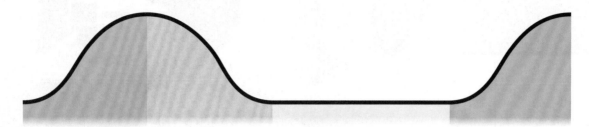

BRINGING IT ALL TOGETHER: CASE STUDY

Moritza is a 20-year-old pregnant female who comes to the prenatal clinic with her boyfriend for her prenatal visit at 39 weeks' gestation. This is her first pregnancy and she has missed several of her previous prenatal office visits. Her pregnancy has been uneventful thus far, but she is concerned today about impending labor and how she will know when to go to the hospital. She feels unprepared for labor and admits she is very afraid of the pain since many of her friends and family members have shared their 'horror' stories about their experiences. She admits she is scared about having an IV in her arm at the hospital. She wants a normal physiologic childbirth.

ASSESSMENT

Moritza has taken good care of herself during this pregnancy, having only gained 22 pounds. She didn't attend any of the prepared childbirth classes offered free through the health department, so she has numerous questions about her labor and birth forthcoming. Fetal heart rate is 140 bpm, fetus active upon palpation, no dependent edema in extremities. Urine specimen was negative for glucose or protein. Today's weight is 138 pounds.

Go to thePoint to find questions to consider about this case.

14

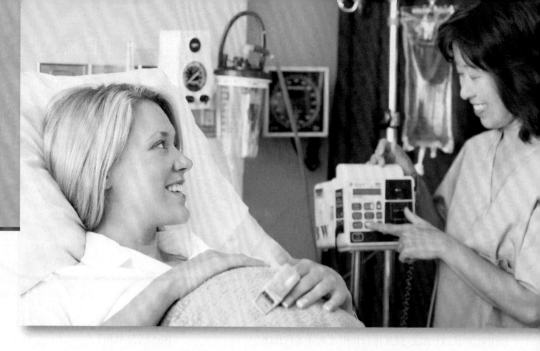

Nursing Management During Labor and Birth

Learning Objectives

Upon completion of the chapter, you will be able to:

1. Examine the measures used to evaluate maternal status during labor and birth.
2. Differentiate the advantages and disadvantages of external and internal fetal monitoring, including the appropriate use for each.
3. Choose appropriate nursing interventions to address nonreassuring fetal heart rate patterns.
4. Outline the nurse's role in fetal assessment.
5. Appraise the various comfort promotion and pain relief strategies used during labor and birth.
6. Summarize the assessment data collected on admission to the perinatal unit.
7. Relate the ongoing assessments involved in each stage of labor and birth.
8. Analyze the nurse's role throughout the labor and birth process.

Sheila was admitted in active labor to the labor and birth unit. She has progressed to the transition phase (dilated 8 cm) and is becoming increasingly more uncomfortable. She is using a patterned-paced breathing pattern now, but is thrashing around in the hospital bed.

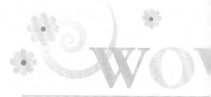

Words of Wisdom
Wise nurses are not always
silent, but they know when to
be during the miracle of birth

INTRODUCTION

The laboring and birthing process is a life-changing event for many women. Nurses need to be respectful, available, encouraging, supportive, and professional in dealing with all women. Nursing management for labor and birth involves assessment, comfort measures, emotional support, information and instruction, advocacy, and support for the partner. Providing the highest quality in maternity care is dependent on nurses valuing the childbirth experience and recognizing it as a life-changing experience for women and their families; caring nurse practice encompasses technical skills and caring behaviors; giving care that protects, promotes, and supports physiologic childbirth; providing optimal, evidence-based care; and recognizing health disparity and cultural diversity in all women cared for to improve their childbirth experience across time, settings, and disciplines. One of the components for evidence-based care and woman-centered care is women preferences to guide care for themselves during the birthing process. In a recent study, women's needs and expectations during labor and birth were assessed. Seven themes emerged—physiologic needs (nutrition, room environment, hygiene, comfort, and privacy); psychologic needs (empathy and advocacy, constant emotional support and encouragement); informational needs (about labor process and hospital policies); communication needs (health care provider and familiar attendant); esteem needs (sense of value, confidence, involvement in decisions); security needs (calming fears); and medical needs (pain relief and prevention of unnecessary interventions during labor and birth) (Iravani et al., 2015). It is important that nurses identify the expectations and needs of women in their care, so as to empower them to fully participate in their childbirth experience.

The health of mothers and their infants is of critical importance, both as a reflection of the current health status of a large segment of our population and as a predictor of the health of the next generation. The United States Department of Health and Human Services [USDHHS] (2010) addresses maternal health in two objectives: reducing maternal deaths and reducing maternal illness and complications due to pregnancy (complications during hospitalized labor and delivery). In addition, two more objectives address increasing the proportion of pregnant women who receive early and adequate prenatal care. A goal in development seeks to increase the proportion of pregnant women who attend a series of prepared childbirth classes. (See Chapter 12 for more information on these objectives.)

This chapter provides information about nursing management during labor and birth. First, the essentials for in-depth assessment of maternal and fetal status during labor and birth are discussed. This is followed by a thorough description of the major methods of promoting comfort and providing pain management during the labor and birth process. The chapter concludes by putting all the information together with a discussion of the nursing care specific to each stage of labor, including the necessary data to be obtained with the admission assessment, methods to evaluate labor progress during the first stage of labor, and key nursing measures that focus on maternal and fetal assessments and pain relief for all stages of labor.

MATERNAL ASSESSMENT DURING LABOR AND BIRTH

During labor and birth, various techniques are used to assess maternal status. These techniques provide an ongoing source of data to determine the woman's response and her progress in labor:

- Assess maternal vital signs, including temperature, blood pressure, pulse, respiration, and pain, which are primary components of the physical examination and ongoing assessment.
- Also review the prenatal record to identify risk factors that may contribute to a decrease in uteroplacental circulation during labor.
- If there is no vaginal bleeding on admission, a vaginal examination is performed to assess cervical dilation, after which it is monitored periodically as necessary to identify progress.
- Evaluate maternal pain and the effectiveness of pain management strategies at regular intervals during labor and birth.

Vaginal Examination

The World Health Organization (WHO) recommends digital vaginal examinations at intervals of 4 hours for routine assessment and identification of a delay in active labor (2014). Although not all nurses perform vaginal examinations on laboring women in all practice settings, most nurses working in community hospitals do so because physicians are not routinely present in labor and birth suites. Since most newborns in the United States are born in community hospitals, nurses are performing vaginal examinations along with midwives and physicians (American Hospital Association, 2015).

 Take Note!

A vaginal examination is an assessment skill that takes time and experience to develop; only by doing it frequently in clinical practice can the practitioner's skill level improve.

The purpose of performing a vaginal examination is to assess the amount of cervical dilation, the percentage of cervical effacement, and the fetal membrane status and to gather information on presentation, position,

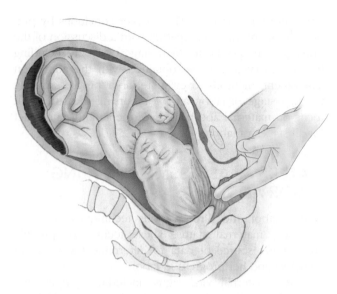

FIGURE 14.1 Vaginal examination to determine cervical dilation and effacement.

station, degree of fetal head flexion, and presence of fetal skull swelling or molding (Fig. 14.1). Prepare the woman by informing her about the procedure, what information will be obtained from it, how she can assist with the procedure, how it will be performed, and who will be performing it.

The woman is typically on her back during the vaginal examination. The vaginal examination is performed gently, with concern for the woman's comfort. If it is the initial vaginal examination to check for membrane status, water is used as a lubricant.

After donning sterile gloves, the examiner inserts his or her index and middle fingers into the vaginal introitus. Next, the cervix is palpated to assess dilation, effacement, and position (e.g., posterior or anterior). If the cervix is open to any degree, the presenting fetal part, fetal position, station, and presence of molding can be assessed. In addition, the membranes can be evaluated and described as intact, bulging, or ruptured.

At the conclusion of the vaginal examination, the findings are discussed with the woman and her partner to bring them up to date about labor progress. In addition, the findings are documented either electronically or in writing and reported to the primary health care provider in charge of the case.

Cervical Dilation and Effacement

The amount of cervical dilation (opening) and the degree of cervical effacement (thinning) are key areas assessed during the vaginal examination as the cervix is palpated with the gloved index finger. Although this finding is somewhat subjective, experienced examiners typically come up with similar findings. The width of the cervical opening determines dilation, and the length of the cervix

assesses effacement. Effacement and dilation are used to assess cervical changes as follows:
- Effacement:
  - 0%: cervical canal is 2 cm long
  - 50%: cervical canal is 1 cm long
  - 100%: cervical canal is obliterated
- Dilation:
  - 0 cm: external cervical os is closed
  - 5 cm: external cervical os is halfway dilated
  - 10 cm: external os is fully dilated and ready for birth passage

The information yielded by this examination serves as a basis for determining which stage of labor the woman is in and what her ongoing care should be.

Fetal Descent and Presenting Part

In addition to cervical dilation and effacement findings, the vaginal examination can also determine fetal descent (station) and presenting part. During the vaginal examination, the gloved index finger is used to palpate the fetal skull (if vertex presentation) through the opened cervix or the buttocks in the case of a breech presentation. Station is assessed in relation to the maternal ischial spines and the presenting fetal part. These spines are not sharp protrusions but rather blunted prominences at the midpelvis. The ischial spines serve as landmarks and have been designated as zero station. If the presenting part is palpated higher than the maternal ischial spines, a negative number is assigned; if the presenting fetal part is felt below the maternal ischial spines, a plus number is assigned, denoting how many centimeters below zero station (see Chapter 13 for a more detailed discussion).

Progressive fetal descent (−5 to +4) is the expected norm during labor—moving downward from the negative stations to zero station to the positive stations in a timely manner. If progressive fetal descent does not occur, a disproportion between the maternal pelvis and the fetus might exist and needs to be investigated.

Rupture of Membranes

The integrity of the membranes can be determined during the vaginal examination. Typically, if intact, the membranes will be felt as a soft bulge that is more prominent during a contraction. If the membranes have ruptured, the woman may have reported a sudden gush of fluid. Membrane rupture also may occur as a slow trickle of fluid. When membranes rupture, the priority focus should be on assessing fetal heart rate (FHR) first to identify a deceleration, which might indicate cord compression secondary to cord prolapse. If the membranes are ruptured when the woman comes to the hospital, the health care provider should ascertain when it occurred. Prolonged ruptured membranes increase the risk of infection as a result of ascending vaginal pathological organisms for both mother and fetus. Signs of intrauterine infection to be alert for include maternal fever, fetal and maternal tachycardia, foul odor of vaginal discharge, and an increase in white blood cell count.

To confirm that membranes have ruptured, a sample of fluid is taken from the vagina via a nitrazine yellow dye swab to determine the fluid's pH. Vaginal fluid is acidic, whereas amniotic fluid is alkaline and turns a nitrazine swab blue. Sometimes, however, false-positive results can occur, especially in women experiencing a large amount of bloody show, because blood is alkaline. The membranes are most likely intact if the nitrazine swab remains yellow to olive green, with pH between 5 and 6. The membranes are probably ruptured if the nitrazine swab turns a blue-green to deep blue, with pH ranging from 6.5 to 7.5 (Tharpe, Farley, & Jordan, 2016).

If the nitrazine test is inconclusive, an additional test, called the *fern test*, can be used to confirm rupture of membranes. With this test, a sample of vaginal fluid is obtained, applied to a microscope slide, and allowed to dry. Using a microscope, the slide is examined for a characteristic fern pattern that indicates the presence of amniotic fluid.

Assessing Uterine Contractions

The primary power of labor is uterine contractions, which are involuntary. Uterine contractions increase intrauterine pressure, causing tension on the cervix. This tension leads to cervical dilation and thinning, which in turn eventually forces the fetus through the birth canal. Normal uterine contractions have a contraction (systole) and a relaxation (diastole) phase. The contraction resembles a wave, moving downward to the cervix and upward to the fundus of the uterus. Each contraction starts with a building up (increment), gradually reaching an acme (peak intensity), and then a letting down (decrement). Each contraction is followed by an interval of rest, which ends when the next contraction begins. At the acme (peak) of the contraction, the entire uterus is contracting, with the greatest intensity in the fundal area. The relaxation phase follows and occurs simultaneously throughout the uterus.

Uterine contractions during labor are monitored by palpation and by electronic monitoring. Assessment of the contractions includes frequency; duration, intensity, and uterine resting tone (see Chapter 13 for a more detailed discussion). Uterine contractions with intensity of 30 mm Hg or greater initiate cervical dilation. During active labor, the intensity usually reaches 50 to 80 mm Hg. Resting tone is normally between 5 and 10 mm Hg in early labor and between 12 and 18 mm Hg in active labor (Hiersch et al., 2015).

To palpate the fundus for contraction intensity, place the pads of your fingers on the fundus and describe how it feels: like the tip of the nose (mild), like the chin

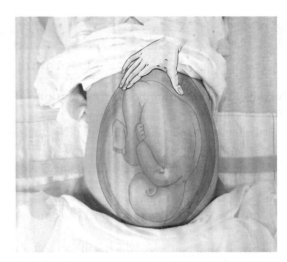

FIGURE 14.2 Nurse palpating the woman's fundus during a contraction.

(moderate), or like the forehead (strong). Palpation of intensity is a subjective judgment of the indentability of the uterine wall; a descriptive term is assigned (mild, moderate, or strong) (Fig. 14.2).

Take Note!

Frequent clinical experience is needed to gain accuracy in assessing the intensity of uterine contractions.

The second method used to assess the intensity of uterine contractions is electronic monitoring, either external or internal. Both methods provide a reasonable measurement of the intensity of uterine contractions. Although the external fetal monitor is sometimes used to estimate the intensity of uterine contractions, it is not as accurate an assessment tool.

Performing Leopold's Maneuvers

Leopold's maneuvers are a method for determining the presentation, position, and lie of the fetus through the use of four specific steps. This method involves inspection and palpation of the maternal abdomen as a screening assessment for malpresentation. A longitudinal lie is expected, and the presentation can be cephalic, breech, or shoulder. Each maneuver answers a question:

- *Maneuver 1*: What fetal part (head or buttocks) is located in the fundus (top of the uterus)?
- *Maneuver 2*: On which maternal side is the fetal back located? (Fetal heart tones are best auscultated through the back of the fetus.)
- *Maneuver 3*: What is the presenting part?
- *Maneuver 4*: Is the fetal head flexed and engaged in the pelvis?

Leopold's maneuvers are described in Nursing Procedure 14.1. Also see Chapter 12.

NURSING PROCEDURE 14.1

Performing Leopold's Maneuvers

Purpose: To Determine Fetal Presentation, Position, and Lie

1. Place the woman in the supine position and stand beside her.

2. Perform the first maneuver to determine presentation.
   a. Facing the woman's head, place both hands on the abdomen to determine fetal position in the uterine fundus.
   b. Feel for the buttocks, which will feel soft and irregular (indicates vertex presentation); feel for the head, which will feel hard, smooth, and round (indicates a breech presentation).

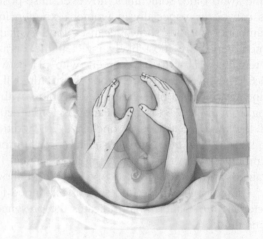

3. Complete the second maneuver to determine position.
   a. While still facing the woman, move hands down the lateral sides of the abdomen to palpate on which side the back is located (feels hard and smooth).
   b. Continue to palpate to determine on which side the limbs are located (irregular nodules with kicking and movement).

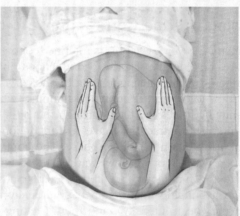

4. Perform the third maneuver to confirm presentation.
   a. Move hands down the sides of the abdomen to grasp the lower uterine segment and palpate the area just above the symphysis pubis.
   b. Place thumb and fingers of one hand apart and grasp the presenting part by bringing fingers together.
   c. Feel for the presenting part. If the presenting part is the head, it will be round, firm, and ballottable; if it is the buttocks, it will feel soft and irregular.

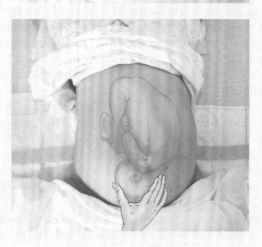

Performing Leopold's Maneuvers (continued)

5. Perform the fourth maneuver to determine attitude.
   a. Turn to face the client's feet and use the tips of the first three fingers of each hand to palpate the abdomen.
   b. Move fingers toward each other while applying downward pressure in the direction of the symphysis pubis. If you palpate a hard area on the side opposite the fetal back, the fetus is in flexion, because you have palpated the chin. If the hard area is on the same side as the back, the fetus is in extension, because the area palpated is the occiput.

Also, note how your hands move. If the hands move together easily, the fetal head is not descended into the woman's pelvic inlet. If the hands do not move together and stop because of resistance, the fetal head is engaged into the woman's pelvic inlet (Walker & Sabrosa, 2014).

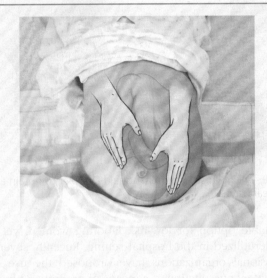

FETAL ASSESSMENT DURING LABOR AND BIRTH

A fetal assessment identifies well-being or signs that indicate compromise. The character of the amniotic fluid is assessed, but the fetal assessment focuses primarily on determining the FHR pattern. Umbilical cord blood analysis and fetal scalp stimulation are additional assessments performed as necessary in the case of questionable FHR patterns.

Analysis of Amniotic Fluid

Amniotic fluid should be clear when the membranes rupture. Rupturing of membranes is either spontaneous or artificial by means of an amniotomy, during which a disposable plastic hook (an amnihook) is used to perforate the amniotic sac. Cloudy or foul-smelling amniotic fluid indicates infection. Green fluid may indicate that the fetus has passed meconium secondary to transient hypoxia, prolonged pregnancy, cord compression, intrauterine growth restriction (IUGR), maternal hypertension, diabetes, or chorioamnionitis; however, it is considered a normal occurrence if the fetus is in a breech presentation. If it is determined that meconium-stained amniotic fluid is due to fetal hypoxia, the maternity and pediatric teams work together to prevent meconium aspiration syndrome. This would necessitate suctioning after the head is born before the infant takes a breath and perhaps direct tracheal suctioning after birth if the Apgar

score is low. In some cases an amnioinfusion (introduction of warmed, sterile normal saline or Ringer's lactate solution into the uterus) is used to dilute moderate to heavy meconium released in utero to assist in preventing meconium aspiration syndrome.

Analysis of the FHR

Analysis of the FHR is one of the primary evaluation tools used to determine fetal oxygen status indirectly. FHR assessment can be done intermittently using a fetoscope (a modified stethoscope attached to a headpiece) or a Doppler (ultrasound) device, or continuously with an electronic fetal monitor applied externally or internally. The object of FHR monitoring is to reduce the mortality/morbidity by ensuring that all fetal hypoxic insults are identified in time to allow removal or alteration of the reason for it, or to enable a safe birth of the fetus before irreversible asphyxia damage occurs (Hastings, 2015).

Intermittent FHR Monitoring

Intermittent FHR monitoring involves auscultation via a fetoscope or a handheld Doppler device that uses ultrasound waves that bounce off the fetal heart, producing echoes or clicks that reflect the rate of the fetal heart (Fig. 14.3). Traditionally, a fetoscope was used to assess FHR, but the handheld Doppler device has been found to have a greater sensitivity than the fetoscope. Intermittent auscultation of the fetal heart rate is an

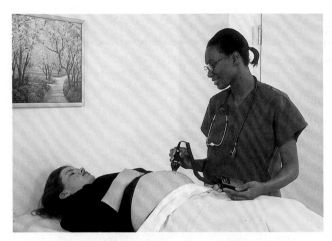

FIGURE 14.3 Nurse using a handheld Doppler to obtain a fetal heart rate.

acceptable option for low-risk laboring women, yet it is underutilized in the hospital setting. Recently several professional organizations have proposed the use of intermittent auscultation as a means of promoting physiologic births (Wisner, 2015); thus, at present it is used in some clinical settings. See Evidence-Based Practice 14.1 for more information.

Take Note!

Doppler devices to detect FHRs are relatively low in cost and are used in hospitals and in home births and birthing centers routinely. Many nurses use them in their work settings.

Intermittent FHR monitoring allows the woman to be mobile in the first stage of labor. She is free to move around and change position at will since she is not attached to a stationary electronic fetal monitor. However, intermittent monitoring does not provide a continuous FHR recording and does not document how the fetus responds to the stress of labor (unless listening is done during the contraction). The best way to assess fetal well-being would be to start listening to the FHR at the end of the contraction (not after one) so that late decelerations could be detected. However, the pressure of the device during a contraction is uncomfortable and can distract the woman from using her paced-breathing patterns.

Intermittent FHR auscultation can be used to detect FHR baseline and rhythm and changes from baseline. However, it cannot detect variability and types of decelerations, as electronic fetal monitoring (EFM) can (Wisner, 2015). During intermittent auscultation to establish a baseline, the FHR is assessed for a full minute after a contraction. From then on, unless there is a problem, listening for 30 seconds and multiplying the value by two is sufficient. If the woman experiences a change in condition during labor, auscultation assessments should be more frequent. Changes in condition include ruptured membranes or the onset of bleeding. In addition, more frequent assessments occur after periods of ambulation, a vaginal examination, administration of pain medications, or other clinically important events (King et al., 2015).

The FHR is heard most clearly at the fetal back. In a cephalic presentation, the FHR is best heard in the lower quadrant of the maternal abdomen. In a breech presentation, it is heard at or above the level of the maternal umbilicus (Fig. 14.4). As labor progresses, the FHR location will change accordingly as the fetus descends into the maternal pelvis for the birthing process. To ensure

---

EVIDENCE-BASED PRACTICE 14.1   INTRAPARTUM FETAL MONITORING

STUDY

Electronic fetal monitoring (EFM) is a widely utilized means of assessing fetal status during labor and has been a central component of intrapartum care. Currently, EFM is the most common method used to evaluate the fetus during labor without substantial evidence to suggest a benefit. Clinicians spend valuable time and energy trying to characterize and distinguish between different types of FHR decelerations even though most of them have been shown to have little association with fetal acidosis. The purpose of this review was to determine if continuous EFM verses intermittent auscultation improved perinatal outcomes.

Findings

A Cochrane review of 13 trials, which included over 37,000 women, found that continuous EFM provided no significant improvement in perinatal death rate (risk rate 0.86; confidence interval 0.59 to 1.23) or cerebral palsy rate (risk rate 1.75; confidence interval 0.84 to 3.63) as compared with intermittent auscultation; however, there was a significant increase in cesarean births (risk rate 1.63; confidence interval 1.29 to 2.07) and operative vaginal births (risk rate 1.15; confidence interval 1.01 to 1.33).

Nursing Implications

Despite the lack of scientific evidence to support routinely using continuous EFM to reduce adverse perinatal outcomes, its use is almost universal in the hospital setting and very likely has contributed to the rise in cesarean birth rates. Nurses are uniquely positioned to influence the monitoring method used in labor by offering intermittent auscultation to low risk women, and requesting orders from the health care providers that include it as an option. The high-touch nature of intermittent auscultation may help nurses reconnect to their clients and to the essence of nursing practice.

Adapted from Cahill, A. G., & Spain, J. (2015). Intrapartum fetal monitoring. *Clinical Obstetrics and Gynecology, 58*(2), 263–268.

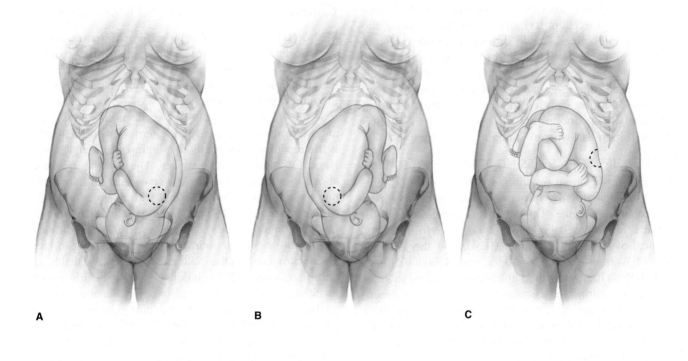

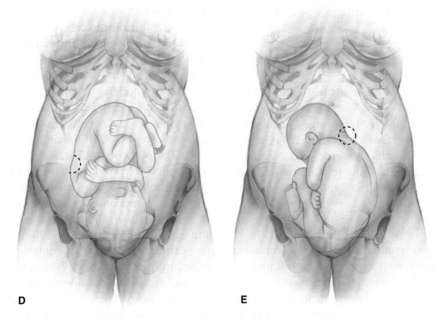

FIGURE 14.4 Locations for auscultating fetal heart rate based on fetal position. **A.** Left occiput anterior (LOA). **B.** Right occiput anterior (ROA). **C.** Left occiput posterior (LOP). **D.** Right occiput posterior (ROP). **E.** Left sacral anterior (LSA).

that the maternal heart rate is not confused with the FHR, palpate the client's radial pulse simultaneously while the FHR is being auscultated through the abdomen.

For low risk women, the FHR and contraction characteristics should be assessed every 15 to 30 minutes in active labor and every 5 to 15 minutes while pushing, as well as before and after any digital vaginal examinations, membrane rupture, medication administered, and ambulation to the restroom (Freeman, 2015).

Nursing Procedure 12.1 lists detailed steps for using a Doppler device to assess FHR. In brief, a small amount of water-soluble gel is applied to the woman's abdomen or ultrasound device before auscultation with the Doppler device to promote sound wave transmission. Usually the FHR is best heard in the woman's lower abdominal quadrants; if the FHR is not found quickly, it may help to locate the fetal back by performing Leopold's maneuvers.

Although the intermittent method of FHR assessment allows the client to move about during labor, the information obtained fails to provide a complete picture of the well-being of the fetus from moment to moment. This leads to the question of what the fetal status is during the times that are not assessed. For women who are considered at low risk for complications, this period of nonassessment is not a problem. However, for the undiagnosed high-risk woman, it might prove ominous.

GUIDELINES FOR ASSESSING FETAL HEART RATE

National professional organizations have provided general guidelines for the frequency of assessments based on existing evidence. The American College of Obstetricians and Gynecologists (ACOG), the Institute for Clinical Systems Improvement (ICSI), and the Association of Women's Health, Obstetric and Neonatal Nurses (AWHONN) have published guidelines designed to assist clinicians in caring for laboring clients. Their recommendations are supported by large controlled studies. They recommend the following guidelines for assessing FHR:

- Initial 10- to 20-minute continuous FHR assessment on entry into labor/birth area
- Completion of a prenatal and labor risk assessment on all clients
- Intermittent auscultation every 30 minutes during active labor for a low-risk woman and every 15 minutes for a high-risk woman
- During the second stage of labor, every 15 minutes for the low-risk woman and every 5 minutes for the high-risk woman and during the pushing stage (Agency for Healthcare Research and Quality [AHRQ, 2014]; Association of Women's Health, Obstetric and Neonatal Nurses [AWHONN], 2015; Institute for Clinical Systems Improvement [ICSI], 2015a).

EVIDENCE-BASED RESULTS: INTERMITTENT VERSUS ELECTRONIC MONITORING

In several randomized controlled studies comparing intermittent auscultation with electronic monitoring in both low- and high-risk clients, no difference in intrapartum fetal death was found. However, in each study a nurse–client ratio of 1:1 was consistently maintained during labor (ICSI, 2015a). This suggests that adequate staffing is essential with intermittent FHR monitoring to ensure optimal outcomes for the mother and fetus. There is insufficient evidence to indicate specific situations where continuous electronic FHR monitoring might result in better outcomes when compared to intermittent assessment. However, in pregnancies involving an increased risk of perinatal death, cerebral palsy, or neonatal encephalopathy and when oxytocin is used for induction or augmentation, it is recommended that continuous EFM be used rather than intermittent fetal auscultation (Society of Obstetricians and Gynecologists of Canada, 2015).

Continuous Electronic Fetal Monitoring

EFM detects the fetal pulse by sensing and analyzing tissue movements via Doppler ultrasound. The machine uses a transducer that is capable of both sending and receiving ultrasound waves. The waves travel through the ultrasound gel, then body tissues, and are eventually reflected by any tissue. The fast reflections are analyzed and software in the machine determines the FHR. EFM is the recommended method of intrapartum fetal surveillance for high-risk pregnancies. Despite the questions about its efficacy and controversy regarding increased rates of surgical births associated with its use, continuous cardiotocography (CTG) remains the predominant method of fetal monitoring today (Nageotte, 2015). The indications for offering women continuous fetal monitoring in labor are documented in the National Institute for Health and Care Excellence (NICE) guidelines. These include women receiving oxytocin infusing; women having epidural analgesia; and a variety of problems related to a compromise in either fetal or maternal health—prolonged rupture of membranes (>24 hours), moderate hypertension (>150/100), confirmed delay in the first or second stage of labor; and the presence of meconium (National Institute for Health and care Excellence [NICE], 2014).

Electronic fetal monitoring (EFM) uses a machine to produce a continuous tracing of the FHR. When the monitoring device is in place, a sound is produced with each heartbeat. In addition, a graphic record of the FHR pattern is produced. The primary objective of EFM is to provide information about fetal oxygenation and prevent fetal injury that could result from impaired fetal oxygenation during labor. The purpose of EFM is to detect FHR changes early before they are prolonged and profound. Fetal hypoxia is demonstrated in a heart rate pattern change and is by far the most common etiology of fetal injury and death that can be prevented with optimal fetal surveillance during labor and early interventions (Cox & King, 2015).

Current methods of continuous EFM were introduced in the United States during the 1970s, specifically for use in clients considered to be at high risk. However, the use of these methods gradually increased and they eventually came to be used for women other than just those at high risk. This increased use has become controversial because it is suspected of being associated with the steadily increasing rates of cesarean births with no decrease in the rate of cerebral palsy (Omo-Aghoja, 2015). Many studies suggest that when compared with standardized intermittent auscultation, the use of intrapartum continuous EFM seems to increase the number of preterm and surgical births but has no significant effect on reducing the incidence of intrapartum death or long-term neurologic injury. When a woman is admitted to the labor unit, a fetal monitor is applied and the FHR is monitored continuously. An impetus for this is the litigious nature of current society, but the benefits have not been proven scientifically. EFM has been given excessive importance in legal cases. Before assigning fault on events at birth, a better understanding of developmental neurobiology and limitations of the present biomarkers is warranted (Freeman, 2015). To date, continuous EFM is not evidence-based for determining fetal health status.

With EFM, there is a continuous record of the FHR: no gaps exist, as they do with intermittent auscultation. The concept of hearing and evaluating every beat of the fetus's heart to allow for early intervention seems logical. On the downside, however, using continuous monitoring can limit maternal movement and encourages the woman to lie in the supine position, which reduces placental perfusion. Despite the criticisms, EFM remains an accurate method for determining fetal health status by providing a moment-to-moment printout of FHR status.

Various groups within the medical community have criticized the use of continuous fetal monitoring for all pregnant clients, whether high risk or low risk. Concerns about the efficiency and safety of routine EFM in labor have led expert panels in the United States to recommend that such monitoring be limited to high-risk pregnancies. However, its use in low-risk pregnancies continues globally (Maso et al., 2015). This remains an important research issue.

Continuous EFM can be performed externally (indirectly), with the equipment attached to the maternal abdominal wall, or internally (directly), with the equipment attached to the fetus. Both methods provide a continuous printout of the FHR, but they differ in their specificity. The efficacy of EFM depends on the accurate interpretation of the tracings, not necessarily which method (external vs. internal) is used.

CONTINUOUS EXTERNAL MONITORING

In external or indirect monitoring, two ultrasound transducers, each of which is attached to a belt, are applied around the woman's abdomen. They are similar to the handheld Doppler device. One transducer is called a tocotransducer, a pressure-sensitive device that is applied against the uterine fundus. It detects changes in uterine pressure and converts the pressure registered into an electronic signal that is recorded on graph paper (Farine, 2015). The tocotransducer is placed over the uterine fundus in the area of greatest contractility to monitor uterine contractions. The other ultrasound transducer records the baseline FHR, long-term variability, accelerations, and decelerations. It is positioned on the maternal abdomen in the midline between the umbilicus and the symphysis pubis. The diaphragm of the ultrasound transducer is moved to either side of the abdomen to obtain a stronger sound and is then attached to the second elastic belt. This transducer converts the fetal heart movements into beeping sounds and records them on graph paper (Fig. 14.5).

Good continuous data are provided on the FHR. External monitoring can be used while the membranes

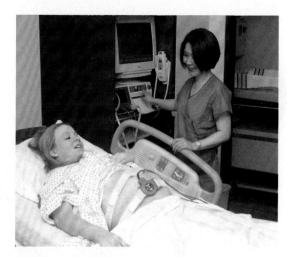

FIGURE 14.5 Continuous external electronic fetal monitoring device applied to the woman in labor.

are still intact and the cervix is not yet dilated, but also can be used with ruptured membranes and a dilating cervix. It is noninvasive and can detect relative changes in abdominal pressure between uterine resting tone and contractions. External monitoring also measures the approximate duration and frequency of contractions, providing a permanent record of FHR (Casanova, 2015).

However, external monitoring can restrict the mother's movements. It also cannot detect short-term variability. Signal disruptions can occur due to maternal obesity, fetal malpresentation, and fetal movement as well as by artifact. The term **artifact** is used to describe irregular variations or absence of the FHR on the fetal monitor record that result from mechanical limitations of the monitor or electrical interference. For instance, the monitor may pick up transmissions from citizen's band (CB) radios used by truck drivers on nearby roads and translate them into a signal. Additionally, gaps in the monitor strip can occur periodically without explanation.

CONTINUOUS INTERNAL MONITORING

Continuous internal monitoring is usually indicated for women or fetuses considered to be at high risk. Possible conditions might include multiple gestation, decreased fetal movement, abnormal FHR on auscultation, IUGR, maternal fever, preeclampsia, dysfunctional labor, preterm birth, or medical conditions such as diabetes or hypertension. It involves the placement of a spiral electrode into the fetal presenting part, usually the head, to assess FHR, and a pressure transducer placed internally within the uterus to record uterine contractions (Fig. 14.6). The fetal spiral electrode is considered the most accurate method of detecting fetal heart characteristics and patterns because it involves receiving a signal directly from the fetus (Nageotte, 2015). Specially trained labor and birth nurses are permitted to place the spiral electrode on the fetal head when the membranes rupture to assess the

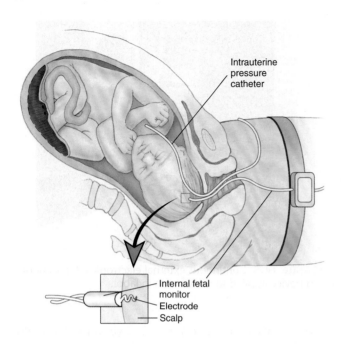

Intrauterine pressure catheter

Internal fetal monitor
Electrode
Scalp

FIGURE 14.6 Continuous internal electronic fetal monitoring.

FHR in some health care facilities, but they do not place the intrauterine pressure catheter in the uterus. Internal monitoring does not have to include both an intrauterine pressure catheter and a scalp electrode. A fetal scalp electrode can be used to monitor the fetal heartbeat without monitoring the maternal intrauterine pressure.

Both the FHR and the duration and interval of uterine contractions are recorded on the graph paper. This method permits evaluation of baseline heart rate and changes in rate and pattern.

Four specific criteria must be met for this type of monitoring to be used:
• Ruptured membranes
• Cervical dilation of at least 2 cm
• Presenting fetal part low enough to allow placement of the scalp electrode
• Skilled practitioner available to insert spiral electrode (ICSI, 2015b)

Compared with external monitoring, continuous internal monitoring can accurately detect both short-term (moment-to-moment) changes and variability (fluctuations within the baseline) and FHR dysrhythmias. In addition, maternal position changes and movement do not interfere with the quality of the tracing.

Determining FHR Patterns

Due to the rising costs of litigations related to birth asphyxia of the newborn and increasing complexity of obstetric populations, it has become absolutely mandatory that all nurses responsible for the care of women in labor are trained adequately in interpretation and documentation of CTG tracings, as well as the guidelines

for interventions based on the assessment of the tracing and overall clinical situation. Assessment parameters of the FHR include baseline FHR and variability, presence of accelerations, periodic or episodic decelerations, and changes or trends of FHR patterns over time. The nurse must be able to interpret the various parameters to determine if the FHR pattern is a *category I*, which is strongly predictive of normal fetal acid–base status at the time of observation and needs no intervention; a *category II*, which is not predictive of abnormal fetal acid–base status and but does require evaluation and continued monitoring; or a *category III*, which is predictive of abnormal fetal acid–base status at the time of observation and requires prompt evaluation and interventions, such as giving maternal oxygen, changing maternal position, discontinuing labor augmentation medication, and/or treating maternal hypotension (Freeman, 2015). Table 14.1 summarizes these categories.

BASELINE FHR

Baseline fetal heart rate refers to the average FHR that occurs during a 10-minute segment that excludes periodic or episodic rate changes, such as tachycardia or bradycardia. It is assessed when the woman has no contractions and the fetus is not experiencing episodic FHR changes. The normal baseline FHR ranges between 110 and 160 beats per minute (bpm) (National Institute of Child Health and Human Development [NICHD], 2015). The normal baseline FHR can be obtained by auscultation, ultrasound, or Doppler, or by a continuous internal direct fetal electrode.

Fetal bradycardia occurs when the FHR is below 110 bpm and lasts 10 minutes or longer (Maso et al., 2015). It can be the initial response of a healthy fetus to asphyxia. Causes of fetal bradycardia might include fetal hypoxia, prolonged maternal hypoglycemia, fetal acidosis, administration of analgesic drugs to the mother, hypothermia, anesthetic agents (epidural), maternal hypotension, fetal hypothermia, prolonged umbilical cord compression, and fetal congenital heart block (Nageotte, 2015). Bradycardia may be benign if it is an isolated event, but it is considered an ominous sign when accompanied by a decrease in baseline variability and late decelerations.

Fetal tachycardia is a baseline FHR greater than 160 bpm that lasts for 10 minutes or longer (NICHD, 2015). It can represent an early compensatory response to asphyxia. Other causes of fetal tachycardia include fetal hypoxia, maternal fever, maternal dehydration, amnionitis, drugs (e.g., cocaine, amphetamines, nicotine), maternal hyperthyroidism, maternal anxiety, fetal anemia, prematurity, fetal infection, chronic hypoxemia, congenital anomalies, fetal heart failure, and fetal arrhythmias. Fetal tachycardia is considered an ominous sign if it is accompanied by a decrease in variability and late decelerations (Yuan, 2015).

TABLE 14.1	INTERPRETING FHR PATTERNS	
Category I: normal	Predictive of normal fetal acid–base status and do not require intervention • Baseline rate (110–160 bpm) • Baseline variability moderate • Present or absent accelerations • Present or absent early decelerations • No late or variable decelerations Can be monitored with intermittent auscultation during labor	
Category II: indeterminate	Not predictive of abnormal fetal acid–base status, but require evaluation and continued surveillance • Fetal tachycardia (>160 bpm) present • Bradycardia (<110 bpm) not accompanied by absent baseline variability • Absent baseline variability not accompanied by recurrent decelerations • Minimal or marked variability • Recurrent late decelerations with moderate baseline variability • Recurrent variable decelerations accompanied by minimal or moderate baseline variability; overshoots, or shoulders • Prolonged decelerations >2 min but <10 min	
Category III: abnormal	Predictive of abnormal fetus acid–base status and require intervention • Fetal bradycardia (<110 bpm) • Recurrent late decelerations • Recurrent variable decelerations—declining or absent • Sinusoidal pattern (smooth, undulating baseline)	

Adapted from Association of Women's Health, Obstetric and Neonatal Nurses [AWHONN]. (2015). *Fetal heart monitoring: Principles and practices*. Washington, D.C.: AWHONN; Cibils, L. A. (2014). *Electronic fetal-maternal monitoring: Antepartum/intrapartum* (2nd ed.). New York, NY: Springer Publishers; Hersh, S., Megregian, M., & Emeis, C. (2014). Intermittent auscultation of the fetal heart rate during labor: An opportunity for shared decision making. *Journal of Midwifery & Women's Health, 59*, 344–349; and Martin, R. J., Fanaroff, A. A., & Walsh, M. C. (2014). *Neonatal-perinatal medicine* (10th ed.). Philadelphia, PA: Elsevier Health Sciences.

BASELINE VARIABILITY

Baseline variability is defined as irregular fluctuations in the baseline fetal heart rate, which is measured as the amplitude of the peak to trough in bpm (Sholapurkar, 2015). It represents the interplay between the parasympathetic and sympathetic nervous systems.

The constant interplay (push-and-pull effect) on the FHR from the parasympathetic and sympathetic systems produces a moment-to-moment change in the FHR. Because variability is in essence the combined result of autonomic nervous system branch function, its presence implies that the both branches are working and receiving adequate oxygen (Timmins & Clark, 2015). Thus, variability is one of the most important characteristics of the FHR. Variability is described in four categories as follows:
• fluctuation range undetectable
• fluctuation range observed at <5 bpm
• fluctuation range from 6 to 25 bpm
• fluctuation range >25 bpm

Absent or minimal variability typically is caused by fetal acidemia secondary to uteroplacental insufficiency, cord compression, a preterm fetus, maternal hypotension, uterine hyperstimulation, abruptio placenta, or a fetal dysrhythmia. Interventions to improve uteroplacental blood flow and perfusion through the umbilical cord include lateral positioning of the mother, increasing the IV fluid rate to improve maternal circulation, administering oxygen at 8 to 10 L/min by mask, considering internal fetal monitoring, documenting findings, and reporting to the health care provider. Preparation for a surgical birth may be necessary if no changes occur after attempting the interventions.

Moderate viability indicates that the autonomic and central nervous systems (CNSs) of the fetus are well developed and well oxygenated. It is considered a good sign of fetal well-being and correlates with the absence of significant metabolic acidosis (Fig. 14.7).

Marked variability occurs when there are more than 25 beats of fluctuation in the FHR baseline. Causes of this include cord prolapse or compression, maternal hypotension, uterine hyperstimulation, and abruptio placenta. Interventions include determining the cause if possible, lateral positioning, increasing intravenous fluid rate, administering oxygen at 8 to 10 L/min by mask, discontinuing oxytocin infusion, observing for changes in tracing, considering internal fetal monitoring, communicating an abnormal pattern to the health care provider, and preparing for a surgical birth if no change in pattern is noted (Freeman, 2015).

FHR variability is an important clinical indicator that is predictive of fetal acid–base balance and cerebral tissue perfusion. It is influenced by fetal oxygenation status, cardiac output, and drug effects (King et al., 2015). As the CNS is desensitized by hypoxia and acidosis, FHR decreases until a smooth baseline pattern appears. Loss of variability may be associated with a poor outcome.

Take Note!

External electronic fetal monitoring cannot assess variability accurately. Therefore, if external monitoring shows a baseline that is smoothing out, use of an internal spiral electrode should be considered to gain a more accurate picture of the fetal health status.

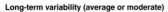
Long-term variability (average or moderate)

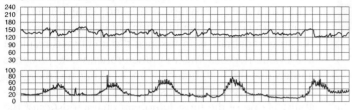

Minimal variability

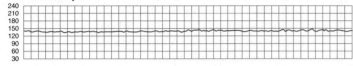

Moderate variability

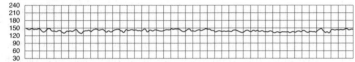

Marked variability

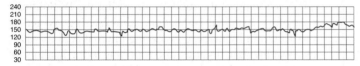

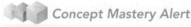

FIGURE 14.7 Examples of fetal monitoring strips.
A. Long-term variability (average or moderate).
B. Minimal variability. **C.** Moderate variability.
D. Marked variability.

PERIODIC BASELINE CHANGES

Periodic baseline changes are temporary, recurrent changes made in response to a stimulus such as a contraction. The FHR can demonstrate patterns of acceleration or deceleration in response to most stimuli. Fetal **accelerations** are transitory abrupt increases in the FHR above the baseline that last <30 seconds from onset to peak. They are associated with sympathetic nervous stimulation. They are visually apparent, with elevations of FHR of more than 15 bpm above the baseline, and their duration is >15 seconds, but less than 2 minutes (NICHD, 2015). They are generally considered reassuring

and require no interventions. Accelerations denote fetal movement and fetal well-being and are the basis for nonstress testing.

> *Concept Mastery Alert*
>
> **Responding to Fetal Heart Rate Distress During Labor**
>
> During possible fetal distress that involves lack of variability, late decelerations, and fetal tachycardia, simply changing the woman's position is inadequate. The nurse should notify the healthcare provider immediately regarding the situation.

Normal Range Pattern

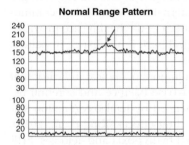

Early Deceleration

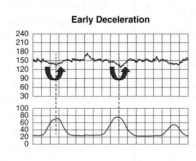

Variable Deceleration

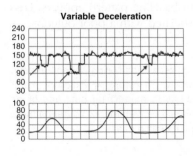

Late Deceleration

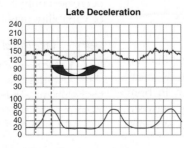

FIGURE 14.8 Decelerations. **A.** Early. **B.** Variable. **C.** Late.

A **deceleration** is a transient fall in FHR caused by stimulation of the parasympathetic nervous system. Decelerations are described by their shape and association to a uterine contraction. They are classified as early, late, and variable only (Fig. 14.8).

Early decelerations are visually apparent, usually symmetrical, and characterized by a gradual decrease in the FHR in which the nadir (lowest point) occurs at the peak of the contraction. They rarely decrease more than 30 to 40 bpm below the baseline. Typically, the onset, nadir, and recovery of the deceleration occur at the same time as the onset, peak, and recovery of the contraction. They are most often seen during the active stage of any normal labor, during pushing, crowning, or vacuum extraction. They are thought to be a result of fetal head compression that results in a reflex vagal response with a resultant slowing of the FHR during uterine contractions. Early decelerations are not indicative of fetal distress and do not require intervention.

Late decelerations are visually apparent, usually symmetrical, transitory decreases in FHR that occur after the peak of the contraction. The FHR does not return to baseline levels until well after the contraction has ended. Delayed timing of the deceleration occurs, with the nadir of the uterine contraction. Late decelerations are associated with uteroplacental insufficiency, which occurs when blood flow within the intervillous space is decreased to the extent that fetal hypoxia or myocardial depression exists (Martin, Fanaroff, & Walsh, 2014). Conditions that may decrease uteroplacental perfusion with resultant decelerations include maternal hypotension, gestational hypertension, placental aging secondary to diabetes and postmaturity, hyperstimulation via oxytocin infusion, maternal smoking, anemia, and cardiac disease. They imply some degree of fetal hypoxia. Recurrent or intermittent late decelerations are always category II (indeterminate) or category III (abnormal) regardless of depth of deceleration. Acute episodes with moderate variability are more likely to be correctable, whereas chronic episodes with loss of variability are less likely to be correctable (Sholapurkar, 2015). Box 14.1 highlights interventions for category III decelerations.

Variable decelerations present as visually apparent abrupt decreases in FHR below baseline and have an unpredictable shape on the FHR baseline, possibly demonstrating no consistent relationship to uterine contractions. The shape of variable decelerations may be U, V, or W, or they may not resemble other patterns (Cahill & Spain, 2015). Variable decelerations usually occur abruptly with quick deceleration. They are the most common deceleration pattern found in the laboring woman and are usually transient and correctable (Ugwumadu, 2015). Variable decelerations are associated with cord compression. However, they are classified either as category II or III depending on the accompanying change in baseline variability (ICSI, 2015a). The pattern of variable

---

BOX 14.1

INTERVENTIONS FOR CATEGORY III PATTERNS

- Notify the health care provider about the pattern and obtain further orders, making sure to document all interventions and their effects on the FHR pattern.
- Discontinue oxytocin or other uterotonic agent as dictated by the facility's protocol, if it is being administered.
- Turn the client on her left or right lateral, knee-chest, or hands and knees to increase placental perfusion or relieve cord compression.
- Administer oxygen via nonrebreather face mask to increase fetal oxygenation.
- Increase the intravenous fluid rate to improve intravascular volume and correct maternal hypotension.
- Assess the client for any underlying contributing causes.
- Provide reassurance that interventions are to effect pattern change.
- Modify pushing in the second stage of labor to improve fetal oxygenation.
- Document any and all interventions and any changes in FHR patterns.
- Prepare for an expeditious surgical birth if the pattern is not corrected in 30 minutes.

Adapted from American College of Obstetricians and Gynecologists [ACOG]. (2014). Safe prevention of the primary cesarean delivery. Obstetric Care Consensus 1, *Obstetrics & Gynecology, 123*, 693–711; Freeman, R. K. (2015). Intrapartum fetal heart rate monitoring. *Protocols for high-risk pregnancies: An evidence-based approach* (pp. 418–422, 6th ed.). John Wiley & Sons; and Cahill, A. G., & Spain, J. (2015). Intrapartum fetal monitoring. *Clinical Obstetrics and Gynecology, 58*(2), 263–268.

---

deceleration consistently related to the contractions with a slow return to FHR baseline warrants further monitoring and evaluation.

Prolonged decelerations are abrupt FHR declines of at least 15 bpm that last longer than 2 minutes, but less than 10 minutes (NICHD, 2015). The rate usually drops to less than 90 bpm. Many factors are associated with this pattern, including prolonged cord compression, abruptio placenta, cord prolapse, supine maternal position, vaginal examination, fetal blood sampling, maternal seizures, regional anesthesia, or uterine rupture (ACOG & SMFM 2014). Prolonged decelerations can be remedied by identifying the underlying cause and correcting it.

A *sinusoidal pattern* is described as having a visually apparent smooth, sinewave-like undulating pattern in the FHR baseline with a cycle frequency of 3 to 5 bpm that persists for >20 minutes. It is attributed to a derangement of CNS control of FHR and occurs when a severe degree of hypoxia secondary to fetal anemia and hypovolemia is present. It is always considered a Category III pattern, and to correct it a fetal intrauterine transfusion would be needed (Nageotte, 2015).

Combinations of FHR patterns obtained by EFM during labor are not infrequent. Category II and III patterns are more significant if they are mixed, persist for long periods, or have frequent prolonged late decelerations, absent or minimal variability, bradycardia or tachycardia, and prolonged variable decelerations lower than 60 bpm. The likelihood of fetal compromise is increased if Category II and III patterns are associated with decreased baseline variability or abnormal contraction patterns (ICSI, 2015a).

Other Fetal Assessment Methods

In situations suggesting the possibility of fetal compromise, such as Category II or Category III FHR patterns, further ancillary testing such as umbilical cord blood analysis and fetal scalp stimulation may be used to validate the FHR findings and assist in planning interventions.

> *Take Note!*
>
> In recent years, the use of fetal scalp sampling has decreased, being replaced by techniques that yield similar information. It has been shown to have a poor positive predictive value for intrapartum hypoxia and recent systematic reviews have reported no evidence of benefit in reducing cesarean section rates (Chandraharan, 2014).

Umbilical Cord Blood Analysis

Neonatal and childhood mortality and morbidity, including cerebral palsy, are often attributed to fetal acidosis, as defined by a low cord pH at birth. Umbilical cord blood acid–base analysis drawn at birth provides an objective method of evaluating a newborn's condition, identifying the presence of intrapartum hypoxia and acidemia. This test is considered a good indicator of fetal oxygenation and acid–base condition at birth (Martin, Fanaroff, & Walsh, 2014). The normal mean pH value range is 7.2 to 7.3. The pH values are useful for planning interventions for the newborn born with low 5-minute Apgar scores, severe FGR, Category II and III patterns during labor, umbilical cord prolapse, uterine rupture, maternal fever, placental abruption, meconium-stained amniotic fluid, and post-term births (Gujral & Nayar, 2015). The interventions needed for the compromised newborn might include providing an optimal extrauterine environment, fluids, oxygen, medications, and other treatments.

Fetal Scalp Stimulation

An indirect method used to evaluate fetal oxygenation and acid–base balance to identify fetal hypoxia is fetal scalp stimulation or vibroacoustic stimulation. If the fetus does not have adequate oxygen reserves, carbon dioxide builds up, leading to acidemia and hypoxemia. These metabolic states are reflected in abnormal FHR patterns as well as fetal inactivity. Fetal stimulation is performed to promote fetal movement with the hope that FHR accelerations will accompany the movement.

Fetal movement can be stimulated with a vibroacoustic stimulator (artificial larynx) applied to the woman's lower abdomen and turned on for 3 to 5 seconds to produce sound and vibration or by placing a gloved finger on the fetal scalp and applying firm pressure. A well-oxygenated fetus will respond when stimulated (tactile or by noise) by moving in conjunction with an acceleration of 15 bpm above the baseline heart rate that lasts at least 15 seconds. This FHR acceleration reflects a pH of more than 7 and a fetus with an intact CNS. Fetal scalp stimulation is not done if the fetus is preterm, or if the woman has an intrauterine infection, a diagnosis of placenta previa (which could lead to hemorrhage), or a fever (which increases the risk of an ascending infection) (King et al., 2015). If no acceleratory response by the fetus is exhibited with either scalp stimulation or vibroacoustic stimulation, further evaluation of the fetus is warranted.

Nurses play an essential role in the evaluation of maternal and fetal status during labor, continued surveillance, initiation of corrective measures when indicated, and reevaluation. A vital attribute of nursing surveillance is that it is a systematic process for assessment, intervention, and evaluation.

PROMOTING COMFORT AND PROVIDING PAIN MANAGEMENT DURING LABOR

Pain during labor is a universal experience, although the intensity of the pain may vary. Labor pain is unique to every woman based on various contributing physiologic, emotional, social, and cultural factors. Although labor and childbirth are viewed as natural processes, both can produce significant pain and discomfort. The physical causes of pain during labor include cervical stretching, hypoxia of the uterine muscle due to a decrease in perfusion during contractions, pressure on the urethra, bladder, and rectum, and distention of the muscles of the pelvic floor (Leonard, 2015).

Pain during labor is a physiological phenomenon. The etiology of pain during the first stage of labor is associated with ischemia of the uterus during contractions. In the second stage, pain is caused by the stretching of the vagina and perineum and compression of the pelvic structures. A woman's pain perception can be influenced by her previous experiences with pain, fatigue, pain anticipation, genetics, positive or negative support system, health care provider's presence and encouragement, labor and birth environment, cultural expectations, and level of emotional stress and anxiety. Pain perception during labor changes in intensity and nature as labor progresses, and this is associated with behavioral changes in the laboring woman (Liu, Fernando, & Mon, 2015).

The techniques used to manage the pain of labor vary according to geography and culture. For example, some Appalachian women believe that placing a hatchet or knife under the bed of a laboring woman may help "cut the pain of childbirth," and a woman from this background may wish to do so in the hospital setting (Bowers, 2015). Asian, Latino, and Orthodox Jewish women may request that their own mothers, not their husbands, attend their births; husbands do not actively participate in the birthing process. Cherokee, Hmong, and Japanese women will often remain quiet during labor and birth and not complain of pain because outwardly expressing pain is not appropriate in their cultures. Never interpret their quietness as freedom from pain. The concept of pain and pain expression during labor has different meanings for women of different cultures. Several points for the nurse to consider when caring for diverse cultural clients include using a qualified interpreter to communicate about pain as needed, offer and support culturally acceptable forms of pain relief, and assess for pain frequently (Wojnar & Narruhn, 2016).

Immigrating to a new country is a stressful process of readjustment and change. Effective verbal communication and understanding nonverbal social cues are invaluable when providing care to diverse cultures. Culturally diverse childbearing families present to the labor and birth suites with the same needs and desires of all families. Give them the same respect and sense of welcome shown to all families. Make sure they have a high-quality birth experience: uphold their religious, ethnic, and cultural values and integrate them into care.

Today, women have many safe nonpharmacologic and pharmacologic choices for the management of pain during labor and birth, which may be used separately or in combination with one another. Pharmacologic approaches are directed at eliminating the physical sensation of labor pain, whereas nonpharmacologic approaches are largely directed at prevention of suffering.

Nurses are in an ideal position to provide childbearing women with balanced, clear, concise information about effective nonpharmacologic and pharmacologic measures to relieve pain. Pain management standards issued by the Joint Commission mandate that pain be assessed in all clients admitted to a health care facility. Attention to the pain that occurs during labor and childbirth should be a priority of care for all nurses (Jones et al., 2015). A pain assessment tool named the *Coping with Labor Algorithm* uses the FOCUS format "Plan, Do, Check, and Act" cycle in laboring women. This tool provides a mechanism for pain documentation and links it to nursing care interventions (Roberts et al., 2010). Thus, it is important for nurses to be knowledgeable about the most recent scientific research on labor pain relief modalities, to make sure that accurate and unbiased information about effective pain relief measures is available to laboring women, to be sure that the woman determines what is an acceptable labor pain level for her, and to allow the woman the choice of pain relief method.

Nonpharmacologic Measures

Nonpharmacologic measures may include continuous labor support, hydrotherapy, hypnosis, ambulation and maternal position changes, transcutaneous electrical nerve stimulation (TENS), acupuncture and acupressure, attention focusing and imagery, therapeutic touch and massage, breathing techniques, and effleurage. Most of these methods are based on the *gate control theory of pain*, which proposes that local physical stimulation can interfere with pain stimuli by closing a hypothetical gate in the spinal cord, thus blocking pain signals from reaching the brain (McGeary, Swanholm, & Gatchel, 2015). It has long been a standard of care for labor nurses to first provide or encourage a variety of nonpharmacologic measures before moving to the pharmacologic interventions.

Nonpharmacologic measures are usually simple, safe, and inexpensive to use. Many of these measures are taught in childbirth classes, and women should be encouraged to try a variety of methods prior to the real labor. Many of the measures need to be practiced for best results and coordinated with the partner/coach. The nurse provides support and encouragement for the woman and her partner using nonpharmacologic methods. Although women cannot consciously direct the labor contractions, they can control how they respond to them, thereby enhancing their feelings of control. See Evidence-Based Practice 14.2 for more information.

Continuous Labor Support

Continuous labor support involves offering a sustained presence to the laboring woman by providing emotional support, comfort measures, advocacy, information and advice, and support for the partner. It is a non-pharmacologic, evidence-based strategy associated with reduced cesarean rates (Jackson & Gregory, 2015). A woman's family, a midwife, a nurse, a doula, or anyone else close to the woman can provide this continuous presence. A support person can assist the woman to ambulate, reposition herself, and use breathing techniques. A support person can also aid with the use of acupressure, massage, music therapy, or therapeutic touch. During the natural course of childbirth, a laboring woman's functional ability is limited secondary to pain, and she often has trouble making decisions. The support person can help make them based on his or her knowledge of the woman's birth plan and personal wishes.

Research has validated the value of continuous labor support versus intermittent support in terms of fewer operative deliveries, cesarean births, and requests for pain medication. Continuous labor support has shown to have beneficial effects on the mother and the newborn

EVIDENCE-BASED PRACTICE 14.2 — EFFECTIVENESS OF AROMATHERAPY AND BIOFEEDBACK IN PROMOTION OF LABOR OUTCOME DURING CHILDBIRTH AMONG PRIMIGRAVIDAS

STUDY

Labor pain is described as the most severe form of pain that every woman may experience during their lifetime. When considering labor analgesia, one is faced with a number of choices each with different advantages and disadvantages depending on the woman's expectations and preferences. Many women would like to avoid taking medications or invasive methods for pain management because of the potential negative impact on their fetus during labor. Severe pain triggers a stress response which may lead to harmful effects on both mother and fetus. The purpose of this study was to evaluate the effect of aromatherapy (essential oils from plants are massaged in the skin and inhaled) and biofeedback (mother was asked to experience both the fetal heart sound and variation in contractions and consciously regulate them) in promotion of labor outcome during childbirth.

Findings

Six hundred nulliparous women were selected randomly and assigned to an Aromatherapy group (n = 200), a biofeedback group (n = 200), or a control group (n = 200). The researchers rated pain by using a visual pain analog scale during their labors. Sixty nine percent of cases in the aromatherapy group expressed it was helpful, provided pain relief and emotional well-being during their labors. Biofeedback was also effective in reducing pain and duration of labor during childbirth compared with the control group.

Nursing Implications

The results of this study indicated that the use of Aromatherapy and Biofeedback, as non-pharmacologic methods were both effective methods of reducing pain perception and duration of labor among women during labor. As a non-pharmacologic nursing intervention, these are easy to administer, cost effective, harmless and appealing to the mother without any apparent maternal or neonatal adverse effects.

Adopted from Janula, R., & Mahipal, S. (2015). Effectiveness of aromatherapy and biofeedback in promotion of labor outcome during childbirth among primigravidas. *Health Science Journal, 9*(1), 1–5.

primarily due to the reduction in anxiety during the laboring experience. Most women expressed greater satisfaction with their childbirth experience (Iravani et al., 2015).

Take Note!

The human presence is of immeasurable value to make the laboring woman feel secure.

Hydrotherapy

Hydrotherapy is a nonpharmacologic measure that may involve showering or soaking in a regular tub or whirlpool bath. When showering is the selected method of hydrotherapy, the woman stands or sits in a shower chair in a warm shower and allows the water to gently glide over her abdomen and back. If a tub or whirlpool is chosen, the woman immerses herself in warm water for relaxation and relief of discomfort. When the woman enters the warm water, the warmth and buoyancy help to release muscle tension and can impart a sense of well-being (Taghavi, Barband, & Khaki, 2015). Warm water provides soothing stimulation of nerves in the skin, promoting vasodilation, reversal of sympathetic nervous response, and a reduction in catecholamines (Dalal, 2015). Contractions are usually less painful in warm water because the warmth and buoyancy of the water have a relaxing effect. Recent research findings reported that women who used hydrotherapy had significantly reduced surgical birth rates, a shorter second stage of labor, reduced analgesic requirements, and a lower incidence of perineal trauma (Taghavi, Barband, & Khaki, 2015). The research concluded that hydrotherapy during labor significantly aids the labor process, minimizes the use of analgesic medications, offers fast- and short-acting pain and anxiety relief, and should he considered as a safe and effective birthing aid (Taghavi, Barband, & Khaki, 2015).

A wide range of hydrotherapy options are available, from ordinary bathtubs to whirlpool baths and showers, combined with low lighting and music. Many hospitals provide showers and whirlpool baths for laboring women for pain relief. However, hydrotherapy is more commonly practiced in birthing centers managed by midwives. The recommendation for initiating hydrotherapy is that the woman be in active labor (more than 5 cm dilated) to prevent the slowing of labor contractions secondary to muscular relaxation. The woman's membranes can be intact or ruptured. Women are encouraged to stay in the bath or shower as long as they feel they are comfortable. The water temperature should not exceed body temperature.

Hydrotherapy is an effective pain management option for many women. Women who are experiencing a healthy pregnancy can be offered this option. The potential risks associated with hydrotherapy including hyperthermia, hypothermia, changes in maternal heart rate, fetal tachycardia, and unplanned underwater birth. The benefits include reducing pain, relieving anxiety, and promoting a sense of control during labor (Nutter, 2016).

Ambulation and Position Changes

Ambulation and position changes during labor are another extremely useful comfort measure. Historically, women adopted a variety of positions during labor, rarely using the recumbent position until during the first half of the twentieth century. The medical profession has favored recumbent positions during labor, but without evidence to demonstrate their appropriateness. A recent Cochrane database systematic review reported there is evidence that walking and upright positions in the first stage of labor reduce the length of labor and do not seem to be associated with increased intervention or negative effects on mothers' and babies' well-being.

In an upright posture, gravity directs the weight of the fetus and amniotic fluid downwards, successively dilating the cervix and the birth canal. Uterine contractions have been shown to be better spaced, stronger and more efficient in dilating the cervix when the mother is in an upright position than when she is supine (Cox & King, 2015). Women should be encouraged to take up whatever position they find most comfortable in the first stage of labor (Cheng & Caughey, 2015a).

Changing position frequently (every 30 minutes or so)—sitting, walking, kneeling, standing, lying down, getting on hands and knees, and using a birthing ball—helps relieve pain (Fig. 14.9). Position changes also may help to speed labor by adding the benefits of gravity and

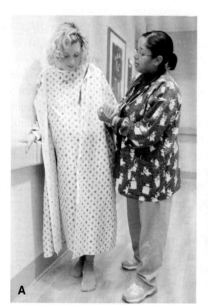
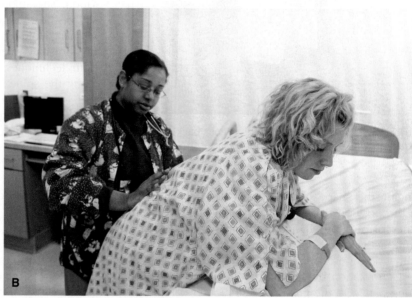
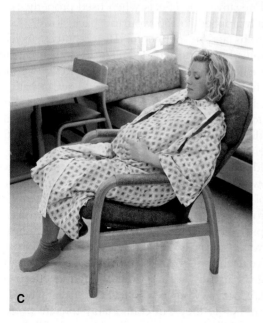
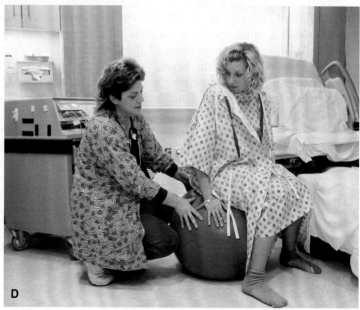

FIGURE 14.9 Various positions for use during labor. **A.** Ambulation. **B.** Leaning forward. **C.** Sitting in a chair. **D.** Using a birthing ball.

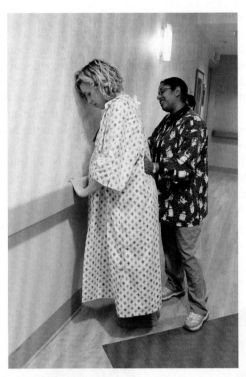

FIGURE 14.10 Nurse massaging the client's back during a contraction while she ambulates during labor.

changing the shape of the pelvis. Research has found that the position that the woman assumes and the frequency of position changes have a profound effect on uterine activity and efficiency. Allowing the woman to obtain a position of comfort frequently facilitates a favorable fetal rotation by altering the alignment of the presenting part with the pelvis. As the mother continues to change position based on comfort, the optimal presentation is afforded (King et al., 2015). Supine positions should be avoided, since they may interfere with labor progress and can cause compression of the vena cava and decrease blood return to the heart.

Swaying from side to side, rocking, or other rhythmic movements may also be comforting. If labor is progressing slowly, ambulating may speed it up again. Upright positions such as walking, kneeling forward, or doing the lunge on the birthing ball give most women a greater sense of control and active movement than just lying down. Table 14.2 highlights some of the more common positions that can be used during labor and birth.

Acupuncture and Acupressure

Acupuncture and acupressure can be used to relieve pain during labor. Although controlled research studies of these methods are limited, there is adequate evidence that both are useful in relieving pain associated with labor and birth. However, both methods require a trained, certified clinician, and such a person is not available in many birth facilities (Halpern & Garg, 2015).

Acupuncture involves stimulating key trigger points with needles. This form of Chinese medicine has been practiced for approximately 3,000 years. Classical Chinese teaching holds that throughout the body there are meridians or channels of energy (*qi*) that when in balance regulate body functions. Pain reflects an imbalance or obstruction of the flow of energy. The purpose of acupuncture is to restore thus diminishing pain (Adams et al., 2015). Stimulating the trigger points causes the release of endorphins, reducing the perception of pain.

Acupressure involves the application of a firm finger or massage used in acupuncture to reduce the pain sensation. The amount of pressure is important. The intensity of the pressure is determined by the needs of the woman. Holding and squeezing the hand of a woman in labor may trigger the point most commonly used for both techniques. Some acupressure points are found along the spine, neck, shoulder, toes, and soles of the feet. Pressure along the side of the spine can help relieve back pain during labor (Fig. 14.10) (Mollart, Adam, & Foureur, 2015). A Cochrane collaboration review found that acupuncture may indeed reduce labor pain, increasing satisfaction with pain management and reduced use of pharmacologic management. However, there is a need for further research (Simkin & Klein, 2015).

Application of Heat and Cold

Superficial applications of heat and/or cold, in various forms, are popular with laboring women. They are easy to use, inexpensive, require no prior practice, and have minimal negative side effects when used properly. Heat is typically applied to the woman's back, lower abdomen, groin, and/or perineum. Heat sources include a hot water bottle, heated rice-filled sock, warm compress (washcloth soaked in warm water and wrung out), electric heating pad, warm blanket, and warm bath or shower. In addition to being used for pain relief, heat is used to relieve chills or trembling, decrease joint stiffness, reduce muscle spasm, and increase connective tissue extensibility (Liu, Fernando, & Mon, 2015).

Cold therapy, or cryotherapy, is usually applied on the woman's back, chest, and/or face during labor. Forms of cold include a bag or surgical glove filled with ice, a frozen gel pack, camper's "ice," a hollow, plastic rolling pin or bottle filled with ice, a washcloth dipped in cold water, soda cans chilled in ice, and even a frozen bag of vegetables. "Instant" cold packs, often available in hospitals, usually are not cold enough to effectively relieve labor pain. Women who feel cold usually need to feel warm before they can comfortably tolerate using a cold pack. Chilled soda cans and rolling pins filled with ice give the added benefit of mechanical pressure when

TABLE 14.2	COMMON POSITIONS FOR USE DURING LABOR AND BIRTH
Standing	• Takes advantage of gravity during and between contractions • Makes contractions feel less painful and be more productive • Helps fetus line up with angle of maternal pelvis • Helps to increase urge to push in second stage of labor
Walking	• Has the same advantages as standing • Causes changes in the pelvic joints, helping the fetus move through the birth canal
Standing and leaning forward on partner, bed, birthing ball	• Has the same advantages as standing • Is a good position for a backrub • May feel more restful than standing • Can be used with electronic fetal monitor
Slow dancing (standing with woman's arms around partner's neck, head resting on his chest or shoulder, with his hands rubbing woman's lower back; sway to music and breathe in rhythm if it helps)	• Has the same advantages as walking • Back pressure helps relieve back pain • Rhythm and music help woman relax and provide comfort
The lunge (standing facing a straight chair with one foot on the seat with knee and foot to the side; bending raised knee and hip, and lunging sideways repeatedly during a contraction, holding each lunge for 5 seconds; partner holds chair and helps with balance)	• Widens one side of the pelvis (the side toward lunge) • Encourages rotation of baby • Can also be done in a kneeling position
Sitting upright	• Helps promote rest • Has more gravity advantage than lying down • Can be used with electronic fetal monitor
Semi-sitting (setting the head of the bed at a 45-degree angle with pillows used for support)	• Has the same advantages as sitting upright • Is an easy position if on a bed
Sitting on toilet or commode	• Has the same advantages as sitting upright • May help relax the perineum for effective bearing down
Rocking in a chair	• Has the same advantages as sitting upright • May help speed labor (rocking movement)
Sitting, leaning forward with support	• Has the same advantages as sitting upright • Is a good position for a backrub
On all fours, on hands and knees	• Helps relieve backache • Assists rotation of baby in posterior position • Allows for pelvic rocking and body movement • Relieves pressure on hemorrhoids • Allows for vaginal examinations • Is sometimes preferred as a pushing position by women with back labor
Kneeling, leaning forward with support on a chair seat, the raised head of the bed, or on a birthing ball	• Has the same advantages as all-fours position • Puts less strain on wrists and hands
Side-lying	• Is a very good position for resting and convenient for many kinds of medical interventions • Helps lower elevated blood pressure • May promote progress of labor when alternated with walking • Is useful to slow a very rapid second stage • Avoids vena cava syndrome • May offer increased control of pushing efforts • Takes pressure off hemorrhoids • Facilitates relaxation between contractions

(continued)

TABLE 14.2	COMMON POSITIONS FOR USE DURING LABOR AND BIRTH (continued)
Squatting	• May relieve backache • Takes advantage of gravity • Requires less bearing-down effort • Widens pelvic outlet by approximately 28% • Pressure is evenly distributed to the perineum, reducing the need for episiotomy • May help fetus turn and move down in a difficult birth • Helps if the woman feels no urge to push • Allows freedom to shift weight for comfort • Offers an advantage when pushing, since upper trunk presses on the top of the uterus
Supported squat (leaning back against partner, who supports woman under the arms and takes the entire woman's weight; standing up between contractions)	• Requires great strength in partner • Lengthens trunk, allowing more room for fetus to maneuver into position • Lets gravity help
Dangle (partner sitting high on bed or counter with feet supported on chairs or footrests and thighs spread; woman leaning back between partner's legs, placing flexed arms over partner's thighs; partner gripping sides with his thighs; woman lowering herself and allowing partner to support her full weight; standing up between contractions)	• Has the same advantages of a supported squat • Requires less physical strength from the partner

Adapted from Gizzo, S., Di Gangi, S., Noventa, M., Bacile, V., Zambon, A., & Nardelli, B. (2014). Women's choice of positions during labor: Return to the past or a modern way to give birth? A cohort study in Italy. *BioMed Research International, 2014*, 638093, doi: http://dx.doi.org/10.1155/2014/638093; Hanson, L., & VandeVusse, L., (2014). Supporting labor progress toward physiologic birth. *Journal of Perinatal & Neonatal Nursing, 28*(2), 101–107; and Magowan, B., Owen, P., & Thomson, A. (2014). *Clinical obstetrics & gynecology* (3rd ed.). St. Louis, MO: Saunders Elsevier.

rolled on the low back. Cold has the additional effects of relieving muscle spasms and reducing inflammation and edema (Tharpe, Farley, & Jordan, 2016).

To date, no randomized controlled studies have evaluated the use of heat and cold, so further study is needed to determine if either approach is efficacious. With appropriate safety precautions, heat and cold offer comfort and relief, and their use should be dictated by the desires and responses of the laboring woman.

Attention Focusing and Imagery

Attention focusing and imagery use many of the senses and the mind to focus on stimuli. The woman can focus on tactile stimuli such as touch, massage, or stroking. She may focus on auditory stimuli such as music, humming, or verbal encouragement. Visual stimuli might be any object in the room, or the woman can imagine the beach, a mountaintop, a happy memory, or even the contractions of the uterine muscle pulling the cervix open and the fetus pressing downward to open the cervix. Some women focus on a particular mental activity such as a song, a chant, counting backwards, or a Bible verse. Breathing, relaxation, positive thinking, and positive visualization work well for mothers in labor. The use of these techniques keeps the sensory input perceived during the contraction from reaching the pain center in the cortex of the brain (Capogna, 2015a).

Effleurage and Massage

Effleurage is a light, stroking, superficial touch of the abdomen, in rhythm with breathing during contractions. It is used as a relaxation and distraction technique from discomfort. External fetal monitor belts may interfere with the ability to accomplish this.

Effleurage and massage use the sense of touch to promote relaxation and pain relief. Massage works as a form of pain relief by increasing the production of endorphins in the body. Endorphins reduce the transmission of signals between nerve cells and thus lower the perception of pain. Because touch receptors go to the brain faster than pain receptors, massage—anywhere on the body—can block the pain message to the brain. In addition, light touch has been found to release endorphins and induce a relaxed state. In addition, touching and massage distract the woman from discomfort. Massage involves manipulation of the body's soft tissues. It is commonly used to help relax tense muscles and to soothe and calm the individual. Massage may help to relieve pain by assisting with relaxation, inhibiting sensory transmission in the pain pathways, or improving blood flow and oxygenation of tissues (Neetu & Panchal, 2015).

Breathing Techniques

Conscious use of breath by the woman has the power to profoundly influence her labor and how she engages with it. The first action anyone takes in any situation is a breath. The breath affects the lungs, immediately cueing the nervous system. The nervous system responds by sending messages, which impact our entire psychophysiologic system. Messages sent from the nervous system affect us physically, emotionally, and mentally. If we alter how we breathe, we alter the constellation of messages and reactions in our entire mind–body experience (Cheng & Caughey, 2015a).

Breathing techniques are effective in producing relaxation and pain relief through the use of distraction. If the woman is concentrating on slow-paced rhythmic breathing, she is not likely to fully focus on contraction pain. Breathing techniques are often taught in childbirth education classes (see Chapter 12 for additional information).

Controlled breathing helps reduce the pain experienced by using stimulus–response conditioning. The woman selects a focal point within her environment to stare at during the first sign of a contraction. This focus creates a visual stimulus that goes directly to her brain. The woman takes a deep cleansing breath, which is followed by rhythmic breathing. Verbal commands from her partner supply an ongoing auditory stimulus to her brain. Benefits of practicing patterned breathing include: breathing

- becomes an automatic response to pain.
- increases relaxation and can be used for deal with life's everyday stresses.
- is calming during labor.
- provides a sense of well-being and a measure of control.
- brings purpose to each contraction, making them more productive.
- provides more oxygen for the mother and fetus (American Pregnancy Association, 2015).

Many couples learn patterned-paced breathing during their childbirth education classes. Three levels may be taught, each beginning and ending with a cleansing breath or sigh after each contraction. In the first pattern, also known as slow-paced breathing, the woman inhales slowly through her nose and exhales through pursed lips. The breathing rate is typically 6 to 9 bpm. In the second pattern, the woman inhales and exhales through her mouth at a rate of four breaths every 5 seconds. The rate can be accelerated to two breaths per second to assist her to relax. The third pattern is similar to the second pattern except that the breathing is punctuated every few breaths by a forceful exhalation through pursed lips. All breaths are kept equal and rhythmic and can increase as contractions increase in intensity (Lindholm & Hildingsson, 2015).

Many childbirth educators do not recommend specific breathing techniques or try to teach parents to breathe the "right" way during labor and birth. Couples are encouraged to find breathing styles that enhance their relaxation and use them. There are numerous benefits to controlled and rhythmic breathing in childbirth (outlined previously), and many women choose these techniques to manage their discomfort during labor.

Pharmacologic Measures

With varying degrees of success, generations of women have sought ways to relieve the pain of childbirth. Pharmacologic pain relief during labor includes systemic analgesia and regional or local anesthesia. Women have seen dramatic changes in pharmacologic pain management options over the years. Methods have evolved from biting down on a stick to control their pain, experiencing 'twilight sleep' during their labors and not remembering what happened, to a more complex pharmacologic approach such as epidural/intrathecal analgesia. Systemic analgesia and regional analgesia/anesthesia have become less common, while newer neuraxial analgesia/anesthesia techniques involving minimal motor blockade have become more popular. **Neuraxial analgesia/anesthesia** is the administration of analgesic (opioids) or anesthetic (capable of producing a loss of sensation in an area of the body) agents, either continuously or intermittently, into the epidural or intrathecal space to relieve pain. Low-dose and ultra-low-dose epidural analgesia, spinal analgesia, and combined spinal–epidural analgesia have replaced the traditional epidural for labor. Neuraxial analgesia does not interfere with the progress or outcome of labor. There is no need to withhold neuraxial analgesia until the active stage of labor (Grant et al., 2015). This shift in pain management techniques allows a woman to be an active participant in labor.

Take Note!

Regardless of which approach is used during labor, the woman has the right to choose the methods of pain control that will best suit her and meet her needs.

Systemic Analgesia

Systemic analgesia involves the use of one or more drugs administered orally, intramuscularly, or intravenously; they become distributed throughout the body via the circulatory system. Depending on which administration method is used, the therapeutic effect of pain relief can occur within minutes and last for several hours. The most important complication associated with the use of this class of drugs is respiratory depression. Therefore, women given these drugs require careful monitoring.

Opioids given close to the time of birth can cause CNS depression in the newborn, necessitating the administration of naloxone (Narcan) to reverse the depressant effects of the opioids.

Several drug categories may be used for systemic analgesia:

- *Opioids*, such as butorphanol (Stadol), nalbuphine (Nubain), meperidine (Demerol), morphine, or fentanyl (Sublimaze)
- *Ataractics*, such as hydroxyzine (Vistaril), promethazine (Phenergan), or prochlorperazine (Compazine)

- *Benzodiazepines*, such as diazepam (Valium) or midazolam (Versed)

Drug Guide 14.1 highlights some of the major drugs used for systemic analgesia.

Systemic analgesics are typically administered parenterally, usually through an existing intravenous line. Nearly all medications given during labor cross the placenta and have a depressant effect on the fetus; therefore, it is important for the woman to receive the least amount of systemic medication that relieves her discomfort so

DRUG GUIDE 14.1 COMMON AGENTS USED FOR SYSTEMIC ANALGESIA

Type	Drug	Comments
Opioids	Morphine 2–5 mg IV	May be given IV or epidurally Rapidly crosses the placenta, causes a decrease in FHR variability Can cause maternal and neonatal CNS depression Decreases uterine contractions
	Meperidine (Demerol) 25–75 mg IV	May be given IV, intrathecally, or epidurally with maximal fetal uptake 2–3 hr after administration Can cause CNS depression Decreases fetal variability
	Butorphanol (Stadol) 1–2 mg IV Q 2–4 hr	Is given IV Is rapidly transferred across the placenta Causes neonatal respiratory depression
	Nalbuphine (Nubain) 10–20 mg IV	Is given IV Causes less maternal nausea and vomiting Causes decreased FHR variability, fetal bradycardia, and respiratory depression
	Fentanyl (Sublimaze) 50–100 mcg IV	Is given IV or epidurally Can cause maternal hypotension, maternal and fetal respiratory depression Rapidly crosses placenta
Antiemetics	Hydroxyzine (Vistaril) 50–100 mg IM	Does not relieve pain but reduces anxiety and potentiates opioid analgesic effects; cannot be given IV Is used to decrease nausea and vomiting
	Promethazine (Phenergan) 25–50 mg IV or IM	Is used for antiemetic effect when combined with opioids Causes sedation and reduces apprehension May contribute to maternal hypotension and neonatal depression
	Prochlorperazine (Compazine) 5–10 mg IV or IM	Frequently given with morphine sulfate for sleep during prolonged latent phase; counteracts the nausea that opioids can produce
Benzodiazepines	Diazepam (Valium) 2–5 mg IV	Is given to enhance pain relief of opioid and cause sedation May be used to stop eclamptic seizures Decreases nausea and vomiting Can cause newborn depression; therefore, lowest possible dose should be used
	Midazolam (Versed) 1–5 mg IV	Is not used for analgesic but amnesia effect Is used as adjunct for anesthesia Is excreted in breast milk

IV, intravenous.
Adapted from Cheng, Y., & Caughey, A. B. (2015a). *Normal labor and delivery.* Retrieved from http://emedicine.medscape.com/article/260036-overview#aw2aab6b2; King, T.L., Brucker, M.C., Kriebs, J. M., Fahey, J. O., Gegor, C. L., & Varney, H. (2015) *Varney's midwifery* (5th ed.). Burlington, MA: Jones & Bartlett Learning; and Skidmore-Roth, L. (2015). *Mosby's 2015 nursing drug reference* (28th ed.). St. Louis, MO: Mosby Elsevier.

that it does not cause any harm to the fetus (Cheng & Caughey, 2015a). Historically opioids have been administered by nurses, but in the past decade there has been increasing use of client-controlled intravenous analgesia (patient-controlled analgesia). With this system, the woman is given a button connected to a computerized pump on the intravenous line. When the woman desires analgesia, she presses the button and the pump delivers a preset amount of medication. This system provides the woman with a sense of control over her own pain management and active participation in the childbirth process.

OPIOIDS

Opioids are morphine-like medications that are most effective for the relief of moderate to severe pain. Opioids typically are administered intravenously. All opioids are lipophilic and cross the placental barrier, but do not affect labor progress in the active phase. Opioids are associated with newborn respiratory depression, decreased alertness, inhibited sucking, and a delay in effective feeding (King et al., 2015).

Opioids decrease the transmission of pain impulses by binding to receptor site pathways that transmit the pain signals to the brain. The effect is increased tolerance to pain and respiratory depression related to a decrease in sensitivity to carbon dioxide (Skidmore-Roth, 2015). All opioids are considered good analgesics. However, respiratory depression can occur in the mother and fetus depending on the dose given. They may also cause a decrease in FHR variability identified on the fetal monitor strip. This FHR pattern change is usually transient. Other systemic side effects include nausea, vomiting, pruritus, delayed gastric emptying, drowsiness, hypoventilation, and newborn depression. To reduce the incidence of newborn depression, birth should occur within 1 hour or after 4 hours of administration to prevent the fetus from receiving the peak concentration (Cheng & Caughey, 2015a).

A recent study reported that parenteral opioids provide some relief from pain in labor, but are associated with neonatal respiratory distress. Maternal satisfaction with opioid analgesia appeared moderate at best (Kerr, Taylor, & Evans, 2015).

Opioid antagonists such as naloxone (Narcan) are given to reverse the effects of the CNS depression, including respiratory depression, caused by opioids. Opioid antagonists also are used to reverse the side effects of neuraxial opioids, such as pruritus, urinary retention, nausea, and vomiting, without significantly decreasing analgesia (Skidmore-Roth, 2015). Consult a current drug guide for more specifics on these drug categories.

ANTIEMETICS

The antiemetic group of medications is used in combination with an opioid to decrease nausea and vomiting and lessen anxiety. These adjunct drugs potentiate the effectiveness of the opioid so that a lesser dose can be given. They may also be used to increase sedation. Promethazine (Phenergan) can be given intravenously, but hydroxyzine (Vistaril) must be given by mouth or by intramuscular injection into a large muscle mass. Neither drug affects the progress of labor, but either may cause a decrease in FHR variability and possible newborn depression (Skidmore-Roth, 2015). Prochlorperazine (Compazine) is typically given intravenously or intramuscularly with morphine sulfate for sleep during a prolonged latent phase. It counteracts the nausea associated with opioids (King et al., 2015).

BENZODIAZEPINES

Benzodiazepines are used for minor tranquilizing and sedative effects. Diazepam (Valium) also is given intravenously to stop seizures resulting from eclampsia. It can be administered to calm a woman who is out of control, thereby enabling her to relax enough so that she can participate effectively during her labor process rather than fighting against it. Lorazepam (Ativan) can also be used for its tranquilizing effect, but increased sedation is experienced with this medication (Skidmore-Roth, 2015). Midazolam (Versed), also given intravenously, produces good amnesia but no analgesia. It is most commonly used as an adjunct for anesthesia. Diazepam and midazolam cause CNS depression for both the woman and the newborn.

Inhaled Analgesics

Nitrous oxide is known by most people as "laughing gas." For labor pain, half nitrous oxide gas (50%) is mixed with half oxygen (50%) and breathed through a mask or mouthpiece. This has been recently introduced in the United States, but has been in widespread use in Europe and Canada for many years. Women have generally reported satisfaction with the use of nitrous oxide for pain relief in labor. An additional factor that may contribute to the decreased perception of pain is maternal control—it is self-administered. Self-administration is not only empowering for women, but it also acts as a safety mechanism because it is almost impossible to overdose when it is self-administered (Halpern & Garg, 2015). Potential side effects of N_2O/O_2 include nausea and vomiting, dizziness, and dysphoria, although these are rare. No FHR abnormalities have been attributed to its use (Badve & Vallejo, 2015).

Regional Analgesia/Anesthesia

Regional analgesia/anesthesia provides pain relief without loss of consciousness. It involves the use of local anesthetic agents, with or without added opioids, to bring about pain relief or numbness through the drug's effects on the spinal cord and nerve roots. Obstetric regional analgesia generally refers to a partial or complete loss of pain sensation below the T8 to T10 level of the spinal cord (Stocks & Griffiths, 2015).

The routes for regional pain relief include epidural block, combined spinal–epidural, local infiltration, pudendal block, and intrathecal (spinal) analgesia/anesthesia. Local and pudendal routes are used during birth for episiotomies (surgical incision into the perineum to facilitate birth); epidural and intrathecal routes are used for pain relief during active labor and birth. The major advantage of regional pain management techniques is that the woman can participate in the birthing process and still have good pain control.

EPIDURAL ANALGESIA

Women requesting epidural analgesia in labor will do so when they feel they need pain relief, and for some it might be quite early in their labor. Epidural analgesia for labor and birth involves the injection of a local anesthetic agent (e.g., lidocaine or bupivacaine) and an opioid analgesic agent (e.g., morphine or fentanyl) into the lumbar epidural space. A small catheter is then passed through the epidural needle to provide continuous access to the epidural space for maintenance of analgesia throughout labor and birth (Fig. 14.11). Epidural analgesia does increase the duration of the second stage of labor and may increase the rate of instrument-assisted vaginal deliveries as well as that of oxytocin administration (Camorcia, 2015). Approximately 60% of laboring women in the United States receive an epidural for pain

relief during labor, but one in eight women who have an epidural during labor still need to use other methods of pain relief In urban areas, many hospitals approach 90% use of epidurals (Capogna, 2015b).

An epidural involves the injection of a drug into the epidural space, which is located outside the dura mater between the dura and the spinal canal. The epidural space is typically entered through the third and fourth lumbar vertebrae with a needle, and a catheter is threaded into the epidural space. An epidural can be used for both vaginal and cesarean births. It has evolved from a regional block producing total loss of sensation to analgesia with minimal blockade. The effectiveness of epidural analgesia depends on the technique and medications used. Theoretically, epidural local anesthetics could block all labor pain if used in large volumes and high concentrations. However, pain relief is balanced against other goals such as walking during the first stage of labor, pushing effectively in the second stage, and minimizing maternal and fetal side effects.

An epidural is contraindicated for women with a previous history of spinal surgery or spinal abnormalities, coagulation defects cardiac disease, obesity, infections, and hypovolemia. It also is contraindicated for the woman who is receiving anticoagulation therapy.

Complications include nausea and vomiting, hypotension, fever, pruritus, intravascular injection, maternal fever, allergic reaction, and respiratory depression. Effects on the fetus during labor include fetal distress secondary to maternal hypotension (Ibrahim et al., 2015). Ensuring

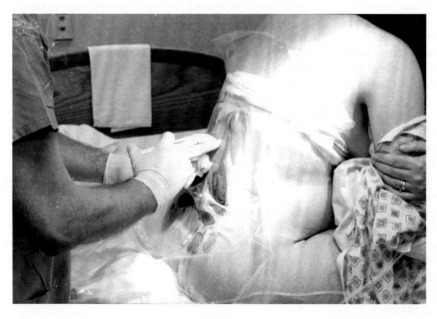

A

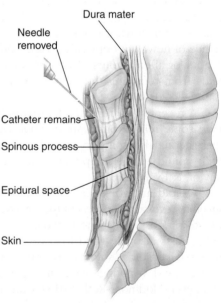

B

FIGURE 14.11 Epidural catheter insertion. **A.** A needle is inserted into the epidural space. **B.** A catheter is threaded into the epidural space; the needle is then removed. The catheter allows medication to be administered intermittently or continuously to relieve pain during labor and childbirth.

that the woman avoids a supine position after an epidural catheter has been placed will help to minimize hypotension.

The addition of opioids, such as fentanyl or morphine, to the local anesthetic helps decrease the amount of motor block obtained. Continuous infusion pumps can be used to administer the epidural analgesia, allowing the woman to be in control and administer a bolus dose on demand (Patkar et al., 2015).

COMBINED SPINAL–EPIDURAL ANALGESIA

Another epidural technique is combined spinal–epidural (CSE) analgesia. This technique involves inserting the epidural needle into the epidural space and subsequently inserting a small-gauge spinal needle through the epidural needle into the subarachnoid space. An opioid, without a local anesthetic, is injected into this space. The spinal needle is then removed and an epidural catheter is inserted for later use.

CSE is advantageous because of its rapid onset of pain relief (within 3 to 5 minutes) that can last up to 3 hours. It also allows the woman's motor function to remain active. Her ability to bear down during the second stage of labor is preserved because the pushing reflex is not lost, and her motor power remains intact. The CSE technique provides greater flexibility and reliability for labor than either spinal or epidural analgesia alone (Stocks & Griffiths, 2015). When compared with traditional epidural or spinal analgesia, which often keeps the woman lying in bed, CSE allows her to ambulate ("walking epidural"). A recent Cochrane review contrasting the CSE analgesia approach with traditional and low-dose epidural analgesia in labor identified that CSE analgesia was associated with a greater incidence of pruritus, but a lower incidence of urinary retention and need for rescue analgesia, than epidural along. In addition, CSE analgesia had a faster onset of pain relief, and there were no differences in labor outcomes (Heesen et al., 2015). Ambulating during labor provides several benefits: it may help control pain better, shorten the first stage of labor, increase the intensity of the contractions, and decrease the possibility of an operative vaginal or cesarean birth.

Although women can walk with CSE, they often choose not to because of sedation and fatigue. Often health care providers do not encourage or assist women to ambulate for fear of injury. Nurses need to evaluate for ambulation safety that includes no postural hypotension and normal leg strength by demonstrating a partial knee bend while standing; they also need to assist with ambulation at all times (Capogna, 2015b). Currently, anesthesiologists are performing walking epidurals using continuous infusion techniques as well as CSE and client-controlled epidural analgesia (Grant et al., 2015).

Complications include maternal hypotension, intravascular injection, accidental intrathecal blockade, postdural puncture headache, pruitis, inadequate or failed

block, maternal fever, and pruritus. Hypotension and associated FHR changes are managed with maternal positioning (semi-Fowler's position), intravenous hydration, and supplemental oxygen (Ibrahim et al., 2015).

PATIENT-CONTROLLED EPIDURAL ANALGESIA

Patient-controlled epidural analgesia (PCEA) involves the use of an indwelling epidural catheter with an infusion of medication and a programmed pump that allows the woman to control the dosing. This method allows the woman to have a sense of control over her pain and reach her own individually acceptable analgesia level. When compared with traditional epidural analgesia, PCEA provides equivalent analgesia with lower anesthetic use, lower rates of supplementation, and higher client satisfaction (Van De Velde, 2015).

With PCEA, the woman uses a handheld device connected to an analgesic agent that is attached to an

Consider This

When I was expecting my first child, I was determined to put my best foot forward and do everything right. I was an experienced OB nurse, and in my mind doing everything right was expected behavior. I was already 2 weeks past my calculated due date and I was becoming increasingly worried. That particular day I went to work with a backache but felt no contractions.

I managed to finish my shift but felt completely wiped out. As I walked to my car outside the hospital, my water broke and I felt the warm fluid run down my legs. I went back inside to be admitted for this much-awaited event.

Although I had helped thousands of women go through their childbirth experience, I was now the one in the bed and not standing alongside it. My husband and I had practiced our breathing techniques to cope with the discomfort of labor, but this "discomfort" in my mind was more than I could tolerate. So despite my best intentions of doing everything right, within an hour I begged for a painkiller to ease the pain. While the medication took the edge off my pain, I still felt every contraction and truly now appreciate the meaning of the word "labor." Although I wanted to use natural childbirth without any medication, I know that I was a full participant in my son's birthing experience, and that is what "doing everything right" was for me!

Thoughts: *Doing what is right varies for each individual, and as nurses we need to support whatever that is. Having a positive outcome from the childbirth experience is the goal; the means it takes to achieve it is less important. How can nurses support women in making their personal choices to achieve a healthy outcome? Are any women "failures" if they ask for pain medication to tolerate labor? How can nurses help women overcome this stigma of being a "wimp"?*

epidural catheter. When she pushes the button, a bolus dose of agent is administered via the catheter to reduce her pain. This method allows her to manage her pain at will without having to ask a staff member to provide pain relief. Evidence supports the use of PCEA which appears to result in greater maternal satisfaction and lower overall medication use (Sng et al., 2015).

LOCAL INFILTRATION

Local infiltration involves the injection of a local anesthetic, such as lidocaine, into the superficial perineal nerves to numb the perineal area. This technique is done by the physician or midwife just before performing an episiotomy or before suturing a laceration. Local infiltration does not alter the pain of uterine contractions, but it does numb the immediate area of the episiotomy or laceration. Local infiltration does not cause side effects for the woman or her newborn.

PUDENDAL NERVE BLOCK

A pudendal nerve block refers to the injection of a local anesthetic agent (e.g., bupivacaine, ropivacaine) into the pudendal nerves near each ischial spine. It provides pain relief in the lower vagina, vulva, and perineum (Fig. 14.12).

A pudendal block is used for the second stage of labor, an episiotomy, or an operative vaginal birth with outlet forceps or vacuum extractor. It must be

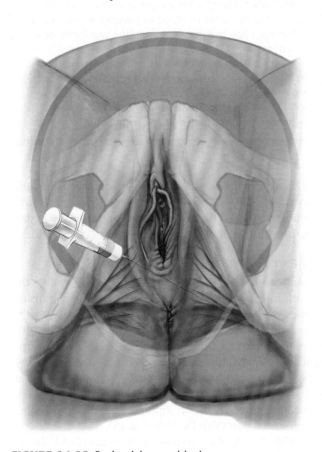

FIGURE 14.12 Pudendal nerve block.

administered about 15 minutes before it would be needed to ensure its full effect. A transvaginal approach is generally used to inject an anesthetic agent at or near the pudendal nerve branch. Neither maternal nor fetal complications are common.

SPINAL (INTRATHECAL) ANALGESIA/ANESTHESIA

The spinal (intrathecal) pain management technique involves injection of an anesthetic "caine" agent, with or without opioids, into the subarachnoid space to provide pain relief during labor or cesarean birth. The subarachnoid space is a fluid-filled area located between the dura mater and the spinal cord. Spinal anesthesia is frequently used for elective and emergent cesarean births. The contraindications are similar to those for an epidural block. Adverse reactions for the woman include hypotension and spinal headache.

The subarachnoid injection of opioids alone, a technique termed intrathecal narcotics, has been gaining popularity since it was introduced in the 1980s. A narcotic is injected into the subarachnoid space, providing rapid pain relief while still maintaining motor function and sensation (Sng, Kwok, & Sia, 2015). An intrathecal narcotic is given during the active phase (more than 5 cm of dilation) of labor. Compared with epidural blocks, intrathecal narcotics are easy to administer, require a smaller volume of medication, produce excellent muscular relaxation, provide rapid-onset pain relief, are less likely to cause newborn respiratory depression, and do not cause motor blockade (Badve & Vallejo, 2015). Although pain relief is rapid with this technique, it is limited by the narcotic's duration of action, which may be only a few hours and not last through the labor. Additional pain measures may be needed to sustain pain management.

General Anesthesia

General anesthesia is typically reserved for emergency cesarean births when there is not enough time to provide spinal or epidural anesthesia or if the woman has a contraindication to the use of regional anesthesia. It can be started quickly and causes a rapid loss of consciousness. General anesthesia can be administered by intravenous injection, inhalation of anesthetic agents, or both. Commonly, thiopental, a short-acting barbiturate, or propofol is given intravenously to produce unconsciousness. This is followed by administration of a muscle relaxant. After the woman is intubated, nitrous oxide and oxygen are administered. A volatile halogenated agent may also be administered to produce amnesia (Cheng & Caughey, 2015a).

All anesthetic agents cross the placenta and affect the fetus. The primary complication with general anesthesia is fetal depression, along with uterine relaxation and potential maternal vomiting and aspiration. General anesthesia complications are usually due to maternal aspiration or the inability to intubate the woman. The incidence of these complications has decreased greatly as a result of improved techniques (Hawkins, 2015).

Although the anesthesiologist or nurse anesthetist administers the various general anesthesia agents, the nurse needs to be knowledgeable about the pharmacologic aspects of the drugs used and must be aware of airway management. Ensure that the woman is not taking anything by mouth (NPO) and has a patent intravenous line. In addition, administer a nonparticulate (clear) oral antacid (e.g., Bicitra or sodium citrate) or a proton pump inhibitor (Protonix) as ordered to reduce gastric acidity. Assist with placement of a wedge under the woman's right hip to displace the gravid uterus and prevent vena cava compression in the supine position. Once the newborn has been removed from the uterus, assist the perinatal team in providing supportive care.

NURSING CARE DURING LABOR AND BIRTH

Childbirth, a physiologic process that is fundamental to all human existence, is one of the most significant cultural, psychological, spiritual, and behavioral events in a woman's life. Although the act of giving birth is a universal phenomenon, it is a unique experience for each woman. Continuous evaluation and appropriate intervention for women during labor are essential to promoting a positive outcome for the family.

The nurse's role in childbirth is to ensure a safe environment for the mother and her newborn. Nurses begin evaluating the mother and fetus during the admission procedures at the health care agency and continue to do so throughout labor. It is critical to provide anticipatory guidance and explain each procedure (fetal monitoring, intravenous therapy, medications given and expected reactions) and what will happen next. This will prepare the woman for the upcoming physical and emotional challenges, thereby helping to reduce her anxiety. Acknowledging members of her support system (family or partner) helps allay their fears and concerns, thereby assisting them in carrying out their supportive role. Knowing how and when to evaluate a woman during the various stages of labor is essential for all labor and birth nurses to ensure a positive maternal experience and a healthy newborn.

A major focus of care for the woman during labor and birth is assisting her with maintaining control over her pain, emotions, and actions while being an active participant. Nurses can help and support women to be actively involved in their childbirth experience by allowing time for discussion, offering companionship, listening to worries and concerns, paying attention to the woman's emotional needs, and offering information to help her understand what is happening in each stage of labor.

Nursing Management During the First Stage of Labor

Depending on how far advanced the woman's labor is when she arrives at the facility; the nurse will determine assessment parameters of maternal-fetal status and plan care accordingly. The nurse will provide high-touch, low-tech supportive nursing care during the first stage of labor when admitting the woman and orienting her to the labor and birth suite. The nurse is usually the primary gatekeeper of observations, interventions, treatments, and often the management of labor in the inpatient perinatal setting. Nursing care during this stage will include taking an admission history (reviewing the prenatal record); checking the results of routine laboratory tests and any special tests such as chorionic villi sampling, amniocentesis, genetic studies, and biophysical profile done during pregnancy; asking the woman about her childbirth preparation (birth plan, classes taken, coping skills); and completing a physical assessment of the woman to establish baseline values for future comparison.

Key nursing interventions include:
- Identifying the estimated date of birth from the client and the prenatal chart
- Validating the client's prenatal history to determine fetal risk status
- Determining fundal height to validate dates and fetal growth
- Performing Leopold's maneuvers to determine fetal position, lie, and presentation
- Checking FHR
- Performing a vaginal examination (as appropriate) to evaluate effacement and dilation progress
- Instructing the client and her partner about monitoring techniques and equipment
- Assessing fetal response and FHR to contractions and recovery time
- Interpreting fetal monitoring strips
- Checking FHR baseline for accelerations, variability, and decelerations
- Repositioning the client to obtain an optimal FHR pattern
- Recognizing FHR problems and initiating corrective measures
- Checking amniotic fluid for meconium staining, odor, and amount
- Comforting client throughout testing period and labor
- Documenting times of notification for team members if problems arise
- Knowing appropriate interventions when abnormal FHR patterns present
- Supporting the client's decisions regarding intervention or avoidance of intervention
- Assessing the client's support system and coping status frequently

In addition to these interventions to promote optimal outcomes for the mother and fetus, the nurse must document care accurately and in a timely fashion. Accurate and timely documentation helps to decrease professional liability exposure, minimize the risk of preventable injuries to women and infants during labor and birth, and preserve families (Simpson, 2015). Guidelines for recording care include documenting:

- All care rendered, to prove that standards were met
- Conversations with all providers, including notification times
- Nursing interventions before and after notifying provider
- Use of the chain of command and response at each level
- All flow sheets and forms, to validate care given
- All education given to client and response to it
- Facts, not personal opinions
- detailed descriptions of any adverse outcome
- Initial nursing assessment, all encounters, and discharge plan
- All telephone conversations (Callahan, 2016).

This standard of documentation is needed to prevent or defend against litigation, which is prevalent in the childbirth arena.

Assessing the Woman Upon Admission

The nurse usually first comes in contact with the woman either by phone or in person. The nurse should ascertain whether the woman is in true or false labor and whether she should be admitted or sent home. Upon admission to the labor and birth suite, the highest priorities include assessing FHR, assessing cervical dilation/effacement, and determining whether membranes have ruptured or are intact. These assessment data will guide the critical thinking in planning care for the client.

If the initial contact is by phone, establish a therapeutic relationship with the woman. Speaking in a calm caring tone facilitates this. Nurses providing a telephone triage service need to have sufficient clinical experience and have clear lines of responsibility to enable sound decision making. When completing a phone assessment, include questions about the following:

- Estimated date of birth, to determine if term or preterm
- Fetal movement (frequency in the past few days)
- Other premonitory signs of labor experienced
- Parity, gravida, and previous childbirth experiences
- Time from start of labor to birth in previous labors
- Characteristics of contractions, including frequency, duration, and intensity
- Appearance of any vaginal bloody show
- Membrane status (ruptured or intact)
- Presence of supportive adult in household or if she is alone

When speaking with the woman over the telephone, review the signs and symptoms that denote true versus false labor, and suggest various positions she can assume to provide comfort and increase placental perfusion. Also suggest walking, massage, and taking a warm shower to promote relaxation. Outline what foods and fluids are appropriate for oral intake in early labor. Throughout the phone call, listen to the woman's concerns and answer any questions clearly.

Reducing the risk of liability exposure and avoiding preventable injuries to mothers and fetuses during labor and birth can be accomplished by adhering to two basic tenets of clinical practice: (1) use applicable evidence and/or published standards and guidelines as the foundation of care, and (2) whenever a clinical choice is presented, choose client safety (Miller, 2014). With these two tenets in mind, advise the woman on the phone to contact her health care provider for further instructions or to come to the facility to be evaluated, since ruling out true labor and possible maternal-fetal complications cannot be done accurately over the phone. Additional nursing responsibilities associated with a phone assessment include:

- Consulting the woman's prenatal record for parity status, estimated date of birth, and untoward events
- Calling the health care provider to inform him or her of the woman's status
- Preparing for admission to the perinatal unit to ensure adequate staff assignment
- Notifying the admissions office of a pending admission

If the nurse's first encounter with the woman is in person, an assessment is completed to determine whether she should be admitted to the perinatal unit or sent home until her labor advances. Recent research findings suggest that women admitted before active labor are approximately twice as likely to be augmented with oxytocin and give birth via cesarean when compared with women admitted in active labor (Neal et al., 2014). Nurses need to make careful assessment of labor progression *prior* to labor admission to decrease early admissions and to improve labor safety and birth outcomes.

Entering a facility is often an intimidating and stressful event for women since it is an unfamiliar environment. Giving birth for the first time is a pivotal event in the lives of most women. Therefore, demonstrate respect when addressing the client; listen carefully and express interest and concern. Nurses must value and respect women and promote their self-worth and sense of control by allowing them to participate in making decisions. Allowing them a fair amount of autonomy in their childbirth decisions, supporting their personal worth, knowing them holistically, and using caring communication will increase client satisfaction (Ivory, 2014).

An admission assessment includes maternal health history, physical assessment, fetal assessment, laboratory studies, and assessment of psychological status. Usually the facility has a form that can be used throughout labor and birth to document assessment findings (Fig. 14.13).

MATERNAL HEALTH HISTORY AND CULTURAL ASSESSMENT

A maternal health history should include typical biographical data such as the woman's name and age and the name of the delivering health care provider. Other information that is collected includes reason for admission, such as labor, cesarean birth, or observation for a complication; the prenatal record data, including the estimated date of birth, a history of the current pregnancy, and the results of any laboratory and diagnostic tests, such as blood type, Rh status, and group B streptococcal status; past pregnancy and obstetric history; past health history and family history; prenatal education; list of medications; risk factors such as diabetes, hypertension, and use of tobacco, alcohol, or illicit drugs; pain management plan; history of potential domestic violence; history of previous preterm births; allergies; time of last food ingestion; method chosen for infant feeding; name of birth attendant (MD or midwife)(s) and pediatrician.

Ascertaining this information is important so that an individualized plan of care can be developed for the woman. If, for example, the woman's due date is still 2 months away, it is important to establish this information so interventions can be initiated to arrest the labor immediately or notify the intensive perinatal team to be available. In addition, if the woman has diabetes, it is critical to monitor her glucose levels during labor, to prepare for a surgical birth if dystocia of labor occurs, and to alert the newborn nursery of potential hypoglycemia in the newborn after birth. By collecting important information about each woman they care for, nurses can help improve the outcomes for all concerned.

Be sure to observe the woman's emotions, support system, verbal interaction, cultural background and language spoken, body language and posture, perceptual acuity, and energy level. This psychosocial information provides cues about the woman's emotional state, culture, and communication systems. For example, if the woman arrives at the labor and birth suite extremely anxious, alone, and unable to communicate in English, how can the nurse meet her needs and plan her care appropriately? It is only by assessing each woman physically and psychosocially that the nurse can make astute decisions regarding proper care. In this case, an interpreter would be needed to assist in the communication process between the staff and the woman to initiate proper care.

It is important to acknowledge and try to understand the cultural differences in women with cultural backgrounds different from that of the nurse. Attitudes toward childbirth are heavily influenced by the culture

---

BOX 14.2

QUESTIONS FOR PROVIDING CULTURALLY COMPETENT CARE DURING LABOR AND BIRTH

- Where were you born? How long have you lived in the United States?
- What languages do you speak and read?
- Who are your major support people?
- What are your religious practices?
- How do you view childbearing?
- Are there any special precautions or restrictions that are important?
- Is birth considered a private or a social experience?
- How would you like to manage your labor discomfort?
- Who will provide your labor support?

Adapted from Bowers, P. (2015). Cultural perspectives in childbearing. Nursing Spectrum. Retrieved from http://ce.nurse.com/ce263-60/cultural-perspectives-in-childbearing; and Anderson, L. (2014). Cultural competence in the nursing practice. Nursetogether. Retrieved from http://www.nursetogether.com/cultural-competence-in-the-nursing-practice

---

in which the woman has been raised. As a result, within every society, specific attitudes and values shape the woman's childbearing behaviors. Be aware of what these are. When carrying out a cultural assessment during the admission process, ask questions (Box 14.2) to help plan culturally competent care during labor and birth.

PHYSICAL EXAMINATION

The physical examination typically includes a generalized assessment of the woman's body systems, including hydration status, vital signs, auscultation of heart and lung sounds, and measurement of height and weight. The physical examination also includes the following assessments:

1. Pain level and coping behaviors demonstrated
2. Uterine activity, including contraction frequency, duration, and intensity
3. Fetal status, including heart rate, position, and station
4. Cervical dilation and degree of effacement
5. Status of membranes (intact or ruptured)
6. Assess vital signs: temperature, pulse, respirations & blood pressure
7. Perform Leopold's maneuvers to determine fetal lie
8. Fundal height measurement
9. Ability to ambulate safely

These assessment parameters form a baseline against which the nurse can compare all future values throughout labor. The findings should be similar to those of the woman's prepregnancy and pregnancy findings, with the exception of her pulse rate, which might be elevated secondary to her anxious state with beginning labor.

ADMISSION ASSESSMENT OBSTETRICS

▲ PATIENT IDENTIFICATION ▲

ADMISSION DATA

Date	Time	Via
		☐ Ambulatory ☐ Wheelchair ☐ Stretcher

Grav.	Term	Pre-term	Ab.	Living	EDC	LMP	GA

Prev. adm. date _____ Reason _____

Obstetrician _____ Pediatrician _____

Ht. _____ Wt. _____ Wt. gain _____

Allergies (meds/food) ☐ None _____ ☐ Hx latex sensitivity

BP _____ T _____ P _____ R _____

FHR _____ Vag exam _____

Reason for Admission

☐ Labor / SROM ☐ Induction _____

☐ Primary C/S _____ ☐ Repeat C/S

☐ Observation _____

☐ OB / Medical complication _____

Onset of labor: ☐ Not in labor

Date _____ Time _____

Membranes: ☐ Intact

☐ Ruptured / Date _____ Time _____

☐ Clear ☐ Meconium ☐ Bloody ☐ Foul

Vaginal bleeding: ☐ None

☐ Normal show ☐ _____

Current Pregnancy Labs   ☐ NPC

☐ POL ☐ PPROM ☐ Cerclage

☐ PIH ☐ Chr. HTN ☐ Other _____

☐ Diabetes _____ Diet _____

☐ Insulin _____

☐ Amniocentesis _____ Results _____

Bld type / RH____Date Rhogam____

Antibody screen ☐ Neg ☐ Pos

Rubella ☐ Non-immune ☐ Immune

Diabetic screen ☐ Normal ☐ Abnormal

Recent exposure to chick pox ☐

Current meds: _____

_____

	Pos	Neg	Tested
Hepatitis B	☐	☐	☐ No
HIV	☐	☐	☐ No
Group B strep	☐	☐	☐ No
GC	☐	☐	☐ No
Chlamydia	☐	☐	☐ No
RPR	☐	☐	☐ No

Previous OB History

☐ POL ☐ Multiple gestation

☐ Prev C/S type _____ Reason _____

☐ PIH ☐ Chronic HTN ☐ Diabetes _____

☐ Stillbirth/demise ☐ Neodeath ☐ Anomalies

☐ Precipitous labor (<3 H) ☐ Macrosomia

☐ PP Hemorrhage

☐ Hx Transfusion reaction ☐ Yes ☐ No

☐ Other _____

Latest risk assessment ☐ None

1. _____ 3. _____

2. _____ 4. _____

Date _____

Signature _____ Time _____

NEUROLOGICAL

☐ WNL

Variance: ☐ HA

☐ Scotoma / visual changes

Reflexes ☐ < 2 + ☐ > 2 +

☐ Clonus ____ bts

☐ Numbness ☐ Tingling

☐ Hx Seizures

☐ _____

RESPIRATORY

☐ WNL

Variance: ☐ Hx Asthma ☐ URI

Respirations: ☐ < 12 ☐ > 24

Effort: ☐ SOB

☐ Shallow ☐ Labored

Auscultation:

☐ Diminished ☐ Crackles

☐ Wheezes ☐ Rhonchi

	No	Yes
Cough for greater than 2 weeks?	☐	☐
Is the cough productive?	☐	☐
Blood in the sputum?	☐	☐
Experiencing any fever or night sweats?	☐	☐
Ever had TB in the past?	☐	☐
Recent exposure to TB?	☐	☐
Weight loss in last 3 weeks?	☐	☐

If the patient answers yes to any three of the above questions implement policy and procedure # 5725-0704.

GASTROINTESTINAL

☐ WNL

Variance: ☐ Heartburn

☐ Epigastric pain   Nausea

☐ Vomiting ☐ Diarrhea

☐ Constipation ☐ Pain

☐ Wt. Gain < 2lbs / month**

☐ Recent change in appetite of < 50% of usual intake for > 5 days

☐ _____

INTEGUMENTARY

☐ WNL

Variance: ☐ Rash ☐ Lacerations

☐ Abrasion ☐ Swelling

☐ Uticaria ☐ Bruising

☐ Diaphoretic/hot

☐ Clammy/cold

☐ Scars

☐ _____

FETAL ASSESSMENT

☐ WNL

Variance:

☐ NRFS

FHR ☐ < 110 ☐ > 160

LTV ☐ Absent ☐ Minimal

☐ Increased

STV Absent

Decelerations: _____

☐ Decreased fetal movement

☐ IUGR

☐ _____

Tobacco use	☐ Denies	☐ Yes	Amt _____
Alcohol use	☐ Denies	☐ Yes	Amt _____
Drug use	☐ Denies	☐ Yes	Amt type _____
Primary language	☐ English	☐ Spanish	☐ _____

CARDIOVASCULAR

☐ WNL

Variance:

☐ MVP

Heart rate: ☐ < 60 ☐ > 100

B/P: Systolic: ☐ < 90 ☐ > 140

Diastolic: ☐ < 50 ☐ > 90

☐ Edema _____

☐ Chest pain / palpitations

☐ _____

MUSCULOSKELETAL

☐ WNL

Variance:

☐ Numbness ☐ Tingling

☐ Paralysis ☐ Deformity

☐ Scoliosis

☐ _____

GENITOURINARY

☐ WNL

Variance: ☐ Albumin _____

Output: ☐ < 30 cc/Hr.

☐ UTI ☐ Rx ☐ Frequency

☐ Dysuria ☐ Hematuria

☐ CVA Tenderness

☐ Hx STD _____

☐ Vag. discharge _____

☐ Rash ☐ Blisters

☐ Warts ☐ Lesions

☐ _____

EARS, NOSE, THROAT, AND EYES

☐ WNL

Variance:

☐ Sore throat ☐ Eyeglasses

☐ Runny nose ☐ Contact lenses

☐ Nasal congestion

PSYCHOSOCIAL

☐ WNL

Variance: ☐ Hx depression

☐ Yes ☐ No

☐ Emotional behavioral care

Affect: ☐ Flat ☐ Anxious

☐ Uncooperative ☐ Combative

Living will ☐ Yes ☐ No

☐ On chart

Healthcare surrogate ☐ Yes ☐ No

☐ On chart

Are you being hurt, hit, frightened by anyone at home or in your life? ☐ Yes ☐ No

Religious preference _____

PAIN ASSESSMENT

1. Do you have any ongoing pain problems? ☐ No ☐ Yes
2. Do you have any pain now? ☐ No ☐ Yes
3. If any of the above questions are answered yes, the patient has a positive pain screening.
4. *Patient to be given pain management education material. Complete pain / symptom assessment on flowsheet.*
5. *Please proceed to complete pain assessment.*

FIGURE 14.13 Sample documentation form used for admission to the perinatal unit. (Used with permission. Briggs Corporation, 2001.)

LABORATORY STUDIES

On admission, laboratory studies typically are done to establish a baseline. Although the exact tests may vary among facilities, they usually include a urinalysis via clean-catch urine specimen and complete blood count. Blood typing and Rh factor analysis may be necessary if the results of these are unknown or unavailable. In addition, if the following test results are not included in the maternal prenatal history, it may be necessary to perform them at this time. They include syphilis screening, hepatitis B (HbsAg) screening, group B streptococcus, human immune deficiency virus (HIV) testing (if woman gives consent), and possible drug screening if the history is positive.

Group B streptococcus (GBS) is a gram-positive organism that colonizes in the female genital tract and rectum and is present in 10% to 30% of all healthy women (King et al., 2015). These women are asymptomatic carriers but can cause GBS disease of the newborn through vertical transmission during labor and horizontal transmission after birth. The mortality rate of infected newborns varies according to time of onset (early or late). Risk factors for GBS include maternal intrapartum fever, prolonged ruptured membranes (>12 to 18 hours), previous birth of an infected newborn, and GBS bacteriuria in the present pregnancy.

The Centers for Disease Control and Prevention (CDC), ACOG and the American Academy of Pediatrics have guidelines that advised universal screening of pregnant women at 35 to 37 weeks' gestation for GBS and intrapartum antibiotic therapy for GBS carriers. These new guidelines reaffirmed the major prevention strategy—universal antenatal GBS screening and intrapartum antibiotic prophylaxis for culture-positive and high-risk women. Also included are new recommendations for laboratory methods for identification of GBS colonization during pregnancy, algorithms for screening and intrapartum prophylaxis for women with preterm labor and premature rupture of membranes, updated prophylaxis recommendations for women with a penicillin allergy, and a revised algorithm for the care of newborn infants (Centers for Disease Control and Prevention [CDC], 2014). Maternal infections associated with GBS include acute chorioamnionitis, endometritis, and urinary tract infection. Neonatal clinical manifestations include pneumonia and sepsis. Identified GBS carriers receive intravenous antibiotic prophylaxis (penicillin G or ampicillin) at the onset of labor or ruptured membranes.

The ACOG, CDC, AWHONN and the United States Preventive Services Task Force all recommend that all pregnant women be offered a screening test for HIV antibodies on their first prenatal visit, again during the third trimester if engaging in high-risk behaviors, and on admission to the labor and birth area. The CDC estimates that 50,000 individuals contract HIV in the United States each year, and 250,000 individuals have undiagnosed HIV infections (CDC, 2015).

If her HIV status is not documented, the woman being admitted to the labor and birth suite should have rapid HIV testing done. To reduce perinatal transmission, women who are HIV-positive are given zidovudine (2 mg/kg intravenously over an hour, and then a maintenance infusion of 1 mg/kg per hour until birth) or a single 200-mg oral dose of nevirapine at the onset of labor; the newborn is given zidovudine orally (2 mg/kg body weight every 6 hours) and should be continued for 6 weeks (Verklan & Walden, 2014). To further reduce the risk of perinatal transmission, ACOG and the United States Public Health Service recommend that women who are infected with HIV and have plasma viral loads of more than 1,000 copies/mL be counseled regarding the benefits of elective cesarean birth. In the absence of any medical intervention, the rate of vertical transmission of HIV to the fetus can range from 15% to 45% (Ashimi et al., 2015).

Additional interventions to reduce the transmission risk would include avoiding use of a scalp electrode for fetal monitoring or doing a scalp blood sampling for fetal pH, delaying amniotomy, encouraging formula feeding after birth, and avoiding invasive procedures such as forceps or vacuum-assisted devices. The nurse stresses the importance of all interventions and the goal to reduce transmission of HIV to the newborn.

Continuing Assessment During the First Stage of Labor

After the admission assessment is complete and the woman and her support person have been orientated to the room, equipment, and procedures, assessment continues for changes that would indicate that labor is progressing as expected. Assess the woman's knowledge, experience, and expectations of labor. Typically, blood pressure, pulse, and respirations are assessed every hour during the latent phase of labor unless the clinical situation dictates that vital signs be taken more frequently. During the active and transition phases, they are assessed every 30 minutes. The temperature is taken every 4 hours throughout the first stage of labor and every 2 hours after membranes have ruptured to detect an elevation indicating an ascending infection.

Vaginal examinations are performed periodically to track labor progress. This assessment information is shared with the woman to reinforce that she is making progress toward the goal of birth. Uterine contractions are monitored for frequency, duration, and intensity every 30 to 60 minutes during the latent phase, every 15 to 30 minutes during the active phase, and every 15 minutes during transition. Note the changes in the character of the contractions as labor progresses, and inform the woman of her progress. Continually determine the woman's level of pain and her ability to cope and use relaxation techniques effectively.

When the fetal membranes rupture, spontaneously or artificially, assess the FHR and check the amniotic fluid for color, odor, and amount. Assess the FHR intermittently or continuously via electronic monitoring. During the latent phase of labor, assess the FHR every 30 to 60 minutes; in the active phase, assess FHR at least every 15 to 30 minutes. Also, be sure to assess the FHR before ambulation, before any procedure, and before administering analgesia or anesthesia to the mother. Table 14.3 summarizes assessments for the first stage of labor.

Remember Sheila from the chapter-opening scenario? What is the nurse's role with Sheila in active labor? What additional comfort measures can the labor nurse offer Sheila?

Nursing Interventions

Nursing interventions during the admission process should include:
- Asking about the client's expectations of the birthing process
- Providing information about labor, birth, pain management options, and relaxation techniques
- Presenting information about fetal monitoring equipment and the procedures needed
- Monitoring FHR and identifying patterns that need further intervention
- Monitoring the mother's vital signs to obtain a baseline for later comparison
- Reassuring the client that her labor progress will be monitored closely and nursing care will focus on ensuring fetal and maternal well-being throughout

As the woman progresses through the first stage of labor, nursing interventions include:
- Encouraging the woman's partner to participate
- Keeping the woman and her partner up to date on the progress of the labor
- Orienting the woman and her partner to the labor and birth unit and explaining all of the birthing procedures
- Providing clear fluids (e.g., ice chips) as needed or requested
- Maintaining the woman's parenteral fluid intake at the prescribed rate if she has an IV
- Initiating or encouraging comfort measures, such as backrubs, cool cloths to the forehead, frequent position changes, ambulation, showers, slow dancing, leaning over a birth ball, side-lying, or counterpressure on lower back (Teaching Guidelines 14.1)

TABLE 14.3	SUMMARY OF ASSESSMENTS DURING THE FIRST STAGE OF LABOR		
Assessments[a]	Latent Phase (0–3 cm)	Active Phase (4–7 cm)	Transition (8–10 cm)
Vital signs (BP, pulse, respirations)	Every 30–60 min	Every 30 min	Every 15–30 min
Temperature	Every 4 hr; more frequently if membranes are ruptured	Every 4 hr; more frequently if membranes are ruptured	Every 4 hr; more frequently if membranes are ruptured
Contractions (frequency, duration, intensity)	Every 30–60 min by palpation or continuously if EFM	Every 15–30 min by palpation or continuously if EFM	Every 15 min by palpation or continuously if EFM
Fetal heart rate	Every hour by Doppler or continuously by EFM	Every 30 min by Doppler or continuously by EFM	Every 15–30 min by Doppler or continuously by EFM
Vaginal examination	Initially on admission to determine phase and as needed based on maternal cues to document labor progression	As needed to monitor labor progression	As needed to monitor labor progression
Behavior/ psychosocial	With every client encounter: talkative, excited, anxious	With every client encounter: self-absorbed in labor; intense and quiet now	With every client encounter: discouraged, irritable, feels out of control, declining coping ability

[a]The frequency of assessments is dictated by the health status of the woman and fetus and can be altered if either one of their conditions changes.
EFM, electronic fetal monitoring.
Adapted from; King, T. L., Brucker, M. C., Kriebs, J. M., Fahey, J. O., Gegor, C. L., & Varney, H. (2015). *Varney's midwifery* (5th ed.). Burlington, MA: Jones & Bartlett Learning; and Green, C. J. (2016). *Maternal newborn nursing care plans* (3rd ed.). Burlington, MA: Jones & Bartlett Learning.

Teaching Guidelines 14.1
POSITIONING DURING THE FIRST STAGE OF LABOR

- Walking with support from the partner (adds the force of gravity to contractions to promote fetal descent)
- Slow-dancing position with the partner holding the woman (adds the force of gravity to contractions and promotes support from and active participation of your partner)
- Side lying with pillows between the knees for comfort (offers a restful position and improves oxygen flow to the uterus)
- Semi-sitting in bed or on a couch leaning against the partner (reduces back pain because fetus falls forward, away from the sacrum)
- Sitting in a chair with one foot on the floor and one on the chair (changes pelvic shape)
- Leaning forward by straddling a chair, a table, or a bed or kneeling over a birth ball (reduces back pain, adds the force of gravity to promote descent; possible pain relief if partner can apply sacral pressure)
- Encourage any position of comfort the woman choses to labor in and give birth.
- Sitting in a rocking chair or on a birth ball and shifting weight back and forth (provides comfort because rocking motion is soothing; uses the force of gravity to help fetal descent)
- Lunge by rocking weight back and forth with foot up on chair during contraction (uses force of gravity by being upright; enhances rotation of fetus through rocking)
- Open knee–chest position (helps to relieve back discomfort) (Gizzo et al., 2014; Tharpe et al., 2016).

- Encouraging the partner's involvement with breathing techniques
- Assisting the woman and her partner to focus on breathing techniques
- Informing the woman that the discomfort will be intermittent and of limited duration; urging her to rest between contractions to preserve her strength; and encouraging her to use distracting activities to lessen the focus on contractions
- Changing bed linens and gown as needed
- Keeping the perineal area clean and dry
- Supporting the woman's decisions about pain management
- Monitoring maternal vital signs frequently and reporting any abnormal values
- Ensuring that the woman takes deep cleansing breaths before and after each contraction to enhance gas exchange and oxygen to the fetus
- Educating the woman and her partner about the need for rest and helping them plan strategies to conserve strength

- Monitoring FHR for baseline, accelerations, variability, and decelerations
- Checking on bladder status and encouraging voiding at least every 2 hours to make room for birth
- Repositioning the woman as needed to obtain optimal heart rate pattern
- Communicating requests from the woman to appropriate personnel
- Respecting the woman's sense of privacy by covering her when appropriate
- Offering human presence by being present with the woman, not leaving her alone for long periods
- Being patient with the natural labor pattern to allow time for change
- Encouraging maternal movement throughout labor to increase the woman's level of comfort
- Dimming the lights in the room when pushing and request softened voices be used to maintain a calm and centered ambiance
- Reporting any deviations from normal to the health care professional so that interventions can be initiated early to be effective (Green, 2016; Lucas et al., 2015; Nagtalon-Ramos, 2014).

See Nursing Care Plan 14.1.

Nursing Management During the Second Stage of Labor

Management of the second stage of labor often follows tradition-based routines rather than evidence-based practices. Current evidence for management of the second stage of labor supports the practices of delayed pushing, spontaneous (nondirected) pushing, and maternal choice positions (Cox & King, 2015). To be able to help women through the second stage of labor requires the nurse to have a comprehensive understanding of physiology and be aware of the latest evidence-based research and apply it to practice (Green, 2016).

Nursing care during the second stage of labor focuses on supporting the woman and her partner in making active decisions about her care and labor management, implementing strategies to prolong the early passive phase of fetal descent, supporting involuntary bearing-down efforts, providing instruction and assistance, and using maternal positions that can enhance descent and reduce pain (King et al., 2015). Women in the past gave birth unaided by following their bodies signals to birth their babies, so the role of the nurse should be to support the woman in her choice of pushing method and to encourage confidence in her maternal instinct of when and how to push.

In the absence of any complications, nurses should not be controlling this stage of labor, but empowering women to achieve a satisfying experience. The primary rationale for directing women to push is to shorten the second stage of labor. Common practice in many labor

Overview of a Woman in the Active Phase of the First Stage of Labor

Candice, a 23-year-old gravida 1, para 0 (G1,P0), is admitted to the labor and birth suite at 39 weeks' gestation having contractions of moderate intensity every 5 to 6 minutes. A vaginal examination reveals that her cervix is 80% effaced and 5 cm dilated. The presenting part (vertex) is at 0 station and her membranes ruptured spontaneously 4 hours ago at home. She is admitted and an intravenous line is started for hydration and vascular access. An external fetal monitor is applied. FHR is 140 bpm and regular. Her partner is present at her bedside. Candice is now in the active phase of the first stage of labor, and her assessment findings are as follows: cervix dilated 7 cm, 80% effaced; moderate to strong contractions occurring regularly, every 3 to 5 minutes, lasting 45 to 60 seconds; at 0 station on pelvic examination; FHR auscultated loudest below umbilicus at 140 bpm; vaginal show—pink or bloody vaginal mucus; currently apprehensive, inwardly focused, with increased dependency; voicing concern about ability to cope with pain; limited ability to follow directions.

NURSING DIAGNOSIS: Anxiety related to labor and birth process and fear of the unknown related to client's first experience

Outcome Identification and Evaluation

The client will remain calm and in control as evidenced by ability to make decisions and use positive coping strategies.

Interventions: *Promoting Positive Coping Strategies*

- Provide instruction regarding the labor process to allay anxiety.
- Orient the woman to the physical environment and equipment as necessary to keep her informed of events.
- Encourage verbalization of feelings and concerns to reduce anxiety.
- Listen attentively to woman and partner to demonstrate interest and concern.
- Inform woman and partner of standard procedures/processes to ensure adequate understanding of events and procedures.

- Frequently update woman of progress and labor status to provide positive reinforcement for actions.
- Reinforce relaxation techniques and provide instruction if needed to aid in coping.
- Encourage participation of the partner in the coaching role; role-model to facilitate partner participation in labor process to provide support and encouragement to the client.
- Provide a presence and remain with the client as much as possible to provide comfort and support.

NURSING DIAGNOSIS: Acute pain related to uterine contractions and stretching of the cervix and birth canal

Outcome Identification and Evaluation

The client will maintain a tolerable level of pain and discomfort as evidenced by statements of pain relief, pain rating of 2 or less on pain rating scale, and absence of adverse effects in client and fetus from analgesia or anesthesia.

Interventions: *Providing Pain Relief*

- Monitor vital signs, observe for signs of pain, and have client rate pain on a scale of 0 to 10 to provide baseline for comparison.
- Encourage client to void every 1 to 2 hours to decrease pressure from a full bladder.
- Assist woman to change positions frequently to increase comfort and promote labor progress.

NURSING CARE PLAN 14.1

Overview of a Woman in the Active Phase of the First Stage of Labor (continued)

- Encourage use of distraction to reduce focus on contraction pain.
- Suggest pelvic rocking, massage, or back counter pressure to reduce pain.
- Assist with use of relaxation and breathing techniques to promote relaxation.
- Use touch appropriately (backrub) when desired by the woman to promote comfort.
- Integrate use of nonpharmacologic measures for pain relief, such as warm water, birthing ball, or other techniques to facilitate pain relief.
- Administer pharmacologic agents as ordered when requested to control pain.
- Provide reassurance and encouragement between contractions to foster self-esteem and continued participation in labor process.

NURSING DIAGNOSIS: Risk of infection related to multiple vaginal examinations following rupture of membranes and tissue trauma

Outcome Identification and Evaluation

The client will remain free of infection as evidenced by the absence of signs and symptoms of infection, vital signs and FHR within acceptable parameters, lab test results within normal limits, and clear amniotic fluid without odor.

Interventions: *Preventing Infection*

- Monitor vital signs (every 2 hours after rupture of membranes [ROM]) and FHR frequently as per protocol to allow for early detection of problems; report fetal tachycardia (early sign of maternal infection) to ensure prompt treatment.
- Provide frequent perineal care and pad changes to maintain good perineal hygiene.
- Change linens and woman's gown as needed to maintain cleanliness.
- Ensure that vaginal examinations are performed only when needed to prevent introducing pathogens into the vaginal vault.
- Monitor lab test results such as white blood cell count to assess for elevations indicating infection.
- Use aseptic technique for all invasive procedures to prevent infection transmission.
- Carry out good handwashing techniques before and after procedures and use standard precautions as appropriate to minimize risk of infection transmission.
- Document amniotic fluid characteristics—color, odor—to establish baseline for comparison.

units is still to coach women to use closed glottis pushing with every contraction, starting at 10 cm of dilation, a practice that is not supported by research. Research suggests that directed pushing during the second stage may be accompanied by a significant decline in fetal pH and may cause maternal muscle and nerve damage if done too early (Reed, 2015). Shortening the phase of active pushing and lengthening the early phase of passive descent can be achieved by encouraging the woman not to push until she has a strong desire to do so and until the descent and rotation of the fetal head are well advanced. Effective pushing can be achieved by assisting the woman to assume a more upright or squatting position. Supporting spontaneous pushing and encouraging women to choose

their own method of pushing should be accepted as best clinical practice (Cheng & Caughey, 2015b).

Perineal lacerations or tears can occur during the second stage when the fetal head emerges through the vaginal introitus. The extent of the laceration is defined by depth: a first-degree laceration extends through the skin; a second-degree laceration extends through the muscles of the perineal body; a third-degree laceration continues through the anal sphincter muscle; and a fourth-degree laceration also involves the anterior rectal wall. Special attention needs to be paid to third- and fourth-degree lacerations to prevent fecal incontinence. Risks for third- or fourth-degree lacerations included nulliparity, being Asian or Pacific Islander, increased birth weight of newborn, operative vaginal birth, episiotomy, and longer second stage of labor. Increasing body mass index was associated with fewer lacerations (Sides et al., 2015). The primary care provider should repair any lacerations during the third stage of labor.

An **episiotomy** is an incision made in the perineum to enlarge the vaginal outlet and theoretically to shorten the second stage of labor. Alternative measures such as warm compresses and continual massage with oil have been successful in stretching the perineal area to prevent cutting it. Certified nurse midwives can cut and repair episiotomies, but they frequently use alternative measures if possible.

Take Note!

Restrictive use of episiotomy has been recommended by ACOG given the risks of the procedure and unclear benefits of routine use (Friedman et al., 2015).

The midline episiotomy has been the most commonly used one in the United States because it can be easily repaired and causes the least amount of pain. The application of warmed compresses and/or intrapartum perineal massage is associated with a decrease in trauma to the perineal area and reduced the need for an episiotomy (Green, 2016). Routine episiotomy has declined since liberal usage has been discouraged by ACOG, except to avoid several maternal lacerations or to expedite difficult births Anal sphincter laceration rates with spontaneous vaginal delivery have decreased, likely reflecting the decreased usage of episiotomy. The decline in operative vaginal delivery corresponds with a sharp increase in cesarean births, which may indicate that health care providers are favoring cesarean births for difficult births (Faisal-Cury et al., 2015). Figure 14.14 shows episiotomy locations.

Continuous Assessment During the Second Stage of Labor

Assessment is continuous during the second stage of labor. Hospital policies dictate the specific type and timing of assessments, as well as the way in which they are documented. Assessment involves identifying the signs typical of the second stage of labor, including:
- Increase in apprehension or irritability
- Spontaneous rupture of membranes
- Sudden appearance of sweat on upper lip
- Increase in blood-tinged show
- Low grunting sounds from the woman
- Complaints of rectal and perineal pressure
- Beginning of involuntary bearing-down efforts

Other ongoing assessments include the contraction frequency, duration, and intensity; maternal vital signs every 5 to 15 minutes; fetal response to labor as indicated by FHR monitor strips; amniotic fluid for color, odor, and amount when membranes are ruptured; and the copying status of the woman and her partner (Table 14.4).

Assessment also focuses on determining the progress of labor. Associated signs include bulging of the perineum, labial separation, advancing and retreating of the newborn's head during and between bearing-down efforts, and **crowning** (fetal head is visible at vaginal opening; Fig. 14.15).

A vaginal examination is completed to determine if it is appropriate for the woman to push. Pushing is appropriate if the cervix has fully dilated to 10 cm and the woman feels the urge to do so.

Nursing Interventions

Nursing interventions during this stage focus on motivating the woman, assisting with positioning and encouraging

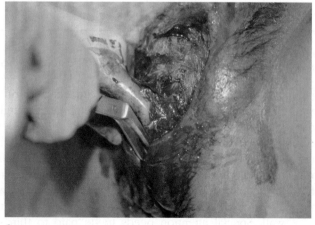

A

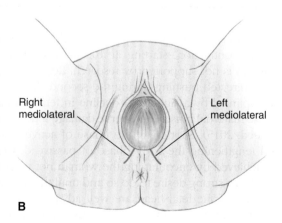

B

FIGURE 14.14 Location of an episiotomy. **A.** Midline episiotomy. **B.** Right and left mediolateral episiotomies.

TABLE 14.4	SUMMARY OF ASSESSMENTS DURING THE SECOND, THIRD, AND FOURTH STAGES OF LABOR		
Assessments[a]	Second Stage of Labor (Birth of Neonate)	Third Stage of Labor (Placenta Expulsion)	Fourth Stage of Labor (Recovery)
Vital signs (BP, pulse, respirations)	Every 5–15 min	Every 15 min	Every 15 min
Fetal heart rate	Every 5–15 min by Doppler or continuously by EFM	Apgar scoring at 1 and 5 min	Newborn—complete head-to-toe assessment; vital signs every 15 min until stable
Contractions/uterus	Palpate every one	Observe for placental separation	Palpating for firmness and position every 15 min for first hour
Bearing down/ pushing	Assist with every effort	None	None
Vaginal discharge	Observe for signs of descent—bulging of perineum, crowning	Assess bleeding after expulsion	Assess every 15 min with fundus firmness
Behavior/ psychosocial	Observe every 15 min: cooperative, focus is on work of pushing newborn out	Observe every 15 min: often feelings of relief after hearing newborn crying; calmer	Observe every 15 min: usually excited, talkative, awake; needs to hold newborn, be close, and inspect body

[a]The frequency of assessments is dictated by the health status of the woman and fetus and can be altered if either one of their conditions changes.
EFM, electronic fetal monitoring.
Adapted from Holvey, N. (2014). Supporting women in the second stage of labor. *British Journal of Midwifery, 22*(3), 182–186; American Hospital Association. (2014). RNs role in labor and delivery. Retrieved from http://www.aha.org/search?q=RNs+role+in+labor+and+delivery&start-date; and Wenner, L. (2015). It's the little things. *Nursing for Women's Health, 19*(2), 203–204.

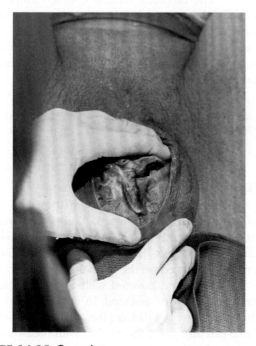

FIGURE 14.15 Crowning.

her to put all her efforts to pushing this newborn to the outside world, and giving her feedback on her progress. If the woman is pushing without progress, suggest that she keep her eyes open during the contractions and look toward where the newborn is coming out. Changing positions frequently will also help in making progress. Positioning a mirror so the woman can visualize the birthing process and how successful her pushing efforts are can help motivate her.

During the second stage of labor, an ideal position would be one that opens the pelvic outlet as wide as possible, provides a smooth pathway for the fetus to descend through the birth canal, takes advantage of gravity to assist the fetus to descend, and gives the mother a sense of being safe and in control of the labor process (Capogna, 2015a). Some suggestions for positions in the second stage include:

• Lithotomy with feet up in stirrups: most convenient position for caregivers, although EBP findings do not support this position physiologically
• Semi-sitting with pillows underneath knees, arms, and back
• Lateral/side-lying with curved back and upper leg supported by partner

- Sitting on birthing stool: opens pelvis, enhances the pull of gravity, and helps with pushing
- Squatting/supported squatting: gives the woman a sense of control
- Kneeling with hands on bed and knees comfortably apart

Other important nursing interventions during the second stage include:

- Providing continuous comfort measures such as mouth care, encouraging position changes, changing bed linen and underpads, and providing a quiet, focused environment
- Instructing the woman on the following bearing-down positions and techniques:
  - Pushing only when she feels an urge to do so
  - Delaying pushing for up to 90 minutes after complete dilation
  - Using abdominal muscles when bearing down
  - Using short pushes of 6 to 7 seconds
  - Focusing attention on the perineal area to visualize the newborn
  - Relaxing and conserving energy between contractions
  - Pushing several times with each contraction
  - Pushing with an open glottis and slight exhalation (Petrocnik & Marshall, 2015)
- Continuing to monitor contraction and FHR patterns to identify problems
- Providing brief, explicit directions throughout this stage
- Continuing to provide psychosocial support by reassuring and coaching
- Facilitating the upright position to encourage the fetus to descend
- Continuing to assess blood pressure, pulse, respirations, uterine contractions, bearing-down efforts, FHR, and coping status of the client and her partner
- Providing pain management if needed
- Providing a continuous nursing presence
- Offering praise for the client's efforts
- Preparing for and assisting with delivery by:
  - Notifying the health care provider of the estimated time frame for birth
  - Preparing the delivery bed and positioning client
  - Preparing the perineal area according to the facility's protocol
  - Offering a mirror and adjusting it so the woman can watch the birth
  - Explaining all procedures and equipment to the client and her partner
  - Setting up delivery instruments needed while maintaining sterility
  - Using standard precautions during the birthing process to avoid body fluid splashes
  - Recording the time of birth, time of placenta, and type of birth

- Receiving newborn and transporting him or her to a warming environment, or covering the newborn with a warmed blanket on the woman's abdomen
- Providing initial care and assessment of the newborn (see the Birth section that follows)

Sheila is completely dilated now and experiencing the urge to push. How can the nurse help Sheila with her pushing efforts? What additional interventions can the labor nurse offer Sheila now? In addition to encouraging Sheila to rest between pushing and offering praise for her efforts, what is the nurse's role during the birthing process?

BIRTH

The second stage of labor ends with the birth of the newborn. The maternal position for birth varies from the standard lithotomy position to side-lying to squatting to standing or kneeling, depending on the birthing location, the woman's preference, and standard protocols. Once the woman is positioned for birth, cleanse the vulva and perineal areas. The primary health care provider then takes charge after donning protective eyewear, masks, gowns, and gloves and performing hand hygiene.

Once the fetal head has emerged, the primary care provider explores the fetal neck to see if the umbilical cord is wrapped around it. If it is, the cord is slipped over the head to facilitate delivery. As soon as the head emerges, the health care provider suctions the newborn's mouth first (because the newborn is an obligate nose breather) and then the nares with a bulb syringe to prevent aspiration of mucus, amniotic fluid, or meconium (Fig. 14.16). The umbilical cord is double-clamped and cut between the clamps by the birth attendant or the woman's partner if desired. With the first cries of the newborn, the second stage of labor ends. For care of the woman undergoing a surgical birth, the reader is referred to Chapter 21.

In addition to encouraging Sheila to rest between pushing and offering praise for her efforts, what is the nurse's role during the birthing process?

IMMEDIATE CARE OF THE NEWBORN

Once birth takes place, the newborn is placed under a radiant warmer, dried, assessed, wrapped in warmed blankets, and placed on the woman's abdomen for warmth and closeness. In some health care facilities, the newborn is placed on the woman's abdomen immediately after birth and covered with a warmed blanket without being dried or assessed. In either scenario, the stability of the newborn dictates the location of aftercare. The nurse can also assist the mother with breast-feeding her newborn for the first time.

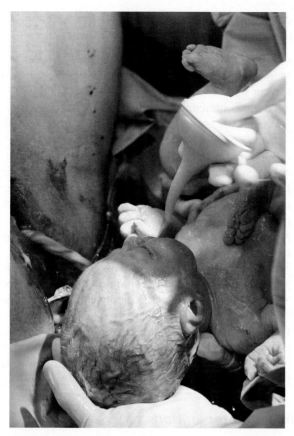

FIGURE 14.16 Suctioning the newborn immediately after birth.

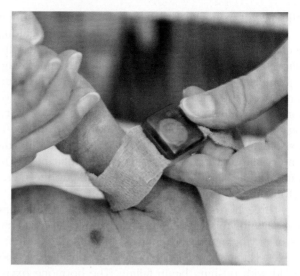

FIGURE 14.17 An example of a security sensor applied to a newborn's arm.

Assessment of the newborn begins at the moment of birth and continues until the newborn is discharged. Drying the newborn and providing warmth to prevent heat loss by evaporation is essential to help support thermoregulation and provide stimulation. Placing the newborn under a radiant heat source and putting on a stockinette/knitted cap will further reduce heat loss after drying.

Assess the newborn by assigning an Apgar score at 1 and 5 minutes. The Apgar score assesses five parameters—(1) heart rate (absent, slow, or fast), (2) respiratory effort (absent, weak cry, or good strong yell), (3) muscle tone (limp, or lively and active), (4) response to irritation stimulus, and (5) color—that evaluate a newborn's cardiorespiratory adaptation after birth. The parameters are arranged from the most important (heart rate) to the least important (color). The newborn is assigned a score of 0 to 2 in each of the five parameters. The purpose of the Apgar assessment is to evaluate the physiologic status of the newborn; see Chapter 18 for additional information on Apgar scoring.

Secure two identification bands on the newborn's wrist and ankle that match the band on the mother's wrist to ensure the newborn's identity. This identification process is completed in the birthing suite before anyone leaves the room. Some health care agencies also take an early photo of the newborn for identification in the event of abduction (National Center for Missing and Exploited Children [NCMEC], 2015).

Other types of newborn security systems can also be used to prevent abduction. Some systems have sensors that are attached to the newborn's identification bracelet or cord clamp. An alarm is set off if the bracelet or clamp activates receivers near exits. Others have an alarm that is activated when the sensor is removed from the newborn (Fig. 14.17). Even with the use of electronic sensors, the parents, nursing staff, and security personnel are responsible for prevention strategies and ensuring the safety and protection of all newborns (NCMEC, 2015). Nurses can help in preventing newborn abduction by educating parents about abduction risks, using identically numbered bands on the baby and parents, by instructing couples to keep their newborn in their direct line of vision within their hospital room at all times, taking color photographs of the infant, wearing color photograph ID badges themselves, discouraging parents/families from publishing birth notices in the public media with mother's name and address, controlling access to nursery/postpartum unit with locked doors, and utilizing infant security tags or abduction alarm systems (NCMEC, 2015).

Sheila gave birth to a healthy 7-lb, 7-oz baby girl. She is eager to hold and nurse her newborn. What is the initial care of the newborn? How can the nurse meet the needs of both the newborn and Sheila, who is exhausted but eager to bond with her newborn?

Nursing Management During the Third Stage of Labor

During the third stage of labor, strong uterine contractions continue at regular intervals under the continuing influence of oxytocin. The uterine muscle fibers shorten, or retract, with each contraction, leading to a gradual decrease in the size of the uterus, which helps shear the placenta away from its attachment site. The third stage is complete when the placenta is delivered. Nursing care during the third stage of labor primarily focuses on immediate newborn care and assessment and observing for signs of placental separation, being available to assist with the delivery of the placenta, recording the time of expulsion and inspecting it for intactness. The nurse should also be assessing by palpating the uterus before and after placental expulsion.

Three hormones play important roles in the third stage. During this stage the woman experiences peak levels of oxytocin and endorphins, while the high adrenaline levels that occurred during the second stage of labor to aid with pushing begin falling. The hormone oxytocin causes uterine contractions and helps the woman to enact instinctive mothering behaviors such as holding the newborn close to her body and cuddling the baby.

Skin-to-skin contact immediately after birth and the newborn's first attempt at breast-feeding further augment maternal oxytocin levels, strengthening the uterine contractions that will help the placenta to separate and the uterus to contract to prevent hemorrhage. Endorphins, the body's natural opiates, produce an altered state of consciousness and aid in blocking out pain. In addition, the drop in adrenaline level from the second stage, which had kept the mother and baby alert at first contact, causes most women to shiver and feel cold shortly after giving birth.

Take Note!

A crucial role for nurses during this time is to protect the natural hormonal process by ensuring unhurried and uninterrupted contact between mother and newborn after birth, providing warmed blankets to prevent shivering, and allowing skin-to-skin contact with initial breast-feeding.

Continuing Assessment During the Third Stage of Labor

Assessment during the third stage of labor includes:
- Monitoring placental separation by looking for the following signs:
  - Firmly contracting uterus
  - Change in uterine shape from discoid to globular ovoid
  - Sudden gush of dark blood from vaginal opening
  - Lengthening of umbilical cord protruding from vagina
- Examining placenta and fetal membranes for intactness the second time (the health care provider assesses the placenta for intactness the first time) (Fig. 14.18)
- Assessing for any perineal trauma, such as the following, before allowing the birth attendant to leave:
  - Firm fundus with bright-red blood trickling: laceration
  - Boggy fundus with red blood flowing: uterine atony
  - Boggy fundus with dark blood and clots: retained placenta
- Inspecting the perineum for condition of episiotomy, if performed
- Assessing for perineal lacerations and ensuring repair by birth attendant

Nursing Interventions

Interventions during the third stage of labor include:
- Describing the process of placental separation to the couple
- Instructing the woman to push when signs of separation are apparent
- Administering an oxytocic agent if ordered and indicated after placental expulsion
- Providing support and information about episiotomy and/or laceration if applicable
- Cleaning and assisting client into a comfortable position after birth, making sure to lift both legs out of stirrups (if used) simultaneously to prevent strain

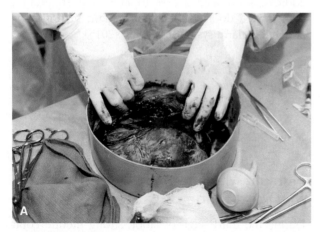 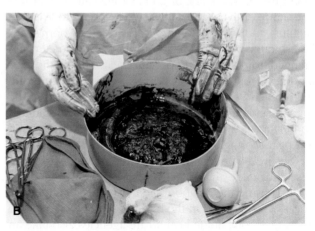

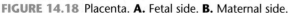
FIGURE 14.18 Placenta. **A.** Fetal side. **B.** Maternal side.

- Assess the woman's knowledge of breast-feeding to determine educational needs
- Instruct her about latching on, positioning, infant sucking and swallowing
- Repositioning the birthing bed to serve as a recovery bed if applicable
- Assisting with transfer to the recovery area if applicable
- Providing warmth by replacing warmed blankets over the woman
- Applying an ice pack to the perineal area to provide comfort to episiotomy if indicated
- Explaining what assessments will be carried out over the next hour and offering positive reinforcement for actions
- Ascertaining any needs
- Monitoring maternal physical status by assessing:
  - Vaginal bleeding: amount, consistency, and color
  - Vital signs: blood pressure, pulse, and respirations taken every 15 minutes
  - Uterine fundus, which should be firm, in the midline, and at the level of the umbilicus
- Recording all birthing statistics and securing primary caregiver's signature
- Documenting birthing event in the birth book (official record of the facility that outlines every birth event), detailing any deviations

Nursing Management During the Fourth Stage of Labor

The fourth stage of labor begins after the placenta is expelled and lasts up to 4 hours after birth, during which time recovery takes place. This recovery period may take place in the same room where the woman gave birth, in a separate recovery area, or in her postpartum room. During this stage, the woman's body is beginning to undergo the many physiologic and psychological changes that occur after birth. The focus of nursing management during the fourth stage of labor involves frequent close observation for hemorrhage, provision of comfort measures, and promotion of family attachment.

Assessment

Assessments during the fourth stage center on the woman's vital signs, status of the uterine fundus and perineal area, comfort level, lochia amount, and bladder status. During the first hour after birth, vital signs are taken every 15 minutes, then every 30 minutes for the next hour if needed. The woman's blood pressure should remain stable and within normal range after giving birth. A decrease may indicate uterine hemorrhage; an elevation might suggest preeclampsia.

The pulse usually is typically slower (60 to 70 bpm) than during labor. This may be associated with a decrease in blood volume following placental separation. An elevated pulse rate may be an early sign of blood loss. The blood pressure usually returns to its prepregnancy level and therefore is not a reliable early indicator of shock. Fever is indicative of dehydration (less than 100.4°F or 38°C) or infection (above 101°F), which may involve the genitourinary tract. Respiratory rate is usually between 16 and 24 breaths per minute and regular. Respirations should be unlabored unless there is an underlying preexisting respiratory condition.

Assess fundal height, position, and firmness every 15 minutes during the first hour following birth. The fundus needs to remain firm to prevent excessive postpartum bleeding. The fundus should be firm (feels like the size and consistency of a grapefruit), located in the midline and below the umbilicus. If it is not firm (boggy), gently massage it until it is firm (see Nursing Procedure 22.1 for more information). Once firmness is obtained, stop massaging.

 Take Note!

If the fundus is displaced to the right of the midline, suspect a full bladder as the cause.

The vagina and perineal areas are quite stretched and edematous following a vaginal birth. Assess the perineum, including the episiotomy if present, for possible hematoma formation. Suspect a hematoma if the woman reports excruciating pain or cannot void or if a mass is noted in the perineal area. Also assess for hemorrhoids, which can cause discomfort.

Assess the woman's comfort level frequently to determine the need for analgesia. Ask the woman to rate her pain on a scale of 1 to 10; it should be less than 3. If it is higher, further evaluation is needed to make sure there aren't any deviations contributing to her discomfort.

Assess vaginal discharge (lochia) every 15 minutes for the first hour and every 30 minutes for the next hour. Palpate the fundus at the same time to ascertain its firmness and help to estimate the amount of vaginal discharge. In addition, palpate the bladder for fullness, since many women receiving an epidural block experience limited sensation in the bladder region. Voiding should produce large amounts of urine (diuresis) each time. Palpating the woman's bladder after each voiding helps in assessing it and ensuring complete emptying. A full bladder will displace the uterus to either side of the midline and potentiate uterine hemorrhage secondary to bogginess.

Nursing Interventions

Nursing interventions during the fourth stage might include:
- Providing support and information to the woman regarding episiotomy repair and related pain relief and self-care measures

- Applying an ice pack to the perineum to promote comfort and reduce swelling
- Assisting with hygiene and perineal care; teaching the woman how to use the perineal bottle after each pad change and voiding; helping the woman into a new gown
- Monitoring for return of sensation and ability to void (if regional anesthesia was used)
- Encouraging the woman to void by ambulating to the bathroom, listening to running water, or pouring warm water over the perineal area with the peribottle
- Monitoring vital signs and fundal and lochia status every 15 minutes and documenting them
- Assessing for postpartum hemorrhage and urinary retention via uterine palpation
- Promoting comfort by offering analgesia for afterpains and warm blankets to reduce chilling
- Offering fluids and nourishment if desired
- Encouraging parent–infant attachment by providing privacy for the family
- Being knowledgeable about and sensitive to typical cultural practices after birth
- Assisting and encouraging the mother to nurse, if she chooses, during the recovery period to promote uterine firmness (the release of oxytocin from the posterior pituitary gland stimulates uterine contractions)
- Teaching the woman how to assess her fundus for firmness periodically and to massage it if it is boggy
- Describing the lochia flow and normal parameters to observe for postpartum
- Teaching safety techniques to prevent newborn abduction
- Demonstrating the use of the portable sitz bath as a comfort measure for her perineum if she had a laceration or an episiotomy repair
- Explaining comfort/hygiene measures and when to use them
- Assisting with ambulation when getting out of bed for the first time
- Providing information about the routine on the mother–baby unit or nursery for her stay
- Observing for signs of early parent–infant attachment: fingertip touch to palm touch to enfolding of the infant (Leonard, 2015; Green, 2016).

The nurse's role in labor and birth is a privileged one, supporting women at one of their most vulnerable times—childbirth. The nurse's focus during this time should be on supporting, protecting, advocating and empowering women. The nurse should also provide informational support, which would allow the woman to realize her aspirations and goals by making decisions through informed choice. Nurses make a long-term difference in the lives of childbearing women with small things they do for their clients that make a big difference to them.

KEY CONCEPTS

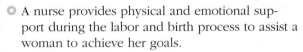

- A nurse provides physical and emotional support during the labor and birth process to assist a woman to achieve her goals.
- When a woman is admitted to the labor and birth area, the admitting nurse must assess and evaluate the risk status of the pregnancy and initiate appropriate interventions to provide optimal care for the client.
- Completing an admission assessment includes taking a maternal health history; performing a physical assessment on the woman and fetus, including her emotional and psychosocial status; and obtaining the necessary laboratory studies.
- The nurse's role in fetal assessment for labor and birth includes determining fetal well-being and interpreting signs and symptoms of possible compromise. Determining the fetal heart rate (FHR) pattern and assessing amniotic fluid characteristics are key.
- FHR can be assessed intermittently or continuously. Although the intermittent method allows the client to move about during labor, the information obtained intermittently does not provide a complete picture of fetal well-being from moment to moment.
- Assessment parameters of the FHR are classified as baseline rate, baseline variability, and periodic changes in the rate (accelerations and decelerations).
- The nurse monitoring the laboring client needs to be knowledgeable about which category the FHR pattern is in so that appropriate interventions can be instituted.
- For a Category III FHR pattern, the nurse should notify the health care provider about the pattern and obtain further orders, making sure to document all interventions and their effects on the FHR pattern.
- In addition to interpreting assessment findings and initiating appropriate inventions for the laboring client, accurate and timely documentation must be carried out continuously.
- Today's women have many safe nonpharmacologic and pharmacologic choices for the management of pain during childbirth. They may be used individually or in combination to complement one another.
- Nursing management for the woman during labor and birth includes comfort measures, emotional support, information and instruction, advocacy, and support for the partner.

- Nursing care during the first stage of labor includes taking an admission history (reviewing the prenatal record), checking the results of routine laboratory work and special tests done during pregnancy, asking the woman about her childbirth preparation (birth plan, classes taken, coping skills), and completing a physical assessment of the woman to establish baseline values for future comparison.

- Nursing care during the second stage of labor focuses on supporting the woman and her partner in making decisions about her care and labor management, implementing strategies to prolong the early passive phase of fetal descent, supporting involuntary bearing-down efforts, providing support and assistance, and encouraging the use of maternal positions that can enhance descent and reduce the pain.

- Nursing care during the third stage of labor primarily focuses on immediate newborn care and assessment and being available to assist with the delivery of the placenta and inspecting it for intactness.

- The focus of nursing management during the fourth stage of labor involves frequently observing the mother for hemorrhage, providing comfort measures, and promoting family attachment.

References and Recommended Readings

Adams, J., Frawley, J., Steel, A., Broom, A., & Sibbritt, D. (2015). Use of pharmacological and non-pharmacological labor pain management techniques and their relationship to maternal and infant birth outcomes: Examination of a nationally representative sample of 1835 pregnant women. *Midwifery, 31*(4), 458–463.

Agency for Healthcare Research and Quality [AHRQ] (2014). Intrapartum fetal heart rate monitoring: nomenclature, and general management principles. Retrieved from http://www.guideline.gov/content.aspx?id=14885

American College of Obstetricians and Gynecologists [ACOG] and Society for Maternal Fetal Medicine [SMFM] (2014). Safe prevention of the primary cesarean delivery. Obstetric Care Consensus 1, *Obstetrics & Gynecology, 123*, 693–711.

American Hospital Association. (2014). RNs role in labor and delivery. Retrieved from http://www.aha.org/search?q=RNs+role+in+labor+and+delivery&start-date

American Hospital Association [AHA] (2015). Prepared to care: The 24/7 role of America's full-service hospitals. Retrieved from http://www.aha.org/content/00-10/PreparedToCareFinal.pdf

American Pregnancy Association. (2015). Patterned breathing during labor. Retrieved from http://www.americanpregnancy.org/labornbirth/patternedbreathing.htm

Anderson, L. (2014). Cultural competence in the nursing practice. *Nursetogether*. Retrieved from http://www.nursetogether.com/cultural-competence-in-the-nursing-practice

Ashimi, O., Hoff, E., Sibai, B., & Hardwicke, R. (2015). 212: Should the current DHHS recommendations for use of antiretroviral drugs in maternal HIV-1 RNA undergo a review? An urban academic experience. *American Journal of Obstetrics & Gynecology, 212*(1), S119–S120.

Association of Women's Health, Obstetric and Neonatal Nurses [AWHONN]. (2015). *Fetal heart monitoring: Principles and practices* (5th ed.). Washington, DC: AWHONN.

Badve, M., & Vallejo, M. C. (2015). Obstetric anesthesia. In *Basic clinical anesthesia* (pp. 501–527). New York, NY: Springer Publishers.

Bowers, P. (2015). Cultural perspectives in childbearing. *Nursing Spectrum*. Retrieved from http://ce.nurse.com/ce263-60/cultural-perspectives-in-childbearing.

Cahill, A. G., & Spain, J. (2015). Intrapartum fetal monitoring. *Clinical Obstetrics and Gynecology, 58*(2), 263–268.

Callahan, T. L. (2016). *Tarascon's OB/GYN pocketbook*. Burlington, MA: Jones & Bartlett Learning.

Camorcia, M. (2015). The second and third stage of labor. In *Epidural labor analgesia* (pp. 103–119). Springer International Publishing.

Capogna, G. (2015a). Humanization of childbirth and epidural analgesia. In *Epidural labor analgesia* (pp. 315–323). Springer International Publishing.

Capogna, G. (2015b). Maintenance of labor analgesia. In *Epidural labor analgesia* (pp. 89–101). Springer International Publishing.

Casanova, R. (2015). *Shelf-life obstetrics and gynecology*. Philadelphia, PA: Lippincott Williams & Wilkins.

Centers for Disease Control and Prevention [CDC] (2014). Group B strep (GBS) guidelines. Retrieved from http://www.cdc.gov/groupbstrep/guidelines/new-differences.html

Centers for Disease Control and Prevention [CDC] (2015). HIV/AIDS testing. Retrieved from http://www.cdc.gov/hiv/basics/testing.html

Chandraharan, E., (2014). Fetal scalp sampling during labor: Is it a useful diagnostic test or a historical test that no longer has a place in modern obstetrics? *BJOG, 121*(9), 1056–1060; discussion 1060–1062.

Cheng, Y., & Caughey, A. B. (2015a). Normal labor and delivery. *eMedicine*. Retrieved from http://emedicine.medscape.com/article/260036-overview#aw2aab6b2.

Cheng, Y. W., & Caughey, A. B. (2015b). Second stage of labor. *Clinical Obstetrics and Gynecology, 58*(2), 227–240.

Cibils, L. A. (2014). *Electronic fetal-maternal monitoring: Antepartum/intrapartum* (2nd ed.). New York, NY: Springer Publishers.

Cox, K. J., & King, T. L. (2015). Preventing primary cesarean births: Midwifery care. *Clinical Obstetrics and Gynecology, 58*(2), 282–293.

Dalal, S. M. (2015). Newer aspects of labor analgesia. *Research Chronicle in Health Sciences, 1*(2), 130–138.

Faisal-Cury, A., Menezes, P. R., Quayle, J., Matijasevich, A., & Diniz, S. G. (2015). The relationship between mode of delivery and sexual health outcomes after childbirth. *The Journal of Sexual Medicine, 12*(5), 1212–1220.

Farine, D. (Ed.). (2015). *New technologies for managing labor*. Boston, MA: Walter de Gruyter GmbH & Co KG.

Freeman, R. K. (2015). Intrapartum fetal heart rate monitoring. *Protocols for high-risk pregnancies: An evidence-based approach* (6th ed., pp. 418–422). John Wiley & Sons.

Friedman, A. M., Ananth, C. V., Prendergast, E., D'Alton, M. E., & Wright, J. D. (2015). Variation in and factors associated with use of episiotomy. *JAMA, 313*(2), 197–199.

Gizzo, S., Di Gangi, S., Noventa, M., Bacile, V., Zambon, A., & Nardelli, B. (2014). Women's choice of positions during labor: Return to the past or a modern way to give birth? A cohort study in Italy. *BioMed Research International, 2014*, 638093.http://dx.doi.org/10.1155/2014/638093.

Grant, E. N., Tao, W., Craig, M., McIntire, D., Leveno, K. (2015). Neuraxial analgesia effects on labor progression: Facts, fallacies, uncertainties and the future. *BJOG, 122*, 288–293.

Green, C. J. (2016). *Maternal newborn nursing care plans* (3rd ed.). Burlington, MA: Jones & Bartlett Learning.

Gujral, K., & Nayar, S. (2015). Current trends in management of fetal growth restriction. *Journal of Fetal Medicine, 1*(3), 125–129.

Halpern, S. H., & Garg, R. (2015). Evidence-based medicine and labor analgesia. In *Epidural labor analgesia* (pp. 285–295). Springer International Publishing.

Hanson, L., & VandeVusse, L., (2014). Supporting labor progress toward physiologic birth. *Journal of Perinatal & Neonatal Nursing, 28*(2), 101–107.

Hastings C. (2015) The role of fetal monitoring in intrapartum care. *British Journal of Healthcare Management, 21*(4), 166–170.

Hawkins, J. L. (2015). Excess in moderation: General anesthesia for cesarean delivery. *Anesthesia & Analgesia, 120*(6), 1175–1177.

Heesen, M., Van de Velde, M., Klöhr, S., Lehberger, J., Rossaint, R., & Straube, S. (2015). Meta-analysis of the success of block following combined spinal-epidural vs epidural analgesia during labor. *Survey of Anesthesiology, 59*(3), 131–133.

Hersh, S., Megregian, M., & Emeis, C. (2014). Intermittent auscultation of the fetal heart rate during labor: An opportunity for shared decision making. *Journal of Midwifery & Women's Health, 59*: 344–349

Hiersch, L., Rosen, H., Salzer, L., Aviram, A., Ben-Haroush, A., & Yogev, Y. (2015). Does artificial rupturing of membranes in the active phase of labor enhance myometrial electrical activity?. *The Journal of Maternal-Fetal & Neonatal Medicine, 28*(5), 515–518.

Holvey, N. (2014) Supporting women in the second stage of labor. *British Journal of Midwifery, 22*(3), 182–186.

Ibrahim, S. E. H., Fridman, M., Korst, L. M., & Gregory, K. D. (2015). Anesthesia complications as a childbirth patient safety indicator. *Survey of Anesthesiology, 59*(3), 127–129.

Institute for Clinical Systems Improvement [ICSI]. (2015a) Fetal monitoring. Retrieved from http://link.springer.com/chapter/10.1007/978-1-4614-8557-5_42#page-1

Institute for Clinical Systems Improvement [ICSI] (2015b). Health care guideline: Management of labor. Retrieved from https://www.icsi.org/_asset/br063k/LaborMgmt.pdf

Iravani, M., Zarean, E., Janghorbani, M., & Bahrami, M. (2015). Women's needs and expectations during normal labor and delivery. *Journal of Education and Health Promotion, 4*, 6.

Ivory, C. H. (2014). Standardizing the words nurses use to document elements of perinatal failure to rescue. *JOGNN: Journal of Obstetric, Gynecologic & Neonatal Nursing, 43*(1), 13–24.

Jackson, S., & Gregory, K. D. (2015). Management of the first stage of labor: Potential strategies to lower the cesarean delivery rate. *Clinical Obstetrics and Gynecology, 58*(2), 217–226.

Janula, R., & Mahipal, S. (2015). Effectiveness of aromatherapy and biofeedback in promotion of labor outcome during childbirth among primigravidas. *Health Science Journal, 9*(1). 1–5.

Jones, L. E., Whitburn, L. Y., Davey, M. A., & Small, R. (2015). Assessment of pain associated with childbirth: Women's perspectives, preferences and solutions. *Midwifery. 31*(7), 708–712.

Kerr, D., Taylor, D., & Evans, B. (2015). Patient-controlled intranasal fentanyl analgesia: A pilot study to assess practicality and tolerability during childbirth. *International Journal of Obstetric Anesthesia, 24*(2), 117–123.

King, T. L., Brucker, M. C., Kriebs, J. M., Fahey, J. O., Gegor, C. L., & Varney, H. (2015). *Varney's midwifery* (5th ed.). Burlington, MA: Jones & Bartlett Learning.

Leonard, P. (2015). Childbirth education: A handbook for nurses. *Nursing Spectrum.* Retrieved from http://ce.nurse.com/60057/childbirth-education-a-handbook-for-nurses

Lindholm, A., & Hildingsson, I. (2015). Women's preferences and received pain relief in childbirth–A prospective longitudinal study in a northern region of Sweden. *Sexual & Reproductive Healthcare, 6*(2), 74–81.

Liu, Y. M., Fernando, R., & Mon, W. Y. (2015). Labor pain. In *Epidural labor analgesia* (pp. 21–37). Springer International Publishing.

Lucas, M. T., da Rocha, M. J., de Medonça Costa, K. M., de Oliveira, G. G., & Melo, J. O. (2015). Nursing care during labor in a model maternity unit: Cross-sectional study. *Online Brazilian Journal of Nursing, 14*(1), 32–40.

Magowan, B., Owen, P., & Thomson, A. (2014). *Clinical obstetrics & gynecology* (3rd ed.). St. Louis, MO: Saunders Elsevier.

Martin, R. J., Fanaroff, A. A., & Walsh, M. C. (2014). *Neonatal-perinatal medicine* (10th ed.). Philadelphia, PA: Elsevier Health Sciences.

Maso, G., Piccoli, M., De Seta, F., Parolin, S., Banco, R., Camacho, M. L., et al. (2015). Intrapartum fetal heart rate monitoring interpretation in labor: A critical appraisal. *Minerva Ginecologica, 67*(1), 65–79.

McGeary, C. A., Swanholm, E., & Gatchel, R. J. (2015). Pain management. *The encyclopedia of clinical psychology* (pp. 1–6). doi: 10.1002/9781118625392.wbecp144.

Miller, L. A. (2014). Ask an expert: Frequently asked questions on nursing liability issues. *Journal of Perinatal & Neonatal Nursing, 28*(1), 9–11.

Mollart, L. J., Adam, J., & Foureur, M. (2015). Impact of acupressure on onset of labor and labor duration: A systematic review. *Women and Birth, 28*(3), 199–206..

Nageotte, M. P. (2015). Fetal heart rate monitoring. *Seminars in Fetal and Neonatal Medicine, 20*(3), 144–148.

Nagtalon-Ramos, J. (2014). *Best evidence-based practices in maternal-newborn nursing care.* Philadelphia, PA: F. A. Davis Company.

National Center for Missing and Exploited Children [NCMEC]. (2015). Infant abductions. Retrieved from http://www.missingkids.com/InfantAbduction

National Institute for Health and care Excellence [NICE]. (2014). *Intrapartum care: Care of healthy women and their babies during childbirth* (CG190). London, UK: NICE.

National Institute of Child Health and Human Development [NICHD]. (2015). NICHD terminology for fetal heart rate characteristics. Retrieved from http://www.nichd.nih.gov/search.cfm?search_string=electronic+fetal+monitoring

Neal, J. L., Lamp, J. M., Buck, J. S., Lowe, N. K., Gillespie, S. L., & Ryan, S. L. (2014). Outcomes of nulliparous women with spontaneous labor onset admitted to hospitals in preactive versus active labor. *Journal of Midwifery & Women's Health, 59*, 28–34.

Neetu, P. S., & Panchal, R. (2015). A study to assess the effectiveness of abdominal effleurage on labor pain intensity and labor outcomes among nullipara mothers during first stage of labor in selected Hospitals of District Ambala, Haryana. *International Journal of Science & Research, 4*(1), 1585–1590.

Nutter, E. (2016). Decreasing vulnerability in childbirth: Waterbirth in military treatment facilities. *Caring for the vulnerable* (4th ed., pp. 253–262). Burlington, MA: Jones & Bartlett Learning.

Omo-Aghoja, L. (2015). Maternal and fetal Acid-base chemistry: A major determinant of perinatal outcome. *Annals of Medical and Health Sciences Research, 4*(1), 8–17.

Patkar, C. S., Vora, K., Patel, H., Shah, V., Modi, M. P., & Parikh, G. (2015). A comparison of continuous infusion and intermittent bolus administration of 0.1% ropivacaine with 0.0002% fentanyl for epidural labor analgesia. *Journal of Anesthesiology, Clinical Pharmacology, 31*(2), 234–238.

Petrocnik, P., & Marshall, J. E. (2015). Hands-poised technique: The future technique for perineal management of second stage of labor? A modified systematic literature review. *Midwifery, 31*(2), 274–279.

Prior, T., & Kumar, S. (2015). Expert review–identification of intrapartum fetal compromise. *European Journal of Obstetrics & Gynecology and Reproductive Biology, 190*, 1–6.

Reed, R. (2015). Supporting women's instinctive pushing behaviour during birth. *The Practicing Midwife, 18*(6), 13–15.

Roberts, L., Gulliver, B., Fisher, J., & Cloyes, K. G. (2010). The coping with labor algorithm: An alternate pain assessment tool for the laboring woman. *Journal of Midwifery & Women's Health, 55*, 107–116.

Sholapurkar, S. (2014). Algorithm for management of category II fetal heart rate tracings: A standardization of right sort? *American Journal of Obstetrics and Gynecology, 210*(2), 175.

Sholapurkar, M. S. L. (2015). *Intrapartum fetal monitoring: Overview, controversies and pitfalls* (pp. 1–8). The Health Foundation.

Sides, C., Rios, A. R., Lam, M. C., Ward, A. R., Stoltzfus, J., & Lucente, V. R. (2015). Above all, do no harm: Modifiable risk factors for high-risk perineal lacerations [139]. *Obstetrics & Gynecology, 125*, 49S.

Simkin, P., & Klein, M. C. (2015). Nonpharmacologic approaches to management of labor pain. *UpToDate,* Retrieved from http://www.uptodate.com/contents/nonpharmacological-approaches-to-management-of-labor-pain.

Simpson, K. R. (2015). Electronic health records. *MCN: The American Journal of Maternal/Child Nursing, 40*(1), 68.

Skidmore-Roth, L. (2015). *Mosby's 2015 nursing drug reference* (28th ed.). St. Louis, MO: Mosby Elsevier.

Sng, B. L., Kwok, S. C., & Sia, A. T. (2015). Modern neuraxial labor analgesia. *Current Opinion in Anesthesiology, 28*(3), 285–289.

Sng, B. L., Zhang, Q., Leong, W. L., Ocampo, C., Assam, P. N., & Sia, A. T. (2015). Incidence and characteristics of breakthrough pain in parturients using computer-integrated patient-controlled epidural analgesia. *Journal of Clinical Anesthesia, 27*(4), 277–284.

Society of Obstetricians and Gynecologists of Canada. (2015). Fetal health surveillance in labor (SOGC Clinical Practice Guidelines). *Journal of Obstetrics and Gynecology in Canada.* Retrieved from http://www.sogc.org.

Stocks, G. M., & Griffiths, S. K. (2015). Initiation of labor analgesia: Epidural, CSE. In *Epidural labor analgesia* (pp. 73–88). Springer International Publishing.

Taghavi, S., Barband, S., & Khaki, A. (2015). Effect of hydrotherapy on pain of labor process. *BALTICA, 28*(1), 116–121.

unit
five

BRINGING IT ALL TOGETHER: CASE STUDY

A 30-year old woman at term presents to the emergency room with abdominal pain. This is her first pregnancy and she is accompanied by her partner and her very anxious sister. She is 40 weeks and 6 days based on her last ultrasound. All pregnancy blood tests have been normal. Earlier in the day she had a mucus-like dark red discharge followed by the onset of irregular period-type cramps. Two hours ago she felt a gush of clear fluid from her vagina and since then she has felt miserable. She took two Tylenol at home for the pain, but she is now in distress and came to the hospital for assessment.

ASSESSMENT

On examination, she is comfortable between pains. Her blood pressure is 130/80 and pulse is 100 bpm. Fetal movement is felt by the nurse. FHR is 142 bpm. Fundal height upon palpation is 37 cm and in a cephalic presentation. Speculum exam shows clear fluid pooled in the posterior vaginal fornix. A ferning pattern is present when fluid is placed on a glass slide. The vaginal exam reveals the cervix to be fully effaced and 4cm dilated. The fetal head is 2 cm above the ischial spines. There is no fetal caput or molding felt during the vaginal exam.

Go to thePoint **to find questions to consider about this case.**

CHAPTER WORKSHEET

MULTIPLE CHOICE QUESTIONS

1. When a client in labor is fully dilated, which instruction would be most effective to assist her in encouraging effective pushing?
   a. Hold your breath and push through entire contraction.
   b. Use chest-breathing with the contraction.
   c. Pant and blow during each contraction.
   d. Wait until you feel the urge to push.

2. During the fourth stage of labor, the nurse assesses the woman at frequent intervals after giving childbirth. What assessment data would cause the nurse the most concern?
   a. Moderate amount of dark red lochia drainage on peripad
   b. Uterine fundus palpated to the right of the umbilicus
   c. An oral temperature reading of 100.6° F
   d. Perineal area bruised and edematous beneath her ice pack

3. When managing a client's pain during labor, nurses should:
   a. Make sure the agents given do not prolong labor
   b. Know that all pain relief measures are similar
   c. Support the client's decisions and requests
   d. Not recommend nonpharmacologic methods

4. When caring for a client during the active phase of labor without continuous electronic fetal monitoring, the nurse would intermittently assess FHR every:
   a. 15 to 30 minutes
   b. 5 to 10 minutes
   c. 45 to 60 minutes
   d. 60 to 75 minutes

5. The nurse notes the presence of transient fetal accelerations on the fetal monitoring strip. Which intervention would be most appropriate?
   a. Reposition the client on the left side.
   b. Begin 100% oxygen via face mask.
   c. Document this as indicating a normal pattern.
   d. Call the health care provider immediately.

6. By the end of the second stage of labor, the nurse would expect which of the following events? The
   a. cervix is fully dilated and effaced
   b. placenta is detached and expelled
   c. fetus is born and on mother's chest
   d. woman to request pain medication

7. Which of the following practices would not be included in a physiologic birth?
   a. Early induction of labor <39 weeks gestation
   b. Freedom of movement for the laboring woman
   c. Continuous presence and support throughout labor
   d. Encouraging spontaneous pushing when urge felt

CRITICAL THINKING EXERCISE

1. A 20-year-old primigravida at term, comes to the birthing center in active labor (dilation 5 cm and 80% effaced, –1 station) with ruptured membranes. She states she wants an "all-natural" birth without medication. Her partner is with her and appears anxious but supportive. On the admission assessment, this client's prenatal history is unremarkable; vital signs are within normal limits; FHR via Doppler ranges between 140 and 144 bpm and is regular.
   a. Based on your assessment data and the woman's request not to have medication, what nonpharmacologic interventions could you offer her?
   b. What positions might be suggested to facilitate fetal descent?

2. Several hours later, the client complains of nausea and turns to her partner and angrily tells him to not touch her and to go away.
   a. What assessment needs to be done to determine what is happening?
   b. What explanation can you offer this client's partner regarding her change in behavior?

STUDY ACTIVITIES

1. Share experiences within a post clinical conference group regarding the pain management interventions of the clients to which you were assigned. Compare and evaluate the effectiveness of different methods used, maternal behavior observed, and neonatal outcome in terms of Apgar scores.

2. On the fetal heart monitor, the nurse notices an elevation of the fetal baseline with the onset of contractions. This elevation would describe _____.

3. Compare and contrast a local birthing center to a community hospital's birthing suite in terms of the pain management techniques and fetal monitoring used.

4. Select a childbirth website for expectant parents and critique the information provided in terms of its educational level and amount of advertising.

Tharpe, N. L., Farley, C. L., & Jordan, R. (2016). *Clinical practice guidelines for midwifery & women's health* (5th ed.). Burlington, MA: Jones and Bartlett.

Timmins, A. E., & Clark, S. L. (2015). How to approach intrapartum category II tracings. *Obstetrics and Gynecology Clinics of North America, 42*(2), 363–375.

Ugwumadu, A. (2015). Author's reply re: Are we (mis)guided by current guidelines on intrapartum fetal heart rate monitoring? Case for a more physiological approach to interpretation. *BJOG: An International Journal of Obstetrics & Gynecology, 122*: 589.

U.S. Department of Health and Human Services. (2010). *Healthy people 2020*. Retrieved from http://www.healthypeople.gov/2020/topicsobjectives2020

Van de Velde, M. (2015). Patient-controlled intravenous analgesia remifentanil for labor analgesia: Time to stop, think and reconsider. *Current Opinion in Anesthesiology, 28*(3), 237–239.

Verklan, T., & Walden, M., (2014). *Core curriculum for neonatal intensive care nursing* (4th ed.). St. Louis, MO: Saunders Elsevier.

Walker, S., & Sabrosa, R. (2014). Assessment of fetal presentation: Exploring a woman-centered approach. *British Journal of Midwifery, 22*(4), 240–244.

Wenner, L. (2015). It's the little things. *Nursing for Women's Health, 19*(2), 203–204.

Wisner, K. (2015). Intermittent auscultation in low-risk labor. *MCN: The American Journal of Maternal/Child Nursing, 40*(1), 58.

Wojnar, D. M., & Narruhn, R. A. (2016). Transcultural aspects of perinatal health care of Somali women. *Caring for the vulnerable* (4th ed., pp. 287–302). Burlington, MA: Jones & Bartlett Learning.

World Health Organization [WHO] (2014). *WHO recommendations for augmentation of labor*. Retrieved from: http://apps.who.int/iris/bitstream/10665/112825/1/9789241507363_eng.pdf

Yuan, S. M. (2015). Fetal cardiac interventions. *Pediatrics & Neonatology, 56*(2), 81–87.

Postpartum Period

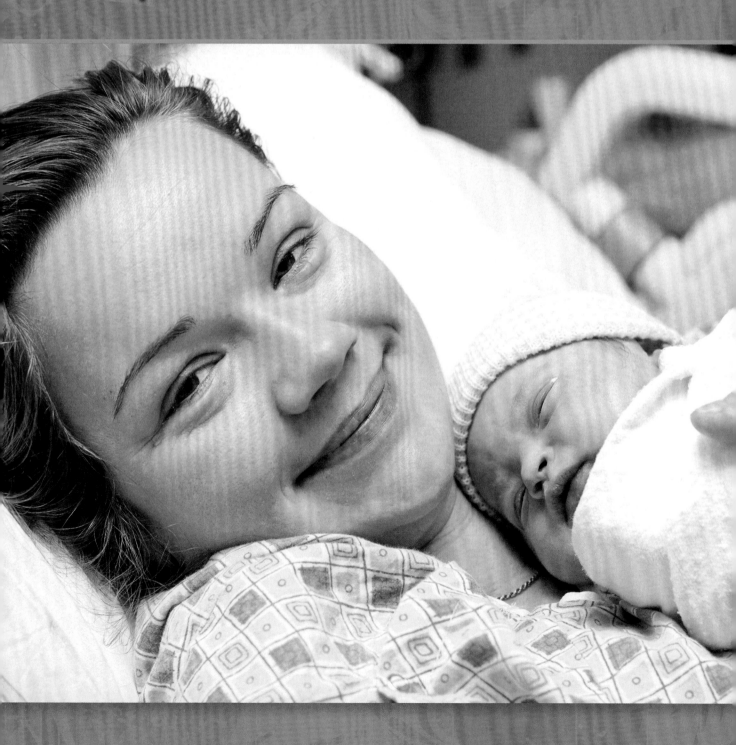

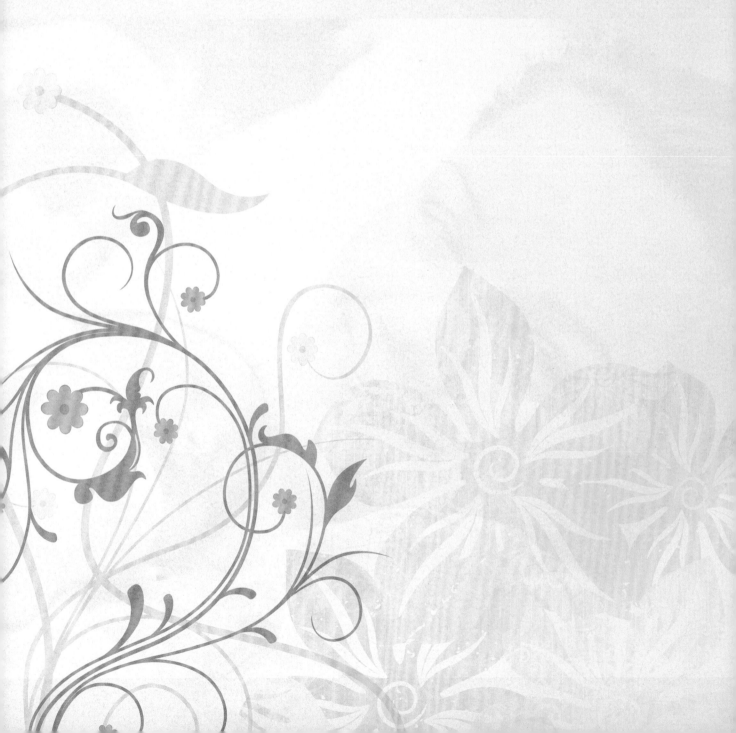

Postpartum Period

15

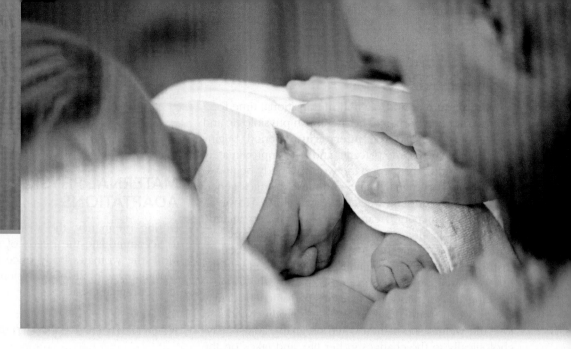

Postpartum Adaptations

Learning Objectives

Upon completion of the chapter, you will be able to:

1. Examine the systemic physiologic changes occurring in the woman after childbirth.
2. Determine the psychological changes that occur in women in the postpartum period.
3. Relate effective maternal self-care measures to be implemented in the postpartum period.
4. Integrate dimensions of postpartum care for the multicultural family.
5. Plan postpartum nursing care with interventions to foster maternal/infant bonding.
6. Assess the phases of maternal role adjustment and accompanying behaviors.
7. Analyze the psychological adaptations occurring in the mother's partner after childbirth.

Betsy had been home only 3 days when she called the OB unit where she had given birth and asked to speak to the lactation consultant. She reported pain in both breasts. Her nipples were tender due to frequent breast-feeding and she described her breasts as heavy, hard, and swollen.

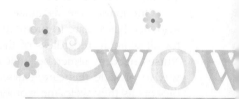

Words of Wisdom
A new mother's expectations are seen through rose-colored glasses, and at times her fantasy is better than the reality.

INTRODUCTION

The postpartum period is a critical transitional time for a woman, her newborn, and her family on physiologic and psychological levels. The **puerperium** period begins after the delivery of the placenta and lasts approximately 6 weeks. During this period the woman's body begins to return to its prepregnant state, and these changes generally resolve by the sixth week after giving birth. However, the postpartum period can also be defined to include the changes in all aspects of the mother's life that occur during the first year after a child is born. Some believe that the postpartum adjustment period lasts well into the first year, making the fourth phase of labor the longest. Keeping this in mind, the true postpartum period may last between 9 and 12 months as the mother works to lose the weight she gained while pregnant, adjusts psychologically to the changes in her life, and takes on the new role of mother.

Nurses caring for childbearing families should consider all aspects of culture, including communication, space, and family roles. Communication encompasses an understanding of not only a person's language, and loudness of speech, but also the meaning of touch and gestures. The concept of personal space and the dimensions of comfort zones differ from culture to culture. Touching, placing clients in proximity to others, and taking away personal possessions can reduce a client's personal security and heighten her anxiety. Nurses must be sensitive to how people respond when being touched and should refrain from touching if the client's response indicates that it is unwelcome. Cultural norms also have an impact on family roles, expectations, and behaviors associated with a member's position in the family. For example, culture may influence whether a man actively participates in the pregnancy and childbirth. Maternity health care professionals in the United States expect men to be involved, but this role expectation may conflict with that of many of the diverse groups now living in the United States. Mexican Americans, Arab Americans, Asian Americans, and Orthodox Jewish Americans, for example, usually view the birthing experience as a woman's affair (Purnell, 2014).

Our major role as nurses is to provide safe and evidence-based care to promote optimal birth outcomes for all women, regardless of their cultural background. Nurses need to remember that there is more than one way to provide this care. Nurses are important cultural brokers as they welcome women and their families into our obstetrical units, where nurses share with those families one of the most intimate experiences of their lives (Bowers & Ceballos, 2015).

This chapter describes the major physiologic and psychological changes that occur in a woman after childbirth. Various systemic adaptations take place throughout the woman's body. In addition, the mother and the family adjust to the new addition psychologically. The birth of a child changes the family structure and the roles of the family members. The adaptations are dynamic and continue to evolve as physical changes occur and new roles emerge.

MATERNAL PHYSIOLOGIC ADAPTATIONS

During pregnancy, the woman's entire body changed to accommodate the needs of the growing fetus. After birth, the woman's body once again undergoes significant changes in all body systems to return her body to its prepregnant state.

Reproductive System Adaptations

The reproductive system goes through tremendous adaptations to return to the prepregnancy state. All organs and tissues of the reproductive system are involved. The female reproductive system is unique in its capacity to remodel itself throughout the woman's reproductive life. The events after birth, with the shedding of the placenta and subsequent uterine involution, involve substantial tissue destruction and subsequent repair and remodeling. For example, the woman's menstrual cycle, interrupted during pregnancy, will begin to return several weeks after childbirth, if the woman is not breast-feeding. Ovulation can return any time, thus breast-feeding should not be considered as a safe contraceptive and other methods should be used to prevent pregnancy. The uterus, which has undergone tremendous expansion during pregnancy to accommodate progressive fetal growth, will return to its prepregnant size over several weeks. The mother's breasts have grown to prepare for lactation and do not return to their prepregnant size as the uterus does.

Uterine Involution

The uterus returns to its normal size through a gradual process of **involution**, which involves retrogressive changes that return it to its nonpregnant size and condition. Involution involves three retrogressive processes:
1. Contraction of muscle fibers to reduce those previously stretched during pregnancy
2. Catabolism, which shrinks enlarged, individual myometrial cells
3. Regeneration of uterine epithelium from the lower layer of the decidua after the upper layers have been sloughed off and shed during lochial discharge (Mattson & Smith, 2016).

The uterus, which weighs approximately 1,000 g (2.2 lb) soon after birth, undergoes physiologic involution as it returns to its nonpregnant state. Approximately

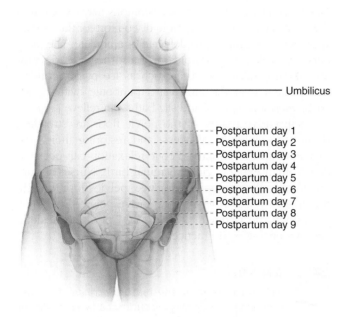

Umbilicus

Postpartum day 1
Postpartum day 2
Postpartum day 3
Postpartum day 4
Postpartum day 5
Postpartum day 6
Postpartum day 7
Postpartum day 8
Postpartum day 9

FIGURE 15.1 Uterine involution.

1 week after birth, the uterus shrinks in size by 50% and weighs about 500 g (1 lb); at the end of 6 weeks, it weighs approximately 60 g (2 oz), about the weight before the pregnancy (Jordan et al., 2014) (Fig. 15.1). During the first few days after birth, the uterus typically descends from the level of the umbilicus at a rate of 1 cm (1 fingerbreadth) per day. By 3 days, the fundus lies 2 to 3 fingerbreadths below the umbilicus (or slightly higher in multiparous women). By the end of 10 days, the fundus usually cannot be palpated because it has descended into the true pelvis.

If these retrogressive changes do not occur as a result of retained placental fragments or infection, then subinvolution of the uterus typically results (delayed or absent involution). Subinvolution is generally responsive to early diagnosis and treatment. Factors that facilitate uterine involution include complete expulsion of amniotic membranes and placenta at birth, a complication-free labor and birth process, breast-feeding, and early ambulation. Factors that inhibit involution include a prolonged labor and difficult birth, incomplete expulsion of amniotic membranes and placenta, uterine infection, overdistention of uterine muscles (such as by multiple gestation, hydramnios, or a large singleton fetus), a full bladder (which displaces the uterus and interferes with contractions), anesthesia (which relaxes uterine muscles), and close childbirth spacing (frequent and repeated distention decreases tone and causes muscular relaxation).

LOCHIA

Lochia is the vaginal discharge that occurs after birth and continues for approximately 4 to 8 weeks. It results from involution, during which the superficial layer of the decidua

basalis becomes necrotic and is sloughed off. Immediately after childbirth, lochia is bright red and consists mainly of blood, fibrinous products, decidual cells, and red and white blood cells. The lochia from the uterus is alkaline but becomes acidic as it passes through the vagina. It is roughly equal to the amount occurring during a heavy menstrual period. The average amount of lochial discharge is 240 to 270 mL (8 to 9 oz) (Bope & Kellerman, 2015).

Women who have had cesarean births tend to have less flow because the uterine debris is removed manually along with delivery of the placenta. Lochia is present in most women for at least 3 weeks after childbirth, but it persists in some women for as long as 6 weeks.

Lochia passes through three stages:
- *Lochia rubra* is a deep-red mixture of mucus, tissue debris, and blood that occurs for the first 3 to 4 days after birth. As uterine bleeding subsides, it becomes paler and more serous.
- *Lochia serosa* is the second stage. It is pinkish brown and is expelled 3 to 10 days postpartum. Lochia serosa primarily contains leukocytes, decidual tissue, red blood cells, and serous fluid.
- *Lochia alba* is the final stage. The discharge is creamy white or light brown and consists of leukocytes, decidual tissue, and reduced fluid content. It occurs from days 10 to 14 but can last 3 to 6 weeks postpartum in some women and still be considered normal.

Lochia at any stage should have a fleshy smell; an offensive odor usually indicates an infection, such as endometritis.

Take Note!

A danger sign is the reappearance of bright-red blood after lochia rubra has stopped. Reevaluation by a health care provider is essential if this occurs.

AFTERPAINS

Part of the involution process involves uterine contractions. Subsequently, many women are frequently bothered by painful uterine contractions termed *afterpains*. All women experience afterpains, but they are more acute in multiparous and breast-feeding women secondary to repeated stretching of the uterine muscles from multiple pregnancies or stimulation during breast-feeding with oxytocin released from the pituitary gland. Primiparous women typically experience mild afterpains because their uterus is able to maintain a contracted state. Breast-feeding and administration of exogenous oxytocin both cause powerful and painful uterine contractions. Afterpains usually respond to oral analgesics.

Take Note!

Afterpains are usually stronger during breast-feeding because oxytocin released by the sucking reflex strengthens the contractions. Mild analgesics can reduce this discomfort.

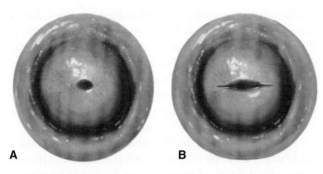

FIGURE 15.2 Appearance of the cervical os. **A.** Before the first pregnancy. **B.** After pregnancy.

Cervix

The cervix typically returns to its prepregnant state by week 6 of the postpartum period. The cervix gradually closes but never regains its prepregnant appearance. Immediately after childbirth, the cervix is shapeless and edematous and is easily distensible for several days. The internal cervical os gradually closes and returns to normal by 2 weeks, whereas the external os widens and never appears the same after childbirth. The external cervical os is no longer shaped like a circle, but instead appears as a jagged slit-like opening, often described as a "fish mouth" (Fig. 15.2).

Vagina

Shortly after birth, the vaginal mucosa is edematous and thin, with few rugae. As ovarian function returns and estrogen production resumes, the mucosa thickens and rugae return in approximately 3 weeks. The vagina gapes at the opening and is generally lax. The vagina returns to its approximate prepregnant size by 6 to 8 weeks postpartum but will always remain a bit larger than it had been before pregnancy.

Normal mucus production and thickening of the vaginal mucosa usually return with ovulation. The vagina gradually decreases in size and regains tone over several weeks. By 3 to 4 weeks, the edema and vascularity have decreased. The vaginal epithelium is generally restored by 6 to 8 weeks postpartum (Mattson & Smith, 2016). Localized dryness and coital discomfort (dyspareunia) usually plague most women until menstruation returns. Water-soluble lubricants can reduce discomfort during intercourse.

Perineum

The perineum is often edematous and bruised for the first day or two after birth. If the birth involved an episiotomy or laceration, complete healing may take as long as 4 to 6 months in the absence of complications at the site, such as hematoma or infection. The muscle tone may or may not return to normal, depending on the extent of injury to muscle, nerve, and connecting tissues (Spiliolpoulos &

Mastrogiannis, 2014). Perineal lacerations may extend into the anus and cause considerable discomfort for the mother when she is attempting to defecate or ambulate. The presence of swollen hemorrhoids may also heighten discomfort. Local comfort measures such as ice packs, pouring warm water over the area via a peribottle, witch hazel pads, anesthetic sprays, and sitz baths can relieve pain.

Supportive tissues of the pelvic floor are stretched during the childbirth process, and restoring their tone may take up to 6 months. Pelvic relaxation can occur in any woman experiencing a vaginal birth. Nurses should encourage all women to practice pelvic floor muscle training exercises (PFMT) to improve pelvic floor tone, strengthen the perineal muscles, and promote healing. See Evidence-Based Practice 15.1

Take Note!

Failure to maintain and restore perineal muscular tone leads to urinary incontinence later in life for many women.

Cardiovascular System Adaptations

The cardiovascular system undergoes dramatic changes after birth. During pregnancy, the heart is displaced slightly upward and to the left. This reverses as the uterus undergoes involution. Cardiac output remains high for the first few days postpartum and then gradually declines to nonpregnant values within 3 months of birth.

Blood volume, which increases substantially during pregnancy, drops rapidly after birth and returns to normal within 4 weeks postpartum. The decrease in both cardiac output and blood volume reflects the birth-related blood loss (an average of 500 mL with a vaginal birth and 1,000 mL with a cesarean birth). The cardiac output deceases to prelabor values 24 to 72 hours postpartum, rapidly falls over the next two weeks and usually returns to nonpregnant levels within 6 to 8 weeks postpartum. Blood plasma volume is further reduced through diuresis, which occurs during the early postpartum period (Cheng & Caughey, 2015). Despite the decrease in blood volume, the hematocrit level remains relatively stable and may even increase, reflecting the predominant loss of plasma. Thus, an acute decrease in hematocrit is not an expected finding and may indicate hemorrhage.

 Concept Mastery Alert

Prioritizing Postpartum Vital Signs

It is not uncommon for women to have a temperature elevation up to 100.4°F in the first 24 hours postpartum. There may also be a slight decrease in blood pressure. The nurse should be most concerned about a blood pressure elevation because preeclampsia may occur during the early postpartum period.

EVIDENCE-BASED PRACTICE 15.1

PELVIC FLOOR MUSCLE TRAINING VERSES NO TREATMENT, OR INACTIVE CONTROL TREATMENTS, FOR URINARY INCONTINENCE IN WOMEN

Stress incontinence is the involuntary leakage of urine with a physical activity that increases intra-abdominal pressure such as coughing or sneezing. This incontinence can occur after childbirth secondary to perineal trauma. Pelvic floor muscle training (PFMT) is the most common intervention for women that experience stress urinary incontinence. The objective of this study was to determine the effects of PFMT for women with urinary incontinence when compared with no treatment, placebo, or other inactive control treatments.

STUDY

Randomized or quasi-randomized trials in women experiencing stress incontinence were reviewed. Twenty-one trials involving 1281 women met the inclusion criteria. Women with stress urinary incontinence who were in the PFMT groups were 8 times more likely than the controls to report that they were cured (46/82 (56.1%) versus 5/83 (6.0%), RR 8.38, 95% CI 3.68 to 19.07) and 17 times more likely to report cure or improvement (32/58 (55%) versus 2/63 (3.2%), RR 17.33, 95% CI 4.31 to 69.64). In trials in women with any type of urinary incontinence, PFMT groups were also more likely to report cure, or more cure and improvement than the women in the control groups, although the effect size was reduced. Women

with stress urinary incontinence were also more satisfied with the active treatment, while women in the control groups were more likely to seek further treatment. Women treated with PFMT leaked urine less often, lost smaller amounts on the short office-based pad test, and emptied their bladders less often during the day.

Findings

The review of trials found that PFMT (muscle-clenching exercises) helps women cure and improve stress urinary incontinence in particular, and all types of incontinence.

Nursing Implications

The review provides support for the widespread recommendation that PFMT be included in first-line conservative management programs for women with stress and any type of urinary incontinence. Long-term effectiveness of PFMT needs to be further researched. The take-away message for nurses working with postpartum women should be to instruct them how to perform PFMT exercises at home to assist in restoring pelvic floor strength and tone. In addition to PFMT exercises, the promotion of healthy weight can also help prevent or reduce incontinence as a woman ages.

Adapted from Dumoulin, C., Hay-Smith, E. J., & Mac Habée-Séguin, G. (2014). Pelvic floor muscle training versus no treatment, or inactive control treatments, for urinary incontinence in women. *Cochrane Database of Systematic Reviews, 2014*(5), CD005654.

Pulse and Blood Pressure

The increase in cardiac output and stroke volume during pregnancy begins to diminish after birth once the placenta has been delivered. This decrease in cardiac output is reflected in bradycardia (40 to 60 bpm) for up to the first 2 weeks postpartum. This slowing of the heart rate is related to the increased blood that flows back to the heart and to the central circulation after it is no longer perfusing the placenta. This increase in central circulation brings about an increased stroke volume and allows a slower heart rate to provide ample maternal circulation. Gradually, cardiac output returns to prepregnant levels by 3 months after childbirth (Mahendru et al., 2014).

Tachycardia (heart rate above 100 bpm) in the postpartum woman warrants further investigation. It may indicate hypovolemia, dehydration, or hemorrhage. However, because of the increased blood volume during pregnancy, a considerable loss of blood may be well tolerated and not cause a compensatory cardiovascular response such as tachycardia. In most instances of postpartum hemorrhage, blood pressure and cardiac output remain increased because of the compensatory increase in heart rate. Thus, a decrease in blood pressure and cardiac output are not expected changes during

the postpartum period. Early identification is essential to ensure prompt intervention.

Blood pressure falls mostly in the first 2 days and then increases 3 to 7 days after childbirth; and returns to prepregnancy levels by 6 weeks (Parpaglioni, 2015). A significant increase accompanied by headache might indicate preeclampsia and requires further investigation. Decreased blood pressure may suggest an infection or a uterine hemorrhage.

Coagulation

Normal physiologic changes of pregnancy, including alterations in hemostasis that favor coagulation, reduced fibrinolysis, and pooling and stasis of blood in the lower limbs, place women at risk for blood clots. These changes, which usually return to prepregnant levels after 3 weeks of postpartum, are important for minimizing blood loss at childbirth. Smoking, obesity, immobility, and postpartum factors such as infection, bleeding, and emergency surgery (including emergency cesarean section) also increase the risk of coagulation disorders (Creasy et al., 2014).

Clotting factors that increased during pregnancy tend to remain elevated during the early postpartum period. Giving birth stimulates this hypercoagulability state further. As a result, these coagulation factors remain elevated for 2 to 3 weeks postpartum (King et al., 2015). This hypercoagulable state, combined with vessel damage during birth and immobility, places the woman at risk for thromboembolism (blood clots) in the lower extremities and the lungs.

Blood Cellular Components

Red blood cell production ceases early in the puerperium, causing mean hemoglobin and hematocrit levels to decrease slightly in the first 24 hours. During the next 2 weeks, both levels rise slowly. The white blood count, which increases in labor, remains elevated for first 4 to 6 days after birth but then falls to 6,000 to 10,000/mm^3. This white blood cell elevation can complicate a diagnosis of infection in the immediate postpartum period.

Urinary System Adaptations

Pregnancy and birth can have profound effects on the urinary system. During pregnancy, the glomerular filtration rate and renal plasma flow increase significantly. Both usually return to normal by 6 weeks after birth. There is a gradual return of bladder tone and normal size and function of the bladder, ureters, and renal pelvis, all of which were dilated during pregnancy.

Many women have difficulty feeling the sensation to void after giving birth if they received an anesthetic block during labor (which inhibits neural functioning of the bladder) or if they received oxytocin to induce or augment their labor (antidiuretic effect). These women will be at risk for incomplete emptying, bladder distention, difficulty voiding, and urinary retention. In addition, urination may be impeded by:

- Perineal lacerations
- Generalized swelling and bruising of the perineum and tissues surrounding the urinary meatus
- Hematomas
- Decreased bladder tone as a result of regional anesthesia
- Diminished sensation of bladder pressure as a result of swelling, poor bladder tone, and numbing effects of regional anesthesia used during labor (Bope & Kellerman, 2015).

Difficulty voiding can lead to urinary retention, bladder distention, and ultimately urinary tract infection. Urinary retention and bladder distention can cause displacement of the uterus from the midline to the right and can inhibit the uterus from contracting properly, which increases the risk of postpartum hemorrhage. Urinary retention is a major cause of uterine atony, which allows excessive bleeding. Frequent voiding of small amounts (less than 150 mL) suggests urinary retention

with overflow, and catheterization may be necessary to empty the bladder to restore tone.

Postpartum diuresis occurs as a result of several mechanisms: the large amounts of intravenous fluids given during labor, a decreasing antidiuretic effect of oxytocin as its level declines, the buildup and retention of extra fluids during pregnancy, and a decreasing production of aldosterone—the hormone that decreases sodium retention and increases urine production (Evans & De Franco, 2014). All of these factors contribute to rapid filling of the bladder within 12 hours of birth. Diuresis begins within 12 hours after childbirth and continues throughout the first week postpartum. Normal function returns within a month after birth (Cunningham et al., 2014).

Consider This

Have you ever felt like a real idiot by not being able to complete a simple task in life? I had a beautiful baby boy after only 6 hours of labor. My epidural worked well and I actually felt very little discomfort throughout my labor. Because it was in the middle of the night when they brought me to my postpartum room, I felt a few hours of sleep would be all I needed to be back to normal. During an assessment early the next morning, the nurse found my uterus had shifted to the right from my midline, and I was instructed to empty my bladder. I didn't understand why the nurse was concerned about where my uterus was located and, besides, I didn't feel any sensation of a full bladder. But I did get up anyway and tried to comply. Despite all the nurse's tricks of running the faucet for sound effects, in addition to having warm water poured over my thighs via the peribottle, I was unable to urinate. How could I not accomplish one of life's simplest tasks?

Thoughts: Women who receive regional anesthesia frequently experience reduced sensation to their perineal area and do not feel a full bladder. The nursing assessment revealed a displaced uterus secondary to a full bladder. What additional "tricks" can be used to assist this woman to void? What explanation should be offered to her regarding why she is having difficulty urinating?

Gastrointestinal System Adaptations

The gastrointestinal system quickly returns to normal after birth because the gravid uterus is no longer filling the abdominal cavity and producing pressure on the abdominal organs. Progesterone levels, which caused relaxation of smooth muscle during pregnancy and diminished bowel tone, also are declining.

Regardless of the type of delivery, most women experience decreased bowel tone and sluggish bowels for several days after birth. Decreased peristalsis occurs in response to analgesics, surgery, diminished intra-abdominal pressure, low-fiber diet, insufficient fluid intake, and diminished muscle tone. In addition, women with an episiotomy, perineal laceration, or hemorrhoids may fear pain or damage to the perineum with their first bowel movement and may attempt to delay it. Subsequently, constipation is a common problem during the postpartum period. A stool softener can be prescribed for this reason.

Most women are hungry and thirsty after childbirth, commonly related to nothing-by-mouth (NPO) restrictions and the energy expended during labor. Their appetite returns to normal immediately after giving birth.

Take Note!

Anticipate the woman's need to replenish her body with food and fluids, and provide both soon after she gives birth.

Musculoskeletal System Adaptations

The effects of pregnancy on the muscles and joints vary widely. Musculoskeletal changes associated with pregnancy, such as increased ligament laxity, weight gain, change in the center of gravity, and carpal tunnel syndrome, revert back during the postpartum period. During pregnancy, the hormones relaxin, estrogen, and progesterone relax the joints. After birth, levels of these hormones decline, resulting in a return of all joints to their prepregnant state, with the exception of the woman's feet. Parous women will note a permanent increase in their shoe size (Jordan et al., 2014).

Woman commonly experience fatigue and activity intolerance and have a distorted body image for weeks after birth secondary to declining relaxin and progesterone levels, which cause hip and joint pain that interferes with ambulation and exercise. Good body mechanics and correct positioning are important during this time to prevent low back pain and injury to the joints. Within 6 to 8 weeks after delivery, joints are completely stabilized and return to normal.

During pregnancy, stretching of the abdominal wall muscles occurs to accommodate the enlarging uterus. This stretching leads to a loss in muscle tone and possibly separation of the longitudinal muscles (rectus abdominis muscles) of the abdomen. Separation of the rectus abdominis muscles, called diastasis recti, is more common in women who have poor abdominal muscle tone before pregnancy. After birth, muscle tone is diminished and the abdominal muscles are soft and flabby. Specific exercises are necessary to help the woman regain muscle tone. Fortunately, diastasis responds well to exercise, and abdominal muscle tone can be improved. (See Chapter 16 for more information about exercises to improve muscle tone.)

Take Note!

If rectus muscle tone is not regained through exercise, support may not be adequate during future pregnancies.

Integumentary System Adaptations

Another system that experiences lasting effects of pregnancy is the integumentary system. As estrogen and progesterone levels decrease, the darkened pigmentation on the abdomen (linea nigra), face (melasma), and nipples gradually fades. Some women experience hair loss during pregnancy and the postpartum periods. Approximately 90% of hairs are growing at any one time, with the other 10% entering a resting phase. Because of the high estrogen levels present during pregnancy, an increased number of hairs go into the resting phase, which is part of the normal hair loss cycle. The most common period for hair loss is within 3 months after birth, when estrogen returns to normal levels and more hairs are allowed to fall out. This hair loss is temporary, and regrowth generally returns to normal levels in 4 to 6 months in two thirds of women and by 15 months in the remainder, although hair may be less abundant than before pregnancy (King et al., 2015).

Striae gravidarum (stretch marks) that developed during pregnancy on the breasts, abdomen, and hips gradually fade to silvery lines. However, these lines do not disappear completely. Although many products on the market claim to make stretch marks disappear, their effectiveness is highly questionable.

The profuse diaphoresis (sweating) that is common during the early postpartum period is one of the most noticeable adaptations in the integumentary system. Many women will wake up drenched with perspiration during the puerperium. This postpartum diaphoresis is a mechanism to reduce the amount of fluids retained during pregnancy and restore prepregnant body fluid levels. It can be profuse at times. It is common, especially at night during the first week after birth. Reassure the client that this is normal and encourage her to change her gown to prevent chilling.

Respiratory System Adaptations

Respirations usually remain within the normal adult range of 16 to 24 breaths per minute. As the abdominal organs resume their nonpregnant position, the diaphragm returns to its usual position. Anatomic changes in the thoracic cavity and rib cage caused by increasing uterine growth resolve quickly. As a result, discomforts such as shortness of breath and rib aches are relieved. Tidal volume, minute volume, vital capacity, and functional residual capacity return to prepregnant values, typically within 1 to 3 weeks of birth (Mattson & Smith, 2016).

Endocrine System Adaptations

The endocrine system rapidly undergoes several changes after birth. Levels of circulating estrogen and progesterone drop quickly with delivery of the placenta. Decreased estrogen levels are associated with breast engorgement and with the diuresis of excess extracellular fluid accumulated during pregnancy (Creasy et al., 2014). Estrogen is at its lowest level a week after birth. For the woman who is not breast-feeding, estrogen levels begin to increase by 2 weeks after birth. For the breast-feeding woman, estrogen levels remain low until breast-feeding frequency decreases.

Other placental hormones (human chorionic gonadotropin [hCG], human placental lactogen [hPL], progesterone) decline rapidly after birth. The hCG levels are nonexistent at the end of the first postpartum week, and hPL is undetectable within 1 day after birth (Mattson & Smith, 2016). Progesterone levels are undetectable by 3 days after childbirth, and production is reestablished with the first menses. Prolactin is a hormone secreted by the anterior pituitary gland involved with lactation and reproduction. Prolactin levels decline within 2 weeks for the woman who is not breast-feeding, but remain elevated for the lactating woman (Jin et al., 2015).

Weight Loss After Childbirth

For all women of reproductive age, excessive weight gain and postpartum weight retention can increase their risk of obesity. Breast-feeding has been shown to have many health benefits for both mother and infant; however, its role in postpartum weight loss is unclear. More research studies are needed to reliably assess the impact of breast-feeding on postpartum weight management (Neville et al., 2014).

The rate and amount of weight loss in the postpartum period seem to be determined by the same factors that determine weight loss at any point in a woman's life, including existing weight/body mass index (BMI), diet, age, and activity level (Nascimento et al., 2014). Thus, there is benefit from overall lifestyle interventions on weight loss in postpartum women which include exercise plus dietary changes to achieve their weight reduction goals. See Evidence-Based Practice 15.2.

Think back to Betsy, the woman experiencing painful changes in her breasts. What is Betsy describing to the lactation consultant? Why has the condition of her breasts changed compared with when she was in the hospital?

EVIDENCE-BASED PRACTICE 15.2   REDUCING POSTPARTUM WEIGHT RETENTION AND IMPROVING BREAST-FEEDING OUTCOMES IN OVERWEIGHT WOMEN: A PILOT RANDOMIZED CONTROLLED TRIAL

Women naturally gain weight during pregnancy and many gradually lose it afterward. Some women, though, find it difficult to lose the pregnancy-related weight during the postpartum period and there is concern that this may be a health risk. The retention of weight gained during pregnancy may contribute to obesity. Obesity in the general population increases the risk of diabetes, heart disease, and high blood pressure. It is suggested that women who return to their prepregnancy weight by about 6 months after childbirth have a lower risk of being overweight 10 years later. Weight gain is also associated with lower rates of breast-feeding initiation and duration. The purpose of this randomized study was to help women reduce their postpartum weight retention and improve breast-feeding outcomes.

STUDY

Thirty-six women with a BMI of >25 were recruited, stratified by BMI and randomized to one of three groups with follow-up to 6 months postpartum. Women received a dietary intervention with or without breast-feeding support from a lactation consultant. All participants initiated breast-feeding, but the group that had lactation support had a longer duration of breast-feeding than the group without the lactation support. In addition, the women with longer breast-feeding duration, also loss the most weight during the 6-month period.

Findings

The study provided evidence to support the feasibility of providing overweight and obese women with targeted dietary advice and breast-feeding support to improve weight and breast-feeding outcomes.

Nursing Implications

Based on the findings of this study, nurses can recommend to their postpartum mothers desiring to lose their pregnancy weight should be encouraged to breast-feed and sustain it for at least 6 months to lose their pregnancy weight gained. Research findings associate breast-feeding with postpartum weight loss due to the increase in women's metabolic rates which burn calories. This information should be reported to postpartum mothers desiring to lose weight and breast-feed. Overall, if gained weight through the pregnancy isn't lost, their risk of cardiovascular diseases, diabetes, hypertension, and cancer will be increased as they age. The weight loss will help prevent these conditions or at the very least reduce their risks.

Adapted from Martin, J., MacDonald-Wicks, L., Hure, A., Smith, R., & Collins, C. E. (2015). Reducing postpartum weight retention and improving breastfeeding outcomes in overweight women: A pilot randomized controlled trial. *Nutrients, 7*(3), 1464–1479.

Global Health of Childbearing Women

Globalization has changed our society in numerous ways, yet the health of women is remaining stagnant or growing worse in many parts of the world. Many women in developing counties are denied their fundamental right to enjoy a complete state of health as defined by the World Health Organization (Boyd-Judson & James, 2014). More than half a million women die each year from complications during and after childbirth (bleeding and infections), the vast majority of them in Africa and Asia (Webber & Chirangi, 2014).

Women throughout the world continue to face enormous obstacles in attempting to access obstetric care. Skilled attendance at childbirth is critical for decreasing maternal and neonatal mortality, yet many women in developing countries give birth outside health facilities, without skilled help. Nurses throughout the world can help advocate for cost-effective, evidence-based interventions to prevent and battle complications from childbirth to save women's lives. The challenge is to guarantee that every pregnant woman who needs care gets it. Nurses can make a difference outside their own country's borders by advocating for all international women through their governmental political systems and encouraging those governments to offer help and save lives.

Lactation

Lactation is the secretion of milk by the breasts. It is thought to be brought about by the interaction of progesterone, estrogen, prolactin, and oxytocin. Breast milk typically appears within 4 to 5 days after childbirth.

BREAST-FEEDING

Breast-feeding is a dynamic process, which requires coupling between periodic motions of the infant's jaws, undulation of the tongue, and breast milk ejection reflex. All mechanisms must be coordinated to be successful. All major health organizations recommend breast-feeding. The American Academy of Pediatrics recommends exclusive breast-feeding for 6 months, followed by the introduction of appropriate complementary foods and continued breast-feeding to 1 year and beyond (American Academy of Pediatrics [AAP], 2015). This recommendation is considered to be the standard of care today. Nurses have an important role in promoting, supporting, and protecting breast-feeding. Proper positioning, latching-on, sucking, and swallowing are the foundation for successful breast-feeding. Although breast-feeding is recommended by international and national organizations, the nurse must respect and support all mothers in either of the infant feeding methods chosen.

During pregnancy, the breasts increase in size and functional ability in preparation for breast-feeding. Estrogen stimulates growth of the milk collection (ductal) system,

whereas progesterone stimulates growth of the milk production system. Within the first month of gestation, the ducts of the mammary glands grow branches, forming more lobules and alveoli. These structural changes make the breasts larger, more tender, and heavy. Each breast gains nearly 1 lb in weight by term, the glandular cells fill with secretions, blood vessels increase in number, and the amounts of connective tissue and fat cells increase (Engel et al., 2015).

Prolactin from the anterior pituitary gland, secreted in increasing levels throughout pregnancy, triggers the synthesis and secretion of milk after the woman gives birth. During pregnancy, prolactin, estrogen, and progesterone cause synthesis and secretion of *colostrum*, which contains protein and carbohydrate but no milk fat. It is only after birth takes place, when the high levels of estrogen and progesterone are abruptly withdrawn, that prolactin is able to stimulate the glandular cells to secrete milk instead of colostrum. This takes place within 4 to 5 days after giving birth.

Oxytocin acts so that milk can be ejected from the alveoli to the nipple. Therefore, sucking by the newborn will release milk. A decrease in the quality of stimulation causes a decrease in prolactin surges and thus a decrease in milk production. Prolactin levels increase in response to nipple stimulation during feedings. Prolactin and oxytocin result in milk production if stimulated by sucking (Stuebe et al., 2015) (Fig. 15.3). If the stimulus (sucking) is not present, as with a woman who is not breast-feeding, breast engorgement and milk production will subside within days postpartum.

Skin-to-skin contact during the first hour following birth is the gold standard to initiate breast-feeding, if the mother decides this is the method of feeding for her newborn. Researchers realized that a newborn's instinct was to seek nourishment after birth. They move on their mother's abdomen up to her breast instinctively. Researchers term this movement the *breast crawl* that helps initiate breast-feeding immediately after childbirth. This instinct occurs when a newborn, left undisturbed and skin-to-skin on the mother's trunk following birth, moves toward her mother's breast for the purpose of locating and self-attaching for the first feeding. From there, the newborn uses leg and arm movements to propel her/himself toward the breast. Upon reaching the sternum, the newborn will bounce her/his head up and down and side to side. As the newborn approaches the nipple, her/his mouth opens and, after several attempts, latch-on and suckling take place. Newborns have senses and skills that enable early initiation of feeding at the breast. Nurses can help facilitate the breast crawl as a continuation of the birthing process. Nurses have a responsibility to promote the health of their childbearing families and provide evidence-based care. Encouraging use of the breast crawl can be the first step in health promotion for every newborn (Zanardo & Straface, 2015).

Breast milk production can be summarized as follows:
• Prolactin levels increase at term with a decrease in estrogen and progesterone levels.

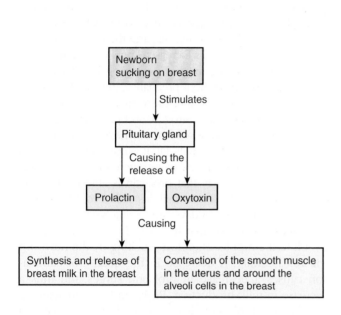

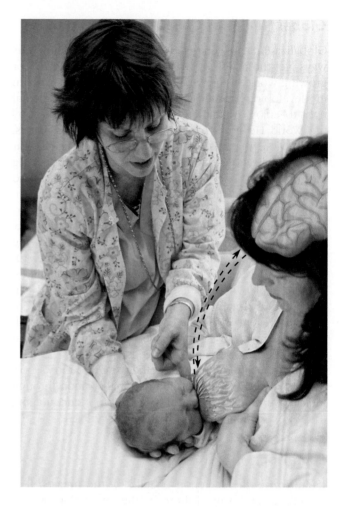

FIGURE 15.3 Physiology of lactation.

• Estrogen and progesterone levels decrease after the placenta is delivered.
• Prolactin is released from the anterior pituitary gland and initiates milk production.
• Oxytocin is released from the posterior pituitary gland to promote milk let-down.
• Infant sucking at each feeding provides continuous stimulus for prolactin and oxytocin release (Wambach & Riordan, 2014).

Typically, during the first 2 days after birth, the breasts are soft and nontender. The woman also may report a tingling sensation in both breasts, which is the "let-down reflex" that occurs immediately before or during breast-feeding. After this time, breast changes depend on whether the mother is breast-feeding or taking measures to prevent lactation.

Engorgement is a postnatal physiologic painful condition in which distension and swelling of the breast tissue occurs as a result of an increase in blood and lymph supply as a precursor to lactation (Fig. 15.4). Breast engorgement usually peaks in 3 to 5 days postpartum and usually subsides within the following 24 to 36 hours

(Alekseev, Vladimir, & Nadezhda, 2015). Engorgement can occur from infrequent feeding or ineffective emptying of the breasts and typically lasts about 24 hours. Breasts increase in vascularity and swell in response to prolactin 2 to 4 days after birth. If engorged, the breasts will be hard and tender to touch. They are temporarily full, tender, and very uncomfortable until the milk supply is ready. Frequent emptying of the breasts helps to minimize discomfort and resolve engorgement. Standing in a warm shower or applying warm compresses immediately before feedings will help to soften the breasts and nipples in order to allow the newborn to latch on more easily.

Treatments to reduce the pain of breast engorgement include heat or cold applications, cabbage leaf compresses, breast massage and milk expression, ultrasound, breast pumping, and anti-inflammatory agents (King et al., 2015). A nonprescription anti-inflammatory medication can also be taken for the breast discomfort and swelling resulting from engorgement. These measures will also enhance the let-down reflex. Between feedings, applying cold compresses to the breasts helps to reduce swelling. To maintain milk supply, the breasts

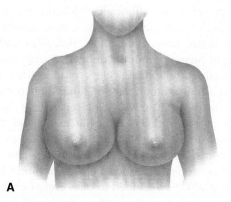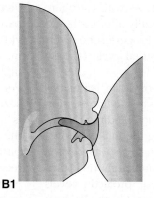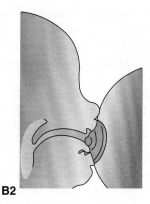

A   B1   B2

FIGURE 15.4 A. Image of engorged breasts. Note swelling and inflammation of both breasts. **B.** Breast engorgement can disrupt breast-feeding: (1) When sucking at a normal breast, the infant's lips compress the areola and fit neatly against the sides of the nipple. The infant also has adequate room to breathe. (2) When a breast is engorged, however, the infant has difficulty grasping the nipple and breathing ability is compromised. (From Pillitteri, A. [2014]. *Maternal and child nursing.* (7th ed.). Philadelphia, PA: Lippincott Williams & Wilkins.)

need to be stimulated by a nursing infant, a breast pump, or manual expression of the milk (Fig. 15.5).

Remember Betsy, with the breast discomfort? The lactation consultant explained that she was experiencing normal breast engorgement and offered several suggestions to help her. What relief measures might she have suggested? What reassurance can be given to Betsy at this time?

SUPPRESSING LACTATION

Various pharmacologic and nonpharmacologic interventions have been used to suppress lactation after childbirth and relieve associated symptoms. Despite the large volume of literature on the subject, there is currently no universal guideline on the most appropriate

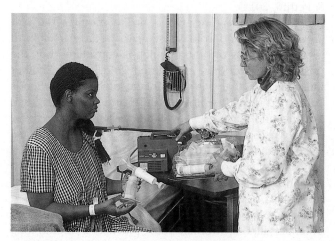

FIGURE 15.5 Nurse instructs the new breast-feeding mother about use of a breast pump. (Copyright B. Proud.)

approach for suppressing lactation in postpartum women (Cunningham et al., 2014). It is estimated that more than 30% of women in the United States do not breast-feed their infants, and a larger proportion discontinues breast-feeding within 2 weeks of childbirth (Senie, 2014). Although physiologic cessation of lactation eventually occurs in the absence of physical stimulus such as infant suckling, a large number of women experience moderate to severe milk leakage and discomfort before lactation ceases.

Up to two thirds of non-breast-feeding women experience moderate to severe engorgement and breast pain when no treatment is applied (Spencer, 2015). If a woman does not desire to breast-feed, some relief measures include wearing a tight, supportive bra 24 hours daily, applying ice to her breasts for approximately 15 to 20 minutes every other hour, avoiding sexual stimulation, and not stimulating the breasts by squeezing or manually expressing milk from the nipples. In addition, avoiding exposing the breasts to warmth (e.g., a hot shower) will help relieve breast engorgement. In women who are not breast-feeding, engorgement typically subsides within 2 to 3 days with application of these measures.

Ovulation and Return of Menstruation

Changing hormone levels constantly interact with one another to produce bodily changes. Four major hormones are influential during the postpartum period: estrogen, progesterone, prolactin, and oxytocin. Estrogen plays a major role during pregnancy, but levels drop profoundly at birth and reach their lowest level a week into the postpartum period. Progesterone quiets the uterus to prevent a preterm birth during pregnancy, and its increasing levels during pregnancy prevent lactation from starting before birth takes place. As with estrogen, progesterone levels decrease dramatically after birth and are undetectable 72 hours after birth. Progesterone levels are reestablished with the first menstrual cycle (Creasy et al., 2014).

During the postpartum period, oxytocin stimulates the uterus to contract during the breast-feeding session and for as long as 20 minutes after each feeding. Oxytocin also acts on the breast by eliciting the milk let-down reflex during breast-feeding. Prolactin is also associated with the breast-feeding process by stimulating milk production. In women who breast-feed, prolactin levels remain elevated into the sixth week after birth (Bope & Kellerman, 2015). The levels of prolactin fluctuate in proportion to nipple stimulation. Prolactin levels decrease in nonlactating women, reaching prepregnant levels by the third postpartum week. High levels of prolactin have been found to delay ovulation by inhibiting ovarian response to follicle-stimulating hormone (Bernard et al., 2015).

The timing of first menses and ovulation after birth differs between women who are breast-feeding and women who are not breast-feeding. For nonlactating women, menstruation may resume as early as 7 to 9 weeks after giving birth, but the majority take up to 3 months, with the first cycle being anovulatory (Barrett et al., 2014). The return of menses in the lactating woman depends on breast-feeding frequency and duration. It can return any time after childbirth, depending on whether the woman is exclusively breast-feeding or supplementing with formula.

Take Note!

Ovulation may occur before menstruation. Therefore, breast-feeding is not a totally reliable method of contraception unless the mother exclusively breast-feeds, has had no menstrual period since giving birth, and whose infant is younger than 6 months old (Alexander et al., 2014).

Betsy tries several of the measures the lactation consultant suggested to relieve her breast discomfort, but is still having heaviness and pain. She feels discouraged and tells the nurse she is thinking of reducing her breast-feeding and using formula to feed her newborn. Is that a good choice? Why or why not? What interventions will help Betsy get through this difficult time?

CULTURAL CONSIDERATIONS FOR THE POSTPARTUM PERIOD

Cultures vary in their postpartum beliefs, practices, and customs. Nurses practice in an increasingly multicultural society. Therefore, they must be open, respectful, nonjudgmental, and willing to learn about ethnically diverse populations. Although childbirth and the postpartum period are unique experiences for each individual woman, how the woman perceives and makes meaning of them is culturally defined. Somali women are highly regarded in Somali society for their roles as mothers. Postpartum women stay at home and refrain from sexual activity for 40 days. At the end of 40 days, there is a celebration and this typically marks the first time the mother and infant have left their home since childbirth. The majority of Somalian and Arab women breastfeed and do so for extended periods of time (Wojnar & Narruhn, 2016). Nurses need to offer early breast feeding instruction to support their efforts while still in the hospital setting before discharge.

Balance of Hot and Cold

Two areas that are significantly different from Western culture involve beliefs about the balance of hot and cold and confinement after childbirth. Vietnamese women view the postpartum period as a cold state (duong) and protect themselves through warmth. Cultural practices include warm water for hygiene and stimulation of lactation, consuming warm foods, and staying indoors. In the United States, childbearing and recovery are viewed as healthy states and mothers receive little formal support for both their recovery and infant care. In China, childbearing and postpartum are viewed as states which disturb the normal health balance between yin and yang. In order to restore balance in health, postpartum women engage in practices for a month related to the maternal role, physical activity, maintenance of body warmth, and certain food consumption that will restore their balance. Recent research findings in a small sample of Chinese women found that postpartum confinement negatively correlated with aerobic endurance and positively correlated with depression. These findings may challenge the assumption that practices of confinement are healthy for Chinese women's recovery after childbirth (Liu, Maloni, & Petrini, 2014).

For many cultures, good health requires the balancing of hot and cold substances. Because childbirth involves the loss of blood, which is considered hot, the postpartum period is considered cold, so the mother must balance that with the intake of hot food. Foods consumed should be hot in nature, and cold foods, such as fruits and vegetables, avoided. Western practices frequently use cold packs or sitz baths to reduce perineal swelling and discomfort. These practices are not acceptable to women of many cultures and can be viewed as harmful. Hot–cold beliefs are common among Latin American, African, and Asian people (Purnell, 2014).

To reduce infant and mother vulnerability and potential illness, women may practice a month-long confinement period after childbirth. During this confinement period, new mothers rest and recuperate. The postpartum period is a time to avoid cold—both in temperature and foods. Women are kept warm, stay inside to prevent becoming chilled, bathe infrequently, and avoid exercise (Rice & Manderson, 2014).

Postpartum Cultural Beliefs

With increasing multiculturalism in the United States, understanding various cultures' views of the postnatal period as it relates to their recovery and well-being after childbirth is important for all nurses. Postpartum nurses need to understand these diverse cultural beliefs and provide creative strategies for encouraging hygiene (sponge baths, perineal care), exercise, and balanced nutrition, while remaining respectful of the cultural significance of these practices. The best approach is to ask each woman to describe what cultural practices are important to her and plan accordingly.

PSYCHOLOGICAL ADAPTATIONS

The process of becoming a mother requires extensive psychological, social, and physical work. Women experience heightened vulnerability and face tremendous challenges as they make this transition. Nurses have a remarkable opportunity to help women learn, gain confidence, and experience growth as they assume the mother identity.

The transition to parenthood, while an exciting time to celebrate the life of their child, causes parents to face new challenges such as physical exhaustion, role overload, and less time for themselves and their partners (Velotti, Castellano, & Zavattini, 2015). Mothers' and fathers' experiences of pregnancy are necessarily different, and this difference continues after childbirth as they both adjust to their new parenting roles. Many couples struggle to adapt to parenthood. Parenting involves caring for infants physically and emotionally to foster the growth and development of responsible, caring adults. A substantial body of research finds no biologic-based differences between mothers and fathers in sensitivity to infants, capacity to provide care or acquisition of parenting skills. Within 15 minutes of holding a newborn, men experience raised levels of oxytocin, cortisol, and prolactin. The increased levels of these nurturing hormones are the same in men and women exposed to infants (Davies, 2015). Other members of the newborn's family, such as siblings and grandparents, also experience changes related to the birth of the newborn (see Chapter 16). Early parent–infant contact after birth improves attachment behaviors.

Parental Attachment Behaviors

The postpartum period is a unique time distinguished by the inseparable relationship parents have with their newborn. To enable an attachment to be built, closeness of this family unit is essential. **Attachment** is the formation of a relationship between a parent and his or her newborn through a process of physical and emotional interactions. Attachment between a woman and her newborn has lifelong implications (King et al., 2015). Maternal attachment has the potential to affect both child development and parenting. The bond between a parent and their newborn is one of strength, power, and potential. Attachment begins before birth, during the prenatal period where acceptance and nurturing of the growing fetus takes place. It continues after giving birth as parents learn to recognize their newborn's cues, adapt to the newborn's behaviors and responses, and meet their newborn's needs.

Several factors take place during the early postpartum period that can have a large influence on the attachment/bonding that occurs during this time. Oxytocin plays an essential role in the chemistry aspect of bonding, and its effects can be enhanced by skin-to-skin contact, breast-feeding, eye contact, social vocalizations, maternal and milk odors, which are soothing for the newborn, and newborn message during the first postpartum hour (Buckley, 2015; Hutcheson & Cheeseman, 2015).

Early and sustained contact between newborns and their parents is vital for initiating their relationship.

Nurses play a crucial role in assisting the attachment process by promoting early parent–newborn interactions. In addition, nurses can facilitate skin-to-skin contact (kangaroo care) by placing the infant onto the bare chests of mothers and fathers to enhance parent–newborn attachment. This activity will enable them to get close to their newborn and experience an intense feeling of connectedness and evoke feelings of being nurturing parents. Encouraging breast-feeding is another way to foster attachment between mothers and their newborns. Finally, nurses can encourage nurturing activities and contact such as touching, talking, singing, comforting, changing diapers, feeding—in short, participating in routine newborn care.

The process of attachment is complex and is influenced by many factors including environmental circumstances, the newborn's health status, and the quality of nursing care (Buckley, 2015). Nurses need to minimize parent–newborn separation by promoting parent–newborn interactions through kangaroo care, breast-feeding, and participation in their newborn care. Nurses who provide positive psychosocial support and clear communication to parents will help support the attachment process within family units.

Maternal Psychological Adaptations

Childbirth is supposed to be the most joyous period in a woman's life and involves the almost spiritual experience of giving birth and being able to give life to another being. For many, this can be a life-changing event and through the centuries has been anticipated with excitement and joy and has even been referred to as a blessing. In reality, childbirth and child rearing are very stressful, financially challenging, and emotionally demanding.

Mood Disorders

Many people consider childbirth a time of happiness and well-being, but it is common for women to experience changes in their mood during this time. This may include being fatigued, irritable or worried, and frequently these mood symptoms become severe enough to need medical intervention. In the postpartum period, mood disorders can be divided into three distinct entities in ascending order of severity: maternal (baby) blues, postpartum depression, and psychosis. These disorders, however, have not been clearly demarcated and it is a matter of much debate whether they are discrete disorders or a single disorder that ranges along a continuum of severity (Finley & Brizendine, 2015).

Up to 85% of new mothers suffer from the short-lived postpartum mood disorder termed "baby blues" or maternal blues, which are characterized by mild depressive symptoms, anxiety, irritability, mood swings, lose their appetite, have trouble sleeping, tearfulness (often for no discernible reason), increased sensitivity, and fatigue (Flynn, 2015). The "blues" typically peak on postpartum days 4 and 5, may last hours to days, and usually resolve by day 10. Although these symptoms may be distressing, they do not reflect psychopathology, and they typically do not affect the mother's ability to function and care for her child.

For additional information, see Chapter 22.

Phases of Maternal Adaptation to Parenthood

Parenthood is a highly anticipated and positive event for most women. Society has constructed many ideal images of motherhood, giving standards for women to live up to, and frequently setting them up for disappointment. Most women are able to experience this mismatch between their ideal and actual self and adapt with minimal discrepancy (Adams, 2015). The woman experiences a variety of responses as she adjusts to a new family member and to postpartum discomforts, changes in her body image, and the reality of change in her life. In the early 1960s, Reva Rubin identified three phases that a mother goes through to adjust to her new maternal role. Rubin's maternal role framework can be used to monitor the client's progress as she "tries on" her new role as a mother. The absence of these processes or inability to progress through the phases satisfactorily may impede the appropriate development of the maternal role (Rubin, 1984). Although Rubin's maternal role development theories are

of value, some of her observations regarding the length of each phase may not be completely relevant for the contemporary woman of the 21st century. Today, many women know their infant's gender, have "seen" their fetus in utero through four-dimensional ultrasound, and have a working knowledge of childbirth and child care. They are less passive than in years past and progress through the phases of attaining the maternal role at a much faster pace than Rubin would have imagined. Still, Rubin's framework is timeless for assessing and monitoring expected role behaviors when planning care and appropriate interventions.

TAKING-IN PHASE

The **taking-in phase** is the time immediately after birth when the client needs sleep, depends on others to meet her needs, and relives the events surrounding the birth process. This phase is characterized by dependent behavior. During the first 24 to 48 hours after giving birth, mothers often assume a very passive role in meeting their own basic needs for food, fluids, and rest, allowing the nurse to make decisions for them concerning activities and care. They spend time recounting their labor experience to anyone who will listen. Such actions help the mother integrate the birth experience into reality—that is, the pregnancy is over and the newborn is now a unique individual, separate from herself. When interacting with the newborn, new mothers spend time claiming the newborn and touching him or her, commonly identifying specific features in the newborn, such as "he has my nose" or "his fingers are long like his father's" (Fig. 15.6).

> **Take Note!**
>
> The taking-in phase typically lasts 1 to 2 days and may be the only phase observed by nurses in the hospital setting because of the shortened postpartum stays that are the norm today.

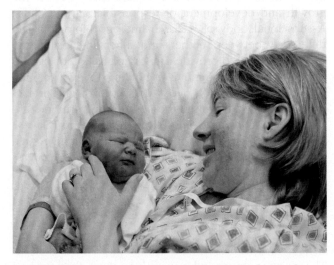

FIGURE 15.6 Mother bonding with newborn during the taking-in phase.

TAKING-HOLD PHASE

The **taking-hold phase**, the second phase of maternal adaptation, is characterized by dependent and independent maternal behavior. This phase typically starts on the second to third day postpartum and may last several weeks.

As the client regains control over her bodily functions during the next few days, she will be taking hold and becoming preoccupied with the present. She will be particularly concerned about her health, the infant's condition, and her ability to care for her or him. She demonstrates increased autonomy and mastery of her own body's functioning, and a desire to take charge with support and help from others. She will show independence by caring for herself and learning to care for her newborn, but she still requires assurance that she is doing well as a mother. She expresses a strong interest in caring for the infant by herself.

LETTING-GO PHASE

In the **letting-go phase**, the third phase of maternal adaptation, the woman reestablishes relationships with other people. She adapts to parenthood through her new role as a mother. She assumes the responsibility and care of the newborn with a bit more confidence now (Edelman, Kudzma, & Mandle, 2014). The focus of this phase is to move forward by assuming the parental role and to separate herself from the symbiotic relationship that she and her newborn had during pregnancy. She establishes a lifestyle that includes the infant. The mother relinquishes the fantasy infant and accepts the real one.

Nurses have recognized the importance of the process of becoming a mother (BAM) to maternal–infant nursing since Rubin's report on maternal role attainment (MRA). Mothers' perceptions of their competence or confidence, or both, in mothering and their expressions of love for their infants included age, relationship with the father, socioeconomic status, birth experience, experienced stress, available support, personality traits, self-concept, child-rearing attitudes, role strain, health status, preparation during pregnancy, relationships with own mother, depression, and anxiety. Infant variables identified as influencing MRA/BAM include appearance, responsiveness, temperament, and health status (DiPietro et al., 2015). More current research has led to renaming the four stages a woman progresses through in establishing a maternal identity in BAM:

1. Commitment, attachment to the unborn baby, and preparation for delivery and motherhood during pregnancy
2. Acquaintance/attachment to the infant, learning to care for the infant, and physical restoration during the first 2 to 6 weeks following birth
3. Moving toward a new normal
4. Achievement of a maternal identity through redefining self to incorporate motherhood (around 4 months).

The mother feels self-confident and competent in her mothering and expresses love for and pleasure interacting with her infant (Mercer & Walker, 2006)

The woman's work in the first stage is to make a commitment to the pregnancy and to the safe birth and care of her unborn child. This commitment is associated with a positive adaptation to motherhood. During the second stage while the mother is placing the infant in her family context and learning how to care for her infant, her attachment and attitude toward her infant, and her self-confidence or sense of competence in mothering, or both, consistently indicate an interdependence of these two variables. The nursing care provided during the first two stages is especially important in assisting mothers as they begin to mother. Follow-up is needed as mothers move toward a new normal and recognize a transformation of self in BAM can continue to reinforce their capabilities (Mercer, 2006).

To foster maternal role attainment, three specific interventions for nurses were identified in a review of the literature (Ferrarello & Hatfield, 2014). First, instructions about infant care and the infant's capabilities are more effective if they are specifically focused on that particular mother's infant. Second, mothers prefer live classes rather than videotapes so they can ask questions. In short, interactive nurse–client relationships are associated with positive maternal growth. Third, identifying barriers that reduce skin-to-skin periods of mother-to-infant during the postpartum hospital stay and intervening to reduce them have implications for both maternal role development and breast-feeding success, if she has chosen this method. Providing times for skin-to-skin mother and infant contact has a positive impact on the long-term health of both. Nurses who interact with clients long term during pregnancy, childbirth and during well child care help build maternal competence. Pregnancy, birth, and becoming a mother collectively represent a critical period of physical and emotional upheaval in a woman's life. The need for a holistic care approach that supports the emotional and physical health of the dyad is imperative (Spiteri et al., 2014).

Transition to motherhood theories (Rubin and Mercer) describe women in a prescribed role; that of being a mother and indeed a predetermined type of mother. In that sense transition to motherhood theory is baby-centered. New theories need to be developed that are woman-centered and conceptualize the woman as an embodied self who is powerful in her own life.

Partner Psychological Adaptations

For partners, whether they are husbands, significant others, boyfriends, same-sex life partners, or just friends, becoming a parent or just sharing the childbirth experience can be a perplexing time as well as a time of great change. This transition is influenced by many factors, including participation in childbirth, relationships with significant others, competence in child care, the family role organization, the individual's cultural background, and the method of infant feeding.

The transition from being merely a partner to being a parent can propel many partners to reorganize their lifestyles. During the postpartum period, partners frequently find themselves struggling to balance personal and work needs with the new demands of parent status and their new self-image. The complexities of the transitional process involved in forging a parenthood identity can be viewed at three different levels: readjustment to a new self-image, formation of a triadic family relationship, and adaptation to redefining themselves and their relationship with their partner: the "more united tag team" (Halford, Petch, & Creedy, 2015).

Nurses can play a key role in supporting a partner's transition to parenthood by keeping partners informed about birth and postpartum routines, reporting on their newborn's health status, and reviewing infant development. They can also contribute by creating participative space for new partners during the postpartum period. This can be achieved, for example, by helping partners take on their new role by supporting and promoting their degree of involvement in the process. They can also be encouraged to actively participate in caring for, and maintaining contact with, their newborns.

> **Take Note!**
> Most research findings stress the importance of early contact between the partner or significant other and the newborn, as well as participation in infant care activities, to foster the relationship (Nolan, 2015).

Infants have a powerful effect on their parents and others, who become intensely involved with them (Fig. 15.7). The father's or significant other's developing bond with the newborn—a time of intense absorption, preoccupation, and interest—is called *engrossment*.

Engrossment

Engrossment is characterized by seven behaviors:
1. Visual awareness of the newborn—the partner perceives the newborn as attractive, pretty, or beautiful.
2. Tactile awareness of the newborn—the partner has a desire to touch or hold the newborn and considers this activity to be pleasurable.
3. Perception of the newborn as perfect—the partner does not "see" any imperfections.
4. Strong attraction to the newborn—the partner focuses all attention on the newborn when they are in the room.
5. Awareness of distinct features of the newborn—the partner can distinguish his/her newborn from others in the nursery.

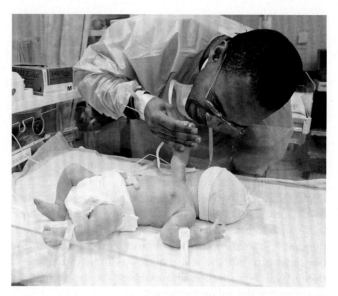

FIGURE 15.7 Engrossment of the father and his newborn.

6. Extreme elation—the partner feels a "high" after the birth of his/her child.
7. Increased sense of self-esteem—the partner feels proud, "bigger," more mature, and older after the birth of his/her child (Sears & Sears, 2015).

Frequently, partners are portrayed as well-meaning but bumbling when caring for newborns. However, they have their own unique way of relating to their newborns and can become as nurturing as mothers. A partner's nurturing responses may be less automatic and slower to unfold than a mother's, but they are capable of a strong bonding attachment to their newborns (Sears & Sears, 2015). Encouraging partners to express their feelings by seeing, touching, and holding their son or daughter and by cuddling, talking to, and feeding him or her will help to cement this new relationship. Reinforcement of this engrossing behavior helps partners to make a positive attachment during this critical period.

Three-Stage Role Development Process

Similar to mothers, partners also go through a predictable three-stage process during the first 3 weeks as they too "try on" their roles as parents. The three stages are expectations, reality, and transition to mastery (Sears & Sears, 2015).

STAGE 1: EXPECTATIONS

New partners pass through stage 1 (expectations) with preconceptions about what home life will be like with a newborn. Many partners may be unaware of the dramatic changes that can occur when this newborn comes home to live with them. For some, it is an eye-opening experience.

STAGE 2: REALITY

Stage 2 (reality) occurs when partners realize that their expectations in stage 1 are not realistic. Their feelings change from elation to sadness, ambivalence, jealousy, and frustration. Many wish to be more involved in the newborn's care and yet do not feel prepared to do so. Some find parenting fun but at the same time do not feel fully prepared to take on that role.

Partner's stress, irritability and frustration in the days, weeks, and months after the birth of their child can turn into depression, just like new maternal experience. Unfortunately, partners rarely discuss their feelings or ask for help, especially during a time when they are supposed to be the "strong one" for the new mother. Depression in partners can cause marital conflicts, reckless or violent behavior, withdrawn parental interactions with the newborn, poor job performance, and substance abuse. In addition, paternal depression following childbirth can have a detrimental effect on a couple's relationship, the parent–child relationship, and on their children's future development (Sethna et al., 2015).

Risk factors for partner postpartum depression include previous history of depression, financial problems, a poor relationship with his/her partner, and an unplanned pregnancy. Symptoms of depression appear 1 to 3 weeks after birth and can include feelings of being very stressed and anxious, being discouraged, fatigued, resentment toward the infant and the attention he or she is getting, and headaches. Partners experiencing these symptoms should understand that it is not a sign of weakness and professional help can be helpful for them.

STAGE 3: TRANSITION TO MASTERY

In stage 3 (transition to mastery), the partner makes a conscious decision to take control and be at the center of his/her newborn's life regardless of his/her preparedness. This adjustment period is similar to that of the mother's letting-go phase, when she incorporates the newest member into the family.

KEY CONCEPTS

- The puerperium period refers to the first 6 weeks after delivery. During this period, the mother experiences many physiologic and psychological adaptations to return her to the prepregnant state.

- Involution involves three processes: contraction of muscle fibers to reduce stretched ones, catabolism (which reduces enlarged, individual cells), and regeneration of uterine epithelium from the lower layer of the decidua after the upper layers have been sloughed off and shed in lochia.

- Lochia passes through three stages: lochia rubra, lochia serosa, and lochia alba during the postpartum period.

- Maternal blood plasma volume decreases rapidly after birth and returns to normal within 4 weeks postpartum.

- Reva Rubin (1984) identified three phases the mother goes through to adjust to her new maternal role: the taking-in, taking-hold, and letting-go phase.

- The transition to fatherhood is influenced by many factors, including participation in childbirth, relationships with significant others, competence in child care, the family role organization, the father's cultural background, and the method of infant feeding.

- Like mothers, partners go through a predictable three-stage process during the first 3 weeks as they too "try on" their roles as f partners. The three stages include expectations, reality, and transition to mastery.

References and Recommended Readings

Adams, M. (2015). Motherhood: A discrepancy theory. *Research and Theory for Nursing Practice, 29*(2), 143–157.

Alekseev, N. P., Vladimir, I. I., & Nadezhda, T. E. (2015). Pathological postpartum breast engorgement: Prediction, prevention, and resolution. *Breastfeeding Medicine, 10*(4), 203–208.

Alexander, L. L., LaRosa, J. H., Bader, H., & Garfield, S. (2014). *New dimensions in women's health* (6th ed.). Sudbury, MA: Jones & Bartlett.

American Academy of Pediatrics [AAP] (2015). *Caring for your baby and young child: Birth to age 5* (6th ed.). Elk Grove Village, Illinois: AAP.

Barrett, E. S., Parlett, L. E., Windham, G. C., & Swan, S. H. (2014). Differences in ovarian hormones in relation to parity and time since last birth. *Fertility & Sterility, 101*(6), 1773–1780.

Bernard, V., Young, J., Chanson, P., & Binart, N. (2015). New insights in prolactin: Pathological implications. *Nature Reviews Endocrinology, 11*(5), 265–275.

Bope, E., & Kellerman, R. (2015). *Conn's current therapy 2015.* Philadelphia, PA: Saunders Elsevier.

Bowers, P., & Ceballos, K. (2015). Cultural perspectives in childbearing. Nurse.com, Retrieved from http://ce.nurse.com/course/ce263-60/cultural-perspectives-in-childbearing/.

Boyd-Judson, L., & James, P. (2014). *Women's global health: Norms and state policies.* Plymouth, UK: Lexington Books.

Buckley, S. (2015). *Hormonal physiology of childbearing: Evidence and implications for women, babies and maternity care.* Washington, D.C.: Childbirth Connection, National Partnership for Women & Families.

Cheng, Y. W., & Caughey, A. B. (2015). Normal labor and delivery. *eMedicine.* Retrieved from http://emedicine.medscape.com/article/260036-overview.

Creasy, R. K., Resnik, R., Iams, J. D., Lockwood, C. J., Moore, T. R., & Greene, M. F. (2014). *Creasy & Resnik's maternal-fetal medicine: Principles and practice* (7th ed.). Philadelphia, PA: Elsevier Saunders.

Cunningham, F. G., Leveno, K. J., Bloom, S. L., Spong, C., Dashe, J. S., Hoffman, B. L., et al. (2014). *William's obstetrics* (24th ed.). New York, NY: McGraw-Hill Publishers.

Davies, J. (2015). Fatherhood Institute: Supporting fathers to play their part. *Community Practitioner, 88*(1), 13–14.

DiPietro, J. A., Goldshore, M. A., Kivlighan, K. T., Pater, H. A., & Costigan, K. A. (2015). The ups and downs of early mothering. *Journal of Psychosomatic Obstetrics & Gynecology, 36*(3)94–102.

Dumoulin C., Hay-Smith, E. J, & Mac Habée-Séguin, G. (2014). Pelvic floor muscle training versus no treatment, or inactive control treatments, for urinary incontinence in women. *Cochrane Database of Systematic Reviews, 2014*(5), CD005654.

Edelman, C. L., Kudzma, E. C., & Mandle, C. L. (2014). *Health promotion throughout the lifespan* (8th ed.). St. Louis, MO: Mosby Elsevier.

Engel, S., Kon, S. K., Mawson, E. H., & Folley, S. J. (2015). Discussion of some recent developments in knowledge of the physiology of the breast. *Proceedings of the Royal Society of Medicine, 40*, 899–906.

Evans, A. T., & De Franco, E. (2014). *Manual of obstetrics* (8th ed.). Philadelphia, PA: Lippincott Williams & Wilkins.

Ferrarello, D., & Hatfield, L. (2014). Barriers to skin-to-skin care during the postpartum stay. *MCN. The American Journal of Maternal Child Nursing, 39*(1), 56–61.

Finley, P. R., & Brizendine, L. (2015). Enhancing our understanding of perinatal depression. *CNS Spectrums, 20*(1), 9–10.

Flynn, R. (2015). Mood disorders during and after pregnancy. *South African Journal of Diabetes, 8*(2), 27–33.

Halford, W. K., Petch, J., & Creedy, D. (2015). Taking baby home. In *Clinical guide to helping new parents* (pp. 87–109). New York, NY: Springer Publishers.

Hutcheson, J. L., & Cheeseman, S. E. (2015). An innovative strategy to improve family–infant bonding. *Neonatal Network, 34*(3), 189–191.

Jin, B., Yu, H., Jin, M., Du, X., & Yang, S. (2015). Measurement of prolactin and estradiol to estimate menses return of breastfeeding mothers. *Reproduction and Contraception, 14*(2), 111–117.

Jordan, R. G., Engstrom, J., Marfell, J., & Farley, C. L. (2014). *Prenatal & postnatal care: A women-centered approach*. Ames, Iowa: John Wiley & Sons.

King, T. L., Brucker, M. C., Kriebs, J. M., Fahey, J. O., Gegor, C. L., & Varney, H. (2015). *Varney's midwifery* (5th ed.). Burlington, MA: Jones & Bartlett Learning.

Liu, Y., Maloni, J. A., & Petrini, M. A. (2014). Effect of postpartum practices of doing the month on Chinese women's physical and psychological health. *Biological Research for Nursing, 16*(1), 55–63.

Mahendru, A., Everett, T., Wilkinson, I., Lees, C., & McEniery, C. (2014). A longitudinal study of maternal cardiovascular function from preconception to the postpartum period. *Journal of Hypertension, 32*(4), 849–856.

Martin, J., MacDonald-Wicks, L., Hure, A., Smith, R., & Collins, C. E. (2015). Reducing postpartum weight retention and improving breastfeeding outcomes in overweight women: A pilot randomized controlled trial. *Nutrients, 7*(3), 1464–1479.

Mattson, S., & Smith, J. (2016). *Core curriculum for maternal-newborn nursing* (5th ed.). St. Louis, MO: Elsevier Saunders.

Mercer, R. (2006). Nursing support of the process of becoming a mother. *Journal of Obstetric, Gynecologic & Neonatal Nursing, 35*(5), 649–651.

Mercer, R., & Walker, L. (2006). A review of nursing interventions to foster becoming a mother. *Journal of Obstetric, Gynecologic & Neonatal Nursing, 35*(5), 568–582.

Nascimento, S., Pudwell, J., Surita, F., Adamo, K., & Smith, G. (2014). The effect of physical exercise strategies on weight loss in postpartum women: a systematic review and meta-analysis. *International Journal of Obesity, 38*(5), 626–635.

Neville, C., McKinley, M., Holmes, V., Spence, D., & Woodside, J. (2014). The relationship between breastfeeding and postpartum weight change—a systematic review and critical evaluation. *International Journal of Obesity, 38*(4), 577–590.

Nolan, M. (2015). Why it is important to involve new fathers in the care of their child: Mary Nolan explores research into the often-neglected role of men and suggests how primary care nurses can develop services to increase their involvement. *Primary Health Care, 25*(3), 18–23.

Norwitz, E. R., & Schorge, J. O. (2015). *Obstetrics & gynecology at a glance* (5th ed.). Oxford, UK: Wiley-Blackwell.

Parpaglioni, R. (2015). Anatomo-physiological changes during labor and after delivery. In *Epidural labor analgesia* (pp. 11–20). Switzerland: Springer International Publishing.

Purnell, L. D. (2014). *Guide to culturally competent health care* (3rd ed.). Philadelphia, PA: F.A. Davis.

Rice, P. L., & Manderson, L. (2014). *Maternity and reproductive health in Asian societies*. Abingdon, Oxon: Routledge.

Rubin, R. (1984). *Maternal identity and the maternal experience*. New York, NY: Springer.

Sears, R. W., & Sears, J. M. (2015). *Ask Dr. Sears: Father-newborn bonding*. Retrieved from http://www.askdrsears.com/topics/pregnancy-childbirth/tenth-month-post-partum/bonding-with-your-newborn/father-newborn-bonding.

Senie, R. T. (2014). *Epidemiology of women's health*. Burlington, MA: Jones & Bartlett Learning.

Sethna, V., Murray, L., Netsi, E., Psychogiou, L., & Ramchandani, P. G. (2015). Paternal depression in the postnatal period and early father–infant interactions. *Parenting, 15*(1), 1–8.

Spencer, B. (2015). Medications and breastfeeding for mothers with chronic illness. *Journal of Obstetric, Gynecologic, & Neonatal Nursing, 44*(4), 543–552.

Spiliopoulos, M., & Mastrogiannis, D. (2014). Normal and abnormal puerperium. *eMedicine*, Retrieved from http://emedicine.medscape.com/article/260187-overview#a1.

Spiteri, G., Borg Xuereb, R., Carrick-Sen, D., Kaner, E., & Martin, C. R. (2014). Preparation for parenthood: a concept analysis. *Journal of Reproductive & Infant Psychology, 32*(2), 148–165.

Stuebe, A. M., Meltzer-Brody, S., Pearson, B., Pedersen, C., & Grewen, K. (2015). Maternal neuroendocrine serum levels in exclusively breastfeeding mothers. *Breastfeeding Medicine, 10*(4), 197–202.

Velotti, P., Castellano, R., & Zavattini, G. C. (2015). Adjustment of couples following childbirth. *European Psychologist, 16*, 1–10

Wambach, K., & Riordan, J. (2014). *Breastfeeding and human lactation* (5th ed.). Burlington, MA: Jones and Bartlett Learning.

Webber, G. C., & Chirangi, B. (2014). Women's health in women's hands: A pilot study assessing the feasibility of providing women with medications to reduce postpartum hemorrhage and sepsis in rural Tanzania. *Health Care for Women International, 35*(7–9), 758–770.

Wojnar, D. M., & Narruhn, R. A. (2016). Transcultural aspects of perinatal health care of Somali women. *Caring for the vulnerable* (4th ed., pp. 287–302). Burlington, MA: Jones & Bartlett Learning.

Zanardo, V., & Straface, G. (2015). The higher temperature in the areola supports the natural progression of the birth to breastfeeding continuum. *PLoS One, 10*(3), e0118774.

MULTIPLE CHOICE QUESTIONS

1. Postpartum breast engorgement occurs 48 to 72 hours after giving birth. What physiologic change influences breast engorgement?
   a. An increase in blood and lymph supply to the breasts
   b. An increase in estrogen and progesterone levels
   c. Colostrum production increases dramatically
   d. Fluid retention in the breasts due to the intravenous fluids given during labor

2. In the taking-in maternal role phase described by Rubin (1984), the nurse would expect the woman's behavior to be characterized as which of the following?
   a. Gaining self-confidence
   b. Adjusting to her new relationships
   c. Being passive and dependent
   d. Resuming control over her life

3. The nurse is explaining to a postpartum woman 48 hours after her giving childbirth that the after-pains she is experiencing can be the result of which of the following?
   a. Abdominal cramping is a sign of endometriosis
   b. A small infant weighing less than 8 lb
   c. Pregnancies that were too closely spaced
   d. Contractions of the uterus after birth

4. The nurse would expect a postpartum woman to demonstrate lochia in which sequence?
   a. Rubra, alba, serosa
   b. Rubra, serosa, alba
   c. Serosa, alba, rubra
   d. Alba, rubra, serosa

5. The nurse is assessing Ms. Smith, who gave birth to her first child 5 days ago. What findings by the nurse would be expected?
   a. Cream-colored lochia; uterus above the umbilicus
   b. Bright-red lochia with clots; uterus 2 fingerbreadths below umbilicus
   c. Light pink or brown lochia; uterus 4 to 5 fingerbreadths below umbilicus
   d. Yellow, mucousy lochia; uterus at the level of the umbilicus

6. Prioritize the postpartum mother's needs 4 hours after giving birth by placing a number 1, 2, 3, or 4 in the blank before each need.
   a. _____ Learn how to hold and cuddle the infant.
   b. _____ Watch a baby bath demonstration given by the nurse.
   c. _____ Sleep and rest without being disturbed for a few hours.
   d. _____ Interaction time (first 30 minutes) with the infant to facilitate bonding.

7. Immediately after childbirth in the recovery area, the nurse observes the mother's partner's fascination and interest in the new son. This behavior is often termed:
   a. Attachment
   b. Engrossment
   c. Bonding
   d. Temperament

8. After the nurse provides instructions to a postpartum woman about postpartum blues, which statement would indicate understanding of it? I will
   a. "Need to take medication daily to treat the anxiety and sadness."
   b. "Call the OB support line only if I start to hear voices."
   c. "Contact my doctor if I become dizzy and fell nauseated."
   d. "Feel like laughing one minute and crying the next minute."

CRITICAL THINKING EXERCISE

1. A new nurse assigned to the postpartum mother–baby unit makes a comment to the oncoming shift that, a 25-year-old primipara, seems lazy and shows no initiative in taking care of herself or her baby. The nurse reported that this new mother talks excessively about her labor and birth experience and seems preoccupied with herself and her needs, not her newborn's care. She wonders if something is wrong with this mother because she seems so self-centered and has to be directed to do everything.
   a. Is there something "wrong" with Ms. Griffin's behavior? Why or why not?
   b. What maternal role phase is being described by the new nurse?
   c. What role can the nurse play to support the mother through this phase?

2. A primipara gave birth to a healthy baby boy yesterday. Her partner seemed elated at the birth, calling their friends and family on his cell phone minutes after the birth. He passed out cigars and praised his wife for her efforts. Today, when the nurse walked into their room, her partner seemed very anxious around his new son and called for the nurse whenever the baby cried or needed a diaper change. He seemed standoffish when asked to hold his son, and he spent time talking to other fathers in the waiting room, leaving his wife alone in the room.
   a. Would you consider Mr. Lenhart's paternal behavior to be normal at this time?
   b. What might Mr. Lenhart be feeling at this time?
   c. How can the nurse help this new father adjust to his new role?

STUDY ACTIVITIES

1. Find an Internet resource that discusses general postpartum care for new mothers who might have questions after discharge. Evaluate the web site's information as to how credible, accurate, and current the information is.

2. Prepare a teaching plan for new mothers, outlining the various physiologic changes that will take place after discharge.

3. The term that describes the return of the uterus to its prepregnant state is _____.

4. A deviated fundus to the right side of the abdomen would indicate a _____.

BRINGING IT ALL TOGETHER: CASE STUDY

A 29-year-old married Latina mother of four children lived with her migrant husband and his parents in a small rural border town. She had given birth to her fourth child 7 weeks ago. She now had four children in the past four years. Her pregnancy, labor, and birth had been uneventful, and an untrained neighbor woman helped conduct the home birth. Because pregnancy was viewed as a normal occurrence that did not require any medical attention, she did not receive any prenatal care for any of her four pregnancies. For the first month after birth, she felt normal, but then began to exhibit restless and anxious behavior. She became isolated from her family, stopped speaking to them, and ceased to care for her newborn or other children. Her family wondered about her isolation, but seemed indifferent to her condition, as they were all busy with their own lives. One day when all of her family members and her children had gone to work in the fields, she ended her life.

Go to the Point **to find questions to consider about this case.**

16

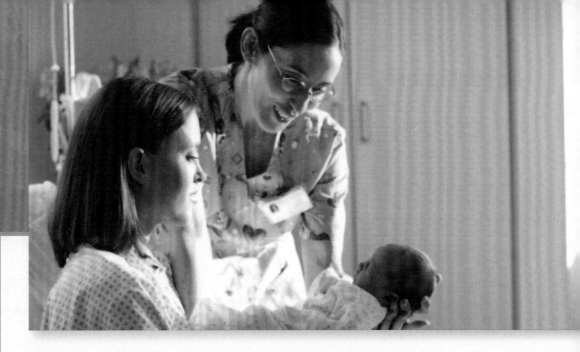

Nursing Management During the Postpartum Period

Learning Objectives

Upon completion of the chapter, you will be able to:

1. Characterize the normal physiologic and psychological adaptations to the postpartum period.

2. Determine the parameters that need to be assessed during the postpartum period.

3. Compare and contrast bonding to the attachment process.

4. Select behaviors that enhance or inhibit the attachment process.

5. Outline nursing management for the woman and her family during the postpartum period.

6. Examine the role of the nurse in promoting successful breast-feeding.

7. Plan areas of health education needed for discharge planning, home care, and follow-up.

A 24-year-old Muslim primipara has just been admitted to the postpartum unit. Her husband sits at the bedside, but doesn't seem to provide her any physical or emotional support after her lengthy labor and difficult birth.

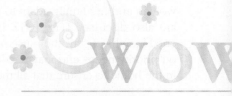

Words of Wisdom
Parenting is an intimate, interactive, continuous, lifelong process.

INTRODUCTION

The postpartum period is a time of major adjustments and adaptations not just for the mother, but for all members of the family. It is during this time that parenting starts and a relationship with the newborn begins. A positive, loving relationship between parents and their newborn promotes the emotional well-being of all. This relationship endures and has profound effects on the child's growth and development.

Take Note!

Parenting is a skill that is often learned by trial and error, with varying degrees of success. Successful parenting, a continuous and complex interactive process, requires the parents to learn new skills and to integrate the new member into the family.

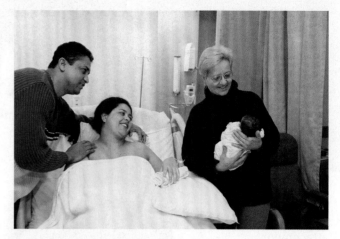

FIGURE 16.1 Parents and grandmother interacting with the newborn.

Once the infant is born, each system in the mother's body takes several weeks to return to its nonpregnant state. The physiologic changes in women during the postpartum period are dramatic. Nurses should be aware of these changes and should be able to make observations and assessments to validate normal occurrences and detect any deviations.

This chapter describes the nursing management of the woman and her family during the postpartum period. (See Chapter 21 for a detailed discussion of the postpartum care of the woman undergoing a surgical birth.) Nursing management during the postpartum period focuses on assessing the woman's ability to adapt to the physiologic and psychological changes occurring at this time (see Chapter 15 for a detailed discussion of these adaptations). The chapter outlines physical assessment parameters for new mothers and newborns. It also focuses on bonding and attachment behaviors; nurses need to be aware of these behaviors so they can perform appropriate interventions. Family members are also assessed to determine how well they are making the transition to this new stage.

Based on assessment findings, the nurse plans and implements care to address the family's needs. Steps to address physiologic needs such as comfort, self-care, nutrition, and contraception are described. Ways to help the woman and her family adapt to the birth of the newborn are also discussed (Fig. 16.1). Because of today's shortened lengths of stay, the nurse may be able to focus only on priority needs and may need to arrange for follow-up in the home to ensure that all the family's needs are met.

SOCIAL SUPPORT AND CULTURAL CONSIDERATIONS

In addition to physical assessment and care of the woman in the postpartum period, strong social support is vital to help her integrate the baby into the family. A key to providing effective postpartum care is to understand the woman in her social and cultural context so that all care

provided is culturally competent and sensitive. In today's mobile society, extended families may live far away and may be unable to help care for the new family. As a result, many new parents turn to health care providers for information as well as physical and emotional support during this adjustment period. Nurses can be an invaluable resource by serving as mentors, teaching about self-care measures and baby care basics, and providing emotional support. Nurses can "mother" the new mother by offering physical care, emotional support, information, and practical help. The nurse's support and care through this critical time can increase the new parents' confidence, giving them a sense of accomplishment in their parenting skills. One important intervention during the postpartum period is promotion of breast-feeding. *Healthy People 2020* includes breast-feeding as a goal for maternal, infant, and child health (U.S. Department of Health and Human Resources [USDHHS], 2010).

As in all nursing care, nurses should provide culturally competent care during the postpartum period. The nurse should engage in ongoing cultural self-assessment and overcome any stereotypes that perpetuate prejudice or discrimination against any cultural group (Bowers & Ceballos, 2015). Providing culturally competent nursing care during the postpartum period requires time, open-mindedness, and patience. The global migration of diverse populations presents nurses with the challenge of providing care to unprecedented numbers of clients and their families with health care beliefs and practices that differ from their own. Sensitivity cannot be assumed; it needs to be nurtured and developed. The skill set needed by nurses to provide culturally competent care to postpartum clients and their families include understanding their beliefs, experiences, and family environment; facilitating their language through appropriate use of interpreters so that the information provided can be understood; and compassionately respecting clients and their human rights. The Chinese culture values traditions and the

Objective	Nursing Significance
Increase the proportion of mothers who breast-feed their babies.	Will provide infants with the most complete form of nutrition, improving their health, growth and development, and immunity.
Increase the number of mothers who breast-feed ever from a baseline of 74% to 81.9%.	Will improve maternal health via breast-feeding's beneficial effects.
Increase the number of mothers who breast-feed at 6 months from a baseline of 43.5% to 60.6%.	Will increase the rate of breast-feeding, particularly among low-income and certain racial and ethnic populations who are less likely to begin breastfeeding in the hospital or to sustain it through the infant's first year.
Increase the number of mothers who breast-feed at 1 year from a baseline of 22.7% to 34.1%.	
Increase the number of mothers who breast-feed exclusively through 3 months from a baseline of 33.6% to 46.2%.	
Increase the number of mothers who breast-feed exclusively through 6 months from a baseline of 14.1% to 25.5%.	

Healthy People objectives based on data from http://www.healthypeople.gov.

involvement of elders in the extended family. Some Chinese women living in the United States practice transnational parenting, a process of sending their American-born child to China to be raised by the extended family there. This obviously has implications for breast-feeding success among these mothers (Lee & Brann, 2015). To promote positive outcomes, the nurse should be sensitive to the woman's and family's culture, religion, and ethnic influences (see "Providing Optimal Cultural Care" in the Nursing Interventions section).

Remember the couple introduced at the beginning of the chapter? When the postpartum nurse comes to examine Raina, her husband quickly leaves the room and returns a short time later after the examination is complete. How do you interpret his behavior toward his wife? What might you communicate to this couple?

NURSING ASSESSMENT IN THE POSTPARTUM PERIOD

Many adaptations and adjustments must be made to accommodate the new family member. The nurse's focus is on assistance for families to maximize their adjustment, surveillance for maladaptation, and education, consultation, collaboration as needed. Comprehensive nursing assessment begins within an hour after the woman gives birth and continues through discharge.

> **Take Note!**
>
> Nurses need a firm grasp of normal findings to be able to recognize abnormal findings and intervene appropriately.

This postpartum assessment includes vital signs and physical and psychosocial assessments. It also includes assessing the parents and other family members, such as siblings and grandparents, for attachment and bonding with the newborn. Although the exact protocol may vary among facilities, postpartum assessment typically is performed as follows:

- During the first hour: every 15 minutes
- During the second hour: every 30 minutes
- During the first 24 hours: every 4 hours
- After 24 hours: every 8 hours (Jordan et al., 2014; Mattson & Smith, 2016).

During each assessment, keep in mind risk factors that may lead to complications, such as infection or hemorrhage, during the recovery period (Box 16.1). Early identification is critical to ensure prompt intervention.

The postpartum period is a time of transition for women. The end of the pregnancy and childbirth initiates physiologic changes as many body systems return to their nonpregnant state. Nurses need to be aware of the normal physiologic and psychological changes that take place in clients' bodies and minds in order to provide comprehensive care during the postpartum period. In addition to client and family teaching, one of the most significant responsibilities of the postpartum nurse is to recognize potential complications after childbirth.

As with any assessment, always review the woman's medical record for information about her pregnancy, labor, and birth. Note any preexisting conditions, any complications that occurred during pregnancy, labor, birth, and immediately afterward, and any treatments provided.

Postpartum assessment of the mother typically includes vital signs, pain level, epidural site inspection for infection, and a systematic head-to-toe review of body systems. The acronym **BUBBLE-EEE—b**reasts, **u**terus, **b**ladder, **b**owels, **l**ochia, **e**pisiotomy/perineum/ epidural site, **e**xtremities, and **e**motional status—can be used as a guide for this head-to-toe review (Cunningham et al., 2014).

FACTORS INCREASING A WOMAN'S RISK FOR POSTPARTUM COMPLICATIONS

Risk Factors for Postpartum Infection
- Operative procedure (forceps, cesarean birth, vacuum extraction)
- History of diabetes, including gestational-onset diabetes
- Prolonged labor (more than 24 hours)
- Use of indwelling urinary catheter
- Anemia (hemoglobin < 10.5 mg/dL)
- Multiple vaginal examinations during labor
- Prolonged rupture of membranes (>24 hours)
- Manual extraction of placenta
- Compromised immune system (HIV positive)

Risk Factors for Postpartum Hemorrhage
- Precipitous labor (less than 3 hours)
- Uterine atony
- Placenta previa or abruptio placenta
- Labor induction or augmentation
- Operative procedures (vacuum extraction, forceps, cesarean birth)
- Retained placental fragments
- Prolonged third stage of labor (more than 30 minutes)
- Multiparity, more than three births closely spaced
- Uterine over distention (large infant, twins, hydramnios)

While assessing the woman and her family during the postpartum period, be alert for danger signs (Box 16.2). Notify the primary health care provider immediately if any are noted.

Vital Signs Assessment

Obtain vital signs and compare them with the previous values, noting and reporting any deviations. Vital sign changes can be an early indicator of complications.

BOX 16.2

POSTPARTUM DANGER SIGNS
- Fever more than 100.4° F (38° C)
- Foul-smelling lochia or an unexpected change in color or amount
- Large blood clots, or bleeding that saturates a peripad in an hour
- Severe headaches or blurred vision
- Visual changes, such as blurred vision or spots, or headaches
- Calf pain with dorsiflexion of the foot
- Swelling, redness, or discharge at the episiotomy, epidural, or abdominal sites
- Dysuria, burning, or incomplete emptying of the bladder
- Shortness of breath or difficulty breathing without exertion
- Depression or extreme mood swings

Temperature

Use a consistent measurement technique (oral, axillary, or tympanic) to get the most accurate readings. Typically, the new mother's temperature during the first 24 hours postpartum is within the normal range or a low-grade elevation. Some women experience a slight fever, up to 100.4° F (38° C), during the first 24 hours. This elevation may be the result of dehydration because of fluid loss during labor. Temperature should be normal after 24 hours with replacement of fluids lost during labor and birth (Green, 2016).

A temperature above 100.4° F (38° C) at any time or an abnormal temperature after the first 24 hours may indicate infection and must be reported. Abnormal temperature readings warrant continued monitoring until an infection can be ruled out through cultures or blood studies. An elevated temperature can identify maternal sepsis, which results in significant maternal morbidity and mortality worldwide. To improve the outcome, it is essential that nurses be vigilant in obtaining accurate values and monitoring their client's temperature.

Pulse

Pulse rates of 60 to 80 beats per minute (bpm) at rest are normal during the first week after birth. This pulse rate is called puerperal bradycardia. During pregnancy, the heavy gravid uterus causes a decreased flow of venous blood to the heart. After giving birth, there is an increase in intravascular volume. The cardiac output is most likely caused by an increased stroke volume from the venous return now. The elevated stroke volume leads to a decreased heart rate (Creasy et al., 2014). Tachycardia in the postpartum woman can suggest anxiety, excitement, fatigue, pain, excessive blood loss or delayed hemorrhage, infection, or underlying cardiac problems. Any pulse rate higher than 100 bpm warrants further investigation to rule out complications.

Respirations

Respiratory rates in the postpartum woman should be within the normal range of 12 to 20 bpm at rest. Pulmonary function typically returns to the prepregnant state after childbirth when the diaphragm descends and the organs revert to their normal positions. Any change in respiratory rate out of the normal range might indicate pulmonary edema, atelectasis, a side effect of epidural anesthesia, or pulmonary embolism and must be reported. Lungs should be clear on auscultation.

Blood Pressure

Assess the woman's blood pressure and compare it with her usual range. Report any deviation from this range. Immediately after childbirth, the blood pressure should remain the same as during labor. An increase in blood pressure could indicate gestational hypertension, whereas a decrease could indicate shock or orthostatic hypotension or dehydration, a side effect of epidural anesthesia. Blood pressure readings should not be higher than 140/90 mm Hg or lower than 85/60 mmHg (King et al., 2015). Blood pressure also may vary based on the woman's position, so assess blood pressure with the woman in the same position every time. Be alert for orthostatic hypotension, which can occur when the woman moves rapidly from a lying or sitting position to a standing one.

Pain

Pain, the fifth vital sign, is assessed along with the other four parameters. Question the woman about the type of pain and its location and severity. Have the woman rate the pain using a numeric scale from 0 to 10 points. Nursing care should focus on providing comfort measures to ease pain which might include perineal care, clean gown, mouth care, providing warm blankets, ensuring adequate fluid intake to facilitate healing, reposition frequently, and encouraging rest between assessments (Nagtalon-Ramos, 2014).

Many postpartum orders will have the nurse premedicate the woman routinely for afterbirth pains rather than wait for her to experience them first. The goal of pain management is to have the woman's pain scale rating maintained between 0 and 2 points at all times, especially after breast-feeding. This can be accomplished by assessing the woman's pain level frequently and preventing pain by administering analgesics. If the woman has severe pain in the perineal region despite use of physical comfort measures, check for a hematoma by inspecting and palpating the area. If one is found, notify the health care provider immediately.

Physical Examination

Physical examination of the postpartum woman focuses on assessing the breasts, uterus, bladder, bowels, lochia, episiotomy/perineum and epidural site and extremities.

Breasts

Inspect the breasts for size, contour, asymmetry, engorgement, or erythema. Check the nipples for cracks, redness, fissures, or bleeding, and note whether they are erect, flat, or inverted. Flat or inverted nipples can make breast-feeding challenging for both mother and infant. Cracked, blistered, fissured, bruised, or bleeding nipples in the breast-feeding woman are generally indications that the baby is improperly positioned on the breast. Palpate the breasts lightly to ascertain if they are soft,

filling, or engorged, and document your findings. For women who are not breast-feeding, use a gentle, light touch to avoid breast stimulation, which would exacerbate engorgement.

Lactogenesis (the onset of milk secretion) is initially triggered by the delivery of the placenta, which results in falling levels of estrogen and progesterone, with the continued presence of prolactin. If the mother is not breast-feeding, the prolactin levels fall and return to normal levels within 2 to 3 weeks. As milk is starting to come in, the breasts become firmer; this is charted as "filling." Engorged breasts are hard, tender, and taut. Ask the woman if she is having any nipple discomfort. Palpate the breasts for any nodules, masses, or areas of warmth, which may indicate a plugged duct that may progress to mastitis if not treated promptly. Any discharge from the nipple should be described and documented if it is not colostrum (creamy yellow) or foremilk (bluish white). Over the first week, the breast milk matures and contains all necessary nutrients in the neonatal period. The breast milk continues to change throughout the period of breast-feeding to meet the changing demands of the growing infant.

Uterus

Assess the fundus (top portion of the uterus) to determine the degree of uterine involution. If possible, have the woman empty her bladder before assessing the fundus and auscultate her bowel sounds prior to uterine palpation. If the client has had a cesarean birth and has a patient-controlled anesthesia (PCA) pump, instruct her to self-medicate prior to fundal assessment to decrease her discomfort.

Using a two-handed approach with the woman in the supine position with her knees flexed slightly and the bed in a flat position or as low as possible, palpate the abdomen gently, feeling for the top of the uterus while the other hand is placed on the lower segment of the uterus to stabilize it (Fig. 16.2).

The fundus should be midline and should feel firm. A boggy or relaxed uterus is a sign of uterine atony (loss of muscle tone in the uterus). This can be the result of bladder distention, which displaces the uterus upward and to the right, or retained placental fragments. Either situation predisposes the woman to hemorrhage.

Once the fundus is located, place your index finger on the fundus and count the number of fingerbreadths between the fundus and the umbilicus (1 fingerbreadth is approximately equal to 1 cm). One to 2 hours after birth, the fundus typically is between the umbilicus and the symphysis pubis. Approximately 6 to 12 hours after birth, the fundus usually is at the level of the umbilicus. If the fundal height is above the umbilicus, which would be an abnormal finding, investigate this immediately to prevent excessive bleeding. Frequently the woman's

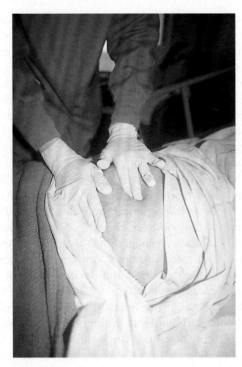

FIGURE 16.2 Palpating the fundus.

bladder is full, thus displacing the uterus up and to either side of the midline. Ask the woman to empty her bladder and reassess the uterus again.

Normally, the fundus progresses downward at a rate of one fingerbreadth (or 1 cm) per day after childbirth and should be nonpalpable by 10 to 14 days postpartum. By day 14, the uterus has descended below the rim of the symphysis pubis and is no longer palpable (Cunningham et al., 2014). On the first postpartum day, the top of the fundus is located 1 cm below the umbilicus and is recorded as u/1. Similarly, on the second postpartum day, the fundus would be 2 cm below the umbilicus and should be recorded as u/2, and so on. Health care agencies differ according to how fundal heights are charted, so follow their protocols for this. If the fundus is not firm, gently massage the uterus using a circular motion until it becomes firm.

Bladder

Considerable diuresis—as much as 3,000 mL/day—begins within 12 hours after childbirth and continues for several days. A single voiding may be 500 mL or more. By 21 days postpartum, the diuresis is usually complete (Jordan et al., 2014). However, many postpartum women do not sense the need to void even if their bladder is full. In this situation the bladder can become distended and displace the uterus upward and to the side, which prevents the uterine muscles from contracting properly and can lead to excessive bleeding. Urinary retention as a result of decreased bladder tone and emptying

can lead to urinary tract infections. It is imperative that nurses monitor clients for signs of urinary tract infections, including fever, urinary frequency and/or urgency, difficult or painful urination, and tenderness over the costovertebral angle (Wilson et al., 2015). Women who received regional anesthesia during labor are at risk for urinary tract infections due to continuous urinary catheterization to prevent urinary retention during labor, which is thought to delay fetal descent. They also experience difficulty voiding and loss of sensation and must wait until it returns to feel a full bladder which might be several hours after childbirth.

Assess for voiding problems by asking the woman the following questions:
- Have you (voided, urinated, gone to the bathroom) yet?
- Have you noticed any burning or discomfort with urination?
- Do you have any difficulty passing your urine?
- Do you feel that your bladder is empty when you finish urinating?
- Do you have any signs of infection such as urgency, frequency, or pain?
- Are you able to control the flow of urine by squeezing your muscles?
- Have you noticed any leakage of urine when you cough, laugh, or sneeze?

Assess the bladder for distention and adequate emptying after efforts to void. Palpate the area over the symphysis pubis. If empty, the bladder is not palpable. Palpation of a rounded mass suggests bladder distention. Also percuss the area: a full bladder is dull to percussion. If the bladder is full, lochia drainage will be more than normal because the uterus cannot contract to suppress the bleeding.

Take Note!

Note the location and condition of the fundus; a full bladder tends to displace the uterus up and to the right.

After the woman voids, palpate and percuss the area again to determine adequate emptying of the bladder. If the bladder remains distended, the woman may be retaining urine in her bladder, and measures to initiate voiding should be instituted. Be alert for signs of infection, including infrequent or insufficient voiding (less than 200 mL), discomfort, burning, urgency, or foul-smelling urine (Mattson & Smith, 2016). Document all urine output.

Bowels

Spontaneous bowel movements may not occur for 1 to 3 days after giving birth because of a decrease in muscle tone in the intestines as a result of elevated progesterone levels. Normal patterns of bowel elimination usually return within a week after birth (Verghese, Futaba, & Latthe, 2015). Often women are hesitant to have a bowel movement due to pain in the perineal area resulting from an episiotomy, lacerations, or hemorrhoids. Some are fearful that they may "rip their stitches" should they strain. Nurses should reassure their clients that stool softeners and/or laxatives to treat constipation have been prescribed for them to reduce discomfort.

Inspect the woman's abdomen for distention, auscultate for bowel sounds in all four quadrants prior to palpating the uterine fundus, and palpate for tenderness. The abdomen typically is soft, nontender, and nondistended. Bowel sounds are present in all four quadrants. Ask the woman if she has had a bowel movement or has passed gas since giving birth, because constipation is a common problem during the postpartum period and many women do not offer this information unless asked about it. Normal assessment findings are active bowel sounds, passing gas, and a nondistended abdomen.

Lochia

Assess lochia in terms of amount, color, odor, and change with activity and time. To assess how much a woman is bleeding, ask her how many perineal pads she has used in the past 1 to 2 hours and how much drainage was on each pad. For example, did she saturate the pad completely, or was only half of the pad covered with drainage? Ask about the color of the drainage, odor, and the presence of any clots. Lochia has a definite musky scent, with an odor similar to that of menstrual flow without any large clots (fist size). Foul-smelling lochia suggests an infection, and large clots suggest poor uterine involution, necessitating additional intervention.

To determine the amount of lochia, observe the amount of lochia saturation on the perineal pad and relate it to time (Fig. 16.3). Also, take into consideration

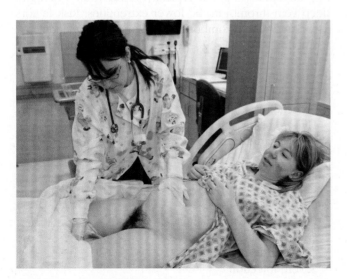

FIGURE 16.3 Assessing lochia.

the specific type of peripad used, because some are more absorbent than others. Lochia flow will increase when the woman gets out of bed (lochia pools in the vagina and the uterus while she is lying down) and when she breast-feeds (oxytocin release causes uterine contractions). A woman who saturates a perineal pad within 30 to 60 minutes is bleeding much more than one who saturates a pad in 2 hours.

Typically, the amount of lochia is described as follows:
- *Scant:* a 1- to 2-in lochia stain on the perineal pad or approximately a 10-mL loss
- *Light or small:* an approximately 4-inch stain or a 10- to 25-mL loss
- *Moderate:* a 4- to 6-in stain with an estimated loss of 25 to 50 mL
- *Large or heavy:* a pad is saturated within 1 hour after changing it (Bope & Kellerman, 2015)

The total volume of lochial discharge varies in women based on their parity, but the amount decreases daily. Check under the woman, by turning her to either side, to make sure additional blood is not hidden and not absorbed on her perineal pad. This also a good time to assess for the presence and condition of hemorrhoids since the nurse is visually inspecting the perineum.

Report any abnormal findings, such as heavy, bright-red lochia with large tissue fragments or a foul odor. If excessive bleeding occurs, the first step would be to massage the boggy fundus until it is firm to reduce the flow of blood. Document all findings.

Women who had a cesarean birth will have less lochia discharge than those who had a vaginal birth, but stages and color changes remain the same. Although the woman's abdomen will be tender after surgery, the nurse must palpate the fundus and assess the lochia to make sure they are within the normal range and that there is no excessive bleeding.

Anticipatory guidance to give the woman at discharge should include information about lochia and the expected changes. Urge the woman to notify her health care provider if lochia rubra returns after the serosa and alba transitions have taken place. This is abnormal and may indicate subinvolution or that the woman is too active and needs to rest more. Lochia is an excellent medium for bacterial growth. Explain to the woman that frequent changing of perineal pads, continued use of her peribottle for rinsing her perineal area, and hand hygiene before and after pad changes are important infection control measures.

Episiotomy/Perineum and Epidural Site

If the woman has an episiotomy, which is not routinely done currently, to assess the episiotomy and perineal area, position the woman on her side with her top leg flexed upward at the knee and drawn up toward her

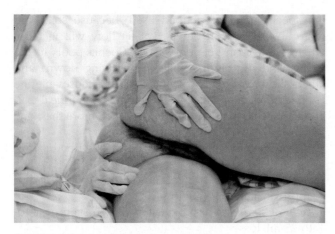

FIGURE 16.4 Inspecting the perineum.

waist. If necessary, use a penlight to provide adequate lighting during the assessment. Wearing gloves and standing at the woman's side with her back to you, gently lift the upper buttock to expose the perineum and anus (Fig. 16.4). Inspect the episiotomy for irritation, ecchymosis, tenderness, or hematomas. Assess for hemorrhoids and their condition.

During the early postpartum period, the perineal tissue surrounding the episiotomy is typically edematous and slightly bruised. The normal episiotomy site should not have redness, discharge, or edema. The majority of healing takes place within the first 2 weeks, but it may take 4 to 6 months for the episiotomy to heal completely (King et al., 2015).

Lacerations to the perineal area sustained during the birthing process that were identified and repaired also need to be assessed to determine their healing status. Lacerations are classified based on their severity and tissue involvement:

- *First-degree laceration:* involves only skin and superficial structures above muscle
- *Second-degree laceration:* extends through perineal muscles
- *Third-degree laceration:* extends through the anal sphincter muscle
- *Fourth-degree laceration:* continues through anterior rectal wall

Assess the episiotomy and any lacerations at least every 8 hours to detect hematomas or signs of infection. Large areas of swollen, bluish skin with complaints of severe pain in the perineal area indicate pelvic or vulvar hematomas. Redness, swelling, increasing discomfort, or purulent drainage may indicate infection. Both findings need to be reported immediately.

A white line running the length of the episiotomy is a sign of infection, as is swelling or discharge. Severe, intractable pain, perineal discoloration, and ecchymosis indicate a perineal hematoma, a potentially dangerous condition. Report any unusual findings. Ice can be applied

to relieve discomfort and reduce edema; sitz baths also can promote comfort and perineal healing (see "Promoting Comfort" in the Nursing Interventions section).

If the woman has had an epidural during her labor, assessment of the epidural wound site is important as well as checking for any side effects of the medication injected such as itching, nausea and vomiting, or urinary retention. Visual inspection of the epidural site and an accurate documentation of intake and output are essential.

Extremities

Pregnancy is associated with an increased risk of venous thromboembolism (VTE), which includes pulmonary embolism and deep vein thrombosis. During pregnancy, the state of hypercoagulability protects the mother against excessive blood loss during childbirth and placental separation. However, this hypercoagulable state can increase the risk of thromboembolic disorders during pregnancy and postpartum. Three factors predispose women to thromboembolic disorders during pregnancy: stasis (compression of the large veins because of the gravid uterus), altered coagulation (state of pregnancy), and localized vascular damage (may occur during the birthing process). All of these factors increase the risk of clot formation and having it travel to the lungs.

While inspecting the woman's extremities, also determine the degree of sensory and motor function return (recovery from anesthesia) by asking the woman if she feels sensation at various areas the nurse touches and also by observing her ambulation stability.

Take Note!
Pulmonary embolism occurs in up to 3 per 1000 births and is a major cause of maternal mortality (Kim et al., 2015).

Pulmonary emboli typically result from dislodged deep vein thrombi in the lower extremities. Risk factors associated with thromboembolic conditions include:
- Anemia
- Diabetes mellitus
- Cigarette smoking
- Obesity
- Preeclampsia
- Hypertension
- Severe varicose veins
- Pregnancy
- Multiple pregnancies
- Cardiovascular disease
- Sickle cell disease
- Postpartum hemorrhage
- Oral contraceptive use
- Cesarean birth
- Severe infection
- Previous thromboembolic disease

- Multiparity
- Bed rest or immobility for 4 days or more
- Advanced maternal age > 35 years (Kline & Kabrhel, 2015)

Because of the subtle presentation of thrombo-embolic disorders, the physical examination may not be enough to detect them. An accurate diagnosis of pulmonary embolism is needed because it requires (1) prolonged therapy (≤9 months of heparin during pregnancy), (2) prophylaxis during future pregnancies, and (3) avoidance of oral contraceptive pills. The woman may report lower extremity tightness or aching when ambulating that is relieved with rest and elevation of the leg. Edema in the affected leg (typically the left), along with warmth and tenderness, and a low-grade fever may also be noted. A duplex ultrasound (two-dimensional ultrasound and Doppler ultrasound that compresses the vein to assess for changes in venous flow) in conjunction with the physical findings frequently is needed for a conclusive diagnosis (Sucker & Zotz, 2015).

Women with an increased risk for this condition during the postpartum period should wear antiembolism stockings or use sequential compression devices to reduce the risk of venous stasis by preventing blood from pooling in the calves of the legs. Encouraging the client to ambulate after childbirth reduces the incidence of thrombophlebitis.

Psychosocial Assessment

Psychosocial assessment of the postpartum woman focuses on emotional status and bonding and attachment.

Emotional Status

Assess the woman's emotional status by observing how she interacts with her family, her level of independence, energy levels, eye contact with her infant (within a cultural context), posture and comfort level while holding the newborn, and sleep and rest patterns. Be alert for mood swings, irritability, or crying episodes.

Remember Raina and her "quiet" husband, the Muslim couple? The postpartum nurse informs Raina that her doctor, Nancy Schultz, has been called away for emergency surgery and won't be available the rest of the day. The nurse explains that Dr. Robert Nappo will be making rounds for her. Raina and her husband become upset. Why? Is culturally competent care being provided to this couple?

Bonding and Attachment

Nurses can be instrumental in promoting attachment by assessing attachment behaviors (positive and negative) and intervening appropriately if needed. Nurses must be able to identify any family discord that might interfere with the attachment process. Remember, however, that mothers from different cultures may behave differently from what is expected in your own culture. For example, Native American mothers tend to handle their newborns less often and use cradle boards to carry them. Native American mothers and many Asian American mothers delay breast-feeding until their milk comes in, because colostrum is considered harmful for the newborn (Bowers & Ceballos, 2015). Do not assume that different behavior is wrong.

Meeting the newborn for the first time after birth can be an exhilarating experience for parents. Although the mother has spent many hours dreaming of her unborn and how he or she will look, it is not until after birth that they meet face to face. They both need to get to know one another and to develop feelings for one another.

Bonding is the close emotional attraction to a newborn by the parents that develops during the first 30 to 60 minutes after birth. It is unidirectional, from parent to infant. It is thought that optimal bonding of the parents to a newborn requires a period of close contact within the first few minutes to a few hours after birth. Bonding is really a continuation of the relationship that began during pregnancy (Sears & Sears, 2015a). It is affected by a multitude of factors, including the parent's socioeconomic status, family history, role models, support systems, cultural factors, and birth experiences. The mother initiates bonding when she caresses her infant and exhibits certain behaviors typical of a mother tending her child. The infant's responses to this, such as body and eye movements, are a necessary part of the process. During this initial period, the infant is in a quiet, alert state, looking directly at the holder.

Take Note!

The length of time necessary for bonding depends on the health of the infant and mother, as well as the circumstances surrounding the labor and birth (Tester-Jones et al., 2015).

Attachment is the development of strong affection between an infant and a significant other (mother, father, sibling, and caretaker). This attachment is reciprocal; both the significant other and the newborn exhibit attachment behaviors. The attachment relationship formed between the infant and primary caregiver influences the child's view of the world and future relationships (Sette, Coppola, & Cassibba, 2015). This tie between two people is psychological rather than biologic, and it does not occur overnight. The process of attachment follows a progressive or developmental course that changes over time. Attachment is an individualized and multifactorial process that differs based on the health of the infant, the mother, environmental circumstances, and the quality of care the infant receives. The newborn responds to the significant other by cooing, grasping, smiling, and crying. Nurses can assess for attachment behaviors by observing the interaction between the newborn and the person holding him or her (Mattson & Smith, 2016). It occurs through mutually satisfying experiences. Maternal attachment begins during pregnancy as the result of fetal movement and maternal fantasies about the infant and continues through the birth and postpartum periods. Attachment behaviors include seeking, physical caretaking behaviors, emotional attentiveness to infant's needs, staying close to, touching, kissing, cuddling, choosing the ***en face*** (face-to-face) **position** while holding or feeding the newborn, expressing pride in the newborn and exchanging gratifying experiences with the infant (McComish, 2015). In a high-risk pregnancy, the attachment process may be complicated by premature birth (lack of time to develop a relationship with the unborn baby) and by parental stress due to the fetal and/or maternal vulnerability.

Bonding is a vital component of the attachment process and is necessary in establishing parent–infant attachment and a healthy, loving relationship. During this early period of acquaintance, mothers touch their infants in a very characteristic manner. Mothers visually and physically "explore" their infants, initially using their fingertips on the infant's face and extremities and progressing to massaging and stroking the infant with their fingers. This is followed by palm contact on the trunk. Eventually, mothers draw their infant toward them and hold the infant (Fig. 16.5).

Generally, research on attachment has found that the process is similar for partners as for mothers, but the pace may be different. Like mothers, partners manifest attachment behaviors during pregnancy. Indeed, Baltes et al. (2014) found that the best predictors of early postnatal attachment for fathers or significant others were

those who viewed the paternal caregiving role as important and also had greater marital quality. Higher levels of paternal sensitivity were associated with better infant–father attachment. Becoming a father or significant partner requires the person to build on the experiences he/she has had throughout childhood and adolescence. Fathers or significant other partners develop an emotional tie with their infants in a variety of ways. They seek and maintain closeness with the infant and can recognize characteristics of the infant. Another study further described paternal attachment as a permanent, cyclical concept characterized by changes in response to the child's developmental stage. When children have a secure, supportive, and sensitive relationship with their fathers or mother's significant other, they are generally better adjusted than those that have a nonsupportive relationship (Lickenbrock & Braungart-Rieker, 2015).

Attachment is a process; it does not occur instantaneously, even though many parents believe in a romanticized version of attachment, which happens right after birth. A delay in the attachment process can occur if a mother's physical and emotional states are adversely affected by exhaustion, pain, and the absence of a support system; if she has an infant in NICU and is separated from it; or had a traumatic birth experience, anesthesia, or an unwanted outcome, such as an ill infant (Lee et al., 2014).

Take Note!

Touch is a basic instinctual interaction between a parent and his or her infant and has a vital role in the infant's early development. Parents provide a variety of tactile stimulation while addressing their infant's daily care routines (Hugill, 2015).

The developmental task for the infant is learning to differentiate between trust and mistrust. If the mother or caretaker is consistently responsive to the infant's care, meeting the baby's physical and psychological needs, the infant will likely learn to trust the caretaker, view the world as a safe place, and grow up to be secure, self-reliant, trusting, cooperative, and helpful. However, if the infant's needs are not met, the child is more likely to face developmental delays, neglect, and child abuse (Klebanov & Travis, 2015).

"Becoming" a parent may take 4 to 6 months. The transition to parenthood, according to Mercer (2006), involves four stages:

1. Commitment, attachment, and preparation for an infant during pregnancy
2. Acquaintance with and increasing attachment to the infant, learning how to care for the infant, and physical restoration during the first weeks after birth
3. Moving toward a new normal routine in the first 4 months after birth
4. Achievement of a parenthood role around 4 months

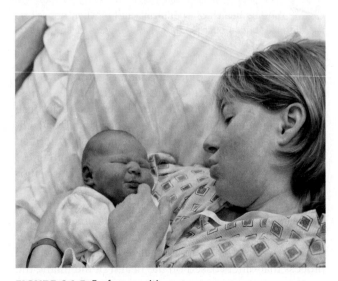

FIGURE 16.5 En face position.

The stages overlap, and the timing of each is affected by variables such as the environment, family dynamics, and the partners (Mercer, 2006).

FACTORS AFFECTING ATTACHMENT

Attachment behaviors are influenced by three major factors:

1. Parents' background (includes the care that the parents received when growing up, cultural practices, relationship within the family, experience with previous pregnancies and planning and course of events during pregnancy, postpartum depression)
2. Infant (includes the infant's temperament and health at birth)
3. Care practices (the behaviors of physicians, midwives, nurses, and hospital personnel, care and support during labor, first day of life in separation of mother and infant, and rules of the hospital or birthing center) (Lewis & Rudolph, 2014).

Attachment occurs more readily with the infant whose temperament, health, appearance, and gender fit the parent's expectations. If the infant does not meet these expectations, attachment can be delayed (Lickenbrock & Braungart-Rieker, 2015).

Factors associated with the health care facility or birthing unit can also hinder attachment. These include:
• Separation of infant and parents immediately after birth and for long periods during the day
• Policies that discourage unwrapping and exploring the infant
• Intensive care environment, restrictive visiting policies
• Staff indifference or lack of support for parent's caretaking attempts and abilities

 Concept Mastery Alert

Grief After Delivery of a Child with Special Needs

It is important for the mother to visit the child in the special care nursery, but the priority is to assist the mother in dealing with the grief that accompanies giving birth to a child with special needs. The mother must first mourn the loss of the "perfect child."

CRITICAL ATTRIBUTES OF ATTACHMENT

The terms *bonding* and *attachment* are often used interchangeably, even though they involve different time frames and interactions. Attachment stages include proximity, reciprocity, and commitment.

Proximity refers to the physical and psychological experience of the parents being close to their infant. This attribute has three dimensions:

1. *Contact:* The sensory experiences of touching, holding, and gazing at the infant are part of proximity-seeking behavior.

2. *Emotional state:* The emotional state emerges from the affective experience of the new parents toward their infant and their parental role.
3. *Individualization:* Parents are aware of the need to differentiate the infant's needs from themselves and to recognize and respond to them appropriately, making the attachment process also, in some way, one of detachment.

Reciprocity is the process by which the infant's abilities and behaviors elicit parental response. Reciprocity is described by two dimensions: complementary behavior and sensitivity. Complementary behavior involves taking turns and stopping when the other is not interested or becomes tired. An infant can coo and stare at the parent to elicit a similar parental response to complement his or her behavior. Parents who are sensitive and responsive to their infant's cues will promote their development and growth. Parents who become skilled at recognizing the ways their infant communicates will respond appropriately by smiling, vocalizing, touching, and kissing.

Commitment refers to the enduring nature of the relationship. The components of this are twofold: centrality and parent role exploration. In centrality, parents place the infant at the center of their lives. They acknowledge and accept their responsibility to promote the infant's safety, growth, and development. Parent role exploration is the parents' ability to find their own way and integrate the parental identity into themselves (Sears & Sears, 2015b).

POSITIVE AND NEGATIVE ATTACHMENT BEHAVIORS

Positive bonding behaviors include maintaining close physical contact, making eye-to-eye contact, speaking in soft, high-pitched tones, and touching and exploring the infant. Table 16.1 highlights typical positive and negative attachment behaviors.

NURSING INTERVENTIONS

In terms of postpartum hospital stays today, "less is more." If the woman had a vaginal delivery, she may be discharged within 48 hours or sooner. If she had a cesarean birth, she may remain hospitalized for up to 72 hours. This shortened stay leaves little time for nurses to prepare the woman and her family for the many changes that will occur when she returns home (see Nursing Care Plan 16.1). Research shows that mothers feel unprepared, uninformed, and unsupported during the postpartum period as they struggle with physical and emotional issues, infant caregiving, breast-feeding concerns, and lifestyle adjustments (Walker, Murphey, & Nichols, 2015). Nurses need to focus on: pain and discomfort, immunizations, nutrition, activity and exercise, infant care, lactation instruction, discharge teaching, sexuality and contraception, and follow-up with the limited

TABLE 16.1	POSITIVE AND NEGATIVE ATTACHMENT BEHAVIORS	
	Positive Behaviors	**Negative Behaviors**
Infant	Smiles; is alert; demonstrates strong grasp reflex to hold parent s finger; sucks well, feeds easily; enjoys being held close; makes eye-to-eye contact; follows parent's face; appears facially appealing; is consolable when crying	Feeds poorly, regurgitates often; cries for long periods, colicky and inconsolable; shows flat affect, rarely smiles even when prompted; resists holding and closeness; sleeps with eyes closed most of time; stiffens body when held; is unresponsive to parents; doesn't pay attention to parents' faces
Parent	Makes direct eye contact; assumes *en face* position when holding infant; claims infant as family member, pointing out common features; expresses pride in infant; assigns meaning to infant's actions; smiles and gazes at infant; touches infant, progressing from fingertips to holding; names infant; requests to be close to infant as much as allowed; speaks positively about infant	Expresses disappointment or displeasure in infant; fails to "explore" infant visually or physically; fails to claim infant as part of family; avoids caring for infant; finds excuses not to hold infant close; has negative self-concept; appears uninterested in having infant in room; frequently asks to have infant taken back to nursery to be cared for; assigns negative attributes to infant and calls infant inappropriate, negative names (e.g., frog, monkey, tadpole)

Adapted from Bope, E., & Kellerman, R. (2015). *Conn's current therapy 2015*. Philadelphia, PA: Saunders Elsevier; Park, S., Kim, S., & Kang, K. (2014). Integrative review of nursing intervention studies on mother-infant interactions. *Child Health Nursing Research*, 20(2), 75–86; and Barnes, D. L. (2014). *Women's reproductive mental health across the lifespan*. New York, NY: Springer Publishers.

time they have with their clients. Planning home visits to reinforce postpartum instructions may enhance maternal-infant wellness (see Evidence-Based Practice 16.1).

Take Note!

Always adhere to standard precautions when providing direct care to reduce the risk of disease transmission.

Providing Optimal Cultural Care

As the face of America is becoming more diverse, nurses must be prepared to care for childbearing families from various cultures. In many cultures, women and their families are cared for and nurtured by their community for weeks and even months after the birth of a new family member. Overall, the culturally competent care for all childbearing families include understanding

---

EVIDENCE-BASED PRACTICE 16.1   ENHANCING NEONATAL WELLNESS WITH HOME VISITATION

STUDY

According to the AAP, there is sufficient evidence that breast-feeding provides the best nutrition for newborns and should be continued for the first 6 months followed by continued breast-feeding during the first year or more, as solid foods are introduced. The purpose of this study was to measure the effectiveness of home visits by RNs on neonatal wellness as measured by the continuance of breast-feeding at 6 months, reduce readmissions for newborn jaundice and identify any maternal or newborn health issues. The home visits were made on days three and seven after discharge from the hospital. A complete physical assessment on both mother and infant was performed at each home visit.

Findings

The study used a longitudinal, mixed method, within-subject design involving 1705 participants. Quantitative

data were compared to regional and national benchmarks. Qualitative data from study participant interviews were analyzed to identify common themes. The data indicated the home visits did help mothers to continue to breast-feed longer when compared to the regional and national statistics and the home visits also effectively identified newborn jaundice with a reduction in the average length of stay for infants readmitted in comparison to benchmarks.

Nursing Implications

The study's results reinforce the need for extended breast-feeding support beyond the hospital setting discharge for new mothers to continue to breast-feed longer. New mothers need to have access to community-based interventions after discharge to reinforce their postpartum education. Nurses can be instrumental in making referrals for home visitations to promote the safe transition from the hospital to the home.

Adapted from Parker, C., Warmuskerken, G., & Sinclair, L. (2015). Enhancing neonatal wellness with home visitation. *Nursing for Women's Health*, 19(1), 36–45.

NURSING CARE PLAN 16.1

Overview of the Postpartum Woman

A 26-year-old G2P2, is a client on the mother–baby unit after giving birth to a term 8-lb, 12-oz baby boy yesterday. The night nurse reports that she has an episiotomy, complains of a pain rating of 7 points on a scale of 1 to 10, is having difficulty breast-feeding, and had heavy lochia most of the night. The nurse also reports that the client seems focused on her own needs and not on those of her infant. Assessment this morning reveals the following:

B: **Breasts** are soft with colostrum leaking; nipples cracked
U: **Uterus** is one fingerbreadth below the umbilicus; deviated to right
B: **Bladder** is palpable; client states she hasn't been up to void yet
B: **Bowels** have not moved; bowel sounds present; passing flatus
L: **Lochia** is moderate; peripad soaked from night accumulation
E: **Episiotomy** site intact; swollen, bruised; hemorrhoids present
E: **Extremities**; no edema over tibia, no warmth or tenderness in calf
E: **Emotional status** is "distressed" as a result of discomfort and fatigue

NURSING DIAGNOSIS: Impaired tissue integrity related to episiotomy

Outcome Identification and Evaluation

The client will remain free of infection, without any signs and symptoms of infection, and exhibit evidence of progressive healing as demonstrated by clean, dry, decreased/absent edema, and an intact episiotomy site.

Interventions: *Promoting Tissue Integrity*

- Monitor episiotomy site for redness, edema, warmth or discharge *to identify infection.*
- Assess vital signs at least every 4 hours *to identify changes suggesting infection.*
- Apply ice pack to episiotomy site *to reduce swelling.*
- Instruct client on use of sitz bath *to promote healing, hygiene, and comfort.*

- Encourage frequent perineal care and peripad changes *to prevent infection.*
- Recommend ambulation *to improve circulation and promote healing.*
- Instruct client on positioning *to relieve pressure on perineal area.*
- Demonstrate use of anesthetic sprays *to numb perineal area.*

NURSING DIAGNOSIS: Pain related to episiotomy, sore nipples, and hemorrhoids

Outcome Identification and Evaluation

The client will experience a decrease in pain as evidenced by reporting that her pain has diminished to a tolerable level and rating it as 2 points or less.

Interventions: *Providing Pain Relief*

- Thoroughly inspect perineum to rule out hematoma as cause of pain.
- Administer analgesic medication as ordered as needed to promote comfort.
- Carry out comfort measures to episiotomy as outlined earlier to reduce pain.
- Explain discomforts and reassure the client that they are time limited to assist in coping with pain.
- Apply Tucks® to swollen hemorrhoids to induce shrinkage and reduce pain.
- Suggest frequent use of sitz bath to reduce hemorrhoid pain.
- Administer stool softener and laxative to prevent straining with first bowel movement.

(continued)

NURSING CARE PLAN 16.1

Overview of the Postpartum Woman (continued)

- Observe positioning and latching-on technique while breast-feeding. Offer suggestions based on observations to correct positioning/latching on to minimize trauma to the breast.
- Suggest air-drying of nipples after breast-feeding and use of plain water to prevent nipple cracking.
- Teach relaxation techniques when breast-feeding to reduce anxiety and discomfort.

NURSING DIAGNOSIS: Risk for ineffective coping related to mood alteration and pain

Outcome Identification and Evaluation

The client will cope with mood alterations, as evidenced by positive statements about newborn and participation in newborn care.

Interventions: *Promoting Effective Coping*

- Provide a supportive, nurturing environment and encourage the mother to vent her feelings and frustrations *to relieve anxiety*.
- Provide opportunities for the mother to rest and sleep *to combat fatigue*.
- Encourage the mother to eat a well-balanced diet *to increase her energy level*.
- Provide reassurance and explanations that mood alterations are common after birth secondary to waning hormones after pregnancy *to increase the mother's knowledge*.
- Allow the mother relief from newborn care *to afford opportunity for self-care*.
- Discuss with partner expected behavior from mother and how additional support and help are needed during this stressful time *to promote partner's participation in care*.
- Make appropriate community referrals for mother–infant support *to ensure continuity of care*.
- Encourage frequent skin-to-skin contact and closeness between mother and infant *to facilitate bonding and attachment behaviors*.
- Encourage client to participate in infant care and provide instructions as needed *to foster a sense of independence and self-esteem*.
- Offer praise and reinforcement of positive mother–infant interactions *to enhance self-confidence in care*.

of traditional folk beliefs; involvement and support by family members; respect; presence of a significant other; breast-feeding and eating healthy; observing the principles of hot and cold; avoidance of sexual intercourse postnatally; encouragement; empowerment; their spiritual dimensions as important; avoidance of evil spirits; and the hope that nurses will anticipate the needs of the mother and infant (McFarland & Wehbe-Alamah, 2015). Box 16.3 highlights some of the major cultural variants during the postpartum period.

Nurses need to remember that childbearing practices and beliefs vary from culture to culture. To provide appropriate nursing care, the nurse should determine the client's preferences before intervening. Cultural practices may include dietary restrictions, certain clothes, taboos, activities for maintaining mental health, and the use of silence, prayer, or meditation. Restoring health may

involve taking folk medicines or conferring with a tribal healer. A language barrier might interfere with communication between the woman and health providers, followed by health care provider's lack of cultural sensitivity, leading to a woman's reluctance in using health services (Santiago & Figueiredo, 2015). Providing culturally diverse care within our global community is challenging for all nurses, because they must remember that one's culture cannot be easily summarized in a reference book, but must be viewed through one's own life experiences.

The Muslim woman and her husband are upset at the thought of having a male doctor care for her because Muslim women are very modest and prefer having a same-sex care provider. What should the nurse do in this situation?

CULTURAL INFLUENCES DURING THE POSTPARTUM PERIOD

African American
- Mother may share care of the infant with extended family members.
- Experiences of older women within the family influence infant care.
- Mothers may protect their newborns from strangers for several weeks.
- Mothers may not bathe their newborns for the first week. Oils are applied to skin and hair to prevent dryness and cradle cap.
- Silver dollars may be taped over the infant's umbilicus in an attempt to flatten the slightly protruding umbilical stump.
- Sleeping with parents is a common practice.

Amish
- Women consider childbearing their primary role in society.
- They generally oppose birth control.
- Pregnancy and childbirth are considered a private matter; they may conceal it from public knowledge.
- Women typically do not respond favorably when hurried to complete a self-care task. Nurses need to take cues from women indicating their readiness to complete morning self-care activities.

Appalachian
- Infant colic is treated by passing the newborn through a leather horse's collar or administering weak catnip tea.
- An *asafetida* bag (a gum resin with a strong odor) is tied around the infant's neck to ward off disease.
- Women may avoid eye contact with nurses and health care providers.
- Women typically avoid asking questions even though they do not understand directions.
- The grandmother may rear the infant for the mother.

Filipino American
- Grandparents often assist in the care of their grandchildren.
- Breast-feeding is encouraged, and some mothers breast-feed their children for up to 2 years.
- Women have difficulty discussing birth control and sexual matters.
- Strong religious beliefs prevail and bedside prayer is common.
- Families are very close-knit and numerous visitors can be expected at the hospital after childbirth.

Japanese American
- Cleanliness and protection from cold are essential components of newborn care. Nurses should bathe the infant daily.

- Newborns routinely are not taken outside the home because it is believed that they should not be exposed to outside or cold air. Infants should be kept in a quiet, clean, warm place for the first month of life.
- Breast-feeding is the primary method of feeding.
- Many women stay in their parents' home for 1 to 2 months after birth.
- Bathing the infant can be the center of family activity at home.

Mexican American
- The newborn's grandmother lives with the mother for several weeks after birth to help with housekeeping and child care.
- Most women will breast-feed for more than 1 year. The infant is carried in a *rebozo* (shawl) that allows easy access for breast-feeding.
- Women may avoid eye contact and may not feel comfortable being touched by a stranger. Nurses need to respect this feeling.
- Some women may bring religious icons to the hospital and may want to display them in their room.

Muslim
- Modesty is a primary concern; nurses need to protect the client's modesty.
- Muslims are not permitted to eat pork; check all food items before serving.
- Muslims prefer a same-sex health care provider; male–female touching is prohibited except in an emergency situation.
- A Muslim woman stays in the house for 40 days after birth, being cared for by the female members of her family.
- Most women will breast-feed, but religious events call for periods of fasting, which may increase the risk of dehydration or malnutrition.
- Women are exempt from obligatory five-times-daily prayers as long as lochia is present.
- Extended family is likely to be present throughout much of the woman's hospital stay. They will need an empty room to perform their prayers without having to leave the hospital.

Native American
- Women are secretive about pregnancies and do not reveal them early.
- Touching is not a typical female behavior and eye contact is brief.
- They resent being hurried and need time for sitting and talking.
- Most mothers breast-feed and practice birth control.

Adapted from Bowers, P., & Caballos, K. (2015). *Cultural perspectives in childbearing*. Retrieved from http://ce.nurse.com/ce263-60/Cultural-Perspectives-in-Childbearing; Dayer-Berenson, L. (2014). *Cultural competencies of nurses: Impact on health and illness* (2nd ed.). Burlington, MA: Jones & Bartlett Learning; and Andrews, M. M., & Boyle, J. S. (2012). *Transcultural concepts in nursing care* (6th ed.). Philadelphia, PA: Wolters Kluwer Health.

Promoting Comfort

The postpartum woman may have discomfort and pain from a variety of sources, such as an episiotomy, perineal lacerations, backache as a result of the epidural, pain from a full bladder, an edematous perineum, inflamed hemorrhoids, engorged breasts, afterbirth pains secondary to uterine contractions in breast-feeding and multiparous mothers, and sore nipples if breast-feeding. Relieving the underlying problem is the first step in pain management. Most practices traditionally employed for postpartum discomforts are not evidence based, so both nonpharmacologic and pharmacologic measures are often used in tandem (King et al., 2015).

Applications of Cold and Heat

COLD

Commonly, an ice pack is the first measure used after a vaginal birth to relieve perineal discomfort from edema, an episiotomy, or a laceration. An ice pack seems to minimize edema, reduce inflammation, decrease capillary permeability, and reduce nerve conduction to the site. It is applied during the fourth stage of labor and can be used for the first 24 hours to reduce perineal edema and to prevent hematoma formation, thus reducing pain and promoting healing. Ice packs are wrapped in a disposable covering or clean washcloth and are applied to the perineal area. Usually the ice pack is applied intermittently for 20 minutes and removed for 10 minutes. Many commercially prepared ice packs are available, but a surgical glove filled with crushed ice and covered can also be used if the mother is not allergic to latex. Ensure that the ice pack is changed frequently to promote good hygiene and to allow for periodic assessments.

HEAT

The **peribottle** is a plastic squeeze bottle filled with warm tap water that is sprayed over the perineal area after each voiding and before applying a new perineal pad. Usually the peribottle is introduced to the woman when she is assisted to the bathroom to freshen up and void for the first time—in most instances, once vital signs are stable after the first hour. Provide the woman with instructions on how and when to use the peribottle. Reinforce this practice each time she changes her pad, voids, or defecates, making sure that she understands to direct the flow of water from front to back. The woman can take the peribottle home and use it over the next several weeks until her lochia discharge stops. The peribottle can be used by women who had either vaginal or cesarean births to provide comfort and hygiene to the perineal area.

After the first 24 hours, a **sitz bath** with room temperature water may be prescribed and substituted for the ice pack to reduce local swelling and promote comfort for an episiotomy, perineal trauma, or inflamed

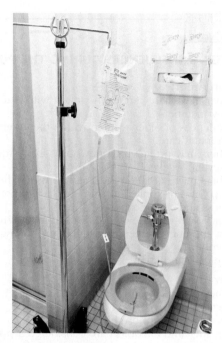

FIGURE 16.6 Sitz bath setup.

hemorrhoids. The change from cold to room temperature therapy enhances vascular circulation and healing. When compared with an infrared light to promote healing and reduce perineal pain, sitz baths were significantly more effective in promoting episiotomy wound healing (Sukhwinder et al., 2014). Before using a sitz bath, the woman should cleanse the perineum with a peribottle or take a shower using mild soap.

Most health care agencies use plastic disposable sitz baths that women can take home. The plastic sitz bath consists of a basin that fits on the commode; a bag filled with warm water is hung on a hook and connected via a tube onto the front of the basin (Fig. 16.6). Teaching Guidelines 16.1 highlights the steps in using a sitz bath.

 Teaching Guidelines 16.1
USING A SITZ BATH

1. Close clamp on tubing before filling bag with water to prevent leakage.
2. Fill sitz bath basin and plastic bag with room-temperature water (comfortable to touch).
3. Place the filled basin on the toilet with the seat raised and the overflow opening facing toward the back of the toilet.
4. Hang the filled plastic bag on a hook close to the toilet or an IV pole.
5. Attach the tubing to the opening on the basin.
6. Sit on the basin positioned on the toilet seat and release the clamp to allow warm water to irrigate the perineum.

7. Remain sitting on the basin for approximately 15 to 20 minutes.
8. Stand up and pat the perineum area dry. Apply a clean peripad.
9. Tip the basin to remove any remaining water and flush the toilet.
10. Wash the basin with warm water and soap and dry it in the sink.
11. Store basin and tubing in a clean, dry area until the next use.
12. Wash hands with soap and water.

Advise the woman to use the sitz bath several times daily to provide hygiene and comfort to the perineal area. Encourage her to continue this measure after discharge. Some facilities have hygienic sitz baths called Suri-Gators in the bathroom that spray an antiseptic, water, or both onto the perineum. The woman sits on the toilet with legs apart so that the nozzle spray reaches her perineal area.

Keep in mind that tremendous hemodynamic changes are taking place within the mother during this early postpartum period, and her safety must be a priority. Fatigue, blood loss, the effects of medications, and lack of food may cause her to feel weak when she stands up. Assisting the woman to the bathroom to instruct her on how to use the peribottle and sitz bath is necessary to ensure her safety. Many women become light-headed or dizzy when they get out of bed and need direct physical assistance. Staying in the woman's room, ensuring that the emergency call light is readily available, and being available if needed during this early period will ensure safety and prevent accidents and falls.

Recent reviews of the use of postpartum local cooling and warming interventions for perineal pain found limited evidence supporting their effectiveness. Additional studies are needed in the area of perineal pain and healing in order to develop evidence-based interventions in the future (Mooventhan & Nivethitha, 2014).

Topical Preparations

Several treatments may be applied topically for temporary relief of perineal pain and discomfort. One such treatment is a local anesthetic spray such as benzocaine topical. These agents numb the perineal area and are used after cleansing the area with water via the peribottle and/or a sitz bath.

Postpartum women are predisposed to hemorrhoid development due to pressure during vaginal birth, constipation, relaxation of the smooth muscles in vein walls, and impaired blood return, all related to increased pressure from the heavy gravid uterus. Nonpharmacologic measures to reduce hemorrhoid discomfort include ice packs, ice sitz baths, and application of cool witch hazel

pads, such as Tucks®. The pads are placed at the rectal area, between the hemorrhoids and the perineal pad. These pads cool the area, help relieve swelling, and minimize itching. Pharmacologic methods used to reduce hemorrhoid pain include local anesthetics (dibucaine) or steroids (hydrocortisone acetate). Prevention or correction of constipation, encouraging the use of the sidelying position, proper toileting habits, assuming positions that minimize putting pressure on the hemorrhoids, and not straining during defecation will be helpful in reducing discomfort (King et al., 2015).

Nipple pain is difficult to treat, although a wide variety of topical creams, ointments, and gels are available to do so. This group includes beeswax, glycerin-based products, petrolatum, lanolin, and hydrogel products. Many women find these products comforting. Beeswax, glycerin-based products, and petrolatum all need to be removed before breast-feeding. These products should be avoided in order to limit infant exposure because the process of removal may increase nipple irritation. Applying expressed breast milk to nipples and allowing it to dry has been suggested to reduce nipple pain. Usually the pain is due to incorrect latch-on and/or removal of the nursing infant from the breast. Early assistance with breast-feeding to ensure correct positioning can help prevent nipple trauma.

Analgesics

Analgesics such as acetaminophen and oral nonsteroidal anti-inflammatory drugs (NSAIDs) such as ibuprofen or naproxen are prescribed to relieve mild postpartum discomfort. For moderate to severe pain, a narcotic analgesic such as codeine or oxycodone in conjunction with aspirin or acetaminophen may be prescribed. Instruct the woman about adverse effects of any medication prescribed. Common adverse effects of oral analgesics include dizziness, light-headedness, nausea and vomiting, constipation, and sedation (Skidmore-Roth, 2015).

Also inform the woman that the drugs are secreted in breast milk. Nearly all medications that the mother takes are passed into her breast milk; however, the mild analgesics (e.g., acetaminophen or ibuprofen) are considered relatively safe for breast-feeding mothers (King et al., 2015). Administering a mild analgesic approximately an hour before breast-feeding will usually relieve afterpains and/or perineal discomfort.

Assisting With Elimination

The bladder is edematous, hypotonic, and congested immediately postpartum. Consequently, bladder distention, incomplete emptying, and inability to void are common. A full bladder interferes with uterine contraction and may lead to hemorrhage, because it will displace the uterus out of the midline. Encourage the woman to void. Often, assisting her to assume the normal voiding position on the commode facilitates this. If the woman has difficulty voiding, pouring warm water over the perineal area, hearing the sound of running tap water, blowing bubbles through a straw, taking a warm shower, drinking fluids, providing her with privacy, or placing her hand in a basin of warm water may stimulate voiding. If these actions do not stimulate urination within 4 to 6 hours after giving birth, catheterization may be needed. Palpate the bladder for distention and ask the woman if she is voiding in small amounts (less than 100 mL) frequently (retention with overflow). If catheterization is necessary, use sterile technique to reduce the risk of infection.

Decreased bowel motility during labor, high iron content in prenatal vitamins, postpartum fluid loss, and the adverse effects of pain medications and/or anesthesia may predispose the postpartum woman to constipation. In addition, the woman may fear that bowel movements will cause pain or injury, especially if she had an episiotomy or a laceration that was repaired with sutures.

Usually a stool softener, such as docusate, with or without a laxative might be helpful if the client has difficulty with bowel elimination. Other measures, such as ambulating and increasing fluid and fiber intake, may also help. Nutritional instruction might include increasing fruits and vegetables in the diet; drinking plenty of fluids (8 to 12 cups daily) to keep the stool soft; drinking small amounts of prune juice and/or hot liquids to stimulate peristalsis; eating high-fiber foods such as bran cereals, whole grains, dried fruits, fresh fruits, and raw vegetables; and walking daily.

Promoting Activity, Rest, and Exercise

The postpartum period is an ideal time for nurses to promote the importance of physical fitness, help women incorporate exercise into their lifestyle, and encourage them to overcome barriers to exercise. The lifestyle changes that occur postpartum may affect a woman's health for decades. Early ambulation is encouraged to reduce the risk of thromboembolism and to improve strengthening.

Many changes occur postpartum, and caring for a newborn alters the woman's eating and sleeping habits, work schedules, and time allocation. Postpartum fatigue is common during the early days after childbirth, and it may continue for weeks or months. Having adequate sleep is critical for new mothers because shorter sleep time, a high percentage of sleep disturbances, and greater fatigue are associated with depressive symptoms in postpartum women (Bhati & Richards, 2015). Working partners with newborns experience fatigue during early parenthood and are unable to recover due to interrupted and poor sleep patterns. This sleep deficit can compromise their work safety (Parfitt & Ayers,

2014). For women, it affects the mother's relationships with significant others and her ability to fulfill household and child care responsibilities. Be sure that the mother recognizes her need for rest and sleep and is realistic about her expectations. Some suggestions include the following:

- Nap when the infant is sleeping, because getting uninterrupted sleep at night is difficult.
- Reduce participation in outside activities and limit the number of visitors.
- Determine the infant's sleep–wake cycles and attempt to increase wakeful periods during the day so the baby sleeps for longer periods at night.
- Eat a balanced diet to promote healing and to increase energy levels.
- Share household tasks to conserve your energy.
- Ask the father or other family members to provide infant care during the night periodically so that mothers can get an uninterrupted night of sleep, if they are not breast-feeding.
- Review your family's daily routine and see if you can "cluster" activities to conserve energy and promote rest.

The demands of parenthood may reduce or prevent exercise in even the most committed person. A targeted exercise program and proper body mechanics can help new mothers deal with the physical challenges of motherhood. Emphasize the benefits of a regular exercise program, which include:

- Helps the woman to lose pregnancy weight
- Reduces the risk of obesity later in life
- Increases overall postpartum well-being
- Increases energy level so the woman can cope with her new responsibilities
- Speeds the return to prepregnant size and shape
- Reduces risk of postpartum depression
- Reduces risk of constipation
- Reduces mental fatigue
- Provides an outlet for stress (Covan, 2015)

Overweight and obesity are epidemic in the United States. Obesity is a risk factor for numerous conditions, including diabetes, hypertension, high cholesterol, stroke, heart disease, cancer and arthritis. More than one third of American women are overweight (ACOG, 2014). Although the average gestational weight gain is small (approximately 25 to 35 lb), excess weight gain and failure to lose weight after pregnancy are important predictors of long-term obesity. The postpartum period is a vulnerable time for excessive weight retention, particularly for the increasing number of women who are overweight at the start of their pregnancy and subsequently find it difficult to lose the additional weight gained during pregnancy. Breast-feeding and exercise may help to control weight in the long term (Neville et al., 2014).

Take Note!

Women who are unable to return to a healthy weight by 6 months postpartum increase their risk factors for the development of chronic diseases including metabolic syndrome, obesity, and cardiovascular disease (Brekke et al., 2014). Encourage women to lose their pregnancy weight by 6 months postpartum, and refer those who don't to community weight-loss programs.

The postpartum woman may face some obstacles to exercising, including physical changes (ligament laxity), competing demands (newborn care), lack of information about weight retention (inactivity equates to weight gain), and stress incontinence (leaking of urine during activity).

A healthy woman with an uncomplicated vaginal birth can resume exercise in the immediate postpartum period. Advise the woman to start slowly and increase the level of exercise over a period of several weeks as tolerated. Infant strollers/carriers may be an option for some women, allowing them to walk with their newborns for exercise. Jogging strollers can be used later when the infant is 6 to 12 months old and can hold his or her head up. Also, exercise videos and home exercise equipment allow mothers to work out while the newborn naps.

Exercising after giving birth promotes feelings of well-being and restores muscle tone lost during pregnancy. Routine exercise should be resumed gradually, beginning with pelvic floor exercises on the first postpartum day and, by the second week, progressing to abdominal, buttock, and thigh-toning exercises. Most postpartum women fail to meet national guidelines for physical activity which may elevate their risk for morbidity and contribute to the intergenerational impact of obesity on their offspring (Downs, Evenson, & Chasan-Taber, 2014). Walking is an excellent form of early exercise as long as the woman avoids jarring and bouncing movements, because joints do not stabilize until 6 to 8 weeks postpartum. Exercising too much too soon can cause the woman to bleed more and her lochia may return to bright red. If this occurs, instruct the woman to stop exercising and rest lying down until the bleeding slows. This increase in bleeding should be a warning to the woman that she is over doing it and needs to slow down her exercise routine.

Recommended exercises for the first few weeks postpartum include abdominal breathing, head lifts, modified sit-ups, double knee roll, and pelvic tilt (Teaching Guidelines 16.2). The number of exercises and their duration is gradually increased as the woman gains strength.

Teaching Guidelines 16.2
POSTPARTUM EXERCISES

Abdominal Breathing
1. While lying on a flat surface (floor or bed), take a deep breath through your nose and expand your abdominal muscles (they will rise up from your midsection).

2. Slowly exhale and tighten your abdominal muscles for 3 to 5 seconds.
3. Repeat this several times.

Head Lift
1. Lie on a flat surface with knees flexed and feet flat on the surface.
2. Lift your head off the flat surface, tuck it onto your chest, and hold for 3 to 5 seconds.
3. Relax your head and return to the starting position.
4. Repeat this several times.

Modified Sit-Ups
1. Lie on a flat surface and raise your head and shoulders 6 to 8 inc so that your outstretched hands reach your knees.
2. Keep your waist on the flat surface.
3. Slowly return to the starting position.
4. Repeat, increasing in frequency as your comfort level allows.

Double Knee Roll
1. Lie on a flat surface with your knees bent.
2. While keeping your shoulders flat, slowly roll your knees to your right side to touch the flat surface (floor or bed).
3. Roll your knees back over your body to the left side until they touch the opposite side of the flat surface.
4. Return to the starting position on your back and rest.
5. Repeat this exercise several times.

Pelvic Tilt
1. Lie on your back on a flat surface with your knees bent and your arms at your side.
2. Slowly contract your abdominal muscles while lifting your pelvis up toward the ceiling.
3. Hold for 3 to 5 seconds and slowly return to your starting position.
4. Repeat several times.

Remember that cultures have different attitudes toward exercise. Some cultures (e.g., Haitian, Arab American, Chinese, and Mexican) expect new mothers to observe a specific period of bed rest or activity restriction; thus, it would be inappropriate to recommend active exercise during the early postpartum period (Bowers & Ceballos, 2015).

Preventing Stress Incontinence

Fifty percent of all parous women develop some degree of pelvic prolapse in their lifetime that is associated with stress incontinence. Stress incontinence causes reduced quality of life and withdrawal from fitness and exercise activities typically. Research suggests that having a vaginal delivery results in direct pelvic muscle trauma and disruption of fascial supports, and also causes damage to the levator ani muscle and pudendal nerve injury.

Offering pelvic floor muscle exercise instruction to all women during their first pregnancy and again after having a vaginal birth is recommended by the National Institute for Health and Care Excellence (NICE) guidelines. Nurses can offer them as a first-line intervention in the prevention of urinary incontinence postpartum (Hall & Woodward, 2015). The more vaginal deliveries a woman has had, the more likely she is to have stress incontinence. Stress incontinence can occur with any activity that causes an increase in intra-abdominal pressure. Postpartum women might consider low-impact activities such as walking, biking, swimming, or low-impact aerobics so they can resume physical activity while strengthening the pelvic floor.

Suggestions to prevent stress incontinence are:

- Start a regular program of pelvic floor muscle exercises after childbirth.
- Lose weight if necessary; obesity is associated with stress incontinence.
- Avoid smoking; limit intake of alcohol and caffeinated beverages, which irritate the bladder.
- Adjust fluid intake to produce a 24-hourly urine output of 1,000 to 2,000 mL.
- Use either an intravaginal or intra-urethral device that puts pressure onto the urethra so that urine will not leak when bladder pressure rises (Laliberte, 2015).

Pelvic floor exercises (Kegel exercises) help to strengthen the pelvic floor muscles if done properly and regularly (Ciaghi, Bianco, & Guarese, 2015). These pelvic floor strengthening exercises were originally developed by Dr. Arnold Kegel in the 1940s as a method of controlling incontinence in women after childbirth. The principle behind these exercises is that strengthening the muscles of the pelvic floor improves urethral sphincter function.

While providing postpartum care, instruct women on primary prevention of stress incontinence by discussing the value and purpose of pelvic floor muscle exercises. Approach the subject sensitively, avoiding the term *incontinent*. The terms *leakage*, *loss of urine*, or *bladder control issues* are more acceptable to most women.

Take Note!

When properly performed, pelvic floor exercises have been effective in preventing or improving urinary continence (Jones & Hawkes, 2015).

Women can perform pelvic floor exercises, doing ten 5-second contractions, whenever they change diapers, talk on the phone, or watch TV. Teach the woman to perform pelvic floor exercises properly; help her to identify the correct muscles by trying to stop and start the flow of urine when sitting on the toilet (Teaching Guidelines 16.3). Pelvic floor exercises can be done without anyone knowing.

Teaching Guidelines 16.3
PERFORMING PELVIC FLOOR MUSCLE EXERCISES

1. Identify the correct pelvic floor muscles by contracting them to stop the flow of urine while sitting on the toilet.
2. Repeat this contraction several times to become familiar with it.
3. Start the exercises by emptying the bladder.
4. Tighten the pelvic floor muscles and hold for 10 seconds.
5. Relax the muscle completely for 10 seconds.
6. Perform 10 exercises at least three times daily. Progressively increase the number that you perform.
7. Perform the exercises in different positions, such as standing, lying, and sitting.
8. Keep breathing during the exercises.
9. Don't contract your abdominal, thigh, leg, or buttocks muscles during these exercises.
10. Relax while doing pelvic floor exercises and concentrate on isolating the right muscles.
11. Attempt to tighten your pelvic muscles before sneezing, jumping, or laughing.
12. Remember that you can perform these exercises anywhere without anyone noticing.

Assisting With Self-Care Measures

Demonstrate and discuss with the woman ways to prevent infection during the postpartum period. Because she may experience lochia drainage for as long as a month after childbirth, describe practices to promote well-being and healing. These measures include:

- Frequently change perineal pads, applying and removing them from front to back to prevent spreading contamination from the rectal area to the genital area.
- Avoid using tampons after giving birth to decrease the risk of infection.
- Shower once or twice daily using a mild soap. Avoid using soap on nipples.
- Use a sitz bath after every bowel movement to cleanse the rectal area and relieve enlarged hemorrhoids.
- Use the peribottle filled with warm water after urinating and before applying a new perineal pad.
- Avoid tub baths for 4 to 6 weeks, until joints and balance are restored, to prevent falls.
- Wash your hands before changing perineal pads, after disposing of soiled pads, and after voiding (Mattson & Smith, 2016).

To reduce the risk of infection at the episiotomy site, reinforce proper perineal care with the client, showing her how to rinse her perineum with the peribottle after she voids or defecates. Stress the importance of always patting gently from front to back and washing her hands thoroughly before and after perineal care. For hemorrhoids, have the client apply witch hazel-soaked pads (Tucks®), ice packs to relieve swelling, or hemorrhoidal cream or ointment if ordered.

Ensuring Safety

One of the safety concerns during the postpartum period is orthostatic hypotension. When the woman rapidly moves from a lying or sitting position to a standing one, her blood pressure can suddenly drop, causing her pulse rate to increase. She may become dizzy and faint. Be aware of this problem and initiate the following safeguards:

• Check blood pressure first before ambulating the client.
• Elevate the head of the bed for a few minutes before ambulating the client.
• Have the client sit on the side of the bed for a few moments before getting up.
• Help the client to stand up, and stay with her.
• Ambulate alongside the client and provide support if needed.
• Frequently ask the client how her head feels.
• Stay close by to assist if she feels light-headed.

Additional topics to address orthostatic hypotension that may concern infant safety include instructing the woman to place the newborn back in the crib on his or her back if she is feeling sleepy to prevent a fall. If the woman falls asleep while holding the infant, she might drop him or her. Also, instruct mothers to keep the door to their room closed when their infant is in their room with them. They should check the identification of anyone who enters their room or who wants to take the infant out of the room. This will prevent infant abduction.

Counseling About Sexuality and Contraception

Pregnancy and childbirth are special periods in a woman's life that involve significant physical, hormonal, psychological, social, and cultural changes that may influence her own sexuality as well as the health of a couple's sexual relationship. This is often a time period filled with excitement, changes, and challenges. Mothers often face changes in their own sexuality in their adjustment to motherhood. Sexuality is an important part of every woman's life. Women want to get back to "normal" as soon as possible after giving birth, but a couple's sexual relationship cannot be isolated from the psychological and psychosocial adjustments that both partners are going through.

Childbirth is a significant life transition that has a measurable impact on postpartum women's sexual function. There are physical (perineal pain), psychological (depression), and contextual factors (motherhood) that contribute to the change in many women's sex lives after

experiencing childbirth. Postpartum women may hesitate to resume sexual relations for a number of reasons. Many postpartum women have fatigue, weakness, loss of sexual desire, perception of decreased attractiveness, change in body appearance, vaginal bleeding, perineal discomfort, hemorrhoids, sore breasts, decreased vaginal lubrication resulting from low estrogen levels, and dyspareunia. Fatigue, the physical demands made by the infant, and the stress of new roles and responsibilities may stress the emotional reserves of couples. New parents may not get much privacy or rest, both of which are necessary for sexual pleasure (Whittock, 2015).

Men may feel they now have a secondary role within the family, and they may not understand their partner's daily routine. The delicate nature of postpartum sexuality makes it difficult for couples to discuss. These issues, combined with the woman's increased investment in the mothering role, can strain the couple's sexual relationship.

Although couples are reluctant to ask, they often want to know when they can safely resume sexual intercourse after childbirth. Typically, sexual intercourse can be resumed once bright-red bleeding has stopped and the perineum is healed from an episiotomy or lacerations. This is usually by the third to the sixth week postpartum. However, there is no set, prescribed time at which to resume sexual intercourse after childbirth. There is no scientific basis for the traditional recommendation to delay sexual activity until the six week postpartum check-up. Each couple must set their own time frame when they feel it is appropriate to resume sexual intercourse. Despite fears and myths about sexual activity during pregnancy, maintaining a couple's sexual interactions throughout pregnancy and the postpartum period can promote sexual health and well-being and a greater depth of intimacy.

Postpartum sexual health and sexual problems are common, which receive little attention from health care providers during the postpartum period, need to be addressed (Halford, Petch, & Creedy, 2015). When counseling the couple about sexuality, determine what knowledge and concerns the couple have about their sexual relationship. Inform the couple that fluctuations in sexual interest are normal. Reassure the breast-feeding mother that she may notice a let-down reflex during orgasm and find her breasts are very sensitive when touched by her partner. Also inform the couple about how to prevent discomfort. Precoital vaginal lubrication may be impaired during the postpartum period, especially in women who are breast-feeding. Use of water-based gel lubricants (K-Y® jelly, Astroglide) can help. Pelvic floor exercises, in addition to preventing stress incontinence, can also enhance sensation.

Initiation of contraception during the postpartum period is important to prevent unintended pregnancy and short birth intervals, which can lead to negative health outcomes for mother and infant. Contraceptive options should be included in the discussions with the couple so that they can make an informed decision before resuming sexual activity. Many couples are overwhelmed with the amount of new information given to them during their brief hospitalization, so many are not ready for a lengthy discussion about contraceptives. Presenting a brief overview of the options, along with literature, may be appropriate. It may be suitable to ask them to think about contraceptive needs and preferences and advise them to use a barrier method (condom with spermicidal gel or foam) until they choose another form of contraception. This advice is especially important if the follow-up appointment will not occur for 4 to 6 weeks after childbirth, because many couples will resume sexual activity before this time. Some postpartum women ovulate before their menstrual period returns and thus need contraceptive protection to prevent another pregnancy.

Recently, the CDC assessed evidence regarding the safety of estrogen-containing contraceptive methods use during the postpartum period. They recommend that postpartum women not use combined hormonal contraceptives during the first 21 days after childbirth because of the high risk for VTE during this period. During days 21 to 42 postpartum, women without risk factors for VTE generally can initiate estrogen-containing contraceptives, but women with risk factors for VTE (e.g., previous VTE or recent cesarean delivery) generally should not use these methods. After 42 days postpartum, no restrictions on the use of combined hormonal contraceptives based on postpartum status apply (Centers for Disease Control and Prevention [CDC], 2015a).

Open and effective communication is necessary for effective contraceptive counseling so that information is clearly understood. Provide clear, consistent information appropriate to the woman and her partner's language, culture, and educational level. This will help the couple select the best contraceptive method. Research supports that postpartum education about contraception leads to more contraception use and fewer unplanned pregnancies and that both short-term and multiple-contact interventions had effects. The use of contraceptives was highest when contraceptive counseling was provided prenatally and again in the postpartum period (Zapata et al., 2015).

Promoting Maternal Nutrition

The postpartum period can be a stressful one for myriad reasons, such as fatigue, the physical stress of pregnancy and birth, and the nonstop work required to take care of the newborn and to meet the needs of other family members. As a result, the new mother may ignore her own nutrition needs. Whether she is breast-feeding or bottle-feeding, encourage the new mother to take good care of herself and eat a healthy diet so that the nutrients lost during pregnancy can be replaced and

she can return to a healthy weight. In general, nutrition recommendations for the postpartum woman include the following:

- Eat a wide variety of foods with high nutrient density.
- Eat meals that require little or no preparation.
- Avoid high-fat fast foods.
- Drink plenty of fluids daily—at least 2,500 mL (approximately 84 oz).
- Avoid fad weight-reduction diets and harmful substances such as alcohol, tobacco, and drugs.
- Avoid excessive intake of fat, salt, sugar, and caffeine.
- Eat the recommended daily servings from each food group (Box 16.4).

Nutrition for the Breast-Feeding Mother

The breast-feeding mother's nutritional needs are higher than they were during pregnancy. The mother's diet and nutritional status influence the quantity and quality of breast milk. Recently, the American Academy of Pediatrics (2014a) recommended that breast-feeding women consume foods that contain iodine, an element that is crucial to healthy brain development and may be lacking in their present diets. Iodine is necessary to

---

BOX 16.4

NUTRITIONAL RECOMMENDATIONS FOR NUTRITION DURING THE POSTPARTUM PERIOD

Recommendations for the Lactating Woman from the Food Guide *MyPlate*
- Fruits: 4 servings
- Vegetables: 4 servings
- Milk: 4 to 5 servings
- Bread, cereal, pasta: 12 or more servings
- Meat, poultry, fish, eggs: 7 servings
- Fats, oils, and sweets: 5 servings (Dudek, 2014).

General Dietary Guidelines for Americans from the Food Guide on *MyPlate* (for the Nonlactating Woman)
- Fruits: Make half of your plate fruits and vegetables.
- Vegetables: Eat red, orange, and dark-green vegetables.
- Milk: Switch to skim milk or 1%.
- Breads, grains, and cereals should be whole grains.
- Meat, poultry, fish, eggs: Eat seafood twice a week and beans, which are high in fiber.
- Eat the right amount of calories for you; enjoy your food, but eat less.
- Be physically active your way in activities that you enjoy.
- Fats, oils, and sweets: Cut back on these.
- Use food labels to help you make better choices (U. S. Department of Agriculture [USDA] & U.S. Department of Health and Human Services [USDHHS], 2014).

produce thyroid hormone, which in turn helps brain development. To meet the needs for breast milk production, the woman's nutritional needs increase as follows:

- *Calories:* +500 cal/day for the first and second 6 months of lactation
- *Protein:* +20 g/day, adding an extra 2 cups of skim milk
- *Calcium:* +400 mg daily—consumption of four or more servings of milk
- *Iodine:* 290 µg daily—dairy products, seafood and iodized salt
- *Fluid:* +2 to 3 quarts of fluids daily (milk, juice, or water); no sodas

Some foods eaten by the breast-feeding mother may affect the flavor of the breast milk or cause gastrointestinal problems for the infant. Not all infants are affected by the same foods. It is suggested that the mother identify the food item that may be causing a problem for the infant and reduce or eliminate her intake of it.

Nutritional needs for breast-feeding mothers are based on the nutritional content of breast milk and the energy expended to produce it. If intake of calories exceeds the energy expended, weight gain occurs. The highest incidence of obesity in women occurs during the childbearing years. Women need to be made aware that weight gained during their reproductive years will have a negative impact on their health as they age. Nurses can assist women in their postpartum weight management program by assessing their readiness to change to lose their pregnancy weight gain; assessing their breast-feeding status, dietary intake, and activity levels; and assessing them for stress and depressive symptoms, which might hinder their weight loss (Green, 2016).

Take Note!

During a woman's brief stay in a health care facility, she may demonstrate a healthy appetite and eat well. Nutritional problems usually start at home when the mother needs to make her own food selections and prepare her own meals. This is a crucial area to address during follow-up.

Supporting the Woman's Choice of Infant Feeding Method

The AAP, WHO, ANA, IOA, USDHHS, ADA, and USP-STF have all released position statements in support of breast-feeding and nurses, should be encouraging it as part of evidence-based practice (Edelman, Kudzma, & Mandle, 2014). Although there is considerable evidence that breast-feeding has numerous health benefits for both mother and infant, many mothers choose to feed their infants formula for the first year of life. Nurses must be able to deliver sound, evidence-based information to help the new mother choose the best way to feed her infant and must support her in her decision. Research findings indicate that parents do listen to nurse's instruction on feeding practices (Stagg & Ustianov, 2015). Many factors affect a woman's choice of feeding method, such as culture, employment demands, support from significant others and family, and knowledge base. Although breast-feeding is encouraged, be sure that couples have the information they need to make an informed decision. Whether a couple chooses to breast-feed or bottle-feed the newborn, support and respect their choice.

Women Who Should Not Breast-Feed

Certain women should not breast-feed. Drugs such as antithyroid drugs, antineoplastic drugs, alcohol, herpes infection on the breasts, or street drugs (methamphetamines, cocaine, PCP, marijuana) enter the breast milk and would harm the infant, so women taking these substances should not breast-feed. To prevent HIV transmission to the newborn, women who are HIV positive should not breast-feed. Other contraindications to breast-feeding include a newborn with an inborn error of metabolism such as galactosemia or phenylketonuria (PKU), active tuberculosis, or a mother with a serious mental health disorder that would prevent her from remembering to feed the infant consistently (Denne, 2015).

Providing Assistance With Breast-Feeding and Bottle-Feeding

First-time mothers often have many questions about feeding, and even women who have had experience with feeding may have questions. Regardless of whether the postpartum woman is breast-feeding or bottle-feeding her newborn, she can benefit from instruction.

PROVIDING ASSISTANCE WITH BREAST-FEEDING

The AAP (2014b) recommends breast-feeding for all full-term newborns. Exclusive breast-feeding is sufficient to support optimal growth and development for approximately the first 6 months of life. Breast-feeding should be continued for at least the first year of life and beyond for as long as mutually desired by mother and child. Educating a mother about breast-feeding will increase the likelihood of a successful breast-feeding experience.

At birth, all newborns should be quickly dried, assessed, and, if stable, placed immediately in uninterrupted skin-to-skin contact (kangaroo care) with their mother. This is good practice whether the mother is going to breast-feed or bottle-feed her infant. Numerous benefits of kangaroo care have been reported related to physiological (thermoregulation, cardiorespiratory stability), behavioral (sleep, breast-feeding duration, and degree of exclusivity), domains, as an effective therapy to relieve procedural pain, and improve neurodevelopment. In addition, kangaroo care provides the newborn with optimal physiologic stability, warmth, and opportunities for the first feed (Campbell-Yeo et al., 2015).

The benefits of breast-feeding for infants are clear (see Chapter 18). To promote breast-feeding, the Baby-Friendly Hospital Initiative, an international program of the World Health Organization and the United Nations International Children's Emergency Fund (UNICEF), was started in 1991. This global health promotion initiative was put forth to improve maternal-infant health by improving rates of exclusive breast-feeding. As part of this program, the hospital or birth center should take the following 10 steps to provide "an optimal environment for the promotion, protection, and support of breast-feeding":

1. Have a written breast-feeding policy that is communicated to all staff.
2. Educate all staff to implement this written policy.
3. Inform all women about the benefits and management of breast-feeding.
4. Show all mothers how to initiate breast-feeding within 30 minutes of birth.
5. Give no food or drink other than breast milk to all newborns.
6. Demonstrate to all mothers how to initiate and maintain breast-feeding.
7. Encourage breast-feeding on demand.
8. Allow no pacifiers to be given to breast-feeding infants.
9. Establish breast-feeding support groups and refer mothers to them.
10. Practice rooming-in 24 hours daily (Cleminson et al., 2015; CDC, 2015a; World Health Organization [WHO], 2014a).

The nurse is responsible for protecting, promoting and supporting breast-feeding when appropriate. For the woman who chooses to breast-feed her infant, the nurse or lactation consultant will need to spend time instructing her about how to do so successfully. Many women have the impression that breast-feeding is simple. Although it is a natural process, women may experience some difficulty in breast-feeding their newborns. Nurses can assist mothers in smoothing out this transition. Assist and provide one-to-one instruction to breast-feeding mothers, especially first-time breast-feeding mothers, to ensure correct technique. Suggestions are highlighted in Teaching Guidelines 16.4 (see Evidence-Based Practice 16.2).

Take Note!

Some newborns "latch on and catch on" right away, and others take more time and patience. Inform new mothers about this to reduce their frustration and uncertainty about their ability to breast-feed.

Tell mothers that they need to believe in themselves and their ability to accomplish this task. They should not panic if breast-feeding does not go smoothly at first; it takes time and practice. Additional suggestions to help mothers relax and feel more comfortable breast-feeding, especially when they return home, include the following:

* Select a quiet corner or room where you won't be disturbed.
* Use a rocking chair to soothe both you and your infant.
* Take long, slow deep breaths to relax before nursing.
* Drink while breast-feeding to replenish body fluids.
* Listen to soothing music while breast-feeding.
* Cuddle and caress the infant while feeding.

EVIDENCE-BASED PRACTICE 16.2   NURSES IMPROVING THE HEALTH OF MOTHERS AND INFANTS BY DANCING THE 10 STEPS TO SUCCESSFUL BREAST-FEEDING

STUDY

The Baby Friendly Hospital Initiative has gained momentum in the United States in recent years. The principles of it are evidence-based and that promoting breast-feeding improves health outcomes and neurocognitive development in infants. The purpose of this study was to implement the Ten Steps to Successful Breast-feeding and see if the rates and duration of breast-feeding improved. The implementation strategies included assessment of current practices, identification of barriers and opportunities, and strategies to support changes in 89 hospitals that participated. The initiative was to increase the number of Baby Friendly designated hospitals over a 2-year process-improvement time frame.

Findings

Results included heightened professional environment of competence, enhanced delivery of client centered care, improved health of mothers and infants, increased client satisfaction, and achievement of benchmarks. The implementation of the Ten Steps to Successful Breast-feeding resulted in improved rates of breast-feeding in all 89 hospitals.

Nursing Implications

This study demonstrated the positive effect of a nurse-led initiative that improved the continuum of care for mothers and infants from the prenatal period through post discharge community care. Nurses can be instrumental by applying principles of evidence-based practices and bring forth change within their health care agencies to improve the outcomes for mothers and their infants.

Adapted from Allen, M., Schafer, D. J. (2015). Nurses improving the health of mothers and infants by dancing the 10 steps to successful breastfeeding. *Journal of Obstetric, Gynecologic, & Neonatal Nursing, 44,* S52

Teaching Guidelines 16.4
BREAST-FEEDING SUGGESTIONS

1. Explain that breast-feeding is a learned skill for both parties.
2. Offer a thorough explanation about the procedure.
3. Instruct the mother to wash her hands before starting.
4. Inform her that her afterpains will increase during breast-feeding.
5. Make sure the mother is comfortable (pain-free) and not hungry.
6. Tell the mother to start the feeding with an awake and alert infant showing hunger signs.
7. Assist the mother to position herself correctly for comfort.
8. Urge the mother to relax to encourage the let-down reflex.
9. Guide the mother's hand to form a "C" to access the breast with thumb on top and other four fingers under the breast.
10. Have the mother lightly tickle the infant's upper lip with her nipple to stimulate the infant to open the mouth wide.
11. Aid her in helping the infant to latch on by bringing the infant rapidly to the breast with a wide-open mouth.
12. Show her how to check that the newborn's mouth position is correct, and tell her to listen for a sucking noise.
13. Demonstrate correct removal from the breast, using her finger to break the suction.
14. Instruct the mother on how to burp the infant before changing from one breast to another.
15. Show her different positions, such as cradle and football holds and side-lying positions (see Chapter 18).
16. Reinforce and praise the mother for her efforts.
17. Allow ample time to answer questions and address concerns.
18. Refer the mother to support groups and community resources.

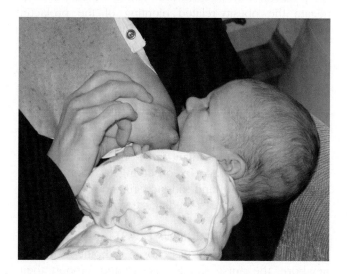

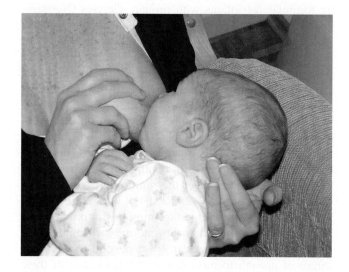

- Set out extra cloth diapers within reach to use as burping cloths.
- Allow sufficient time to enjoy each other in an unhurried atmosphere.
- Involve other family members in all aspects of the infant's care from the start.
- Contact a local La Leche or Nursing Mother's group for continued guidance/support.

Because obesity in America is increasing in all walks of life, it is important for nurses to be knowledgeable about how it impacts breast-feeding and ways to support the obese mother. Research shows that mothers who are obese (BMI > 30) are less likely to initiate lactation, have difficulties with latching on, have delayed lactogenesis, experience mechanical challenges, and are prone to early cessation of breast-feeding (Shannon, Chao, & Ramos, 2015). Obesity rates are highest among African American women, who have the lowest rate of breast-feeding initiation and shortest duration when compared with Hispanic and White women. Women who are overweight and obese have lowered prolactin responses to infant sucking, thus milk production may be inhibited. Lactation plays a significant role in preventing future obesity in both the mother and the infant (Masho, Cha, & Morris, 2015).

Nurses can assist in managing obesity-related lactation challenges by keeping the mother and newborn together to facilitate early and frequent sucking to trigger prolactin and oxytocin production, which will help negate the obesity-related blunting of the prolactin response. Suggesting a sandwich technique to insert the mother's breast into the newborn's mouth to elicit sucking might be helpful for the mother with large breasts. In the sandwich technique, the mother is taught to grasp her breast by making a "C" with her thumb and index finger. The thumb stabilizes the top of the breast while the remaining four fingers support her breast from below. Massage or pumping the breast may soften and extend the nipple for easier infant latch-on. In short, nurses can make a difference by observing lactation, assessing infant hydration and satisfaction, and reassuring the mother about her breast-feeding capacity.

PROVIDING ASSISTANCE WITH BOTTLE-FEEDING

If the mother or couple has chosen to bottle-feed their newborn, the nurse should respect and support their decision. Discuss with the parents what type of formula they will use. Commercial formulas are classified as cow's milk-based (Enfamil, Similac), soy protein-based (Isomil, Prosobee, Nursoy), or specialized or therapeutic formulas for infants with protein allergies (Nutramigen, Pregestimil, Alimentum). Commercial formulas can also be purchased in various forms: powdered (must be mixed with water), condensed liquid (must be diluted with equal amounts of water), ready to use (poured directly into bottles), and prepackaged (ready to use in disposable bottles).

Breast milk is a dynamic fluid with compositional changes occurring throughout the period of lactation that reflects the growth rate and developmental needs of the infant. Infant formula, in contrast, has a static composition, intended to meet the nutritional requirements of infants from birth to 12 months of age (Lönnerdal & Hernell, 2015). Nurses need to bring this information to the attention of mothers who choose to formula feed their infants that changes may be needed in different stages of growth to meet the nutritional needs of their infant.

Newborns need about 108 cal/kg or approximately 650 cal/day (Dudek, 2014). Therefore, explain to parents that a newborn will need 2 to 4 ounces to feel satisfied at each feeding. Until about age 4 months, most bottle-fed infants need six feedings a day. After this time, the number of feedings declines to accommodate other foods in the diet, such as fruits, cereals, and vegetables (Dudek, 2014). For more information on newborn nutrition and bottle feeding, see Chapter 18.

When teaching the mother about bottle-feeding, provide the following guidelines:
• Wash hands with soap and water and dry using a clean or disposable cloth.
• Make sure all bottles, nipples and other utensils are clean.
• Make feeding a relaxing time, a time to provide both food and comfort to your newborn.
• Use the feeding period to promote bonding by smiling, singing, making eye contact, and talking to the infant.
• Powdered formula mixes more easily and the lumps dissolve faster if you use room-temperature water.
• Store any formula prepared in advance in the refrigerator to keep bacteria from growing.
• Do not microwave formula; the microwave won't heat it evenly, causing hot spots.
• Always hold the newborn when feeding. Never prop the bottle.
• Use a comfortable position when feeding the newborn. Place the newborn in your dominant arm, which is supported by a pillow. Or have the newborn in a semi-upright position supported in the crook of your arm. (This position reduces choking and the flow of milk into the middle ear.)
• Tilt the bottle so that the nipple and the neck of the bottle are always filled with formula. This prevents the infant from taking in too much air.
• Stimulate the sucking reflex by touching the nipple to the infant's lips.
• Refrigerate any powdered formula that has been combined with tap water.
• Discard any formula not taken; do not keep it for future feedings.
• Burp the infant frequently, and place the baby on his or her back for sleeping.
• Use only iron-fortified infant formula for the first year (Moses, 2014).

Teaching About Breast Care

Regardless of whether or not the mother is breast-feeding her newborn, urge her to wear a very supportive, snug bra 24 hours a day to support enlarged breasts and promote comfort. A woman who is breast-feeding should wear a supportive bra throughout the lactation period. A woman who is not nursing should wear it until engorgement ceases, and then should wear a less restrictive one. The bra should fit snugly while still allowing the mother to breathe without restriction. All new mothers should use plain water to clean their breasts, especially the nipple area; soap is drying and should be avoided.

Assessing the Breasts

Instruct the mother how to examine her breasts daily. Daily assessment includes the milk supply (breasts will feel full as they are filling), the condition of the nipples (red, bruised, fissured, or bleeding), and the success of breast-feeding. The fullness of the breasts may progress to engorgement in the breast-feeding mother if feedings are delayed or breast-feeding is ineffective. Palpating both breasts will help identify whether the breasts are soft, filling, or engorged. A similar assessment of the breasts should be completed on the nonlactating mother to identify any problems, such as engorgement or mastitis.

Alleviating Breast Engorgement

Breast engorgement usually occurs during the first week postpartum. It is a common response of the breasts to the sudden change in hormones and the presence of an increased amount of milk. Reassure the woman that this condition is temporary and usually resolves within 72 hours.

ALLEVIATING BREAST ENGORGEMENT IN THE BREAST-FEEDING WOMAN

If the mother is breast-feeding, encourage frequent feedings, at least every 2 to 3 hours, using manual expression just before feeding to soften the breast so the newborn can latch on more effectively. Advise the mother to allow the newborn to feed on the first breast until it softens before switching to the other side. See Chapter 18 for more information on alleviating breast engorgement and other common breast-feeding concerns.

ALLEVIATING BREAST ENGORGEMENT AND SUPPRESSING LACTATION IN THE BOTTLE-FEEDING WOMAN

If the woman is bottle-feeding, explain that breast engorgement is a self-limiting phenomenon that disappears as increasing estrogen levels suppress milk formation (i.e., lactation suppression). Encourage the woman to use ice packs, to wear a snug, supportive bra 24 hours a day, and to take mild analgesics such as acetaminophen. Encourage her to avoid any stimulation to the breasts that might foster milk production, such as warm showers or pumping or massaging the breasts. Medication is no longer given to hasten lactation suppression because these agents had limited effectiveness and adverse side effects. Teaching Guidelines 16.5 provides tips on lactation suppression.

Teaching Guidelines 16.5
SUPPRESSING LACTATION

1. Wear a supportive, snugly fitting bra 24 hours daily, but not one that binds the breasts too tightly or interferes with your breathing.
2. Suppression may take 5 to 7 days to accomplish.
3. Take mild analgesics to reduce breast discomfort.
4. Let shower water flow over your back rather than your breasts.
5. Avoid any breast stimulation in the form of sucking or massage.

6. Drink to quench your thirst. Restricting your fluid intake will not dry up your milk.
7. Reduce your salt intake to decrease fluid retention.
8. Use ice packs or cool compresses (e.g., cool cabbage leaves) inside the bra to decrease local pain and swelling; change them every 30 minutes (King et al., 2015).

Promoting Family Adjustment and Well-Being

The postpartum period involves extraordinary physiologic, psychological, and sociocultural changes in the life of a woman and her family. Adapting to the role of a parent is not an easy process. The postpartum period is a "getting-to-know-you" time when parents begin to integrate the newborn into their lives as they reconcile the fantasy child with the real one. This can be a very challenging period for families. Nurses play a major role in assisting families to adapt to the changes, promoting a smooth transition into parenthood. Appropriate and timely interventions can help parents adjust to the role changes and promote attachment to the newborn (Fig. 16.7).

For couples who already have children, the addition of a new member may bring role conflict and challenges. The nurse should provide anticipatory guidance about siblings' responses to the new baby, increased emotional tension, child development, and meeting the multiple needs of the expanding family. Although the multiparous woman has had experience with newborns, do not assume that her knowledge is current and accurate, especially if some time has elapsed since her previous child was born. Reinforcing information is important for all families.

Promoting Parental Roles

Parents' roles develop and grow when they interact with their newborn (see Chapter 15 for information on maternal and paternal adaptation). The pleasure they derive from this interaction stimulates and reinforces this behavior. With repeated, continued contact with the newborn, parents learn to recognize cues and understand the newborn's behavior. This positive interaction contributes to family harmony.

Nurses need to know the stages parents go through as they make their new parenting roles fit into their life experience. Assess the parents for attachment behaviors (normal and deviant), adjustment to the new parental role, family member adjustment, social support system, and educational needs. To promote parental role adaptation and parent–newborn attachment, provide the following nursing interventions:

• Provide as many opportunities as possible for parents to interact with their newborn. Encourage parents to explore, hold, and provide care for their newborn. Praise them for their efforts.

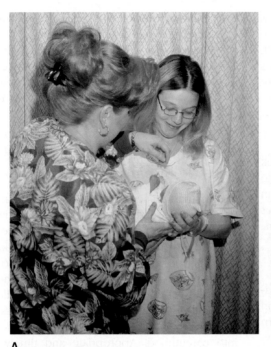

A

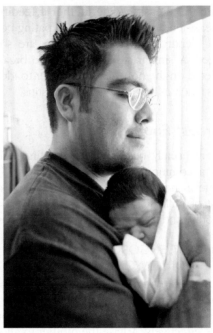

B

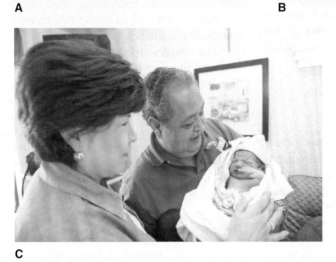

C

FIGURE 16.7 Examples of family members carrying out roles to promote adjustment and well-being. **A.** An aunt admiring the newest member of the family. **B.** A father holding his newborn closely on his chest. **C.** Grandparents welcoming the newest little one to the family circle.

- Model behaviors by holding the newborn close, calling the newborn's name, and speaking positively.
- Speak directly to the newborn in a calm voice, while pointing out the newborn's positive features to the parents.
- Evaluate the family's strengths and weaknesses and readiness for parenting.
- Assess for risk factors such as lack of social support and the presence of stressors.
- Observe the effect of culture on the family interaction to determine healthy family dynamics.
- Monitor parental attachment behaviors to determine whether alterations require referral. Positive behaviors include holding the newborn closely or in an *en face* position, talking to or admiring the newborn, or demonstrating closeness. Negative behaviors include avoiding contact with the newborn, calling it names,

or showing a lack of interest in caring for the newborn (see Table 16.1).
- Monitor the parents' coping behaviors to determine alterations that need intervention. Positive coping behaviors include positive conversations between the partners, both parents wanting to be involved with newborn care, and lack of arguments between the parents. Negative behaviors include not visiting, limited conversations or periods of silence, and heated arguments or conflict.
- Identify the support systems available to the new family and encourage them to ask for help. Ask direct questions about home or community support. Make referrals to community resources to meet the family's needs.
- Arrange for community home visits in high-risk families to provide positive reinforcement of parenting skills and nurturing behaviors with the newborn.

- Provide anticipatory guidance about the following before discharge to reduce the new parents' frustration:
  - Newborn sleep–wake cycles (they may be reversed)
  - Variations in newborn appearance and developmental milestones (growth spurts)
  - How to interpret crying cues (hunger, wet, discomfort) and what to do about them
  - Sensory enrichment/stimulation (colorful mobile)
  - Signs and symptoms of illness and how to assess for fever
  - Important phone numbers, follow-up care, and needed immunizations
  - Physical and emotional changes associated with the postpartum period
  - Need to integrate siblings into care of the newborn; stress that sibling rivalry is normal and offer ways to reduce it
  - Ways to make time together for the couple

In addition, nurses can help fathers to feel more competent in assuming their parental role by teaching and providing information (Fig. 16.8). Education can dispel any unrealistic expectations they may have, helping them to cope more successfully with the demands of fatherhood and thereby fostering a nurturing family relationship.

Explaining Sibling Roles

It can be overwhelming to a young child to have another family member introduced into his or her small, stable world. Although most parents try to prepare siblings for the arrival of their new little brother or sister, many young children experience stress. They may view the new infant as competition, or fear that they will be replaced in the parents' affection. All siblings need extra attention from their parents and reassurance that they are loved and important. Many parents need reassurance that sibling rivalry is normal. Suggest the following to help parents minimize sibling rivalry:

- Expect and tolerate some regression (thumb sucking, bedwetting).
- Explain childbirth in an appropriate way for the child's age.
- Encourage discussion about the new infant during relaxed family times.
- Encourage the sibling(s) to participate in decisions, such as the baby's name and toys to buy.
- Take the sibling on a tour of the maternity suite.
- Buy a T-shirt that says "I'm the [big brother or big sister]."
- Spend "special time" with the child.
- Read with the child. Some suggested titles include: *Things to Do With a New Baby* (Ormerod, 1984); *Betsy's Baby Brother* (Wolde, 1975); *The Berenstain Bears' New Baby* (Berenstain, 1974); and *Mommy's Lap* (Horowitz & Sorensen, 1993).
- Plan time for each child throughout the day.
- Role-play safe handling of a newborn, using a doll. Give the preschooler or school-age child a doll to care for.
- Encourage older children to verbalize emotions about the newborn.
- Purchase a gift that the child can give to the newborn.
- Purchase a gift that can be given to the child by the newborn.
- Arrange for the child to come to the hospital to see the newborn (Fig. 16.9).
- Move the sibling from his or her crib to a youth bed months in advance of the birth of the newborn.
- Show the older sibling photos of the baby growing in mommy's belly. Let them pat the baby beneath the bulge, talk to baby, and feel the baby kick.
- Make the older sibling feel important by giving them a title "mommy's helper."

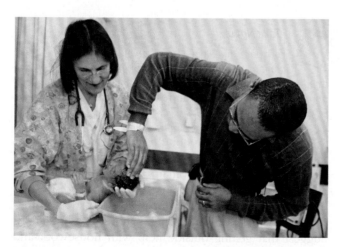

FIGURE 16.8 Father participating in newborn care.

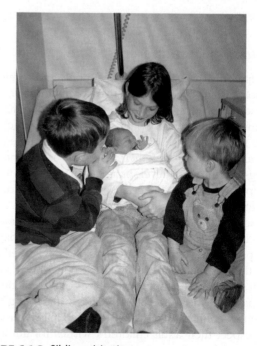

FIGURE 16.9 Sibling visitation.

- Encourage grandparents to pay attention to the older child when visiting.
- Tell the older sibling that their friends come and go, but siblings are forever.
- Encourage "Do unto others as you would have them do unto you" (Sears & Sears, 2015c).

Consider This

Katie and Molly have been excited about having a new baby sister ever since they were told about their mother's pregnancy. The 6-year-old twins are eagerly looking out the front window, waiting for their parents to bring their new sister, Jessica, home. The girls are big enough to help their mother care for their new sibling, and for the past few months they have been fixing up the new nursery and selecting baby clothes. They practiced diapering their dolls—their mother was specific about not using any powder or lotion on Jessica's bottom—and holding them correctly to feed them bottles. Finally, their mother arrives home from the hospital with Jessica in her arms!

The girls notice that their mother is very protective of Jessica and watches them carefully when they care for her. They fight over the opportunity to hold her or feed her. What is special to both of them is the time they spend alone with their parents. Although a new family member has been added, the twins still feel special and loved by their parents.

Thoughts: Bringing a new baby into an established family can cause conflict and jealousy. What preparation did the older siblings have before Jessica arrived? Why is it important for parents to spend time with each sibling separately?

Discussing Grandparents' Role

Grandparents can be a source of support and comfort to the postpartum family if effective communication skills are used and roles are defined. The grandparents' role and involvement will depend on how close they live to the family, their willingness to become involved, and cultural expectations of their role. Just as parents and siblings go through developmental changes, so too do grandparents. These changes can have a positive or negative effect on the relationship.

Newborn care, feeding, and child-rearing practices have changed since the grandparents raised the parents. New parents may lack parenting skills but nonetheless want their parents' support without criticism. A grandparent's "take-charge approach" may not be welcome by new parents who are testing their own parenting roles, and family conflict may ensue. However, many grandparents respect their adult children's wishes for autonomy and remain "resource people" for them when requested.

Take Note!

Grandparents' involvement can enrich the lives of the entire family if accepted in the right context and dose by the family.

Nurses can assist in the grandparents' role transition by assessing their communication skills, role expectations, and support skills during the prenatal period. Find out whether the grandparents are included in the couple's social support network and whether their support is wanted or helpful. If they are, and it is, then encourage the grandparents to learn about the parenting, feeding, and child-rearing skills their children have learned in childbirth classes. This information is commonly found in "grandparenting" classes, which introduce new parenting concepts and bring the grandparents up to date on today's childbirth practices.

Teaching About Postpartum Blues

The postpartum period is typically a happy yet stressful time, because the birth of an infant is accompanied by enormous physical, social, and emotional changes. The postpartum woman may report feelings of emotional lability, such as crying one minute and laughing the next (see Chapter 15 for postpartum blues discussion). Although postpartum blues is usually benign and self-limited, these mood changes can be frightening to the woman. It is prudent to ask two questions—about having pleasure and interest in things, or feeling predominately down, depressed, or hopeless. Once postpartum blues are determined to be the likely cause of her mood symptoms, the nurse can offer anticipatory guidance that these mood swings are commonly experienced and usually resolve spontaneously within a week and offer reassurance. Women should also be counseled to seek further evaluation if these moods do not resolve within two weeks, as postpartum depression may be developing (King et al., 2015).

Take Note!

Postpartum blues have been regarded as brief, benign, and without clinical significance, but several studies have proposed a link between blues and subsequent depression in the 6 months following childbirth (Cristescu et al., 2015).

Postpartum blues require no formal treatment other than support and reassurance because they do not usually interfere with the woman's ability to function and care for her infant. Nurses can ease a mother's distress by encouraging her to vent her feelings and by demonstrating patience and understanding with her and her family. Suggest that getting outside help with housework and infant care might help her to feel less overwhelmed until the blues ease. Provide telephone numbers she can call when she feels down during the day. Making women aware of this disorder while they are pregnant will increase their knowledge about this mood disturbance, which may lessen their embarrassment and increase their willingness to ask for and accept help if it does occur.

The postpartum woman also is at risk for postpartum depression and postpartum psychosis; these conditions are discussed in Chapter 22.

Preparing for Discharge

The World Health Organization (WHO) recommends that the length of stay in the health care facility should be individualized for each mother and baby, but should be at least 24 hours after birth (2014b). A shortened hospital stay may be indicated if the following criteria are met:

- Mother is afebrile and vital signs are within normal range.
- Lochia is appropriate amount and color for stage of recovery.
- Hemoglobin and hematocrit values are within normal range.
- Uterine fundus is firm; urinary output is adequate.
- ABO blood groups and RhD status are known and, if indicated, anti-D immunoglobulin has been administered.
- Surgical wounds are healing and no signs of infection are present.
- Mother is able to ambulate without difficulty.
- Food and fluids are taken without difficulty.
- Self-care and infant care are understood and demonstrated.
- Family or other support system is available to care for both.
- Mother is aware of possible complications (WHO, 2014b).

Providing Immunizations

Prior to discharge, check the immunity status for rubella for all mothers and give a subcutaneous injection of rubella vaccine if they are not serologically immune (titer less than 1:8). Be sure that the client signs a consent form to receive the vaccine. The rubella vaccine should not be given to any woman who is immune compromised, and the immune status of her close contacts needs to be determined before any vaccine is administered to her to prevent a more virulent case of the vaccine-preventable illness or potential death. With the recent increase in the number of pertussis in infants younger than three months of age, the CDC is also recommending vaccination with (Tdap) (combination of diphtheria, pertussis, and tetanus vaccines) for the mother during her postpartum stay (CDC, 2015b). Nursing mothers can be vaccinated because the live,

attenuated rubella virus is not communicable. Inform all mothers receiving immunization about adverse effects (rash, joint symptoms, and a low-grade fever 5 to 21 days later) and the need to avoid pregnancy for at least 28 days after being vaccinated because of the risk of teratogenic effects (CDC, 2015b).

Rh Status

If the client is Rh negative, check the Rh status of the newborn. Verify that the woman is Rh negative and has not been sensitized, that her indirect Coombs' test (antibody screen) is negative, and that the newborn is Rh positive. Mothers who are Rh negative and have given birth to an infant who is Rh positive should receive an injection of Rh immunoglobulin within 72 hours after birth to prevent a sensitization reaction in the Rh-negative woman who received Rh-positive blood cells during the birthing process. Administering RhoGAM prevents initial isoimmunization in Rh-negative mothers by destroying fetal erythrocytes in the maternal system before maternal antibodies can develop and maternal memory cells become sensitized. This is a classic passive immunization technique. The usual protocol for the Rh-negative woman is to receive two doses of Rh immunoglobulin (RhoGAM), one at 28 weeks' gestation and the second dose within 72 hours after childbirth. The standard dose of Rho(D) immune globulin (RhoGAM) is 300 mcg given intramuscularly, which prevents the development of antibodies for an exposure of up to 15 mL of fetal red blood cells (King et al., 2015). A signed consent form is needed after a thorough explanation is provided about the procedure, including its purpose, possible adverse effects, and effect on future pregnancies.

RhoGam contains actual Rh antibodies produced by people who have become sensitized. It is therefore, a blood product. Each dose contains enough Anti-D to suppress the immune response of 15 mL of Rh positive red blood cells (Jordan et al., 2014). Jehovah's Witnesses and others who belong to religions prohibiting the use of blood products should consult their conscience and possibly ecclesiastical leaders about the use of RhoGam. Nurses need to respect whatever their decision is.

Ensuring Follow-Up Care

New mothers and their families need to be attended to over an extended period of time by nurses knowledgeable about mother care, infant feeding (breast-feeding and bottle-feeding), infant care, and nutrition. Although continuous nursing care stops on discharge from the hospital or birthing center, extended episodic nursing care needs to be provided at home. Some of the challenges faced by families after discharge are described in Box 16.5.

Many new mothers are reluctant to "cut the cord" after their brief stay in the health care facility and need

---

BOX 16.5

CHALLENGES FACING FAMILIES AFTER DISCHARGE

- Lack of role models for breast-feeding and infant care
- Lack of support from the new mother's own mother if she did not breast-feed
- Increased mobility of society, which means that extended family may live far away and cannot help care for the newborn and support the new family
- Feelings of isolation and limited community ties for women who work full time
- Shortened hospital stays: parents may be over-whelmed by all the information they are given in the brief hospital stay
- Prenatal classes usually focus on the birth itself rather than on skills needed to care for themselves and the newborn during the postpartum period
- Limited access to education and support systems for families from diverse cultures

Adapted from Bope, E., & Kellerman, R. (2015). *Conn's current therapy 2015*. Philadelphia, PA: Saunders Elsevier; and Bang, K., Huh, B., & Kwon, M. (2014). The effect of a postpartum nursing intervention program for immigrant mothers. *Child Health Nursing Research, 20*(1), 11–19.

---

expanded community services. Women who are discharged too early from the hospital run the risk of uterine subinvolution, discomfort at an episiotomy or cesarean site, infection, fatigue, and maladjustment to their new role. Postpartum nursing care should include a range of family-focused care, including telephone calls, outpatient clinics, and home visits. Typically, public health nurses, community and home health nurses, and the health care provider's office staff will provide postpartum care after hospital discharge.

PROVIDING TELEPHONE FOLLOW-UP

Telephone follow-up typically occurs during the first week after discharge to check on how things are going at home. Calls can be made by perinatal nurses within the agency as part of follow-up care or by the local health department nurses. One disadvantage of a phone call assessment is that the nurse cannot see the client and thus must rely on the mother or the family's observations. The experienced nurse needs to be able to recognize distress and give appropriate advice and referral information if needed.

PROVIDING OUTPATIENT FOLLOW-UP

For mothers with established health care providers such as private pediatricians and obstetricians, visits to the office are arranged soon after discharge. For the woman with an uncomplicated vaginal birth, an office visit is usually scheduled for 4 to 6 weeks after childbirth. A woman who had a cesarean birth frequently is seen within 2

weeks after hospital discharge. Hospital discharge orders will specify when these visits should be made. Newborn examinations and further diagnostic laboratory studies are scheduled within the first week.

Take Note!

The hospital stay of the mother and her healthy term newborn should be long enough to allow identification of early problems and to ensure that the family is able and prepared to care for the infant at home (WHO, 2014b).

Outpatient clinics are available in many communities. If family members run into a problem, the local clinic is available to provide assessment and treatment. Clinic visits can replace or supplement home visits. Although these clinics are open during daytime hours only and the staff members are unfamiliar with the family, they can be a valuable resource for the new family with a problem or concern.

PROVIDING HOME VISIT FOLLOW-UP

Home visits are usually made within the first week after discharge to assess the mother and newborn. During the home visit, the nurse assesses for and manages common physical and psychosocial problems. In addition, the home nurse can help the new parents adjust to the change in their lives. The postpartum home visit usually includes the following:

- *Maternal assessment:* general well-being, vital signs, breast health and care, abdominal and musculoskeletal status, voiding status, fundus and lochia status, psychological and coping status, family relationships, proper feeding technique, environmental safety check, newborn care knowledge, and health teaching needed (Fig. 16.10 shows sample assessment forms.)
- *Infant assessment:* physical examination, general appearance, vital signs, home safety check, child development status, any education needed to improve parents' skills

The home care nurse must be prepared to support and educate the woman and her family in the following areas:

- Breast-feeding or bottle-feeding technique and procedures
- Appropriate parenting behavior and problem solving
- Maternal/newborn physical, psychosocial, and culture–environmental needs
- Emotional needs of the new family
- Warning signs of problems and how to prevent or eliminate them
- Sexuality issues, including contraceptive use
- Immunization needs for both mother and infant
- Family dynamics for smooth transition
- Links to health care providers and community resources

Maternal Assessment
Maternal/Newborn Record System

Page 1 of 2

Date _MO_ / _DAY_ / _YR_ Time begin: _____ Date of delivery _MO_ / _DAY_ / _YR_

Time end: _____

Medication allergy   ☐ None   Identify_____
Significant health history ☐ None   Identify_____

PHYSICAL

TEMP.	PULSE	RESP.	BP /

Breasts   ☐ Nursing   ☐ Non-nursing
Color   ☐ Normal   ☐ Reddened
Condition   ☐ Soft   ☐ Firm   ☐ Engorged   ☐ Blocked ducts
Secretion   ☐ Colostrum   ☐ Milk   ☐ Other_____
Support bra   ☐ No   ☐ Yes, fit ☐ Appropriate
                                        ☐ Inappropriate

Nipples (If nursing) ☐ Erect ☐ Flat   ☐ Inverted
    Condition ☐ Intact   ☐ Bruised ☐ Blistered
              ☐ Fissured   ☐ Bleeding ☐ Scabbed
    Care   ☐ Water only ☐ Soap   ☐ Air dry
              ☐ Topical agent (type/frequency) _____

              ☐ Other _____
Self-exam   ☐ Accurate   ☐ Inaccurate/instructed

Abdomen
Diastasis recti ☐ Absent   ☐ Present_____cm
                 ☐ Exercise taught
Incision   ☐ None
    Type   ☐ Transverse ☐ Vertical ☐ Umbilical
    Closure   ☐ Staples   ☐ Sutures   ☐ Steri-strips
    Condition   ☐ Approximated   ☐ Open_____cm
                 ☐ Redness _____
                 ☐ Swelling _____
                 ☐ Discharge _____
                 ☐ Other _____

Reproductive Tract
Uterus   ☐ Firm ☐ Firm with massage   ☐ Boggy
            Height_____ ☐ Midline   ☐ Displaced L R
            ☐ Non tender   ☐ Tender   ☐ With touch ☐ Constant
Lochia   ☐ Rubra ☐ Serosa ☐ Alba
            ☐ Clots (describe)_____
            ☐ Fleshy odor ☐ Foul odor
            Pads   Type _____ Number/day _____
            Saturation % ├──┼──┼──┼──┤
                         0 25 50 75 100
Perineum   ☐ Intact ☐ Laceration
            ☐ Episiotormy   Type _____ Extension _____
    Condition ☐ Redness _____
              ☐ Edema _____
              ☐ Eccymosis _____
              ☐ Discharge _____
              ☐ Approximation _____
    Care   ☐ Front-to-back cleansing ☐ Peri-bottle
              ☐ Soap/water
              ☐ Ice ☐ Sitz bath ☐ Warm ☐ Cool
              ☐ Topical agent (type/frequency) _____

              ☐ Other _____

Elimination
Urinary tract
    Voiding pattern   ☐ Normal   ☐ Incontinence
                      ☐ Bladder distention ☐ Catheter (type)
    Signs of infection ☐ None/reviewed ☐ Urgency ☐ Frequency
                       ☐ Dysuria ☐ CVA tenderness L R
Gastrointestinal tract
    Bowel pattern   ☐ Normal   ☐ No BM
                      ☐ Constipation ☐ Diarrhea
                      ☐ Meds/treatments (type, frequency, effect) _____

    Hemorrhoids   ☐ No ☐ Yes (describe) _____
                      ☐ Meds/treatments (type, frequency, effect) _____

Lower Extremities
Edema   ☐ None ☐ Pedal ☐ Ankle ☐ Pretibial ☐ Thigh
        ☐ Pitting (describe)
Signs of thrombophlebitis   ☐ None

	L	R		L	R
Homan's sign	☐	☐	Redness	☐	☐
Pain	☐	☐	Warmth	☐	☐
Swelling	☐	☐			

Pain

	No	Yes Managed	Problematic
Abdominal incision	☐	☐	☐
Back	☐	☐	☐
Breasts	☐	☐	☐
Headache	☐	☐	☐
Hemorrhoid	☐	☐	☐
Nipple	☐	☐	☐
Perineum	☐	☐	☐
Uterine cramping	☐	☐	☐
Other _____	☐	☐	☐

Analgesic ☐ No
           ☐ Yes (type/dose/frequency) _____

Reportable danger signs ☐ Aware ☐ Unaware/instructed

TESTS ☐ None
           ☐ Urinalysis
           ☐ CBC
           ☐ _____

IDENTIFIED NEEDS
_____
_____
_____
_____
_____
_____
_____
_____

Signature _____

A

FIGURE 16.10 Sample postpartum home visit assessment form. **A.** Maternal assessment. **B.** Newborn assessment. (Used with permission: Copyright Briggs Corporation. Professional Nurse Associates.) (*continued*)

Maternal Assessment
Maternal/Newborn Record System

Page 2 of 2

PATIENT IDENTIFICATION
Record No. _____

Name _____
Home address _____
STREET
CITY   STATE   ZIP

ACTIVITIES OF DAILY LIVING - 24 HOUR HISTORY

Date __MO__ / __DAY__ / __YR__

Nutrition

Appetite	☐ Good	☐ Fair	☐ Poor
Usual pattern	☐ Yes	☐ No	
Special diet	☐ No	☐ Yes _____
Food intolerance/allergy	☐ No	☐ Yes _____
Vitamin/mineral supplement	☐ No	☐ Yes _____
Fluid intake (type/amount) _____			

BREAKFAST	LUNCH	DINNER	SNACKS

General Hygiene ☐ Adequate ☐ Inadequate (describe)

Sleep/Activity

Amount of Activity

Night, uninterrupted _____ hrs

Naps ☐ No ☐ Yes _____ hrs

Fatigue ☐ None ☐ Minimal ☐ Moderate ☐ Exhausted

Activities

Limitations ☐ None Identify _____

	Appropriate	Inappropriate/instructed
☐ Self-care	☐ Infant care	
Stair climbing	☐	☐
Lifting	☐	☐
Household tasks	☐	☐
Outside home	☐	☐
Other _____		

Exercise

☐ None

	Accurate	Inaccurate/instructed
Kegel	☐	☐
Postpartum	☐	☐
Other _____		

PSYCHOLOGICAL

Review of Labor and Birth

Missing pieces	☐ No	☐ Yes
Unmet expectations	☐ No	☐ Yes
Unresolved feelings	☐ No	☐ Yes
Pertinent data _____		

Postpartum Timetable (Key on reverse side)
☐ Taking in ☐ Taking hold ☐ Letting go

Emotional Status ☐ Happy ☐ Ambivalent ☐ Anxious
☐ Sad ☐ Other _____

Postpartum-depression (Key on reverse side)
☐ 0 ☐ 1 ☐ 2 ☐ 3 ☐ 4
☐ Signs/Symptoms Reviewed

General Comments (body image, role changes, concerns) _____

SEXUALITY

	Aware	Unaware/instructed
Relationship with partner		
Adjustment	☐	☐
Expressions of affection	☐	☐
Resuming Intercourse		
Timing (lack of lochia, comfort)	☐	☐
Vaginal dryness	☐	☐
Milk ejection (if lactating)	☐	☐
Position variation	☐	☐
Libidinal changes	☐	☐
Return of Menses	☐	☐

Contraceptive Method

☐ None   ☐ Undecided/aware of options
☐ Natural family planning
☐ Cervical cap
☐ Condom
☐ Diaphragm
☐ Hormones ☐ Pill ☐ Injection ☐ Implant
☐ IUD
☐ Spermicide
☐ Sterilization ☐ Female ☐ Male
☐ Other _____

Accurate use ☐ Yes ☐ No/instructed

IDENTIFIED NEEDS

_____

Signature _____

FIGURE 16.10 (continued)

Maternal Assessment
Maternal/Newborn Record System

Date MO / DAY / YR   Time begin: _____   Date of Birth MO / DAY / YR
Time end: _____
Significant history ☐ None   Identify_____

PHYSICAL
Temp _____ Pulse (rate/rhythm) _____ Resp _____
Weight _____ Birth weight _____ % Change _____
Length_____ Head _____ Chest _____

HEAD/NECK
1. Fontanels   Level   Bulging   Depressed
   Anterior   ☐   ☐   ☐
   Posterior   ☐   ☐   ☐
   Sutures   ☐ Open ☐ Closed ☐ Overriding
2. Variations ☐ Molding ☐ Caput ☐ Cephalhematoma

NORMAL ABNORMAL   DETAIL VARIATIONS/ABNORMAL FINDINGS

3. Face (symmetry)   ☐ ☐
4. Eyes (symmetry, conjunctiva, sciera, eyelids, PERL)   ☐ ☐
5. Ears (shape, position, auditory response)   ☐ ☐
6. Nose (patency)   ☐ ☐
7. Mouth (lip, mucous membranes, tongue, palate)   ☐ ☐
8. Neck (ROM, symmetry)   ☐ ☐

Chest
9. Appearance (shape, breasts, nipples)   ☐ ☐
10. Breath sounds   ☐ ☐
11. Clavicles   ☐ ☐

Cardiovascular
12. Heart sounds   ☐ ☐
13. Brachial/femoral pulses (compare strength, equality)   ☐ ☐

Abdomen
14. Appearance (shape, size)   ☐ ☐
15. Cord (condition)   ☐ ☐
16. Liver (less than or equal to 3 cm ↓ ®costal margin)   ☐ ☐

Genitalia
17. Female (labia, introitus, discharge)   ☐ ☐
18. Male (meatus, scrotum, testes)   ☐ ☐
19. Circumcision ☐ No ☐ Yes   ☐ ☐

Musculoskeletal
20. Muscle tone   ☐ ☐
21. Extremities (symmetry, digits, ROM)   ☐ ☐
22. Hips (symmetry, ROM)   ☐ ☐
23. Spine (alignment, integrity)   ☐ ☐

Neurologic
24. Reflexes (presence, symmetry)
    Moro   ☐ ☐
    Grasp   ☐ ☐
    Babinski   ☐ ☐
25. Cry (presence, quality)   ☐ ☐

PHYSICAL (CONT'D)
Skin
Turgor ☐ Good ☐ Poor
Condition ☐ Smooth ☐ Dry, cracked ☐ Peeling
Color ☐ Pink ☐ Ruddy ☐ Cyanotic ☐ Pale
☐ Jaundice (note levels)
   ☐ Head (3 mg/dl)
   ☐ Head and upper chest (6 mg/dl)
   ☐ Head and entire chest (9 mg/dl)
   ☐ Head, chest and abdomen to umbilicus (12 mg/dl)
   ☐ Head, chest and entire abdomen (15 mg/dl)
   ☐ Head, chest, abdomen, legs and feet (18 mg/dl)
Variations (Rashes, lesions, birthmarks). _____

NUTRITION
Feeding
Reflexes ☐ Root ☐ Suck ☐ Swallow
Hunger cues identified ☐ Yes ☐ No/instructed

BREAST	FORMULA
Frequency___ times in ___ hours	Type _____
Time per breast___ min ___min	Amount _____ oz.
Positioning ☐ Correct	Frequency _____
☐ Incorrect_____	Preparation ☐ Correct
Latch ☐ Correct	☐ Incorrect
☐ Incorrect _____	
Appropriate audible swallows	☐ Correct
☐ Yes ☐ No_____	☐ _____

Satiation demonstrated ☐ Yes
   ☐ No (describe)_____
Regurgitation ☐ No ☐ Yes (describe)_____
Pacifier use ☐ No ☐ Yes (type/pattern)_____

Stool (number/day, color, consistency)_____
Urine (number/day, color)_____

BEHAVIOR
Sleep/Activity Pattern (24 hours)
Sleep (16–20 hrs)   ☐ Yes ☐ No (describe)_____
Awake-alert (2–3 hrs)   ☐ Yes ☐ No (describe)_____
Awake-crying (2–4 hrs)   ☐ Yes ☐ No (describe)_____

Consolability (Key on reverse) ☐ 0 ☐ 1 ☐ 2 ☐ 3 ☐ 4

TESTS ☐ None   Time
☐ Metabolic screen kit no. _____ _____
☐ Bilirubin   _____
☐ Hematocrit   _____
☐ _____ _____
☐ _____ _____

INENTIFIED NEEDS _____
_____
_____
_____
Signature _____

B

FIGURE 16.10 (continued)

KEY CONCEPTS

- The transitional adjustment period between birth and parenthood includes education about baby care basics, the role of the new family, emotional support, breast-feeding or bottle-feeding support, and maternal mentoring.

- Sensitivity to how childbearing practices and beliefs vary for multicultural families and how best to provide appropriate nursing care to meet their needs are important during the postpartum period.

- A thorough postpartum assessment is key to preventing complications as is frequent hand hygiene by the nurse, especially between handling mothers and infants.

- The postpartum assessment that uses the acronym BUBBLE-EE (breasts, uterus, bowel, bladder, lochia, episiotomy/perineum/epidural site, extremities, and emotions) is a helpful guide in performing a systematic head-to-toe postpartum assessment.

- Lochia is assessed according to its amount, color, and change with activity and time. It proceeds from lochia rubra to serosa to alba.

- Because of shortened agency stays, nurses must use this brief time with the client to address areas of comfort, elimination, activity, rest and exercise, self-care, sexuality and contraception, nutrition, family adaptation, discharge, and follow-up.

- The AAP advocates breast-feeding for all full-term newborns, maintaining that, ideally, breast milk should be the sole nutrient for the first 6 months and continued with foods until 12 months of life or longer.

- Successful parenting is a continuous and complex interactive process that requires the acquisition of new skills and the integration of the new member into the existing family unit.

- Bonding is a vital component of the attachment process and is necessary in establishing parent–infant attachment and a healthy, loving relationship; attachment behaviors include seeking and maintaining proximity to, and exchanging gratifying experiences with, the infant.

- Nurses can be instrumental in facilitating attachment by first understanding attachment behaviors (positive and negative) of newborns and parents, and intervening appropriately to promote and enhance attachment.

- New mothers and their families need to be attended to over an extended period of time by nurses knowledgeable about mother care, newborn feeding (breast-feeding and bottle-feeding), newborn care, and nutrition.

References and Recommended Readings

Allen, M., & Schafer, D. J. (2015). Nurses improving the health of mothers and infants by dancing the 10 steps to successful breast-feeding. *Journal of Obstetric, Gynecologic, & Neonatal Nursing, 44*, S52.

American Academy of Pediatrics [AAP]. (2014a). Iodine deficiency: Pregnant and breastfeeding women need supplementation. *AAP News*. Retrieved from http://aapnews.aappublications.org/content/35/6/11.1.extract

American Academy of Pediatrics [AAP]. (2014b). *Ten steps to support parent's choice to breastfeed their baby*. Retrieved from http://www2.aap.org/breastfeeding/files/pdf/tenstepsposter.pdf

American College of Obstetricians & Gynecologists [ACOG]. (2014). Challenges for overweight and obese women. *Obstetrics & Gynecology, 1234*(3), 726–730.

Andrews, M. M., & Boyle, J. S. (2012). *Transcultural concepts in nursing care* (6th ed.). Philadelphia, PA: Wolters Kluwer Health.

Baltes, P. B., Featherman, D. L., & Lerner, R. M. (2014). *Life-span development and behavior* (10th ed.). New York, NY: Psychology Press.

Bang, K., Huh, B., & Kwon, M. (2014). The effect of a postpartum nursing intervention program for immigrant mothers. *Child Health Nursing Research, 20*(1), 11–19.

Barnes, D. L. (2014). *Women's reproductive mental health across the lifespan*. New York, NY: Springer Publishers.

Bhati, S., & Richards, K. (2015). A systematic review of the relationship between postpartum sleep disturbance and postpartum depression. *JOGNN: Journal of Obstetric, Gynecologic & Neonatal Nursing, 44*(3), 350–357.

Bope, E., & Kellerman, R. (2015). *Conn's current therapy 2015*. Philadelphia, PA: Saunders Elsevier.

Bowers, P., & Ceballos, K. (2015). *Cultural perspectives in childbearing*. Retrieved from http://ce.nurse.com/ce263-60/Cultural-Perspectives-in-Childbearing.

Brekke, H. K., Bertz, F., Rasmussen, K. M., Bosaeus, I., Ellegård, L., & Winkvist, A. (2014). Diet and exercise interventions among overweight and obese lactating women: Randomized trial of effects on cardiovascular risk factors. *PLoS One, 9*(2), 1–8.

Campbell-Yeo, M. L., Disher, T. C., Benoit, B. L., & Johnston, C. C. (2015). Understanding kangaroo care and its benefits to preterm infants. *Pediatric Health, Medicine & Therapeutics, 6*, 15–33.

Centers for Disease Control and Prevention [CDC]. (2015a). *Reproductive health*. Retrieved from http://www.cdc.gov/reproductivehealth/unintendedpregnancy/usmec.htm.

Centers for Disease Control and Prevention [CDC]. (2015b). *Tdap for pregnant women: Information for providers*. Retrieved from http://www.cdc.gov/vaccines/vpd-vac/pertussis/tdap-pregnancy-hcp.htm

Ciaghi, F., Bianco, A. D., & Guarese, O. (2015). Prevalence of pelvic floor disorders during the post-partum period. A prospective study and a proposal of a multidisciplinary prevention strategy. *Scienza Riabilitativa, 17*(1), 5–15.

Cleminson, J., Oddie, S., Renfrew, M. J., & McGuire, W. (2015). Being baby friendly: Evidence-based breastfeeding support. *Archives of Disease in Childhood-Fetal and Neonatal Edition, 100*(2), 173–178.

Covan, E. K. (2015). Benefits of exercise for body, mind, and spirit. *Health Care for Women International, 36*(3), 255.

Creasy, R. K., Resnik, R., Iams, J. D., Lockwood, C. J., Moore, T. R., & Greene, M. F. (2014). *Creasy & Resnik's maternal-fetal medicine: Principles and practice* (7th ed.). Philadelphia, PA: Elsevier Saunders.

Cristescu, T., Behrman, S., Jones, S. V., Chouliaras, L., & Ebmeier, K. P. (2015). Be vigilant for perinatal mental health problems. *The Practitioner, 259*(1780), 19–23.

Cunningham, F. G., Leveno, K. J., Bloom, S. L., Spong, C., Dashe, J. S., Hoffman, B. L., et al. (2014). *Williams' obstetrics* (24th ed.). New York, NY: McGraw-Hill Publishers.

Dayer-Berenson, L. (2014). *Cultural competencies of nurses: Impact on health and illness* (2nd ed.). Berlington, MA: Jones & Bartlett Learning

Denne, S. C. (2015). Neonatal nutrition. *Pediatric Clinics of North America, 62*(2), 427–438.

Downs, D. S., Evenson, K. R., & Chasan-Taber, L. (2014). Obesity and physical activity during pregnancy and postpartum: Evidence, guidelines, and recommendations. In *Obesity during pregnancy in clinical practice* (pp. 183–227). London, England: Springer.

Dudek, S. G. (2014). *Nutrition essentials for nursing practice* (7th ed.). Philadelphia, PA: Lippincott Williams & Wilkins.

Edelman, C. L., Kudzma, E. C., & Mandle, C. L. (2014). *Health promotion throughout the lifespan* (8th ed.). St. Louis, MO: Elsevier Mosby.

Green, C. J. (2016). *Maternal-newborn nursing care plans* (3rd ed.). Burlington, MA: Jones & Bartlett Learning.

Halford, W. K., Petch, J., & Creedy, D. (2015). Caring and sexuality. In *Clinical guide to helping new parents* (pp. 131–150). New York, NY: Springer Publishers.

Hall, B., & Woodward, S. (2015). Pelvic floor muscle training for urinary incontinence postpartum. *British Journal of Nursing, 24*(11), 576–579.

Hugill, K. (2015). The senses of touch and olfaction in early mother-infant interaction. *British Journal of Midwifery, 23*(4), 238–243.

Jones, C., & Hawkes, R. (2015). Managing pregnancy-related pelvic floor dysfunction. *Primary Health Care, 25*(1), 24–28.

Jordan, R. G., Engstrom, J., Marfell, J., & Farley, C. L. (2014). *Prenatal & postnatal care: A women-centered approach*. Ames, Iowa: John Wiley & Sons.

Kim, Y. K., Kim, K. B., Kim, C. H., & Ha, H. (2015). Pulmonary embolism and uterine venous plexus thrombosis in the postpartum period. *Korean Journal of Legal Medicine, 39*(2), 41–44.

King, T. L., Brucker, M. C., Kriebs, J. M., Fahey, J. O., Gegor, C. L., & Varney, H. (2015). *Varney's midwifery* (5th ed.). Burlington, MA: Jones & Bartlett Learning.

Klebanov, M. S., & Travis, A. D. (2015). *The critical role of parenting in human development*. New York, NY: Routledge, Taylor & Francis Group.

Kline, J. A., & Kabrhel, C. (2015). Emergency evaluation for pulmonary embolism, Part 1: Clinical factors that increase risk. *The Journal of Emergency Medicine, 49*(1), 104–117.

Laliberte, R. (2015). Leaky bladder. *Prevention, 67*(7), 52–54.

Lee, A., & Brann, L. (2015). Influence of cultural beliefs on infant feeding, postpartum and childcare practices among Chinese-American mothers in New York City. *Journal of Community Health, 40*(3), 476–483.

Lee, L. A., Carter, M., Stevenson, S. B., & Harrison, H. (2014). Improving family-centered care practices in the NICU. *Neonatal Network, 33*(3), 125–132.

Lewis, M., & Rudolph, K. D. (2014). *Handbook of developmental psychopathology* (3rd ed.). New York, NY: Springer Publishers.

Lickenbrock, D. M., & Braungart-Rieker, J. M. (2015). Examining antecedents of infant attachment security with mothers and fathers: An ecological systems perspective. *Infant Behavior & Development, 39*, 173–187.

Lönnerdal, B., & Hernell, O. (2015). An opinion on "staging" of infant formula – A developmental perspective on infant feeding. *Journal of Pediatric Gastroenterology and Nutrition, 62*(1):9–21.

Mattson, S., & Smith, J. E. (2016). *Core curriculum for maternal-newborn nursing* (5th ed.). St. Louis, MO: Saunders Elsevier.

Masho, S. W., Cha, S., & Morris, M. R. (2015). Prepregnancy obesity and breastfeeding non-initiation in the United States: An examination of racial and ethnic differences. *Breastfeeding Medicine, 10*(5), 253–262.

McComish, J. F. (2015). Infant mental health and attachment. *Journal of Child & Adolescent Psychiatric Nursing, 28*(2), 63–64. doi: 10.1111/jcap.12114

McFarland, M. R. & Wehbe-Alamah, H. B. (2015). *Leininger's cultural care and diversity and universality: A worldwide nursing theory* (3rd ed.). Burlington, MA: Jones & Bartlett Learning.

Mercer, R. T. (2006). Nursing support of the process of becoming a mother. *Journal of Obstetric, Gynecologic, and Neonatal Nursing, 35*(5), 649–651.

Mooventhan, A., & Nivethitha, L. (2014). Scientific evidence-based effects of hydrotherapy on various systems of the body. *North American Journal of Medical Sciences, 6*(5), 199–209.

Moses, S. (2014). Formula feeding. *Family practice notebook.* Retrieved from http://www.fpnotebook.com/pharm/NICU/FrmlFdng.htm

Nagtalon-Ramos, J. (2014). *Best evidence-based practices in maternal-newborn nursing care*. Philadelphia, PA: F. A. Davis Company.

Neville, C., McKinley, M., Holmes, V., Spence, D., & Woodside, J. (2014). The effectiveness of weight management interventions in breastfeeding women – A systematic review and critical evaluation. *Birth, 41*(3), 223–236.

Parfitt, Y., & Ayers, S. (2014). Transition to parenthood and mental health in first-time parents. *Infant Mental Health Journal, 35*, 263–273.

Park, S., Kim, S., & Kang, K. (2014). Integrative review of nursing intervention studies on mother-infant interactions. *Child Health Nursing Research, 20*(2), 75–86.

Parker, C., Warmuskerken, G., & Sinclair, L. (2015). Enhancing neonatal wellness with home visitation. *Nursing for Women's Health, 19*(1), 36–45.

Purnell, L. D. (2014). *Guide to culturally competent health care* (3rd ed.). Philadelphia, PA: F. A. Davis.

Santiago, M., & Figueiredo, M. (2015). Immigrant women's perspective on prenatal and postpartum care: Systematic review. *Journal of Immigrant & Minority Health, 17*(1), 276–284.

Sears, R. W., & Sears, J. M. (2015a). Bonding – What it means. Retrieved from http://www.askdrsears.com/topics/pregnancy-childbirth/tenth-month-post-partum/bonding-with-your-newborn/bonding-what-it-means.

Sears, R. W., & Sears, J. M. (2015b). Attachment parenting. Retrieved from http://www.askdrsears.com/topics/parenting/attachment-parenting.

Sears, R. W., & Sears, J. M. (2015c). Introducing a new baby: 11 smooth-entry tips. Retrieved from http://www.askdrsears.com/topics/parenting/discipline-behavior/bothersome-behaviors/sibling-rivalry/introducing-new-baby-11

Sette, G., Coppola, G., & Cassibba, R. (2015). The transmission of attachment across generations: The state of art and new theoretical perspectives. *Scandinavian Journal of Psychology, 56*(3), 315–326.

Shannon, C., Chao, M., & Ramos, D. E. (2015). A gap analysis of effective interventions for postpartum weight loss in obese new mothers. *Obstetrics & Gynecology, 125*, 56–59..

Skidmore-Roth, L. (2015). *Mosby's 2015 nursing drug reference* (28th ed.). St. Louis, MO: Mosby Elsevier.

Stagg, J., & Ustianov, J. (2015). Improving and sustaining breastfeeding practices through a statewide learning collaborative. *Journal of Obstetric, Gynecologic, & Neonatal Nursing, 44*, S55.

Sucker, C., & Zotz, R. B. (2015). Prophylaxis and treatment of venous thrombosis and pulmonary embolism in pregnancy. *Reviews in Vascular Medicine, 3*(2), 24–30.

Sukhwinder, K., Poonam, S., Sulakshna, C., & Jodibala, H. (2014). Comparison of infrared light therapy vs sitz bath on episiotomy in terms of wound healing and intensity of pain among postnatal mothers. *International Journal of Nursing Care, 2*(1), 37–41.

Tester-Jones, M., O'Mahen, H., Watkins, E., & Karl, A. (2015). The impact of maternal characteristics, infant temperament and contextual factors on maternal responsiveness to infant. *Infant Behavior & Development, 40*, 1–11.

U.S. Department of Agriculture [USDA] & U.S. Department of Health and Human Services [USDHHS]. (2014). *Choose MyPlate*. Center for Nutrition Policy and Promotion. Retrieved from http://www.DietaryGuidelines.gov

U.S. Department of Health and Human Resources [USDHHS]. (2010). *Healthy people 2020*. Retrieved from http://www.healthypeople.gov/2020/topicsobjectives2020

Verghese, T. S., Futaba, K., & Latthe, P. (2015). Constipation in pregnancy. *The Obstetrician & Gynecologist, 17*(2), 111–115.

Walker, L. O., Murphey, C. L., & Nichols, F. (2015). The broken thread of health promotion and disease prevention for women during the postpartum period. *Journal of Perinatal Education, 24*(2), 81–92.

Wilson, B. L., Passante, T., Rauschenbach, D., Yang, R., & Wong, B. (2015). Bladder management with epidural anesthesia: A randomized controlled trial. *MCN. The American Journal of Maternal Child Nursing, 40*(4), 234–242. doi: 10.1097/NMC.0000000000000156

Whittock, J. (2015). Promoting sexual health: Sex after childbirth. *MIDIRS Midwifery Digest, 25*(1), 77–80.

World Health Organization [WHO]. (2014a). Implementation of the baby-friendly hospital initiative. Retrieved from http://www.who.int/elena/bbc/implementation_bfhi/en/

World Health Organization [WHO]. (2014b). WHO recommendations on postnatal care of the mother and newborn. Retrieved from http://apps.who.int/iris/bitstream/10665/97603/1/9789241506649_eng.pdf

Zapata, L. B., Murtaza, S., Whiteman, M. K., Jamieson, D. J., Robbins, C. L., Marchbanks, P. A., et al. (2015). Contraceptive counseling and postpartum contraceptive use. *American Journal of Obstetrics and Gynecology, 212*(2), 171–179.

MULTIPLE CHOICE QUESTIONS

1. When assessing a postpartum woman, which of the following would lead the nurse to suspect postpartum blues?
   a. Panic attacks and suicidal thoughts
   b. Anger toward self and infant
   c. Periodic crying and insomnia
   d. Obsessive thoughts and hallucinations

2. Which of these activities would best help the postpartum nurse to provide culturally sensitive care for the childbearing family?
   a. Taking a transcultural course
   b. Caring for only families of his or her cultural origin
   c. Teaching Western beliefs to culturally diverse families
   d. Educating himself or herself about diverse cultural practices

3. Which of the following suggestions would be most appropriate to include in the teaching plan for a postpartum woman who needs to lose weight?
   a. Increase fluid intake and acid-producing foods in her diet.
   b. Avoid empty-calorie foods, breastfeed, increase exercise.
   c. Start a high-protein, low carbohydrate diet and restrict fluids.
   d. Eat no snacks or carbohydrates after dinner.

4. After teaching a group of breast-feeding women about nutritional needs, the nurse determines that the teaching was successful when the women state that they need to increase their intake of which nutrients?
   a. Carbohydrates and fiber
   b. Fats and vitamins
   c. Calories and protein
   d. Iron-rich foods and minerals

5. Which of the following would lead the nurse to suspect that a postpartum woman was developing a complication?
   a. Fatigue and irritability
   b. Perineal discomfort and pink discharge
   c. Pulse rate of 60 bpm
   d. Swollen, tender, hot area on breast

6. Which of the following would the nurse assess as indicating positive bonding between the parents and their newborn?
   a. Holding the infant close to the body
   b. Having visitors hold the infant
   c. Buying expensive infant clothes
   d. Requesting that the nurses care for the infant

7. Which activity would the nurse include in the teaching plan for parents with a newborn and an older child to reduce sibling rivalry when the newborn is brought home?
   a. Punishing the older child for bedwetting behavior
   b. Sending the sibling to the grandparents' house
   c. Planning a daily "special time" for the older sibling
   d. Allowing the sibling to share a room with the infant

8. The major purpose of the first postpartum homecare visit is to:
   a. Identify complications that require interventions
   b. Obtain a blood specimen for PKU testing
   c. Complete the official birth certificate
   d. Support the new parents in their parenting roles

9. The nurse is instructing the postpartum client who plans to bottle-feed her newborn about measures to prevent breast engorgement when she is discharged. Which of the following measures should the nurse include in the teaching plan?
   a. Decreasing her fluid intake for the first week at home
   b. Wearing a tight-fitting supportive bra 24 hours daily
   c. Take a diuretic to release the extra fluid in the breasts
   d. Manually express the milk that is accumulating

10. A new mother was brought to the postpartum unit who gave birth 12 hours ago. Because this is her first child, which of the following goals by the nurse is most appropriate?
    a. Early discharge for the mother and newborn
    b. Rapid transition into her role of being a parent/caretaker
    c. Minimal need for expression of her feelings now
    d. Effective education of both parents before discharge

CRITICAL THINKING EXERCISES

1. As a nurse working on a postpartum unit, you enter the room of, a 22-year-old primipara, and find her chatting on the phone while her newborn is crying loudly in the bassinette, which has been pushed into the bathroom. You pick up and comfort the newborn. While holding the baby, you ask the client if she was aware her newborn was crying. She replies, "That's about all that monkey does since she was born!" You hand the newborn to her and she places the newborn on the bed away from her and continues her phone conversation.

a. What is your nursing assessment of this encounter?

b. What nursing interventions would be appropriate?

c. What specific discharge interventions may be needed?

2. A 34-year-old single primipara, left the hospital after a 36-hour stay with her newborn son. She lives alone in a one-bedroom walk-up apartment. As the postpartum home health nurse visiting her 2 days later, you find the following:

- Tearful client pacing the floor holding her crying son
- Home cluttered and in disarray
- Fundus firm and displaced to right of midline
- Moderate lochia rubra; episiotomy site clean, dry, and intact
- Vital signs within normal range; pain rating less than 3 points on scale of 1 to 10
- Breasts engorged slightly; supportive bra on
- Newborn assessment within normal limits
- Distended bladder upon palpation; reporting urinary frequency

a. Which of these assessment findings warrants further investigation?

b. What interventions are appropriate at this time, and why?

c. What health teaching is needed before you leave this home?

3. The nurse walks into the room of a 24-year-old primigravida. She asks the nurse to hand her the bottle sitting on the bedside table, stating, "I'm going to finish it off because my baby only ate half of it 3 hours ago when I fed him."

a. What response by the nurse would be appropriate at this time?

b. What action should the nurse take?

c. What health teaching is needed for this new mother prior to discharge?

STUDY ACTIVITIES

1. Identify two questions that a nurse would ask a postpartum woman to assess for postpartum blues.

2. Find a web site that offers advice to new parents about breast-feeding. Critique the site, the author's credentials, and the accuracy of the content.

3. Outline instructions you would give to a new mother on how to use her peribottle.

4. Breast tissue swelling secondary to vascular congestion after childbirth and preceding lactation describes _____.

5. Listen to the postpartum story of one of your assigned clients and share it with your peers in class or as part of online discussion.

BRINGING IT ALL TOGETHER: CASE STUDY

A 26-year-old African American woman gave birth to a healthy term neonate yesterday and is preparing for discharge. The mother is illiterate and lives in a poor agricultural area of town not far from the hospital. This is her fourth infant in five years. The postpartum nurse comes into the room and observes that this mother has wrapped a piece of unclean cloth tightly around the infant's abdomen with a quarter which covers the cord stump. The take-home infant outfit is not clean and not appropriate for the weather conditions outside. The mother is waiting for a ride home from a friend. The postpartum nurse is here to provide her with discharge instructions.

ASSESSMENT

Client's general appearance is healthy, but appears fatigued. Vital signs are as follows: BP 120/74; Pulse 78; Temp 98.2F; Respirations 20 bpm. Her breasts are soft upon palpation, no engorgement present. She plans to bottle-feed her infant. Her abdominal exam is without significant findings and involution is proceeding normally. Fundus is at the level of the umbilicus and firm. Lochia rubra is moderate, with no clots. Voiding well and has had a bowel movement this morning. No episiotomy site to assess. Newborn physical exam was normal per pediatrician's notes.

Go to thePoint **to find questions to consider about this case.**

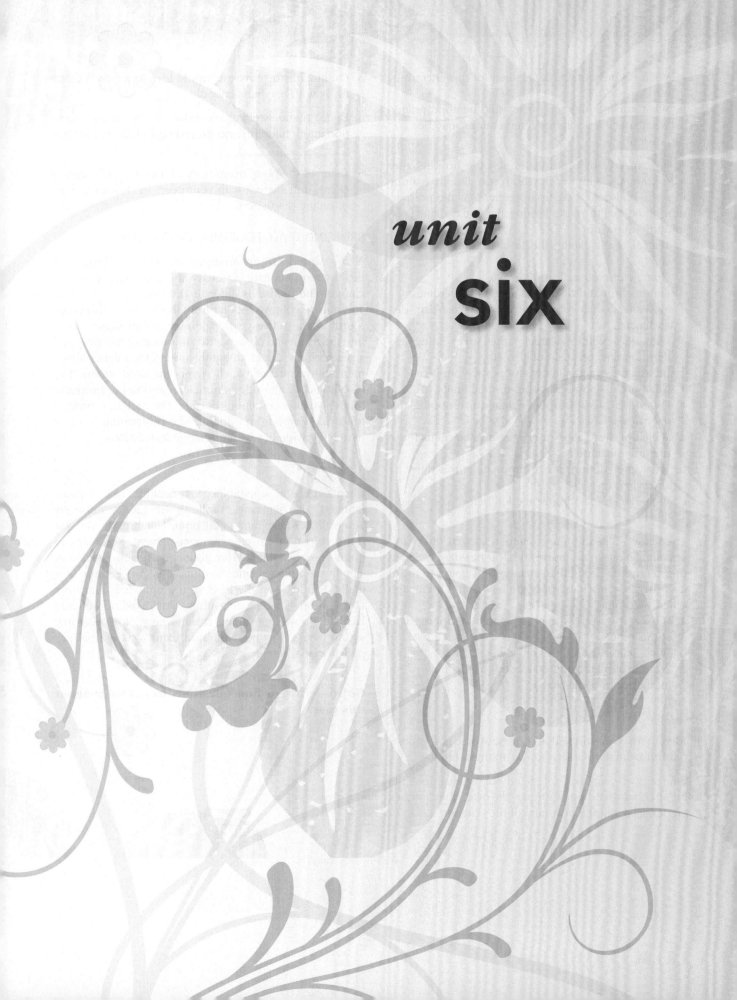

unit
six

The Newborn

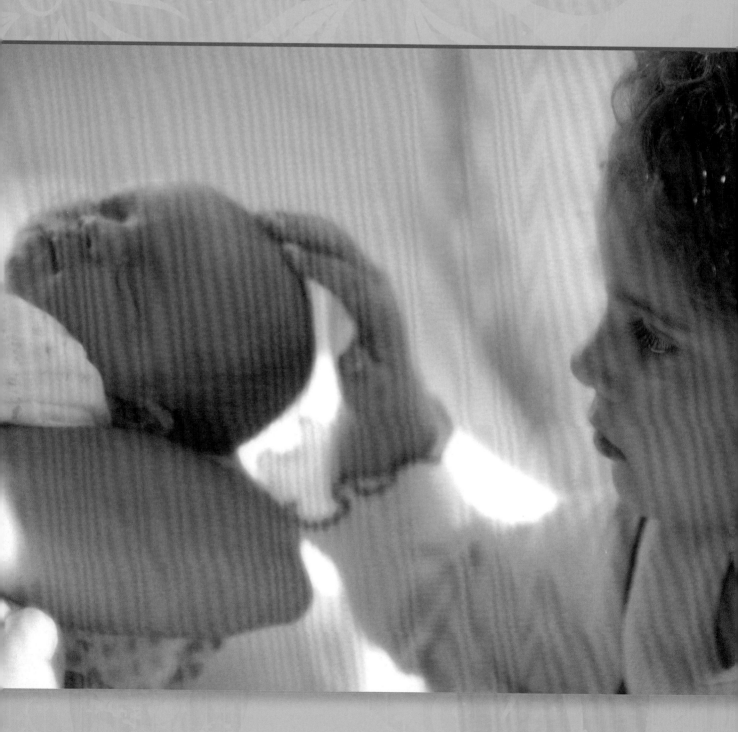

17

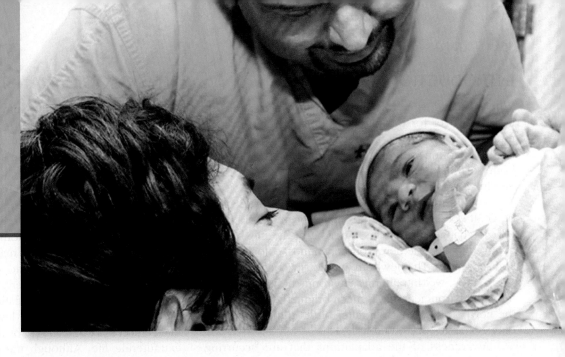

Newborn Transitioning

Learning Objectives

Upon completion of the chapter, you will be able to:

1. Examine the major physiologic changes that occur as the newborn transitions to extrauterine life.

2. Determine the primary challenges faced by the newborn during the transition to extrauterine life.

3. Interpret the factors that influence the initiation of newborn respirations.

4. Compare and contrast the cardiovascular changes that take place from fetal circulation to extrauterine circulation after birth.

5. Relate three characteristics that predispose newborns to heat loss after birth.

6. Distinguish three primary immunoglobulins that help strengthen the newborn's immunologic system.

7. Differentiate the three behavioral patterns that newborns progress through after birth.

8. Assess the five typical behavioral responses triggered by external stimuli of the newborn.

The Healthy Start home care nurse reviewed the client's file in her car before she got out: 18-year-old primipara, 1 week postpartum with a term newborn girl weighing 7 lb. The new mother, Maria, greeted the nurse at the door and let her inside the house. After performing a postpartum assessment on Maria and an assessment of her newborn daughter, the nurse asked Maria if she had any questions or concerns. Maria's eyes welled up with tears: she is worried that her daughter can't see.

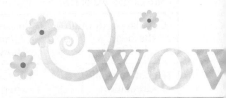

Words of Wisdom
Newborns can't always be judged by their outer wrapping; rather, we should focus on the awesome gift inside.

INTRODUCTION

When a child is born, the exhaustion and stress of labor are over for the parents, but now the newborn must begin the work of physiologically and behaviorally adapting to the new environment. The first 24 hours of life can be the most precarious (Swanson & Sinkin, 2015).

The **neonatal period** is defined as the first 28 days of life. It is a period of the most dramatic and rapid physiologic changes in humans. After birth, the newborn is exposed to a whole new world of sounds, colors, smells, and sensations. The newborn, previously confined to the warm, dark, wet intrauterine environment, is now thrust into an environment that is much brighter and cooler. As the newborn adapts to life after birth, numerous physiologic changes occur (Table 17.1).

Awareness of the adaptations that are occurring forms the foundation for providing support to the newborn during this crucial time. Physiologic and behavioral changes occur quickly during this transition period. Being aware of any deviations from the norm is crucial to ensure early identification and prompt intervention.

This chapter describes the physiologic changes of the newborn's major body systems. It also discusses the behavioral adaptations, including behavioral patterns and the newborn's behavioral responses, which occur during this transition period.

PHYSIOLOGIC TRANSITIONING

The adaptation from the intrauterine to extrauterine environment is complex and difficult, but required for all humans. Maternal medical and fetal conditions can have a profound effect on the successful transition. The mechanics of birth require a change in the newborn for survival outside the uterus. Immediately at birth, respiratory gas exchange, along with circulatory modifications, must occur to sustain extrauterine life. During this time, as newborns strive to attain homeostasis, they also experience complex changes in major organ systems. The newborn's most dramatic and most rapid extrauterine transitions occur in four interdependent areas: respiratory, circulatory, thermoregulation, and their ability to stabilize their blood glucose levels. All four areas must make successful transitions for the newborn to adapt to extrauterine life. Although the transition usually takes place within the first 6 to 10 hours of life, many adaptations take weeks to attain full maturity.

Cardiovascular System Adaptations

During fetal life, the heart relies on certain unique structures that assist it in providing adequate perfusion of vital body parts. The umbilical vein carries oxygenated blood from the placenta to the fetus. The ductus venosus allows the majority of the umbilical vein blood to bypass the liver and merge with blood moving through the vena

TABLE 17.1	ANATOMIC AND PHYSIOLOGIC COMPARISON OF THE FETUS AND NEWBORN	
Topic of Comparison	**Fetus**	**Newborn**
Respiratory system	Fluid-filled, high-pressure system causes blood to be shunted from the lungs through the ductus arteriosus to the rest of the body	Air-filled, low-pressure system encourages blood flow through the lungs for gas exchange; increased oxygen content of blood in the lungs contributes to the closing of the ductus arteriosus (becomes a ligament)
Site of gas exchange	Placenta	Lungs
Circulation through the heart	Pressures in the right atrium are greater than in the left, encouraging blood flow through the foreman ovale	Pressures in the left atrium are greater than in the right, causing the foreman ovale to close
Hepatic portal circulation	Ductus venosus bypasses; maternal liver performs filtering functions	Ductus venosus closes (becomes a ligament); hepatic portal circulation begins
Thermoregulation	Body temperature is maintained by maternal body temperature and the warmth of the intrauterine environment	Body temperature is maintained through a flexed posture and brown fat

Adapted from Sharma, A., Ford, S., & Calvert, J. (2014). Adaptation for life: A review of neonatal physiology. *Anesthesia & Intensive Care Medicine*, *15*(3), 89–95; Stave, U. (2014). *Perinatal physiology*. New York, NY: Springer Publishers; and King, T. L., Brucker, M. C., Kriebs, J. M., Fahey, J. O., Gegor, C. L., & Varney, H. (2015). *Varney's midwifery*. (5th ed.). Burlington, MA: Jones & Bartlett Learning.

cava, bringing it to the heart sooner. The foramen ovale allows more than half the blood entering the right atrium to cross immediately to the left atrium, bypassing the pulmonary circulation. The ductus arteriosus connects the pulmonary artery to the aorta, which allows bypassing of the pulmonary circuit. Only a small portion of blood passes through the pulmonary circuit for the main purpose of perfusion of the structure, rather than for oxygenation. The fetus depends on the placenta to provide oxygen and nutrients and to remove waste products.

At birth, the circulatory system must switch from fetal to newborn circulation and from placental to pulmonary gas exchange. Successful transition from fetal to postnatal circulation requires increased pulmonary blood flow, removal of the placenta, and closure of the intracardiac (foramen ovale) and extracardiac shunts (ductus venosus and ductus arteriosus). These changes are needed to equalize the right ventricular output with that of the left (Stark & Eichenwald, 2016). The physical forces of the contractions of labor and birth, mild asphyxia, increased intracranial pressure as a result of cord compression and uterine contractions, and the cold stress experienced immediately after birth lead to an increased release of catecholamines that is critical for the changes involved in the transition to extrauterine life. The increased levels of epinephrine and norepinephrine stimulate increased cardiac output and contractility, surfactant release, and promotion of pulmonary fluid clearance (Sharma, Ford, & Calvert, 2014).

Fetal to Neonatal Circulation Changes

Changes in circulation occur immediately at birth as the fetus separates from the placenta (Fig. 17.1). When the umbilical cord is clamped, the first breath is taken and the lungs begin to function. As a result, systemic vascular resistance increases and blood return to the heart via the inferior vena cava decreases. Concurrently with these changes, there is a rapid decrease in pulmonary vascular resistance and an increase in pulmonary blood flow (Cuneo, 2014). The foramen ovale functionally closes with a decrease in pulmonary vascular resistance, which leads to a decrease in right-sided heart pressures. An increase in systemic pressure, after clamping of the cord, leads to an increase in left-sided heart pressures. The ductus arteriosus, ductus venosus, and umbilical vessels that were vital during fetal life are no longer needed. Over a period of months these fetal vessels form nonfunctional ligaments.

Before birth, the foramen ovale allowed most of the oxygenated blood entering the right atrium from the inferior vena cava to pass into the left atrium of the heart. With the newborn's first breath, air pushes into the lungs, triggering an increase in pulmonary blood flow and pulmonary venous return to the left side of the heart. As a result, the pressure in the left atrium becomes higher than in the right atrium. The increased left atrial

pressure causes the foramen ovale to close, thus allowing the output from the right ventricle to flow entirely to the lungs. With closure of this fetal shunt, oxygenated blood is now separated from nonoxygenated blood. The subsequent increase in tissue oxygenation further promotes the increase in systemic blood pressure and continuing blood flow to the lungs. The foramen ovale normally closes functionally at birth when left atrial pressure increases and right atrial pressure decreases. Permanent anatomic closure, though, really occurs throughout the next several weeks.

During fetal life, the ductus arteriosus, located between the aorta and the pulmonary artery, protected the lungs against circulatory overload by shunting blood (right to left) into the descending aorta, bypassing the pulmonary circulation. Its patency during fetal life is promoted by continual production of prostaglandin E2 (PGE2) by the ductus arteriosus (van Vonderen et al., 2014). The ductus arteriosus becomes functionally closed within the first few hours after birth. Oxygen is the most important factor in controlling its closure. Closure depends on the high oxygen content of the aortic blood that results from aeration of the lungs at birth. At birth, pulmonary vascular resistance decreases, allowing pulmonary blood flow to increase and oxygen exchange to occur in the lungs. It occurs secondary to an increase in PO_2 coincident with the first breath and umbilical cord occlusion when it is clamped.

The ductus venosus shunted blood from the left umbilical vein to the inferior vena cava during intrauterine life. It closes within a few days after birth because this shunting is no longer needed as a result of activation of the liver. The activated liver now takes over the functions of the placenta (which was expelled at birth). The ductus venosus becomes a ligament in extrauterine life.

The two umbilical arteries and one umbilical vein begin to constrict at birth because with placental expulsion, blood flow ceases. In addition, peripheral circulation increases. Thus, the vessels are no longer needed and they too become ligaments. Successful transition and closure of the three fetal shunts creates a neonatal circulation where deoxygenated blood returns to the heart through the inferior and superior vena cava. Deoxygenated blood enters the right atrium then into the right ventricle and travels through the pulmonary artery to the pulmonary vascular bed. Oxygenated blood returns through pulmonary veins to the left atrium, the left ventricle, and through the aorta to the systemic circulation (Stave, 2014). Box 17.1 provides a summary of fetal to neonatal circulation.

Heart Rate

During the first few minutes after birth, the newborn's heart rate is approximately 110 to 160 bpm. Thereafter, it begins to decrease to an average of 120 to 130 bpm (Creasy et al., 2014). The newborn is highly dependent

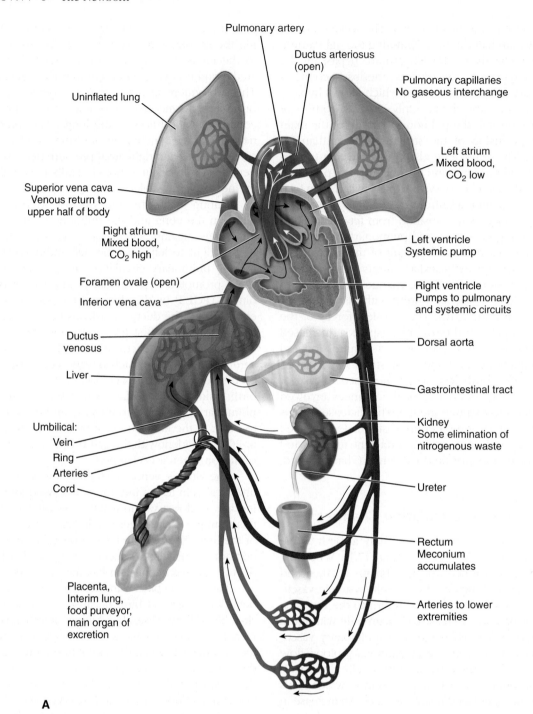

Pulmonary artery

Ductus arteriosus (open)

Pulmonary capillaries
No gaseous interchange

Uninflated lung

Left atrium
Mixed blood,
CO_2 low

Superior vena cava
Venous return to
upper half of body

Right atrium
Mixed blood,
CO_2 high

Left ventricle
Systemic pump

Foramen ovale (open)

Right ventricle
Pumps to pulmonary
and systemic circuits

Inferior vena cava

Ductus
venosus

Dorsal aorta

Liver

Gastrointestinal tract

Kidney
Some elimination of
nitrogenous waste

Umbilical:
Vein
Ring
Arteries
Cord

Ureter

Rectum
Meconium
accumulates

Placenta,
Interim lung,
food purveyor,
main organ of
excretion

Arteries to lower
extremities

A

FIGURE 17.1 Cardiovascular adaptations of the newborn. Note the changes in oxygenation between (**A**) prenatal circulation and (**B**) postnatal (pulmonary) circulation.

on heart rate for maintenance of cardiac output and blood pressure. Although blood pressure is not taken routinely in the healthy term newborn, it is usually highest after birth and reaches a plateau within a week after birth. Cardiac defects may be identified in the newborn nursery by conducting a thorough and systematic physical assessment, including inspection, palpation, auscultation, and measurement of blood pressure and oxygen saturations. The ability of the nurse to identify irregular findings during physical assessment aids rapid identification and treatment.

Take Note!

Transient functional cardiac murmurs may be heard during the neonatal period as a result of the changing dynamics of the cardiovascular system at birth (Fillipps & Bucciarelli, 2015).

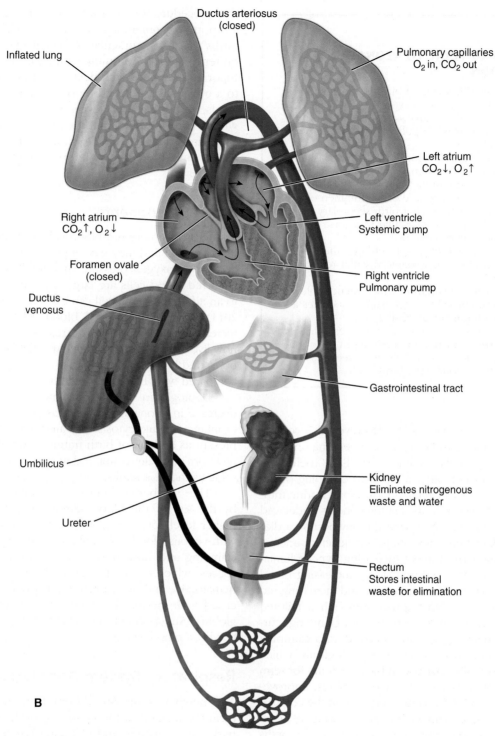

Inflated lung

Ductus arteriosus
(closed)

Pulmonary capillaries
O_2 in, CO_2 out

Left atrium
$CO_2\downarrow$, $O_2\uparrow$

Right atrium
$CO_2\uparrow$, $O_2\downarrow$

Left ventricle
Systemic pump

Foramen ovale
(closed)

Right ventricle
Pulmonary pump

Ductus
venosus

Gastrointestinal tract

Umbilicus

Kidney
Eliminates nitrogenous
waste and water

Ureter

Rectum
Stores intestinal
waste for elimination

B

FIGURE 17.1 *(continued)*

The fluctuations in both the heart rate and blood pressure tend to follow the changes in the newborn's behavioral state. An increase in activity, such as wakefulness, movement, or crying, corresponds to an increase in heart rate and blood pressure. In contrast, the compromised newborn demonstrates markedly less physiologic variability overall. Tachycardia may be found with volume depletion, cardiorespiratory disease, drug withdrawal, and hyperthyroidism. Bradycardia is often associated with apnea and is often seen with hypoxia.

Blood Volume

The blood volume of the newborn depends on the amount of blood transferred from the placenta at birth. It is usually estimated to be 80 to 85 mL/kg of body weight

BOX 17.1

SUMMARY OF FETAL TO NEONATAL CIRCULATION

- Clamping umbilical cord at birth eliminates the placenta as a reservoir for blood.
- Onset of respirations causes a rise in PO_2 in the lungs and a decrease in pulmonary vascular resistance, *which…*
- Increases pulmonary blood flow and increases pressure in the left atrium, *which…*
- Decreases pressure in the right atrium of the heart, which causes closure of the foramen ovale (closes within minutes after birth secondary to a decreased pulmonary vascular resistance and increased left heart pressure).
- With an increase in oxygen levels after the first breath, an increase in systemic vascular resistance occurs, *which…*
- Decreases vena cava return, which reduces blood flow in the umbilical vein (constricts, becomes a ligament with functional closing).
- Closure of the ductus venosus (becomes a ligament) causes an increase in pressure in the aorta, which forces closure of the ductus arteriosus within 10 to 15 hours after birth.

in the term infant (Stave, 2014). However, the volume may vary by as much as 25% to 40%, depending on when clamping of the umbilical cord occurs. Early (before 30 to 40 seconds) or late (after 3 minutes) clamping of the umbilical cord changes circulatory dynamics during transition. Recent studies indicate that the benefits of delayed cord clamping include improving the newborn's cardiopulmonary adaptation, preventing iron-deficient anemia in full-term newborns without increasing hypervolemia-related risks and increased iron stores, increasing blood pressure, improving oxygen transport, and increasing red blood cell flow (McAdams, 2014). Although a tailored approach is required in the case of cord clamping, current available data suggests that delayed cord clamping offers the newborn many benefits physiologically, which include at least a 30% increase in blood volume for term infants and a 50% increase in preterm infants, improvement of systemic blood pressure, increase in the cerebral oxygen index, higher hemoglobin levels at 24 to 48 hours of age, and increased serum iron levels at 4 to 6 months (Kluckow & Hooper, 2015; Leslie, 2015). Cord blood has also been described as "nature's first stem cell transplant" because it possesses regenerative properties and can grow into different types of cells in the body (van Vonderen et al., 2014).

Professional organizations American Academy of Pediatrics (AAP) (2013) and American College of Obstetricians & Gynecologists (ACOG) (2014) have released opinions that support delayed cord clamping for preterm infants, but endorse further research on

this procedure for term infants. WHO (2014) released a report recommending delayed cord clamping for "all births" as a best practice. A recent Cochrane Review on term infants and timing of umbilical cord clamping reported that those with delayed cord clamping had up to a 60% increase in red blood cells, high hemoglobin levels, and higher iron levels at 4 to 6 months. Infants whose cords were clamped early were twice as likely to be iron deficit at 3 to 6 months (Leslie, 2015). So, at this time, there is no uniform agreement about this practice.

Blood Components

The fetus has more red blood cells per cubic millimeter than an adult and they have a greater affinity for oxygen at a lower oxygen pressure than adult red blood cells. Fetal red blood cells are larger in size when compared to an adult, thus each cell can carry more oxygen (Stave, 2014). After birth, the red blood cell count gradually increases as the cell size decreases, because the cells now live in an environment with much higher PO_2. A newborn's red blood cells have a life span of 80 to 100 days, compared with 120 days in adults.

Hemoglobin initially declines as a result of a decrease in neonatal red cell mass (physiologic anemia of infancy). Leukocytosis (elevated white blood cells) is present as a result of birth trauma soon after birth. The newborn's platelet count and aggregation ability are the same as those of adults.

The newborn's hematologic values are affected by the site of the blood sample (capillary blood has higher levels of hemoglobin and hematocrit compared with venous blood), placental transfusion (delayed cord clamping and normal shift of plasma to extravascular spaces, which causes higher levels of hemoglobin and hematocrit), and gestational age (increased age is associated with increased numbers of red cells and hemoglobin) (Andersson et al., 2014). Table 17.2 lists normal newborn blood values.

Respiratory System Adaptations

The newborn's transition from fetal to neonatal life includes aeration of the lungs, establishment of pulmonary gas exchange, and changing the fetal circulation into the adult type. Lung aeration leads to the establishment of functional residual capacity, allowing pulmonary gas exchange to start. The first breath of life is a gasp that generates an increase in transpulmonary pressure and results in diaphragmatic descent. Hypercapnia, hypoxia, and acidosis resulting from normal labor become stimuli for initiating respirations. Inspiration of air and expansion of the lungs allow for an increase in tidal volume (amount of air brought into the lungs). **Surfactant** is a surface tension–reducing lipoprotein

TABLE 17.2	NORMAL NEWBORN BLOOD VALUES	
Lab Data	**Normal Range**	
Hemoglobin	16–18 g/dL	
Hematocrit	46–68%	
Platelets	150,000–350,000/µL	
Red blood cells	4.5–7.0 (1,000,000/µL)	
White blood cells	10–30,000/mm^3	

Adapted from Fischbach, F., & Dunning, M. B. *Manual of laboratory and diagnostic tests.* (9th ed.). Philadelphia, PA: Lippincott Williams & Wilkins; Verklan, T., & Walden, M. *Core curriculum for neonatal intensive care nursing.* (4th ed.). St. Louis, MO: Saunders Elsevier; and Davidson, M. R. (2014). *Fast facts for the neonatal nurse: A nursing orientation and care guide in a nutshell.* New York, NY: Springer.

found in the newborn's lungs that prevents alveolar collapse at the end of expiration and loss of lung volume. It lines the alveoli to enhance aeration of gas-free lungs, thus reducing surface tension and lowering the pressure required to open the alveoli. Normal lung function depends on surfactant, which permits a decrease in surface tension at end expiration (to prevent atelectasis) and an increase in surface tension during lung expansion (to facilitate elastic recoil on inspiration). Surfactant provides the lung stability needed for gas exchange. The newborn's first breath, in conjunction with surfactant, overcomes the surface forces to permit aeration of the lungs. The chest wall of the newborn is floppy because of the high cartilage content and poorly developed musculature. Thus, accessory muscles to help in breathing are ineffective.

One of the most crucial adaptations that the newborn makes at birth is adjusting from a fluid-filled intrauterine environment to a gaseous extrauterine environment. During fetal life, the lungs are expanded with an ultrafiltrate of the amniotic fluid. During and after birth, this fluid must be removed and replaced with air. Passage through the birth canal allows intermittent compression of the thorax, which helps eliminate the fluid in the lungs. Pulmonary capillaries and the lymphatics remove the remaining fluid.

If fluid is removed too slowly or incompletely (e.g., with decreased thoracic squeezing during birth or diminished respiratory effort), transient tachypnea (respiratory rate above 60 bpm) of the newborn occurs. Examples of situations involving decreased thoracic compression and diminished respiratory effort include cesarean birth and sedation in newborns. Research findings support the need for thoracic compression because the absence of the neonate's exposure to labor contractions, which may occur with cesarean births or heavy sedation during the labor process or general anesthesia administered during the surgical birth, is associated with an increased risk of transient tachypnea at term, with oxygen supplementation being needed for a longer duration (Hooper, Polglase, & Roehr, 2015).

Take Note!

A neonate born by cesarean section does not have the same benefit of the birth canal squeeze as does the newborn born by vaginal delivery. Closely observe the respirations of the newborn after cesarean delivery.

Lungs

Before the newborn's lungs can maintain respiratory function, the following events must occur:
- Initiation of respiratory movement
- Expansion of the lungs
- Establishment of functional residual capacity (ability to retain some air in the lungs on expiration)
- Increased pulmonary blood flow
- Redistribution of cardiac output (Bope & Kellerman, 2015)

Initial breathing is probably the result of a reflex triggered by pressure changes, noise, light, temperature changes, touching, compression of the fetal chest during the birthing process, and high carbon dioxide and low oxygen concentrations of the newborn's blood. Central chemoreceptors stimulated by hypoxia and hypercapnia further increase the respiratory drive. Many theories address the initiation of respiration in the newborn, but most are based on speculation from observations rather than on empirical research (Sharma et al., 2014). Research continues to search for answers to these questions.

Respirations

After respirations are established in the newborn, they are shallow and irregular, ranging from 30 to 60 breaths per minute, with short periods of apnea (less than 15 seconds). The newborn's respiratory rate varies according to his or her activity; the more active the newborn, the higher the respiratory rate, on average. Signs of respiratory distress to observe for include cyanosis, tachypnea, expiratory grunting, sternal retractions, and nasal flaring. Respirations should not be labored, and the chest movements should be symmetric. In some cases, **periodic breathing** may occur, which is the cessation of breathing that lasts 5 to 10 seconds without changes in color or heart rate (Davidson, 2014). Periodic breathing may be observed in newborns within the first few days of life and requires close monitoring.

> **Take Note!**
> Apneic periods lasting more than 15 seconds with cyanosis and heart rate changes require further evaluation (Mattson & Smith, 2015).

Body Temperature Regulation

Newborns are dependent on their environment for the maintenance of body temperature, much more so immediately after birth than later in life. One of the most important elements in a newborn's survival is obtaining a stable body temperature to promote an optimal transition to extrauterine life. On average, a newborn's temperature ranges from 97.9° to 99.7°F (36.6° to 37.6°C). Since newborns lose heat easily after birth, having skin-to-skin contact with their mothers is recommended as the initial method for maintaining newborn body temperature. Skin-to-skin contact should be the first line of treatment for hypothermia and as a measure to reduce discomfort from painful procedures. See Evidence-Based Practice 17.1.

Thermoregulation is the process of maintaining the balance between heat loss and heat production in order to maintain the body's core internal temperature. It is a critical physiologic function that is closely related to the transition and survival of the newborn. An appropriate thermal environment is essential for maintaining a normal body temperature. Compared with adults, newborns tolerate a narrower range of environmental temperatures and are extremely vulnerable to both under heating and

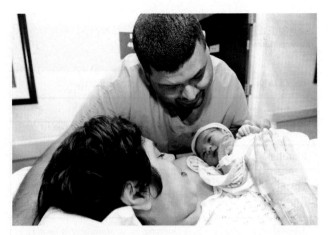

FIGURE 17.2 Father and mother looking at their newborn after birth. Note the newborn's hat and warm blanket to preserve body heat.

overheating. Nurses play a key role in providing an appropriate environment to help newborns maintain thermal stability (Fig. 17.2).

Heat Loss

Newborns have several characteristics that predispose them to heat loss:
- Thin skin with blood vessels close to the surface
- Lack of shivering ability to produce heat until 3 months old

---

EVIDENCE-BASED PRACTICE 17.1   **EFFECT OF EARLY MATERNAL/NEWBORN SKIN-TO-SKIN CONTACT AFTER BIRTH ON THE DURATION OF THIRD STAGE OF LABOR AND INITIATION OF BREAST-FEEDING**

STUDY

The holding of a newborn with vertical skin-to-skin contact typically in an upright position with the swaddled newborn on the chest of the mother, is commonly referred to as kangaroo care. It has been recommended that this skin-to-skin contact is a feasible, natural, and cost-effective intervention for breast-feeding initiation and thermoregulation. The aim of this study was to determine the effect of early maternal–newborn skin-to-skin contact after birth on the duration of the third stage of labor and initiation of breast-feeding.

Findings

A nonrandomized controlled clinical trial was conducted using a sample of 100 laboring women. The project included a study group (50) who had skin-to-skin contact and a control group (50) who received routine hospital care. Tools used to collect data included a structured interview, assessment of mothers during the third stage of labor, and an outcome assessment of first breast-feeding. The results revealed that success in

first-time breast-feeding during the complete separation of the placenta and immediate contraction of the uterus was higher in the study group compared to the control group. There were statistically significant differences between the study and control groups in third stage of labor duration (9 minutes shorter), complete placental separation, and immediate contraction of the uterus or excessive bleeding. The study concluded that mothers who practice early mother/newborn skin-to-skin contact immediately after giving birth experienced a shorter third stage duration and early successful initiation of breast-feeding.

Nursing Implications

Based on these findings, it would make sense to incorporate early skin-to-skin contact immediately post birth and delay routine infant care until the success of the first breast-feeding process for the benefits it provides both mother and newborn. Nurses need to apply evidence-based research into their care since this application would improve maternal and child health outcomes.

Adapted from Essa, R. M., & Ismail, N. I. Effect of early maternal/newborn skin-to-skin contact after birth on the duration of third stage of labor and initiation of breastfeeding. *Journal of Nursing Education and Practice*, 5(4), 98–107.

- Limited stores of metabolic substrates (glucose, glycogen, fat)
- Limited use of voluntary muscle activity or movement to produce heat
- Large body surface area relative to body weight
- Lack of subcutaneous fat, which provides insulation
- Little ability to conserve heat by changing posture (fetal position)
- No ability to adjust their own clothing or blankets to achieve warmth
- Inability to communicate that they are too cold or too warm

Every newborn struggles to maintain body temperature from the moment of birth, when the newborn's wet body is exposed to the much cooler environment of the birthing room. The amniotic fluid covering the newborn cools as it evaporates rapidly in the low humidity and air conditioning of the room. The newborn's temperature may decrease 3 to 5 degrees within minutes after leaving the warmth of the mother's uterus (99.6°F [37.5°C]). The skin of newborns adjusts quickly to the challenging environmental conditions of extrauterine

Consider This

When I look down at my little miracle of life in my arms, I can't help but beam with pride at this great accomplishment. She seems so vulnerable and defenseless, and yet is equipped with everything she needs to survive at birth. When the nurse brought my daughter in for the first time after birth, I wanted to see and feel every part of her. Much to my dismay, she was wrapped up like a mummy in a blanket and she had a pink knit cap on her head. I asked the nurse why all the babies had to look like they were bound for the North Pole with all these layers on. Wasn't the nurse aware it was summertime and probably at least 85 degrees outside?

The nurse explained that newborns lose body heat easily and need to be kept warm until their temperature stabilizes. Even though I wanted to get up close and personal with my baby, I decided to keep the pink polar bear outfit on her.

Thoughts: *Newborns may be born with "everything they need to survive" on the outside, but they still experience temperature instability and lose heat through radiation, evaporation, convection, and conduction. Because the newborn's head is the largest body part, a great deal of heat can be lost if a cap is not kept on the head. What guidance can be given to this mother before discharge to stabilize her daughter's temperature while at home? What simple examples can be used to demonstrate your point?*

life. However, certain functions, for example, microcirculation, continue to develop even beyond the neonatal period (McCall et al., 2014).

The transfer of heat depends on the temperature of the environment, air speed, and water vapor pressure or humidity. Heat exchange between the environment and the newborn involves the same mechanisms as those with any physical object and its environment. Heat can be lost by four mechanisms including conduction (3%), convection (34%), evaporation (24%), and radiation (39%) (Sharma et al., 2014). Prevention of heat loss is a key nursing intervention (Fig. 17.3).

CONDUCTION

Conduction involves the transfer of heat from one object to another when the two objects are in direct contact with each other. Conduction refers to heat fluctuation between the newborn's body surface when in contact with other solid surfaces, such as a cold mattress, scale, or circumcision restraining board. Heat loss by conduction can also occur when touching a newborn with cold hands or when the newborn has direct contact with a colder object such as a metal scale. Using a warmed cloth diaper or blanket to cover any cold surface touching a newborn directly helps to prevent heat loss through conduction. Placing the newborn skin-to-skin with the mother also helps prevent heat loss through conduction.

CONVECTION

Convection involves the flow of heat from the body surface to cooler surrounding air or to air circulating over a body surface. An example of convection-related heat loss would be a cool breeze that flows over the newborn. To prevent heat loss by this mechanism, keep the newborn out of direct cool drafts (open doors, windows, fans, air conditioners) in the environment, work inside an isolette as much as possible and minimize opening portholes that allow cold air to flow inside, and warm any oxygen or humidified air that comes in contact with the newborn. Using clothing and blankets in isolettes is an effective means of reducing the newborn's exposed surface area and providing external insulation. Also, transporting the newborn to the nursery in a warmed isolette, rather than carrying him or her, helps to maintain warmth and reduce exposure to the cool air.

EVAPORATION

Evaporation involves the loss of heat when a liquid is converted to vapor. Evaporative loss may be insensible (such as from skin and respiration) or sensible (such as from sweating). Insensible loss occurs, but the individual is not aware of it. Sensible loss is objective and can be noticed. It depends on air speed and the absolute humidity of the

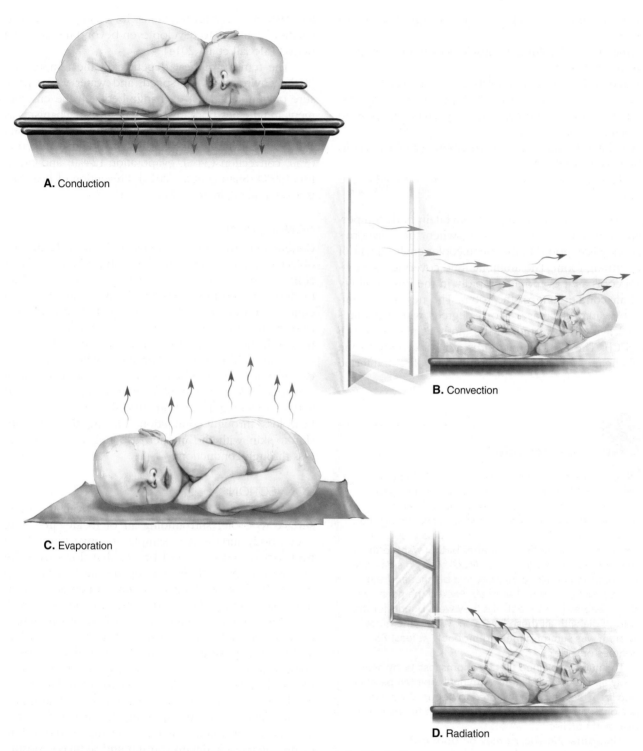

A. Conduction

B. Convection

C. Evaporation

D. Radiation

FIGURE 17.3 The four mechanisms of heat loss in the newborn. **A.** Conduction. **B.** Convection. **C.** Evaporation. **D.** Radiation.

air. For example, when the baby is born, the body is covered with amniotic fluid. The fluid evaporates into the air, leading to heat loss. Heat loss via evaporation also occurs when bathing a newborn. Drying newborns immediately after birth with warmed blankets and placing a cap on their head will help to prevent heat loss through evaporation. In addition, drying the newborn after bathing will help prevent heat loss through evaporation. Promptly changing wet linens, clothes, or diapers will also reduce heat loss and prevent chilling.

RADIATION

Radiation involves the loss of body heat to cooler, solid surfaces that are in proximity but not in direct contact with the newborn. The amount of heat loss depends on the size of the cold surface area, the surface temperature of the newborn's body, and the temperature of the receiving surface area. For example, when a newborn is placed in a single-wall isolette next to a cold window, heat loss from radiation occurs. Newborns will become cold even though they are in a heated isolette. To reduce heat loss by radiation, keep cribs and isolettes away from outside walls, cold windows, and air conditioners. Also, using radiant warmers for transporting newborns and when performing procedures that may expose the newborn to the cooler environment will help reduce heat loss.

A warmed transporter is an enclosed isolette on wheels. A radiant warmer is an open bed with a radiant heat source above. This type of environment allows health care providers to reach the newborn to carry out procedures and treatments.

Overheating

The newborn is also prone to overheating. Limited insulation and limited sweating ability can predispose any newborn to overheating. Control of body temperature is achieved via a complex negative feedback system that creates a balance between heat production, heat gain, and heat loss. The primary heat regulator is located in the hypothalamus and the central nervous system. The immaturity of the newborn's central nervous system makes it difficult to create and maintain this balance. Therefore, the newborn can become overheated easily. For example, an isolette that is too warm or one that is left too close to a sunny window may lead to hyperthermia. Although heat production can substantially increase in response to a cool environment, basal metabolic rate and the resultant heat produced cannot be reduced. Overheating increases fluid loss, the respiratory rate, and the metabolic rate considerably.

Thermoregulation

Humans have the ability to regulate their body temperature within a narrow range. Newborns have a decreased ability to regulate their body temperature, producing heat through nonshivering thermogenesis. Thermoregulation, the balance between heat loss and heat production, is related to the newborn's rate of metabolism and oxygen consumption. The newborn attempts to conserve heat and increase heat production by increasing the metabolic rate, increasing muscular activity through movement, increasing peripheral vasoconstriction, and assuming a fetal position to hold in heat and minimize exposed body surface area.

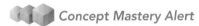
Concept Mastery Alert

Effects of Cold Stress in the Newborn's Brown Fat Metabolism

The newborn first experiences an increase in norepinephrine in response to a cold environment. This then influences the triglycerides to stimulate brown fat metabolism.

An environment in which body temperature is maintained without an increase in metabolic rate or oxygen use is called a **neutral thermal environment**. Within a neutral thermal environment, the rates of oxygen consumption and metabolism are minimal, and internal body temperature is maintained because of thermal balance. A neutral thermal environment promotes growth and stability, conserves energy for basic bodily functions, and minimizes heat (energy) and water loss (Knobel, 2014). Because newborns have difficulty maintaining their body heat through shivering or other mechanisms, they need a higher environmental temperature to maintain a neutral thermal environment. If the environmental temperature decreases, the newborn responds by consuming more oxygen. The respiratory rate increases (tachypnea) in response to the increased need for oxygen. As a result the newborn's metabolic rate increases.

As noted earlier, the newborn's primary method of heat production is through nonshivering thermogenesis. This is a process in which brown fat (adipose tissue) is oxidized in response to cold exposure. Brown fat is a special kind of highly vascular fat found only in newborns. Brown adipose tissue is a unique tissue that is able to convert chemical energy directly into heat when activated by the sympathetic nervous system. It is produced during the third trimester; ordinarily disappears by 3 to 5 weeks after birth and is vital for thermogenesis. The brown coloring is derived from the fat's rich supply of blood vessels and nerve endings. These fat deposits, which are capable of intense metabolic activity—and thus can generate a great deal of heat—are found between the scapulae, axillae, at the nape of the neck, in the mediastinum, and in areas surrounding the kidneys and adrenal glands. Brown fat makes up about 6% of term body weight in the full-term newborn (Betz & Enerback, 2015). When the newborn experiences a cold environment, norepinephrine is released. This in turn stimulates brown fat metabolism by breaking down triglycerides. Cardiac output increases, increasing blood flow through the brown fat tissue. Subsequently, this blood becomes warmed as a result of the increased metabolic activity of the brown fat (Fig. 17.4).

Newborns can experience heat loss through all four mechanisms, ultimately resulting in cold stress. **Cold stress** is excessive heat loss that requires a newborn

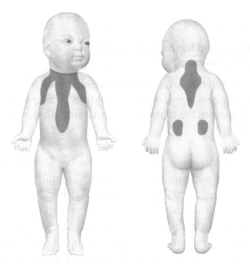

FIGURE 17.4 Areas of brown fat in a newborn.

to use compensatory mechanisms (such as nonshivering thermogenesis and tachypnea) to maintain core body temperature (Davidson, 2014). The consequences of cold stress can be quite severe. As the body temperature decreases, the newborn becomes less active, lethargic, hypotonic, and weaker. All newborns are at risk for cold stress, particularly within the first 12 hours of life. However, preterm newborns are at the greatest risk for cold stress and experience more profound effects than full-term newborns because they have fewer fat stores, poorer vasomotor responses, and less insulation to cope with a hypothermic event.

Cold stress in the newborn can lead to the following problems if not reversed: depleted brown fat stores, increased oxygen needs, respiratory distress, increased glucose consumption leading to hypoglycemia, metabolic acidosis, jaundice, hypoxia, and decreased surfactant production (Mattson & Smith, 2015).

Take Note!

Nurses must be aware of the thermoregulatory needs of the newborn and must ensure that these needs are met to provide the newborn with the best start possible. Maintenance of temperature stability should be focused on preventative measures.

To minimize the effects of cold stress and maintain an NTE, the following interventions are helpful:
• Prewarming blankets and hats to reduce heat loss through conduction
• Keeping the infant transporter (warmed isolette) fully charged and heated at all times
• Drying the newborn completely after birth to prevent heat loss from evaporation
• Encouraging skin-to-skin contact with the mother if the newborn is stable
• Promoting early breast-feeding to provide fuels for nonshivering thermogenesis

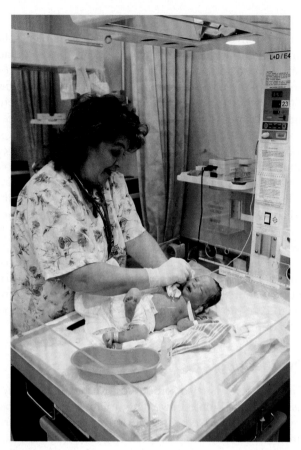

FIGURE 17.5 Bathing a newborn under a radiant warmer to prevent heat loss.

• Using heated and humidified oxygen
• Always using radiant warmers and double-wall isolettes to prevent heat loss from radiation
• Deferring bathing until the newborn is medically stable, and using a radiant heat source while bathing (Fig. 17.5)
• Avoiding the placement of a skin temperature probe over a bony area or one with brown fat, because it does not give an accurate assessment of the whole body temperature (most temperature probes are placed over the liver when the newborn is supine or side-lying)

The preceding interventions allow the newborn to minimize his or her metabolic rate and oxygen consumption, thereby conserving vital energy stores required for optimum growth.

Hepatic System Function

The liver has an essential role in the synthesis, degradation, and regulation of pathways involved in the metabolism of carbohydrates, proteins, lipids, trace elements, and vitamins. At birth, the newborn's liver slowly assumes the functions that the placenta handled during fetal life. Most enzymatic pathways are present in the newborn, but are inactive at birth and generally become fully active at 3 months of age. These functions include blood coagulation, and also iron storage, carbohydrate metabolism, and conjugation of bilirubin, as discussed next. Glycogen reserves provide energy and may become depleted if the metabolic needs of the newborn increase, such as during cold or respiratory stress.

Iron Storage

As red blood cells are destroyed after birth, their iron is released and stored by the liver until new red cells need to be produced. Newborn iron stores are determined by total body hemoglobin content and length of gestation. If the mother's iron intake was adequate during pregnancy, sufficient iron has been stored in the newborn's liver for use during the first 6 months of age.

Carbohydrate Metabolism

Glucose is an essential fuel for brain metabolism. When the placenta is lost at birth, the maternal glucose supply is cut off. Initially, the newborn's serum glucose levels decline. Newborns must learn to regulate their blood glucose concentration and adjust to an intermittent feeding schedule. Usually, a term newborn's blood glucose level is 70% to 80% of the maternal blood glucose level at birth. Hypoglycemia is one of the most frequent problems encountered, and maintaining glucose homeostasis is one of the important physiologic events during the fetal-to-newborn transition. During the first 24 to 48 hours of life, as normal neonates transition from intrauterine to extrauterine life, their plasma glucose levels are usually lower than later in life (Thornton et al., 2015).

Glucose is the main source of energy for the first several hours after birth. With the newborn's increased energy needs after birth, the liver releases glucose from glycogen stores for the first 24 hours. Initiating early breast-feeding or bottle feeding helps to stabilize the newborn's blood glucose levels. No evidence supports universal invasive routine measurement of glucose in healthy term newborns. Selective screening of at-risk newborns is more appropriate (Adamkin, 2015).

Bilirubin Conjugation

The liver is also responsible for the conjugation of bilirubin—a yellow-to-orange bile pigment produced by the breakdown of red blood cells. In utero, elimination of bilirubin in the blood is handled by the placenta and the mother's liver. However, once the cord is cut, the newborn must now assume this function.

Bilirubin normally circulates in plasma, is taken up by liver cells, and is changed to a water-soluble pigment that is excreted in the bile. This conjugated form of bilirubin is excreted from liver cells as a constituent of bile.

The principal source of bilirubin in the newborn is the hemolysis of erythrocytes. This is a normal occurrence after birth, when fewer red blood cells are needed to maintain extrauterine life. When red blood cells die after approximately 80 days of life, the heme in their hemoglobin is converted to bilirubin. Bilirubin is released in an unconjugated form called indirect bilirubin, which is fat soluble. Enzymes, proteins, and different cells in the reticuloendothelial system and liver process the unconjugated bilirubin into conjugated bilirubin or direct bilirubin. This form is water soluble and now enters the gastrointestinal system via the bile and is eventually excreted through feces. The kidneys also excrete a small amount.

Newborns produce bilirubin at a rate of approximately 6 to 8 mg/kg/day. This is more than twice the production rate in adults, primarily because of relative polycythemia and increased red blood cell turnover. Bilirubin production typically declines to the adult level within 10 to 14 days after birth (Bhutani et al., 2015). In addition, the metabolic pathways of the liver are relatively immature and thus cannot conjugate bilirubin as quickly as needed.

Failure of the liver cells to break down and excrete bilirubin can cause an increased amount of bilirubin in the bloodstream, leading to jaundice (Sharma et al., 2014). Bilirubin is toxic to the body and must be excreted. Blood tests ordered to determine bilirubin levels measure bilirubin in the serum. Total bilirubin is a combination of indirect (unconjugated) and direct (conjugated) bilirubin. When unconjugated bilirubin pigment is deposited in the skin and mucous membranes as a result of increased bilirubin levels, **jaundice**, also known as icterus, develops, with a yellowing of the skin, sclera, and mucous membranes. Visible jaundice as a result of increased blood bilirubin levels occurs in more than half of all healthy newborns. Even in healthy term newborns, extremely elevated blood levels of bilirubin during the first week of life can cause bilirubin encephalopathy, a permanent and devastating form of brain damage (Wong & Bhutani, 2015).

Common risk factors for the development of jaundice include fetal–maternal blood group incompatibility, prematurity, asphyxia at birth, an insufficient intake of milk during breast-feeding, drugs (such as diazepam [Valium], oxytocin [Pitocin], sulfisoxazole/erythromycin [Pediazole], and chloramphenicol [Chloromycetin]), maternal gestational diabetes, infrequent feedings, male gender, trauma during birth, resulting in cephalhematoma, cutaneous bruising from birth trauma, polycythemia, previous sibling with hyperbilirubinemia, intrauterine infections such as TORCH (toxoplasmosis, other viruses, rubella, cytomegalovirus, herpes simplex viruses), and ethnicity such as Asian or Native American (Moses, 2015).

The causes of newborn jaundice can be classified into three groups based on the mechanism of accumulation:

1. Bilirubin overproduction, such as from blood incompatibility (Rh or ABO), drugs, trauma at birth, polycythemia, delayed cord clamping, and breast milk jaundice
2. Decreased bilirubin conjugation, as seen in physiologic jaundice, hypothyroidism, and breast-feeding
3. Impaired bilirubin excretion, as seen in biliary obstruction (biliary atresia, gallstones, neoplasm), sepsis, hepatitis, chromosomal abnormality (Turner syndrome, trisomies 18 and 21), and drugs (aspirin, acetaminophen, sulfa, alcohol, steroids, antibiotics) (Nagtalon-Ramos, 2014)

Jaundice in the newborn is discussed in more detail in Chapter 24.

Gastrointestinal System Adaptations

The full-term newborn has the capacity to swallow, digest, metabolize, and absorb food taken in soon after birth. At birth, the pH of the stomach contents is mildly acidic, reflecting the pH of the amniotic fluid. The once-sterile gut changes rapidly, depending on what feeding is received. Bowel sounds are normally heard shortly after birth, but may be hypoactive on the first day.

Mucosal Barrier Protection

Humans start their development in a sterile intrauterine environment, but from the very moment of birth all epithelial surfaces in direct contact with the environment (skin, respiratory, gastrointestinal, and urogenital tract) are colonized by microorganisms. An important adaptation of the gastrointestinal system is the development of a mucosal barrier to prevent the penetration of harmful substances (bacteria, toxins, and antigens) present within the intestinal lumen. At birth, the newborn must be prepared to deal with bacterial colonization of the gut. Colonization is dependent on oral intake. Nutrition, be it breast milk or formula, plays a major role in early colonization patterns in the neonatal gut. It usually occurs within 24 hours of age and is required for the production of vitamin K (Gritz & Bhandari, 2015). After birth, environmental, oral, and cutaneous microbes from the mother will be mechanically transferred to the newborn by several processes including suckling, kissing, and caressing. Thus, the proximity of the birth canal and the anus, as well as parental expression of neonatal care, are effective methods of ensuring transmission of microbes from one generation to the next. If harmful substances are allowed to penetrate the mucosal epithelial barrier

under pathologic conditions, they can cause inflammatory and allergic reactions (Nylund et al., 2014).

Take Note!

Human breast milk provides a passive mechanism to protect the newborn against the dangers of a deficient intestinal defense system. It contains antibodies, viable leukocytes, and many other substances that can interfere with bacterial colonization and prevent harmful penetration.

Stomach and Digestion

The newborn must rapidly adapt from receiving all nutrient and energy requirements via the placenta to obtaining them orally after birth. The physiologic capacity of the newborn stomach is considerably less than its anatomic capacity. There is a rapid gain in physiologic capacity during the first 4 days of life. After the first 4 days, the anatomic and physiologic capacities more closely approximate each other. Researchers have found that for the first 24 hours after birth, the newborn's small stomach does not stretch to hold more, as it will within a day or two later (Batchelor, 2014). This explains the experience of countless hospital nurses who have learned the hard way that when newborns are fed an ounce or two by bottle during the first day of life, most of it tends to come right back up. The walls of the newborn stomach stay firm, expelling extra milk rather than stretching to hold it.

For bottle-fed newborns, small, frequent feedings set up a healthy eating pattern right from the start (breast-fed newborns self-regulate how much they consume). Experts now advise adults that it is healthier to eat smaller amounts more often and the same is true for babies and children. Coaxing an infant to take more milk leads to overfeeding. If feeling overfull at feedings becomes the norm for a young infant, this may lead to unhealthy eating habits that contribute to childhood and adult obesity later. Early onset obesity is a precursor to a life-long weight struggle and numerous comorbidities (Redsell et al., 2015; Reilly & Hughes, 2015).

The cardiac sphincter and nervous control of the stomach is immature, which may lead to uncoordinated peristaltic activity and frequent regurgitation. Immaturity of the pharyngoesophageal sphincter and absence of lower esophageal peristaltic waves also contribute to the reflux of gastric contents. Avoiding overfeeding and stimulating frequent burping may minimize regurgitation. Most digestive enzymes are available at birth, allowing newborns to digest simple carbohydrates and protein. However, they have limited ability to digest complex carbohydrates and fats, because amylase and lipase levels are low at birth. As a result, newborns excrete a fair amount of lipids, resulting in fatty stools.

Adequate digestion and absorption are essential for newborn growth and development. Normally, term newborns lose 5% to 10% of their birth weight as a result of insufficient caloric intake within the first week after birth, shifting of intracellular water to extracellular space, and insensible water loss. To gain weight, the term newborn requires an intake of 108 kcal/kg/day from birth to 6 months of age. Understanding the role and importance of nutrition in early postnatal life on growth and development is vital, but how it links to later health has the potential of health benefits for all future generations (Robinson, 2015).

Bowel Elimination

The frequency, consistency, and type of stool passed by newborns vary widely. The evolution of a stool pattern begins with a newborn's first stool, which is meconium. **Meconium** is composed of amniotic fluid, shed mucosal cells, intestinal secretions, and blood. It is greenish black, has a tarry consistency, and is usually passed within 12 to 24 hours of birth. The first meconium stool passed is semisterile, but this changes rapidly with ingestion of bacteria through feedings. After feedings are initiated, a transitional stool develops, which is greenish brown to yellowish brown, thinner in consistency, and seedy in appearance. If breast-fed, the stools will resemble light mustard with seed-like particles. If formula-fed, the stools will be tan or yellow in color and firmer. The frequency of bowel movements varies widely from one infant to another.

Take Note!

Newborns that are fed early pass stools sooner, which helps to reduce bilirubin buildup (Mattson & Smith, 2015).

The last development in the stool pattern is the milk stool. Its characteristics differ in breast-fed and formula-fed newborns. The stools of the breast-fed newborn are yellow-gold, loose, and stringy to pasty in consistency, and typically sour-smelling. The stools of the formula-fed newborn vary depending on the type of formula ingested. They may be yellow, yellow-green, or greenish and loose, pasty, or formed in consistency, and they have an unpleasant odor.

Renal System Changes

A full complement of one million nephrons is present by 34 weeks gestation. The glomeruli and nephrons are functionally immature at birth, resulting in a reduced glomerular filtration rate (GFR) and limited concentrating ability. A limited ability to concentrate urine and the reduced GFR make the newborn susceptible to both dehydration and fluid overload (Sharma et al.,

2014). Frequently the newborn's kidneys are described as immature, but they are able to carry out their usual responsibilities and can handle the challenge of excretion and maintaining acid–base balance. Only when the newborn is faced with unexpected imbalances of water, electrolytes, or a disruption of acid–base status secondary to a preterm birth or illness does it lack the ability to handle the body's fluid homeostasis. A newborn infant's body mass is 75% water, the highest proportion of body water at any stage of a person's life. The majority of term newborns void immediately after birth, indicating adequate renal function. Although the newborn's kidneys can produce urine, they are limited in their ability to concentrate it until about 3 months of age, when the kidneys mature more. Until that time, a newborn voids frequently and the urine has a low specific gravity (1.001 to 1.020). About six to eight voidings daily is average for most newborns; this indicates adequate fluid intake (Harshman & Brophy, 2014).

The renal cortex is relatively underdeveloped at birth and does not reach maturity until 12 to 18 months of age. The GFR is the amount of fluid filtered each minute by all the glomeruli of both kidneys and is one index of kidney function. At birth, the newborn's GFR is approximately 30% of normal adult values, reaching approximately 50% of normal adult values by the 10th day of life and full adult values by the first year of life (Chishti, 2014). The low GFR and the limited excretion and conservation capability of the kidney affect the newborn's ability to excrete salt, water loads, and drugs.

Take Note!

The possibility of fluid overload is increased in newborns; keep this in mind when administering intravenous therapy to a newborn.

Immune System Adaptations

Essential to the newborn's survival is the ability to respond effectively to hostile environmental forces. The newborn's immune system begins working early in gestation, but many of the responses do not function adequately during the early neonatal period. The newborn is protected from certain infections, in part because of maternal antibodies circulating in their system until about 6 months of age. Immunoglobulin G (IgG) crosses the placenta to the fetus while in utero. Newborns who are breast-fed receive antibodies from the breast milk, which includes IgE, IgA, IgM, and IgG (Nagtalon-Ramos, 2014). The risk of acquiring an infection is great because a newborn's immune system is immature and is not able to respond for long periods of time to fight infections. The intrauterine environment usually protects the fetus from harmful microorganisms and the need for defensive immunologic responses. With exposure to a wide variety of microorganisms at birth, the newborn must develop a balance between its host defenses and the hostile environmental organisms to ensure a safe transition to the outside world. Healthy infants begin to produce their own antibodies, starting at 2 to 3 months of age.

Responses of the immune system serve three purposes: defense (protection from invading organisms), homeostasis (elimination of worn-out host cells), and surveillance (recognition and removal of enemy cells). The newborn's immune system response involves recognition of the pathogen or other foreign material, followed by activation of mechanisms to react against and eliminate it. All immune responses primarily involve leukocytes (white blood cells).

The immune system's responses can be divided into two categories: natural and acquired immunity. These mechanisms are interrelated and interdependent; both are required for immunocompetency.

Natural Immunity

Natural immunity includes responses or mechanisms that do not require previous exposure to the microorganism or antigen to operate efficiently. Physical barriers (such as intact skin and mucous membranes), chemical barriers (such as gastric acids and digestive enzymes), and resident nonpathologic organisms make up the newborn's natural immune system. Natural immunity involves the most basic host defense responses: ingestion and killing of microorganisms by phagocytic cells.

Acquired Immunity

Acquired immunity involves two primary processes: (1) the development of circulating antibodies or immunoglobulins capable of targeting specific invading agents (antigens) for destruction and (2) formation of activated lymphocytes designed to destroy foreign invaders. Acquired immunity is absent until after the first invasion by a foreign organism or toxin.

Immunologic ability depends heavily on immunoglobulins such as IgG, IgM, and IgA. The newborn depends largely on these three immunoglobulins for defense against microorganisms associated with illness. Newborns remain very susceptible to infections for months.

IgG is the major immunoglobulin and the most abundant, making up about 80% of all circulating antibodies (Martin, Fanaroff, & Walsh, 2014). It is found in serum and interstitial fluid. It is the only class able to cross the placenta, with active placental transfer beginning at approximately 20 to 22 weeks' gestation. IgG produces antibodies against bacteria, bacterial toxins, and viral agents.

IgA is the second most abundant immunoglobulin in the serum. IgA does not cross the placenta, and maximum levels are reached during childhood. This immunoglobulin is believed to protect mucous membranes from viruses and bacteria. IgA is predominantly found in the gastrointestinal and respiratory tracts, tears, saliva, colostrum, and breast milk.

Take Note!

A major source of IgA is human breast milk, so breast-feeding is believed to have significant immunologic advantages over formula feeding (Walker, 2014).

IgM is found in blood and lymph fluid and is the first immunoglobulin to respond to infection. It does not cross the placenta, and levels are generally low at birth unless a congenital intrauterine infection is present. IgM offers a major source of protection from blood-borne infections. The predominant antibodies formed during neonatal or intrauterine infection are of this class.

Integumentary System Adaptations

The newborn skin is critical to its transition from intrauterine to extrauterine environments and to the journey to self-sufficiency. The newborn's skin is a large organ, making up approximately 13% of body weight in contrast to 3% of body weight in an adult. It is sensitive, fragile, with a neutral pH on the surface, lower lipid content, and higher water content when compared with adults. Because of these characteristics, newborn skin is vulnerable to injury and infections (Visscher, et al., 2015). The most important function of the skin is to provide a protective barrier between the body and the environment. It limits the loss of water, prevents absorption of harmful agents, protects thermoregulation and fat storage, and protects against physical trauma. The epidermal barrier begins to develop during midgestation and is fully formed by about 32 weeks' gestation. Although the neonatal epidermis is similar to the adult epidermis in thickness and lipid composition, skin development is not complete at birth (King et al., 2015). Although the basic structure is the same as that of an adult, the less mature the newborn, the less mature the skin functions. Fewer fibrils connect the dermis and epidermis in the newborn compared with the adult. Also in a newborn, the risk of injury producing a break in the skin from the use of tapes and monitors and from handling is greater than for an adult. Improper handling of the newborn during daily skin care practices, such as bathing, can cause damage, prevent healing, and interfere with the normal maturation process.

Newborns vary greatly in appearance. Many of the variations are temporary and reflect the physiologic adaptations that the newborn is experiencing. Skin coloring varies, depending on the newborn's age, race, or ethnic group; temperature; and whether he or she is crying. Skin color changes with both the environment and health status. At birth, the newborn's skin is dark red to purple. As the newborn begins to breathe air his or her skin color changes to red. This redness normally begins to fade the first day.

Neurologic System Adaptations

The nervous system is immature and continues to develop to achieve a full complement of cortical and brainstem cells by 1 year of age. The brain increases its size threefold during the first year of life. The nervous system consists of the brain, spinal cord, 12 cranial nerves, and a variety of spinal nerves that come from the spinal cord. Neurologic development follows cephalocaudal (head-to-toe) and proximal–distal (center-to-outside) patterns. Myelin develops early on in sensory impulse transmitters. Thus, the newborn has an acute sense of hearing, smell, and taste. The newborn's sensory capabilities include:

- *Hearing*—well developed at birth, responds to noise by turning to sound.
- *Taste*—ability to distinguish between sweet and sour by 72 hours old.
- *Smell*—ability to distinguish between mother's breast milk and breast milk from others.
- *Touch*—sensitivity to pain, responds to tactile stimuli.
- *Vision*—is incomplete at birth. Maturation is dependent on nutrition and visual stimulation. Newborns have ability to focus only on close objects (8 to 10 inches away) with a visual acuity of 20/140; they can track objects in midline or beyond (90 inches). This is the least mature sense at birth. The ability to fix, follow, and be alert is indicative of an intact CNS (King et al., 2015).

Remember Maria, the new mother who is worried that her daughter can't see? What might the new mother notice about her daughter's behavior? What might be the new mother's expectations?

Congenital Reflexes

Successful adaptations demonstrated by the respiratory, circulatory, thermoregulatory, and musculoskeletal systems indirectly indicate the central nervous system's successful transition from fetal to extrauterine life, because the central nervous system plays a major role in all these adaptations. In the newborn, congenital reflexes are the hallmarks of maturity of the central nervous system, viability, and adaptation to extrauterine life.

The presence and strength of a reflex is an important indication of neurologic development and function. A **reflex** is an involuntary muscular response to a sensory stimulus. It is built into the nervous system and does not need the intervention of conscious thought to take effect. The physical assessment of the neurologic system

of the newborn includes evaluating the major reflexes (gag, Babinski, Moro, and Galant) and minor ones (finger grasp, toe grasp, rooting, sucking, head righting, stepping, and tonic neck).

To assess each reflex, the nurse progresses methodically, taking care to document each finding (Weber & Kelly, 2014). Many neonatal reflexes disappear with maturation, although some remain throughout adulthood. The arcs of these reflexes end at different levels of the spine and brain stem, reflecting the function of the cranial nerves and motor systems. The ways newborns blink, move their limbs, focus on a caretaker's face, turn toward sound, suck, swallow, and respond to the environment are all indications of their neurologic abilities. Congenital defects within the central nervous system are frequently not overt but may be revealed in abnormalities in tone, posture, or behavior (Davidson, 2014). Damage to the nervous system (birth trauma, perinatal hypoxia) during the birthing process can cause delays in the normal growth, development, and functioning of the newborn. Early identification may help to identify the cause and to start early intervention to decrease long-term complications or permanent sequelae.

Newborn reflexes are assessed to evaluate neurologic function and development. Absent or abnormal reflexes in a newborn, persistence of a reflex past the age when it is normally lost, or redevelopment of an infantile reflex in an older child or adult may indicate neurologic pathology. (See Chapter 18 for a description of newborn reflex assessment.)

The Healthy Start nurse explained to Maria that all newborns are born with some degree of myopia (inability to see distances) and that 20/20 vision is not generally achieved until 2 years of age. What developmental information should the nurse discuss with Maria?

BEHAVIORAL ADAPTATIONS

In addition to adapting physiologically, the newborn also adapts behaviorally. All newborns progress through a specific pattern of events after birth, regardless of their gestational age or the type of birth they experienced.

Behavioral Patterns

The newborn usually demonstrates a predictable pattern of behavior during the first several hours after birth, characterized by two periods of reactivity separated by a sleep phase. Behavioral adaptation is a defined progression of events triggered by stimuli from the extrauterine environment after birth.

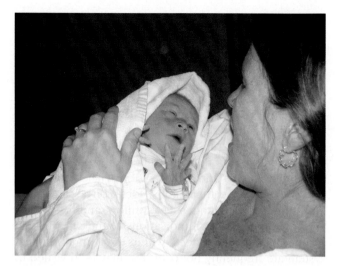

FIGURE 17.6 The first period of reactivity is an optimal time for interaction.

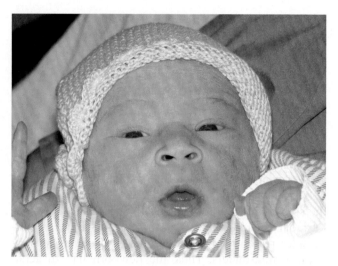

FIGURE 17.7 Newborn during the second period of reactivity. Note the newborn's wide-eyed interest.

First Period of Reactivity

The first period of reactivity begins at birth and may last from 30 minutes up to 2 hours. The newborn is alert and moving and may appear hungry. This period is characterized by myoclonic movements of the eyes, spontaneous Moro reflexes, sucking motions, chewing, rooting, and fine tremors of the extremities. Muscle tone and motor activity are increased (Healy & Fallon, 2014). Respiration and heart rate are elevated but gradually begin to slow as the next period begins.

This period of alertness allows parents to interact with their newborn and to enjoy close contact with their new baby (Fig. 17.6). The appearance of sucking and rooting behaviors provides a good opportunity for initiating breast-feeding. Many newborns latch on the nipple and suck well at this first experience.

Period of Decreased Responsiveness

At 30 to 120 minutes of age, the newborn enters the second stage of transition—that of the *sleep period* or a decrease in activity. This phase is referred to as a period of decreased responsiveness. Movements are less jerky and less frequent. Heart and respiratory rates decline as the newborn enters the sleep phase. The muscles become relaxed, and responsiveness to outside stimuli diminishes. During this phase, it is difficult to arouse or interact with the newborn. No interest in sucking is shown. This quiet time can be used for both mother and newborn to remain close and rest together after labor and the birthing experience.

Second Period of Reactivity

The second period of reactivity begins as the newborn awakens and shows an interest in environmental stimuli. This period lasts 2 to 8 hours in the normal newborn (Davidson, 2014). Heart and respiratory rates increase. Peristalsis also increases. Thus, it is not uncommon for the newborn to pass meconium or void during this period. In addition, motor activity and muscle tone increase in conjunction with an increase in muscular coordination (Fig. 17.7).

Interaction between the mother and the newborn during this second period of reactivity is encouraged if the mother has rested and desires it. This period also provides a good opportunity for the parents to examine their newborn and ask questions.

 Take Note!

Teaching about feeding, positioning for feeding, and diaper-changing techniques can be reinforced during this time.

Behavioral Responses

Newborn development is a reflection of the dynamic relationship between endowment and environment. Newborns demonstrate several predictable responses when interacting with their environment. How they react to the world around them is termed a **neurobehavioral response**. It comprises predictable periods that are probably triggered by external stimuli. Expected newborn behaviors include orientation, habituation, motor maturity, self-quieting ability, and social behaviors. Any deviation in behavioral responses requires further assessment, because it may indicate a complex neurobehavioral problem.

Orientation

The response of newborns to stimuli is called *orientation*. They become more alert when they sense a new stimulus in their environment. Orientation reflects newborns' response to auditory and visual stimuli, demonstrated by their movement of head and eyes to focus on that stimulus. Newborns prefer the human face and bright shiny objects. As the face or object comes into their line of vision, newborns respond by staring at the object intently. Newborns use this sensory capacity to become familiar with people and objects in their surroundings.

Remember Maria, who was concerned about her newborn daughter's vision? She told the nurse that her daughter did not show any interest in her pastel-colored homemade mobile she had hung across the room from her crib. What suggestions can the nurse make to Maria regarding the placement of the mobile and the types and colors of objects used to promote orientation in her newborn daughter?

Habituation

Habituation is the newborn's ability to process and respond to visual and auditory stimuli. It is a measure of how well and appropriately an infant responds to the environment. Habituation is the ability to block out external stimuli after the newborn has become accustomed to the activity. During the first 24 hours after birth, newborns should increase their ability to habituate to environmental stimuli and sleep. Habituation provides a useful indicator of their neurobehavioral intactness.

Motor Maturity

Motor maturity depends on gestational age and involves evaluation of posture, tone, coordination, and movements. These activities enable newborns to control and coordinate movement. When stimulated, newborns with good motor organization demonstrate movements that are rhythmic and spontaneous. Bringing the hand up to the mouth is an example of good motor organization. As newborns adapt to their new environment, smoother movements should be observed. Such motor behavior is a good indicator of the newborn's ability to respond and adapt accordingly; it indicates that the central nervous system is processing stimuli appropriately.

Self-Quieting Ability

Self-quieting ability (also called self-soothing) refers to newborns' ability to quiet and comfort themselves. Newborns vary in their ability to console themselves or to be consoled. "Consolability" is how newborns are able to change from the crying state to an active alert, quiet alert, drowsy, or sleep state. They console themselves by hand-to-mouth movements and sucking, alerting to external stimuli, and motor activity (Karp, 2014). Recent research outlines five things (the five "**S**'s") that parents can do to calm a fussy infant:

1. **S**waddling tightly
2. **S**ide/stomach position on the lap of the caretaker
3. **S**hushing loudly or continuous white noise
4. **S**winging using any rhythmic movement
5. **S**ucking (Karp, 2014)

Assisting parents to identify consoling behaviors to quiet their newborn if the newborn is not able to self-quiet is important.

Social Behaviors

Newborns begin extrauterine life able to engage in it with their sensory capabilities and communicate with their environment through a complex repertoire of behaviors. Social behaviors include cuddling and snuggling into the arms of the parent when the newborn is held. Usually newborns are very sensitive to being touched, cuddled, and held. Cuddliness is very important to parents because they frequently gauge their ability to care for their newborn by the newborn's acceptance or positive response to their actions. This can be assessed by the degree to which the newborn nestles into the contours of the holder's arms. Most newborns cuddle, but some will resist. Assisting parents to assume comforting behaviors (e.g., by cooing while holding their newborn) and praising them for their efforts can help foster cuddling behaviors.

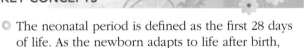

KEY CONCEPTS

- The neonatal period is defined as the first 28 days of life. As the newborn adapts to life after birth, numerous physiologic changes occur.

- At birth, the cardiopulmonary system must switch from fetal to neonatal circulation and from placental to pulmonary gas exchange.

- One of the most crucial adaptations that the newborn makes at birth is the adjustment of a fluid medium exchange from the placenta to the lungs and that of a gaseous environment.

- Neonatal red blood cells have a life span of 80 to 100 days in comparison with the adult red blood cell life span of 120 days. This difference in red blood cell life span causes several adjustment problems.

- Thermoregulation is the maintenance of balance between heat loss and heat production. It is a critical physiologic function that is closely related to the transition and survival of the newborn.

- The newborn's primary method of heat production is through nonshivering thermogenesis, a process in which brown fat (adipose tissue) is oxidized in response to cold exposure. Brown fat is a special kind of highly vascular fat found only in newborns.

- Heat loss in the newborn is the result of four mechanisms: conduction, convection, evaporation, and radiation.

- Responses of the immune system serve three purposes: defense (protection from invading organisms), homeostasis (elimination of worn-out host cells), and surveillance (recognition and removal of enemy cells).

- In the newborn, congenital reflexes are the hallmarks of maturity of the CNS, viability, and adaptation to extrauterine life.

- The newborn usually demonstrates a predictable pattern of behavior during the first several hours after birth, characterized by two periods of reactivity separated by a sleep phase.

References and Recommended Readings

Adamkin, D. H. (2015). Metabolic screening and postnatal glucose homeostasis in the newborn. *Pediatric Clinics of North America, 62*(2), 385–409.

American Academy of Pediatrics [AAP]. (2013). Statement of endorsement: Timing of umbilical cord clamping after birth. *Pediatrics, 131*(4), e1323.

American College of Obstetricians & Gynecologists [ACOG]. (2012). Committee Opinion No. 543: Timing of umbilical cord clamping after birth. *Obstetrics & Gynecology, 120*(6), 1522–1526.

Andersson, O., Domellöf, M., Andersson, D., & Hellström-Westas, L. (2014). Effect of delayed vs early umbilical cord clamping on iron status and neurodevelopment at age 12 months: A randomized clinical trial. *JAMA pediatrics, 168*(6), 547–554.

Batchelor, H. (2014). Pediatric development: Gastrointestinal. In *Pediatric formulations* (pp. 43–54). New York, NY: Springer.

Betz, M. J., & Enerbäck, S. (2015). Human brown adipose tissue: What we have learned so far. *Diabetes, 64*(7), 2352–2360.

Bhutani, V. K., Wong, R. J., Vreman, H. J., & Stevenson, D. K. (2015). Bilirubin production and hour-specific bilirubin levels. *Journal of Perinatology, 35*(9), 735–738.

Bope, E. T., & Kellerman, R. D. (2015). *Conn's current therapy 2015*. Philadelphia, PA: Elsevier.

Chishti, A. S. (2014). Assessment of renal function. In *Kidney and urinary tract diseases in the newborn* (pp. 117–126). Berlin, Heidelberg, Germany: Springer.

Creasy, R. K., Resnik, R., Iams, J. D., Lockwood, C. J., Moore, T. R., & Greene, M. F. (2014). *Creasy & Resnik's maternal-fetal medicine: Principles and practice* (7th ed.). St. Louis, MO: Elsevier.

Cuneo, B. (2014). Transition from fetal to neonatal circulation. In *Pediatric and congenital cardiology, cardiac surgery and intensive care,*(pp. 179–199). Berlin, Heidelberg, Germany: Springer.

Davidson, M. R. (2014). *Fast facts for the neonatal nurse: A nursing orientation and care guide in a nutshell*. New York, NY: Springer.

Essa, R. M., & Ismail, N. I. (2015). Effect of early maternal/newborn skin-to-skin contact after birth on the duration of third stage of labor and initiation of breastfeeding. *Journal of Nursing Education and Practice, 5*(4), 98–107.

Fillipps, D. J., & Bucciarelli, R. L. (2015). Cardiac evaluation of the newborn. *Pediatric Clinics of North America, 62*(2), 471–489.

Fischbach, F., & Dunning, M. B. (2014). *Manual of laboratory and diagnostic tests* (9th ed.). Philadelphia, PA: Lippincott Williams & Wilkins.

Gritz, E. C., & Bhandari, V. (2015). The human neonatal gut microbiome: a brief review. *Frontiers in Pediatrics, 3*. 17–26.

Harshman, L. A., & Brophy, P. D. (2014). Development of renal function in the fetus and newborn. In *Kidney and urinary tract diseases in the newborn* (pp. 59–76). Berlin, Heidelberg, Germany: Springer.

Healy, P., & Fallon, A. (2014). Developments in neonatal care and nursing responses. *British Journal of Nursing, 23*(1), 21–24.

Hooper, S. B., Polglase, G. R., & Roehr, C. C. (2015). Cardiopulmonary changes with aeration of the newborn lung. *Pediatric Respiratory Reviews, 16*(3), 147–150.

Karp, H. (2014). *The happiest baby on the block*. New York, NY: Bantam Dell.

King, T. L., Brucker, M. C., Kriebs, J. M., Fahey, J. O., Gegor, C. L., & Varney, H. (2015). *Varney's midwifery* (5th ed.). Burlington, MA: Jones & Bartlett Learning.

Kluckow, M., & Hooper, S. B. (2015). Using physiology to guide time to cord clamping. *Seminars in Fetal and Neonatal Medicine, 20*(4), 225–231.

Knobel, R. B. (2014). Fetal and neonatal thermal physiology. *Newborn and Infant Nursing Reviews, 14*(2), 45–49.

Leslie, M. S. (2015). Perspectives on implementing delayed cord clamping. *Nursing for Women's Health, 19*(2), 164–176.

Martin, R. J., Fanaroff, A. A., & Walsh, M. C. (2014). *Neonatal-perinatal medicine* (10th ed.). Philadelphia, PA: Elsevier.

Mattson, S., & Smith, J. (2015). *Core curriculum for maternal-newborn nursing* (5th ed.). Philadelphia, PA: Elsevier.

McAdams, R. M. (2014). Time to implement delayed cord clamping. *Obstetrics & Gynecology, 123*(3), 549–552.

McCall, E., Alderdice, F., Halliday, H., Johnston, L., & Vohra, S. (2014). Challenges of minimizing heat loss at birth: A narrative overview of evidence-based thermal care interventions. *Newborn and Infant Nursing Reviews, 14*(2), 56–63.

Moses, S. (2015). Jaundice in newborns. *Family Practice Notebook*, Retrieved June 2015, from http://www.fpnotebook.com/NICU/GI/JndcInNwbrns.htm

Nagtalon-Ramos, J. (2014). *Maternal-newborn nursing care: Best evidence-based practices*. Philadelphia, PA: F.A. Davis Company.

Nylund, L., Satokari, R., Salminen, S., & de Vos, W. M. (2014). Intestinal microbiota during early life–impact on health and disease. *Proceedings of the Nutrition Society, 73*(04), 1–13.

Redsell, S. A., Edmonds, B., Swift, J. A., Siriwardena, A. N., Weng, S., Nathan, D., et al. (2015). Systematic review of randomized controlled trials of interventions that aim to reduce the risk, either directly or indirectly, of overweight and obesity in infancy and early childhood. *Maternal & Child Nutrition, 12*(1), 24–38. doi: 10.1111/mcn.12184

Reilly, J. J., & Hughes, A. R. (2015). Early life risk factors for childhood obesity. In L. Stewart & J. Thompson (Eds.), *Early years nutrition and healthy weight* (pp. 40–45). Hoboken, NJ: Wiley Blackwell Publishers.

Robinson, S. M. (2015). Infant nutrition and lifelong health: Current perspectives and future challenges. *Journal of Developmental Origins of Health and Disease, 6*(5), 384–389.

Sharma, A., Ford, S., & Calvert, J. (2014). Adaptation for life: A review of neonatal physiology. *Anesthesia & Intensive Care Medicine, 15*(3), 89–95.

Stave, U. (2014). *Perinatal physiology*. New York, NY: Springer.

Stark, A. R., & Eichenwald, E. C. (2016). Persistent pulmonary hypertension of the newborn. *UpToDate*, Retrieved from http://www.uptodate.com/contents/persistent-pulmonary-hypertension-of-the-newborn

Swanson, J. R., & Sinkin, R. A. (2015). Transition from fetus to newborn. *Pediatric Clinics of North America, 62*(2), 329–343.

Thornton, P. S., Stanley, C. A., De Leon, D. D., Harris, D., Haymond, M. W., Hussain, K., et al. (2015). Recommendations from the Pediatric Endocrine Society for evaluation and management of persistent hypoglycemia in neonates, infants, and children. *The Journal of Pediatrics, 167*(2), 238–245.

van Vonderen, J. J., Roest, A. A., Siew, M. L., Walther, F. J., Hooper, S. B., & te Pas, A. B. (2014). Measuring physiological changes during the transition to life after birth. *Neonatology, 105*(3), 230–242.

Verklan, T., & Walden, M. (2014). *Core curriculum for neonatal intensive care nursing* (4th ed.). St. Louis, MO: Elsevier.

Visscher, M. O., Adam, R., Brink, S., & Odio, M. (2015). Newborn infant skin: Physiology, development, and care. *Clinics in Dermatology, 33*(3), 271–280.

Walker, M. (2014). *Breastfeeding management for the clinician: Using the evidence* (3rd ed.). Burlington, MA: Jones & Bartlett Learning.

Weber, J., & Kelley, J. (2014). *Health assessment in nursing* (5th ed.). Philadelphia, PA: Lippincott Williams & Wilkins.

Wong, R. J., & Bhutani, V. K. (2016). Clinical manifestations of unconjugated hyperbilirubinemia in term and late preterm infants. *UpToDate*, Retrieved May 2016, from: http://www.uptodate.com/contents/clinical-manifestations-of-unconjugated-hyperbilirubinemia-in-term-and-late-preterm-infants

World Health Organization [WHO]. (2014). *Delayed clamping of the umbilical cord to reduce infant anemia* (Doc. No. WHO/RHR/14.19 ed.). Geneva, Switzerland: Author.

MULTIPLE-CHOICE QUESTIONS

1. When assessing the term newborn, the following are observed: newborn is alert, heart and respiratory rates have stabilized, and meconium has been passed. The nurse determines that the newborn is exhibiting behaviors indicating:
   a. Initial period of reactivity
   b. Second period of reactivity
   c. Decreased responsiveness period
   d. Sleep period for newborns

2. A nurse observes a 3-day-old term newborn that is starting to appear mildly jaundiced. What might explain this condition?
   a. Physiologic jaundice secondary to breast-feeding
   b. Hemolytic disease of the newborn due to blood incompatibility
   c. Exposing the newborn to high levels of oxygen
   d. Overfeeding the newborn with too much glucose water

3. After teaching a group of nursing students about thermoregulation and appropriate measures to prevent heat loss by evaporation, which of the following student behaviors would indicate successful teaching?
   a. Transporting the newborn in an isolette
   b. Maintaining a warm room temperature
   c. Placing the newborn on a warmed surface
   d. Drying the newborn immediately after birth

4. After birth, the nurse would expect which fetal structure to close as a result of increases in the pressure gradients on the left side of the heart?
   a. Foramen ovale
   b. Ductus arteriosus
   c. Ductus venosus
   d. Umbilical vein

5. Which of the following newborns could be described as breathing normally?
   a. Newborn A is breathing deeply, with a regular rhythm, at a rate of 20 bpm.
   b. Newborn B is breathing diaphragmatically with sternal retractions, at a rate of 70 bpm.
   c. Newborn C is breathing shallowly, with 40-second periods of apnea and cyanosis.
   d. Newborn D is breathing shallowly, at a rate of 36 bpm, with short periods of apnea.

6. When assessing a term newborn (6 hours old), the nurse auscultates bowel sounds and documents recent passing of meconium. These findings would indicate:
   a. Abnormal gastrointestinal newborn transition and needs to be reported
   b. An intestinal anomaly that needs immediate surgery
   c. A patent anus with no bowel obstruction and normal peristalsis
   d. A malabsorption syndrome, resulting in fatty stools

7. A nursing student questions the nursery nurse why they do not bathe the newborn immediately upon admission to the nursery observation area after birth. The nurse states that this would increase the risk of:
   a. Jaundice
   b. Infection
   c. Hypothermia
   d. Anemia

8. Because the newborn's red blood cells breakdown much sooner than those of an adult, what might result?
   a. Anemia
   b. Bruising
   c. Apnea
   d. Jaundice

9. The nurse performs a physical examination on a newborn 2 hours after birth. Which of the following findings indicate a need for a pediatric consultation? Select all that apply:
   a. Respiratory rate of 50 breaths per minute
   b. Intermittent episodes of apnea, lasting <10 seconds each
   c. Absent Moro reflex when startled
   d. Preauricular skin tag noted on left ear
   e. White raised bumps noted on nose and face
   f. Yellow blanching of the skin when pressure applied to the nose

CRITICAL THINKING EXERCISES

1. As the nurse manager, you have been orienting a new nurse in the nursery for the past few weeks. Although she has been demonstrating adequacy with most procedures, today you observe her bathing several newborns without covering them, weighing them on the scale without a cover, leaving the storage door open with the transporter nearby, and leaving the newborns' head covers and blankets off after showing them to family members through the nursery observation window.
   a. What is your impression of this behavior?
   b. What principles concerning thermoregulation need to be reinforced?
   c. How will you evaluate whether your instructions have been effective?

2. The most important adaptations for the newborn to make after birth are to establish respirations, make cardiovascular adjustments, and establish thermoregulation. Nursing care focuses on monitoring and supporting adjustments to extrauterine adaptation. Write appropriate nursing interventions to help achieve the following newborn adaptations:
   a. Respiratory adaptation
   b. Safety, including prevention of infection
   c. Thermoregulation

STUDY ACTIVITIES

1. While in the nursery clinical setting, identify the period of behavioral reactivity (first, inactivity, or second period) for two newborns born at different times. Share your findings during the post conference for that clinical day.

2. Dramatic changes occur in the cardiovascular system at birth. When the umbilical cord is clamped and the placenta is separated, there is a resultant increase in systemic blood pressure and changes to the three major fetal shunts (ductus venosus, foramen ovale, and ductus arteriosus) occur. Outline what happens to cause their functional closures during this period of transition.

3. Find two web sites about the transition to extrauterine life that can be shared with other nursing students as well as nursery nurses. Critique the information presented in terms of how accurate and current it is.

4. The most common mechanism of heat loss in the newborn is _____.

5. The newborn creates heat in three ways—by shivering, through muscle activity, and through thermogenesis by the metabolism of brown adipose tissue. Which is the most effective?

BRINGING IT ALL TOGETHER: CASE STUDY

An 18-year-old woman gave birth to her first infant 3 days ago, but she does not smile when the *Healthy Start* nurse greets her at a home visit. The nurse questions her about what has happened since she was discharged from the hospital 2 days ago. She tells the nurse that her breasts are swollen, hot, and very painful when touched. She states she knows that breast-feeding is best for her child, but she is not sure she wants to continue to breast-feed because of the pain. Her infant is lying on the bare kitchen table in only a diaper crying.

ASSESSMENT

On examining the woman's breasts, the nurse finds that they are both very swollen and hot to the touch, but there is no redness or palpated lump. (The client bites her lip and a tear falls from her eye when the nurse palpates her breasts). Milk drips freely from both nipples. Temperature is 37.7°C. The nurse examines the infant girl weighing 2,580 g. Her extremities are cyanotic and cold to touch. The infant has lost 100 g since birth and appears hungry. The nurse requests the client to breast-feed her infant so that she can observe the infant, and finds that the infant is having trouble grasping the very swollen areola. When the infant finally latches on, she does not seem to suck very vigorously.

Go to thePoint **to find questions to consider about this case.**

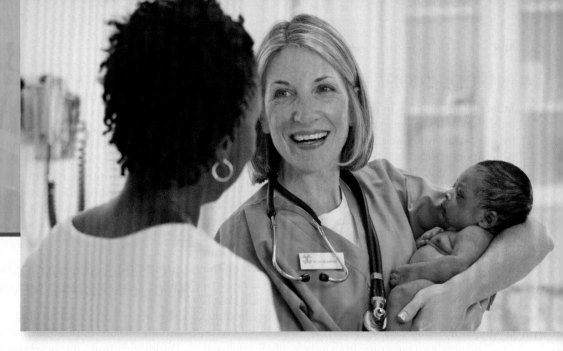

18

KEY TERMS

acrocyanosis

Apgar score

caput succedaneum

cephalhematoma

circumcision

Epstein's pearls

erythema toxicum

gestational age

harlequin sign

immunizations

infant abduction

milia

molding

Mongolian spots

nevus flammeus

nevus vasculosus

ophthalmia
   neonatorum

phototherapy

pseudo-
   menstruation

stork bites

vernix caseosa

Nursing Management of the Newborn

Learning Objectives

Upon completion of the chapter, you will be able to:

1. Perform the assessments needed during the immediate newborn period.

2. Employ interventions that meet the immediate needs of the term newborn.

3. Demonstrate the components of a typical physical examination of a newborn.

4. Distinguish common variations that can be noted during a newborn's physical examination.

5. Characterize common concerns in the newborn and appropriate interventions.

6. Compare the importance of the newborn screening tests.

7. Plan for common interventions that are appropriate during the early newborn period.

8. Analyze the nurse's role in meeting the newborn's nutritional needs.

9. Outline discharge planning content and education needed for the family with a newborn.

Kelly, a 16-year-old first-time mother, calls the hospital maternity unit 3 days after being discharged home. She tells the nurse that her newborn son "looks yellow, like a canary" and "isn't nursing well." She wonders what is wrong.

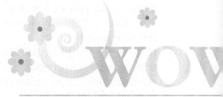

Words of Wisdom
You can send a more powerful message with your actions and behavior than with words alone.

INTRODUCTION

Immediately after the birth of a newborn, all mother and father/support persons/significant others are faced with the task of learning and understanding as much as possible about caring for this new family member, even if the parents already have other children. In their new or expanded role as parents, they will face many demands and challenges. For most, this is a wonderful, exciting time filled with many discoveries and much information.

Mother and father/support persons or significant others learn as they watch the nurse interacting with their newborn. Nurses play a major role in teaching the newborn's caretakers about normal newborn characteristics and about ways to foster optimal growth and development. This role is even more important today because of limited hospital stays.

The newborn has come from a dark, small, enclosed space in the mother's uterus into the bright, cold, extrauterine environment. Nurses can easily forget that they are caring for a small human being who is experiencing his or her first taste of human interaction outside the uterus. The newborn period is an extremely important one, and two national health goals have been developed to address this critical period (see the *Healthy People*

2020 feature; U.S. Department of Health and Human Services [USDHHS], 2010).

It is also easy to overlook the intensity with which mother and father/support persons/significant others and visitors observe the actions of nurses as they care for the new family member. Nurses need to serve as a model for giving nurturing care to newborns. This chapter provides information about assessment and interventions in the period immediately following the birth of a newborn and during the early newborn period.

NURSING MANAGEMENT DURING THE IMMEDIATE NEWBORN PERIOD

The period of transition from intrauterine to extrauterine life occurs during the first several hours after birth. During this time, the newborn is undergoing numerous adaptations, many of which are occurring simultaneously (see Chapter 17 for more information on the newborn's adaptation). The neonate's temperature, respirations, and cardiovascular dynamics stabilize during this period. Close observation of the newborn's status is essential. Careful examination of the newborn at birth allows for detection of anomalies, birth injuries, and disorders that

---

HEALTHY PEOPLE 2020 • 18.1

Objective	Nursing Significance
• Increase the proportion of mothers who breast-feed their babies during the early postpartum period from a baseline of 74% to 81.9%. • Increase the proportion of mothers who breast-feed at 6 months from a baseline of 43.5% to 60.6%. • Increase the proportion of mothers who breast-feed at 1 year from a baseline of 22.7% to 34.1%. • Ensure appropriate newborn bloodspot screening and follow-up testing. • Increase the number of states and the District of Columbia that verify through linkage with vital records that all newborns are screened shortly after birth for conditions mandated by their state-sponsored screening program. • Increase the proportion of screen-positive children who receive follow-up testing within the recommended time period. • (Developmental) Increase the proportion of children with a diagnosed condition identified through newborn screening who have an annual assessment of services needed and received. • Increase the proportion of newborns who are screened for hearing loss by no later than age 1 month, have audiologic evaluation by age 3 months, and are enrolled in appropriate intervention service no later than age 6 months.	• Will emphasize the importance of breast milk as the most complete form of nutrition for infants. • Will help promote infant health, growth, immunity, and development throughout the newborn and infant periods. • Will help foster early detection and prompt treatment for conditions, thereby lessening the incidence of illness, disability, and death associated with these conditions and their overall effects on the newborn, infant, and family.

Healthy People objectives based on data from http://www.healthypeople.gov.

can compromise adaptation to extrauterine life. Problems that occur during this critical time can have a life-long impact.

Assessment

The initial newborn assessment is completed in the birthing area to determine whether the newborn is stable enough to stay with the parents or whether resuscitation or other immediate interventions are necessary. Recently, an easy, rapid newborn assessment tool, the RAPP, has been developed to enhance the nurse's ability to quickly and accurately assess the newborn's physiologic condition. The RAPP assessment (**r**espiratory **a**ctivity, **p**erfusion, and **p**osition) provides a method to swiftly evaluate the newborn's condition so that decisions can be made regarding newborn stability (Ludington-Hoe & Morgan, 2014). A second assessment may be performed within the first 2 to 4 hours, when the newborn is admitted to the nursery or the labor and birth room. A third assessment is usually completed before discharge, according to the hospital policy. The purpose of these assessments is to determine the newborn's overall health status, to provide information to the mother and father/support persons/significant others about their newborn, and to identify apparent physical abnormalities (Davidson, 2014).

During the initial newborn assessment, look for signs that might indicate a problem, including:

1. Nasal flaring
2. Chest retractions
3. Grunting on exhalation
4. Labored breathing
5. Generalized cyanosis
6. Abnormal breath sounds: rhonchi, crackles (rales), wheezing, and stridor
7. Abnormal respiratory rates (tachypnea, more than 60 breaths/minute; bradypnea, less than 25 breaths/minute)
8. Flaccid body posture
9. Pallor
10. Apneic episodes
11. Abnormal heart rates (tachycardia, more than 160 bpm; bradycardia, less than 100 bpm)
12. Abnormal newborn size: small or large for gestational age

If any of these findings is noted, medical intervention may be necessary.

Apgar Scoring

The **Apgar score**, introduced in 1952 by Dr. Virginia Apgar, is used worldwide to evaluate a newborn's physical condition at 1 minute and 5 minutes after birth. An additional Apgar assessment is done at 10 minutes if the 5-minute score is less than 7 points. The heart rate was found to be the most important diagnostic and prognostic

of the five signs (Apgar, 2015). It can be used as a rapid method for assessing the survival of a neonate. Assessment of the newborn at 1 minute provides data about the newborn's initial adaptation to extrauterine life. Assessment at 5 minutes provides a clearer indication of the newborn's overall central nervous system status.

Five parameters are assessed with Apgar scoring. A quick way to remember the parameters of Apgar scoring is as follows:

- **A**: appearance (color)
- **P**: pulse (heart rate)
- **G**: grimace (reflex irritability)
- **A**: activity (muscle tone)
- **R**: respiratory (respiratory effort)

Each parameter is assigned a score ranging from 0 to 2 points. A score of 0 points indicates an absent or poor response; a score of 2 points indicates a normal response (Table 18.1). A normal newborn's score should be 8 to 10 points. The higher the score indicates the better condition of the newborn. If the Apgar score is 8 points or higher, no intervention is needed other than supporting normal respiratory efforts and maintaining thermoregulation. Scores of 4 to 7 points signify moderate difficulty and scores of 0 to 3 points represent severe distress in adjusting to extrauterine life. The Apgar score is influenced by the presence of infection, newborn maturity, mother's age, congenital anomalies, physiologic immaturity, maternal sedation via medications, labor management, and neuromuscular disorders (Rudiger & Konstantelos, 2015).

When the newborn experiences physiologic depression, the Apgar score characteristics disappear in a predictable manner: first the pink coloration is lost, next the respiratory effort, and then the tone, followed by the reflex irritability and finally heart rate (Apgar, 2015).

> ### Take Note!
> Although Apgar scoring is done at 1 and 5 minutes, it can also be used as a guide during the immediate newborn period to evaluate the newborn's status for any changes because it focuses on critical parameters that must be assessed throughout the early transition period.

Length and Weight

Parents are eager to know their newborn's length and weight. These measurements are taken soon after birth. A disposable tape measure or a built-in measurement board located on the side of some scales can be used. Length is measured from the head of the newborn to the heel with the newborn unclothed (Fig. 18.1). Because of the flexed position of the newborn after birth, place the newborn in a supine position and extend the leg completely when measuring the length. The expected length range of a full-term newborn is usually 44 to 55 cm

TABLE 18.1	APGAR SCORING FOR NEWBORNS		
Parameter (Assessment Technique)	**0 Point**	**1 Point**	**2 Points**
Heart rate (auscultation of apical heart rate for 1 full minute)	Absent	Slow (<100 bpm)	>100 bpm
Respiratory effort (observation of the volume and vigor of the newborn's cry; auscultation of depth and rate of respirations)	Apneic	Slow, irregular, shallow	Regular respirations (usually 30–60 breaths/minute), strong, good cry
Muscle tone (observation of the extent of flexion in the newborn's extremities and newborn's resistance when the extremities are pulled away from the body)	Limp, flaccid	Some flexion, limited resistance to extension	Tight flexion, good resistance to extension with quick return to flexed position after extension
Reflex irritability (flicking of the soles of the feet or suctioning of the nose with a bulb syringe)	No response	Grimace or frown when irritated	Sneeze, cough, or vigorous cry
Skin color (inspection of trunk and extremities with the appropriate color for ethnicity appearing within minutes after birth)	Cyanotic or pale	Appropriate body color; blue extremities (acrocyanosis)	Completely appropriate color (pink on both trunk and extremities)

Data from Cunningham, F. G., Leveno, K. J., Bloom, S. L., Spong, C. Y., Dashe, J. S., Hoffman, B. L., et al. (2014). *William's obstetrics* (24th ed.). New York, NY: McGraw-Hill Medical; and Marcdante, K. J., & Kliegman, R. M. (2014). *Nelson essentials of pediatrics* (7th ed.). Philadelphia, PA: Elsevier Science Health.

(17 to 22 in). Molding can affect measurement (Weber & Kelley, 2014).

Most often, newborns are weighed using a digital scale that reads the weight in grams. Typically, the term newborn weighs 2,500 to 4,000 g (5 lb, 8 oz to 8 lb, 14 oz; Fig. 18.2). Birth weights less than 10% or more than 90% on a growth chart are outside the normal range and need further investigation. Weights taken at later times are compared with previous weights and are documented with regard to gain or loss on a nursing flow sheet. Newborns can lose up to 10% of their initial birth weight by 3 to 4 days of age secondary to loss of meconium, extracellular fluid, and limited food intake. This weight loss is usually regained by the 10th day of life (Fonseca et al., 2014).

Newborns can be classified by their birth weight regardless of their gestational age (American Academy of Pediatrics [AAP], 2015a) as follows:
- Low birth weight: >2,500 g (>5.5 lb)
- Very low birth weight: >1,500 g (>3.5 lb)
- Extremely low birth weight: >1,000 g (>2.5 lb)

Vital Signs

Heart rate and respiratory rate are assessed immediately after birth with Apgar scoring. Heart rate, obtained by taking an apical pulse for 1 full minute, typically is 110 to 160 bpm. Newborns' respirations are assessed when they are quiet or sleeping. Place a stethoscope on the right side of the chest and count the breaths

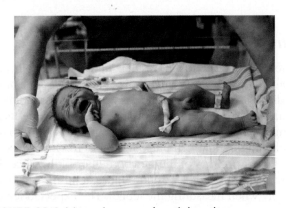

FIGURE 18.1 Measuring a newborn's length.

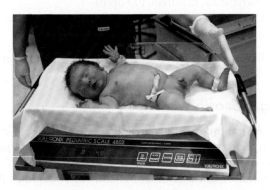

FIGURE 18.2 Weighing the newborn. Note how the nurse guards the newborn with her hand to prevent falling.

for 1 full minute to identify any irregularities. The newborn respiratory rate is 30 to 60 breaths/minute with symmetric chest movement. Heart and respiratory rates are usually assessed every 30 minutes until stable for 2 hours after birth. Once stable, the heart rate and respiratory rates are checked every 8 hours. These assessment time frames may vary per hospital protocols, so nurses should follow the facility's procedures (Nagtalon-Ramos, 2014).

Vital signs are assessed at birth, within 1 to 4 hours after birth according to hospital policy. Vital signs are used for identifying a variety of complications and for ensuring well-being of the newborn. In some health care agencies, temperatures are taken immediately after the Apgar score has been taken to allow for identification of hypothermia, which then requires a glucose check, but nurses need to follow their hospital protocols on this assessment timing. In term newborns, the normal axillary temperature range should be maintained at 97.7° to 99.5° F (36.5° to 37.5° C). Rectal temperatures are no longer taken because of the risk of perforation (AAP, 2015b). The thermometer or temperature probe is held in the midaxillary space according to manufacturer's directions and hospital protocol. Blood pressure is not usually assessed as part of a normal newborn examination unless there is a clinical indication or low Apgar scores. If assessed, an oscillometer (Dinamap) is used. The typical range is 50 to 75 mm Hg (systolic) and 30 to 45 mm Hg (diastolic). Crying, moving, and late clamping of the umbilical cord will increase systolic pressure (Weber & Kelley, 2014). Typical values for newborn vital signs are provided in Table 18.2.

Gestational Age Assessment

To determine a newborn's **gestational age** (the stage of maturity), physical signs and neurologic characteristics are assessed. Typically, gestational age is determined by using a tool such as the Ballard gestational age assessment or Ballard Scale. It determines a newborn's gestational age between 20 and 44 weeks. A score is assigned to the various parameters, and the total score corresponds to a maturity rating in weeks of gestation (Fig. 18.3). This scoring system provides an objective estimate of gestational age by scoring the specific parameters of physical as well as neuromuscular maturity. Points are given for each assessment parameter, with a low score of –1 point or –2 points for extreme immaturity to 4 or 5 points for postmaturity. The scores from each section are added to correspond to a specific gestational age in weeks.

The physical maturity section of the examination is done during the first 2 hours after birth. The physical maturity assessment section of the Ballard examination evaluates physical characteristics that appear different at different stages depending on a newborn's gestational maturity. Newborns who are physically mature have higher scores than those who are not. The areas assessed on the physical maturity examination include:

- *Skin texture*—typically ranges from sticky and transparent to smooth, with varying degrees of peeling and cracking, to parchment-like or leathery with significant cracking and wrinkling
- *Lanugo*—soft downy hair on the newborn's body, which is absent in preterm newborns, appears with maturity, and then disappears again with postmaturity
- *Plantar creases*—creases on the soles of the feet, which range from absent to covering the entire foot, depending on maturity (the greater the number of creases, the greater the newborn's maturity)
- *Breast tissue*—the thickness and size of breast tissue and areola (the darkened ring around each nipple), which range from being imperceptible to full and budding
- *Eyes and ears*—eyelids can be fused or open and ear cartilage and stiffness determine the degree of maturity (the greater the amount of ear cartilage with stiffness, the greater the newborn's maturity)
- *Genitals*—in males, evidence of testicular descent and appearance of scrotum (which can range from smooth to covered with rugae) determine maturity; in females, appearance and size of clitoris and labia determine maturity (a prominent clitoris with flat labia suggests prematurity, whereas a clitoris covered by labia suggests greater maturity)

The neuromuscular maturity section typically is completed within 24 hours after birth. Six activities or maneuvers that the newborn performs with various body parts are evaluated to determine the newborn's degree of maturity:

1. *Posture*—How does the newborn hold his or her extremities in relation to the trunk? The greater the degree of flexion, the greater the maturity. For example,

TABLE 18.2	NEWBORN VITAL SIGNS	
Newborn Vital Signs	**Ranges of Values**
Temperature	97.7–99.5° F (36.5–37.5° C)
Heart rate (pulse) to 180 during crying	110 –160 bpm; can increase
Respirations	30–60 breaths/minute at rest; will increase with crying
Blood pressure	50–75 mm Hg systolic, 30–45 mm Hg diastolic

Data from Moses, S. (2015). Pediatric vital signs. *Family Practice Notebook*. Retrieved from http://www.fpnotebook.com/cv/exam/pdtrcvtlsgns.htm; and Kliegman, R. M., Behrman, R. E., Jenson, H. B., & Stanton, B. F. (2014). *Nelson's textbook of pediatrics* (20th ed.). St. Louis, MO: Saunders Elsevier.

NEUROMUSCULAR MATURITY

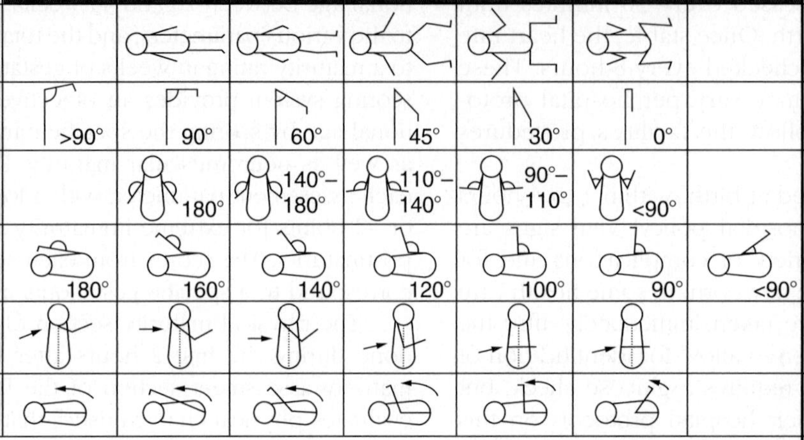

NEUROMUSCULAR MATURITY SIGN	SCORE							RECORD SCORE HERE
	−1	0	1	2	3	4	5	
POSTURE								
SQUARE WINDOW (Wrist)	>90°	90°	60°	45°	30°	0°		
ARM RECOIL		180°	140°–180°	110°–140°	90°–110°	<90°		
POPLITEAL ANGLE	180°	160°	140°	120°	100°	90°	<90°	
SCARF SIGN								
HEEL TO EAR								
						TOTAL NEUROMUSCULAR MATURITY SCORE		

SCORE
Neuromuscular ____
Physical ____
Total ____

MATURITY RATING

Score	Weeks
−10	20
−5	22
0	24
5	26
10	28
15	30
20	32
25	34
30	36
35	38
40	40
45	42
50	44

PHYSICAL MATURITY

PHYSICAL MATURITY SIGN	SCORE							RECORD SCORE HERE
	−1	0	1	2	3	4	5	
SKIN	sticky, friable, transparent	gelatinous, red, translucent	smooth, pink, visible veins	superficial peeling and/or rash, few veins	cracking pale areas, rare veins	parchment, deep cracking, no vessels	leathery, cracked, wrinkled	
LANUGO	none	sparse	abundant	thinning	bald areas	mostly bald		
PLANTAR SURFACE	heel-toe 40–50 mm:−1 <40 mm:−2	>50 mm no crease	faint red marks	anterior transverse crease only	creases ant. 2/3	creases over entire sole		
BREAST	impercep-tible	barely perceptible	flat areola no bud	stippled areola 1–2 mm bud	raised areola 3–4 mm bud	full areola 5–10 mm bud		
EYE-EAR	lids fused loosely: −1 tightly: −2	lids open pinna flat stays folded	sl. curved pinna; soft; slow recoil	well-curved pinna; soft but ready recoil	formed and firm instant recoil	thick cartilage, ear stiff		
GENITALS (Male)	scrotum flat, smooth	scrotum empty, faint rugae	testes in upper canal, rare rugae	testes descending, few rugae	testes down, good rugae	testes pendulous, deep rugae		
GENITALS (Female)	clitoris prominent and labia flat	prominent clitoris and small labia minora	prominent clitoris and enlarging minora	majora and minora equally prominent	majora large, minora small	majora cover clitoris and minora		
						TOTAL PHYSICAL MATURITY SCORE		

FIGURE 18.3 Gestational age assessment tool. The New Ballard Score (2014). Adapted from http://www.ballardscore.com

extension of arms and legs is scored as 0 points and full flexion of arms and legs is scored as 4 points.

2. *Square window*—How far can the newborn's hands be flexed toward the wrist? The angle is measured and scored from more than 90 degrees to 0 degrees to determine the maturity rating. As the angle decreases, the newborn's maturity increases. For example, an angle of more than 90 degrees is scored as −1 point and an angle of 0 degrees is scored as 4 points.

3. *Arm recoil*—How far do the newborn's arms "spring back" to a flexed position? This measure evaluates the degree of arm flexion and the strength of recoil. The reaction of the arm is then scored from 0 to 4 points based on the degree of flexion as the arms are returned

to their normal flexed position. The higher the points assigned, the greater the neuromuscular maturity (for example, recoil less than a 90-degree angle is scored as 4 points).

4. *Popliteal angle*—How far will the newborn's knees extend? The angle created when the knee is extended is measured. An angle of less than 90 degrees indicates greater maturity. For example, an angle of 180 degrees is scored as –1 point and an angle of less than 90 degrees is scored as 5 points.

5. *Scarf sign*—How far can the elbows be moved across the newborn's chest? An elbow that does not reach midline indicates greater maturity. For example, if the elbow reaches or nears the level of the opposite shoulder, this is scored as –1 point; if the elbow does not cross the proximate axillary line, it is scored as 4 points.

6. *Heel to ear*—How close can the newborn's feet be moved to the ears? This maneuver assesses hip flexibility: the lesser the flexibility, the greater the newborn's maturity. The heel-to-ear assessment is scored in the same manner as the scarf sign.

After the scoring is completed, the 12 scores are totaled and then compared with standardized values to determine the appropriate gestational age in weeks. Scores range from very low in preterm newborns to very high for mature and postmature newborns.

Typically newborns are also classified according to their gestational age as:

• *Preterm or premature*—born prior to 37 completed weeks' gestation, regardless of birth weight
• *Term*—born between 38 and 42 weeks' gestation
• *Post-term or postdates*—born after completion of week 42 of gestation
• *Postmature*—born after 42 weeks and demonstrating signs of placental aging

Using the information about gestational age and then considering birth weight, newborns can also be classified as follows:

• *Small for gestational age (SGA)*—weight less than the 10th percentile on standard growth charts (usually <5.5 lb)
• *Appropriate for gestational age (AGA)*—weight between 10th and 90th percentiles
• *Large for gestational age (LGA)*—weight more than the 90th percentile on standard growth charts (usually >9 lb)

Chapter 23 describes these variations in birth weight and gestational age in greater detail.

Take Note!

Gestational age assessment is important because it allows the nurse to plot growth parameters and to anticipate problems related to prematurity, postmaturity, and growth abnormalities.

Nursing Interventions

During the immediate newborn period, care focuses on helping the newborn to make the transition to extrauterine life. The nursing interventions include maintaining airway patency, ensuring proper identification, administering prescribed medications, and maintaining thermoregulation.

Maintaining Airway Patency

Immediately after birth, a newborn is suctioned to remove fluids and mucus from the mouth and nose (Fig. 18.4). Typically, the newborn's mouth is suctioned first with a bulb syringe to remove debris and then the nose is suctioned. Suctioning in this manner helps prevent aspiration of fluid into the lungs by an unexpected gasp. Recent studies, along with recommendations from leading maternal health experts and the WHO, support using a towel to wipe secretions from the mouth and nose of newborns for stable newborns. Routine suctioning of the mouth and airways is not required. Despite evidence showing that the use of routine suctioning shows no benefit and may produce harm, the practice remains commonplace (Bond, 2015; Saugstad, 2015).

When suctioning a newborn with a bulb syringe, compress the bulb before placing it into the oral or nasal cavity. Release bulb compression slowly, making sure the tip is placed away from the mucous membranes to draw up the excess secretions. Remove the bulb syringe from the mouth or nose, and then, while holding the bulb syringe tip over an emesis basin lined with paper towel or tissue, compress the bulb to expel the secretions. Repeat the procedure several times until all secretions are removed or use a towel to wipe away secretions per hospital policy.

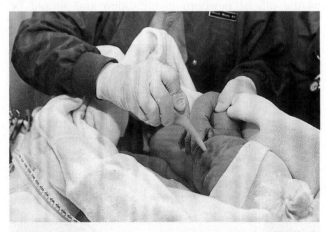

FIGURE 18.4 A newborn is suctioned by means of a bulb syringe to remove mucus from the mouth and nose. The head-down-and-to-the-side position facilitates drainage. Care is given with the infant under a radiant heat source. (Copyright Caroline Brown, RNC, MS, DEd.)

Take Note!

Always keep a bulb syringe near the newborn in case he or she develops sudden choking or a blockage in the nose. It may be lifesaving.

Ensuring Proper Identification

Infant abduction continues to be a threat in hospitals and health care organizations across the country. The abduction by nonfamily members of newborns from health care facilities has clearly become a subject of concern for parents, maternal-child care nurses, health care security and risk management administrators, law enforcement officials, and the National Center for Missing & Exploited Children (NCMEC). Staff identification (ID) badges, training, video surveillance, access control and tagging systems can help prevent a newborn from being abducted from the hospital. Proactive security measures must become everyone's responsibility to ensure the safety of all newborns and their families in all hospital settings.

Before the newborn and family leave the birthing area, be sure that agency policy about identification has been followed. Typically, the mother, the newborn, and the father or any significant other or support person of the mother's choosing receive ID bracelets. The newborn commonly receives two ID bracelets, one on a wrist and one on an ankle. The mother receives a matching one, usually on her wrist. The ID bands usually state name, gender, date and time of birth, and identification number. The same identification number is on the bracelets of all family members.

These ID bracelets are provided for the safety of the newborn and must be secured before the mother and newborn leave the birthing area. The ID bracelets are checked by all nurses to validate that the correct newborn is brought to the right mother if they are separated for any period of time (Fig. 18.5). They also serve as the official newborn identification and should be

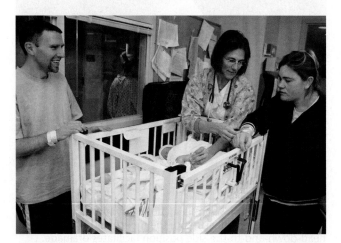

FIGURE 18.5 The nurse checks the newborn's identification band against the mother's.

checked before initiating any procedure on that newborn and on discharge from the unit (NCMEC, 2015). Taking the newborn's picture within 2 hours after birth with a color camera or color video/digital image also helps prevent mix-ups and abduction. Many facilities use electronic devices that sound an alarm if a newborn is taken beyond a certain point on the unit or removed from the area.

Newborns' footprints may also be taken, using a form that includes the mother's fingerprint, name, date, and time of the birth. Some states require footprints of the newborn, although many studies point out that birthing room staff does not take consistently legible footprints suitable for identification purposes (Goyal, Nagar, & Kumar, 2014). Many states have stopped requiring newborn footprints, and thus other means of identification are needed, such as collecting cord blood at the time of birth for DNA testing; facial biometric recognition, and live scans to capture digital forensic-quality prints that are suitable for identification purposes (Otsuka, 2014).

Prevention of infant abductions has been successful through a combination of increased security measures in hospitals, including video cameras and alarm devices, and education of staff and parents about precautions to take while in the hospital. It is critical not to allow anyone without identification to take an infant for any reason and to keep the infant within the sight of the parent or nursery staff at all times. These measures should be largely invisible and create a sense of security rather than increasing parental fears about abduction.

Although infant abduction rates are rare, the safety and security of mothers and infants should remain a high priority for nurses. By being aware of physical security of maternity units, educating expectant parents on the methods used by potential abductors, and working with community resources, these tragic incidents can be prevented.

Administering Prescribed Medications

During the immediate newborn period, two medications are commonly ordered: vitamin K and eye prophylaxis with either erythromycin or tetracycline ophthalmic ointment (Drug Guide 18.1).

VITAMIN K

Prophylactic treatment of newborns with intramuscular vitamin K has been the standard of care for decades in the United States. Vitamin K, a fat-soluble vitamin, promotes blood clotting by increasing the synthesis of prothrombin by the liver. A deficiency of this vitamin delays clotting and might lead to hemorrhage. Newborns are at risk for vitamin K deficiency and subsequent bleeding unless supplemented at birth. Vitamin K deficiency is an acquired coagulopathy in newborn infants because of an

DRUG GUIDE 18.1   DRUGS FOR THE NEWBORN

Drug	Action/Indication	Nursing Implications
Phytonadione (vitamin K [Aqua-MEPHYTON, Konakion, Mephyton])	Provides the newborn with vitamin K (necessary for production of adequate clotting factors II, VII, IX, and X by the liver) during the first week of birth until newborn can manufacture it Prevents vitamin K deficiency bleeding (VKDB) of the newborn	• Administer within 1 to 2 hours after birth. • Give as an IM injection at a 90-degree angle into the outer middle third of the vastus lateralis muscle. • Use a 25-gauge, 5/8-in needle for injection. • Hold the leg firmly and inject medication slowly. • Adhere to standard precautions. • Assess for bleeding at injection site after administration.
Erythromycin ophthalmic ointment 0.5% or tetracycline ophthalmic ointment 1%	Provides bactericidal and bacteriostatic actions to prevent *Neisseria gonorrhoeae* and *Chlamydia trachomatis* conjunctivitis Prevents ophthalmia neonatorum	• Be alert for chemical conjunctivitis for 1 to 2 days. • Wear gloves, and open eyes by placing the thumb and finger above and below the eye. • Gently squeeze the tube or ampoule to apply medication into the conjunctival sac from the inner canthus to the outer canthus of each eye. • Do not touch the tip to the eye. • Close the eye to make sure the medication permeates. • Wipe off excess ointment after 1 minute.

Adapted from King, T. L., Brucker, M. C., Kriebs, J. M., Fahey, J. O., Gegor, C. L., & Varney, H. (2015). *Varney's midwifery* (5th ed.). Burlington, MA: Jones & Bartlett Learning; and Skidmore-Roth, L. (2015). *Mosby's 2015 nursing drug reference* (28th ed.). St. Louis, MO: Elsevier Health Sciences.

accumulation of inactive vitamin K coagulation factors, which leads to an increased bleeding tendency. Supplementation of vitamin K at birth has been recommended in the United States since 1961 and successfully reduces the risk of bleeding in newborns (Bellini, 2015).

Generally, the bacteria of the intestine produce vitamin K in adequate quantities. However, the newborn's bowel is sterile, so vitamin K is not produced in the intestine until after microorganisms have been introduced, such as with the first feeding. Usually, it takes about a week for the newborn to produce enough vitamin K to prevent vitamin K deficiency bleeding. An oral vitamin K preparation is also being given to newborns outside the United States, but at least three doses are needed over a 1-month period (Abrams & Savelli, 2014).

The efficacy of vitamin K in preventing early vitamin K deficiency bleeding is firmly established and has been the standard of care since the AAP recommended it in the early 1960s. The AAP (2015c) recommends that vitamin K be administered to all newborns soon after birth in a single intramuscular dose of 0.5 to 1 mg (Fig. 18.6). The AAP also suggests that additional research is needed to validate the efficacy and safety of oral forms of vitamin K, which have been used in many parts of the world, but currently are not recommended in the United States.

EYE PROPHYLAXIS

All newborns in the United States, whether delivered vaginally or by cesarean birth, must receive an installation of a prophylactic agent in their eyes within an hour or two of birth. This is mandated in all 50 states to prevent **ophthalmia neonatorum**, which can cause neonatal blindness (Centers for Disease Control and Prevent [CDC], 2015a). Ophthalmia neonatorum is a hyperacute purulent conjunctivitis occurring during the first 10 days of life. It is usually contracted during birth when

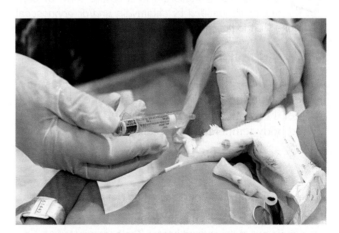

FIGURE 18.6 The nurse administers vitamin K IM to the newborn.

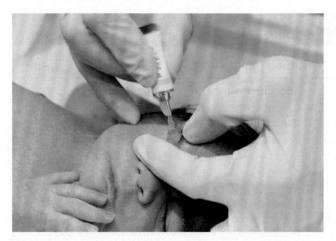

FIGURE 18.7 The nurse administers eye prophylaxis.

the baby comes in contact with vaginal discharge of the mother infected with gonorrhea and chlamydia (CDC, 2015a). Most often both eyelids become swollen and red with purulent discharge.

Prophylactic agents that are currently recommended (and in most states legally required) include erythromycin 0.5% ophthalmic ointment or tetracycline 1% ophthalmic ointment in a single application. Silver nitrate solution was formerly used but has little efficacy in preventing chlamydial eye disease (Moore & MacDonald, 2015).

Regardless of which agent is used, instillation should be done as soon as possible after birth (Fig. 18.7). If instillation is delayed to allow visualization and bonding, the nursery staff should make sure the agent is administered when the newborn reaches the nursery for observation and assessment.

Inform all parents about the eye treatment, including why it is recommended, what problems may arise if the treatment is not given, and possible adverse effects of the treatment.

 Take Note!

Ophthalmia neonatorum is a severe form of conjunctivitis caused by chlamydia and/or gonococcal infections that is potentially a blinding condition in newborns.

Maintaining Thermoregulation

Newborns have trouble regulating their temperature; especially during the first few hours after birth (see Chapter 17 for a complete discussion). Therefore, maintaining body temperature is crucial.

Concept Mastery Alert

Use of a Radiant Heater in Preventing Newborn Heat Loss

A 1-day-old infant should have adequate thermoregulation to remain out of the radiant heater. The best way to prevent heat loss is to ensure that the infant does not come in contact with cold surfaces.

Assess body temperature frequently during the immediate newborn period. The baby's temperature should be taken every 30 minutes for the first 2 hours or until the temperature has stabilized, and then every 8 hours until discharge or follow hospital protocols (King et al., 2015). Commonly a thermistor probe (automatic sensor) is attached to the newborn to record body temperature on a monitoring device. The probe is taped to the newborn's abdomen, usually in the right upper quadrant, which allows for position changes without having to readjust the probe. The other end of the thermistor probe is inserted into the radiant heat control panel. Temperature parameters are set on an alarm system connected to the heat panel that will sound if the newborn's temperature falls out of the set range. Check the probe connection periodically to make sure that it remains secure. Remember the potential for heat loss in newborns, and perform all nursing interventions in a way that minimizes heat loss and prevents hypothermia.

Axillary temperatures can also be used to assess the newborn's body temperature. Place a thermometer under the newborn's axilla and place the arm over the chest to keep the thermometer in place and provide comfort to the newborn.

Nursing interventions to help maintain body temperature include:
- Dry the newborn immediately after birth to prevent heat loss through evaporation.
- Wrap the baby in warmed blankets to reduce heat loss via convection.
- Skin-to-skin contact with mother as soon as stabilized.
- Use a warmed cover on the scale to weigh the unclothed newborn.
- Warm stethoscopes and hands before examining the baby or providing care.
- Avoid placing newborns in drafts or near air vents to prevent heat loss through convection.
- Delay the initial bath until the baby's temperature has stabilized to prevent heat loss through evaporation.
- Avoid placing cribs near cold outer walls to prevent heat loss through radiation.
- Put a cap on the newborn's head after it is thoroughly dried after birth.
- Place the newborn under a temperature-controlled radiant warmer (Fig. 18.8).

NURSING MANAGEMENT DURING THE EARLY NEWBORN PERIOD

The early newborn period is a time of great adjustment for both the mother and the newborn; both of them are adapting to many physiologic and psychological changes. In the past, mothers and newborns remained in the health care facility while these dramatic changes were taking place, with nurses and doctors readily available. However, today shorter hospital

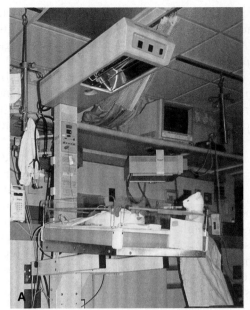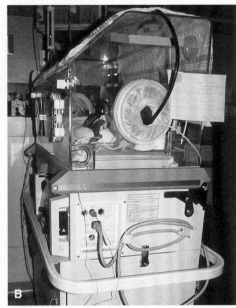

FIGURE 18.8 Maintaining thermoregulation. **A.** Radiant warmer. **B.** Isolette.

stays are the norm, and new mothers can easily be overwhelmed by having to go through all of these changes in such a short time: the woman gives birth, experiences marked physiologic and psychological changes, and must adapt to her newborn and learn the skills needed to care for herself and the baby, all within 24 to 48 hours.

The nurse's role is to assist the mother and her newborn through this dramatic transition period. The newborn needs continued health assessment, and the mother needs to be taught to care for the new baby. At discharge, the new mother may panic and feel insecure about her role as a primary caretaker. Nurses play a major role in promoting the newborn's transition by providing ongoing assessment and care and in promoting the woman's confidence by serving as a role model and teaching about proper newborn care.

Assessment

The newborn requires ongoing assessment after leaving the birthing area to ensure that his or her transition to extrauterine life is progressing without problems. The nurse uses the data gathered during the initial assessment as a baseline for comparison.

Perinatal History

Pertinent maternal and fetal data are vital to formulate a plan of care for the mother and her newborn. Historical information is obtained from the medical record and from interviewing the mother. Review the maternal history because it provides pertinent information, such as the presence of certain risk factors that could affect the newborn. Keep in mind that a comprehensive maternal history may not be available, especially if the mother has

had limited or no prenatal care. Historical information usually includes the following:

- Mother's name, medical record number, blood type, serology result, rubella and hepatitis status, and history of substance abuse
- Other maternal tests that are relevant to the newborn and care, such as human immunodeficiency virus (HIV) and group B streptococcus status
- Intrapartum maternal antibiotic therapy (type, dose, and duration)
- Maternal illness that can affect the pregnancy, evidence of chorioamnionitis, maternal use of medications such as steroids
- Prenatal care, including timing of first visit and subsequent visits
- Risk for blood group incompatibility, including Rh status and blood type
- Fetal distress or any nonreassuring fetal heart rate patterns during labor
- Known inherited conditions such as sickle cell anemia and phenylketonuria (PKU)
- Birth weights of previous live-born children, along with identification of any newborn problems
- Social history, including tobacco, alcohol, and recreational drug use
- History of depression or domestic violence
- Cultural factors, including primary language and educational level
- Pregnancy complications associated with abnormal fetal growth, fetal anomalies, or abnormal results from tests of fetal well-being
- Information on the progress of labor, birth, labor complications, duration of ruptured membranes, and presence of meconium in the amniotic fluid
- Medications given during labor, at birth, and immediately after birth

- Time and method of delivery, including presentation and the use of forceps or a vacuum extractor
- Status of the newborn at birth, including Apgar scores at 1 and 5 minutes, the need for suctioning, weight, gestational age, vital signs, and umbilical cord status
- Medications administered to the newborn
- Postbirth maternal information, including placental findings, positive cultures, and presence of fever

Newborn Physical Examination

The initial newborn physical examination, which may demonstrate subtle differences related to the newborn's age, is carried out within the first 24 hours after birth. For example, a newborn who is 30 minutes old has not yet completed the normal transition from intrauterine to extrauterine life, and thus variability may exist in vital signs and in respiratory, neurologic, gastrointestinal, skin, and cardiovascular systems. Therefore, a comprehensive examination should be delayed until after the newborn has completed the transition.

The physical examination should not be initiated if the newborn is crying or appears to be upset. Instead, it is best to postpone the assessment until the newborn is calm. In a quiet newborn, begin the examination with the least invasive and noxious elements of the examination (auscultation of heart and lungs). Then examine the areas most likely to irritate the newborn (e.g., examining the hips and eliciting the Moro reflex). A general visual assessment provides an enormous amount of information about the well-being of a newborn. Initial observation gives an impression of a healthy (stable) versus an ill newborn and a term versus a preterm newborn.

A typical physical examination of a newborn includes a general survey of skin color, posture, state of alertness, head size, overall behavioral state, respiratory status, gender, and any obvious congenital anomalies. Check the overall appearance for anything unusual. Then complete the examination in a systematic fashion.

Remember Kelly, who called the home health nurse and said her newborn son "looks like a canary"? What additional information is needed about the baby? What might be causing his yellow color?

ANTHROPOMETRIC MEASUREMENTS

Shortly after birth, after the gender of the child is revealed, most women and their partners/significant others want to know the vital statistics of their newborn—length and weight—to report to their family and friends. Additional measurements, including head and chest circumference, are also taken and recorded. Abdominal measurements are not routinely obtained unless there is a suspicion of pathology that causes abdominal distention. The newborn's progress from that point onward will be validated based on these early measurements. These measurements will be compared with future serial measurements to determine growth patterns, which are plotted on growth charts to evaluate normalcy. Therefore, accuracy is paramount.

Length. The average length of most newborns is 50 cm (20 in), but it can range from 44 to 55 cm (17 to 22 in). Measure length with the unclothed newborn lying on a warmed blanket placed on a flat surface with the knees held in an extended position. Then run a tape measure down the length of the newborn—from the head to the soles of the feet—and record this measurement in the newborn's record (see Fig. 18.1).

Weight. At birth the average newborn weighs 3,400 g (7.5 lb), but normal birth weights can range from 2,500 to 4,000 g (5 lb, 8 oz to 8 lb, 13 oz). Newborns are weighed immediately after birth and then daily. Newborns usually lose up to 6% of their birth weight within the first few days of life, but regain it in approximately 10 days.

Newborns are weighed on admission to the nursery or are taken to a digital scale to be weighed and returned to the mother's room. First, balance the scale if it is not balanced. Place a warmed protective cloth or paper as a barrier on the scale to prevent heat loss by conduction; recalibrate the scale to zero after applying the barrier. Next, place the unclothed newborn in the center of the scale. Keep a hand above the newborn for safety (see Fig. 18.2).

Weight is affected by racial origin, genetics, maternal age, size of the parents, maternal nutrition, maternal weight prenatally, and placental perfusion (Tawia & McGuire, 2014). Weight should be correlated with gestational age. A newborn who weighs more than normal might be LGA or an infant of a diabetic mother; a newborn who weighs less than normal might be SGA, preterm, or have a genetic syndrome. It is important to identify the cause for the deviation in size and to monitor the newborn for complications common to that etiology.

Head Circumference. The average newborn head circumference is 32 to 38 cm (13 to 15 in). Measure the circumference at the head's widest diameter (the occipitofrontal circumference). Wrap a flexible or paper measuring tape snugly around the newborn's head and record the measurement (Fig. 18.9A).

Take Note!

Head circumference may need to be remeasured at a later time if the shape of the head is altered from birth.

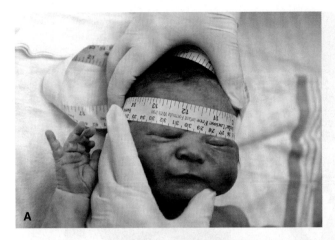
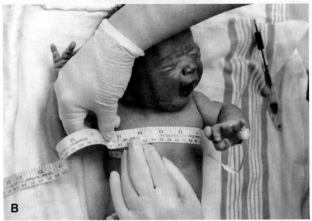

FIGURE 18.9 A. Measuring head circumference.
B. Measuring chest circumference.

The head circumference should be approximately one fourth of the newborn's length or about half the infant's body length plus 10 cm. Expected head circumference for a term infant is between 32 and 37 cm (12.5 to 14.5 in) (Nagtalon-Ramos, 2014). A small head might indicate microcephaly caused by rubella, toxoplasmosis, or SGA status; an enlarged head might indicate hydrocephalus or increased intracranial pressure. Both need to be documented and reported for further investigation.

Chest Circumference. The average chest circumference is 30 to 36 cm (12 to 14 in). It is generally equal to or about 2 to 3 cm less than the head circumference (Weber & Kelley, 2014). Place a flexible or paper tape measure around the unclothed newborn's chest just below the nipple line without pulling it taut (see Fig. 18.9B).

Take Note!

The head and chest circumferences are usually equal by about 1 year of age.

VITAL SIGNS

In the newborn, temperature, pulse, and respirations are monitored frequently and compared with baseline data obtained immediately after birth. Generally, vital signs (excluding blood pressure) are taken:

• On admission to the nursery or in the labor and birth room after the woman/parents are allowed to hold and bond with the newborn
• Once every 30 minutes until the newborn has been stable for 2 hours
• Then once every 4 to 8 hours until discharge (Davidson, 2014)

Blood pressure is not routinely assessed in a normal newborn unless the baby's clinical condition warrants it. This schedule can change depending on the baby's health status.

Obtain a newborn's temperature by placing an electronic temperature probe in the midaxillary area or by monitoring the electronic thermistor probe that has been taped to the abdominal skin (applied when the newborn was placed under a radiant heat source). Monitor the newborn's temperature frequently per hospital protocol for changes until it stabilizes. If the temperature is higher, adjust the environment, such as removing some clothing or blankets. If the temperature is lower, check the radiant warmer setting or add a warmed blanket. Report any abnormalities to the primary health care provider if simple adjustments to the environment do not change the baby's temperature.

Obtain an apical pulse by placing the stethoscope over the fourth intercostal space on the chest. Listen for a full minute, noting rate, rhythm, and abnormal sounds such as murmurs. In the typical newborn, the heart rate is 110 to 160 bpm, with wide fluctuations with activity and sleep. Sinus arrhythmia is a normal finding. Murmurs detected during the newborn period do not necessarily indicate congenital heart disease, but they need to be evaluated further if they persist. Also palpate the apical, femoral, and brachial pulses for presence and equality (Fig. 18.10). Report any abnormalities to the primary health care provider for evaluation.

Assess respirations by observing the rise and fall of the chest for 1 full minute. Respirations should be symmetric, slightly irregular, shallow, and unlabored at a rate of 30 to 60 breaths/minute. The newborn's respirations are predominantly diaphragmatic, but they are synchronous with abdominal movements. Also auscultate breath sounds. Note any abnormalities, such as tachypnea, bradypnea, grunting, gasping, periods of apnea lasting longer than 20 seconds, asymmetry or decreased chest expansion, abnormal breath sounds (rhonchi and crackles), or sternal retractions. Some variations might exist early after birth, but if the abnormal pattern persists, notify the primary health care provider.

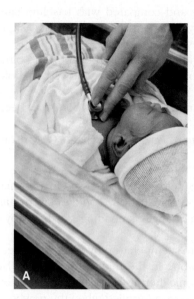
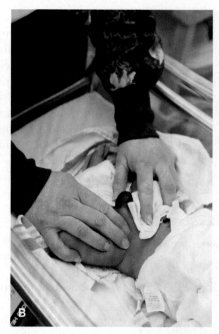
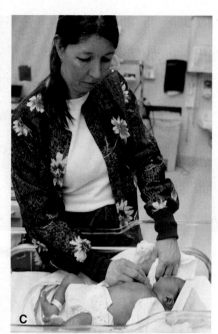

FIGURE 18.10 Assessing the newborn's vital signs. **A.** Assessing the apical pulse. **B.** Palpating the femoral pulse. **C.** Palpating the brachial pulse.

SKIN

The newborn's skin is similar in structure to the adult's, but many of the functions are not fully developed. Observe the overall appearance of the skin, including color, texture, turgor, and integrity. The newborn's skin should be smooth and flexible, and the color should be consistent with genetic background.

Skin Condition and Color. Check skin turgor by pinching a small area of skin over the chest or abdomen and note how quickly it returns to its original position. In a well-hydrated newborn, the skin should return to its normal position immediately. Skin that remains "tented" after being pinched may indicate dehydration. A small amount of lanugo (fine downy hair) may be observed over the shoulders and on the sides of the face and upper back. There may be some cracking and peeling of the skin. The skin should be warm to the touch and intact.

The newborn's skin often appears blotchy or mottled, especially in the extremities. Persistent cyanosis of fingers, hands, toes, and feet with mottled blue or red discoloration and coldness is called **acrocyanosis** (Fig. 18.11). It may be seen in newborns during the first few weeks of life in response to exposure to cold. Acrocyanosis is normal and intermittent. Any change in color of the newborn skin needs further investigation.

Newborn Skin Variations. While assessing the skin, make note of any rashes, ecchymoses or petechiae, nevi, or dark pigmentation. Skin lesions can be congenital or transient; they may be a result of infection or may

result from the mode of birth. If any of them are present, observe the anatomic location, arrangement, type, and color. Bruising may result from the use of devices such as a vacuum extractor during delivery. Petechiae may be the result of pressure on the skin during the birth process. Forceps marks may be observed over the cheeks and ears. A small puncture mark may be seen if internal fetal scalp electrode monitoring was used during labor.

Common skin variations include vernix caseosa, stork bites or salmon patches, milia, Mongolian spots, erythema toxicum, harlequin sign, nevus flammeus, and nevus vasculosus (Fig. 18.12).

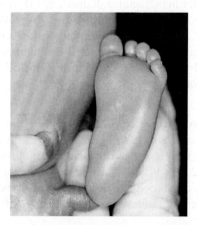

FIGURE 18.11 Acrocyanosis. This commonly appears on the feet and hands of babies shortly after birth. This infant is a 32-week newborn. (From Fletcher M. [1998]. Physical diagnosis in neonatology. Philadelphia, PA: Lippincott-Raven Publishers.)

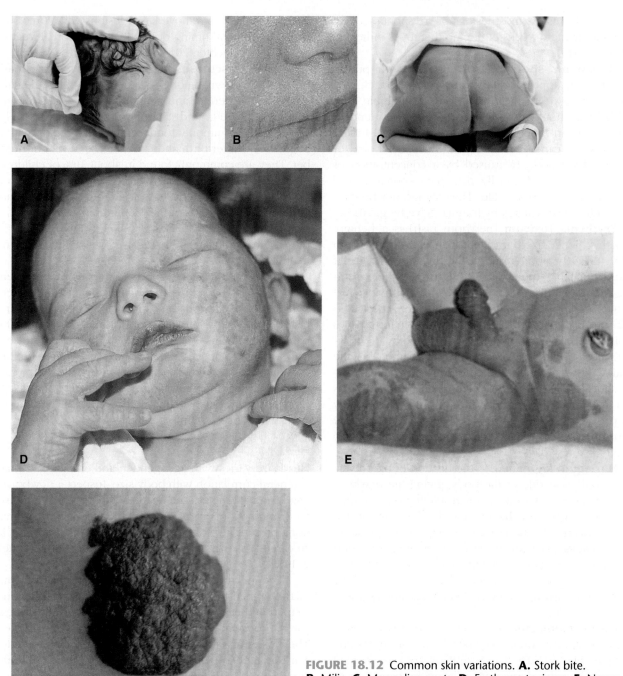

FIGURE 18.12 Common skin variations. **A.** Stork bite. **B.** Milia. **C.** Mongolian spots. **D.** Erythema toxicum. **E.** Nevus flammeus (port-wine stain). **F.** Strawberry hemangioma.

Vernix caseosa is a thick white substance that protects the skin of the fetus. It is formed by secretions from the fetus's oil glands and is found during the first 2 or 3 days after birth in body creases and the hair. It does not need to be removed because it will be absorbed into the skin.

Stork bites or salmon patches are superficial vascular areas found on the nape of the neck, on the eyelids, and between the eyes and upper lip (see Fig. 18.12A). The name comes from the marks on the back of the neck where, as myth goes, a stork may have picked up the

baby. They are caused by a concentration of immature blood vessels and are most visible when the newborn is crying. They are considered a normal variant, and most fade and disappear completely within the first year.

Milia are multiple pearly-white or pale yellow unopened sebaceous glands frequently found on a newborn's nose. They may also appear on the chin and forehead (see Fig. 18.12B). They form from oil glands and disappear on their own within 2 to 4 weeks. When they occur in a newborn's mouth and gums, they are termed **Epstein's pearls**. They occur in approximately

80% of newborns. As most lesions break spontaneously within the first few weeks of life, no therapy is indicated (El-Radhi, 2015).

Mongolian spots are benign blue or purple splotches that appear solitary on the lower back and buttocks of newborns, but may occur as multiple over the legs and shoulders (see Fig. 18.12C). They tend to occur in African American, Asian, Hispanic, and Indian newborns but can occur in dark-skinned newborns of all races. The spots are caused by a concentration of pigmented cells and usually disappear spontaneously within the first 4 years of life. They should not be confused with bruises caused by trauma (Silverberg, 2015).

Erythema toxicum (newborn rash) is a benign, idiopathic, generalized, transient rash that occurs in up to 70% of all newborns during the first week of life. It consists of small papules or pustules on the skin resembling flea bites. It is often mistaken for staphylococcal pustules. The rash is common on the face, chest, and back (see Fig. 18.12D). One of the chief characteristics of this rash is its lack of pattern. It is caused by the newborn's eosinophils reacting to the environment as the immune system matures. Histologically, erythema toxicum shows an abundance of eosinophils. Although it has been recognized and described for centuries, its etiology and pathogenesis remain unclear (Gloster, Gebauer, & Mistur, 2016a). It does not require any treatment and disappears in a few days.

Harlequin sign refers to the dilation of blood vessels on only one side of the body, giving the newborn the appearance of wearing a clown suit. It gives a distinct midline demarcation, which is described as pale on the nondependent side and red on the opposite, dependent side. It results from immature autoregulation of blood flow and is commonly seen in low-birth-weight newborns when there is a positional change (Lomax, 2015). It is transient, lasting as long as 20 minutes, and no intervention is needed.

Nevus flammeus, also called a port-wine stain, commonly appears on the newborn's face or other body areas (see Fig. 18.12E). It is a capillary angioma located directly below the dermis. It is flat with sharp demarcations and is purple red. This skin lesion is made up of mature capillaries that are congested and dilated. It ranges in size from a few millimeters to large, occasionally involving as much as half the body surface. Although it does not grow in area or size, it is permanent and will not fade. Although they may occur anywhere on the body, the majority are located in the head and neck areas. Port-wine stains may be associated with structural malformations, bony or muscular overgrowth, and certain cancers. Recent studies have noted an association between port-wine birthmarks and childhood cancer, so newborns with these lesions should be monitored with periodic eye examinations, neurologic imaging, and extremity measurements. Lasers and intense pulsed light

have been used to remove larger lesions with some success. The optimal timing of treatment is before 1 year of age (Giese & Richter, 2015).

Nevus vasculosus, also called a strawberry mark or strawberry hemangioma, is a benign capillary hemangioma in the dermal and subdermal layers. It is raised, rough, dark red, and sharply demarcated (see Fig. 18.12F). It is commonly found in the head region within a few weeks after birth and can increase in size or number. They are commonly found in about 10% of children. This type of hemangioma may be very subtle or even absent in the first few weeks of life, but they proliferate in the first few months of life. Commonly seen in premature infants weighing less than 1,500 g (El-Radhi, 2015), these hemangiomas tend to resolve by age 3 without any treatment.

The most important aspects of nursing management related to newborn skin variations include: adequate recognition of the lesions and knowledge of their natural history so that accurate information can be offered to the parents/significant other or partner. The majority of the skin lesions do not require any therapeutic intervention, but referral is necessary if there is: visual, airway or ear-canal obstruction, extensive growth, severe facial disfigurement, recurrent bleeding, infection, or ulceration, or excessive concern by the parents.

HEAD

Head size varies with age, gender, and ethnicity and has a general correlation with body size. Inspect a newborn's head from all angles. The head should appear symmetric and round. As many as 90% of the congenital malformations present at birth are visible on the head and neck, so careful assessment is very important (Pfister & Ramel, 2014).

The newborn has two fontanels at the juncture of the cranial bones. The anterior fontanel is diamond shaped and closes by 18 to 24 months. Typically it measures 4 to 6 cm at the largest diameter (bone to bone). The posterior one is triangular, smaller than the anterior fontanel (usually fingertip size or 0.5 to 1 cm), and closes by 6 to 12 weeks. Palpate both fontanels, which should be soft, flat, and open. Then palpate the skull. It should feel somewhat smooth and fused, except at the area of the fontanels, over molding areas, and sutures. Also assess the size of the head and the anterior and posterior fontanels, and compare them with appropriate standards.

Variations in Head Size and Appearance. During inspection and palpation, be alert for common variations that may cause asymmetry. These include molding, caput succedaneum, and cephalhematoma.

Molding is the elongated shaping of the fetal head to accommodate passage through the birth canal (Fig. 18.13). It occurs with a vaginal birth from a vertex

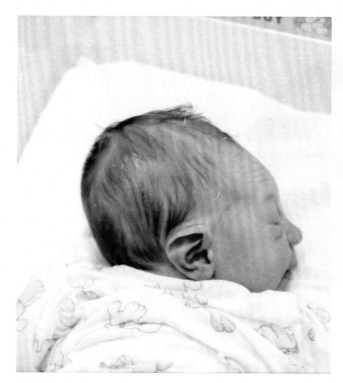

FIGURE 18.13 Molding in a newborn's head.

position in which elongation of the fetal head occurs with prominence of the occiput and overriding sagittal suture line. It typically resolves within a week after birth without intervention.

Caput succedaneum describes localized edema on the scalp that occurs from the pressure of the birth process. It is commonly observed after prolonged labor. Clinically, it appears as a poorly demarcated soft tissue swelling that crosses suture lines. Pitting edema and overlying petechiae and ecchymosis are noted (Fig. 18.14A). The swelling will gradually dissipate in about 3 days without any treatment. Newborns who were delivered via vacuum extraction usually have a caput in the area where the cup was used.

Cephalhematoma is a localized subperiosteal collection of blood of the skull which is always confined by one cranial bone. This condition is due to pressure on the head and disruption of the vessels during birth. It occurs after prolonged labor and use of obstetric interventions such as low forceps or vacuum extraction. The clinical features include a well-demarcated, often fluctuant swelling with no overlying skin discoloration. The swelling does not cross suture lines and is firmer to the touch than an edematous area (see Fig. 18.14B). Aspiration is not required for resolution and is likely to increase the risk of infection. Hyperbilirubinemia occurs following the breakdown of the red blood cells within the hematoma. This type of hyperbilirubinemia occurs later than classic physiologic hyperbilirubinemia. Cephalhematoma usually appears on the second or third day

after birth and disappears within weeks or months. Large cephalhematomas can lead to increased bilirubin levels and subsequent jaundice (Lomax, 2015).

Common Abnormalities in Head or Fontanel Size. Common abnormalities in head or fontanel size that may indicate a problem include:

- *Microcephaly*—a head circumference more than 2 standard deviations below average or less than 10% of normal parameters for gestational age, caused by failure of brain development. There is a reduced production of neurons leading to a reduction of brain volume and as a consequence of that a reduced skull size. Microcephaly is common, affecting more than 25,000 infants in the United States each year. Children with severe microcephaly, defined as more than 3 standard deviations below the mean for age and sex, are more likely to have imaging abnormalities and more severe developmental impairments than those with milder microcephaly. About 40% of children with microcephaly also have epilepsy, 20% have cerebral palsy, 50% have intellectual disability, and 20% to 50% have ophthalmologic and hearing disorders (Boom, 2015a). It can be familial, with autosomal dominant or recessive inheritance, and it may be associated with infections (cytomegalovirus), rubella, toxoplasmosis, and syndromes such as trisomy 13, 18, or 21 and fetal alcohol syndrome. Genetic counseling and clinical management through carrier detection/prenatal diagnosis in families can help reduce the incidence of these disorders (Alcantara & O'Driscoll, 2014).
- *Macrocephaly*—a head circumference more than 90% of normal, typically related to hydrocephalus (Boom, 2015b). It is often familial (with autosomal dominant inheritance) and can be either an isolated anomaly or a manifestation of other anomalies, including hydrocephalus and skeletal disorders (achondroplasia).
- *Large fontanels*—more than 6 cm in the anterior diameter bone to bone or more than a 1-cm diameter in the posterior fontanel; possibly associated with malnutrition, hydrocephaly, congenital hypothyroidism, trisomies 13, 18, and 21, and various bone disorders such as osteogenesis imperfecta.
- *Small or closed fontanels*—smaller-than-normal anterior and posterior diameters or fontanels that are closed at birth. Craniosynostosis and abnormal brain development are associated with a small fontanel or early fontanel closure associated with microcephaly (Sheth, Ranalli, & Aldana, 2014).

FACE

Observe the newborn's face for fullness and symmetry. The face should have full cheeks and should be symmetric when the baby is resting and crying. If forceps were used during birth, the newborn may have bruising and reddened areas over both cheeks and parietal bones

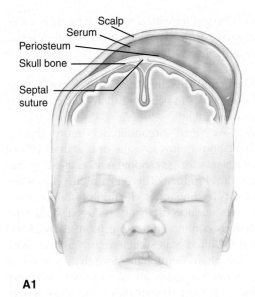

Scalp
Serum
Periosteum
Skull bone
Septal
suture

A1

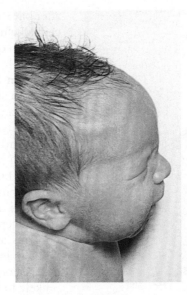

A2

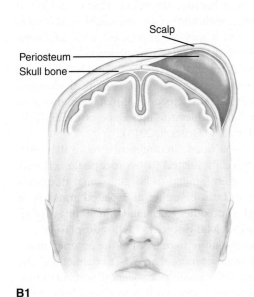

Scalp
Periosteum
Skull bone

B1

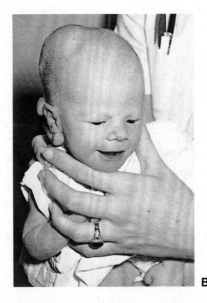

B2

FIGURE 18.14 A1 and A2. Caput succedaneum involves the collection of serous fluid and often crosses the suture line. (**A2.** From Chung, *Visual diagnosis and treatment in pediatrics* (2nd ed.). Philadelphia: LWW.) **B1 and B2.** Cephalhematoma involves the collection of blood and does not cross the suture line. (Photos, except for (A2), from O'Doherty, N. (1979). *Atlas of the newborn.* Philadelphia: J B Lippincott, 1979:136, and 1979:117, 143, with permission.)

secondary to the pressure of the forceps blades. Reassure the parents that this resolves without treatment, and point out improvement each day.

Problems with the face can also involve facial nerve paralysis caused by trauma from the use of forceps. Paralysis is usually apparent on the first or second day of life. Typically, the newborn will demonstrate asymmetry of the face with an inability to close the eye and move the lips on the affected side. Newborns with facial nerve paralysis have difficulty making a seal around the nipple, and consequently milk or formula drools from the paralyzed side of the mouth. Most facial nerve palsies resolve spontaneously within days, although full recovery may require weeks to months. Attempt to determine the cause from the newborn's history.

Nose. Inspect the nose for size, symmetry, position, and lesions. The newborn's nose is small and narrow. The nose should have a midline placement, patent nares, and an intact septum. The nostrils should be of equal size and should be patent. A slight mucous discharge may be present, but there should be no actual drainage. The newborn is a preferential nose breather and will use sneezing to clear the nose if needed. The newborn can smell after the nasal passages are cleared of amniotic fluid and mucus (Clark-Gambelunghe & Clark, 2015).

Mouth. Inspect the newborn's mouth, lips, and interior structures. The lips should be intact with symmetric movement and positioned in the midline; there should not be any lesions. Inspect the lips for pink color, moisture, and cracking. The lips should encircle the examiner's finger to form a vacuum. Variations involving the lip might include cleft upper lip (separation extending up to the nose) or thin upper lip associated with fetal alcohol syndrome.

Assess the inside of the mouth for alignment of the mandible, intact soft and hard palate, sucking pads inside the cheeks, a midline uvula, a free-moving tongue, and working gag, swallow, and sucking reflexes. The mucous membranes lining the oral cavity should be pink and moist, with minimal saliva present.

Normal variations might include Epstein's pearls (small, white epidermal cysts on the gums and hard palate that disappear in weeks), erupted natal teeth that may need to be removed to prevent aspiration (Fig. 18.15), and thrush (white plaque inside the mouth caused by exposure to *Candida albicans* during birth), which cannot be wiped away with a cotton-tipped applicator.

Eyes. Inspect the external eye structures, including the eyelids, lashes, conjunctiva, sclera, iris, and pupils, for position, color, size, and movement. There may be marked edema of the eyelids and subconjunctival hemorrhages due to pressure during birth. The eyes should be clear and symmetrically placed. Test the blink reflex by bringing an object close to the eye; the newborn should respond quickly by blinking. Also test the newborn's pupillary reflex: pupils should be equal, round, and reactive to light bilaterally. Assess the newborn's gaze: he or she should be able to track objects to the midline. Movement may be uncoordinated during the first few weeks of life. Many newborns have transient strabismus (deviation or wandering of eyes

independently) and searching nystagmus (involuntary repetitive eye movement), which is caused by immature muscular control. These are normal for the first 3 to 6 months of age.

Examine the internal eye structures. A red reflex (luminous red appearance seen on the retina) should be seen bilaterally on retinoscopy. The red reflex normally shows no dullness or irregularities.

Chemical conjunctivitis commonly occurs within 24 hours of instillation of eye prophylaxis after birth. There is lid edema with sterile discharge from both eyes. Usually it resolves within 48 hours without treatment.

Ears. Inspect the ears for size, shape, skin condition, placement, amount of cartilage, and patency of the auditory canal. The ears should be soft and pliable and should recoil quickly and easily when folded and released. Ears should be aligned with the outer canthi of the eyes. Low-set ears and abnormally shaped ears are characteristic of many syndromes and genetic abnormalities, such as trisomy 13 or 18, and internal organ abnormalities involving the renal system. Findings of sinuses or preauricular skin tags should prompt further evaluation for possible renal abnormalities since both systems develop at the same time.

An otoscopic examination is not typically done because the newborn's ear canals are filled with amniotic fluid and vernix caseosa, which would make visualization of the tympanic membrane difficult.

Newborn hearing screening is required by law in most states (discussed later in the chapter). Hearing loss is the most common birth defect in the United States: One in 1,000 newborns are profoundly deaf and 3 in 1,000 have some degree of hearing impairment (March of Dimes, 2015a). Delays in identification and intervention may affect the child's cognitive, verbal, behavioral, and emotional development. Screening at birth has reduced the age at which newborns with hearing loss are identified and has improved early intervention rates dramatically.

Available treatments include cochlear implantation, hearing augmentation, and follow-up by an audiologist, otolaryngologist, pediatrician, geneticist, and deaf education specialist (Nikolopoulos, 2015). Prior to universal newborn screening, children were usually older than 2 years before significant congenital hearing loss was detected; by this time it had already affected their speech and language skills (CDC, 2015b).

Causes of hearing loss can be conductive, sensorineural, or central. Risk factors for congenital hearing loss include cytomegalovirus infection and preterm birth necessitating a stay in the neonatal intensive care unit.

To assess for hearing ability generally, observe the newborn's response to noises and conversations. The newborn typically turns toward these noises and startles with loud ones.

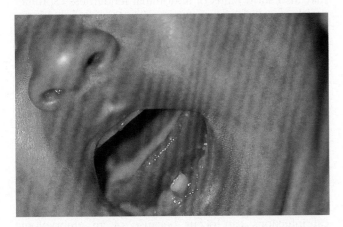

FIGURE 18.15 A natal tooth in a 16-day-old neonate. Natal teeth can be present at birth and are usually considered benign. No treatment is needed if they don't interfere with feeding.

NECK

Inspect the newborn's neck for movement and ability to support the head. The newborn's neck will appear almost nonexistent because it is so short. Creases are usually noted. The neck should move freely in all directions and should be capable of holding the head in a midline position. The newborn should have enough head control to be able to hold it up briefly without support. Report any deviations such as restricted neck movement or absence of head control.

Also inspect the clavicles (collarbone), which should be straight and intact. The clavicles are the bones mostly commonly broken in infants, especially large ones experiencing difficult births, in operative vaginal births, abnormal fetal positions, and in maternal obesity. In most cases, the fractured clavicle is asymptomatic, but edema, crepitus, and decreased or absent movement and pain or tenderness on movement of the arm on the affected side may be noted. Major risk factors for clavicle fractures are typically vacuum births and large newborn birth weights (Ahn et al., 2015). If the newborn with clavicular fracture is in pain, the affected arm should be immobilized, with the arm abducted more than 60 degrees and the elbow flexed more than 90 degrees. In addition to immobilization, treatment involves minimizing pain overall.

CHEST

Inspect the newborn's chest for size, shape, and symmetry. The newborn's chest should be round, symmetric, and 2 to 3 cm smaller than the head circumference. The xiphoid process may be prominent at birth, but it usually becomes less apparent when adipose tissue accumulates. Nipples may be engorged and may secrete a white discharge. This discharge, which occurs in both boys and girls, is a result of exposure to high levels of maternal estrogen while in utero. This enlargement and milky discharge usually dissipates within a few weeks. Some newborns may have extra nipples, called supernumerary nipples. They are typically small, raised, pigmented areas vertical to the main nipple line, 5 to 6 cm below the normal nipple. Supernumerary nipples may be unilateral or bilateral, and they may include an areola, nipple, or both. They tend to be familial and do not contain glandular tissue. Supernumerary nipples are generally thought to be benign. Some studies have suggested an association with renal or urogenital anomalies, whereas other studies have failed to show this association. There is insufficient evidence to recommend imaging studies or removal in the absence of other clinical concerns or physical findings (Gloster, Gebauer, & Mistur, 2016b). Reassure parents that these extra small nipples are harmless.

The newborn chest is usually barrel shaped, with equal anteroposterior and lateral diameters, and symmetric. Auscultate the lungs bilaterally for equal breath sounds. Normal breath sounds should be heard, with little difference between inspiration and expiration. Fine crackles can be heard on inspiration soon after birth as a result of amniotic fluid being cleared from the lungs. Diminished breath sounds might indicate atelectasis or pneumonia (Weber & Kelley, 2014).

Listen to the heart when the newborn is quiet or sleeping. S1 and S2 heart sounds are accentuated at birth. The point of maximal impulse is a lateral to midclavicular line located at the fourth intercostal space. A displaced point of maximal impulse may indicate tension pneumothorax or cardiomegaly. Murmurs are common during the first few hours as the foramen ovale is closing. Although cardiac murmurs in the neonatal period do not necessarily indicate heart disease, they should be evaluated if they persist (Fillipps & Bucciarelli, 2015).

ABDOMEN

Inspect the abdomen for shape and movement. Typically, the newborn's abdomen is protuberant but not distended. This contour is a result of the immaturity of the abdominal muscles. Abdominal movements are synchronous with respirations because newborns are, at times, abdominal breathers.

Auscultate bowel sounds in all four quadrants and then palpate the abdomen for consistency, masses, and tenderness. Perform auscultation and palpation systematically in a clockwise fashion until all four quadrants have been assessed. Palpate gently to feel the liver, the kidneys, and any masses. The liver is normally palpable 1 to 3 cm below the costal margin in the midclavicular line. The kidneys are 1 to 2 cm above and to both sides of the umbilicus. Normal findings would include bowel sounds in all four quadrants and no masses or tenderness on palpation. Absent or hyperactive bowel sounds might indicate an intestinal obstruction. Abdominal distention might indicate ascites, obstruction, infection, masses, or an enlarged abdominal organ. The newborn may also show signs of abdominal tenderness (Springer & Glasser, 2015). Imaging is a mainstay to diagnosis abdominal pathology and should be readily performed in a newborn with abdominal distention to determine the underlying etiology.

Inspect the umbilical cord area for the correct amount of blood vessels (two arteries and one vein). The umbilical vein is larger than the two umbilical arteries. Evidence of only a single umbilical artery is associated with renal and gastrointestinal anomalies. Also inspect the umbilical area for signs of bleeding, infection, inflammation, redness, swelling, purulent drainage or bleeding, erythema around the umbilicus, granuloma, or abnormal communication with the intra-abdominal organs. Umbilical infections can occur because of an embryologic remnant or poor hygiene. Traditionally, gram-positive organisms, such as *Staphylococcus aureus* and *Streptococcus pyogenes,* were most commonly identified, but gram-negative and polymicrobial infections are seen today. An umbilical cord infection (omphalitis) can spread to adjacent tissue, causing peritonitis, hepatic vein thrombosis and hepatic abscess. Immediate evaluation and referral is needed (Lomax, 2015).

GENITALIA

Male. Inspect the penis and scrotum in the male. In the circumcised male newborn, the glans should be smooth, with the meatus centered at the tip of the penis. It will appear reddened until it heals. For the uncircumcised male, the foreskin should cover the glans. Check the position of the urinary meatus: it should be in the midline at the glans' tip. If it is on the ventral surface of the penis, the condition is termed hypospadias; if it is on the dorsal surface of the penis, it is termed epispadias. In either case, circumcision should be avoided until further evaluation.

Inspect the scrotum for size, symmetry, color, presence of rugae, and location of testes. The scrotum usually appears relatively large with well-formed rugae and that should cover the scrotal sac. There should not be bulging, edema, or discoloration (Fig. 18.16A).

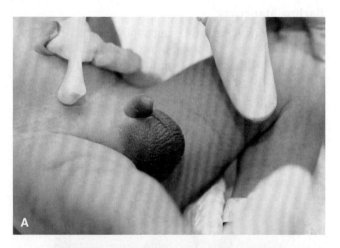

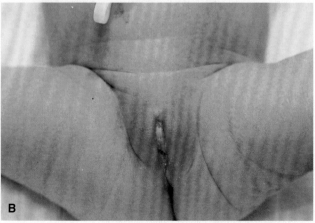

FIGURE 18.16 Newborn genitalia. **A.** Male genitalia. Note the darkened color of the scrotum. **B.** Female genitalia.

Palpate the scrotum for evidence of the testes, which should be in the scrotal sac. The testes should feel firm and smooth and should be of equal size on both sides of the scrotal sac in the term newborn. Undescended testes (cryptorchidism) might be palpated in the inguinal canal in preterm infants; they can be unilateral or bilateral. If the testes are not palpable within the scrotal sac, further investigation is needed.

Female. In the female newborn, inspect the external genitalia. The urethral meatus is located below the clitoris in the midline (Mutter & Prat, 2014). In contrast to the male genitalia, the female genitalia will be engorged: the labia majora and minora may both be edematous. The labia majora is large and covers the labia minora. The clitoris is large and the hymen is thick. These findings are due to the maternal hormones estrogen and progesterone (see Fig. 18.16B). A vaginal discharge composed of mucus mixed with blood may also be present during the first few weeks of life. This discharge, called **pseudomenstruation**, requires no treatment. Explain this phenomenon to the parents.

Variations in female newborns may include a labial bulge, which might indicate an inguinal hernia, ambiguous genitalia, a rectovaginal fistula with feces present in the vagina, and an imperforate hymen.

Male and Female. Inspect the anus in both male and female newborns for position and patency. Passage of meconium indicates patency. If meconium is not passed, a lubricated rectal thermometer can be inserted or a digital examination can be performed to determine patency. Abnormal findings would include anal fissures or fistulas and no meconium passed within 24 hours after birth.

EXTREMITIES AND BACK

Upper Extremities. Inspect the newborn's upper extremities for appearance and movement. Inspect the hands for shape, number, and position of fingers and presence of palmar creases. The newborn's arms and hands should be symmetric and should move through the range of motion without hesitation. Observe for spontaneous movement of the extremities. Each hand should have five digits. Note any extra digits (polydactyly) or fusing of two or more digits (syndactyly). Most newborns have three palmar creases on the hand. A single palmar crease, called a simian line, is frequently associated with Down syndrome.

A brachial plexus injury can occur during a difficult birth involving shoulder dystocia. Erb palsy is an injury resulting from damage to the upper plexus, and palsies associated with the lower brachial plexus are termed Klumpke palsies. Factors associated with obstetric brachial plexus paralysis include large birth weight, breech delivery, labor anomalies, operative vaginal birth, and shoulder dystocia. Obstetric brachial plexus paralysis results from excessive lateral traction on the head away from the shoulder. This force on the brachial plexus can cause varying degrees of injury to the nerves. The affected arm hangs limp alongside the body, and the affected shoulder and arm are adducted, extended, and internally rotated with a pronated wrist. The Moro reflex is absent on the affected side in brachial palsy. Complete recovery may take 6 months or longer. Current research studies support endogenous labor forces as the etiology of this injury. Despite training in the management of shoulder dystocia and a rising institutional cesarean section rate, the incidence of brachial plexus injuries has remained unchanged compared with 10 years earlier (Tung & Moore, 2015).

Lower Extremities. Assess the lower extremities in the same manner. They should be of equal length, with symmetric skinfolds. Inspect the feet for clubfoot (a turning-inward position), which is secondary to intrauterine positioning. This may be positional or structural. Perform the Ortolani and Barlow maneuvers to identify congenital hip dislocation, commonly termed developmental dysplasia of the hip. Nursing Procedure 18.1 highlights the steps for performing these maneuvers. Table 18.3 summarizes the newborn assessment.

NEUROLOGIC STATUS

Assess the newborn's state of alertness, posture, muscle tone, and reflexes.

Newborn Alertness, Posture, and Muscle Tone. The newborn should be alert and not persistently lethargic. The normal posture is hips abducted and partially flexed, with knees flexed. Arms are adducted and flexed at the

---

NURSING PROCEDURE 18.1

Performing Ortolani and Barlow Maneuvers

Purpose: To Detect Congenital Developmental Dysplasia of the Hip

Ortolani Maneuver

1. Place the newborn in the supine position and flex the hips and knees to 90 degrees at the hip.

2. Grasp the inner aspect of the thighs and abduct the hips (usually to approximately 180 degrees) while applying upward pressure.

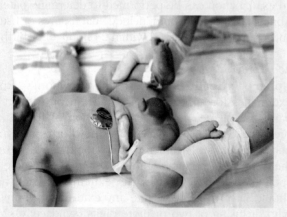

3. Listen for any sounds during the maneuver. There should be no "cluck" or "click" heard when the legs are abducted. Such a sound indicates the femoral head hitting the acetabulum as the head reenters the area. This suggests developmental hip dysplasia.

Barlow Maneuver

1. With the newborn still lying supine and grasping the inner aspect of the thighs (as just mentioned), adduct the thighs while applying outward and downward pressure to the thighs.

2. Feel for the femoral head slipping out of the acetabulum; also listen for a click.

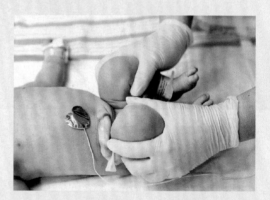

Inspect the back. The spine should appear straight and flat and should be easily flexed when the baby is held in a prone position. Observe for the presence of a tuft of hair, a pilonidal dimple in the midline, a cyst, or a mass along the spine. These abnormal findings should be documented and reported to the primary health care provider.

Adapted from Tamai, J., & McCarthy, J. J. (2015). Developmental dysplasia of the hip. *eMedicine*. Retrieved from http://emedicine. medscape.com/article/1248135-overview; and Weber, J., & Kelley, J. (2014). *Health assessment in nursing* (5th ed.). Philadelphia, PA: Lippincott Williams & Wilkins.

TABLE 18.3	NEWBORN ASSESSMENT SUMMARY	
Assessment	**Usual Findings**	**Variations and Common Problems**
Anthropometric measurements	Head circumference: 33–37 cm (13–14 in) Chest circumference: 30–33 cm (12–13 in) Weight: 2,500–4,000 g (5.5–8.5 lb) Length: 45–55 cm (19–21 in.)	SGA, LGA, preterm, post-term
Vital signs	Temperature: 97–99° F (36.5–37.5° C) Apical pulse: 110–160 bpm Respirations: 30–60 breaths/minute	
Skin	Normal: smooth, flexible, good skin turgor, well hydrated, warm	Jaundice, acrocyanosis, milia, Mongolian spots, stork bites
Head	Normal: varies with age, gender, and ethnicity	Microcephaly, macrocephaly, enlarged fontanels
Face	Normal: full cheeks, facial features symmetric	Facial nerve paralysis, nevus flammeus, nevus vasculosus
Nose	Normal: small, placement in the midline and narrow, ability to smell	Malformation or blockage
Mouth	Normal: aligned in midline, symmetric, intact soft and hard palate	Epstein's pearls, erupted precocious teeth, thrush
Neck	Normal: short, creased, moves freely, baby holds head in midline	Restricted movement, clavicular fractures
Eyes	Normal: clear and symmetrically placed on face; online with ears	Chemical conjunctivitis, subconjunctival hemorrhages
Ears	Normal: soft and pliable with quick recoil when folded and released	Low-set ears, hearing loss
Chest	Normal: round, symmetric, smaller than head	Nipple engorgement, whitish discharge
Abdomen	Normal: protuberant contour, soft, three vessels in umbilical cord	Distended, only two vessels in umbilical cord
Genitals	Normal male: smooth glans, meatus centered at tip of penis Normal female: swollen female genitals as a result of maternal estrogen	Edematous scrotum in males, vaginal discharge in females
Extremities and spine	Normal: extremities symmetric with free movement	Congenital hip dislocation; tuft or dimple on spine

Data from Davidson, M. R. (2014). *Fast facts for the neonatal nurse: A nursing orientation and care guide in a nutshell.* New York, NY: Springer Publishing Company; and Weber, J., & Kelley, J. (2014). *Health assessment in nursing* (5th ed.). Philadelphia, PA: Lippincott Williams & Wilkins.

elbow. Fists are often clenched, with fingers covering the thumb.

To assess for muscle tone, support the newborn with one hand under the chest. Observe how the neck muscles hold the head. The neck extensors should be able to hold the head in line briefly. There should be only slight head lag when pulling the newborn from a supine position to a sitting one.

Newborn Reflexes. Assess the newborn's reflexes to evaluate neurologic function and development. Absent or abnormal reflexes in a newborn, persistence of a reflex past the age when the reflex is normally lost, or return of an infantile reflex in an older child or adult may indicate neurologic pathology (Table 18.4). Reflexes commonly assessed in the newborn include sucking, Moro, stepping, tonic neck, rooting, Babinski, palmar grasp and plantar grasp reflexes. Spinal reflexes tested include truncal incurvation (Galant reflex) and anocutaneous reflex (anal wink).

The *sucking reflex* is elicited by gently stimulating the newborn's lips by touching them. The newborn will

TABLE 18.4	NEWBORN REFLEXES: APPEARANCE AND DISAPPEARANCE	
Reflex	Appearance	Disappearance
Blinking	Newborn	Persists into adulthood
Moro	Newborn	3–6 mo
Grasp	Newborn	3–4 mo
Stepping	Birth	1–2 mo
Tonic neck	Newborn	3–4 mo
Sneeze	Newborn	Persists into adulthood
Rooting	Birth	4–6 mo
Gag reflex	Newborn	Persists into adulthood
Cough reflex	Newborn	Persists into adulthood
Babinski sign	Newborn	12 mo

spread to form a C shape. The newborn initially appears startled and then relaxes to a normal resting position (see Fig. 18.17B).

Assess the *stepping reflex* by holding the newborn upright and inclined forward with the soles of the feet touching a flat surface. The baby should make a stepping motion or walking, alternating flexion and extension with the soles of the feet (see Fig. 18.17C).

The *tonic neck reflex* resembles the stance of a fencer and is often called the fencing reflex. Test this reflex by having the newborn lie on the back. Turn the baby's head to one side. The arm toward which the baby is facing should extend straight away from the body with the hand partially open, whereas the arm on the side away from the face is flexed and the fist is clenched tightly. Reversing the direction to which the face is turned reverses the position (see Fig. 18.17D).

Elicit the *rooting reflex* by stroking the newborn's cheek. The newborn should turn toward the side that was stroked and should begin to make sucking movements (see Fig. 18.17E).

The *Babinski reflex* should be present at birth and disappears at approximately 1 year of age. It is elicited by stroking the lateral sole of the newborn's foot from the heel toward and across the ball of the foot. The toes should fan out. A diminished response indicates a neurologic problem and needs follow-up (see Fig. 18.17F).

The newborn exhibits two grasp reflexes: *palmar grasp* and *plantar grasp*. Elicit the palmar grasp reflex by placing a finger on the newborn's open palm. The baby's hand will close around the finger. Attempting to remove the finger causes the grip to tighten. Newborns have strong grasps and can almost be lifted from a flat

typically open the mouth and begin a sucking motion. Placing a gloved finger in the newborn's mouth will also elicit a sucking motion (Fig. 18.17A).

The *Moro reflex*, also called the embrace reflex, occurs when the neonate is startled. To elicit this reflex, place the newborn on his or her back. Support the upper body weight of the supine newborn by the arms, using a lifting motion, without lifting the newborn off the surface. Then release the arms suddenly. The newborn will throw the arms outward and flex the knees; the arms then return to the chest. The fingers also

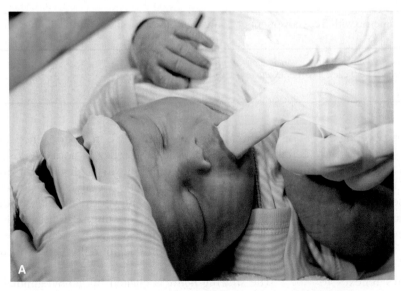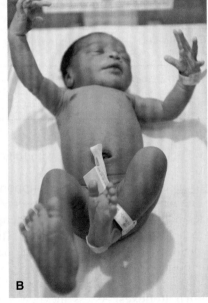

FIGURE 18.17 Newborn reflexes. **A.** Sucking reflex. **B.** Moro reflex.

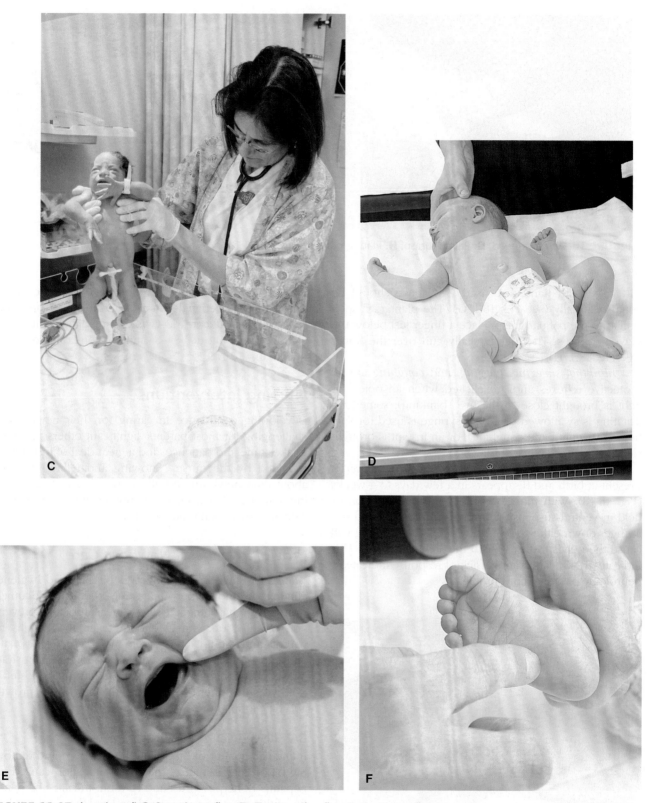

FIGURE 18.17 *(continued)* **C.** Stepping reflex. **D.** Tonic neck reflex. **E.** Rooting reflex. **F.** Babinski reflex. *(continued)*

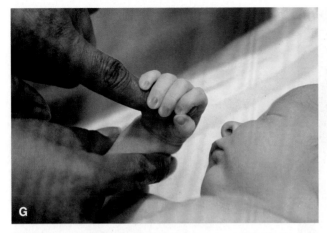

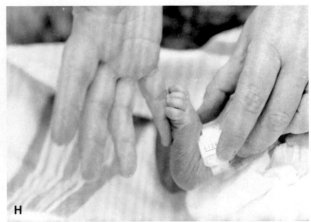

FIGURE 18.17 *(continued)* **G.** Palmar grasp. **H.** Plantar grasp.

surface if both hands are used. The grasp should be equal bilaterally (see Fig. 18.17G). The plantar grasp is similar to the palmar grasp. Place a finger just below the newborn's toes. The toes typically curl over the finger (see Fig. 18.17H).

Blinking, sneezing, gagging, and *coughing* are all protective reflexes and are elicited when an object or light is brought close to the eye (blinking); something irritating is swallowed or a bulb syringe is used for suctioning (gagging and coughing); or an irritant is brought close to the nose (sneezing).

The *truncal incurvation reflex* (*Galant reflex*) is present at birth and disappears in a few days to 4 weeks (Fig. 18.18). With the newborn in a prone position or held in ventral suspension, apply firm pressure and run a finger down either side of the spine. This stroking will cause the pelvis to flex toward the stimulated side. This indicates T2–S1 innervation. Lack of response indicates a neurologic or spinal cord problem.

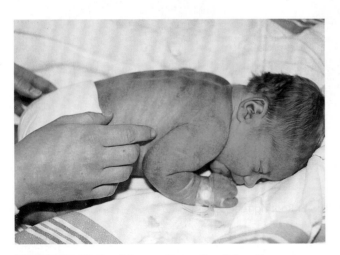

FIGURE 18.18 Trunk incurvation reflex. When the paravertebral area is stroked, the newborn flexes his or her trunk toward the direction of the stimulation. (Copyright Caroline Brown, RNC, MS, DEd.)

The *anocutaneous reflex* (*anal wink*) is elicited by stimulating the perianal skin close to the anus. The external sphincter will constrict (wink) immediately with stimulation. This indicates S4–S5 innervations (Marcdante & Kliegman, 2014).

Nursing Interventions

Developing confidence in caring for their newborn is challenging for most parents/significant others/partners. It takes time and patience, and a great deal of instruction provided by the nurse. "Showing and telling" parents about their newborn and all the procedures (e.g., feeding, bathing, changing, and handling) involved in daily care are key nursing interventions.

Providing General Newborn Care

Generally, newborn care involves bathing and hygiene, elimination and diaper area care, cord care, circumcision care, environmental safety measures, and prevention of infection. Nurses should teach these skills to parents and should serve as role models for appropriate and consistent interaction with newborns. Demonstrating respect for the newborn and family helps foster a positive atmosphere to promote the newborn's growth and development.

BATHING AND HYGIENE

Immediately after birth, drying the newborn and removing blood may minimize the risk of infection caused by hepatitis B, herpes virus, and HIV, but the specific benefits of this practice remain unclear. Until the newborn has been thoroughly bathed, standard precautions should be used when handling the newborn. Nurses need to follow their hospital policies regarding the timing and procedures for newborn bathing and hygiene.

Newborns are bathed primarily for aesthetic reasons, and bathing is postponed until thermal and cardiorespiratory stability is ensured. Traditional reasons why nurses bathe the newborn are so they can conduct a physical assessment, reduce the effect of hypothermia, and allow the mother to rest (Davidson, 2014). However, recent research suggests that nurses do not need to give the newborn an initial bath to reduce heat loss; rather, the parents could be given this opportunity, supported by nurses. A study found that the amount of heat loss was similar in newborns bathed by parents versus newborns who were bathed by nurses (Davidson, 2014).

Nursing Procedure 18.2 explains the steps for bathing the newborn. It is important for the nurse to wear gloves, because of potential exposure to maternal blood on the newborn, and perform the bath quickly, drying the baby thoroughly to prevent heat loss by evaporation.

After bathing, place the newborn under the radiant warmer and wrap him or her securely in blankets to prevent chilling. Check the baby's temperature within an hour to make sure it is within normal limits. If it is low, place the newborn under a radiant heat source again.

After the initial bath, the newborn may not receive another full one during the stay in the birthing unit. The diaper area will be cleansed at each diaper change, and any milk spilled into the newborn's neck folds from breast-feeding or formula will be cleaned. Clear water and a mild soap are appropriate to cleanse the diaper area. The use of lotions, baby oil, and powders is not encouraged because oils and lotions can lead to skin irritation and can cause rashes. Powders should not be used because they can be inhaled, causing respiratory distress. If the parents want to use oils and lotions, have them apply a small amount onto their hand first, away from the newborn; this warms the lotion. Then the parents should apply the lotion or oil sparingly.

Encourage the parents to gather all items needed before starting the bath: a soft, clean washcloth; two cotton balls to clean the eyes; mild, unscented soap and shampoo; towels or blankets; a tub or basin with warm water; a clean diaper; and a change of clothes. Instruct parents that a bath two or three times weekly is sufficient for the first year; more frequent bathing may dry the skin. Parents should not fully immerse the newborn into water until the umbilical cord area is healed—up to 2 weeks after birth. Encourage parents to give the infant a sponge bath until the umbilical cord falls off and the navel area is healed completely. If the newborn has been circumcised, advise parents to wait until that area has also healed (usually 1 to 2 weeks). Until then, clean the penis with mild soap and water and apply a small amount of petroleum jelly to the tip to prevent the diaper from adhering to the penis. Instruct parents to apply the diaper loosely and place the newly circumcised male infant on his side or back to prevent pressure and irritation on the penis.

Other guidelines for bathing newborns are given in Teaching Guidelines 18.1.

Teaching Guidelines 18.1
BATHING A NEWBORN

• Select a warm room with a flat surface at a comfortable working height.
• Before the bath, gather all supplies needed so they will be within reach.
• Never leave the newborn alone or unattended at any time during the bath.
• Undress the newborn down to shirt and diaper.
• Always support the newborn's head and neck when moving or positioning him or her.
• Place a blanket or towel underneath the newborn for warmth and comfort.
• In this order, progressing from the cleanest to the dirtiest areas:
  • Wipe eyes with plain water, using either cotton balls or a washcloth. Wipe from the inner corner of the eyes to the outer with separate wipes.
  • Wash the rest of the face, including ears, with plain water.
  • Using baby shampoo, gently wash the hair and rinse with water.
  • Pay special attention to body creases, and dry thoroughly.
  • Wash extremities, trunk, and back. Wash, rinse, dry, cover.
  • Wash diaper area last, using soap and water, and dry; observe for rash.
• Put on a clean diaper and clean clothes after the bath.

ELIMINATION AND DIAPER AREA CARE

Newborn elimination patterns are highly individualized. Usually the urine is light amber in color. Soaking 6 to 12 diapers a day indicates adequate hydration. Stools can change in color, texture, and frequency without signaling a problem. Meconium is passed for the first 48 hours after birth; the stools appear thick, tarry, sticky, and dark green. Transitional stools (thin, brown to green, less sticky than meconium) typically appear by day 3 after initiation of feeding. The stool characteristics after transitional stool depend on whether the newborn is breast-fed or bottle-fed. Breast-fed newborns typically pass mustard-colored, soft stool with a seedy consistency; formula-fed newborns pass yellow to brown, soft stools with a pasty consistency. As long as the newborn seems content, is eating normally, and shows no signs of illness, minor changes in bowel movements should not be a concern.

The newborn needs to be checked frequently to see whether a diaper change is needed, especially after feeding. Adhere to standard precautions when providing diaper area care. Instruct parents to keep the top edge of the diaper folded down below the umbilical cord area to

NURSING PROCEDURE 18.2

Bathing the Newborn

It is important that the nurse wear gloves, because of potential exposure to maternal blood on the newborn, and performs the bath quickly, drying the baby thoroughly to prevent heat loss by evaporation. Keep the newborn covered to prevent heat loss during the bathing procedure.

1. Begin the newborn bath starting from the cleanest area (the eyes) and proceeding to the most soiled area (the diaper area) to prevent cross-contamination. Use plain warm water on the face and eyes, adding a mild soap (e.g., Dove) to cleanse the remainder of the body. Wash, rinse, and dry each area before proceeding to the next one.

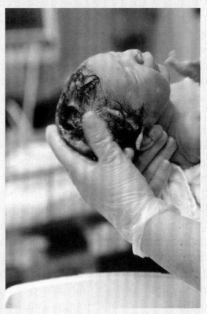

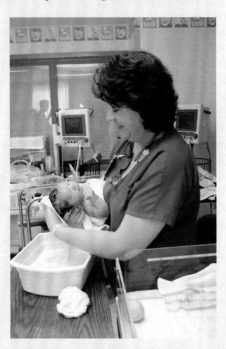

3. Make sure to cleanse all body creases, especially the neck folds to remove any milk that may have dripped into these areas.

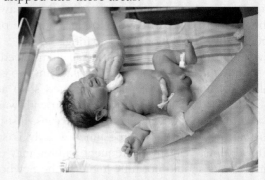

2. Wash the hair using running water so that the scalp can be thoroughly rinsed. A mild shampoo or soap can be used. Wash both fontanel areas. Frequently, parents avoid these "soft spots" because they fear that they will "hurt the baby's brain" if they rub too hard. Reassure parents that there is a strong membrane providing protection. Urge the parents to clean and rinse these areas well. If the anterior fontanel is not rinsed well after shampooing, cradle cap (dry flakes on the scalp) can develop. Avoid getting water in ears to prevent infection.

4. Continue downward washing the trunk and extremities ending up with the diaper area last.

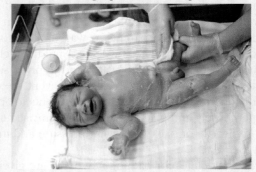

prevent irritation and to allow air to help dry the cord. For a male infant, point the penis down to prevent urine from wetting the top of the diaper where the umbilicus is located.

Meconium can be difficult to remove from the skin. Use plain water or special cleansing wipes if necessary to clean the area. Teach parents how to clean the diaper area properly and how to prevent skin irritation. Encourage them to avoid products such as powder and fragranced items, which could irritate the newborn's skin.

Discuss the pros and cons of using cloth diapers versus disposable diapers so that the parents can make informed decisions. Regardless of the type of diapers used, up to 10 diapers a day, or about 70 a week, will be needed.

Additional information about diapering might include:

- Before diapering, make sure all supplies are within reach, including clean diaper, cleaning agent or wipes, and ointment.
- Lay the newborn on a changing table and remove the dirty diaper.
- Use water and mild soap or wipes to gently wipe the genital area clean; wipe from front to back for girls to avoid urinary tract infections.
- Wash your hands thoroughly before and after changing diapers.

While performing diaper area care, parents should observe the area closely for irritation or rash. Tips for preventing or healing a diaper rash include:

- Change diapers frequently, especially after bowel movements.
- Apply a "barrier" cream, such as A&D ointment or Desitin, after cleaning with mild soap and water.
- Use dye- and fragrance-free detergents to wash cloth diapers.
- Avoid the use of plastic pants, because they tend to hold in moisture.
- Expose the newborn's bottom to air several times a day.
- Place the newborn's buttocks in warm water after he or she has had a diaper on all night.

Take Note!

Advise parents that a rash that persists for more than 3 days may be fungal in origin and may require additional treatment. Encourage the parents to notify the health care provider.

CORD CARE

The umbilical cord begins drying within hours after birth and is shriveled and blackened by the second or third day. Within 7 to 10 days, it sloughs off and the umbilicus heals. During this transition, frequent assessments of the area are necessary to detect any bleeding or signs of infection. Cord bleeding is abnormal and may occur if the cord clamp is loosened. Any cord drainage is also abnormal and is generally caused by infection, which requires immediate treatment.

The only care necessary for the umbilical cord stump is to keep it clean and dry. Keep the cord stump area dry and clean with water only daily. Expect to remove the cord clamp approximately 24 hours after birth by using a cord-cutting clamp. However, if the cord is still moist, keep the clamp in place and ensure a referral to home health care so that the home care nurse can remove it after discharge. Always adhere to agency policies regarding cord care; changes in policy may be necessary based on new research findings.

Many parents avoid contact with the cord site to make sure they don't "bother" it. Teach them how to care for the cord site when they go home to prevent complications (Teaching Guidelines 18.2).

Teaching Guidelines 18.2
UMBILICAL CORD CARE

- Observe for bleeding, redness, drainage, or foul odor from the cord stump and report it to your newborn's primary care provider immediately.
- Avoid tub baths until the cord has fallen off and the area has healed.
- Expose the cord stump to the air as much as possible throughout the day.
- Fold diapers below the level of the cord to prevent contamination of the site and to promote air-drying of the cord.
- Observe the cord stump, which will change color from yellow to brown to black. This is normal.
- Never pull the cord or attempt to loosen it; it will fall off naturally.

CIRCUMCISION AND CARE OF THE PENIS

Circumcision is one of the oldest and most common surgical procedures performed worldwide, but remains controversial. It is performed for medical, religious, cultural, and social reasons. **Circumcision** is the surgical removal of all or part of the foreskin (prepuce) of the penis (Freedman & Hurwitz, 2015). This has been traditionally done for hygiene and medical reasons and is the oldest known religious rite. In the Jewish faith, circumcision is a ritual that is performed by a *mohel* (ordained circumciser) on the eighth day after birth if possible. The circumcision is followed by a *bris* (the Jewish religious ceremony), typically in the home, during which the newborn is named and symbolically enters the Jewish religious community.

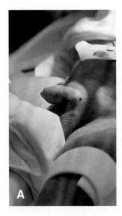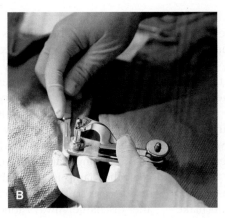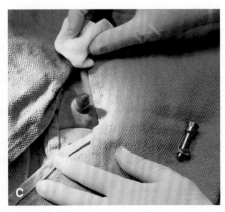

FIGURE 18.19 Circumcision. **A.** Before the procedure. **B.** Clamp applied and foreskin removed. **C.** Appearance after circumcision.

Most other circumcisions are performed in the hospital before the newborn is discharged as this is convenient for parents or taken to the doctor's outpatient office after discharge, is practical, and has a demonstrated record of safety. There are three commonly used methods of circumcision: the Gomco clamp, the Hollister Plastibell device, and the Mogen clamp. During the circumcision procedure, part of the foreskin is removed by clamping and cutting with a scalpel (Gomco or Mogen clamp) or by using a Plastibell. The Plastibell is fitted over the glans, and the excess foreskin is pulled over the plastic ring. A suture is tied around the rim to apply pressure to the blood vessels, creating hemostasis. The excess foreskin is cut away. The plastic rim remains in place until healing occurs. The plastic ring typically loosens and falls off in approximately 1 week. Petroleum jelly should be applied to the circumcised area after the procedure is done with the Gomco or Mogen clamp (Sinkey et al., 2015) (Fig. 18.19).

The debate over routine newborn circumcision continues in the United States. For many years, the purported benefits and harms of circumcision have been debated in the medical literature and society at large, with no clear consensus to date. Despite the controversy, circumcision is the most common surgical procedure performed on newborns, and almost two thirds (61%) of American male newborns are circumcised (CDC, 2015c).

Policy Statement by American Academy of Pediatrics.
A policy statement by the AAP indicates that newborn circumcision has potential disadvantages and risks as well as medical benefits and advantages. Risks to the newborn include infection, hemorrhage, skin dehiscence, adhesions, urethral fistula, and pain. Benefits to the newborn include the following:
• Urinary tract infections are slightly less common in circumcised boys. However, rates are low in both circumcised and uncircumcised boys and are easily treated without long-term sequelae.

• Sexually transmitted infections are less common in circumcised males, but the risk is believed to be related more to behavioral factors than to circumcision status. However, circumcised males have a 50% lower risk of acquiring HIV infection, herpes simplex virus, human papillomavirus (HPV), genital ulcer disease, bacterial vaginosis, and trichomoniasis (Tobian, Kacker, & Quinn, 2014).
• There appears to be a slightly lower rate of penile cancer in circumcised males. However, penile cancer is rare and risk factors such as genital warts, infection with HPV, multiple sex partners, and cigarette smoking seem to play a much larger role in causing penile cancer than circumcision status (Marcdante & Kliegman, 2014).

The new AAP recommendations state that if parents decide to circumcise their newborn, pain relief must be provided. Research has found that newborns circumcised without analgesia experience pain and stress, indicated by changes in heart rate, blood pressure, oxygen saturation, and cortisol levels (Morrison et al., 2014). Analgesic methods may include EMLA® cream (a topical mixture of local anesthetics, lidocaine and prilocaine), a dorsal penile nerve block with buffered lidocaine, acetaminophen, skin-to-skin contact, a sucrose pacifier, and swaddling (Cunningham et al., 2014).

The AAP (2015e) recommends that parents be given accurate and unbiased information about the risks and benefits of circumcision. As with other newborn procedures, research continues. Nurses must keep informed about current medical research to allow parents to make informed decisions. The absence of compelling medical evidence in favor of or against newborn circumcision makes informed consent of parents of paramount importance. The circumcision discussion involves cultural, religious, medical, and emotional considerations. Nurses may have difficulty remaining unbiased and unemotional as they present the facts to parents. Circumcision is a very personal decision for parents, and the nurse's major responsibility is to inform the parents of the risks and benefits of the procedure and to address concerns so that the parents can reach a fully informed decision.

Take Note!

The decision to circumcise the male newborn is often a social one, with the strongest factor being whether the newborn's father is himself circumcised (Mielke, 2014).

Preoperative circumcision preparation should include confirmation of the following:

- Infant is at least 12 hours old or older
- Infant has received standard vitamin K prophylaxis
- Infant has voided normally at least once since birth
- Infant has not eaten for at least an hour prior to the procedure
- Written parental consent has been obtained
- Correct identification of the infant brought to the procedure room

Immediately after circumcision, the tip of the penis is usually covered with petroleum-jelly–coated gauze to keep the wound from sticking to the diaper. Continued care of this site includes:

- Assess for bleeding every 30 minutes for at least 2 hours.
- Document the first voiding to evaluate for urinary obstruction or edema.
- Squeeze soapy water over the area daily and then rinse with warm water. Pat dry.
- Apply a small amount of petroleum jelly with every diaper change if the Plastibell was used; clean with mild soap and water if other techniques were used.
- Fasten the diaper loosely over the penis and avoiding placing the newborn on his abdomen to prevent friction.

If a Plastibell has been used, it will fall off by itself in about a week. Inform parents of this and advise them not to pull it off sooner. Also instruct the parents to check daily for any foul-smelling drainage, bleeding, or unusual swelling.

If the newborn is uncircumcised, wash the penis with mild soap and water after each diaper change and do not force the foreskin back; it will retract normally over time.

SAFETY

Newborns are completely dependent on those around them to ensure their safety. Their safety must be ensured while in the health care facility and after they are discharged. Parental education is key, especially as the newborn grows and develops and begins to respond to and explore his or her surroundings (Teaching Guidelines 18.3).

Teaching Guidelines 18.3
GENERAL NEWBORN SAFETY

- Have emergency telephone numbers readily available, such as those for emergency medical assistance and the poison control center.
- Keep small or sharp objects out of reach to prevent them from being aspirated.
- Put safety plugs in wall sockets within the child's reach to prevent electrocution.
- Do not leave the infant alone in any room without a portable intercom on.
- Always supervise the newborn in the tub: a newborn can drown in 2 in of water.
- Make sure the crib or changing table is sturdy, without any loose hardware, and is painted with lead-free paint.
- Avoid placing the crib or changing table near blinds or curtain cords.
- Provide a smoke-free environment for all infants.
- Place all infants on their backs to sleep to prevent sudden infant death syndrome.
- To prevent falls, do not leave the newborn alone on any elevated surface.
- Use sun shields on strollers and hats to avoid overexposing the newborn to the sun.
- To prevent infection, thoroughly wash your hands before preparing formula.
- Thoroughly investigate any infant care facility before using it.

Adapted from Centers for Disease Control and Prevention [CDC]. (2015d). *Infants and toddlers—safety in the home and community.* Retrieved from http://www.cdc.gov/parents/infants/safety.html

Environmental Safety. People who enter a health care facility for treatment expect to be safe there until they return home, but ensuring a safe environment can be a daunting challenge to a health care facility.

Consider this scenario: A woman dressed in nurse's clothing entered the hospital room of a new mother soon after she had given birth. This "nurse" told the mother that she needed to take her newborn to the nursery to have him weighed. Sometime later, a staff nurse making her routine rounds realized something was wrong when she saw that the newborn's bassinet in the mother's room was empty and the mother was sound asleep in her bed. The staff nurse called security immediately because she suspected that a newborn abduction had taken place.

This is a typical abduction scenario that is repeated many times throughout the United States each year. In **infant abduction**, someone who is not a family member takes a child less than 1 year old (NCMEC, 2015). Infant abductions are traumatic for the parents, the community, and the health care facility. The facility may also face huge financial liability if a lawsuit is filed by the parents.

Abductions typically occur during the day and are usually carried out by women who are not criminally sophisticated. Many of these women experienced a pregnancy loss in the past; they are often emotionally immature and compulsive, with low self-esteem. Most female abductors can play the role of a hospital employee convincingly. Infants usually are abducted when taken for testing, during return to the nursery, when left unattended in the nursery, or while a mother was napping or showering (Joint Commission, 2015).

Health care agencies are challenged to prevent infant abduction by instituting sound security practices and systems (Joint Commission, 2015). Such measures include the following:

- All newborns must be transported in cribs and not carried.
- Nurses must respond immediately to any security alarm that sounds on the unit.
- Newborns must never be unattended at any time, especially in hallways.
- All staff must wear appropriate identification at all times.
- Encourage mothers to keep their baby/bassinet on their far side, away from the door.
- Personnel should be wary of visitors who do not seem to be visiting a specific mother.
- The electronic security system should be checked to make sure it works.
- Footprint the newborn, take a color photograph, and record the newborn's physical examination within 2 hours of birth.
- Discontinue publication of birth notices in local newspapers.
- Develop and implement a proactive infant abduction prevention plan.
- Ensure the proper functioning and placement of any electronic sensors used on newborns.
- Parents should be taught what infant abduction is; why infant security is important; the schedule of nursery, feeding, and visiting hours; rules about visitor access; the facility's security policies and procedures; what parents can do to protect their infant in the hospital; which staff members are allowed to handle the newborn; and what a proper ID looks like.

Educating staff, educating mothers, and access control are the three key steps to preventing abductions from any health care facility. Providing a safe and secure environment is a shared responsibility of the facility, staff, and parents. Preventing abductions requires everyone to learn and follow the rules and policies.

Car Safety. Every state requires the use of car seats for infants and children, because motor vehicle accidents are still the leading cause of unintentional injury and death in children under age 5. National Highway Traffic Safety Administration statistics show that nearly one half of deaths and injuries in infants occurred because they were not properly restrained. Child safety seats, when installed and used properly, can prevent injuries and save lives (AAP, 2015f).

Despite evidence that the use of car seats can reduce the morbidity and mortality of motor vehicle crashes, parents who lack knowledge about them may underuse or misuse them (Hodges & Smith, 2014). Make sure that both parents understand the importance of safely transporting their newborn in a federally approved safety car seat every time the infant rides in a car. Do not release any newborn unless the parents have a car seat in place for their newborn's ride home (Fig. 18.20). If they cannot afford one, many community organizations will provide one for them. According to the AAP's policy statement on child passenger safety (AAP, 2015f), no one car seat is considered to be the "safest" or the "best," but rather consistent and proper use is the key to preventing injuries and deaths. Instruct parents in the following:

- Select a car seat that is appropriate for the child's size and weight.
- Caution caregivers against the placement of car seats on elevated or soft surfaces outside the car to prevent falling.
- Use the car seat correctly, every time the child is in the car.
- Use rear-facing car safety seats for most infants up to 2 years of age or until they reach the highest weight or height allowed by the manufacturer of their CSS.
- Make sure the harness (most seats have a three- to five-point harness) is in the slots at or below the shoulders.

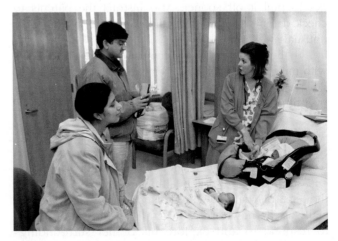

FIGURE 18.20 Newborn in a properly secured car seat.

INFECTION PREVENTION

The nurse plays a major role in preventing infection in the newborn environment. Ways to control infection are as follows:

- Minimize exposure of newborns to organisms.
- Wash your hands before and after providing care, and insist that all personnel wash their hands before handling any newborn.
- Do not allow ill staff or visitors to visit or handle newborns.
- Avoid sharing any infant supplies with another infant
- Monitor the umbilical cord stump and circumcision site for signs of infection.
- Provide eye prophylaxis by instilling prescribed medication soon after birth.
- Educate parents about appropriate home measures that will prevent infections, such as practicing good hand hygiene before and after diaper changes, keeping the newborn well hydrated, avoiding taking the infant into crowds (which may expose him or her to colds and flu viruses), observing for early signs of infection (fever, vomiting, loss of appetite, lethargy, labored breathing, green watery stools, and drainage from umbilical cord site or eyes), and keeping pediatrician appointments for routine immunizations.

Promoting Sleep

Although many parents feel their newborns need them every minute of the day, babies actually need to sleep much of the day initially. Usually newborns sleep up to 15 hours daily. They sleep for 2 to 4 hours at a time but do not sleep through the night because their stomach capacity is too small to go long periods without nourishment.

Take Note!

All newborns develop their own sleep patterns and cycles, but it may take several months before the newborn sleeps through the night. Frequently, newborns have their day and night hours reversed and tend to sleep more during the daytime and less during the night.

Parents should place the newborn on his or her back to sleep. To prevent suffocation, all fluffy bedding, quilts, sheepskins, stuffed animals, and pillows should be removed from the crib. Parents should be informed that the practice of "co-sleeping" (sharing a bed) is not safe. For example, infants who sleep in adult beds are up to 40 times more likely to suffocate than those who sleep in cribs (AAP, 2015g). Suffocation can occur when the infant gets entangled in bedding or caught under pillows, or slips between the bed and the wall or the headboard and mattress. The parent may accidentally roll against or on top of the baby. The safest place for a newborn to sleep is in a crib, without any movable objects close by. Benefits versus risks of co-bedding, bed sharing, or co-sleeping include the following:

- *Benefits*—Promotes breast-feeding practices; increases bonding time between the infant and mother; promotes skin-to-skin contact; and increases maternal vigilance over infant.
- *Risks*—Increases risk for SIDS for infants younger than 4 months; risk of death if parent rolls over the infant; interrupts infant sleeping patterns; risk of asphyxia due to entrapment or airway obstruction; and unsafe design of adult beds for infants (Gaydos et al., 2014).

Teach parents to avoid other unsafe conditions, such as placing the newborn in the prone position, using a crib that does not meet federal safety guidelines, allowing window cords to hang loose and in proximity to the crib, placing blankets and pillows in the crib (can potentially smother infant), exposure to tobacco smoke, alcohol, and illicit drugs or setting the room temperature too high (can cause overheating) (CDC, 2015d). Recommendations for safe infant sleeping practices are an important aspect of education for new parents. It is important for nurses to assess families' cultural beliefs and their prior practices to fully understand how to make recommendations in a culturally sensitive manner.

The *Safe to Sleep Campaign* (NICHD, 2014) recommends the following to reduce the risk of SIDS:

- Always place the baby on his or her back to sleep for all sleep times, including naps.
- Room share—keep baby's sleep area in the same room next to where you sleep.
- Use a firm sleep surface, free from soft objects, toys, blankets, and crib bumpers.

Enhancing Bonding

Encourage and enhance parent–newborn interaction by involving both parents with the baby and demonstrating appropriate nurturing behaviors:

- Say "hello" and introduce yourself to the newborn.
- Ask the parents' permission to care for and hold their newborn. This helps parents to realize that they are responsible for their child and reminds nurses of their role.
- Show parents the power of a soothing voice to calm the newborn (Fig. 18.21).
- Provide care to the newborn in the least stressful way.
- Demonstrate ways to gently wake up the newborn for better feeding.
- Tell parents what you are doing, why you are doing it, and how they can duplicate what you are doing at home.
- Offer the opportunity for parents to perform care while you observe them. Support their efforts to soothe the newborn throughout the care process.

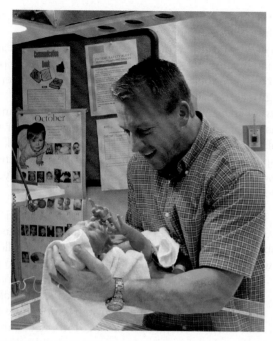

FIGURE 18.21 The father uses a soothing voice to calm the newborn.

- Help parents to interpret the communication cues the newborn uses.
- Point out the efforts the newborn is making to connect with the parents (e.g., alerting to the familiar voice, following the parents while they are speaking, quieting when held securely).

One of the most pleasurable aspects of newborn care is being close to them. Bonding begins soon after birth when parents cradle their newborn and gently stroke him or her with their fingers. Provide parents with opportunities for "skin-to-skin" contact with the newborn, holding the baby against their own skin when feeding or cradling. Many newborns respond very positively to gentle massage. If necessary, recommend books and videos that cover the subject.

For newborns, crying is their only way to communicate that something is wrong. Try to find out the reason why: Is the diaper wet? Is the room too hot or too cold? Is the baby uncomfortable (e.g., diaper rash or tight clothing)? Suggest the following ways in which parents can soothe an upset newborn:

- Try feeding or burping to relieve air or stomach gas.
- Lightly rub the newborn's back and speak softly to him or her.
- Gently sway side to side, or rock back and forth in a rocking chair.
- Talk with the newborn while making eye contact.
- Take the newborn for a walk in a stroller or carriage to get fresh air.
- Change the baby's position from back to side or vice versa.

- Try singing, reciting poetry and nursery rhymes, or reading to the baby.
- Turn on a musical mobile above the newborn's head.
- Give more physical contact by walking, rocking, or patting the newborn.
- Swaddle the newborn to provide a sense of security and comfort. To do this:
  - Spread out a receiving blanket, with one corner folded slightly.
  - Lay the newborn face up with head at the folded corner.
  - Wrap the left corner over the baby's body and tuck it beneath the baby.
  - Bring the bottom corner over the baby's feet.
  - Wrap the right corner around the baby, leaving only the head exposed.
  - Arms can be released from the blanket to allow for self-comforting.

Assisting With Screening Tests

Newborn screening has been among the most successful public health programs of the 21st century. Approximately 4 million infants are screened annually in the United States (Adamkin, 2015). Screening newborns for problems is important because some potentially life-threatening metabolic diseases may not be obvious at birth. Newborn screening tests that are required in most states before discharge are used to check for certain genetic and inborn errors of metabolism and hearing. Early identification and initiation of treatment can prevent significant complications and can minimize the negative effects of untreated disease.

GENETIC AND INBORN ERRORS OF METABOLISM SCREENING

Although each state mandates which conditions must be tested, the most common screening tests are for PKU, hypothyroidism, galactosemia, and sickle cell disease (Table 18.5).

The trend toward early discharge of newborns can affect the timing of screening and the accuracy of some test results. For example, the newborn needs to ingest enough breast milk or formula to elevate phenylalanine levels for the screening test to identify PKU accurately, so newborn screening for PKU testing should not be performed before 24 hours of age.

Screening tests for genetic and inborn errors of metabolism require a few drops of blood taken from the newborn's heel (Fig. 18.22). These tests are usually performed shortly before discharge. Newborns that are discharged before 24 hours of age need to have repeat tests done within a week in an outpatient facility.

Be aware of which conditions your state regularly screens for at birth to ensure that the parents are taught about the tests and the importance of early treatment.

TABLE 18.5 | **SELECTED CONDITIONS SCREENED FOR IN THE NEWBORN**

Condition	Description	Clinical Picture/ Effect If not Treated	Treatment	Timing of Screening
PKU	Autosomal recessive inherited deficiency in one of the enzymes necessary for the metabolism of phenylalanine to tyrosine—essential amino acids found in most foods	Irritability, vomiting of protein feedings, and a musty odor to the skin or body secretions of the newborn; if not treated, mental and motor retardation, seizures, microcephaly, and poor growth and development	Lifetime diet of foods low in phenylalanine (low protein) and monitoring of blood levels; special newborn formulas available: Phenex and Lofenalac	Universally screened for in the United States; testing is done 24–48 hours after protein feeding (PKU)
Congenital hypo- thyroidism	Deficiency of thyroid hormone necessary for normal brain growth, calorie metabolism, and development; may result from maternal hypothyroidism	Increased risk in newborns with birth weight <2,000 g or >4,500 g, and those of Hispanic and Asian ethnic groups; feeding problems, growth and breathing problems; if not treated, irreversible brain damage and intellectual disability before age 1	Lifelong thyroid replacement therapy	Testing (measures thyroxin [T_4] and TSH) is done between days 4 and 6 of life
Galactosemia	Absence of the enzyme needed for the conversion of the milk sugar galactose to glucose	Poor weight gain, vomiting, jaundice, mood changes, loss of eyesight, seizures, and intellectual disability; if untreated, galactose buildup causing permanent damage to the brain, eyes, and liver, and eventually death	Eliminate milk from diet; substitute soy milk	First test done on discharge from the hospital with a follow-up test within 1 mo
Sickle cell anemia	Recessively inherited abnormality in hemoglobin structure, most commonly found in African American newborns	Anemia developing shortly after birth; increased risk for infection, growth restriction, vaso-occlusive crisis	Maintenance of hydration and hemodilution, rest, electrolyte replacement, pain management, blood replacement, and antibiotics	Bloodspot obtained at same time of other newborn screening tests or prior to 3 months of age

Adapted from Bhattacharya, K., Wotton, T., & Wiley, V. (2014). The evolution of blood-spot newborn screening. *Translational Pediatrics*, *3*(2), 63–70; Boyle, C. A., Bocchini, J. A., & Kelly, J. (2014). Reflections on 50 years of newborn screening. *Pediatrics*, *133*(6), 961–963; and Greene, C. L., & Matern, D. (2014). Newborn screening for inborn errors of metabolism. In *Physician's guide to the diagnosis, treatment, and follow-up of inherited metabolic diseases* (pp. 719–735). Berlin, Germany: Springer.

Also be familiar with the optimal time frame for screening and conditions that could affect the results. Ensure that a satisfactory specimen has been obtained at the appropriate time and that circumstances that could cause false results have been minimized. Send out specimens and completed forms within 24 hours of collection to the appropriate laboratory (Nagtalon-Ramos, 2014).

HEARING SCREENING

Hearing loss is the most common birth disorder in the United States: approximately 3 to 5 newborns out of every 1,000 live births have some degree of hearing loss. Unlike a physical deformity, hearing loss is not clinically detectable at birth and thus remains difficult to assess (CDC, 2015b). Factors associated with an increased risk of hearing loss include the following:

- Family history of hereditary childhood sensory hearing loss
- Congenital infections such as cytomegalovirus, rubella, toxoplasmosis, or herpes
- Craniofacial anomalies involving the pinna or ear canal

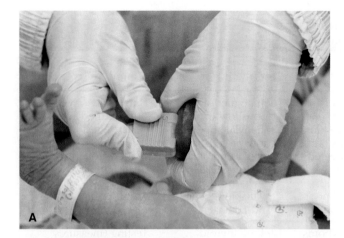

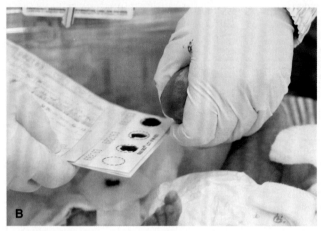

FIGURE 18.22 Screening for PKU. **A.** Performing a heel stick. **B.** Applying the blood specimen to the card for screening.

- Low birth weight (less than 1,500 g)
- Postnatal infections such as bacterial meningitis
- Head trauma
- Hyperbilirubinemia requiring an exchange transfusion
- Exposure to ototoxic drugs, especially aminoglycosides
- Perinatal asphyxia (Nikolopoulos, 2015)

Delays in identification and intervention may affect the child's language development, academic performance, and cognitive development. Detection before 3 months greatly improves outcomes. Because of this, auditory screening programs for all newborns are recommended by the AAP (2015d) and are mandated by law in over 30 states. Screening only infants with risk factors is not enough, because as many as 50% of infants born with hearing loss have no known risk factors (CDC, 2015b). Early identification and intervention can prevent severe psychosocial, educational, and language development delays.

The current goals of *Healthy People 2020* (USDHHS, 2010) are to screen all infants by 1 month of age, confirm hearing loss with an audiologic examination by 3 months of age, and treat with comprehensive early

---

NEWBORN HEARING SCREENING METHODS

Newborn hearing screening is the standard of care in hospitals nationwide. The primary purpose of newborn hearing screening is to identify newborns who are likely to have a hearing loss and who require further evaluation. A newborn's hearing can be screened in one of two ways: otoacoustic emission (OAE) or automated auditory brainstem response (ABR).

In OAE, an earphone is placed in the infant's ear canal and the sounds produced by the newborn's inner ear are measured in response to certain tones or clicks presented through the earphone. Preset parameters in the equipment decide whether the OAEs are sufficient for the newborn to pass or whether a referral is necessary for further evaluation.

In ABR, an earphone is placed in the ear canal or an earmuff is placed over the newborn's ear, and a soft, rapid tapping noise is presented. Electrodes placed around the newborn's head, neck, and shoulders record neural activity from the infant's brainstem in response to the tapping noises. The ABR tests how well the ear and the nerves leading to the brain work. Like OAEs, automated ABR screening is sensitive to more than mild degrees of hearing loss, but a "pass" does not guarantee normal hearing.

Adapted from Mersch, J., Kibby, J. E., & Bredenkamp, J. K. (2014). Newborn infant hearing screening. *MedicineNet.com,* Retrieved from http://www.medicinenet.com/newborn_infant_hearing_screening/article.htm; American Speech-Language-Hearing Association [ASHA]. (2014). *Newborn infant hearing screening.* Retrieved from http://www.asha.org/Practice-Portal/Professional-Issues/Newborn-Infant-Hearing-Screening/; and American Academy of Pediatrics [AAP]. (2015d). *Purpose of newborn hearing screening.* Retrieved from http://www.healthychildren.org/English/ages-stages/baby/Pages/Purpose-of-Newborn-Hearing-Screening.aspx

---

intervention services before 6 months of age (see the *Healthy People 2020* feature earlier in this chapter and Box 18.1 for screening methods). All newborns should be screened prior to discharge to ensure that any newborn with a hearing loss is not missed. Those with suspected hearing loss should be referred for follow-up assessment. In addition, nurses should ensure that testing is accurate to facilitate early diagnosis and intervention services and to optimize the newborn's developmental potential. The implementation of newborn hearing screenings has lowered the mean age of hearing loss identification and many deaf children are now diagnosed in the early age of months old.

Common Concerns

During the newborn period of transition, certain conditions can develop that require intervention. These conditions, although not typically life threatening, can be a source of anxiety for the parents. Common concerns include transient tachypnea of the newborn, physiologic jaundice, and hypoglycemia.

TRANSIENT TACHYPNEA OF THE NEWBORN

Transient tachypnea of the newborn appears soon after birth. It occurs when the fetal liquid in the lungs is removed slowly or incompletely. This can be due to the lack of thoracic squeezing that occurs during a cesarean birth or diminished respiratory effort if the mother received central nervous system depressant medication. Prolonged labor, macrosomia of the fetus, and maternal asthma also have been associated with this condition. A vaginal birth appears to be protective against transient tachypnea of the newborn (Cunningham et al., 2014).

Transient tachypnea is accompanied by retractions; expiratory grunting or cyanosis and is relieved by low-dose oxygen therapy. Mild or moderate respiratory distress typically is present at birth or within 6 hours of birth. Transient tachypnea of the newborn is generally a self-limited disorder without significant morbidity. Transient tachypnea of the newborn resolves over a 24-hour to 72-hour period.

Nursing interventions include providing supportive care: giving oxygen, ensuring warmth, observing respiratory status frequently, and allowing time for the pulmonary capillaries and the lymphatics to remove the remaining fluid. The clinical course is relatively benign, but any newborn respiratory issue can be very frightening to the parents. Provide a thorough explanation and reassure them that the condition will resolve over time.

PHYSIOLOGIC JAUNDICE

Physiologic jaundice is very common in newborns, with the majority demonstrating yellowish skin, mucous membranes, and sclera within the first 3 days of life. In any given year, approximately 65% of the newborns in the United States will experience clinical jaundice (King et al., 2015). Jaundice is the visible manifestation of hyperbilirubinemia. It typically results from the deposition of unconjugated bilirubin pigment in the skin and mucous membranes.

Physiologic jaundice can be best understood as an imbalance between the production and elimination of bilirubin, with a multitude of factors and conditions affecting each of these processes. When an imbalance results because of an increase in circulating bilirubin (or the bilirubin load) to significantly high levels, it may go on to cause acute neurologic sequelae (acute bilirubin encephalopathy). In most infants, an increase in bilirubin production (e.g., due to hemolysis) is the primary cause of physiologic jaundice, and thus reducing bilirubin production is a rational approach for its management.

Factors that contribute to the development of physiologic jaundice in the newborn include an increased bilirubin load because of relative polycythemia, a shortened erythrocyte life span (80 days compared with the adult 120 days), and immature hepatic uptake and conjugation processes (Chu, 2014). Normally the liver removes bilirubin from the blood and changes it into a form that can be excreted. As the red blood cell breakdown continues at a fast pace, the newborn's liver cannot keep up with bilirubin removal. Thus, bilirubin accumulates in the blood, causing a yellowish discoloration on the skin.

AAP Guidelines for Prevention and Management of Hyperbilirubinemia in Newborns. The AAP has recently released guidelines for the prevention and management of hyperbilirubinemia in newborns:

- Promote and support successful breast-feeding practices to make sure the newborn is well hydrated and stooling frequently to promote elimination of bilirubin.
- Advise mothers to nurse their infants at least 8 to 12 times per day for the first several days.
- Avoid routine supplementation of nondehydrated breast-fed infants with water or dextrose water because that will not lower bilirubin levels.
- Ensure that all infants are routinely monitored for the development of jaundice and that nurseries have established protocols for the assessment of jaundice. Jaundice should be assessed whenever the infant's vital signs are measured but no less than every 8 to 12 hours.
- Before discharge, complete a systematic assessment for the risk of severe hyperbilirubinemia.
- Provide early and focused follow-up based on the risk assessment.
- When indicated, treat newborns with phototherapy or exchange transfusion to prevent acute bilirubin encephalopathy (AAP, 2015h).

In newborn infants, jaundice can be detected by blanching the skin with digital pressure on the bridge of the nose, sternum, or forehead, revealing the underlying color of the skin and subcutaneous tissue. If jaundice is present, the blanched area will appear yellow before the capillary refill. The assessment of jaundice must be performed in a well-lit room or, preferably, in daylight at a window. Jaundice is usually seen first in the face and progresses caudally to the trunk and extremities (AAP, 2015h).

Measures that parents can take to reduce the risk of jaundice include exposing the newborn to natural sunlight for short periods of time throughout the day to help oxidize the bilirubin deposits on the skin, providing breast-feeding on demand to promote elimination of bilirubin through urine and stooling, and avoiding glucose water supplementation, which hinders elimination.

If or when the levels of unconjugated serum bilirubin increase and do not return to normal levels with increased hydration, phototherapy is used. The serum level of bilirubin at which phototherapy is initiated is a matter of clinical judgment by the physician, but it is often begun when bilirubin levels reach 12 to 15 mg/dL in the first 48 hours of life in a term newborn (Davidson, 2014). **Phototherapy** involves exposing the newborn to ultraviolet light, which converts unconjugated bilirubin into products that can be excreted through feces and urine. Phototherapy is the most common treatment for hyperbilirubinemia and has virtually eliminated the need for exchange transfusions in newborns now.

Take Note!

Exposure of newborns to sunlight represents the first documented use of phototherapy in the medical literature. Sister J. Ward, a charge nurse in Essex, England, recognized in 1956 that when jaundiced newborns were exposed to the sun they became less yellow. This observation changed the entire treatment of jaundice in newborns (Maisels, 2015).

Phototherapy reduces bilirubin levels in the blood by breaking down unconjugated bilirubin into colorless compounds. These compounds can then be excreted in the bile. Phototherapy aims to curtail the increase in bilirubin blood levels; thereby preventing kernicterus, a condition in which unconjugated bilirubin enters the brain. If not treated, kernicterus can lead to brain damage and death.

During the past several decades, phototherapy has generally been administered with either banks of fluorescent lights or spotlights. Factors that determine the dosage of phototherapy include spectrum of light emitted, irradiance of light source, design of light unit, surface area of newborn exposed to the light, and distance of the newborn from the light source (McDermott, 2015). For phototherapy to be effective, the rays must penetrate as much of the skin as possible. Thus, the newborn must be naked and turned frequently to ensure maximum exposure of the skin. Several side effects of standard phototherapy have been identified: frequent loose stools, increased insensible water loss, transient rash, and potential retinal damage if the newborn's eyes are not covered sufficiently.

Recently, fiberoptic pads (Biliblanket or Bilivest) have been developed that can be wrapped around the newborn or on which the newborn can lie. The light is delivered from a tungsten–halogen bulb through a fiber-optic cable and is emitted from the sides and ends of the fibers inside a plastic pad (Plavskii, Tret'yakova, & Mostovnikova, 2014). These products work on the premise that phototherapy can be improved by delivering higher-intensity therapeutic light to decrease bilirubin levels. The pads do not produce appreciable heat like the banks of lights or spotlights do, so insensible water loss is not increased. Eye patches also are not needed; thus, parents can feed and hold their newborns continuously to promote bonding.

When caring for newborns receiving phototherapy for jaundice, nurses must do the following:

- Closely monitor body temperature and fluid and electrolyte balance.
- Document frequency, character, and consistency of stools.
- Monitor hydration status (weight, specific gravity of urine, and urine output).
- Turn frequently to increase the infant's skin exposure to phototherapy.
- Observe skin integrity (as a result of exposure to diarrhea and phototherapy lights).
- Provide eye protection to prevent corneal injury related to phototherapy exposure.
- Encourage parents to participate in their newborn's care to prevent parent–infant separation.

See Chapter 24 for a more detailed discussion of hyperbilirubinemia.

The home health nurse made a postpartum visit to Kelly to assess the situation. Kelly's son was slightly jaundiced when the home health nurse pressed gently over his sternum, but Kelly said he was nursing better compared with the previous 2 days. What home suggestions can the nurse make to Kelly to reduce the jaundice? What specific education about physiologic jaundice is needed?

HYPOGLYCEMIA

During the first 24 to 48 hours of life, as normal newborns transition from intrauterine to extrauterine life, their plasma glucose levels are typically lower than later in life. Hypoglycemia affects as many as 40% of all full-term newborns. It is defined as a blood glucose level of less than 30 mg/dL or a plasma concentration of less than 40 mg/dL in the first 72 hours of life (Thornton et al., 2015). From a physiologic perspective, a newborn may be said to be hypoglycemic when glucose supply is inadequate to meet demand. In newborns, blood glucose levels fall to a low point during the first few hours of life because the source of maternal glucose is removed when the placenta is expelled. This period of transition is usually smooth, but certain newborns are at greater risk for hypoglycemia: infants of mothers who have diabetes, preterm newborns, and newborns with intrauterine growth restriction (IUGR), inadequate caloric intake, sepsis, asphyxia, hypothermia, polycythemia, glycogen storage disorders, and endocrine deficiencies (Adamkin, 2015).

Most newborns experience transient hypoglycemia and are asymptomatic. The symptoms, when present, are nonspecific and include jitteriness, lethargy, cyanosis, apnea, seizures, high-pitched or weak cry, hypothermia, and poor feeding. If hypoglycemia is prolonged or is left untreated, serious, long-term adverse neurologic sequelae such as learning disabilities and intellectual disabilities can occur (Stanley et al., 2015).

Treatment of hypoglycemia in the newborn includes administration of a rapid-acting source of glucose such as a sugar/water mixture or early formula-feeding. In acute, severe cases, intravenous administration of glucose may be required. Continuous monitoring of glucose levels is not only prudent but mandatory in high-risk newborns. Although there is no specific means of preventing hypoglycemia in newborns, it is wise and cautious to monitor for symptoms and intervene as soon as symptoms are noted. Subsequently, early diagnosis and appropriate intervention are essential for all newborns.

Nursing care of the hypoglycemic newborn includes monitoring for signs of hypoglycemia or identifying high-risk newborns prone to this disorder based on their perinatal history, physical examination, body measurements, and gestational age. Glucose screening should be performed only on at-risk infants and those with clinical symptoms compatible with hypoglycemia (National Guideline Clearinghouse, 2015).

Prevent hypoglycemia in newborns at risk by initiating early feedings with breast milk or formula. If hypoglycemia persists despite feeding, notify the primary health care provider for orders such as intravenous therapy with dextrose solutions. Anticipate hypoglycemia in certain high-risk newborns and begin assessments immediately on nursery admission.

Promoting Nutrition

Several physiologic changes dictate the type and method of feeding throughout the newborn's first year. Some of these changes include the following:

• Stomach capacity is limited at birth. The emptying time is short (2 to 3 hours) and peristalsis is rapid. Therefore, small, frequent feedings are needed at first, with amounts progressively increasing with maturity.
• The immune system is immature at birth, so the baby is at a high risk for food allergies during the first 4 to 6 months of life. Introducing solid foods prior to this time increases the risk of developing food allergies.
• Pancreatic enzymes and bile to assist in digestion of fat and starch are in limited supply until about 3 to 6 months of age. Infants cannot digest cereal prior to this time.
• The kidneys are immature and unable to concentrate urine until about 4 to 6 weeks of age. Excess protein and mineral intake can place a strain on kidney function and can lead to dehydration. Infants need to consume more water per unit of body weight than adults do as a result of their high body weight from water.
• Immature muscular control at birth changes over time to assist in the feeding process by improving head and

neck control, hand–eye coordination, swallowing, and ability to sit, grasp, and chew. At about 4 to 6 months, inborn reflexes disappear, head control develops, and the infant can sit to be fed, making spoon-feeding possible (Dudek, 2014)

NEWBORN NUTRITIONAL NEEDS

As newborns grow, their energy and nutrient requirements change to meet their body's changing needs. During infancy, energy, protein, vitamin, and mineral requirements per pound of body weight are higher than at any other time of life. These high levels are needed to fuel the rapid growth and development during this stage of life. Generally, an infant's birth weight doubles in the first 4 to 6 months of life and triples within the first year (Walker, 2014).

A newborn's caloric needs range from 110 to 120 cal/kg body weight. Breast milk and formulas contain approximately 20 cal/oz, so the caloric needs of young infants can be met if several feedings are given throughout the day. Most term infants need a basic formula if the mother chooses not to breast-feed. These formulas are modeled after breast milk, which contains 20 cal/oz. There is no evidence to recommend one brand over the other since all of them are nutritionally interchangeable. All formulas are classified based on three parameters: caloric density, carbohydrate source, and protein composition (see Table 18.6).

Fluid requirements for the newborn and infant range from 100 to 150 mL/kg daily. This requirement can be met through breast- or bottle-feeding. Additional water supplementation is not necessary. Adequate carbohydrates, fats, protein, and vitamins are achieved through consumption of breast milk or formula. The AAP (2015i) recommends that bottle-fed infants be given iron supplementation, because iron levels are low in all types of formula milk. This can be achieved by giving iron-fortified formula from birth. The breast-fed infant draws on iron reserves for the first 6 months and then needs iron-rich foods or supplementation added at 6 months of age. The AAP (2015i) also has recommended that all infants (breast- and bottle-fed) receive a daily supplement of 400 IU of vitamin D starting within the first few days of life to prevent rickets and vitamin D deficiency. It is also recommended that fluoride supplementation be given to infants not receiving fluoridated water after the age of 6 months (AAP, 2015i). Recently, the AAP recommended that all pregnant and lactating women use iodized salt and take a supplement of 150 μg of iodine daily. An iodine deficiency can affect fetal and early childhood neurocognitive development (AAP, 2015j).

SUPPORTING THE CHOICE OF FEEDING METHOD

The benefits of breast-feeding are significant and well documented. Numerous health-related professional

TABLE 18.6 COMPARISON OF BREAST MILK WITH SELECTED FORMULA COMPOSITION

Type	Brand Names	Calories per Ounce	Carbohydrate Source	Protein Source	Indications
Breast milk	None	20	Lactose	Human milk	Preferred for all infants
Term formula	Enfamil; Similac; Carnation Good Start	20	Lactose	Cow's milk	Appropriate for all term infants
Term formula with DHA and ARA	Enfamil Lipil; Good Start DHA and ARA; Similac Advance	20	Lactose	Cow's milk	Marketed to promote good vision and brain development; to make them more like breast milk.
Preterm formula	Enfamil 24 Premature; Preemie SMA 24	24	Lactose	Cow's milk	Usually given to preterm infants <34 weeks' gestation
Soy formula	Enfamil Prosobee; Good Start Soy	20	Corn based	Soy	For infants with galactosemia
Hypoallergenic formula	Similac Alimentum; Enfamil Nutramigen; Enfamil Pregestimil	20	Corn or sucrose	Extensively hydrolyzed	For infants with a milk protein allergy
Nonallergenic formula	Neocate; Nutramigen AA	20	Corn or sucrose	Amino acids	For infants with a milk protein allergy
Antireflux formula	Enfamil AR; Similac Sensitive RS	20	Lactose thickened with rice starch	Cow's milk	For infants with gastric reflux disorder

Adapted from Lönnerdal, B. (2014). Infant formula and infant nutrition: bioactive proteins of human milk and implications for composition of infant formulas. *The American Journal of Clinical Nutrition, 99*(3), 712S–717S; Kent, G. (2014). Regulating fatty acids in infant formula: critical assessment of US policies and practices. *International Breastfeeding Journal, 9*(1), 2–10; and Abrams, S. A., & Schanler, R. J. (2014). Data do not support claims that "supplement formulas" are better than standard formulas for breastfed infants. *AAP News, 35*(6), 26–27.

organizations promote breast-feeding because of the health benefits for both the mother and infant. Nurses should encourage and advocate breast-feeding for their clients and provide support for the family throughout their breast-feeding experiences. Parents typically decide about the method of feeding well before the infant is born. Prenatal and childbirth classes present information about breast-feeding versus bottle-feeding and allow the parents to make up their minds about which method is best for them. Various factors can influence their decision, including socioeconomic status, culture, sexual objectification, fear of a negative community reaction, personal inconvenience, dietary restrictions, lack of social support, lack of self-efficacy, high frequency of violence, employment, level of education, lack of access to breast pumps, lack of time, free formula provided by government programs, range of care interventions provided during pregnancy, childbirth, and the early postpartum period, and especially partner support (Dunn et al., 2015). Nurses can provide evidence-based information to assist the couple in making their decision. Regardless of which method is chosen, the nurse needs to respect and support the couple's decision.

FEEDING THE NEWBORN

The newborn can be fed at any time during the transition period if assessments are normal and a desire is demonstrated. Before the newborn can be fed, determine his or her ability to suck and swallow. Clear any mucus in the nares or mouth with a bulb syringe before initiating feeding. Auscultate bowel sounds, check for abdominal distention, and inspect the anus for patency. If these parameters are within normal limits, newborn feeding may be started. Most newborns are on demand feeding schedules and are allowed to feed when they awaken. When they go home, mothers are encouraged to feed their newborns every 2 to 4 hours during the day and only when the newborn awakens during the night for the first few days after birth.

Parents often have many questions about feeding. Generally, newborns should be fed on demand whenever they seem hungry. Most newborns will give clues about their hunger status by crying, placing their fingers or fist in their mouth, rooting around, and sucking.

Newborns differ in their feeding needs and preferences, but most breast-fed ones need to be fed every 2 to 3 hours, nursing for 10 to 20 minutes on each breast. The length of feedings is up to the mother and newborn. Encourage the mother to respond to cues from her infant and not feed according to a standard or preset schedule.

Formula-fed newborns usually feed every 3 to 4 hours, finishing a bottle in 30 minutes or less. Daily formula intake for an infant should be 1.5 to 2 oz/lb of body weight, but growth is a better measure of health than the amount of formula consumed (Schlenker & Gilbert, 2015). If the newborn seems satisfied, wets 6 to 10 diapers daily, produces several stools a day, sleeps well, and is gaining weight regularly, then he or she is probably receiving sufficient breast milk or formula.

Newborns swallow air during feedings, which causes discomfort and fussiness. Parents can prevent this by burping them frequently throughout the feeding. Tips about burping include:

- Hold the newborn upright with his or her head on the parent's shoulder (Fig. 18.23A).
- Support the head and neck while the parent gently pats or rubs the newborn's back (Fig. 18.23B).
- Have the newborn sit on the parent's lap, while supporting the baby's chest and head. Gently rub the newborn's back with the other hand.
- Lay the newborn on the parent's lap with the baby's back facing up.
- Support the newborn's head in the crook of the parent's arm and gently pat or rub the back.

Take Note!

It is the upright position, not the strength of the patting or rubbing that allows the newborn to release air accumulated in the stomach.

Stress to parents that feeding time is more than an opportunity to get nutrients into their newborn; it is also a time for closeness and sharing. Feedings are as much for the baby's emotional pleasure as his or her physical well-being. Encourage parents to maintain eye contact with the newborn during the feeding, hold him or her comfortably close to them, and talk softly during the feeding to promote closeness and security.

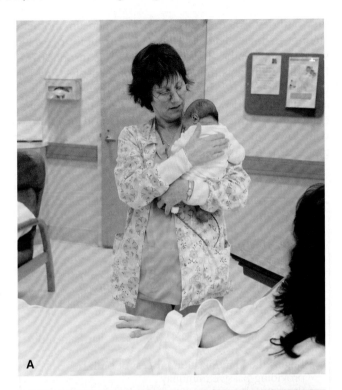

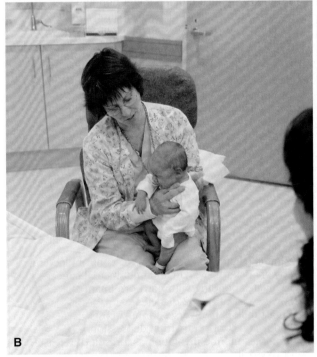

FIGURE 18.23 The nurse demonstrates (**A**) holding the newborn upright over the shoulder and (**B**) sitting the newborn upright, supporting the neck and chin.

BREAST-FEEDING

There is consensus in the medical community that breast-feeding is optimal for all newborns. The AAP and the American Dietetic Association recommend breast-feeding exclusively for the first 6 months of life, continuing it in conjunction with other food at least until the newborn's first birthday. An estimated 75% of American mothers attempt to breast-feed, but just 13% are able to exclusively by 6 months (Busch, Logan, & Wilkinson, 2014). Box 18.2 highlights the advantages of breast-feeding for the mother and newborn. In addition, breast-feeding is associated with lower incidence of necrotizing enterocolitis and diarrhea during the early period of life and with lower incidence of inflammatory bowel diseases, type 2 diabetes, and obesity later in life (Martin, Fanaroff,

---

BOX 18.2

ADVANTAGES OF BREAST-FEEDING

Advantages for the Newborn
- Contributes to the development of a strong immune system
- Stimulates growth of positive bacteria in digestive tract
- Reduces incidence of stomach upset, diarrhea, and colic
- Begins the immunization process at birth by providing passive immunity
- Promotes optimal mother–infant bonding
- Reduces risk of newborn constipation
- Promotes greater developmental gains in preterm infants
- Provides easily tolerated and digestible formula that is sterile, at proper temperature, and readily available with no artificial colorings, flavorings, or preservatives
- Is less likely to result in overfeeding, leading to obesity
- Promotes better tooth and jaw development as a result of sucking hard
- Provides protection against food allergies
- Lowers health care costs due to fewer illnesses
- Is associated with avoidance of type 1 diabetes and heart disease

Advantages for the Mother
- Can facilitate postpartum weight loss by burning extra calories
- Stimulates uterine contractions to control bleeding
- Lowers risk for ovarian and endometrial cancers
- Facilitates bonding with newborn infant
- Lowers risk of type 2 diabetes
- Breast milk is free verses formula costs.
- Reduces risk of postpartum depression
- Promotes uterine involution as a result of release of oxytocin
- Lowers the risk of breast cancer and osteoporosis
- Affords some protection against conception, although it is not a reliable contraceptive method

Data from Schlenker, E., & Gilbert, J. A. (2015). *William's essentials of nutrition and diet therapy* (11th ed.). St. Louis, MO: Mosby Elsevier; Christopher, G. C., & Krell, J. K. (2014). Changing the breastfeeding conversation and our culture. *Breastfeeding Medicine, 9*(2), 53–55; and Walker, M. (2014). *Breastfeeding management for the clinician: Using the evidence* (3rd ed.). Burlington, MA: Jones & Bartlett Learning.

& Welsh, 2014). Mothers should continue to breast-feed during mild illnesses such as colds or flu. However, in the United States mothers with HIV are advised not to breast-feed.

The composition of breast milk changes over time from colostrum to transitional milk, and finally to mature milk. Colostrum is a thick, yellowish substance secreted during the first few days after birth. It is high in protein, minerals, and fat-soluble vitamins. It is rich in immunoglobulins A, which help protect the newborn's gastrointestinal tract against infections. It is a natural laxative that helps rid the intestinal tract of meconium quickly (Gephart & Weller, 2014).

Transitional milk occurs between colostrum and mature milk and contains all the nutrients in colostrum, but it is thinner and less yellow than colostrum. This transitional milk is replaced by true or mature milk around day 10 after birth. Mature milk appears bluish and is not as thick as colostrum. It provides 20 cal/oz and contains the following:

- *Protein*—Although the content is lower than formula, it is ideal to support growth and development for the newborn. The majority of the protein is whey, which is easy to digest.
- *Fat*—Approximately 58% of total calories are fat, but they are easy to digest. Essential fatty acid content is high, as is the level of cholesterol, which helps develop enzyme systems capable of handling cholesterol later in life.
- *Carbohydrate*—Approximately 35% to 40% of total calories are in the form of lactose, which stimulates the growth of natural defense bacteria in the gastrointestinal system and promotes calcium absorption.
- *Water*—Water, the major nutrient in breast milk, makes up 85% to 95% of the total volume. Total milk volume varies with the age of the infant and demand.
- *Minerals*—Breast milk contains calcium, phosphorus, chlorine, potassium, and sodium, with trace amounts of iron, copper, and manganese. Iron absorption is about 50%, compared with about 4% for iron-fortified formulas.
- *Vitamins*—All vitamins are present in breast milk; vitamin D is the lowest in amount. Vitamin D supplementation is recommended by the AAP now.
- *Enzymes*—Lipase and amylase are found in breast milk to assist with digestion (Dudek, 2014).

Breast-Feeding Assistance. Breast-feeding can be initiated immediately after birth. If the newborn is healthy and stable, wipe the newborn from head to toe with a dry cloth and place him or her skin to skin on the mother's abdomen. Then cover the newborn and mother with another warmed blanket to hold in the warmth. Immediate mother–newborn contact takes advantage of the newborn's natural alertness after a vaginal birth and fosters bonding. This immediate contact also reduces maternal bleeding and stabilizes the newborn's temperature, blood glucose level, and respiratory rate (Khan et al., 2015).

Left alone on the mother's abdomen, a healthy newborn scoots upward, pushing with the feet, pulling with the arms, and bobbing the head until finding and latching on to the mother's nipple. A newborn's sense of smell is highly developed, which also helps in finding the nipple. As the newborn moves to the nipple, the mother produces high levels of oxytocin, which contracts the uterus, thereby minimizing bleeding. Oxytocin also causes the breasts to release colostrum when the newborn sucks on the nipple. Colostrum is rich in antibodies and thus provides the newborn with her "first immunization" against infection.

Keys to successful breast-feeding include:
- Initiating breast-feeding within the first hour of life if the newborn is stable
- Placing the newborn on the mother's chest/abdomen immediately after birth
- Following the newborn's feeding schedule—8 to 12 times in 24 hours
- Providing unrestricted periods of breast-feeding
- Offering no supplement unless medically indicated
- Having a lactation consultant observe a feeding session
- Avoiding artificial nipples and pacifiers except during a painful procedure
- Increasing fluid intake to encourage greater milk production (Evidence-Based Practice Box 18.1)
- Feeding from both breasts over each 24-hour period
- Watching for indicators of sufficient intake from infant:
  - Six to ten wet diapers daily
  - Waking up hungry 8 to 12 times in 24 hours
  - Acting content and falling asleep after feeding
- Keeping the newborn with the mother throughout the hospital stay
- The nurse or lactation consultant should be available to guide and support the breast-feeding mother while on the postpartum unit

Help position the newborn so that latching-on is effective and is not painful for the mother. Placing pillows or a folded blanket under the mother's head may help, or rolling her to one side and tucking the newborn next to her. Assess both the mother and newborn

EVIDENCE-BASED PRACTICE 18.1   **PRIMARY CARE SETTING: A COMMUNITY PILOT PROJECT APPLYING THE TRI-CORE BREAST-FEEDING MODEL: BEYOND THE BASICS**

STUDY

Ongoing evidence-based practice findings strongly indicate that the lifelong health and economic benefits of breast-feeding contributes greatly to the health status of the infant, the mother, the family, and the society at large. Promotional lactation interventions are needed in the community to initiate and foster breast-feeding efforts beyond the hospital after discharge. The purpose of this study was to develop a primary care breast-feeding support program, bridging the gap from hospital discharge into primary care to improve breast-feeding rates. The study incorporated the three core interventions of the Tri-Core model: (1) Improving lactation support; (2) enhancing maternal and staff lactation education; and (3) fostering maternal confidence in their ability to breast-feed.

Findings

The study population ($N = 50$) included middle- to low-income families that had recently given birth to a healthy full-term infant who desired to breast-feed within the early postpartum period. Outcomes were measured by the assessment of breast-feeding rates, durations, and reported maternal self-efficacy levels at 1 month, and a 2-month visit. Ongoing office support was provided with lactation visits and phone calls. Findings indicated significant gains in all three areas especially in overall breast-feeding rates when compared to previous rates, especially in rates of exclusive breast-feeding.

Nursing Implications

Based on the results of this study, nurses should remain instrumental in promoting successful breast-feeding practices by initiating breast-feeding as soon as possible after birth, assisting the mother to find a comfortable position for breast-feeding, assessing the infant's latch on to the mother's breast, and reassuring her that the infant is getting adequate amount of breast milk. In addition, utilizing multiprofessional community resources to encourage and support continued breast-feeding efforts is essential. Community referrals are important to help support the novice breast-feeding mother to reinforce breast-feeding instruction once she is discharged from the hospital. Nurses involved in improving breast-feeding rates benefits all ages and its greatest impact will be improving short- and long-term health care outcomes for all families.

Adapted from Busch, D., Nassar, L., & Silbert-Flagg, J. (2015). The necessity of breastfeeding–promoting breastfeeding in the primary care setting; A community pilot project applying the Tri-Core Breastfeeding Model: Beyond the basics. *Journal of Pregnancy & Child Health, 2*(3), 2–7.

during this initial session to determine needs for assistance and education. One tool used frequently in this assessment is the LATCH scoring tool (Abbas & Hasan, 2015). The LATCH scoring tool is a breast-feeding charting system that provides a systematic method for gathering information about individual breast-feeding sessions. The system assigns a numerical score of 0, 1, or 2 to five key components of breast-feeding. Each letter of the acronym LATCH denotes an area of assessment: "L" is for how well the infant latches onto the breast; "A" is for the amount of audible swallowing noted; "T" is for the mother's nipple type; "C" is for the mother's level of comfort; "H" is for the amount of help the mother needs to hold her infant to the breast. The system is visually represented in the same form as the Apgar scoring grid, and the numbers are handled in the same way. With the LATCH system, the nurse can assess maternal and infant variables, define areas of needed intervention, and determine priorities in providing client care and teaching (Table 18.7). The higher the score, the lesser the nursing intervention needed by the mother and baby.

Breast-Feeding Positioning. The mother and infant must be in comfortable positions to ensure breast-feeding success. The four most common positions for breast-feeding are the football, cradle, across-the-lap, and side-lying holds. Each mother, on experimentation, can decide which positions feel most comfortable for her (Fig. 18.24).

- In the *football hold*, the mother holds the infant's back and shoulders in her palm and tucks the infant under her arm. Remind the mother to keep the infant's ear, shoulder, and hip in a straight line. The mother supports the breast with her hand and brings it to the infant's lips to latch on. She continues to support the breast until the infant begins to nurse. This position allows the mother to see the infant's mouth as she guides her infant to the nipple. This is a good choice for mothers who have had a cesarean birth because it avoids pressure on the incision.
- The *cradling position* is the one most commonly used. The mother holds the baby in the crook of her arm, with the infant facing the mother. The mother supports the breast with her opposite hand.
- In the *across-the-lap position*, the mother places a pillow across her lap, with the infant facing the mother. The mother supports the infant's back and shoulders with her palm and supports her breast from underneath. After the infant is in position, the infant is pulled forward to latch on.
- In the *side-lying position*, the mother lies on her side with a pillow supporting her back and another pillow supporting the newborn in the front. To start, the mother props herself up on an elbow and supports the newborn with that arm, while holding her breast with the opposite hand. Once nursing is started, the mother lies down in a comfortable position.

To promote latching-on, instruct the mother to make a C or a V shape with her fingers. In the C hold, the

TABLE 18.7	THE LATCH SCORING TOOL		
Parameters	0 Point	1 Point	2 Points
L: latch	Sleepy infant, no sustained latch achieved	Must hold nipple in infant's mouth to sustain latch and suck; must stimulate infant to continue to suck	Grasps nipple; tongue down; rhythmic sucking
A: audible swallowing	None	A few observed with stimulation	Spontaneous and intermittent both <24 hours old and afterward
T: type of nipple	Inverted (drawn inward into breast tissue)	Flat (not protruding)	Everted or protruding out after stimulation
C: comfort of nipple	Engorged, cracked bleeding; severe discomfort	Filling; reddened, small blisters or bruises; mild to moderate discomfort	Soft, nontender
H: hold (positioning)	Nurse must hold infant to breast	Minimal assistance; help with positioning, then mother takes over	No assistance needed by nurse

Adapted from Walker, M. (2014). *Breastfeeding management for the clinician: Using the evidence* (3rd ed.). Burlington, MA: Jones & Bartlett Learning; Altuntas, N., Turkyilmaz, C., Yildiz, H., Kulali, F., Hirfanoglu, I., Onal, E., et al . (2014). Validity and reliability of the infant breastfeeding assessment tool, the mother baby assessment tool, and the LATCH scoring system. *Breastfeeding Medicine, 9*(4), 191–195; and Lauwers & Swisher (2016). Cultivating better outcomes for mothers and newborns through integrated best practice models. In *Association of women's health, obstetric and neonatal nurses (June 14–18, 2014).* AWHONN.

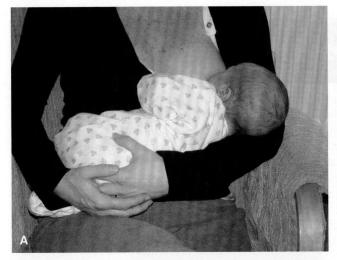

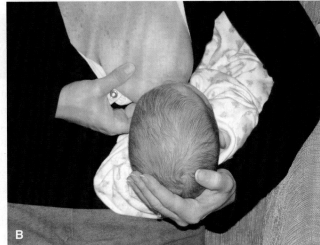

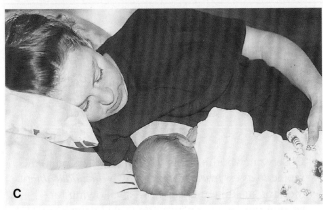

FIGURE 18.24 Breast-feeding positions. **A.** Cradling position. **B.** Football hold position. **C.** Side-lying position.

mother places her thumb well above the areola and the other four fingers below the areola and under the breast. In the V hold, the mother places her index finger above the areola and her other three fingers below the areola and under the breast. Either method can be used as long as the mother's hand is well away from the nipple so the infant can latch on.

Breast-Feeding Education. Breast-feeding is not an innate skill in human mothers. Almost all women have the potential to breast-feed successfully, but many fail because of inadequate knowledge. Nursing Care Plan 18.1 gives typical nursing diagnoses, outcomes, and interventions. For many mothers and newborns, breast-feeding goes smoothly from the start, but for others it is a struggle. Nurses can help throughout the experience by not being judgmental and by demonstrating techniques and offering encouragement and praise for success. Correct positioning will enhance good attachment and will ensure effective milk transfer. Nurses should emphasize that the key to successful breast-feeding is correct positioning and latching-on.

Teaching by nurses has been shown to have a significant effect on both the ability to breast-feed successfully

and the duration of lactation (Dudek, 2014). During the first few breast-feeding sessions, mothers want to know how often they should be nursing, whether breast-feeding is going well, if the newborn is getting enough nourishment, and what problems may ensue and how to cope with them. Education for the breast-feeding mother is highlighted in Teaching Guidelines 18.4.

Take Note!

Remember that the supply of milk is equal to the demand—the more sucking, the more milk.

Remember Kelly, who was concerned about jaundice in her newborn son? At her son's 2-week well-baby checkup at the clinic, his bilirubin level came back within normal limits. Kelly still felt he was not getting enough to eat and stated that she might switch to formula-feeding her son. What information can the nurse present to promote and reinforce breast-feeding? Should the nurse make a referral to the lactation consultant?

Overview of the Mother and Newborn Having Difficulty With Breast-Feeding

Baby boy James, weight 7 lb, 4 oz, was born a few hours ago. His mother, is a 19-year-old gravida 1, para 1. His Apgar scores were 9 points at both 1 and 5 minutes. Labor and birth were unremarkable, and James was admitted to the nursery for assessment. After stabilization, James was brought to his mother, who had said she wished to breast-feed. The postpartum nurse assisted the new mother with positioning and latching-on and left the room for a few minutes. On returning, the mother was upset, James was crying, and she stated she wanted a bottle of formula to feed him since she didn't have milk and her nipples hurt.

Assessment reveals a young, inexperienced mother placed in an uncomfortable situation with limited knowledge of breast-feeding. Anxiety from the mother transferred to James, resulting in crying. The mother, apprehensive about breast-feeding, needs additional help.

NURSING DIAGNOSIS: Ineffective breast-feeding related to pain and limited skill

Outcome Identification and Evaluation

The mother will demonstrate understanding of breast-feeding skills as evidenced by use of correct positioning and technique, and verbalization of appropriate information related to breast-feeding.

Interventions: *Providing Education*

- Instruct the mother on proper positioning for breast-feeding; suggest use of football hold, side-lying position, modified cradle, and across-the-lap position *to ensure comfort and to promote ease in breast-feeding.*
- Review breast anatomy and milk letdown reflex *to enhance mother's understanding of lactation.*

- Observe newborn's ability to suck and latch on to the nipple *to assess whether newborn has adequate ability.*
- Monitor sucking and newborn swallowing for several minutes *to ensure adequate latching on and to assess intake.*
- Reinforce nipple care with water and exposure to air *to maintain nipple integrity.*

NURSING DIAGNOSIS: Anxiety related to breast-feeding ability and irritable, crying newborn

Outcome Identification and Evaluation

The mother will verbalize increased comfort with breast-feeding as evidenced by positive statements related to breast-feeding and verbalization of desire to continue to breast-feed newborn.

Interventions: *Reducing Anxiety*

- Ensure that the environment is calm and soothing without distractions *to promote maternal and newborn relaxation.*
- Show the mother correct latching-on technique *to promote breast-feeding.*
- Assist in calming newborn by holding and talking *to ensure that the newborn is relaxed prior to latching on.*
- Reassure the mother she can be successful at breast-feeding *to enhance her self-esteem and confidence.*
- Encourage frequent trials and attempts *to enhance confidence.*
- Encourage the mother to verbalize her anxiety/fears *to reduce anxiety.*

NURSING CARE PLAN 18.1

Overview of the Mother and Newborn Having Difficulty With Breast-Feeding (continued)

NURSING DIAGNOSIS: Pain related to breast-feeding and incorrect latching-on technique

Outcome Identification and Evaluation

The mother will experience a decrease in pain during breast-feeding as evidenced by statements of less nipple pain.

Interventions: *Reducing Pain*

- Suggest several alternate positions for breast-feeding *to increase comfort.*
- Demonstrate how to break suction before removing infant from breast *to minimize trauma to nipple.*
- Inspect nipple area *to promote early identification of trauma.*
- Reinforce correct latching-on technique *to prevent nipple trauma.*
- Administer pain medication if indicated *to relieve pain.*
- Instruct about nipple care between feedings *to maintain nipple integrity.*

Teaching Guidelines 18.4
BREAST-FEEDING

- Set aside a quiet place where you can be relaxed and won't be disturbed. Relaxation promotes milk letdown.
- Sit in a comfortable chair or rocking chair or lie on a bed. Try to make each feeding calm, quiet, and leisurely. Avoid distractions.
- Listen to soothing music and sip a nutritious drink during feedings.
- Initially, nurse the newborn every few hours to stimulate milk production. Remember that the supply of milk is equal to the demand—the more sucking, the more milk.
- Watch for signals from the infant to indicate that he or she is hungry, such as:
  - Nuzzling against the mother's breasts
  - Demonstrating the rooting reflex by making sucking motions
  - Placing fist or hands in mouth to suck on
  - Crying and squirming
  - Smacking the lips
- Stimulate the rooting reflex by touching the newborn's cheek to initiate sucking.
- Look for signs indicating that the newborn has latched on correctly: wide-open mouth with the nipple and much of the areola in the mouth, lips rolled outward, and tongue over lower gum, visible jaw movement drawing milk out, rhythmic sucking with an audible swallowing (soft "ka" or "ah" sound indicates the infant is swallowing milk).
- Hold the newborn closely, facing the breast, with the newborn's ear, shoulder, and hip in direct alignment.

- Nurse the infant on demand, not on a rigid schedule. Feed every 2 to 3 hours within a 24-hour period for a total of 8 to 12 feedings.
- Alternate the breast you offer first; identify with a safety pin on bra.
- Vary your position for each feeding to empty breasts and reduce soreness.
- Look for signs that the newborn is getting enough milk:
  - At least six wet diapers and two to five loose yellow stools daily
  - Steady weight gain after the first week of age
  - Pale-yellow urine, not deep yellow or orange
  - Sleeping well, yet looks alert and healthy when awake
- Wake up the newborn if he or she has nursed less than 5 minutes by unwrapping him or her.
- Before removing the baby from the breast, break the infant's suction by inserting a finger.
- Burp the infant to release air when changing breasts and at the end of the breast-feeding session.
- Avoid supplemental formula feedings unless indicated for a medical reason. Do not take drugs or medications unless approved by the health care provider.
- Avoid drinking alcohol or caffeinated drinks because they pass through milk.
- Do not smoke while breast-feeding; it increases the risk of sudden infant death syndrome.
- Always wash your hands before expressing or handling milk to store.
- Wear nursing bras and clothes that are easy to undo.

Adapted from Dyson, L., McCormick, F. M., & Renfrew, M. J. (2014). Interventions for promoting the initiation of breastfeeding. *Sao Paula Medical Journal, 132*(1), 68–72; La Leche League. (2015a). *Lactation support and health care providers.* Retrieved from http://www.llli.org/resources/providers.html?m=0,2; and Walker, M. (2014). *Breastfeeding management for the clinician: Using the evidence* (3rd ed.). Sudbury, MA: Jones & Bartlett.

Breast Milk Storage and Expression. If the breast-feeding mother becomes separated from the newborn for any reason (e.g., work, travel, or illness), she needs instruction on how to express and store milk safely. Expressing milk can be done manually (hand compression of breast) or by using a breast pump. Manual or handheld pumps are inexpensive and can be used by mothers who occasionally need an extra bottle if they are going out (Fig. 18.25A). Electric breast pumps are used for mothers who experience a lengthy separation from their infants and need to pump their breasts regularly, e.g., while at the work place (Fig. 18.25B).

To ensure the safety of expressed breast milk, instruct the mother as follows:

• Wash your hands before expressing milk or handling breast milk.
• Find a quiet, clean place to express milk if returned to workplace
• Use clean containers to store expressed milk.
• Use sealed and chilled milk within 24 hours.
• Discard any milk that has been refrigerated for more than 24 hours.
• Use any frozen expressed milk within 3 months.
• Do not use microwave ovens to warm chilled milk.
• Discard any used milk; never refreeze it.

• Store milk in quantities to be used for each feeding (2 to 4 oz).
• Thaw milk in warm water before using (La Leche League, 2015b).

Common Breast-Feeding Concerns. Breast-feeding women may experience problems such as cracked nipples, engorgement (the painful overfilling of the breasts with milk), or mastitis (inflammation of the breast). Breast-feeding should not be painful for the mother. If she has sore, cracked nipples, the first step is to find the cause. Incorrect positioning or latching-on, removing the infant from the breast without first breaking the suction, or wearing a bra that is too tight can cause cracked or sore nipples. Cracked nipples can increase the risk of mastitis because a break in the skin may allow *Staphylococcus aureus* or other organisms to enter the body.

Sore nipples usually are caused by improper infant attachment, which traumatizes the tissue. The nurse should review techniques for proper positioning and latching-on. It is important to get this correct from the first feed to assist in the prevention of incorrect attachment and associated nipple trauma. Recommend the following to the mother:

• Use only warm water, not soap, to clean the nipples to prevent dryness.

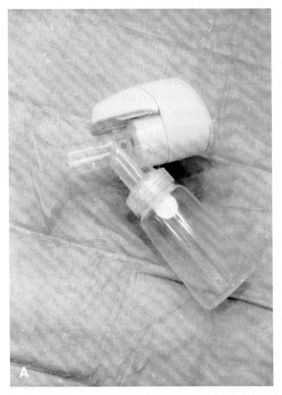
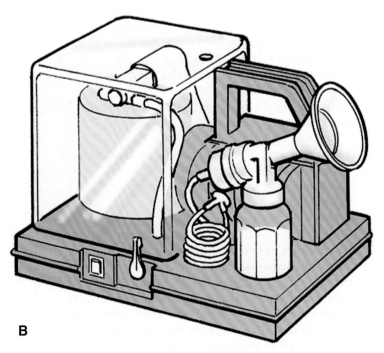

FIGURE 18.25 A. Hand-held breast pump. **B**. Electric breast pump. (Part B from Lippincott (2015). *Lippincott Nursing Procedures* (7th ed.), Philadelphia, PA: Wolters Kluwer).

- Express some milk before feeding to stimulate the milk ejection reflex.
- Avoid using breast pads with plastic liners, and change pads when they are wet.
- Wear a comfortable bra that is not too tight.
- Apply a few drops of breast milk to the nipples after feeding.
- Take systemic anti-inflammatory such as ibuprofen for discomfort.
- Rotate positions when feeding the infant to promote complete breast emptying.
- Leave the nursing bra flaps down after feeding to allow nipples to air-dry.
- Inspect the nipples daily for redness or cracks (Walker, 2014).

To ease nipple pain and trauma, reinforce appropriate latching-on techniques and remind the woman about the need to break the suction at the breast before removing the newborn from the breast. Additional measures may include applying cold compresses over the area and massaging breast milk onto the nipple after feeding.

Engorgement may occur as the milk comes in around day 3 or 4 after birth of the newborn. Explain to the mother that engorgement, though uncomfortable, is self-limited and will resolve as the newborn continues to nurse. The mother should continue to nurse during engorgement to avoid a plugged milk duct, which could lead to mastitis. Provide the following tips for relieving engorgement:

- Take warm to hot showers to encourage milk release.
- Express some milk manually before breast-feeding.
- Wear a supportive nursing bra 24 hours a day to provide support.
- Feed the newborn in a variety of positions—sitting up and then lying down.
- Massage the breasts from under the axillary area down toward the nipple.
- Increase the frequency of feedings.
- Apply warm compresses to the breasts prior to nursing.
- Stay relaxed while breast-feeding.
- Use a breast pump if nursing or manual expression is not effective.
- Remember that this condition is temporary and resolves quickly.

Mastitis, or inflammation of the breast, causes flu-like symptoms, chills, fever, and malaise. These symptoms may occur before the development of soreness, aching, swelling, and redness in the breast (usually the upper outer quadrant). This condition usually occurs in just one breast when a milk duct becomes blocked, causing inflammation, or through a cracked or damaged nipple, allowing bacteria to infect a portion of the breast. Treatment consists of rest, warm compresses,

antibiotics, breast support, and continued breast-feeding (the infection will not pass into the breast milk). Explain to the mother that it is important to keep the milk flowing in the infected breast, whether it is through nursing or manual expression or with a breast pump.

FORMULA-FEEDING

Despite the general acknowledgment that breast-feeding is the most desirable means of feeding infants, many mothers choose formula-feeding and need education about this procedure. Formula-fed infants grow more rapidly than breast-fed infants not only in weight but also in length.

Formula-feeding requires more than just opening, pouring, and feeding. Parents need information about the types of formula available, preparation and storage of formula, equipment, feeding positions, and the amount to feed their newborn. The mother also needs to know how to prevent lactation (see Chapter 16 for more information).

Commercially prepared formulas are regulated by the Food and Drug Administration (FDA), which sets minimum and maximum levels of nutrients. Formulas are manufactured by numerous manufacturers in the United States. Normal full-term infants usually receive conventional cow milk-based formula, but the health care provider makes this decision. If the infant shows signs of a reaction or lactose intolerance, a switch to another formula type is recommended.

The general recommendation is for all infants to receive iron-fortified formula until the age of 1 year. The latest generation of infant formulas includes some fortification with docosahexaenoic acid (DHA) and arachidonic acid (ARA), two natural components of breast milk. Many feel the FDA does not adequately regulate the use of fatty acid additives (DHA and ARA) to infant formula before they are marketed, and there is no systematic assessment after marketing is underway. Researchers are calling for more FDA regulation over additives in infant formulas (Kent, 2014). Commercial formulas come in three forms: powder, concentrate, and easy to feed or ready to use. All are similar in terms of nutritional content but differ in expense. Powdered formula is the least expensive, with concentrated formula the next most expensive. Both must be mixed with water before using. Ready-to-feed formula is the most expensive; it can be opened and poured into a bottle and fed directly to the infant.

Parents need information about the equipment needed for formula-feeding. Basic supplies are four to six 4-oz bottles, eight to ten 8-oz bottles, eight to ten nipple units, a bottle brush, and a nipple brush. A key area of instruction is assessing for flow of formula through the nipple and checking for any nipple damage. When the bottle is filled and turned upside down, the flow from the nipple should be approximately one drop per second. If the parents are using bottles with disposable bags, instruct them to make sure they have a tight-fitting nipple to prevent leaks. Frequent observation of the flow rate from the nipple and the condition of the nipple will prevent choking and aspiration associated with too fast a rate of delivery. Ask the parents to fill a bottle with formula and then turn it upside down and observe the rate at which the formula drips from the bottle. If it is too fast (more than one drop per second), then the nipple should be replaced.

Correct formula preparation is critical to the newborn's health and development. Mistakes in dilution may result if the parents do not understand how to prepare the formula or make measurement errors. The safety of the water supply should be considered. If well water is used, parents should sterilize the water by boiling it or should use bottled water. Many health care providers still recommend that all water used in formula preparation be brought to a rolling boil for 1 to 2 minutes and then cooled to room temperature before use.

Opened cans of ready-made or concentrated formula should be covered and refrigerated after being prepared for the day (24 hours). Instruct parents to discard any unused portions after 48 hours.

Take Note!

Any formula left in the bottle after feeding should also be discarded, because the infant's saliva has been mixed with it.

To warm refrigerated formula, advise the parents to place the bottle in a pan of hot water or an electric bottle warmer and test the temperature by letting a few drops fall on the inside of the wrist. If it is comfortably warm to the mother, it is the correct temperature.

Formula-Feeding Assistance. The process of feeding a newborn formula from a bottle should mirror breast-feeding as closely as possible. Although nutrition is important, so are the emotional and interactive components of feeding. Encourage parents to cuddle their newborn closely and position him or her so that the head is in a comfortable position, not too far back or turned, which makes swallowing difficult (Fig. 18.26). Also urge parents to communicate with their newborn during the feedings by talking and singing to him or her.

Although it may seem that bottle-feeding is not a difficult task, many new parents find it awkward. At first glance, holding an infant and a bottle appears simple enough, but both the position of the baby and the angle of the bottle must be correct.

Formula-Feeding Positions. Advise mothers to feed their newborns in a relaxed and quiet setting to create a sense of calm for themselves and the baby. Make sure that

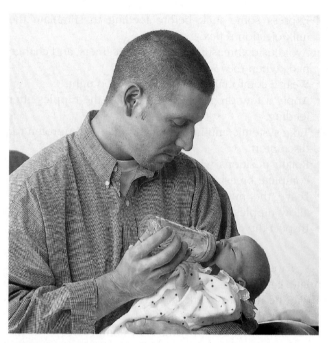

FIGURE 18.26 Father holding his newborn securely while feeding.

comfort is a priority for both mother and newborn. The mother can sit in a comfortable chair, using a pillow to support the arm in which she is holding the baby. The mother can cradle the newborn in a semi-upright position, supporting the newborn's head in the crook of her arm. Holding the newborn close during feeding provides stimulation and helps prevent choking. Holding the newborn's head raised slightly will help prevent formula from washing backward into the eustachian tubes in the ears, which can lead to an ear infection.

Formula-Feeding Education. Parents require teaching about the correct preparation and storage of formula as well as the techniques for feeding; refer to Teaching Guidelines 18.5.

Teaching Guidelines 18.5
FORMULA-FEEDING

* Wash your hands with soap and water before preparing formula.
* Mix the formula and water amounts exactly as the label specifies.
* Always hold the newborn and bottle during feedings; never prop the bottle.
* Never freeze formula or warm it in the microwave.
* Place refrigerated formula in a pan of hot water for a few minutes to warm.
* Test the temperature of the formula by shaking a few drops on the wrist.

- Hold the bottle like a pencil, keeping it tipped to prevent air from entering. Position the bottle so that the nipple remains filled with milk.
- Burp the infant after every few ounces to allow air swallowed to escape.
- Move the nipple around in the infant's mouth to stimulate sucking.
- Always keep a bulb syringe close by to use if choking occurs.
- Avoid putting the infant to bed with a bottle to prevent "baby bottle tooth decay."
- Feed the newborn approximately every 3 to 4 hours.
- Use an iron-fortified formula for the first year.
- Prepare enough formula for the next 24 hours.
- Check nipples regularly and discard any that are sticky, cracked, or leaking.
- Store unmixed, open liquid formula in the refrigerator for up to 48 hours.
- Throw away any formula left in the bottle after each feeding.

Proper positioning makes bottle-feeding easier and more enjoyable for both the mother and newborn. As in breast-feeding, frequent burping is key. Advise the parents to hold the bottle so that formula fills the nipple, thus allowing less air to enter. Infants get fussy when they swallow air during feedings and need to be relieved of it every 2 to 3 oz.

Emphasize to parents that an electrolyte imbalance can occur in infants who are fed formula that has been incorrectly mixed. Mixing the formula with too *little* water (i.e., too thickly) can cause hypernatremia because the high concentration of sodium is too much for the baby's immature kidneys to handle. As a result, sodium is excreted along with water, leading to dehydration. Mixing the formula with too *much* water in an effort to save money can lead to failure to thrive, diminished nutrition, fluoride overdose, and lack of weight gain (Monahan, 2014).

WEANING AND INTRODUCTION OF SOLID FOODS

Weaning. Eventually, breast-feeding or formula-feeding comes to an end. Weaning involves the transition from breast to bottle, from breast or bottle to cup, or from liquids to solids. Weaning from breast-feeding to cup has several advantages over weaning to a bottle because it eliminates the step of weaning first to a bottle and then to a cup. Another advantage is that the bottle does not become a security object for the infant.

Weaning can be done because the mother is returning to work and cannot keep breast-feeding, or because the infant is losing interest in breast-feeding and showing signs of independence. There is no "right" time to wean; it depends on the desires of the mother and infant. Weaning represents a significant change in the way the mother and infant interact, and each mother must decide for herself when she and her infant are ready to take that step. Either one can start the weaning process, but usually it occurs between 6 months and 1 year of age.

To begin weaning from the breast, instruct mothers to substitute breast-feeding with a cup or a bottle. Often the midday feeding is the easiest feeding to replace. A trainer cup with two handles and a snap-on lid with a spout is appropriate and minimizes spilling. Because weaning is a gradual process, it may take months. Instruct parents to proceed slowly and let the infant's willingness and interest guide them.

Weaning from the bottle to the cup also needs to be timed appropriately for mother and infant. Typically, the night bottle is the last to be given up, with cup drinking substituted throughout the day. Slowly diluting the formula with water over a week can help in this process; the final result is an all-water bottle. To prevent the baby from sucking on the bottle during the night, remove it from the crib after the infant falls asleep.

Introduction of Solid Foods. When infants double their birth weight and weigh at least 13 lb, it is time to consider introducing solid foods. Readiness cues include:
- Consumption of 32 oz of formula or breast milk daily (estimated)
- Ability to sit up with minimal support and turn head away to indicate fullness
- Reduction of protrusion reflex so cereal can be propelled to back of throat
- Demonstration of interest in food others around them are eating
- Ability to open mouth automatically when food approaches it

When introducing solid foods, certain principles apply:
- New foods should be introduced one at a time and a week apart so that if a problem develops, the responsible item can be identified.
- Infants should be allowed to set the pace regarding how much they wish to eat.
- New foods should not be introduced more frequently than every 3 to 5 days.
- Fruits are added after cereals; then vegetables and meats are introduced; eggs are introduced last.
- A relaxed, unhurried, calm atmosphere for meals is important.
- A variety of foods are provided to ensure a balanced diet.
- Infants should never be force-fed (Schlenker & Gilbert, 2015).

Nurses can promote good feeding practices by actively listening to new mothers, helping them clarify their feelings, and discussing solutions. A warm, sincere manner and tone of voice will put an anxious mother at ease. Giving accurate information, making suggestions, and presenting options will enable the mother to decide what is best for her and her infant. Nurses should be sensitive to the individual, family, and economic and cultural differences among mothers before offering suggestions for feeding practices that may not be appropriate.

Preparing for Discharge

Preparing the parents for discharge is an essential task for the nurse. Because of today's shorter hospital stays, the nurse must identify the major teaching topics that need to be covered. Nurses should assess the parents' baseline knowledge and learning needs and plan how to meet them. Using the following principles fosters a learner-centered approach:

- Make the environment conducive to learning. Encourage the parents to feel comfortable during this stressful time by using support and praise.
- Allow the parents to provide input about the content and the process of learning. What do they want and need to learn?
- Build the parents' self-esteem by confirming that their responses to the entire birthing process and aftercare are legitimate, and others have felt the same way.
- Ensure that what the parents learn is relevant to their day-to-day home situation.
- Encourage responsibility by reinforcing that their emotional and physical responses are within the normal range.
- Respect cultural beliefs and practices that are important to the family by taking into account their heritage and health beliefs regarding newborn care. Examples include placing a bellyband over the newborn's navel (Hispanics and African Americans), delaying naming the newborn (Asian Americans and Haitians), and delaying breast-feeding (Native Americans; they regard colostrum as "bad") (Bowers, 2015).

While in the hospital, women have ready access to support and hands-on instruction regarding feeding and newborn care. When the new mother is discharged, this close supervision and support by nurses should not end abruptly. Providing the new parents with the phone number of the mother–baby unit will help them through this stressful transitional period. Giving the new family information and offering backup support via the telephone will increase parenting success (see Evidence-Based Practice 18.1).

ENSURING FOLLOW-UP CARE

Most newborns are scheduled for their first health follow-up appointment within 2 to 4 days after discharge so they can have additional laboratory work done as part of the newborn screening series, especially if they

Consider This

I have always prided myself on being very organized and in control in most situations, but survival at home after childbirth wasn't one of them. I left the hospital 24 hours after giving birth to my son because my doctor said I could. The postpartum nurse encouraged me to stay longer, but wanting to be in control and sleeping in my own bed again won out. I thought my baby would be sleeping while I sent out birth announcements to my friends and family—wrong! What happened instead was my son didn't sleep as I imagined and my nipples became sore after breast-feeding every few hours. I was weary and tired and wanted to sleep, but I couldn't. Somehow I thought I would be getting a full night's sleep because I was up throughout the day, but that was a fantasy too. At 2 o'clock in the morning when you are up feeding your baby, you feel you are the only one in the world up at that time and feel very much alone. My feelings of being organized and in control all the time have changed dramatically since I left the hospital. I have learned to yield to the important needs of my son and derive satisfaction from being able to bring comfort to him and to let go of my control.

Thoughts: It is interesting to see how a newborn changed this woman's need to organize and control her environment. What "tips of survival" could the nurse offer this woman to help in her transition to home with her newborn? How can friends and family help when women arrive home from the hospital with their newborns?

were discharged within 48 hours. After this first visit, the typical schedule of health care visits is as follows: 2 to 4 weeks of age; 2, 4, and 6 months of age for checkups and vaccines; 9 months of age for a checkup; 12 months for a checkup and tuberculosis testing; 15 and 18 months for checkups and vaccines; and 2 years of age for a checkup. These appointments provide an opportunity for parents to ask questions and receive anticipatory guidance as their newborn grows and develops.

In addition to encouraging parents to keep follow-up appointments, advise parents to call their health care provider if they notice signs of illness in their newborn. They should know which over-the-counter medicines should be kept on hand. Review the following warning signs of illness with parents:

- Temperature of 101° F (38.3° C) or higher
- Forceful, persistent vomiting, not just spitting up
- Refusal to take feedings
- Two or more green, watery diarrheal stools
- Infrequent wet diapers and change in bowel movements from normal pattern
- Lethargy or excessive sleepiness
- Inconsolable crying and extreme fussiness
- Abdominal distention
- Difficult or labored breathing

Figure 1. Recommended immunization schedule for persons aged 0 through 18 years – United States, 2016.
(FOR THOSE WHO FALL BEHIND OR START LATE, SEE THE CATCH-UP SCHEDULE [FIGURE 2]).

These recommendations must be read with the footnotes that follow. For those who fall behind or start late, provide catch-up vaccination at the earliest opportunity as indicated by the green bars in Figure 1. To determine minimum intervals between doses, see the catch-up schedule (Figure 2). School entry and adolescent vaccine age groups are shaded.

Vaccine	Birth	1 mo	2 mos	4 mos	6 mos	9 mos	12 mos	15 mos	18 mos	19–23 mos	2-3 yrs	4-6 yrs	7-10 yrs	11-12 yrs	13–15 yrs	16–18 yrs
Hepatitis B[1] (HepB)	1st dose	←------ 2nd dose ------→			←---------------------- 3rd dose ----------------------→											
Rotavirus[2] (RV) RV1 (2-dose series); RV5 (3-dose series)			1st dose	2nd dose	See footnote 2											
Diphtheria, tetanus, & acellular pertussis[3] (DTaP: <7 yrs)			1st dose	2nd dose	3rd dose		←------ 4th dose ------→					5th dose				
Haemophilus influenzae type b[4] (Hib)			1st dose	2nd dose	See footnote 4		←-- 3rd or 4th dose, See footnote 4 --→									
Pneumococcal conjugate[5] (PCV13)			1st dose	2nd dose	3rd dose		←-- 4th dose --→									
Inactivated poliovirus[6] (IPV: <18 yrs)			1st dose	2nd dose	←---------------------- 3rd dose ----------------------→							4th dose				
Influenza[7] (IIV; LAIV)					←----- Annual vaccination (IIV only) 1 or 2 doses -----→					Annual vaccination (LAIV or IIV) 1 or 2 doses				Annual vaccination (LAIV or IIV) 1 dose only		
Measles, mumps, rubella[8] (MMR)					See footnote 8		←------ 1st dose ------→					2nd dose				
Varicella[9] (VAR)							←------ 1st dose ------→					2nd dose				
Hepatitis A[10] (HepA)						←------- 2-dose series, See footnote 10 -------→										
Meningococcal[11] (Hib-MenCY ≥ 6 weeks; MenACWY-D ≥9 mos; MenACWY-CRM ≥ 2 mos)				←------------------------ See footnote 11 ------------------------→										1st dose		Booster
Tetanus, diphtheria, & acellular pertussis[12] (Tdap: ≥7 yrs)														(Tdap)		
Human papillomavirus[13] (2vHPV: females only; 4vHPV, 9vHPV: males and females)														(3-dose series)		
Meningococcal B[11]															See footnote 11	
Pneumococcal polysaccharide[5] (PPSV23)												←---------------- See footnote 5 ----------------→				

| Range of recommended ages for all children | Range of recommended ages for catch-up immunization | Range of recommended ages for certain high-risk groups | Range of recommended ages for non-high-risk groups that may receive vaccine, subject to individual clinical decision making | No recommendation |

This schedule includes recommendations in effect as of January 1, 2016. Any dose not administered at the recommended age should be administered at a subsequent visit, when indicated and feasible. The use of a combination vaccine generally is preferred over separate injections of its equivalent component vaccines. Vaccination providers should consult the relevant Advisory Committee on Immunization Practices (ACIP) statement for detailed recommendations, available online at http://www.cdc.gov/vaccines/hcp/acip-recs/index.html. Clinically significant adverse events that follow vaccination should be reported to the Vaccine Adverse Event Reporting System (VAERS) online (http://www.vaers.hhs.gov) or by telephone (800-822-7967). Suspected cases of vaccine-preventable diseases should be reported to the state or local health department. Additional information, including precautions and contraindications for vaccination, is available from CDC online (http://www.cdc.gov/vaccines/recs/vac-admin/contraindications.htm) or by telephone (800-CDC-INFO [800-232-4636]).

This schedule is approved by the Advisory Committee on Immunization Practices (http://www.cdc.gov/vaccines/acip), the American Academy of Pediatrics (http://www.aap.org), the American Academy of Family Physicians (http://www.aafp.org), and the American College of Obstetricians and Gynecologists (http://www.acog.org).

NOTE: The above recommendations must be read along with the footnotes of this schedule.

FIGURE 18.27 Recommended childhood immunization schedule.

PROVIDING IMMUNIZATION INFORMATION

In the last century, vaccinations have been the most effective medical intervention to reduce mortality and morbidity caused by communicable diseases. It is believed that vaccines save at least two to three million lives annually worldwide (Delany, Rappuoli, & De Gregorio, 2014). Parents also need instructions about immunizations for their newborn. **Immunization** is the process of rendering an individual immune or of becoming immune to certain communicable diseases (Verklan & Walden, 2015). The purpose of the immune system is to identify unknown (nonself) substances in the body and develop a defense against these invaders. Disease prevention by immunization is a public health priority and is one of the leading health indicators as part of *Healthy People 2020*. Despite many advances in vaccine delivery, the goal of universal immunization has not been reached (Davidson, 2014). Nurses can help meet this national goal by educating new parents about the importance of disease prevention through immunizations.

Immunity can be provided either passively or actively. Passive immunity is protection transferred via already formed antibodies from one person to another. Passive immunity includes transplacental passage of antibodies from a mother to her newborn, immunity passed through breast milk, and immunity from immunoglobulins. Passive immunity provides limited protection and decreases over a period of weeks or months (Chu & Englund, 2014). Active immunity is protection produced by an individual's own immune system. It can be obtained by having the actual disease or by receiving a vaccine that produces an immunologic response by that person's body. Active immunity may be lifelong either way; see Chapter 17.

Young infants and children are susceptible to various illnesses because their immune systems are not yet mature. Many of these illnesses can be prevented by following the recommended schedule of childhood immunizations. Figure 18.27 shows the *2015 Childhood Immunization Schedule*. Refer to *thePoint* website for information about how to view the latest CDC immunization schedule. The schedule for immunizations should be reviewed with parents, stressing the importance of continued follow-up health care to preserve their infant's health.

The newborn's first immunization (hepatitis B) is received in the hospital soon after birth. The first dose can also be given by age 2 months if the mother is HbsAg negative. If the mother is HbsAg positive, then the newborn should receive hepatitis B vaccine and hepatitis B immunoglobulin within 12 hours of birth (Cunningham et al., 2014).

Education for the parents should include the risks and benefits for each vaccine and possible adverse effects. Federal law requires a consent form to be signed before administering a vaccine. Parents have the right to refuse immunizations based on their religious beliefs and can sign a waiver noting their decision. When consent has been received, the nurse administering the vaccine must document the date and time it was given, name and manufacturer, lot number and expiration date of the vaccine given, site and route of administration, and the name and title of the nurse who administered the vaccine. Despite overwhelming evidence of vaccine safety, suspicion and misconception continues in small groups of hesitant or resistant parents/partners/significant others, often leading to outbreaks of vaccine-preventable infections. On the front lines of vaccinations, nurses can improve vaccination rates by developing trust with parents/partners/significant others and arming them with information based on sound evidence.

KEY CONCEPTS

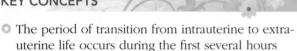

- The period of transition from intrauterine to extrauterine life occurs during the first several hours after birth. It is a time of stabilization for the newborn's temperature, respiration, and cardiovascular dynamics.

- The newborn's bowel is sterile at birth. It usually takes about a week for the newborn to produce vitamin K in sufficient quantities to prevent VKDB.

- It is recommended that all newborns in the United States receive an installation of a prophylactic agent (erythromycin or tetracycline ophthalmic ointment) in their eyes within an hour or two of being born.

- Nursing measures to maintain newborns' body temperature include drying them immediately after birth to prevent heat loss through evaporation, wrapping them in prewarmed blankets, putting a hat on their head, and placing them under a temperature-controlled radiant warmer.

- The specific components of a typical newborn examination include a general survey of skin color, posture, state of alertness, head size, overall behavioral state, respiratory status, gender, and any obvious congenital anomalies.

- Gestational age assessment is pertinent because it allows the nurse to plot growth parameters and to anticipate potential problems related to prematurity/postmaturity and growth abnormalities such as SGA/LGA.

- After the newborn has passed the transitional period and stabilized, the nurse needs to complete ongoing assessments, vital signs, weight and measurements, cord care, hygiene measures, newborn screening tests, and various other tasks until the newborn is discharged home from the birthing unit.

- Important topics about which to educate parents include environmental safety, newborn characteristics, feeding and bathing, circumcision and cord care, sleep and elimination patterns of newborns, safe infant car seats, holding/positioning, and follow-up care.

- Newborn screening tests consist of hearing and certain genetic and inborn errors of metabolism tests required in most states for newborns before discharge from the birth facility.

- The AAP and the American Dietetic Association recommend breast-feeding exclusively for the first 6 months of life and that it continue along with other food at least until the first birthday.

- Parents who choose not to breast-feed need to know what types of formula are available, preparation and storage of formula, equipment, feeding positions, and how much to feed their infant.

- Common problems associated with the newborn include transient tachypnea, physiologic jaundice, and hypoglycemia.

- Transient tachypnea of the newborn appears soon after birth; is accompanied by retractions, expiratory grunting, or cyanosis; and is relieved by low-dose oxygen.

- Physiologic jaundice is a very common condition in newborns, with the majority demonstrating yellowish skin, mucous membranes, and sclera within the first 3 days of life. Newborns undergoing phototherapy in the treatment of jaundice require close monitoring of their body temperature and fluid and electrolyte balance; observation of skin integrity; eye protection; and parental participation in their care.

- The newborn with hypoglycemia requires close monitoring for signs and symptoms of hypoglycemia if present. In addition, newborns at high risk need to be identified based on their perinatal history, physical examination, body measurements, and gestational age.

- The schedule for immunizations should be reviewed with parents, stressing the importance of continual follow-up health care to preserve their infant's health.

References and Recommended Readings

Abbas, I. M., & Hasan, R. T. (2015). Assessment of LATCH tool regarding initiation of breastfeeding among women after childbirth. *Assessment, 5*(05), 38–44.

Abrams, S., & Savelli, S. L. (2014). Be prepared to address parents' concerns about vitamin K injection. *AAP News, 35*(5), 1–1.

Abrams, S. A., & Schanler, R. J. (2014). Data do not support claims that 'supplement formulas' are better than standard formulas for breastfed infants. *AAP News, 35*(6), 26–27.

Adamkin, D. H. (2015). Metabolic screening and postnatal glucose homeostasis in the newborn. *Pediatric Clinics of North America, 62*(2), 385–409.

Ahn, E. S., Jung, M. S., Lee, Y. K., Ko, S. Y., Shin, S. M., & Hahn, M. H. (2015). Neonatal clavicular fracture: Recent 10 year study. *Pediatrics International, 57*(1), 60–63.

Alcantara, D., & O'Driscoll, M. (2014). Congenital microcephaly. *American Journal of Medical Genetics Part C: Seminars in Medical Genetics, 166C*, 124–139.

Altuntas, N., Turkyilmaz, C., Yildiz, H., Kulali, F., Hirfanoglu, I., Onal, E., et al. (2014). Validity and reliability of the infant breastfeeding assessment tool, the mother baby assessment tool, and the LATCH scoring system. *Breastfeeding Medicine, 9*(4), 191–195.

American Academy of Pediatrics [AAP]. (2015a). A recommendation for the definition of "late preterm" and the birth weight-gestational age classification system. Retrieved from http://www.aap.org/en-us/search/pages/results.aspx?k=newborn birth weight classification&s=Clinical Support

American Academy of Pediatrics [AAP]. (2015b). *Pediatric clinical practice guidelines & policies: A compendium of evidence-based research for pediatric practice* (14th ed.). Elk Grove Village, IL: American Academy of Pediatrics.

American Academy of Pediatrics [AAP]. (2015c). *Where we stand: Administration of vitamin K*. Retrieved from http://www.healthychildren.org/English/ages-stages/prenatal/delivery-beyond/Pages/Where-We-Stand-Administration-of-Vitamin-K.aspx

American Academy of Pediatrics [AAP]. (2015d). *Purpose of newborn hearing screening*. Retrieved from http://www.healthychildren.org/English/ages-stages/baby/Pages/Purpose-of-Newborn-Hearing-Screening.aspx

American Academy of Pediatrics [AAP]. (2015e). *Circumcision*. Retrieved from http://www.healthychildren.org/English/ages-stages/prenatal/decisions-to-make/Pages/Circumcision.aspx

American Academy of Pediatrics [AAP]. (2015f). *Car seats: Information for families for 2014*. Retrieved from http://www.healthychildren.org/English/safety-prevention/on-the-go/Pages/Car-Safety-Seats-Information-for-Families.aspx

American Academy of Pediatrics [AAP]. (2015g). *Co-sleeping*. Retrieved from http://www.aap.org/en-us/search/pages/results.aspx?k=co-sleeping

American Academy of Pediatrics [AAP]. (2015h). *Jaundice*. Retrieved from http://www.healthychildren.org/English/ages-stages/baby/Pages/Jaundice.aspx

American Academy of Pediatrics [AAP]. (2015i). *Vitamins and iron supplements*. Retrieved from http://www.healthychildren.org/English/ages-stages/baby/feeding-nutrition/Pages/Vitamin-Iron-Supplements.aspx

American Academy of Pediatrics [AAP]. (2015j). Iodine deficiency: Pregnant, breastfeeding women need supplementation, AAP says. *AAP News, 35*(6), Retrieved from http://aapnews.aappublications.org/content/35/6/11.1.extract

American Speech-Language-Hearing Association [ASHA] (2014). *Newborn infant hearing screening*. Retrieved from http://www.asha.org/Practice-Portal/Professional-Issues/Newborn-Infant-Hearing-Screening/

Apgar, V. (2015). A proposal for a new method of evaluation of the newborn infant. *Anesthesia & Analgesia, 120*(5), 1056–1059.

Bellini, S. (2015). What parents need to know about vitamin K administration at birth. *Nursing for Women's Health, 19*(3), 261–265.

Bhattacharya, K., Wotton, T., & Wiley, V. (2014). The evolution of blood-spot newborn screening. *Translational Pediatrics, 3*(2), 63–70.

Bond, S. (2015). Rethinking old practices: Evidence supports wiping, not suctioning, newborn secretions at birth. *Journal of Midwifery & Women's Health, 60*(2), 220–224.

Boom, J. A. (2015a). Microcephaly in infants and children: Etiology and evaluation. UpToDate. Retrieved from http://www.uptodate.com/contents/microcephaly-in-infants-and-children-etiology-and-evaluation

Boom, J. A. (2015b). Macrocephaly in infants and children: Etiology and evaluation. UpToDate. Retrieved from http://www.uptodate.com/contents/macrocephaly-in-infants-and-children-etiology-and-evaluation

Boyle, C. A., Bocchini, J. A., & Kelly, J. (2014). Reflections on 50 years of newborn screening. *Pediatrics, 133*(6), 961–963.

Bowers, P. (2015). Cultural perspectives of childbearing. Nursing Spectrum. Retrieved from http://ce.nurse.com/ce263-60/CoursePage

Busch, D., Nassar, L., & Silbert-Flagg, J. (2015). The necessity of breastfeeding–promoting breastfeeding in the primary care setting; A community pilot project applying the Tri-Core Breastfeeding Model: Beyond the basics. *Journal of Pregnancy & Child Health, 2*(3), 2–7.

Busch, D. W., Logan, K., & Wilkinson, A. (2014). Clinical practice breastfeeding recommendations for primary care: Applying a tri-core breastfeeding conceptual model. *Journal of Pediatric Health Care, 28*(6), 486–496.

Centers for Disease Control and Prevention [CDC]. (2015a). *Conjunctivitis in newborns*. Retrieved from http://www.cdc.gov/conjunctivitis/newborns.html

Centers for Disease Control and Prevention [CDC]. (2015b). *Hearing loss in children: Recommendations and guidelines*. Retrieved from http://www.cdc.gov/ncbddd/hearingloss/recommendations.html

Centers for Disease Control and Prevention [CDC]. (2015c). *Trends in circumcision for male newborns in U.S. Hospitals*. Retrieved from http://www.cdc.gov/nchs/data/hestat/circumcision_2013/circumcision_2013.htm

Centers for Disease Control and Prevention [CDC]. (2015d). *Infants and toddlers—safety in the home and community*. Retrieved from http://www.cdc.gov/parents/infants/safety.html

Christopher, G. C., & Krell, J. K. (2014). Changing the breastfeeding conversation and our culture. *Breastfeeding Medicine, 9*(2), 53–55.

Chu, J. (2014). Approach to jaundice in infancy. In *Mount sinai expert guides: Hepatology* (pp. 374–381), doi: 10.1002/9781118748626.ch36

Chu, H. Y., & Englund, J. A. (2014). Maternal immunization. *Clinical Infectious Diseases, 59*(4), 560–568..

Clark-Gambelunghe, M. B., & Clark, D. A. (2015). Sensory development. *Pediatric Clinics of North America, 62*(2), 367–384.

Cunningham, F. G., Leveno, K. J., Bloom, S. L., Spong, C. Y., Dashe, J. S., Hoffman, B. L., et al. (2014). *William's obstetrics* (24th ed.). New York, NY: McGraw-Hill Medical.

Davidson, M. R. (2014). *Fast facts for the neonatal nurse: A nursing orientation and care guide in a nutshell*. New York, NY: Springer Publishing Company.

Delany, I., Rappuoli, R., & De Gregorio, E. (2014). Vaccines for the 21st century. *EMBO Molecular Medicine, 6*(6), 708–720.

Dudek, S. G. (2014). *Nutrition essentials for nursing practice* (7th ed.). Philadelphia, PA: Lippincott Williams & Wilkins.

Dunn, R. L., Kalich, K. A., Henning, M. J., & Fedrizzi, R. (2015). Engaging field-based professionals in a qualitative assessment of barriers and positive contributors to breastfeeding using the social ecological model. *Maternal and Child Health Journal, 19*(1), 6–16.

Dyson, L., McCormick, F. M., & Renfrew, M. J. (2014). Interventions for promoting the initiation of breastfeeding. *Sao Paulo Medical Journal, 132*(1), 68–72.

El-Radhi, A. S. (2015). Management of common neonatal problems. *British Journal of Nursing, 24*(5), 258–266.

Fillipps, D. J., & Bucciarelli, R. L. (2015). Cardiac evaluation of the newborn. *Pediatric Clinics of North America, 62*(2), 471–489.

Fonseca, M. J., Severo, M., Barros, H., & Santos, A. C. (2014). Determinants of weight changes during the first 96 hours of life in full-term newborns. *Birth, 41*(2), 160–168.

Freedman, A. L., & Hurwitz, R. S. (2015). Complications of newborn circumcision: Prevention, diagnosis and treatment, In P. P. Godbole, M. A. Koyle, & D. T. Wilcox(Eds.), *Pediatric urology: surgical complications and management, 2*, Hoboken, NJ: John Wiley & Sons. doi: 10.1002/9781118473382.ch25

Gaydos, L. M., Blake, S. C., Gazmararian, J. A., Woodruff, W., Thompson, W. W., & Dalmida, S. G. (2014). Revisiting safe sleep recommendations for African-American Infants: Why current counseling is insufficient. *Maternal and Child Health Journal,* 1–8 (Online: June 3, 2014).

Gephart, S. M., & Weller, M. (2014). Colostrum as oral immune therapy to promote neonatal health. *Advances in Neonatal Care, 14*(1), 44–51.

Giese, R. A., & Richter, G. T. (2015). Capillary malformations. In G. T. Richter & J. Y. Suen (Eds.), *Head and neck vascular anomalies: A practical case-based approach* (pp. 127–128). San Diego, CA: Plural Publishing.

Gloster, H. M Jr, Gebauer, L. E., & Mistur, R. L. (Eds.) (2016a). Erythema toxicum neonatorum. In H. M. Gloster, Jr., L. E. Gebauer, & R. L. Mistur *Absolute dermatology review* (pp. 87–89). Springer International Publishing.

Gloster, H. M Jr, Gebauer, L. E., & Mistur, R. L. (Eds.) (2016b). Supernumerary nipples. In *Absolute dermatology review* (pp. 355–356). Springer International Publishing.

Goyal, D., Nagar, S., & Kumar, B. (2014). An enhanced approach for face recognition of newborns using HMM and SVD coefficients. *International Journal of Computer Applications, 88*(14), 17–23.

Greene, C. L., & Matern, D. (2014). Newborn screening for inborn errors of metabolism. In *Physician's guide to the diagnosis, treatment, and follow-up of inherited metabolic diseases* (pp. 719–735). Berlin Heidelberg, Germany: Springer Publishers

Joint Commission. (2015). Infant abductions: Preventing future occurrences. Retrieved from http://www.jointcommission.org/SentinelEvents/SentinelEventAlert/sea_9.htm

Kent, G. (2014). Regulating fatty acids in infant formula: critical assessment of US policies and practices. *International Breastfeeding Journal, 9*(1), 2–10.

Khan, J., Vesel, L., Bahl, R., & Martines, J. C. (2015). Timing of breastfeeding initiation and exclusivity of breastfeeding during the first month of life: Effects on neonatal mortality and morbidity—A systematic review and meta-analysis. *Maternal and Child Health Journal,* 19(3), 468–479.

King, T. L., Brucker, M. C., Kriebs, J. M., Fahey, J. O., Gegor, C. L., & Varney, H. (2015). *Varney's midwifery* (5th ed.). Burlington, MA: Jones & Bartlett Learning.

Kliegman, R. M., Behrman, R. E., Jenson, H. B., & Stanton, B. F. (2014). *Nelson's textbook of pediatrics* (20th ed.). St. Louis, MO: Elsevier.

La LecheLeague. (2015a). *Lactation support and health care providers.* Retrieved from http://www.llli.org/resources/providers.html?m=0,2

La LecheLeague. (2015b). *Expressing and storing milk.* Retrieved from http://www.llli.org/nb/nbjulaug07p168.html

Lauwers, J., & Swisher, A. (2016). *Counseling the nursing mother: A lactation consultant's guide.* (6th ed.), Burlington, MA: Jones & Bartlett Learning.

Lomax, A. (2015). *Examination of the newborn: An evidence-based guide* (2nd ed.). West Sussex, UK: John Wiley & Sons.

Lönnerdal, B. (2014). Infant formula and infant nutrition: bioactive proteins of human milk and implications for composition of infant formulas. *The American Journal of Clinical Nutrition, 99*(3), 712S–717S

Ludington-Hoe, S. M., & Morgan, K. (2014). Infant assessment and reduction of sudden unexpected postnatal collapse risk during skin-to-skin contact. *Newborn and Infant Nursing Reviews, 14*(1), 28–33.

Maisels, M. J. (2015). Sister Jean Ward, phototherapy, and jaundice: A unique human and photochemical interaction. *Journal of Perinatology, 35*(9):671–675.

Marcdante, K. J., & Kliegman, R. M. (2014) *Nelson essentials of pediatrics* (7th ed.). Philadelphia, PA: Elsevier.

March of Dimes (2015a). *Hearing loss.* Retrieved from http://www.marchofdimes.com/baby/hearing-impairment.aspx

Martin, R. J., Fanaroff, A. A., & Walsh, M. C. (2014). *Fanaroff & Martin's neonatal-perinatal medicine* (10th ed.). Philadelphia, PA: Elsevier.

McDermott, J. L. (2015). G586 (P) Phototherapy management in jaundiced babies: Jaundice management tool. *Archives of Disease in Childhood, 100*(Suppl 3), A268–A269.

Mersch, J., Kibby, J. E., & Bredenkamp, J. K. (2104). Newborn infant hearing screening. *MedicineNet.com,* Retrieved from http://www.medicinenet.com/newborn_infant_hearing_screening/article.htm

Mielke, R. T. (2014). Counseling parents who are considering newborn male circumcision. *Journal of Midwifery & Women's Health, 59*(2), 225.

Monahan, E. (2014). What are the dangers of diluted baby formula? *Livestrong.* Retrieved from http://www.livestrong.com/article/97662-dangers-diluted-baby-formula/

Moore, D. L., & MacDonald, N. E. (2015). Preventing ophthalmia neonatorum. *Pediatrics & Child Health, 20*(2), 93–96.

Morrison, K., Herbst, K., Corbett, S., & Herndon, C. D. (2014). Pain management practice patterns for common pediatric urology procedures. *Urology, 83*(1), 206–210.

Moses, S. (2015).) Pediatric vital signs. *Family Practice Notebook.* Retrieved from http://www.fpnotebook.com/cv/exam/pdtrcvtlsgns.htm

Nagtalon-Ramos, J. (2014). *Maternal-newborn nursing care: Best evidence-based practices.* Philadelphia, PA: F.A. Davis.

National Center for Missing & Exploited Children [NCMEC]. (2015). *Infant abductions.* Retrieved from http://www.missingkids.com/InfantAbduction

National Guideline Clearinghouse. (2015). *Guidelines for glucose monitoring and treatment of hypoglycemia in neonates.* Retrieved from http://www.guideline.gov/content.aspx?id=11218&search=glucose+monitoring+of+hypoglycemia+in+neonates

National Institute of Child Health and Human Development [NICHD]. (2014). *Safe to sleep public education campaign.* Retrieved from http://www.nichd.nih.gov/sts/news/downloadable/Pages/infographic_horizontal.aspx

Nikolopoulos, T. P. (2015). Neonatal hearing screening: What we have achieved and what needs to be improved. *International Journal of Pediatric Otorhinolaryngology, 79*(5), 635–637.

Otsuka, Y. (2014). Face recognition in infants: A review of behavioral and near-infrared spectroscopic studies. *Japanese Psychological Research, 56*(1), 76–90.

Pfister, K. M., & Ramel, S. E. (2014). Linear growth and neurodevelopmental outcomes. *Clinics in Perinatology, 41*(2), 309–321.

Plavskii, V. Y., Tret'yakova, A. I., & Mostovnikova, G. R. (2014). Phototherapeutic systems for the treatment of hyperbilirubinemia of newborns. *Journal of Optical Technology, 81*(6), 341–348.

Rüdiger, M., & Konstantelos, D. (2015). Apgar score and risk of cause-specific infant mortality. *The Lancet, 385*(9967), 505–506.

Saugstad, O. D. (2015). Delivery room management of term and preterm newly born infants. *Neonatology, 107*(4), 365–371.

Schlenker, E., & Gilbert, J. A. (2015). *William's essentials of nutrition and diet therapy* (11th ed.). St. Louis, MO: Elsevier.

Sheth, R. D., Ranalli, N., & Aldana, P. (2014). Pediatric craniosynostosis. *eMedicine,* Retrieved from http://emedicine.medscape.com/article/1175957-overview

Silverberg, N. B. (2015). Normal color variations in children of color. In N. B. Silverberg, C. Duran-McKinster, & Y-K. Tay (Eds.), *Pediatric skin of color* (pp. 63–68). New York, NY: Springer.

Sinkey, R. G., Eschenbacher, M. A., Walsh, P. M., Doerger, R. G., Lambers, D. S., Sibai, B. M., et al. (2015). The GoMo study: A randomized clinical trial assessing neonatal pain with Gomco vs Mogen clamp circumcision. *American Journal of Obstetrics and Gynecology, 212*(5), 664–e1.

Skidmore-Roth, L. (2015). *Mosby's 2015 nursing drug reference* (28th ed.). St. Louis, MO: Elsevier.

Springer, S. C., & Glasser, J. G. (2015). Bowel obstruction in the newborn. *eMedicine*. Retrieved from http://emedicine.medscape.com/article/980360-overview

Stanley, C. A., Rozance, P. J., Thornton, P. S., De Leon, D. D., Harris, D., Haymond, M. W., et al. (2015). Re-evaluating "transitional neonatal hypoglycemia": mechanism and implications for management. *The Journal of Pediatrics, 166*(6), 1520—1525.

Tamai, J., & McCarthy, J. J. (2015). Developmental dysplasia of the hip. *eMedicine*. Retrieved from http://emedicine.medscape.com/article/1248135-overview

Tawia, S., & McGuire, L. (2014). Early weight loss and weight gain in healthy, full-term, exclusively-breastfed infants. *Breastfeeding Review, 22*(1), 31–42

Thornton, P. S., Stanley, C. A., De Leon, D. D., Harris, D., Haymond, M. W., Hussain, K., et al. (2015). Recommendations from the Pediatric Endocrine Society for evaluation and management of persistent hypoglycemia in neonates, infants, and children. *The Journal of Pediatrics, 167*(2), 238–245.

Tobian, A. A., Kacker, S., & Quinn, T. C. (2014). Male circumcision: a globally relevant but under-utilized method for the prevention of HIV and other sexually transmitted infections. *Annual Review of Medicine, 65*, 293–306.

Tung, T. H., & Moore, A. M. (2015). 14 Brachial plexus injuries. In S. E. Mackinnon (Ed.), *Nerve surgery* (pp. 391–479). New York, NY: Thieme Medical Publishers.

U.S. Department of Health and Human Services [USDHHS]. (2010). *Healthy people 2020*. Retrieved from http://www.healthypeople.gov/2020/topicsobjectives2020

Verklan, M. T., & Walden, M. (2015). *Core curriculum for neonatal intensive care nursing* (5th ed.). St. Louis, MO: Elsevier.

Walker, M. (2014). *Breastfeeding management for the clinician: Using the evidence* (3rd ed.). Burlington, MA: Jones & Bartlett Learning.

Weber, J., & Kelley, J. (2014). *Health assessment in nursing* (5th ed.). Philadelphia, PA: Lippincott Williams & Wilkins.

MULTIPLE CHOICE QUESTIONS

1. At birth, a newborn's assessment reveals the following: heart rate of 140 bpm, loud crying, some flexion of extremities, crying when bulb syringe is introduced into the nares, and a pink body with blue extremities. The nurse would document the newborn's Apgar score as:
   a. 5 points
   b. 6 points
   c. 7 points
   d. 8 points

2. The nurse is explaining phototherapy to the parents of a newborn. The nurse would include which of the following as the purpose?
   a. Increase surfactant levels
   b. Stabilize the newborn's temperature
   c. Destroy Rh-negative antibodies
   d. Oxidize bilirubin on the skin

3. The nurse administers a single dose of vitamin K intramuscularly to a newborn after birth to promote:
   a. Conjugation of bilirubin
   b. Blood clotting
   c. Foreman ovale closure
   d. Digestion of complex proteins

4. A prophylactic agent is instilled in both eyes of all newborns to prevent which of the following conditions?
   a. Gonorrhea and chlamydia
   b. Thrush and enterobacter
   c. *Staphylococcus* and syphilis
   d. Hepatitis B and herpes

5. The AAP recommends that all newborns be placed on their backs to sleep to reduce the risk of:
   a. Respiratory distress syndrome
   b. Bottle mouth syndrome
   c. Sudden infant death syndrome
   d. GI regurgitation syndrome

6. Which one of the following immunizations is most commonly received by newborns before hospital discharge?
   a. Pneumococcus
   b. Varicella
   c. Hepatitis A
   d. Hepatitis B

7. Which condition would be missed if a newborn were screened before he had tolerated protein feedings for at least 48 hours?
   a. Hypothyroidism
   b. Cystic fibrosis
   c. Phenylketonuria
   d. Sickle cell disease

8. Which of the following findings in a newborn would the nurse document as abnormal when assessing the newborn head?
   a. Two soft spots palpated between the cranial bones
   b. A spongy area of edema outlined on the head
   c. Head circumference 32 cm, chest 34 cm
   d. Asymmetry of the head with overriding bones

9. Which of the following findings in a newborn would be considered normal?
   a. Passage of meconium within the first 24 hours
   b. Respiratory rate of 80 breaths/minute
   c. Yellow skin tones at 10 hours after birth
   d. Bleeding from the umbilicus area

CRITICAL THINKING EXERCISE

1. An African American mother who delivered her first baby, and is on the mother–baby unit, calls the nursery nurse into her room and expresses concern about how her daughter looks. The mother tells the nurse that her baby's head looks like a "banana" and is mushy to the touch, and she has "white spots" all over her nose. In addition, there appear to be "big bluish bruises" all over her baby's buttocks. She wants to know what is wrong with her baby and whether these problems will go away.
   a. How should the nurse respond to this mother's questions?
   b. What additional newborn instruction might be appropriate at this time?
   c. What reassurance can be given to this new mother regarding her daughter's appearance?

2. At approximately 12:30 am on a Friday, a woman enters a hospital through a busy emergency department. She is wearing a white uniform and a lab coat with a stethoscope around her neck. She identifies herself as a new nurse coming back to check on something she had left on the unit on an earlier shift. She enters a postpartum client's room containing the mother's newborn, pushes the open crib down a hallway, and escapes through an exit. The security cameras aren't working. The infant isn't discovered missing until the 2 am check by the nurse.
   a. What impact does an infant abduction have on the family and the hospital?
   b. What security measure was the weak link in the chain of security?
   c. What can hospitals do to prevent infant abduction?

STUDY ACTIVITIES

1. Obtain a set of vital signs (temperature, pulse, and respiration) of a newborn on admission to the nursery. Repeat this procedure and compare changes in the values several hours later. Discuss what changes in the vital signs you would expect during this transitional period.

   The discussion of newborn changes noticed will vary from student to student, depending on the interview information obtained from the new mother.

2. Interview a new mother on the postpartum unit on her second day about the changes she has noticed in her newborn's appearance and behavior within the past 24 hours. Discuss your interview findings at postconference. This discussion will vary depending on questions asked during the bath demonstration as well as each individual mother's response to it.

3. Demonstrate a newborn bath to a new mother in her room, using the principle of bathing from the cleanest to the dirtiest body part. Discuss the questions asked by the mother and her reaction to the demonstration in postconference.

4. Go to the La Leche League web site (refer to thePoint website). Review the information it provides on breast-feeding. How helpful would it be to a new mother?

   The La Leche League website is filled with helpful information with pictures to assist new mothers with breast-feeding. Each student will have his or her own opinion about how helpful the website is and what educational level it addresses.

5. Debate the risks and benefits of neonatal circumcision within your nursing group at postconference. Did either side present a stronger position? What is your opinion, and why?

   The risks of neonatal circumcision include hemorrhage, infection, adhesions, dehiscence, urethral fistula, meatal stenosis, and pain. The benefits of neonatal circumcision include prevention of penile cancer, decreased incidence of UTIs and STIs, and preservation of male body consistent with father and peers where the procedure is common. Students will express their own opinions about their thoughts based on their value systems and cultural backgrounds.

BRINGING IT ALL TOGETHER: CASE STUDY

Two days after having a difficult birth of her first child at 37 weeks' gestation, 25-year-old Molly and her partner took their son home from the hospital. That evening while she was breast-feeding him, Molly noticed that the whites of her son's eyes seemed slightly yellow, a condition that worsened noticeably by the next day. Molly called the *Healthy Start* Home Health nurse and requested a visit to evaluate her newborn.

ASSESSMENT

Upon examining the 3-day-old newborn, the nurse noted that there were a few areas of bruising on the newborn's head and a yellow hue on the infant's skin when she pressed on boney prominent areas. When questioning the mother about her breast-feeding, the mother stated that her son didn't seem all that interested at times, so she let him sleep instead.

Go to thePoint **to find questions to consider about this case.**

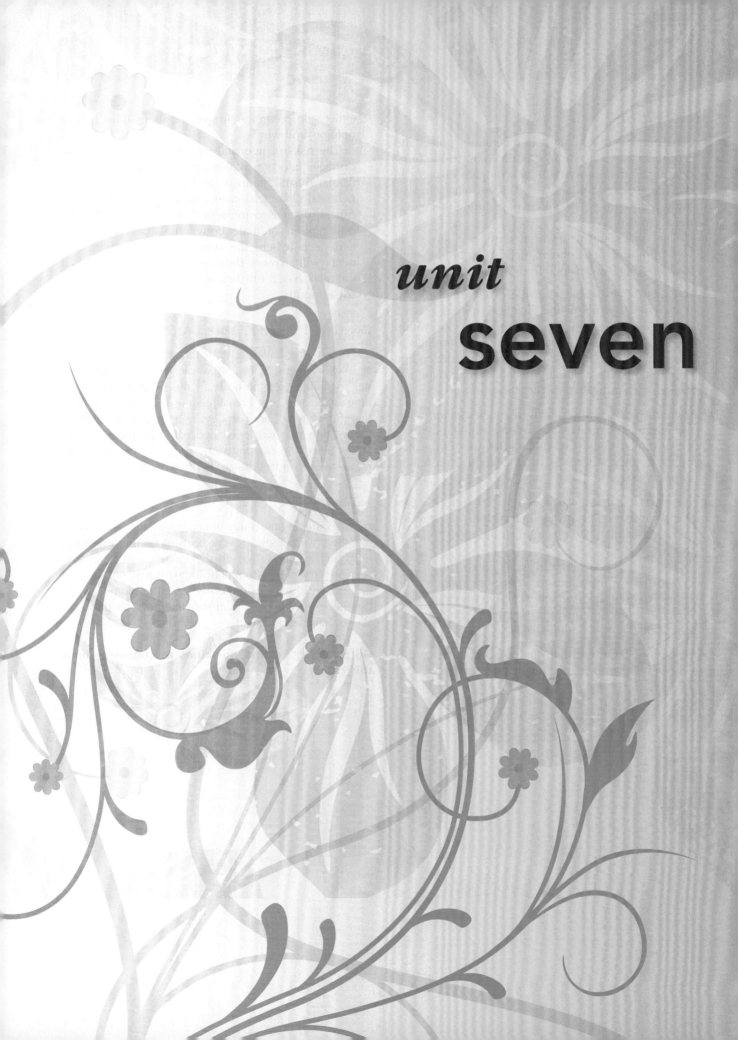

unit
seven

Childbearing at Risk

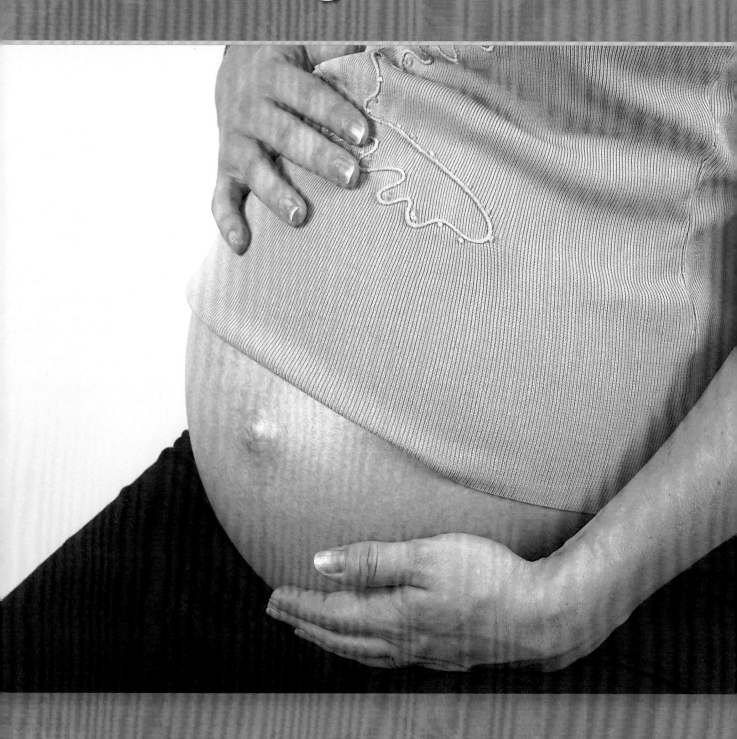

19

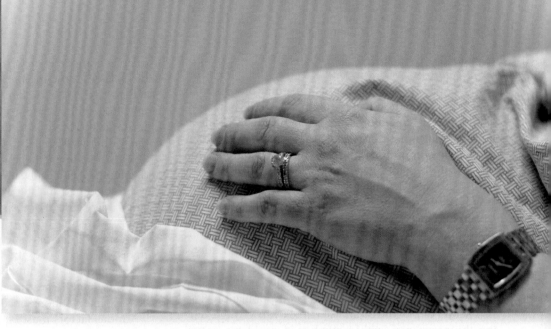

Nursing Management of Pregnancy at Risk: Pregnancy-Related Complications

Learning Objectives

Upon completion of the chapter, you will be able to:

1. Compare and contrast a normal pregnancy to a high risk one. Determine the common factors that might place a pregnancy at high risk.

2. Detect the causes of vaginal bleeding during early and late pregnancy.

3. Outline nursing assessment and management for the pregnant woman experiencing vaginal bleeding.

4. Develop a plan of care for the woman experiencing preeclampsia, eclampsia, and HELLP syndrome.

5. Examine the pathophysiology of hydramnios and subsequent management.

6. Evaluate factors in a woman's prenatal history that place her at risk for premature rupture of membranes (PROMs).

7. Formulate a teaching plan for maintaining the health of pregnant women experiencing a high-risk pregnancy.

Helen, a 35-year-old G5 P4, presents to the labor and birth suite with severe abdominal pain. She reports that the pain began suddenly about an hour ago while she was resting. She has had two prior cesarean births and thus far has had an uneventful past 32 weeks. Helen appears distressed and is moaning. What additional assessments do you need to do to care for Helen? What might be your immediate nursing action?

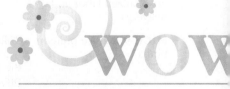

Words of Wisdom
Detours and bumps along the road of life can be managed, but many cannot be entirely cured.

INTRODUCTION

Most people view pregnancy as a natural process with a positive outcome—the birth of a healthy newborn. Unfortunately, conditions can occur that may result in negative outcomes for the fetus, mother, or both. A **high-risk pregnancy** is one in which a condition exists that jeopardizes the health of the mother, her fetus, or both. The condition may result from the pregnancy, or it may be a condition that was present before the woman became pregnant.

Approximately, one in four pregnant women is considered to be at high risk or diagnosed with complications (Nagtalon-Ramos, 2014). Women who are considered to be at high risk have a higher morbidity and mortality compared with mothers in the general population. The risk status of a woman and her fetus can change during the pregnancy, with a number of problems occurring during labor, birth, or afterward, even in women without any known previous antepartal risk. Examples of high-risk conditions include gestational diabetes and ectopic pregnancy. Many obstetric complications and conditions are life-threatening emergencies with high morbidity and mortality rates. It is essential that these be identified early to ensure the best possible outcome for the mother and infant. These conditions are specifically addressed in *Healthy People 2020* (U.S. Department of Health and Human Services, 2010). Early identification of the woman at risk is essential to ensure that appropriate interventions are instituted promptly, increasing the opportunity to change the course of events and provide a positive outcome.

The term *risk* may mean different things to different groups. For example, health care providers may focus on the disease processes and treatments to prevent complications. Nurses may focus on nursing care and on the psychosocial impact on the woman and her family.

Insurance companies may concentrate on the economic issues related to the high-risk status. The woman's attention may be focused on her own needs and those of her family. Together, working as a collaborative team, the ultimate goal of care is to ensure the best possible outcome for the woman, her fetus, and her family.

Risk assessment begins at the first antepartal visit and continues with each subsequent visit because factors may be identified in later visits that were not apparent during earlier visits. For example, as the nurse and client develop a trusting relationship, previously unidentified or unsuspected factors (such as drug abuse or intimate partner violence) may be revealed. Through education and support, the nurse can encourage the client to inform her health care provider of these concerns, and necessary interventions or referrals can be made.

Various factors must be considered when determining a woman's risk for adverse pregnancy outcomes, and a comprehensive approach to high-risk pregnancy is needed. For example, prenatal stress and distress have been shown to have significant consequences for the mother, child, and family. Pregnancy-specific stress such as depression, anxiety, and perceived stress may increase the risk for adverse birth outcomes and is associated with preterm births (Staneva et al., 2015). Risks are grouped into broad categories based on threats to health and pregnancy outcome. Current categories of risk are biophysical, psychosocial, sociodemographic, and environmental (Box 19.1) (Cunningham et al., 2014).

This chapter describes the major conditions directly related to pregnancy that can complicate a pregnancy, possibly affecting maternal and fetal outcomes. These include bleeding during pregnancy (spontaneous abortion, ectopic pregnancy, gestational trophoblastic disease, cervical insufficiency, placenta previa, abruptio placentae, and placenta accreta), hyperemesis gravidarum, gestational hypertension, HELLP syndrome, gestational diabetes, blood incompatibility, amniotic fluid imbalances (polyhydramnios and oligohydramnios), multiple gestation, and premature rupture of membranes. Chapter 20 addresses preexisting conditions that can complicate a woman's pregnancy as well as populations that are considered to be at high risk.

BLEEDING DURING PREGNANCY

Bleeding at any time during pregnancy is potentially life threatening. Every minute of every day, a woman dies in pregnancy or childbirth. The biggest killer is obstetric hemorrhage, the successful treatment of which is a challenge for both the developed and developing worlds. The presence of an attendant at every birth and access to emergency obstetric care are strategic to reducing maternal morbidity and mortality (World Health Organization [WHO], 2015). Management of obstetric hemorrhage involves early recognition, assessment, and resuscitation.

HEALTHY PEOPLE *2020* • *19.1*

Objective	Nursing Significance
MICH-6 Reduce maternal illness and complications due to pregnancy (complications during hospitalized labor and delivery).	Will reduce perinatal morbidity and mortality and optimize pregnancy outcomes.
MICH-9 Reduce preterm births.	Will help to preserve the health and well-being of the growing fetus if the pregnancy goes to term.

Healthy People objectives based on data from
http://www.healthypeople.gov.

BOX 19.1

FACTORS PLACING A WOMAN AT RISK DURING PREGNANCY

Biophysical Factors
- Genetic conditions
- Chromosomal abnormalities
- Multiple pregnancy
- Defective genes
- Inherited disorders
- ABO incompatibility
- Large fetal size
- Medical and obstetric conditions
- Preterm labor and birth
- Cardiovascular disease
- Chronic hypertension
- Cervical insufficiency
- Placental abnormalities
- Infection
- Diabetes
- Maternal collagen diseases
- Thyroid disease
- Asthma
- Post-term pregnancy
- Hemoglobinopathies
- Nutritional status
- Inadequate dietary intake
- Food fads
- Excessive food intake
- Under- or overweight status
- Hematocrit value less than 33%
- Eating disorder

Psychosocial Factors
- Smoking
- Caffeine
- Alcohol and substance abuse
- Maternal obesity
- Inadequate support system
- Situational crisis
- History of violence
- Emotional distress
- Unsafe cultural practices

Sociodemographic Factors
- Poverty status
- Lack of prenatal care
- Age younger than 15 years or older than 35 years
- Parity—All first pregnancies and more than five pregnancies
- Marital status—Increased risk for unmarried women
- Accessibility to health care
- Ethnicity—Increased risk in non-White women

Environmental Factors
- Infections
- Radiation
- Pesticides
- Illicit drugs
- Industrial pollutants
- Second-hand cigarette smoke
- Personal stress

Adapted from Martin, R. J., Fanaroff, A. A., & Walsh, M. C. (2014). *Fanaroff & Martin's neonatal-perinatal medicine* (10th ed.). Philadelphia, PA: Elsevier Health Sciences; Foley, M., Strong, T. M., & Garite, T. (2014). *Obstetric intensive care manual* (4th ed.). New York, NY: McGraw-Hill Publishers; and Cunningham, F. G., Leveno, K. J., Bloom, S. L., Spong, C. Y., Dashe, J. S., Hoffman, B. L., Casey, B. M., & Sheffield, J. S. (2014). *Williams' obstetrics* (24th ed.). New York, NY: McGraw-Hill Education.

Various methods are available to try to stop the bleeding, ranging from pharmacologic methods to aid uterine contraction (e.g., oxytocin, ergometrine, and prostaglandins) to surgical methods to stem the bleeding (e.g., balloon tamponade, compression sutures, or arterial ligation). Bleeding can occur early or late in the pregnancy and may result from numerous conditions. Bleeding is experienced by approximately 20% of women during the first trimester of pregnancy (Knez, Day, & Jurkovic, 2014). Conditions commonly associated with early bleeding (first half of pregnancy) include spontaneous abortion, uterine fibroids, ectopic pregnancy, gestational trophoblastic disease, and cervical insufficiency. Conditions associated with late bleeding include placenta previa, abruptio placentae, and placenta accreta, which usually occur after the 20th week of gestation.

Spontaneous Abortion

Abortion is considered not only a major reproductive health matter, but also a health risk factor for women's well-being. Spontaneous abortion is the most common complication of early pregnancy (Tulandi & Al-Fozan,

2014). An **abortion** is the loss of an early pregnancy, usually before week 20 of gestation. Abortion can be spontaneous or induced. A spontaneous abortion refers to the loss of a fetus resulting from natural causes, that is, not elective or therapeutically induced by a procedure. A stillbirth is the loss of a fetus after the 20th week of development, whereas a miscarriage refers to a loss before the 20th week. Nonmedical people often use the term *miscarriage* to denote an abortion that has occurred spontaneously. A miscarriage can occur during early pregnancy, and many women who miscarry may not even be aware that they are pregnant. About 80% of spontaneous abortions occur within the first trimester. The terms *stillbirth* and *miscarriage* can sometimes be confusing. Both refer to the loss of an early pregnancy; however, stillbirth occurs later in pregnancy. Some stillbirths can occur right up to the time of labor and delivery. Stillbirths are much less common than miscarriages, occurring in only 1 out of every 160 pregnancies (March of Dimes, 2015a).

The overall rate for spontaneous abortion in the United States is reported to be 15% to 20% of recognized pregnancies in the United States. However, with the development of highly sensitive assays for human chorionic gonadotropin (hCG) levels that detect pregnancies prior to the expected next menses, the incidence of pregnancy loss increases significantly—to about 60% to 70% (King et al., 2015). The frequency of spontaneous abortion increases further with maternal age.

Pathophysiology

The causes of spontaneous abortion are varied and often unknown. The most common cause for first-trimester abortions is fetal genetic abnormalities, usually unrelated to the mother. Chromosomal abnormalities are more likely causes in the first trimester and maternal disease is more likely in the second trimester. Those occurring during the second trimester are more likely related to maternal conditions, such as cervical insufficiency, congenital, or acquired anomaly of the uterine cavity (uterine septum or fibroids), hypothyroidism, diabetes mellitus, chronic nephritis, use of crack cocaine, inherited and acquired thrombophilias, lupus, polycystic ovary syndrome, severe hypertension, and acute infection such as rubella virus, cytomegalovirus, herpes simplex virus, bacterial vaginosis, and toxoplasmosis (Jones & Lopez, 2014).

Women experiencing a first-trimester abortion at home without a dilation and curettage (D&C) to resolve it require frequent monitoring of hCG levels to validate that all the conceptus tissues have been expelled. Women going through a second-trimester abortion are admitted to the hospital to have an augmented labor and delivery. Nursing care would focus on care of the laboring women with tremendous attention paid to providing emotional support to the woman and her family.

Nursing Assessment

When a pregnant woman calls and reports vaginal bleeding, she must be seen as soon as possible by a health care professional to ascertain the etiology. Varying degrees of vaginal bleeding, low back pain, abdominal cramping, and passage of products of conception tissue may be reported. Ask the woman about the color of the vaginal bleeding (bright red is significant) and the amount—for example, question her about the frequency with which she is changing her peripads (saturation of one peripad hourly is significant) and the passage of any clots or tissue. Instruct her to save any tissue or clots passed and bring them with her to the health care facility. Also, obtain a description of any other signs and symptoms the woman may be experiencing, along with a description of their severity and duration. It is important to remain calm and listen to the woman's description.

When the woman arrives at the health care facility, assess her vital signs and observe the amount, color, and characteristics of the bleeding. Ask her to rate her current pain level, using an appropriate pain assessment tool. Also, evaluate the amount and intensity of the woman's abdominal cramping or contractions, and assess the woman's level of understanding about what is happening to her. A thorough assessment helps in determining the type of spontaneous abortion, such as threatened abortion, inevitable abortion, incomplete abortion, complete abortion, missed abortion, and habitual abortion, that the woman may be experiencing (Table 19.1).

Nursing Management

Nursing management of the woman with a spontaneous abortion focuses on providing continued monitoring and psychological support, for the family is experiencing acute loss and grief. An important component of this support is reassuring the woman that spontaneous abortions usually result from an abnormality and that her actions did not cause the abortion.

PROVIDING CONTINUED MONITORING

Continued monitoring and ongoing assessments are essential for the woman experiencing a spontaneous abortion. Monitor the amount of vaginal bleeding through pad counts and observe for passage of products of conception tissue. Assess the woman's pain and provide appropriate pain management to address the cramping discomfort.

Assist in preparing the woman for procedures and treatments such as surgery to evacuate the uterus or medications such as misoprostol or PGE2. If the woman is Rh negative and not sensitized, expect to administer RhoGAM within 72 hours after the abortion is complete. Drug Guide 19.1 gives more information about these medications.

PROVIDING SUPPORT

A woman's emotional reaction may vary depending on her desire for this pregnancy and her available support network. Provide both physical and emotional support. In addition, prepare the woman and her family for the assessment process and answer their questions.

Explaining some of the causes of spontaneous abortions can help the woman to understand what is happening and may allay her fears and guilt that she did something to cause the pregnancy loss. Most women experience an acute sense of loss and go through a grieving process with a spontaneous abortion. Providing sensitive listening, counseling, and anticipatory guidance to the woman and her family will allow them to verbalize their feelings and ask questions about future pregnancies.

The grieving period may last as long as two years after a pregnancy loss, with each person grieving in his or her own way. Encourage friends and family to be supportive but give the couple space and time to work through their loss. Referral to a community support group for parents who have experienced a miscarriage can be very helpful during this grief process.

TABLE 19.1	CATEGORIES OF ABORTION		
Category	Assessment Findings	Diagnosis	Therapeutic Management
Threatened abortion	Vaginal bleeding (often slight) early in a pregnancy No cervical dilation or change in cervical consistency Mild abdominal cramping Closed cervical os No passage of fetal tissue	Vaginal ultrasound to confirm if sac is empty Declining maternal serum hCG and progesterone levels to provide additional information about viability of pregnancy	Conservative supportive treatment Possible reduction in activity in conjunction with nutritious diet and adequate hydration
Inevitable abortion	Vaginal bleeding (greater than that associated with threatened abortion) Rupture of membranes Cervical dilation Strong abdominal cramping Possible passage of products of conception	Ultrasound and hCG levels to indicate pregnancy loss	Vacuum curettage if products of conception are not passed, to reduce risk of excessive bleeding and infection Prostaglandin analogs such as misoprostol to empty uterus of retained tissue (only used if fragments are not completely passed)
Incomplete abortion (passage of some of the products of conception)	Intense abdominal cramping Heavy vaginal bleeding Cervical dilation	Ultrasound confirmation that products of conception still in uterus	Client stabilization Evacuation of uterus via D&C or prostaglandin analog
Complete abortion (passage of all products of conception)	History of vaginal bleeding and abdominal pain Passage of tissue with subsequent decrease in pain and significant decrease in vaginal bleeding	Ultrasound demonstrating an empty uterus	No medical or surgical intervention necessary Follow-up appointment to discuss family planning
Missed abortion (nonviable embryo retained in utero for at least 6 weeks)	Absent uterine contractions Irregular spotting Possible progression to inevitable abortion	Ultrasound to identify products of conception in uterus	Evacuation of uterus (if inevitable abortion does not occur): suction curettage during first trimester, dilation and evacuation during second trimester Induction of labor with intravaginal PGE2 suppository to empty uterus without surgical intervention
Habitual abortion	History of three or more consecutive spontaneous abortions Not carrying the pregnancy to viability or term	Validation via client's history	Identification and treatment of underlying cause (possible causes such as genetic or chromosomal abnormalities, reproductive tract abnormalities, chronic diseases or immunologic problems) Cervical cerclage in second trimester if incompetent cervix is the cause

Ectopic Pregnancy

An **ectopic pregnancy** is any pregnancy in which the fertilized ovum implants outside the uterine cavity. The term *ectopic* is derived from the Greek word *ektopos,* meaning "out of place," and refers to the implantation of a fertilized egg in a location outside of the uterine cavity, including the fallopian tubes, cervix, ovary, and the abdominal cavity. This abnormally implanted embryo grows and draws its blood supply from the site of abnormal implantation. As the embryo enlarges, it creates the potential for organ rupture because only the uterine

DRUG GUIDE 19.1 MEDICATIONS RELATED TO ABORTIONS

Medication	Action/Indications	Nursing Implications
Misoprostol (Cytotec)	Stimulates uterine contractions to terminate a pregnancy; to evacuate the uterus after abortion to ensure passage of all the products of conception.	• Monitor for side effects such as diarrhea, abdominal pain, nausea, vomiting, and dyspepsia. • Assess vaginal bleeding and report any increased bleeding, pain, or fever. • Monitor for signs and symptoms of shock, such as tachycardia, hypotension, and anxiety.
Mifepristone (RU-486)	Acts as progesterone antagonist, allowing prostaglandins to stimulate uterine contractions; causes the endometrium to slough; may be followed by administration of misoprostol within 48 hours.	• Monitor for headache, vomiting, diarrhea, and heavy bleeding. • Anticipate administration of antiemetic prior to use to reduce nausea and vomiting. • Encourage client to use acetaminophen to reduce discomfort from cramping.
PGE2, dinoprostone (Cervidil, Prepidil Gel, Prostin E2)	Stimulates uterine contractions, causing expulsion of uterine contents; to expel uterine contents in fetal death or missed abortion during second trimester, or to efface and dilate the cervix in pregnancy at term.	• Bring gel to room temperature before administering. • Avoid contact with skin. • Use sterile technique to administer. • Keep client supine for 30 min after administering. • Document time of insertion and dosing intervals. • Remove insert with retrieval system after 12 hours or at the onset of labor. • Explain purpose and expected response to client.
Rh(D) immuno-globulin (Gamulin, HydroRho-D, Rho-GAM, MICRhoGAM)	Suppresses immune response of nonsensitized Rh-negative clients who are exposed to Rh-positive blood; to prevent isoimmunization in Rh-negative women exposed to Rh-positive blood after abortions, miscarriages, and pregnancies.	• Administer intramuscularly in deltoid area. • Give only MICRhoGAM for abortions and miscarriages <12 weeks unless fetus or father is Rh negative (unless client is Rh positive, Rh antibodies are present). • Educate woman that she will need this after subsequent deliveries if newborns are Rh positive; also check lab study results prior to administering the drug.

Adapted from King, T. L., Brucker, M. C., Kriebs, J. M., Fahey, J. O., Grgor, C. L., & Varney, H. (2015). *Varney's midwifery* (5th ed.). Burlington, MA: Jones & Bartlett Learning; and Skidmore-Roth, L. (2015). *Mosby's 2015 nursing drug reference* (28th ed.). Philadelphia, PA: Elsevier.

cavity is designed to expand and accommodate fetal development. Ectopic pregnancy can lead to massive hemorrhage, infertility, or death.

Ectopic pregnancies occur in 1 in every 50 pregnancies in the United States or roughly 2% of all pregnancies are diagnosed as ectopic; this rate has increased dramatically during the past 30 years (March of Dimes, 2015b). It is a major health concern for women of reproductive age and is the primary cause of death during the first trimester of pregnancy in the United States (Szypulski, 2015). The discovery of ectopic pregnancies prior to rupture has increased dramatically in the past few decades as a result of improved diagnostic techniques such as the development of sensitive and specific radioimmunoassays for hCG, high-resolution ultrasonography, and the widespread availability of laparoscopy (Desai et al., 2014).

With an ectopic pregnancy, rupture and hemorrhage may occur due to the growth of the embryo. A ruptured ectopic pregnancy is a medical emergency; therefore prediction of any tubal rupture before its occurrence is extremely important. It is a potentially life-threatening condition and involves pregnancy loss. Even in the United States, women can and do still die from ectopic pregnancy, although early diagnosis has helped prevent that.

Pathophysiology

Normally, the fertilized ovum implants in the uterus. In ectopic pregnancy, the journey along the fallopian tube is arrested or altered in some way. With an ectopic pregnancy, the ovum implants outside the uterus. The most common site for implantation is the fallopian tubes, but some ova may implant in the ovary, the intestine, the

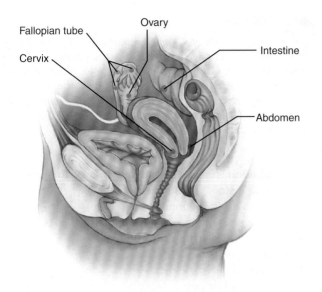

FIGURE 19.1 Possible sites for implantation with an ectopic pregnancy.

Fallopian tube
Cervix
Ovary
Intestine
Abdomen

cervix, or the abdominal cavity (Fig. 19.1) (Sepilian & Wood, 2015). None of these anatomic sites can accommodate placental attachment or a growing embryo.

Risk Factors

Ectopic pregnancies usually result from conditions that obstruct or slow the passage of the fertilized ovum through the fallopian tube to the uterus. This may be a physical blockage in the tube, or failure of the tubal epithelium to move the zygote (the cell formed after the egg is fertilized) down the tube into the uterus. In the general population, most cases are the result of tubal scarring secondary to pelvic inflammatory disease (PID). Organisms such as *Neisseria gonorrhea* and *Chlamydia trachomatis* preferentially attack the fallopian tubes, producing silent infections. A recent study reported a twofold increased risk for ectopic pregnancy in women with a history of a chlamydia infection, secondary to tubal damage (Randall & LaMontagne, 2015). Other associated risk factors for ectopic pregnancy include previous tubal surgery, infertility, PID, previous pregnancy loss (induced or spontaneous, use of an intrauterine contraceptive system, previous ectopic pregnancy, uterine fibroids, sterilization, smoking (which alters tubal motility), history of multiple sexual partners, use of progestin-only oral contraceptives, douching, and exposure to diethylstilbestrol (DES) (Ardehali & Casikar, 2015).

Therapeutic Management

The diagnosis of ectopic pregnancy can be challenging because many women are asymptomatic before tubal rupture. The classic clinical triad of ectopic pregnancy includes abdominal pain, amenorrhea, and vaginal bleeding. Unfortunately, only about half of women present with all three symptoms.

Diagnostic procedures used for a suspected ectopic pregnancy include a urine pregnancy test to confirm the pregnancy, beta-hCG concentrations to exclude a false-negative urine test, and a transvaginal ultrasound to visualize the misplaced pregnancy (Bourne, 2015).

Historically, the treatment of ectopic pregnancy was limited to surgery. The therapeutic management of ectopic pregnancy depends on whether the tube is intact or has ruptured, creating a medical emergency. In the event of a surgical intervention, preservation of the affected fallopian tube is attempted (King et al., 2015).

MEDICAL INTERVENTION

With early diagnosis, most women with ectopic pregnancy could be treated with methotrexate. The overall success rate of medical treatment in properly selected women is nearly 90%. To be eligible for medical therapy, the client must be hemodynamically stable, with no signs of active bleeding in the peritoneal cavity, low beta-hCG levels (<5,000 mIU/mL) and the mass (which must measure less than 4 cm as determined by ultrasound) must be unruptured.

Contraindications to medical treatment include an unstable client, severe persistent abdominal pain, renal or liver disease, immunodeficiency, active pulmonary disease, peptic ulcer, suspected intrauterine pregnancy, and poor client compliance (Tulandi, 2015). The potential advantages include avoidance of surgery, the preservation of tubal patency and function, and a lower cost.

The medical approach today for an unruptured tubal pregnancy most often consists of a single-dose IM injection of methotrexate (Rheumatrex; Trexall) with outpatient follow-up. Medical management with methotrexate, though not approved by the Food and Drug Administration for this purpose, has been endorsed by the American College of Obstetricians and Gynecologists. Prostaglandins, misoprostol, and actinomycin have also been used in the medical (nonsurgical) management of ectopic pregnancy, with a reported success rate of approximately 90%. Methotrexate is a folic acid antagonist that inhibits cell division in the developing embryo. It typically has been used as a chemotherapeutic agent in the treatment of leukemia, lymphomas, and carcinomas. It has been shown to produce results similar to that for surgical therapy in terms of high success rate, low complication rate, and good reproductive potential (Dalia et al., 2014). Adverse effects associated with methotrexate include nausea, vomiting, stomatitis, diarrhea, gastric upset, increased abdominal pain, and dizziness. Methotrexate for an ectopic pregnancy is ordered based on the client's body surface area. The administration of methotrexate should be limited to people who have had education and training in the handling and administration of hazardous drugs. In some facilities internal policies require that only nurses who have completed a chemotherapy certification and/ or hazardous drug competency program can administer this product (Cohen et al., 2015).

Prior to receiving the single-dose intramuscular injection to treat unruptured pregnancies, the woman needs to be counseled on the risks, benefits, adverse effects, and the possibility of failure of medical therapy, which would result in tubal rupture, necessitating surgery (Tulandi, 2015). The woman is then instructed to return weekly for follow-up laboratory studies for the next several weeks until beta-hCG titers decrease. Beta-hCG level changes between days 0 and 4 after methotrexate therapy have clinical significance and predictive value. A decreasing beta-hCG level is highly predictive of treatment success (Agarwal & Odejinmi, 2014).

SURGICAL INTERVENTION

Surgical management for the unruptured fallopian tube might involve a linear salpingostomy to preserve the tube—an important consideration for the woman wanting to preserve her future fertility. It may also be considered when medical treatment is considered unsuitable.

With a ruptured ectopic pregnancy, surgery is necessary as a result of possible uncontrolled hemorrhage. A laparotomy with a removal of the tube (salpingectomy) may be necessary. With earlier diagnosis and medical management, the focus has changed from preventing maternal death to facilitating rapid recovery and preserving fertility.

Regardless of the treatment approach (medical or surgical), the woman's beta-hCG level is monitored until it is undetectable to ensure that any residual trophoblastic tissue that forms the placenta is gone. Also, all Rh-negative unsensitized clients are given Rh immunoglobulin to prevent isoimmunization in future pregnancies.

Nursing Assessment

Nursing assessment focuses on determining the existence of an ectopic pregnancy and whether or not it has ruptured. A woman with a suspected ectopic pregnancy may have to undergo several diagnostic tests, some of which are invasive. Consider how she might feel during all of these tests, anticipate her questions, and offer her thorough explanations and reassurances.

HEALTH HISTORY AND PHYSICAL EXAMINATION

Assess the client thoroughly for signs and symptoms that may suggest an ectopic pregnancy. The onset of signs and symptoms varies, but they usually begin at about the seventh or eighth week of gestation. A missed menstrual period, adnexal fullness, and tenderness may indicate an unruptured tubal pregnancy. As the tube stretches, the pain increases. Pain may be unilateral, bilateral, or diffuse over the abdomen.

Take Note!

The hallmark of ectopic pregnancy is abdominal pain with spotting within 6 to 8 weeks after a missed menstrual period. Although this is the classic triad, all three of these signs and symptoms occur in only about 50% of cases. Many women have symptoms typical of early pregnancy, such as breast tenderness, nausea, fatigue, shoulder pain, and low back pain.

In addition, review the client's history for possible contributing factors. These may include:
- Previous ectopic pregnancy
- History of sexually transmitted infections (STIs)
- Fallopian tube scarring from PID
- In utero exposure to DES
- Endometriosis
- Previous tubal or pelvic surgery
- Infertility and infertility treatments, including use of fertility drugs
- Uterine abnormalities such as fibroids
- Presence of intrauterine contraception
- Use of progestin-only mini pill (slows ovum transport)
- Postpartum or postabortion infection
- Altered estrogen and progesterone levels (interferes with tubal motility)
- Increasing age (older than 35 years)
- Cigarette smoking (Ardehali & Casikar, 2015).

If rupture or hemorrhage occurs before treatment begins, symptoms may worsen and include severe, sharp, and sudden pain in the lower abdomen as the tube tears open and the embryo is expelled into the pelvic cavity; feelings of faintness; referred pain to the shoulder area, indicating bleeding into the abdomen, caused by phrenic nerve irritation; hypotension; marked abdominal tenderness with distention; and hypovolemic shock (Cunningham et al., 2014).

LABORATORY AND DIAGNOSTIC TESTING

The use of transvaginal ultrasound to visualize the misplaced pregnancy and low levels of serum beta-hCG assist in diagnosing an ectopic pregnancy. The ultrasound determines whether the pregnancy is intrauterine, assesses the size of the uterus, and provides evidence of fetal viability. The visualization of an adnexal mass and the absence of an intrauterine gestational sac are diagnostic of ectopic pregnancy (Kao et al., 2014). In a normal intrauterine pregnancy, beta-hCG levels typically double every 2 to 4 days until peak values are reached 60 to 90 days after conception. Concentrations of hCG decrease after 10 to 11 weeks and reach a plateau at low levels by 100 to 130 days (Ko & Cheung, 2014).). Therefore, low beta-hCG levels are suggestive of an ectopic pregnancy or impending abortion. Additional tests may be done to rule out other conditions such as spontaneous abortion, ruptured ovarian cyst, appendicitis, and salpingitis.

Nursing Management

Nursing management for the woman with an ectopic pregnancy focuses on preparing the woman for treatment, providing support, and providing education about preventive measures.

PREPARING THE WOMAN FOR TREATMENT

Administer analgesics as ordered to promote comfort and relieve discomfort from abdominal pain. Although the intensity of the pain can vary, women often report a great deal of pain. If the woman is treated medically, explain the medication that will be used and what she can expect. Also review signs and symptoms of possible adverse effects. If treatment will occur on an outpatient basis, outline the signs and symptoms of ectopic rupture (severe, sharp, stabbing, unilateral abdominal pain; vertigo/fainting; hypotension; and increased pulse) and advise the woman to seek medical help immediately if they occur.

If surgery is needed, close assessment and monitoring of the client's vital signs, bleeding (peritoneal or vaginal), and pain status are critical to identify hypovolemic shock, which may occur with tubal rupture. Prepare the client physiologically and psychologically for surgery or any procedure. Provide a clear explanation of the expected outcome. Astute vigilance and early referral will help reduce short- and long-term morbidity.

PROVIDING EMOTIONAL SUPPORT

The woman with an ectopic pregnancy requires support throughout diagnosis, treatment, and aftercare. A woman's psychological reaction to an ectopic pregnancy is unpredictable. However, it is important to recognize she has experienced a pregnancy loss in addition to undergoing treatment for a potentially life-threatening condition. The woman may find it difficult to comprehend what has happened to her because events occur so quickly. In the woman's mind, she had just started a pregnancy and now it has ended abruptly. Bleeding during any pregnancy is traumatic because of the uncertainty of the outcome. Help her to make this experience more "real" by encouraging her and her family to express their feelings and concerns openly, and by validating that this is a loss of pregnancy and that it is okay to grieve over the loss. Although the woman may have physically recovered following an ectopic pregnancy, she may still experience significant emotional distress for a long time.

Provide emotional support, spiritual care, and information about community support groups (such as *Resolve through Sharing*) as the client grieves for the loss of her unborn child and comes to terms with the medical complications of the situation. Acknowledge the client's pregnancy and allow her to discuss her feelings about what the pregnancy means. Also, stress the need for follow-up blood testing for several weeks to monitor hCG titers until they return to zero, indicating resolution of the ectopic pregnancy. Ask about her feelings and concerns about her future fertility, and provide teaching about the need to use contraceptives for at least three menstrual cycles to allow her reproductive tract to heal and the tissue to be repaired. Include the woman's partner in this discussion to make sure both parties understand what has happened, what intervention is needed, and what the future holds regarding childbearing.

EDUCATING THE CLIENT

Preventing ectopic pregnancies through screening and client education is essential. Many can be prevented by avoiding conditions that might cause scarring of the fallopian tubes. In addition, a contributing factor to the development of ectopic pregnancy is a previous ectopic pregnancy. Therefore, educating the woman is crucial. Prevention education may include the following:

- Reduce risk factors such as sexual intercourse with multiple partners or intercourse without a condom.
- Avoid contracting STIs that lead to PID.
- Obtain early diagnosis and adequate treatment of STIs.
- If an intrauterine contraceptive system is chosen, descriptions of the signs of PID should be included to reduce the risk of repeat ascending infections, which can be responsible for tubal scarring.
- Avoid smoking during childbearing years since a correlation and increase in risk exists.
- Use condoms to decrease the risk of infections that cause tubal scarring.
- Seek prenatal care early to confirm the location of pregnancy.

Gestational Trophoblastic Disease

Gestational trophoblastic disease (GTD) comprises a spectrum of neoplastic disorders that originate in the placenta. There is abnormal hyperproliferation of trophoblastic cells that normally would develop into the placenta during pregnancy. GTDs encompass hydatidiform mole (complete and partial), invasive mole, gestational choriocarcinoma, placental-site trophoblastic tumor, and epithelioid trophoblastic tumor (Nguyen & Slim, 2014). Gestational tissue is present, but the pregnancy is not viable. The incidence is hard to determine due to uncommon diagnosis and inaccuracy of documentation of pregnancy loss, but it is thought to occur in about 1 in 1,000 pregnancies in the United States; in Asian countries, the rate is 1 of every 120 pregnancies American Cancer Society (ACS, 2015). The two most common types of GTD are hydatidiform mole (partial or complete) and choriocarcinoma.

Pathophysiology

The pathogenesis is unique because the maternal tumor arises from gestational rather than maternal tissue.

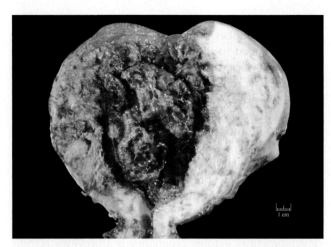

FIGURE 19.2 Complete hydatidiform mole as seen in a cutaway of a uterus. The chorionic villi degenerate and become filled with a viscid fluid, forming transparent vesicles. (From Reichert (2011). Diagnostic Gynecologic and Obstetric Pathology. Courtesy of Dr. Enrique Higa. Philadelphia, PA: LWW.)

Hydatidiform mole is a benign neoplasm of the chorion in which the chorionic villi degenerate and become transparent vesicles containing clear, viscid fluid. Hydatidiform mole is classified as complete or partial, distinguished by differences in clinical presentation, pathology, genetics, and epidemiology (Strohl & Lurain, 2014). The complete mole contains no fetal tissue and develops from an "empty egg," which is fertilized by a normal sperm (the paternal chromosomes replicate, resulting in 46 all-paternal chromosomes) (Fig. 19.2). The embryo is not viable and dies. No circulation is established, and no embryonic tissue is found. The complete mole is associated with the development of choriocarcinoma. Surgery can totally remove most complete moles, but as many as one in five women will have some persistent molar tissue and require further treatment (ACS, 2015). Most women with a classic complete mole present with vaginal bleeding, anemia, excessively enlarged uterus, preeclampsia, and hyperemesis.

The partial mole has a triploid karyotype (69 chromosomes), because two sperm have provided a double contribution by fertilizing the ovum. Women with a partial mole usually present with the clinical features of a missed or incomplete abortion, including vaginal bleeding and a small- or normal-size for date uterus (Dickson & Mullany, 2015).

The exact cause of molar pregnancy is unknown, but researchers are looking into a genetic basis. Other theories include an ovular defect, stress, or a nutritional deficiency (carotene). Although the etiology remains uncertain, at some point in the pregnancy trophoblastic cells that normally would form the placenta proliferate and the chorionic villi become edematous. The latter changes become the grape-like clusters that characterize the molar pregnancy (King et al., 2015). Studies have revealed some remarkable features about molar pregnancies, including:

- Ability to invade into the wall of the uterus
- Tendency to recur in subsequent pregnancies
- Possible development into choriocarcinoma, a virulent cancer with metastasis to other organs
- Influence of nutritional factors, such as protein deficiency
- Tendency to affect older women more often than younger women

Having a molar pregnancy (partial or complete) results in the loss of the pregnancy and the possibility of developing choriocarcinoma, a chorionic malignancy from the trophoblastic tissue. Typically asymptomatic, the first symptoms of choriocarcinoma in 80% of cases are shortness of breath, indicative of metastasis to the lungs. Choriocarcinoma affects women of all ages and can occur during pregnancy, after childbirth, or even years remote from the antecedent pregnancy. The most frequent sites of metastases are the lungs, lower genital tract, brain, and liver. Choriocarcinoma is highly responsive to chemotherapy, with an overall remission rate greater than 90% (Hensley & Shviraga, 2014). Partial moles rarely transform into choriocarcinoma.

Therapeutic Management

Treatment consists of immediate evacuation of the uterine contents as soon as the diagnosis is made and long-term follow-up of the client to detect any remaining trophoblastic tissue that might become malignant. D&C is used to empty the uterus. The tissue obtained is sent to the laboratory for analysis to evaluate for choriocarcinoma. Serial levels of hCG are used to detect residual trophoblastic tissue for 1 year. If any tissue remains, hCG levels will not regress. In 80% of women with a benign hydatidiform mole, serum hCG titers steadily drop to normal within 8 to 12 weeks after evacuation of the molar pregnancy. In the other 20% of women with a malignant hydatidiform mole, serum hCG levels begin to rise (Berkowitz, Goldstein, & Horowitz, 2014).

As a result of the increased risk for cancer, the client is advised to receive extensive follow-up therapy for the next 12 months. The follow-up protocol may include:

- Baseline hCG level, chest radiograph, and pelvic ultrasound
- Quantitative hCG levels every week until undetectable for 3 consecutive weeks; then serial hCG levels monthly for 1 year
- Chest radiograph every 6 months to detect pulmonary metastasis
- Regular pelvic examinations to assess uterine and ovarian regression
- Systemic assessments for symptoms indicative of lung, brain, liver, or vaginal metastasis

- Strong recommendation to avoid pregnancy for 1 year because the pregnancy can interfere with the monitoring of hCG levels
- Use of a reliable contraceptive for at least 1 year (Cunningham et al., 2014)

Nursing Assessment

The nurse plays a crucial role in identifying and bringing this condition to the attention of the health care provider based on sound knowledge of the typical clinical manifestations and through astute antepartal assessments.

Clinical manifestations of GTD are very similar to those of spontaneous abortion at about 12 weeks of pregnancy. Assess the woman for potential clinical manifestations at each antepartal visit. Be alert for the following:
- Report of early signs of pregnancy, such as amenorrhea, breast tenderness, fatigue
- Brownish vaginal bleeding/spotting
- Anemia
- Inability to detect a fetal heart rate after 10 to 12 weeks' gestation
- Fetal parts not evident with palpation
- Bilateral ovarian enlargement caused by cysts and elevated levels of hCG
- Persistent, often severe, nausea and vomiting (due to high hCG levels)
- Fluid retention and swelling
- Uterine size larger than expected for pregnancy dates
- Extremely high hCG levels present; no single value considered diagnostic
- Early development of preeclampsia (usually not present until after 24 weeks)
- Absence of fetal heart rate or fetal activity
- Expulsion of grapelike vesicles (possible in some women)

The diagnosis is made by very high hCG levels and the characteristic appearance of the vesicular molar pattern in the uterus via transvaginal ultrasound.

Nursing Management

Nursing management of the woman with GTD focuses on preparing her for a D&C, providing emotional support to deal with the loss and potential risks, and educating her about the risk that cancer may develop after a molar pregnancy and the strict adherence needed with the follow-up program. The woman must understand the need for the continued follow-up care regimen to improve her chances of future pregnancies and to ensure her continued quality of life.

PREPARING THE CLIENT

Upon diagnosis, the client will need an immediate evacuation of the uterus. Perform preoperative care, preparing the client physically and psychologically for the procedure.

PROVIDING EMOTIONAL SUPPORT

To aid the client and her family in coping with the loss of the pregnancy and the possibility of a cancer diagnosis, use the following interventions:
- Listen to their concerns and fears.
- Allow them time to grieve for the pregnancy loss.
- Acknowledge their loss and sad feelings (say you are sorry for their loss).
- Encourage them to express their grief; allow them to cry.
- Provide them with as much factual information as possible to help them make sense of what is happening.
- Enlist support from additional family and friends as appropriate and with the client's permission.

EDUCATING THE CLIENT

After GTD is diagnosed, teach the client about the condition and appropriate interventions that may be necessary to save her life. Explain each phase of treatment accurately and provide support for the woman and her family as they go through the grieving process.

Consider This

We had lived across the dorm hall from each other during nursing school but really did not get to know each other except for a casual hello in passing. When we graduated, Rose went to work in the emergency room and I worked in OB. We saw each other occasionally in the employee cafeteria, but a quick hello was all that we usually exchanged. I heard she married one of the paramedics who worked in the ER and was soon pregnant. I finally got to say more than hello when she was admitted to the OB unit bleeding during her fourth month of pregnancy. Gestational trophoblastic disease was discovered instead of a normal pregnancy. I remember holding her in my arms as she wept. She was told she had a complete molar pregnancy after surgery, and she would need extensive follow-up for the next year. I lost track of her that summer as my life became busier. Around Thanksgiving time, I heard she had died from choriocarcinoma. I attended her funeral, finally, to get the time to say a final hello and good-bye, but this time with sadness and tears.

Thoughts: Rose was only 26 years old when she succumbed to this very virulent cancer. I think back and realize I missed knowing this brave young woman and wished that I had taken the time to say more than hello. Could her outcome have been different? Why wasn't it recognized earlier? Did she not follow up after her diagnosis? I can only speculate regarding the whom, what, and where. She lived a short but purposeful life, and hopefully continued research will change other women's outcomes in the future.

As with any facet of health care, be aware of the latest research and new therapies. Inform the client about her follow-up care, which will probably involve close clinical surveillance for approximately 1 year, and reinforce its importance in monitoring the client's condition. Tell the client that serial serum beta-hCG levels are used to detect residual trophoblastic tissue. Continued high or increasing hCG titers are abnormal and need further evaluation.

Inform the client about the possible use of chemotherapy, such as methotrexate, which may be started prophylactically. Strongly urge the client to use a reliable contraceptive to prevent pregnancy for 1 year, because a pregnancy would interfere with tracking the serial beta-hCG levels used to identify a potential malignancy. Stress the need for the client to cooperate and adhere to the plan of therapy throughout this yearlong follow-up period.

Cervical Insufficiency

Cervical insufficiency, also called premature dilation of the cervix, describes a weak, structurally defective cervix that spontaneously dilates in the absence of uterine contractions in the second trimester, or early third trimester, resulting in the loss of the pregnancy. Since this typically occurs in the fourth or fifth month of gestation before the point of fetal viability, the fetus dies unless the dilation can be arrested. The incidence of cervical insufficiency is less than 1% in the obstetrical population (AHRQ, 2015).

Pathophysiology

The exact mechanism contributing to cervical insufficiency is not known. The cervix may have less elastin, less collagen, and greater amounts of smooth muscle than the normal cervix, and thus results in loss of sphincter tone (Magowan, Owen, & Thomson, 2014). Several theories have been proposed that focus on damage to the cervix as a key component of hormonal factors, such as increased amounts of relaxin. When the pressure of the expanding uterine contents becomes greater than the ability of the cervical sphincter to remain closed, the cervix suddenly relaxes, allowing effacement and dilation to proceed. The cervical dilation is typically rapid, relatively painless, and accompanied by minimal bleeding (Norwitz & Conroy, 2015).

Cervical insufficiency is likely to be the clinical end point of many pathologic processes, such as congenital cervical hypoplasia, in utero DES exposure that caused cervical hypoplasia, or trauma to the cervix (conization, amputation, obstetric laceration, or forced cervical dilation [may occur during elective pregnancy termination]). Other conditions such as previous precipitous birth, a prolonged second stage of labor, increased amounts of relaxin and progesterone, or increased uterine volume (multiple gestation, hydramnios) are associated with cervical insufficiency (Berghella, 2014). However, the exact etiology of cervical insufficiency is not known.

Cervical length also has been associated with cervical insufficiency and, subsequently, preterm birth. Recent studies have examined the association between a short cervical length and the risk of preterm birth. Some have demonstrated a continuum of risk between a shorter cervix on ultrasound and a higher risk of preterm birth, leading to the hypothetical argument that women with a short cervix on ultrasound might benefit from cervical cerclage (the sewing closed of the cervix). The American Congress of Obstetricians and Gynecologists (ACOG) does not recommend cerclage placement for women with a short cervix who do not have a history of preterm birth, as it has not been shown to be beneficial in this population (2014a).

Therapeutic Management

Cervical insufficiency may be treated in a variety of ways: bed rest; pelvic rest; avoidance of heavy lifting; progesterone supplementation in women at risk for preterm birth; placement of a cervical pessary (a round, silicone device at the mouth of the cervix) or surgically, via a cervical cerclage procedure in the second trimester. Cerclage was devised more than 50 years ago based on the hypothesis that for some women, weakness or malfunction of the cervix has a causative role in the pathway to preterm birth. It can either be performed transvaginally or transabdominally. Cervical cerclage involves using a heavy purse-string suture to secure and reinforce the internal os of the cervix (Fig. 19.3).

According to the American College of Obstetricians and Gynecologists (ACOG) (2014a), if a short cervix is identified at or after 20 weeks and no infection (chorioamnionitis) is present, the decision to proceed with cerclage should be made with caution. ACOG recommends the following indications for cervical cerclage: history of second trimester pregnancy loss with painless dilation; prior cerclage placement for cervical insufficiency; history of spontaneous preterm birth prior to 34 weeks' gestation; and painless cervical dilatation on physical examination in the second trimester (2014a). Complications associated with cerclage placement are suture displacement, rupture of membranes, and chorioamnionitis, and their incidence varies widely in relation to the timing and indications for the cerclage (Abu Hashim, Al-Inany, & Kilani, 2014). The optimal timing for cerclage removal is unclear, but ACOG (2014a) supports cerclage placement up to 28 weeks' gestation. A recent meta-analysis of randomized controlled trials concluded that either vaginal progesterone or cerclage are equally efficacious in the prevention of preterm birth in women with a short cervix in the mid trimester, singleton gestation, and previous preterm birth (Jena et al., 2015).

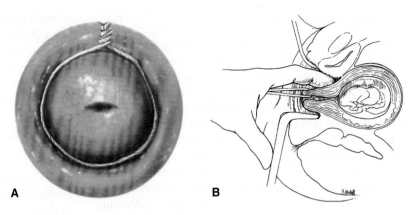

FIGURE 19.3 A. Cervical cerclage. **B.** Suturing the cervix for cervical insufficiency.

Nursing Assessment

RISK FACTORS

Nursing assessment focuses on obtaining a thorough history to determine any risk factors that might have a bearing on this pregnancy: previous cervical trauma, preterm labor, fetal loss in the second trimester, or previous surgeries, or procedures involving the cervix. History may reveal a previous loss of pregnancy around 20 weeks.

Also be alert for complaints of vaginal discharge or pelvic pressure. Commonly with cervical insufficiency the woman will report a pink-tinged vaginal discharge or an increase in low pelvic pressure, cramping to vaginal bleeding, and loss of amniotic fluid. Cervical dilation also occurs. If this continues, rupture of the membranes, release of amniotic fluid, and uterine contractions occur, subsequently resulting in delivery of the fetus, often before it is viable.

> **Take Note!**
>
> The diagnosis of cervical insufficiency remains difficult in many circumstances. The cornerstone of diagnosis is a history of a pregnancy loss during the second or early third trimester associated with painless cervical dilation without evidence of uterine activity.

DIAGNOSTIC TESTS

Transvaginal Ultrasound. Transvaginal ultrasound typically is done between 16 and 24 weeks' gestation to determine cervical length, evaluate for shortening, and attempt to predict an early preterm birth. Cervical shortening occurs from the internal os outward and can be viewed on ultrasound as funneling. The amount of funneling can be determined by dividing funnel length by cervical length. The most common time at which a short cervix or funneling develops is 16 to 24 weeks, so ultrasound screening should be performed during this interval (Herrera & Lewis, 2014). A cervical length of less than 25 mm is abnormal between 16 and 24 weeks and may increase the risk of preterm labor. Among clients with a short cervix, provide education concerning the signs and symptoms of preterm labor, especially

as the pregnancy approaches potential viability. Prenatal visits/contacts may be scheduled at more frequent intervals to increase client interaction with the care provider, especially between 20 and 34 weeks' gestation, which may decrease the rate of extremely early preterm births.

Expect the woman (particularly a woman with pelvic pressure, backache, or increased mucoid discharge) to undergo serial transvaginal ultrasound evaluations every few days to avoid missing rapid changes in cervical dilation or until the trend in cervical length can be characterized (Cunningham et al., 2014).

Home Uterine Activity Monitoring. For a woman at risk for preterm birth, home uterine activity monitoring can be used to screen for prelabor uterine contractility so that escalating contractility can be identified, allowing earlier intervention to prevent preterm birth. The home uterine activity monitor consists of a pressure sensor attached to a belt that is held against the abdomen and a recording/storage device that is carried on a belt or hung from the shoulder. Uterine activity is typically recorded by the woman for 1 hour twice daily, while she is performing routine activities. The stored data are transmitted via telephone to a perinatal nurse, and a receiving device prints out these data. The woman is contacted if there are any problems.

Although in theory identifying early contractions to initiate interventions to arrest the labor sounds reasonable, a recent Cochrane Review study found that uterine activity monitoring in asymptomatic high-risk women is inadequate for predicting preterm birth. There was no impact on maternal or perinatal outcomes or prediction of preterm births (Urquhart et al., 2015). This practice continues even though numerous randomized trials have found no relationship between monitoring and actual reduction of preterm labor. In more recent research findings, cervical length is predictive of preterm birth in all populations studied. A cervical length of less than 25 mm warrants intervention to improve the health outcomes of pregnant women and their infants (Boots et al., 2014).

Nursing Management

Nursing management focuses on monitoring the woman very closely for signs of preterm labor: backache, increase in vaginal discharge, rupture of membranes, and uterine contractions. Provide emotional support and education to allay the couple's anxiety about the well-being of their fetus. Provide preoperative care and teaching as indicated if the woman will be undergoing cerclage. Teach the client and her family about the signs and symptoms of preterm labor and the need to report any changes immediately. Also reinforce the need for activity restrictions (if appropriate) and continued regular follow-up. Continuing surveillance throughout the pregnancy is important to promote a positive outcome for the family. The nurse can play a pivotal role in identifying preterm labor through risk assessment, physical examination, and client advocacy.

Placenta Previa

Placenta previa is a bleeding condition that occurs during the last two trimesters of pregnancy. In placenta previa (literally, "afterbirth first"), the placenta implants over the cervical os. It may cause serious morbidity and mortality to the fetus and mother. The risk of placenta previa in a first pregnancy is 1 in 400, but it rises to 1 in 160 after one cesarean section; 1 in 60 after two; 1 in 30 after three; and 1 in 10 after four cesarean sections and is associated with potentially serious consequences from hemorrhage, abruption (separation) of the placenta, or emergency cesarean birth (Joy & Temming, 2015). With the rising incidence of cesarean section operations combined with increasing maternal age and more infertility treatments, the number of cases of placenta previa is increasing dramatically. The cesarean section rate must be reduced to decrease maternal; morbidity and mortality. Comprehensive risk assessment, combined with advances in ultrasound, can provide earlier detection of this impaired placental implantation (Wiedaseck & Monchek, 2014).

Pathophysiology

The exact cause of placenta previa is unknown. It is initiated by implantation of the embryo in the lower uterus, perhaps due to uterine endometrial scarring or damage in the upper segment, which may incite placental growth in the unscarred lower uterine segment. Uteroplacental underperfusion may also be present, which may increase the surface area required for placental attachment and may cause the placenta to encroach on the lower uterine segment. With placental attachment and growth, the cervical os may become covered by the developing placenta. Placental vascularization is defective, allowing the placenta to attach directly to the myometrium (accreta), deeply attach to the myometrium (increta), or infiltrate the myometrium (percreta).

Placenta previa is generally classified according to the degree of coverage or proximity to the internal os, as follows (Fig. 19.4):
- Total placenta previa: the internal cervical os is completely covered by the placenta
- Partial placenta previa: the internal os is partially covered by the placenta
- Marginal placenta previa: the placenta is at the margin or edge of the internal os
- Low-lying placenta previa: the placenta is implanted in the lower uterine segment and is near the internal os but does not reach it

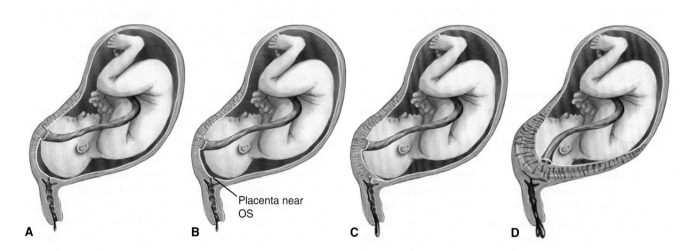

| Low-lying | Marginal | Partial | Complete |

A   **B**   **C**   **D**

Placenta near OS

FIGURE 19.4 Classification of placenta previa. **A.** Low-lying. **B.** Marginal. **C.** Partial. **D.** Complete.

Therapeutic Management

Therapeutic management depends on the extent of bleeding, the amount of placenta over the cervical os, whether the fetus is developed enough to survive outside the uterus, the position of the fetus, the mother's parity, and the presence or absence of labor (Cunningham et al., 2014). With the increase in the rate of previous cesarean sections, the frequency of placenta previa has increased. Most women continue to present in emergency departments, therefore the associated morbidity due to hemorrhage remains high. Efforts should be made to avoid primary cesarean section where possible. In addition, prenatal care and timely diagnosis of placenta previa on ultrasound can decrease the associated morbidity.

If the mother and fetus are both stable, therapeutic management may involve expectant ("wait-and-see" or watchful waiting) care. This care can be carried out at home or on an antepartal unit in the health care facility. If there is no active bleeding and the client has ready access to reliable transportation, can maintain bed rest at home, and can comprehend instructions, expectant care at home is appropriate. However, if the client requires continuous care and monitoring and cannot meet the home care requirements, the antepartal unit is the best environment.

Nursing Assessment

Nursing assessment involves a thorough history, including possible risk factors, and physical examination. Evaluate the client closely for these risk factors:
- Advancing maternal age (more than 35 years)
- Previous cesarean birth
- Multiparity
- Uterine insult or injury
- Cocaine use
- Prior placenta previa
- Infertility treatment
- Multiple gestations
- Previous induced surgical abortion
- Smoking
- Previous myomectomy to remove fibroids
- Short interval between pregnancies
- Hypertension or diabetes (Archibong & Ahmed, 2015).

HEALTH HISTORY AND PHYSICAL EXAMINATION

Ask the client if she has any problems associated with bleeding, now or in the recent past. The classical clinical presentation is painless, bright-red vaginal bleeding occurring during the second or third trimester. The initial bleeding usually is not profuse and it ceases spontaneously, only to recur again. The first episode of bleeding occurs (on average) at 27 to 32 weeks' gestation. The bleeding is thought to arise secondary to the thinning of the lower uterine segment in preparation for the onset of labor. When the bleeding occurs at the implantation site

in the lower uterus, the uterus cannot contract adequately and stop the flow of blood from the open vessels. Typically with normal placental implantation in the upper uterus, minor disruptive placental attachment is not a problem, because there is a larger volume of myometrial tissue able to contract and constrict bleeding vessels.

Assess the client for uterine contractions, which may or may not occur with the bleeding. Palpate the uterus; typically it is soft and nontender on examination. Auscultate the fetal heart rate; it commonly is within normal parameters. Fetal distress is usually absent but may occur when cord problems arise, such as umbilical cord prolapse or cord compression, or when the client has experienced blood loss to the extent that maternal shock or placental abruption has occurred (King et al., 2015).

LABORATORY AND DIAGNOSTIC TESTING

To validate the position of the placenta, a transvaginal ultrasound is done. In addition, MRI may be ordered when preparing for delivery because it allows identification of placenta accreta (placenta abnormally adherent to the myometrium), increta (placenta accreta with penetration of the myometrium), or percreta (placenta accreta with invasion of the myometrium to the peritoneal covering, causing rupture of the uterus) in addition to placenta previa. These placental abnormalities, although rare, carry a very high morbidity and mortality rate, possibly necessitating a hysterectomy at delivery.

Nursing Management

Whether the care setting is in the client's home or in the health care facility, the nurse focuses on monitoring the maternal–fetal status, including assessing for signs and symptoms of vaginal bleeding and fetal distress and providing support and education to the client and her family, including providing information about the diagnostic studies and procedures that are performed. For the majority of women, a cesarean birth will be planned. Nursing Care Plan 19.1 discusses the nursing process for the woman with placenta previa.

MONITORING MATERNAL–FETAL STATUS

Assess the degree of vaginal bleeding; inspect the perineal area for blood that may be pooled underneath the woman. Estimate and document the amount of bleeding. Perform a peripad count on an ongoing basis, making sure to report any changes in amount or frequency to the health care provider. If the woman is experiencing active bleeding, prepare for blood typing and cross-matching in the event a blood transfusion is needed.

 Take Note!

Avoid doing vaginal examinations in the woman with placenta previa because they may disrupt the placenta and cause hemorrhage.

NURSING CARE PLAN 19.1

Overview of the Woman with Placenta Previa

A 39-year-old G5, P4, multigravida client at 32 weeks' gestation, was admitted to the labor and birth suite with sudden vaginal bleeding. She had no further active bleeding and did not complain of any abdominal discomfort or tenderness. She did complain of occasional "tightening" in her stomach. Her abdomen palpated soft. Fetal heart rates were in the 140s with accelerations with movement. She was placed on bed rest with bathroom privileges. Ultrasound identified a low-lying placenta with a viable, normal-growth fetus. She was diagnosed with placenta previa and admitted for observation and surveillance of fetal well-being. Her history revealed two previous cesarean births, smoking half a pack of cigarettes per day, and endometritis infection after birth of her last newborn. Additional assessment findings included painless, bright-red vaginal bleeding with initial bleeding ceasing spontaneously; irregular, mild, and sporadic uterine contractions; fetal heart rate and maternal vital signs within normal range; fetus in transverse lie; anxiety related to the outcome of pregnancy; and expression of feelings of helplessness.

NURSING DIAGNOSIS: Risk for injury (fetal and maternal) related to threat to uteroplacental perfusion and hemorrhage

Outcome Identification and Evaluation

The client will maintain adequate tissue perfusion as evidenced by stable vital signs, decreased blood loss, few or no uterine contractions, normal fetal heart rate patterns and variability, and positive fetal movement.

Interventions: *Maintaining Adequate Tissue Perfusion*

- Establish intravenous access to allow for administration of fluids, blood, and medications as necessary.
- Obtain type and cross-match for at least two units blood products to ensure availability should bleeding continues.
- Obtain specimens as ordered for blood studies, such as CBC and clotting studies, to establish a baseline and use for future comparison.
- Monitor output to evaluate adequacy of renal perfusion.
- Administer intravenous fluid replacement therapy as ordered to maintain blood pressure and blood volume.
- Palpate for abdominal tenderness and rigidity to determine bleeding and evidence of uterine contractions.
- Institute bed rest to reduce oxygen demands.
- Assess for rupture of membranes to evaluate for possible onset of labor.
- Avoid vaginal examinations to prevent further bleeding episodes.
- Complete an Rh titer to identify the need for RhoGAM.

- Avoid nipple stimulation to prevent uterine contractions.
- Continuously monitor for contractions or PROM to allow for prompt intervention.
- Administer tocolytic agents as ordered to stall preterm labor.
- Monitor vital signs frequently to identify possible hypovolemia and infection.
- Assess frequently for active vaginal bleeding to minimize risk of hemorrhage.
- Continuously monitor fetal heart rate with electronic fetal monitor to evaluate fetal status.
- Assist with fetal surveillance tests as ordered to aid in determining fetal well-being.
- Observe for abnormal fetal heart rate patterns, such as loss of variability, decelerations, tachycardia, to identify fetal distress.
- Position client in side-lying position with wedge for support to maximize placental perfusion.
- Assess fetal movement to evaluate for possible fetal hypoxia.
- Teach woman to monitor fetal movement to evaluate well-being.
- Administer oxygen as ordered to increase oxygenation to mother and fetus.

NURSING CARE PLAN 19.1

Overview of the Woman with Placenta Previa (continued)

NURSING DIAGNOSIS: Anxiety related to threat to self and fetus, unknown future.

Outcome Identification and Evaluation

The client will experience a decrease in anxiety as evidenced by verbal reports of less anxiety, use of effective coping measures, and calm demeanor.

Interventions: *Minimizing Anxiety*

- Provide factual information about diagnosis and treatment, and explain interventions and the rationale behind them *to provide client with understanding of her condition.*
- Answer questions about health status honestly *to establish a trusting relationship.*
- Speak calmly to client and family members *to minimize environmental stress.*
- Encourage the use of past effective techniques for coping *to promote relaxation and feelings of control.*
- Acknowledge and facilitate the woman's spiritual needs *to promote effective coping.*
- Involve the woman and family in the decision-making process *to foster self-confidence and control over situation.*
- Maintain a presence during stressful periods *to allay anxiety.*
- Use the sense of touch if appropriate *to convey caring and concern.*
- Encourage talking as a means *to release tension.*

Monitor maternal vital signs and uterine contractility frequently for changes. Have the client rate her level of pain using an appropriate pain rating scale. Assess fetal heart rates via Doppler or electronic monitoring to detect fetal distress. Monitor the woman's cardiopulmonary status, reporting any difficulties in respirations, changes in skin color, or complaints of difficulty in breathing. Have oxygen equipment readily available should fetal or maternal distress develop. Encourage the client to lie on her side to enhance placental perfusion.

If the woman has an intravenous (IV) line inserted, inspect the IV site frequently. Alternately, anticipate the insertion of an intermittent IV access device such as a saline lock, which can be used if quick access is needed for fluid restoration and infusion of blood products. Obtain laboratory tests as ordered, including complete blood count (CBC), coagulation studies, and Rh status if appropriate.

Administer pharmacologic agents as necessary. Give Rh immunoglobulin if the client is Rh negative at 28 weeks' gestation. Monitor tocolytic (anticontraction) medication if prevention of preterm labor is needed.

PROVIDING SUPPORT AND EDUCATION

Determine the woman's level of understanding about placenta previa and the associated procedures and treatment plan. Doing so is important to prevent confusion and gain her cooperation. Provide information about the condition and make sure that all information related is consistent with information from the primary care provider. Explain all assessments and treatment measures as needed.

Act as a client advocate in obtaining information for the family. Teach the woman how to perform and record daily fetal movement. This action serves two purposes: (1) It provides valuable information about the fetus and (2) it is an activity in which the client can participate, thereby fostering some feeling of control over the situation.

If the woman will require prolonged hospitalization or home bed rest, assess the physical and emotional impact that this may have on her. Evaluate her coping mechanisms to help determine how well she will be able to adjust and adhere to the treatment plan. Allow the client to verbalize her feelings and fears, and provide emotional support. Also, provide opportunities for distraction—educational videos, arts and crafts, computer games, reading books—and evaluate the client's response.

In addition to the emotional impact of prolonged bed rest, thoroughly assess the woman's skin to prevent skin breakdown and to help alleviate her discomfort secondary to limited physical activity. Instruct the woman in appropriate skin care measures. Encourage her to eat a balanced diet with adequate fluid intake to ensure adequate nutrition and hydration and prevent complications associated with urinary and bowel elimination secondary to bed rest.

Teach the client and family about any signs and symptoms that should be reported immediately. In addition, prepare the woman for the possibility of a cesarean birth. The woman must notify her health care provider about any bleeding episodes or backaches (may indicate preterm labor contractions) and must adhere to the prescribed bed rest regimen. To ensure adherence to the plan and a positive outcome, the client needs to be aware of and understand the rationales for the ongoing observations.

Abruptio Placentae

Abruptio placentae is the premature separation of a normally implanted placenta after the 20th week of gestation prior to birth, which leads to hemorrhage. It is a significant cause of third-trimester bleeding, with a high mortality rate. It occurs in about 1% of all pregnancies throughout the world, or approximately 1 in 100 pregnancies. There is a 10 to 20 times greater risk of reoccurrence in a subsequent pregnancy. It typically peaks between 24 and 26 weeks' gestation.

Maternal risks include obstetric hemorrhage, need for blood transfusions, emergency hysterectomy, disseminated intravascular coagulopathy (DIC), and renal failure. Maternal death is rare, but seven times higher than the overall maternal mortality rate. Perinatal consequences include low birth weight, preterm delivery, asphyxia, stillbirth, and perinatal death. In developed countries, approximately 10% of all preterm births and 10% to 20% of all perinatal deaths are caused by placental abruption (Mukherjee et al., 2014). The overall fetal mortality rate for placental abruption is up to 50%, depending on the extent of the abruption. Maternal mortality is approximately 6% in abruptio placentae and is related to cesarean birth and/or hemorrhage/coagulopathy (Jaju, Kulkarni, & Mundada, 2014).

Pathophysiology

The etiology of this condition is unknown; however, it has been proposed that abruption starts with degenerative changes in the small maternal blood vessels, resulting in blood clotting, degeneration of the decidua (uterine lining), and possible rupture of a vessel. Bleeding from the blood vessel forms a blood clot between the placenta and the uterine wall. The continued bleeding causes increased pressure behind the placenta and results in separation from the uterine wall (Moses, 2015a). Fetal blood supply is compromised and fetal distress develops in proportion to the degree of placental separation. This is caused by the insult of the abruption itself and by issues related to prematurity when early birth is required to alleviate maternal or fetal distress.

Abruptio placentae is classified according to the extent of separation and the amount of blood loss from the maternal circulation. Classifications include:

- Mild (grade 1): Minimal bleeding (less than 500 mL), marginal separation (10% to 20%), tender uterus, no coagulopathy, no signs of shock, no fetal distress
- Moderate (grade 2): Moderate bleeding (1,000 to 1,500 mL), moderate separation (20% to 50%), continuous abdominal pain, mild shock, normal maternal blood pressure, maternal tachycardia
- Severe (grade 3): Absent to moderate bleeding (more than 1,500 mL), severe separation (more than 50%), profound shock, dark vaginal bleeding, agonizing abdominal pain, decreased maternal blood pressure, significant maternal tachycardia and development of DIC(Atkinson et al., 2015).

Abruptio placentae also may be classified as partial or complete, depending on the degree of separation. Alternately, it can be classified as concealed or apparent, by the type of bleeding (Fig. 19.5).

Remember Helen, the pregnant woman with severe abdominal pain? Electronic fetal monitoring revealed uterine hypertonicity with absent fetal heart sounds. Palpation of her abdomen

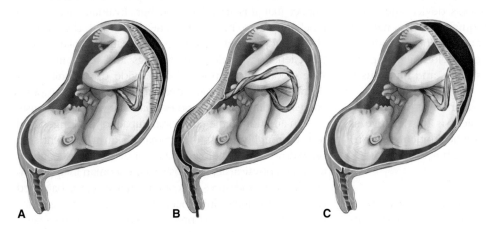

A Partial abruption, concealed hemorrhage

B Partial abruption, apparent hemorrhage

C Complete abruption, concealed hemorrhage

FIGURE 19.5 Classifications of abruptio placentae. **A.** Partial abruption with concealed hemorrhage. **B.** Partial abruption with apparent hemorrhage. **C.** Complete abruption with concealed hemorrhage.

revealed rigidity and extreme tenderness in all four quadrants. Her vital signs were as follows: temperature, afebrile; pulse, 94; respirations, 22; blood pressure, 130/90 mm Hg. What might you suspect as the cause of Helen's abdominal pain? What course of action would you anticipate for Helen?

Therapeutic Management

Treatment of abruptio placentae is designed to assess, control, and restore the amount of blood lost; provide a positive outcome for both mother and newborn; and prevent coagulation disorders, such as DIC (Box 19.2). Emergency measures include starting two large-bore

---

BOX 19.2

DISSEMINATED INTRAVASCULAR COAGULATION

DIC is a bleeding disorder characterized by an abnormal reduction in the elements involved in blood clotting resulting from their widespread intravascular clotting (Davis & Kessler, 2014).). This disorder can occur secondary to abruptio placentae, amniotic fluid embolism, endotoxin sepsis, retained dead fetus, posthemorrhagic shock, hydatidiform mole, and gynecologic malignancies.

The clinical and pathologic manifestations of DIC can be described as a loss of balance between the clot-forming activity of thrombin and the clot-lysing activity of plasmin. Therefore, too much thrombin tips the balance toward the prothrombic state and the client develops clots. Alternately, too much clot lysis (fibrinolysis) results from plasmin formation and the client hemorrhages. Small clots form throughout the body, and eventually the blood-clotting factors are used up, rendering them unavailable to form clots at sites of tissue injury. Clot-dissolving mechanisms are also increased, which results in bleeding (possibly severe).

DIC is usually associated with high mortality and morbidity rates. No single laboratory test is sensitive or specific enough to diagnose DIC definitively, but it can be diagnosed by using a combination of multiple clinical and laboratory tests that reflect the pathophysiology of the syndrome.

Laboratory studies that assist in the diagnosis include:
• Decreased fibrinogen and platelets
• Prolonged PT and aPTT
• Positive D-dimer tests and fibrin (split) degradation products (objective evidence of the simultaneous formation of thrombin and plasmin) (ARUP Laboratories, 2016)

Adapted from Davis, S. J., & Kessler, C. M. (2014). Disseminated intravascular coagulation: Diagnosis and management. In *Hemostasis and thrombosis: Practical guidelines in clinical management* (pp. 151–168). Hoboken, NJ: Wiley Blackwell; and Kobayashi, T. (2014). Obstetrical disseminated intravascular coagulation score. *Journal of Obstetrics and Gynecology Research*, 40(6), 1500–1506.

---

intravenous lines with normal saline or lactated Ringer's solution to combat hypovolemia, obtaining blood specimens for evaluating hemodynamic status values and for typing and cross-matching, and frequently monitoring fetal and maternal well-being. After the severity of abruption is determined and appropriate blood and fluid replacement is given, cesarean birth is done immediately if fetal distress is evident. If the fetus is not in distress close monitoring continues, with delivery planned at the earliest signs of fetal distress. Because of the possibility of fetal blood loss through the placenta, a neonatal intensive care team should be available during the birth process to assess and treat the newborn immediately for shock, blood loss, and hypoxia.

If the woman develops DIC, treatment focuses on determining the underlying cause of DIC and correcting it. Replacement therapy of the coagulation factors is achieved by transfusion of fresh-frozen plasma along with cryoprecipitate to maintain the circulating volume and provide oxygen to the cells of the body. Anticoagulant therapy (low-molecular-weight heparin), packed red cells, platelet concentrates, antithrombin concentrates, and nonclotting protein-containing volume expanders, such as plasma protein fraction or albumin, are also used to combat this serious condition. The use of blood products must be dictated by the clinical picture and not simply to normalize laboratory test results (Holt, 2015). Prompt identification and early intervention are essential for a woman with acute DIC associated with abruptio placentae to treat DIC and possibly save her life.

Nursing Assessment

Abruptio placentae is a medical emergency. The nurse plays a critical role in assessing the pregnant woman presenting with abdominal pain and/or experiencing vaginal bleeding, especially in a concealed hemorrhage, in which the extent of bleeding is not recognized. Rapid assessment is essential to ensure prompt, effective interventions to prevent maternal and fetal morbidity and mortality. Comparison Chart 19.1 compares placenta previa with abruptio placentae.

HEALTH HISTORY AND PHYSICAL EXAMINATION

Abruptio placentae produces a wide range of clinical effects, depending on the extent of placental separation and the amount of maternal blood loss. Begin the health history by assessing the woman for risk factors that may predispose her to abruptio placentae, such as advanced maternal age (over 35 years old), poor nutrition, multiple gestation, excessive intrauterine pressure caused by polyhydramnios, chronic hypertension, cigarette smoking, severe trauma (e.g., auto accident, intimate partner violence), history of abruption in a previous pregnancy, placental abnormalities, cocaine or methamphetamine abuse, thrombophilia, alcohol ingestion, and multiparity

COMPARISON CHART 19.1   PLACENTA PREVIA VERSUS ABRUPTIO PLACENTAE

Manifestation	Placenta Previa	Abruptio Placentae
Onset	Insidious	Sudden
Type of bleeding	Always visible; slight, then more profuse	Can be concealed or visible
Blood description	Bright red	Dark
Discomfort/pain	None (painless)	Constant; uterine tenderness on palpation
Uterine tone	Soft and relaxed	Firm to rigid
Fetal heart rate	Usually in normal range	Fetal distress or absent
Fetal presentation	May be breech or transverse lie; engagement is absent	No relationship

(Deering, 2015). In addition, be alert for other notable risk factors, such as male fetal gender, chorioamnionitis, prolonged premature ruptured membranes (more than 24 hours), oligohydramnios, preeclampsia, and low socioeconomic status (Nagtalon-Ramos, 2014).

Assess the woman for bleeding. As the placenta separates from the uterus, hemorrhage ensues. It can be apparent, appearing as vaginal bleeding, or it can be concealed. Vaginal bleeding is present in 80% of women diagnosed with abruptio placentae and may be significant enough to jeopardize both maternal and fetal health within a short time frame. The remaining 20% of abruptions are associated with a concealed hemorrhage and the absence of vaginal bleeding. Monitor the woman's level of consciousness, noting any signs or symptoms that may suggest shock.

Take Note!

Vital signs can be within normal range, even with significant blood loss, because a pregnant woman can lose up to 40% of her total blood volume without showing signs of shock (Schultz & McConachie, 2015).

Assess the woman for complaints of pain, including the type, onset, and location. Ask if she has had any contractions. Palpate the abdomen, noting any contractions, uterine tenderness, tenseness, or rigidity. Ask if she has noticed any changes in fetal movement and activity. Decreased fetal movement may be the presenting complaint, resulting from fetal jeopardy or fetal death (Cunningham et al., 2014). Assess fetal heart rate and continue to monitor it electronically.

Take Note!

Classic manifestations of abruptio placentae include painful, dark-red vaginal bleeding (port-wine color) because the bleeding comes from the clot that was formed behind the placenta; "knife-like" abdominal pain; uterine tenderness; contractions; and decreased fetal movement. Rapid assessment is essential to ensure prompt, effective interventions to prevent maternal and fetal morbidity and mortality.

LABORATORY AND DIAGNOSTIC TESTING

Laboratory and diagnostic tests may be helpful in diagnosing the condition and guiding management. These studies may include:

- *CBC:* Determines the current hemodynamic status; however, it is not reliable for estimating acute blood loss.
- *Fibrinogen levels:* Typically are increased in pregnancy (hyperfibrinogenemia); thus, a moderate dip in fibrinogen levels might suggest DIC and, if profuse bleeding occurs, the clotting cascade might be compromised.
- *Prothrombin time (PT)/activated partial thromboplastin time (aPTT):* Determines the client's coagulation status, especially if surgery is planned.
- *Type and cross-match:* Determines blood type if a transfusion is needed
- *Nonstress test:* Demonstrates findings of fetal jeopardy manifested by late decelerations or bradycardia.
- *Biophysical profile:* Aids in evaluating clients with chronic abruption; a low score (less than 6 points) suggests possible fetal compromise (Creasy et al., 2014).

Ultrasound is not useful for making a definitive diagnosis because the clot is sonographically visible in less than 50% of the cases. A CT scan is a more reliable method for evaluation of placental abruption (Hosein, Abdel-Kariem, & Shriki, 2014).

Nursing Management

Nursing management of the woman with abruptio placentae warrants immediate care to provide the best outcome for both mother and fetus.

ENSURING ADEQUATE TISSUE PERFUSION

When the woman arrives at the facility, place her on strict bed rest and in a left lateral position to prevent pressure on the vena cava. This position provides uninterrupted perfusion to the fetus. Expect to administer oxygen therapy via nasal cannula to ensure adequate tissue perfusion. Monitor oxygen saturation levels via pulse oximetry to evaluate the effectiveness of interventions.

Obtain maternal vital signs frequently, as often as every 15 minutes as indicated, depending on the woman's status and amount of blood loss. Observe for changes in vital signs suggesting hypovolemic shock and report them immediately. Also expect to insert an indwelling urinary (Foley) catheter to assess hourly urine output and initiate an intravenous infusion for fluid replacement using a large-bore catheter.

Assess fundal height for changes. An increase in size would indicate bleeding. Monitor the amount and characteristics of any vaginal bleeding as frequently as every 15 to 30 minutes. Be alert for signs and symptoms of DIC, such as bleeding gums, tachycardia, oozing from the intravenous insertion site, and petechiae, and administer blood products as ordered if DIC occurs.

Institute continuous electronic fetal monitoring. Assess uterine contractions and report any increased uterine tenseness or rigidity. Also observe the tracing for tetanic uterine contractions or changes in fetal heart rate patterns suggesting that the fetus has been compromised.

PROVIDING SUPPORT AND EDUCATION

A woman diagnosed with abruptio placentae may be filled with a sense of heightened anxiety and apprehension for her own health as well as for the health of her fetus. Communicate empathy and understanding of the client's experience, and provide emotional support throughout this frightening time. Remain with the woman and her partner, acknowledge their emotions and fears, and address their spiritual and cultural needs. Answer their questions about the status of their fetus openly and honestly, being sure to explain indicators of fetal well-being. Provide information about the various diagnostic tests, treatments, and procedures that may be done, including the possible need for a cesarean birth. Depending on the client's status, extent of bleeding, and length of gestation, the fetus may not survive. If the fetus does survive, he or she most likely will require neonatal intensive care. Assist the client and family to deal with the loss or with the birth of a newborn in the neonatal intensive care unit.

Although abruptio placentae is not a preventable condition, client education is important to help reduce the risk for a recurrence of this condition. Encourage the woman to avoid drinking, smoking, or using drugs during pregnancy. Urge her to seek early and continuous prenatal care and to receive prompt health care if any signs and symptoms occur in future pregnancies.

Think back to Helen, the pregnant woman described at the beginning of the chapter. She was diagnosed with abruptio placentae and was prepared for an emergency cesarean birth. On exploration, there was almost a 75% abruption, with approximately 800 mL of concealed blood between the uterus and the placenta. In addition, she lost an additional 500 mL during surgery. What in Helen's history may have placed her at increased risk for abruption? What assessments and interventions would be essential during her postpartum recovery secondary to her large blood loss? What psychosocial interventions would be necessary due to her fetal loss?

Placenta Accreta

Placenta accreta is a potentially life-threatening obstetrical hemorrhagic condition that requires a multidisciplinary approach to management. The incidence of placenta accreta has increased and seems to parallel the increasing cesarean birth rate or intrauterine procedures. Placenta accreta is a condition in which the placenta attaches itself too deeply into the wall of the uterus but does not penetrate the uterine muscle. It is further subcategorized as *placenta increta*, when the placenta invades the myometrium, and *placenta percreta*, when it has extended through the myometrium and uterine serosa and adjacent tissue. A common risk of placenta accreta during the birthing process is the possibility of hemorrhaging during manual attempts to detach the placenta. According to the March of Dimes (2015c), 1 in 530 births results in this condition. The specific cause of placenta accreta is unknown, but it can be related to placenta previa, advanced maternal age, smoking, and previous cesarean births. According to the literature, a cesarean birth increases the possibility of a future placenta accreta; the more cesarean births that are done, the greater the incidence.

According to ACOG (2014b), postpartum hemorrhage is a complication associated with placenta accreta. Ninety percent of accretas have postpartum hemorrhage, and 50% of these will result in a hysterectomy (ACOG, 2014b). Women at highest risk of emergency hysterectomy are those who are multiparous, had a cesarean birth in either a previous or the present pregnancy, or had abnormal placentation. The essential management issues are early detection and immediate and appropriate intervention. If a placenta accreta diagnosis is made, the client should be counseled that a cesarean section and possible hysterectomy may be necessary interventions (Creasy et al., 2014).

Placenta accreta is typically diagnosed after birth when the placenta fails to normally separate from the uterine wall. A prenatal screening diagnosis via ultrasound and magnetic resonance imaging (MRI) would decrease maternal and fetal morbidities and mortalities. A profuse hemorrhage may result because the uterus cannot contract to close off the open blood vessels. Management will depend on the severity of the bleeding and frequently necessitates a prompt hysterectomy (Humphrey, 2015). Nurses need to be prepared to assist in this emergency situation as dictated by the health care provider.

HYPEREMESIS GRAVIDARUM

Hyperemesis gravidarum is a severe form of nausea and vomiting of pregnancy associated with significant costs and psychosocial impacts. At least 70% to 85% of women experience nausea and vomiting during their pregnancy (Castillo & Phillippi, 2015). The term *morning sickness* is often used to describe this condition when symptoms are relatively mild. Studies have shown that nausea and vomiting of pregnancy is associated with improved fetal outcomes, such as lower rates of miscarriage (Ayyavoo et al., 2014). Such symptoms usually disappear after the first trimester. This mild form mostly affects the quality of life of the woman and her family, whereas the severe form—**hyperemesis gravidarum**—results in dehydration, weight loss, electrolyte imbalance, and the need for hospitalization (Taylor, 2014).

Unlike morning sickness, hyperemesis gravidarum is a complication of pregnancy characterized by persistent, uncontrollable nausea and vomiting that begins in the first trimester and causes dehydration, ketosis, and weight loss of more than 5% of prepregnancy body weight. Risk factors for hyperemesis include previous pregnancy complicated by hyperemesis, molar pregnancies, history of helicobacter pylori infection, multiple gestation, prepregnancy history of genitourinary disorders, clinical hyperthyroid disorders, and prepregnancy psychiatric diagnosis (King et al., 2015).

Hyperemesis (uncontrollable vomiting) is estimated to occur in approximately 2% of pregnant women. The prevalence increases in molar pregnancies and multiple gestations. The peak incidence is at 8 to 12 weeks of pregnancy, and symptoms usually resolve by week 20 (Maltepe et al., 2015).

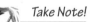

Take Note!

Every pregnant woman needs to be instructed to report any episodes of severe nausea and vomiting or episodes that extend beyond the first trimester.

Pathophysiology

Although the exact cause of nausea and vomiting is unknown, its effects—decreased placental blood flow, decreased maternal blood flow, and acidosis—can threaten the health of the mother and fetus. Dehydration can also lead to preterm labor (Smith et al., 2016).

Numerous theories abound, but few studies have produced scientific evidence to identify the etiology of this condition. It is likely that multiple factors contribute to it.

Elevated levels of hCG are present in all pregnant women during early pregnancy, usually declining after 12 weeks. This corresponds to the usual duration of morning sickness. In hyperemesis gravidarum, the hCG levels are often higher and extend beyond the first trimester. Symptoms exacerbate the disease. Decreased fluid intake and prolonged vomiting cause dehydration; dehydration increases the serum concentration of hCG, which in turn exacerbates the nausea and vomiting—a vicious cycle. A few other theories that have been proposed to explain its etiology include:
- *Endocrine theory*—High levels of hCG and estrogen during pregnancy.
- *Metabolic theory*—Vitamin B_6 deficiency.
- *Genetic factors* that may predispose the woman to this condition.
- *Psychological theory*—psychological stress increases the symptoms.

Therapeutic Management

Hyperemesis gravidarum is a diagnosis of exclusion. Careful consideration of other conditions must be assessed when a client experiences nausea and vomiting for the first time after 9 weeks' gestation.

Conservative management in the home is the first line of treatment for the woman with hyperemesis gravidarum. This usually focuses on dietary and lifestyle changes. If conservative management fails to alleviate the client's symptoms and nausea and vomiting continue, hospitalization is necessary to reverse the effects of severe nausea and vomiting.

On admission to the hospital, blood tests are ordered to assess the severity of the client's dehydration, electrolyte imbalance, ketosis, and malnutrition. Parenteral fluids and drugs are ordered to rehydrate the woman and reduce the symptoms. The first choice for fluid replacement is generally normal saline, which aids in preventing hyponatremia, with vitamins (pyridoxine [B_6]) and electrolytes added. Oral food and fluids are withheld for the first 24 to 36 hours to allow the gastrointestinal tract to rest. Antiemetics may be administered rectally or intravenously to control the nausea and vomiting initially because the woman is considered NPO (not able to ingest anything by mouth). Once her condition stabilizes and she is allowed oral intake, medications may be administered orally.

If the client does not improve after several days of bed rest, "gut rest," intravenous fluids, and antiemetics, total parenteral nutrition or feeding through a percutaneous endoscopic gastrostomy tube is instituted to prevent malnutrition. Administering antiemetics intravenously or intramuscularly is typically the second pillar of treatment for hyperemesis gravidarum. Finding a drug that works for any given client is largely a matter of trial and error. If one drug is ineffective, another class of drugs with a different mechanism of action may help. Promethazine (Phenergan) and prochlorperazine (Compazine) are among the older preparations usually tried first. If they fail to relieve symptoms, newer drugs such as ondansetron (Zofran) may be tried. Most drugs are given intravenously or intramuscularly. There is no evidence that any antiemetic class is superior to another with respect to effectiveness (King et al., 2015) (Drug Guide 19.2).

Few women receive complete relief of symptoms from any one therapy. Complementary and alternative medicine therapies appeal to many women as supplements to traditional ones. Some popular therapies include acupressure, massage, therapeutic touch, ginger, and the wearing of Sea-Bands to prevent nausea and vomiting. Recent research has reported a positive effect of using acupressure (provided by Sea-Bands) over the *nei guan* acupoint on the wrist to control nausea and vomiting associated with pregnancy (Matthews et al., 2014).

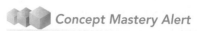 *Concept Mastery Alert*

Priority Interventions in Hyperemesis Gravidarum

Hyperemesis gravidarum is nausea and vomiting in early pregnancy that prevents the woman from ingesting adequate nutrition. IV fluids may be required for rehydration, but the priority is to stop all intake of food and fluid for a period of time until vomiting has stopped.

Nursing Assessment

Nursing assessment of the woman with hyperemesis gravidarum requires a thorough history and physical examination to identify signs and symptoms associated with this disorder. The client is extremely uncomfortable. She may experience many hours of lost work productivity and sleep, and hyperemesis may damage family relationships. If hyperemesis progresses untreated, it may cause neurologic disturbances, renal damage, dehydration, ketosis, alkalosis from loss of hydrochloric acid, hypokalemia, retinal hemorrhage, or death (Peled et al.,

---

DRUG GUIDE 19.2 MEDICATIONS USED FOR HYPEREMESIS GRAVIDARUM

Medication	Action/Indications	Nursing Implications
Promethazine (Phenergan)	Diminishes vestibular stimulation and acts on the chemoreceptor trigger zone (CTZ) Symptomatic relief of nausea and vomiting, and motion sickness.	Be alert for urinary retention, dizziness, hypotension, and involuntary movements. Institute safety measures to prevent injury secondary to sedative effects. Offer hard candy and frequent rinsing of mouth for dryness.
Prochlorperazine (Compazine)	Acts centrally to inhibit dopamine receptors in the CTZ and peripherally to block vagus nerve stimulation in the gastrointestinal tract. Controls severe nausea and vomiting.	Be alert for abnormal movements and for neuroleptic malignant syndrome such as seizures, hyper/hypotension, tachycardia, and dyspnea. Assess mental status, intake/output. Caution client not to drive as a result of drowsiness or dizziness. Advise to change position slowly to minimize effects of orthostatic hypotension.
Ondansetron (Zofran)	Blocks serotonin release, which stimulates the vagal afferent nerves, thus stimulating the vomiting reflex	Monitor for possible side effects such as diarrhea, constipation, abdominal pain, headache, dizziness, drowsiness, and fatigue. Monitor liver function studies as ordered.

Adapted from King, T. L., Brucker, M. C., Kriebs, J. M., Fahey, J. O., Grgor, C. L., & Varney, H. (2015). *Varney's midwifery* (5th ed.). Burlington, MA: Jones & Bartlett Learning; and Ogunyemi, D. A., Fong, A., & Herrero, T. C. (2015). Hyperemesis gravidarum. *eMedicine.* Retrieved from http://emedicine.medscape.com/article/254751-overview

2014). Laboratory and diagnostic tests aid in determining the severity of the disorder.

Health History and Physical Examination

Begin the history by asking the client about the onset, duration, and course of her nausea and vomiting. Ask her about any medications or treatments she used and how effective they were in relieving her nausea and vomiting. Obtain a diet history from the client, including a dietary recall for the past week. Note the client's knowledge of nutrition and need for appropriate nutritional intake. Be alert for patterns that may contribute to or trigger her distress. Also ask about any complaints of ptyalism (excessive salivation), anorexia, indigestion, and abdominal pain or distention. Ask if she has noticed any blood or mucus in her stool.

Review the client's history for possible risk factors, such as young age, nausea and vomiting with previous pregnancy, history of intolerance of oral contraceptives, nulliparity, trophoblastic disease, multiple gestation, emotional or psychological stress, gastroesophageal reflux disease, primigravida status, obesity, hyperthyroidism, and *Helicobacter pylori* seropositivity (Ogunyemi, Fong, & Herrero, 2015). Weigh the client and compare this weight with her weight before she began experiencing symptoms and to her prepregnancy weight to estimate the degree of loss. With hyperemesis, weight loss usually exceeds 5% of body mass.

Inspect the mucous membranes for dryness and check skin turgor for evidence of fluid loss and dehydration. Assess blood pressure for changes, such as hypotension, that may suggest a fluid volume deficit. Also note any complaints of weakness, fatigue, activity intolerance, dizziness, or sleep disturbances.

Assess the client's perception of the situation. Note any evidence of depression, anxiety, irritability, mood changes, and decreased ability to concentrate, which can add to her emotional distress. Much of the psychological distress is self-limiting in this condition and probably in the causal pathway (Tan et al., 2014). Determine the woman's support systems that are available for help.

Laboratory and Diagnostic Testing

The results of laboratory and diagnostic tests may provide clues to the severity or etiology of the disorder. These may include:

- *Liver enzymes:* To rule out hepatitis, pancreatitis, and cholestasis; elevations of aspartate aminotransferase (AST) and alanine aminotransferase (ALT) are usually present.
- *CBC:* Elevated levels of red blood cells and hematocrit, indicating dehydration.
- *Urine ketones:* Positive when the body breaks down fat to provide energy in the absence of adequate intake.

- *TSH and T4* to rule out thyroid disease.
- *Blood urea nitrogen:* Increased in the presence of salt and water depletion
- *Urine specific gravity*—greater than 1.025, possibly indicating concentrated urine linked to inadequate fluid intake or excessive fluid loss; ketonuria.
- *Serum electrolytes:* Decreased levels of potassium, sodium, and chloride resulting from excessive vomiting and loss of hydrochloric acid in stomach.
- *Ultrasound:* Evaluation for molar pregnancy or multiple gestation (Cunningham et al., 2014).

Nursing Management

Nursing management for the client with hyperemesis gravidarum focuses on promoting comfort by controlling the client's nausea and vomiting and promoting adequate nutrition. In addition, the nurse plays a major role in supporting and educating the client and her family.

Promoting Comfort and Nutrition

During the initial period, expect to withhold all oral food and fluids, maintaining NPO status to allow the gastrointestinal tract to rest. In addition, administer prescribed antiemetics to relieve the nausea and vomiting and intravenous fluids to replace fluid losses. Monitor the rate of infusion to prevent overload and assess the intravenous insertion site to prevent infiltration or infection. Also administer electrolyte replacement therapy as ordered to correct any imbalances, and periodically check serum electrolyte levels to evaluate the effectiveness of therapy.

Provide physical comfort measures such as hygiene measures and oral care. Pay special attention to the environment, making sure to keep the area free of pungent odors. As the client's nausea and vomiting subside, gradually introduce oral fluids and foods in small amounts. Monitor intake and output and assess the client's tolerance to the increase in intake.

Providing Support and Education

Women with hyperemesis gravidarum commonly are fatigued physically and emotionally. Many are exhausted, frustrated, and anxious. Offer reassurance that all interventions are directed toward promoting positive pregnancy outcomes for both the woman and her fetus. Providing information about the expected plan of care may help to alleviate the client's anxiety. Listen to her concerns and feelings, answering all questions honestly. Educate the woman and her family about the condition and its treatment options (Teaching Guidelines 19.1). Teach the client about therapeutic lifestyle changes, such as avoiding stressors and fatigue that may trigger nausea and vomiting. Offer ongoing support and encouragement and promote active participation in care decisions, thereby empowering the client and her family. Attempting to provide the client with a sense of control may help her overcome the feeling that she has lost control. If necessary, refer the client to a spiritual advisor or counseling. Also suggest possible local or national support groups that the client may contact for additional information. Arrange for possible home care follow-up for the client and reinforce discharge instructions to promote understanding. Timely counseling, balanced nutrition, pharmacotherapy, and emotional support are associated with favorable outcomes for the woman with this condition. Collaborate with community resources to ensure continuity of care.

Teaching Guidelines 19.1
TEACHING TO MINIMIZE NAUSEA AND VOMITING

- Avoid noxious stimuli—such as strong flavors, perfumes, or strong odors such as frying bacon—that might trigger nausea and vomiting.
- Avoid tight waistbands to minimize pressure on abdomen.
- Eat small, frequent meals throughout the day—six small meals.
- Separate fluids from solids by consuming fluids in between meals.
- Avoid lying down or reclining for at least 2 hours after eating.
- Use high-protein supplement drinks.
- Avoid foods high in fat.
- Increase your intake of carbonated beverages.
- Increase your exposure to fresh air to improve symptoms.
- Eat when you are hungry, regardless of normal mealtimes.
- Drink herbal teas containing peppermint or ginger.
- Avoid fatigue and learn how to manage stress in life.
- Schedule daily rest periods to avoid becoming overtired.
- Eat foods that settle the stomach, such as dry crackers, toast, or soda.

HYPERTENSIVE DISORDERS OF PREGNANCY

Hypertension remains the most commonly encountered medical condition in pregnant women, complicating up to 15% of all pregnancies. It results in frequent hospital admissions, maternal morbidity and mortality, and preterm births with concomitant neonatal morbidity and mortality. Hypertensive disorders of pregnancy comprise a spectrum of severity ranging from a mild elevation of blood pressure to severe preeclampsia and hemolysis. Recent data show that hypertensive disorders of pregnancy are associated with long-term cardiovascular risks in women (Miller & Carpenter, 2015).

Hypertensive disorders of pregnancy include chronic hypertension, gestational hypertension, preeclampsia, eclampsia, and chronic hypertension with superimposed preeclampsia. Preeclampsia complicates about 3% to 5% of pregnancies. All hypertensive disorders, which affect up to 15% of pregnancies, are on the rise. Hypertensive disorders are associated with higher rates of maternal, fetal, and infant mortality and with severe morbidity, especially in cases of severe preeclampsia, eclampsia, and HELLP syndrome (ACOG, 2014c).

ACOG (2010c) and the National High Blood Pressure Education Program Working Group on High Blood Pressure in Pregnancy (2002) have identified a classification system for hypertensive disorders. Hypertension may be a preexisting condition (chronic hypertension) or it may present for the first time during pregnancy (gestational hypertension). Both chronic hypertension and preeclampsia can be subclassified as either mild or severe. For chronic hypertension, subclassification is dependent on systolic and diastolic values. For preeclampsia, subclassification is dependent on the severity of end organ involvement (Foley, Strong, & Garite, 2014). Regardless of its onset or subclassification, hypertension jeopardizes the well-being of the mother as well as the fetus.

The classification of hypertensive disorders in pregnancy currently consists of five categories:
1. *Chronic hypertension*: Hypertension that exists prior to pregnancy or that develops before 20 weeks' gestation.
2. *Gestational hypertension*: Blood pressure elevation (140/90 mm Hg) identified after 20 weeks' gestation without proteinuria. Blood pressure returns to normal by 12 weeks' postpartum.
3. *Preeclampsia*: most common hypertensive disorder of pregnancy, which develops with proteinuria after 20 weeks' gestation. It is a multisystem disease process, which is classified as mild or severe, depending on the severity of the organ dysfunction.
4. *Eclampsia*: Onset of seizure activity in a woman with preeclampsia
5. *Chronic hypertension with superimposed preeclampsia*: Occurs in approximately 20% of pregnant women with increased maternal and fetal morbidity rates (King et al., 2015).

Population-based data indicate that approximately 1% of pregnancies are complicated by chronic hypertension, 5% to 6% by gestational hypertension (without proteinuria), and 3% to 5% by preeclampsia (Carson & Gibson, 2015). Worldwide, 50,000 to 60,000 women die from preeclampsia each year, corresponding to 12% of all maternal deaths (Clausen & Bergholt, 2014).

Chronic Hypertension

Chronic hypertension is defined as blood pressure exceeding 140/90 mm Hg before pregnancy or before 20 weeks' gestation. When hypertension is first identified during a woman's pregnancy and she is less than 20 weeks' gestation, blood pressure elevations usually represent chronic hypertension. Chronic hypertension occurs in about 20% of women of childbearing age, with the prevalence varying according to age, race, and body mass index (BMI). As our nation's obesity rate rises, more women will start pregnancies with elevated blood pressures. About 25% of women with chronic hypertension develop preeclampsia during pregnancy (Clausen & Bergholt, 2014). Women with chronic hypertension in pregnancy should be monitored for the development of worsening hypertension and/or the development of superimposed preeclampsia.

Women with mild chronic hypertension often do not require antihypertensive therapy during most of pregnancy. Pharmacologic treatment of mild hypertension does not reduce the likelihood of developing preeclampsia later in gestation and increases the likelihood of intrauterine growth restriction. If maternal blood pressure exceeds 160/100 mm Hg, however, drug treatment is recommended (Magee et al., 2015). Nurses can play a large role in educating their hypertensive clients to help them understand potential complications and how simple changes in their lifestyles might be helpful in influencing the pregnancy outcome positively.

Gestational Hypertension

The gestational hypertension category is used in women with nonproteinuric hypertension of pregnancy, in which the pathophysiologic disturbances of the preeclampsia syndrome do not develop before giving birth. Gestational hypertension is a temporary diagnosis for hypertensive pregnant women who do not meet the criteria for preeclampsia (both hypertension and possibly proteinuria) or chronic hypertension (hypertension first detected before the 20th week of pregnancy).

Gestational hypertension is characterized by hypertension (>140/90) without proteinuria after 20 weeks' gestation resolving by 12 weeks' postpartum (Magowan, Owen, & Thomson, 2014). Previously, gestational hypertension was known as pregnancy-induced hypertension or toxemia of pregnancy, but these terms are no longer used. Gestational hypertension is defined as systolic blood pressure > 140 mm Hg and/or diastolic > 90 mm Hg on at least two occasions at least 4 to 6 hours apart after the 20th week of gestation, in women known to be normotensive prior to this time and prior to pregnancy (King et al., 2015). Gestational hypertension can be differentiated from chronic hypertension, which appears before the 20th week of gestation; or

hypertension before the current pregnancy, which continues after the woman gives birth.

A recent study found that progesterone supplementation during the first trimester significantly reduced the incidence of gestational hypertension and fetal distress in primigravida women. This supplementation might be a future therapy with addition studies to validate it (Zainul et al., 2014).

Preeclampsia and Eclampsia

Normal physiologic adaptations to pregnancy are altered in the woman who develops preeclampsia. **Preeclampsia** can be described as a multisystem, vasopressive disorder that targets the cardiovascular, hepatic, renal, and central nervous systems (CNSs). Preeclampsia can be classified as mild or severe with a potential progression to eclampsia. Each is associated with specific criteria. Comparison Chart 19.2 highlights these classifications.

Pathophysiology

Preeclampsia remains an enigma. The condition can be devastating to both the mother and fetus, yet the etiology still remains a mystery to medical science despite decades of research. Many theories exist, but none has truly explained the widespread pathologic changes that result in pulmonary edema, oliguria, seizures, thrombocytopenia, and abnormal liver enzymes (Cunningham et al., 2014). Despite the results of several research studies, the use of aspirin or supplementation with calcium, magnesium, zinc, or antioxidant therapy (vitamin C and E), salt restriction, diuretic therapy, or fish oils has not proved to prevent this destructive condition.

Preeclampsia is a two-stage event; .the underlying mechanisms involved are vasospasm and hypoperfusion. In the first stage, the key feature is widespread vasospasm. In addition, endothelial injury occurs, leading to platelet adherence, fibrin deposition, and the presence of schistocytes (fragment of an erythrocyte). The second stage of preeclampsia is the woman's response to abnormal placentation, when symptoms appear, i.e., hypertension, proteinuria, and edema due to hypoperfusion.

The first stage of generalized vasospasm results in elevation of blood pressure and reduced blood flow to the brain, liver, kidneys, placenta, and lungs. Decreased liver perfusion leads to impaired liver function and subcapsular hemorrhage. This is demonstrated by epigastric pain and elevated liver enzymes in the maternal serum. Decreased brain perfusion leads to small cerebral hemorrhages and symptoms of arterial vasospasm such as headaches, visual disturbances, blurred vision, and hyperactive deep tendon reflexes (DTRs). A thromboxane/prostacyclin imbalance leads to increased thromboxane (potent vasoconstrictor and stimulator of

COMPARISON CHART 19.2	PREECLAMPSIA VERSUS ECLAMPSIA		
	Mild Preeclampsia	Severe Preeclampsia	Eclampsia
Blood pressure	>140/90 mm Hg after 20 weeks' gestation	>160/110 mm Hg	>160/110 mm Hg
Proteinuria	300 mg/24 hours or greater than 1+ protein on a random dipstick urine sample	>500 mg/24 hours; greater than 3+ on random dipstick urine sample	Marked proteinuria
Seizures/coma	No	No	Yes
Hyperreflexia	No	Yes	Yes
Other signs and symptoms	Mild facial or hand edema Weight gain	Headache Oliguria Blurred vision, scotomata (blind spots) Pulmonary edema Thrombocytopenia (platelet count <100,000 platelets/mm^3) Cerebral disturbances Epigastric or RUQ pain HELLP	Severe headache Generalized edema RUQ or epigastric pain Visual disturbances Cerebral hemorrhage Renal failure HELLP

platelet aggregation) and decreased prostacyclin (potent vasodilator and inhibitor of platelet aggregation), which contribute to the hypertensive state. Decreased kidney perfusion reduces the glomerular filtration rate, resulting in decreased urine output and increased serum levels of sodium, BUN, uric acid, and creatinine, further increasing extracellular fluid and edema. Increased capillary permeability in the kidneys allows albumin to escape, which reduces plasma colloid osmotic pressure and moves more fluid into extracellular spaces; this leads to pulmonary edema and generalized edema. Poor placental perfusion resulting from prolonged vasoconstriction helps to contribute to intrauterine growth restriction, premature separation of the placenta (abruptio placentae), persistent fetal hypoxia, and acidosis. In addition, hemoconcentration (resulting from decreased intravascular volume) causes increased blood viscosity and elevated hematocrit (ACOG, 2014c).

Therapeutic Management

Management of the woman with preeclampsia varies depending on the severity of her condition and its effects on the fetus. Typically the woman is managed conservatively if she is experiencing mild symptoms. However, if the condition progresses, management becomes more aggressive. The "cure" for preeclampsia/eclampsia is always delivery of the placenta. The resolution following expulsion of the placenta supports theories related to the placental influence on the disease (Dekker, 2014). According to recent studies, prevention of preeclampsia should be considered with daily low-dose aspirin from 12 weeks' gestation and onward to women identified at high risk for it. While women with chronic hypertension or a personal history of preeclampsia should receive aspirin during pregnancy, further research should be ongoing to predict preeclampsia in low risk women (Bujold, 2015).

MANAGEMENT FOR MILD PREECLAMPSIA
Conservative strategies for mild preeclampsia are used if the woman exhibits no signs of renal or hepatic dysfunction or coagulopathy. A woman with mild elevations in blood pressure may be placed on bed rest at home. She is encouraged to rest as much as possible in the lateral recumbent position to improve uteroplacental blood flow, reduce her blood pressure, and promote diuresis. In addition, antepartal visits and diagnostic testing—such as CBC, clotting studies, liver enzymes, and platelet levels—increase in frequency. The woman will be asked to monitor her blood pressure daily (every 4 to 6 hours while awake) and report any increased readings; she will also measure the amount of protein found in urine using a dipstick and will weigh herself for any weight gain. She also should take daily fetal movement counts, and if there is any decrease in movement, she needs to be evaluated by her health care provider that day. A balanced, nutritional diet with no sodium restriction is advised. In addition, she is encouraged to drink six to eight 8-oz glasses of water daily. If home management fails to reduce the blood pressure, admission to the hospital is warranted and the treatment strategy is individualized based on the severity of the condition and the gestational age at the time of diagnosis.

During the hospitalization, the woman with mild preeclampsia is monitored closely for signs and symptoms of severe preeclampsia or impending eclampsia (e.g., persistent headache, hyperreflexia). Blood pressure measurements are frequently recorded along with daily weights to detect excessive weight gain resulting from edema. Fetal surveillance is instituted in the form of daily fetal movement counts, nonstress testing, and serial ultrasounds to evaluate fetal growth and amniotic fluid volume to confirm fetal well-being. Expectant management (watchful waiting) usually continues until the pregnancy reaches term, fetal lung maturity is documented, or complications develop that warrant immediate birth. Women with mild preeclampsia are at greatest risk for postpartum hypertension (King et al., 2015).

Prevention of disease progression is the focus of treatment during labor. Blood pressure is monitored frequently and a quiet environment is important to minimize the risk of stimulation and to promote rest. Intravenous magnesium sulfate is infused to prevent any seizure activity, along with antihypertensives if blood pressure values begin to rise. Calcium gluconate is kept at the bedside in case the magnesium level becomes toxic. Continued close monitoring of neurologic status is warranted to detect any signs or symptoms of hypoxemia, impending seizure activity, or increased intracranial pressure. An indwelling urinary (Foley) catheter usually is inserted to allow for accurate measurement of urine output.

MANAGEMENT FOR SEVERE PREECLAMPSIA

Severe preeclampsia may develop suddenly and bring with it high blood pressure of more than 160/110 mm Hg, proteinuria of more than 5 g in 24 hours, oliguria of less than 400 mL in 24 hours, cerebral and visual symptoms, and rapid weight gain. This clinical picture signals severe preeclampsia, and immediate hospitalization is needed.

Treatment is highly individualized and based on disease severity and fetal age. Birth of the infant is the only cure, because preeclampsia depends on the presence of trophoblastic tissue. Therefore, the exact age of the fetus is assessed to determine viability.

Severe preeclampsia is treated aggressively because hypertension poses a serious threat to mother and fetus. The goal of care is to stabilize the mother–fetus dyad and prepare for birth. Therapy focuses on controlling hypertension, preventing seizures, preventing long-term morbidity, and preventing maternal, fetal, or newborn death (Foo et al., 2015). Intense maternal and fetal surveillance starts when the mother enters the hospital and continues throughout her stay.

The woman in labor with severe preeclampsia typically receives oxytocin to stimulate uterine contractions and magnesium sulfate to prevent seizure activity. Oxytocin and magnesium sulfate can be given simultaneously via infusion pumps to ensure both are administered at the prescribed rate. Magnesium sulfate is given intravenously via an infusion pump. A loading dose of 4 to 6 g is given over 5 minutes. Then, a maintenance dose of 2 g/hr is given.

The client is evaluated closely for magnesium toxicity. If at all possible, a vaginal delivery is preferable to a cesarean birth for better maternal outcomes and less risk associated with a surgical birth. PGE2 gel may be used to ripen the cervix. A cesarean birth may be performed if the client is seriously ill. A pediatrician/neonatologist or neonatal nurse practitioner should be available in the birthing room to care for the newborn. A newborn whose mother received high doses of magnesium sulfate needs to be monitored for respiratory depression, hypocalcemia, and hypotonia. Decreased fetal heart rate variability may occur but, in general, magnesium sulfate does not pose a risk to the fetus. The newborn may exhibit respiratory depression, loss of reflexes, muscle weakness, and neurologic depression (Martin, Fanaroff, & Walsh, 2014).

MANAGEMENT OF ECLAMPSIA

In the woman who develops an eclamptic seizure, the convulsive activity begins with facial twitching, followed by generalized muscle rigidity. The woman's face initially may become distorted, with protrusion of the eyes, and foaming at the mouth may occur. Respirations cease for the duration of the seizure, resulting from muscle spasms, thus compromising fetal oxygenation. Seizure complications can include tongue biting, head trauma, broken bones, and aspiration. Coma usually follows the seizure activity, with respiration resuming. Eclamptic seizures are life-threatening emergencies and require immediate treatment to decrease maternal morbidity and mortality.

As with any seizure, the initial management is to clear the airway and administer adequate oxygen. Positioning the woman on her left side and protecting her from injury during the seizure are the key. Suction equipment must be readily available to remove secretions from her mouth after the seizure is over. Intravenous fluids are administered after the seizure at a rate to replace urine output and additional insensible losses. Fetal heart rate is monitored closely. Magnesium sulfate is administered intravenously to prevent further seizures. Serum magnesium levels, respiratory rate, reflexes, and urine output in women receiving magnesium sulfate are closely monitored to avoid magnesium toxicity and prevent cardiac arrest. Calcium gluconate (1 g intravenously) is typically ordered to counteract magnesium toxicity. Hypertension is controlled with antihypertensive medications. After the woman's seizures are controlled, her stability is assessed. If she is found stable, birth via induction or cesarean birth is performed (Amorim et al., 2015). If the woman's condition remains stable, she will be transferred to the postpartum unit for care. If she becomes unstable after giving birth, she may be transferred to the critical care unit for closer observation.

Nursing Assessment

Preventing complications related to preeclampsia requires the use of assessment, advocacy, and counseling skills. Assessment begins with the accurate measurement of the client's blood pressure at each encounter. In addition, nurses need to assess for subjective complaints that may indicate progression of the disease—visual changes, severe headaches, unusual bleeding or bruising, or epigastric pain (Nagtalon-Ramos, 2014). The significant signs of preeclampsia—proteinuria and hypertension—occur without the woman's awareness. Unfortunately, by the time symptoms are noticed, gestational hypertension can be severe.

Take Note!

The absolute blood pressure (value that validates elevation) of 140/90 mm Hg should be obtained on two occasions 4 to 6 hours apart to be diagnostic of preeclampsia. Proteinuria is defined as 300 mg or more of urinary protein per 24 hours or more than 1+ protein by chemical reagent strip or dipstick of at least two random urine samples collected at least 4 to 6 hours apart with no evidence of urinary tract infection (ACOG, 2014c).

HEALTH HISTORY AND PHYSICAL EXAMINATION

Take a thorough history during the first antepartal visit to identify whether the woman is at risk for preeclampsia. Risk factors include:
- Primigravida status
- Chromosomal abnormalities
- Structural congenital anomalies
- Multiple gestation
- History of preeclampsia in a previous pregnancy
- Excessive placental tissue, as is seen in women with GTD
- Chronic stress
- Use of ovulation drugs
- Family history of preeclampsia (mother or sister)
- Lower socioeconomic status
- History of diabetes, hypertension, or renal disease
- Poor nutrition
- Lower socioeconomic status
- African–American ethnicity
- Age extremes (younger than 20 or older than 35)
- Obesity (Ross, 2015).

In addition, complete a nutritional assessment that includes the woman's usual intake of protein, calcium, daily calories, and fluids.

Women at risk for preeclampsia require more frequent prenatal visits throughout their pregnancy, and they require teaching about problems so that they can report them promptly.

Blood pressure must be measured carefully and consistently. Obtain all measurements with the woman in the same position (blood pressure is highest in the sitting position and lowest in the side-lying position) and by using the same technique (automated vs. manual). This standardization in position and technique will yield the most accurate readings (Norwitz, 2015).

Obtain the client's weight (noting gain since last visit), and assess for amount and location of edema. Asking questions such as "Do your rings still fit on your fingers?" or "Is your face puffy when you get up in the morning?" will help to determine whether fluid retention is present or if the woman's status has changed since her last visit.

Take Note!

Although edema is not a cardinal sign of preeclampsia, weight should be monitored frequently to identify sudden gains in a short time span. Current research relies less on the classic triad of symptoms (hypertension, proteinuria, and edema or weight gain) and more on decreased organ perfusion, endothelial dysfunction (capillary leaking and proteinuria), and elevated blood pressure as key indicators (Carson & Gibson, 2015).

If edema is present, assess the distribution, degree, and pitting. Document your findings and identify whether the edema is dependent or pitting. Dependent edema is present on the lower half of the body if the client is ambulatory, where hydrostatic pressure is greatest. It is usually observed in the feet and ankles or in the sacral area if the client is on bed rest. Pitting edema is edema that leaves a small depression or pit after finger pressure is applied to a swollen area (Carson & Gibson, 2014). Record the depth of pitting demonstrated when pressure is applied. Although subjective, the following is used to record relative degrees:
- 1+ pitting edema = 2-mm depression into skin; disappears rapidly
- 2+ pitting edema = 4-mm skin depression; disappears in 10 to 15 seconds
- 3+ pitting edema = 6-mm depression into skin; lasts more than 1 minute
- 4+ pitting edema = 8-mm depression into skin; lasts 2 to 3 minutes

At every antepartal visit, assess the fetal heart rate with a Doppler device. Also check a clean-catch urine specimen for protein using a dipstick.

LABORATORY AND DIAGNOSTIC TESTING

Various laboratory tests may be performed to evaluate the woman's status. Typically these include a CBC, serum electrolytes, BUN, creatinine, and hepatic enzyme levels. Urine specimens are checked for protein; if levels are 1 to 2+ or greater, a 24-hour urine collection is completed.

Nursing Management

Nursing management of the woman with preeclampsia focuses on close monitoring of blood pressure and ongoing assessment for evidence of disease progression. Throughout the client's pregnancy, fetal surveillance is essential.

INTERVENING FOR PREECLAMPSIA

The woman with mild preeclampsia requires frequent monitoring to detect changes because preeclampsia can progress rapidly. Instruct all women in the signs and symptoms of preeclampsia and urge them to contact their health care professional for immediate evaluation should any occur.

Typically, women with mild preeclampsia can be managed at home if they have a good understanding of the disease process, blood pressure and vital signs are stable, there are no abnormal laboratory test results, and if good fetal movement is demonstrated (Teaching Guidelines 19.2). The home care nurse makes frequent visits and follow-up phone calls to assess the woman's condition, to assist with scheduling periodic evaluations of the fetus (such as nonstress tests), and to evaluate any changes that might suggest a worsening of the woman's condition.

Teaching Guidelines 19.2
TEACHING FOR THE WOMAN WITH MILD PREECLAMPSIA

- Rest in a quiet environment to prevent cerebral disturbances.
- Drink 8 to 10 glasses of water daily.
- Consume a balanced, high-protein diet including high-fiber foods.
- Obtain intermittent bed rest to improve circulation to the heart and uterus.
- Limit your physical activity to promote urination and subsequent decrease in blood pressure.
- Enlist the aid of your family so that you can obtain appropriate rest time.
- Perform self-monitoring as instructed, including:
  - Taking your own blood pressure twice daily
  - Checking and recording weight daily
  - Performing urine dipstick twice daily
  - Recording the number of fetal kicks daily
- Contact the home health nurse if any of the following occurs:
  - Increase in blood pressure
  - Protein present in urine
  - Gain of more than 1 lb in 1 week
  - Burning or frequency when urinating
  - Decrease in fetal activity or movement
  - Headache (forehead or posterior neck region)
  - Dizziness or visual disturbances
  - Increase in swelling in hands, feet, legs, and face
  - Stomach pain, excessive heartburn, or epigastric pain
  - Decreased or infrequent urination
  - Contractions or low back pain
  - Easy or excessive bruising
  - Sudden onset of abdominal pain
  - Nausea and vomiting

Early detection and management of mild preeclampsia is associated with the greatest success in reducing progression of this condition. As long as the client carries out the guidelines of care as outlined by the health care provider and remains stable, home care can continue to maintain the pregnancy until the fetus is mature. If disease progression occurs, hospitalization is required.

INTERVENING FOR SEVERE PREECLAMPSIA

The woman with severe preeclampsia requires hospitalization. Maintain the client on complete bed rest in the left lateral lying position. Ensure that the room is dark and quiet to reduce stimulation. Give sedatives as ordered to encourage quiet bed rest. The client is at risk for seizures if the condition progresses. Therefore, institute and maintain seizure precautions, such as padding the side rails and having oxygen, suction equipment, and call light readily available to protect the client from injury.

Take Note!

Preeclampsia increases the risk of placental abruption, preterm birth, intrauterine growth restriction, and fetal distress during childbirth. Always be prepared if you see symptoms of preeclampsia!

Closely monitor the client's blood pressure. Administer antihypertensives as ordered to reduce blood pressure (Drug Guide 19.3). Assess the client's vision and level of consciousness. Report any changes and any complaints of headache or visual disturbances. Offer a high-protein diet with 8 to 10 glasses of water daily. Monitor the client's intake and output every hour and administer fluid and electrolyte replacements as ordered. Assess the woman for signs and symptoms of pulmonary edema, such as crackles and wheezing heard on auscultation, dyspnea, decreased oxygen saturation levels, cough, neck vein distention, anxiety, and restlessness. The treatment of acute pulmonary edema is symptomatic and includes the administration of vasodilating agents and of diuretics. The development of acute pulmonary edema in women with hypertension during pregnancy is associated with high levels of intravenous fluid administration (Pauli & Repke, 2015).

To achieve a safe outcome for the fetus, prepare the woman for possible testing to evaluate fetal status as preeclampsia progresses. Testing may include the nonstress test, serial ultrasounds to track fetal growth, amniocentesis to determine fetal lung maturity, Doppler velocimetry to screen for fetal compromise, and biophysical profile to evaluate ongoing fetal well-being (Mattson & Smith, 2016).

Other laboratory tests may be performed to monitor the disease process and to determine if it is progressing into HELLP syndrome. These include liver enzymes such as lactic dehydrogenase (LDH), ALT, and AST; chemistry panel, such as creatinine, BUN, uric acid, and glucose;

DRUG GUIDE 19.3   MEDICATIONS USED WITH PREECLAMPSIA AND ECLAMPSIA

Medication	Action/Indications	Nursing Implications
Magnesium sulfate	Blockage of neuromuscular transmission, vasodilation Prevention and treatment of eclamptic seizures	Loading dose of 4 to 6 g by IV in 100 mL of fluid administered over 15 to 20 minutes, followed by a maintenance dose of 2 g as a continuous intravenous infusion. Monitor serum magnesium levels closely. Assess DTRs and check for ankle clonus. Have calcium gluconate readily available in case of toxicity. Monitor for signs and symptoms of toxicity, such as flushing, sweating, hypotension, and cardiac and central nervous system depression.
Hydralazine hydrochloride (Apresoline)	Vascular smooth muscle relaxant, thus improving perfusion to renal, uterine, and cerebral areas Reduction in blood pressure	Administer 5 to 10 mg by slow intravenous bolus every 20 minutes as needed. Use parenteral form immediately after opening ampule. Withdraw drug slowly to prevent possible rebound hypertension. Monitor for adverse effects such as palpitations, headache, tachycardia, anorexia, nausea, vomiting, and diarrhea.
Labetalol hydrochloride (Normodyne)	Alpha-1 and beta blocker Reduction in blood pressure	Be aware that drug lowers blood pressure without decreasing maternal heart rate or cardiac output. Administer IV dose of 20 to 40 mg every 15 minutes as needed and then administer intravenous V infusion of 2 mg/min until desired blood pressure value achieved. Monitor for possible adverse effects such as gastric pain, flatulence, constipation, dizziness, vertigo, and fatigue.
Nifedipine (Procardia)	Calcium channel blocker/dilation of coronary arteries, arterioles, and peripheral arterioles Reduction in blood pressure, stoppage of preterm labor	Administer 10 to 20 mg orally for three doses and then every 4 to 8 hours. Monitor for possible adverse effects such as dizziness, peripheral edema, angina, diarrhea, nasal congestions, cough.
Sodium nitroprusside	Rapid vasodilation (arterial and venous) Severe hypertension requiring rapid reduction in blood pressure	Administer via continuous IV infusion with dose titrated according to blood pressure levels. Wrap intravenous infusion solution in foil or opaque material to protect from light. Monitor for possible adverse effects, such as apprehension, restlessness, retrosternal pressure, palpitations, diaphoresis, abdominal pain.
Furosemide (Lasix)	Diuretic action, inhibiting the reabsorption of sodium and chloride from the ascending loop of Henle Pulmonary edema (used only if condition is present)	Administer via slow IV bolus at a dose of 10 to 40 mg over 1 to 2 minutes. Monitor urine output hourly. Assess for possible adverse effects such as dizziness, vertigo, orthostatic hypotension, anorexia, vomiting, electrolyte imbalances, muscle cramps, and muscle spasms.

Adapted from King, T. L., Brucker, M. C., Kriebs, J. M., Fahey, J. O., Grgor, C. L., & Varney, H. (2015). *Varney's midwifery* (5th ed.). Burlington, MA: Jones & Bartlett Learning; and Skidmore-Roth, L. (2015). *Mosby's 2015 nursing drug reference* (28th ed.). Philadelphia, PA: Elsevier Health Science.

CBC, including platelet count; coagulation studies, such as PT, PTT, fibrinogen, and bleeding time; and a 24-hour urine collection for protein and creatinine clearance.

Administer parenteral magnesium sulfate as ordered to prevent seizures. Assess DTRs to evaluate the effectiveness of therapy. Clients with preeclampsia commonly present with hyperreflexia. Severe preeclampsia causes changes in the cortex, which disrupts the equilibrium of impulses between the cerebral cortex and the spinal cord. Brisk reflexes (hyperreflexia) are the result of an irritable cortex and indicate CNS involvement (Marik, 2015). Diminished or absent reflexes occur when the client develops magnesium toxicity. Because magnesium is a potent neuromuscular blockade, the afferent and efferent nerve pathways do not relay messages properly and hyporeflexia develops. Common sites used to assess DTRs are biceps reflex, triceps reflex, patellar reflex, Achilles reflex, and plantar reflex. Nursing Procedure 19.1 highlights the steps for assessing the patellar reflex.

The National Institute of Neurological Disorders and Stroke, a division of the National Institutes of Health, published a scale in the early 1990s that, although subjective, is used widely today. It grades reflexes from 0 to 4+. Grades 2+ and 3+ are considered normal, whereas grades 0 and 4 may indicate pathology (Table 19.2). Because these are subjective assessments, to improve communication of reflex results, condensed descriptor categories such as absent, average, brisk, or clonus should be used rather than numeric codes (Magowan, Owen, & Thomson, 2014).

Clonus is the presence of rhythmic involuntary contractions, most often at the foot or ankle. Sustained clonus confirms CNS involvement. Nursing Procedure 19.2 highlights the steps when testing for ankle clonus.

With magnesium sulfate administration, the client is at risk for magnesium toxicity. Closely assess the client for signs of toxicity, which include a respiratory rate of less than 12 breaths per minute, absence of DTRs, and a decrease in urinary output (<30 mL/hr). Also monitor serum magnesium levels. Although exact levels may vary among agencies, serum magnesium levels ranging from 4 to 7 mEq/L are considered therapeutic, whereas levels more than 8 mEq/dL are generally considered toxic. As levels increase, the woman is at risk for severe problems:
- 10 mEq/L: Possible loss of DTRs
- 15 mEq/L: Possible respiratory depression
- 25 mEq/L: Possible cardiac arrest (Skidmore-Roth, 2015).

If signs and symptoms of magnesium toxicity develop, expect to administer calcium gluconate as the antidote.

Throughout the client's stay, closely monitor her for signs and symptoms of labor. Perform continuous electronic fetal monitoring to assess fetal well-being. Note trends in baseline rate and presence or absence of accelerations or decelerations. Also observe for signs

NURSING PROCEDURE 19.1

Assessing the Patellar Reflex

Purpose: To Evaluate for Nervous System Irritability Related to Preeclampsia

1. Place the woman in the supine position (or sitting upright with the legs dangling freely over the side of the bed or examination table).

2. If lying supine, have the woman flex her knee slightly.

3. Place a hand under the knee to support the leg and locate the patellar tendon. It should be midline just below the knee cap.

4. Using a reflex hammer or the side of your hand, strike the area of the patellar tendon firmly and quickly.

5. Note the movement of the leg and foot. A patellar reflex occurs when the leg and foot move (documented as 2+).

6. Repeat the procedure on the opposite leg.

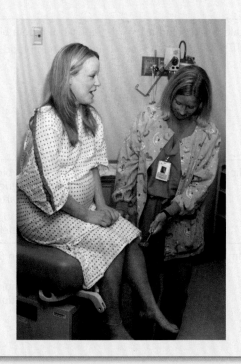

of fetal distress and report them immediately. Administer glucocorticoid treatment as ordered to enhance fetal lung maturity and prepare for labor induction if the mother's condition warrants.

Keep the client and family informed of the woman's condition and educate them about the course of treatment. Provide emotional support for the client and family. Severe preeclampsia is very frightening for the client and her family, and most expectant mothers are very

TABLE 19.2	GRADING DEEP TENDON REFLEXES	
Description of Finding		**Grade**
Reflex absent, none elicited		0
Hypoactive response, sluggish		1
Reflex in lower half of normal range		2
Reflex in upper half of normal range		3
Hyperactive, brisk, clonus present		4

Adapted from King, T. L., Brucker, M. C., Kriebs, J. M., Fahey, J. O., Grgor, C. L., & Varney, H. (2015). *Varney's midwifery.* (5th ed.), Burlington, MA: Jones & Bartlett Learning; Nagtalon-Ramos, J. (2014). *Maternal-newborn nursing care: Best evidence-based practices.* Philadelphia, PA: F. A. Davis Company.

anxious about their own health as well as that of the fetus. To allay anxiety, use light touch to comfort and reassure her that the necessary actions are being taken. Actively listening to her concerns and fears and communicating them to the health care provider are important to keep open the lines of communication. Offering praise for small accomplishments can provide positive reinforcement for effective behaviors.

INTERVENING FOR ECLAMPSIA

The onset of seizure activity identifies **eclampsia**. Typically, eclamptic seizures are generalized and start with facial twitching. The body then becomes rigid, in a state of tonic muscular contraction. The clonic phase of the seizure involves alternating contraction and relaxation of all body muscles. Respirations stop during seizure activity and resume shortly after it ends. Client safety is the primary concern during eclamptic seizures. If possible, turn the client to her side and remain with her. Make sure that the side rails are up and padded. Dim the lights and keep the room quiet.

Document the time and sequence of events as soon as possible. After the seizure activity has ceased, suction the nasopharynx as necessary and administer oxygen. Continue the magnesium sulfate infusion to prevent further seizures. Ensure continuous electronic fetal monitoring, evaluating fetal status for changes. Also assess the client for uterine contractions. After the client is stabilized, prepare her for the birthing process as soon as possible to reduce the risk of perinatal mortality.

PROVIDING FOLLOW-UP CARE

After delivery of the newborn, continue to monitor the client for signs and symptoms of preeclampsia/eclampsia for at least 48 hours. Expect to continue to administer

---

NURSING PROCEDURE 19.2

Testing for Ankle Clonus

Purpose: To Evaluate for Nervous System Irritability Related to Preeclampsia

1. Place the woman in the supine position.
2. Have the client slightly bend her knee and place a hand under the knee to support it.
3. Dorsiflex the foot briskly and then quickly release it.

4. Watch for the foot to rebound smoothly against your hand. If the movement is smooth without any rapid contractions of the ankle or calf muscle, then clonus is not present; if the movement is jerky and rapid, clonus is present.
5. Repeat on the opposite side.

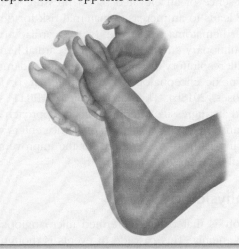

magnesium sulfate infusion for 24 hours to prevent seizure activity, and monitor serum magnesium levels for toxicity.

Assess vital signs at least every 4 hours, along with routine postpartum assessments: fundus, lochia, breasts, bladder, bowels, and the woman's emotional state. Monitor urine output closely. Diuresis is a positive sign that, along with a decrease in proteinuria, signals resolution of the disease.

HELLP SYNDROME

HELLP syndrome is an acronym for hemolysis, elevated liver enzymes, and low platelet count. It is a variant of the preeclampsia/eclampsia syndrome that occurs in 10% to 20% of clients whose conditions are labeled as severe. Women with HELLP syndrome are at increased risk for complications such as cerebral hemorrhage, retinal detachment, hematoma/liver rupture, acute renal failure, disseminated intravascular coagulation (DIC), placental abruption, and maternal death (Vigil-De Gracia, 2015). It is a life-threatening obstetric complication considered by many to be a severe form of preeclampsia involving hemolysis, thrombocytopenia, and liver dysfunction.

Both HELLP and preeclampsia occur during the later stages of pregnancy, and sometimes after childbirth. HELLP syndrome is a clinically progressive condition. Early diagnosis is critical to prevent liver distention, rupture, and hemorrhage and the onset of DIC. If the condition presents prenatally, morbidity and mortality can affect both mother and baby.

HELLP syndrome occurs in up to 20% of pregnant women diagnosed with severe preeclampsia. It is unique, as it is a laboratory-value specific diagnosis. Women with HELLP usually have fewer signs of abnormalities consistent with the metabolic syndrome and a lower prevalence of thrombophilia as compared with preeclampsia women without HELLP (Sibai, 2015). Although it has been reported as early as 17 weeks' gestation, most of the time it is diagnosed between 22 and 36 weeks' gestation (Cunningham et al., 2014). It can present prior to the presence of an elevated blood pressure. HELLP syndrome leads to an increased maternal risk for developing liver hematoma or rupture, stroke, cardiac arrest, seizure, pulmonary edema, DIC, subendocardial hemorrhage, adult respiratory distress syndrome, renal damage, sepsis, hypoxic encephalopathy, and maternal, or fetal death (Moses, 2015b). The recognition of HELLP syndrome and an aggressive multidisciplinary approach and prompt transfer of these women to obstetric centers with expertise in this field are required for the improvement of maternal–fetal prognosis.

Pathophysiology

The hemolysis that occurs is termed microangiopathic hemolytic anemia. This cascade of events is thought to happen when red blood cells become fragmented as they pass through small, damaged blood vessels. Elevated liver enzymes are the result of reduced blood flow to the liver secondary to obstruction from fibrin deposits. At the same time, endothelial damage and fibrin deposition in the liver may lead to liver impairment and can result in hemorrhagic necrosis, indicated by right upper quadrant tenderness, nausea, and vomiting. Hyperbilirubinemia and jaundice result from liver impairment. Low platelets result from vascular damage, the result of vasospasm, and platelets aggregate at sites of damage, resulting in thrombocytopenia in multiple sites (Khan & Meirowitz, 2015).

Therapeutic Management

The treatment for HELLP syndrome is based on the severity of the disease, the gestational age of the fetus, and the condition of the mother and fetus. The mainstay of treatment is lowering of high blood pressure with rapid-acting antihypertensive agents, prevention of convulsions or further seizures with magnesium sulfate, and use of steroids for fetal lung maturity if necessary, followed by the birth of the infant and placenta (Foley, Strong, & Garite, 2014). The client should be admitted or transferred to a tertiary center with a neonatal intensive care unit. Additional treatment includes correction of the coagulopathies that accompany HELLP syndrome. After this syndrome is diagnosed and the woman's condition is stable, birth of the infant is indicated.

Magnesium sulfate is used prophylactically to prevent seizures. Antihypertensives such as hydralazine or labetalol are given to control blood pressure. Blood component therapy—such as fresh-frozen plasma, packed red blood cells, or platelets—is transfused to address the microangiopathic hemolytic anemia. Birth may be delayed up to 96 hours so that betamethasone or dexamethasone can be given to stimulate lung maturation in the preterm fetus.

Nursing Assessment

Nursing assessment of the woman with HELLP is similar to that for the woman with severe preeclampsia. Be alert for complaints of nausea (with or without vomiting), malaise, epigastric or right upper quadrant pain, and demonstrable edema. Perform systematic assessments frequently, as indicated by the woman's condition and response to therapy.

A diagnosis of HELLP syndrome is made based on laboratory test results, including:

• Low hematocrit that is not explained by any blood loss
• Elevated LDH (liver impairment)
• Elevated AST (liver impairment)
• Elevated ALT (liver impairment)
• Elevated BUN

- Elevated bilirubin level
- Elevated uric acid and creatinine levels (renal involvement)
- Low platelet count (less than 100,000 cells/mm^3)

Nursing Management

Nursing management of the woman diagnosed with HELLP syndrome is the same as that for the woman with severe preeclampsia. If possible, the woman with HELLP syndrome should be transferred to a tertiary care center once she has been assessed and stabilized. Closely monitor the client for changes and provide ongoing support throughout this experience.

GESTATIONAL DIABETES

Gestational diabetes is a condition involving glucose intolerance that occurs during pregnancy. It is discussed in greater detail in Chapter 20.

BLOOD INCOMPATIBILITY

Blood incompatibility most commonly involves one of two issues: blood type or the Rh factor. *Blood type incompatibility*, also known as ABO incompatibility, arises when a mother with blood type O becomes pregnant with a fetus with a different blood type (type A, B, or AB). The mother's serum contains naturally occurring anti-A and anti-B, which can cross the placenta and hemolyze fetal red blood cells. It is usually less severe than Rh incompatibility. One reason is that fetal red blood cells express less of the ABO blood group antigens compared with adult levels. In addition, in contrast to the Rh antigens, the ABO blood group antigens are expressed by a variety of fetal (and adult) tissues, reducing the chances of anti-A and anti-B binding their target antigens on the fetal red blood cells. ABO incompatibility rarely causes significant hemolysis, and prenatal treatment is not warranted.

Rh isoimmunization occurs when a pregnant woman's immune system creates antibodies against fetal Rh blood factors. Although the mother will exhibit no symptoms of Rh incompatibility, Rh antibodies adversely affect fetal health. Rh antibodies can cause fetal heart problems, breathing difficulties, jaundice, and a form of anemia known as hemolytic disease of the newborn. Rh sensitization occurs in approximately 1 in 1,000 births to Rh-negative women (March of Dimes, 2015d). Today RH isoimmunization in pregnant women and hemolytic disease of the newborn are rarely seen, primarily because women who are Rh negative are given anti-D immune globulin prophylaxis (RhoGAM) in the third trimester of pregnancy and after childbirth if the newborn is Rh positive.

Pathophysiology

ABO Incompatibility

Hemolysis associated with ABO incompatibility is limited to type O mothers with fetuses who have type A or B blood. In mothers with type A and B blood, naturally occurring antibodies are of the IgM class, which do not cross the placenta, whereas in type O mothers, the antibodies are predominantly IgG in nature. Because A and B antigens are widely expressed in a variety of tissues besides red blood cells, only a small portion of the antibodies crossing the placenta is available to bind to fetal red cells. In addition, fetal red cells appear to have less surface expression of A or B antigen, resulting in few reactive sites—hence the low incidence of significant hemolysis in affected neonates.

With ABO incompatibility, usually the mother is blood type O, with anti-A and anti-B antibodies in her serum; the infant is blood type A, B, or AB. The incompatibility arises as a result of the interaction of antibodies present in maternal serum and the antigen sites on the fetal red cells.

Rh Incompatibility

Rh incompatibility is a condition that develops when a woman with Rh-negative blood type is exposed to Rh-positive blood cells and subsequently develops circulating titers of Rh antibodies. Individuals with Rh-positive blood type have the D antigen present on their red cells, whereas individuals with an Rh-negative blood type do not. The presence or absence of the Rh antigen on the RBC membrane is genetically controlled.

In the United States, about 15% of the White population, 5% to 8% of the African American and Hispanic populations, and 1% to 2% of the Asian and Native American populations are Rh negative. The vast majority (85%) of individuals is considered Rh positive (March of Dimes, 2015d).

Rh incompatibility most commonly arises with exposure of an Rh-negative mother to Rh-positive fetal blood during pregnancy or birth, during which time erythrocytes from the fetal circulation leak into the maternal circulation. Isoimmunization can also occur during an amniocentesis, ectopic pregnancy, placenta previa, placenta abruption, in utero fetal death, spontaneous abortion, or abdominal/pelvic trauma. After a significant exposure, alloimmunization or sensitization occurs. As a result, maternal antibodies are produced against the foreign Rh antigen.

Theoretically, fetal blood and maternal blood do not mix during pregnancy. In reality, however, small placental accidents (transplacental bleeds secondary to minor separation), abortions, ectopic pregnancy, abdominal trauma, trophoblastic disease, amniocentesis, placenta previa, and abruptio placentae allow fetal blood to enter the maternal circulation and initiate the production of antibodies to destroy Rh-positive blood. The amount of fetal blood necessary to produce Rh incompatibility varies. In one study, less than 1 mL of Rh-positive blood was shown to result in sensitization of women who are Rh negative (Salem & Singer, 2015).

Once sensitized, it takes approximately a month for Rh antibodies in the maternal circulation to cross over into the fetal circulation. In 90% of cases, sensitization occurs during delivery (Cunningham et al., 2014). Thus, most firstborn infants with Rh-positive blood type are not affected because the short period from first exposure of Rh-positive fetal erythrocytes to the birth of the infant is insufficient to produce a significant maternal IgG antibody response.

The risk and severity of alloimmune response increase with each subsequent pregnancy involving a fetus with Rh-positive blood. A second pregnancy with an Rh-positive fetus often produces a mildly anemic infant, whereas succeeding pregnancies produce infants with more serious hemolytic anemia.

Nursing Assessment

At the first prenatal visit, determine the woman's blood type and Rh status. Also obtain a thorough health history, noting any reports of previous events involving hemorrhage to delineate the risk for prior sensitization. When the client's history reveals an Rh-negative mother who may be pregnant with an Rh-positive fetus, prepare the client for an antibody screen (indirect Coombs test) to determine whether she has developed isoimmunity to the Rh antigen. This test detects unexpected circulating antibodies in a woman's serum that could be harmful to the fetus (Davidson, 2014).

Nursing Management

If the indirect Coombs test is negative (meaning no antibodies are present), then the woman is a candidate for RhoGAM. If the test is positive, RhoGAM is of no value because isoimmunization has occurred. In this case, the fetus is carefully monitored for hemolytic disease.

The incidence of isoimmunization has declined dramatically as a result of prenatal and postnatal RhoGAM administration after any event in which blood transfer may occur. The standard dose is 300 mcg, which is effective for 15 mL of fetal blood cells. Rh immunoglobulin helps to destroy any fetal cells in the maternal circulation before sensitization occurs, thus inhibiting maternal antibody production. This provides temporary passive immunity, thereby preventing maternal sensitization.

The current recommendation is for every Rh-negative nonimmunized woman to receive RhoGAM at some point between 28 and 32 weeks' gestation and again within 72 hours after giving birth. Other indications for RhoGAM include:

- Ectopic pregnancy
- Chorionic villus sampling
- Amniocentesis
- Prenatal hemorrhage
- Molar pregnancy
- Maternal trauma
- Percutaneous umbilical sampling
- Therapeutic or spontaneous abortion
- Fetal death
- Fetal surgery (King et al., 2015).

Despite the availability of RhoGAM and laboratory tests to identify women and newborns at risk, isoimmunization remains a serious clinical reality that continues to contribute to perinatal and neonatal mortality. Nurses, as client advocates, are in a unique position to make sure test results are brought to the health care provider's attention so appropriate interventions can be initiated. In addition, nurses must stay abreast of current literature and research regarding isoimmunization and its management. Stress to all women that early prenatal care can help identify and prevent this condition. Because Rh incompatibility is preventable with the use of RhoGAM, prevention remains the best treatment. Nurses can make a tremendous impact to ensure positive outcomes for the greatest possible number of pregnancies through education.

AMNIOTIC FLUID IMBALANCES

Amniotic fluid develops from several maternal and fetal structures, including the amnion, chorion, maternal blood, fetal lungs, gastrointestinal tract, kidneys, and skin. Any alteration in one or more of the various sources will alter the amount of amniotic fluid. Polyhydramnios and oligohydramnios are two imbalances associated with amniotic fluid.

Polyhydramnios

Polyhydramnios, also called hydramnios, is a condition in which there is too much amniotic fluid (more than 2,000 mL) surrounding the fetus between 32 and 36 weeks. It occurs in approximately 2% of all pregnancies and is associated with fetal anomalies of development such as upper gastrointestinal obstruction or atresias, neural tube defects, and anterior abdominal-wall defects, together with impaired swallowing in fetuses with chromosomal anomalies, such as trisomy 13 and 18 (Carter & Boyd, 2015). Approximately 18% of all women with diabetes will develop polyhydramnios during their pregnancy. There is an increase in cesarean births for fetal labor intolerance, low 5-min Apgar scores, increased neonatal birth weight, congenital anomalies, and newborn intensive care unit admissions for women with too much amniotic fluid at term (Moore, 2015). Overall, it is associated with poorer fetal outcomes because of the increased incidence of preterm births, fetal malpresentation, and cord prolapse.

There are several causes of polyhydramnios. Generally, too much fluid is being produced, there is a problem with the fluid being taken up, or both. It can be associated with maternal disease and fetal anomalies, but it can also be idiopathic (of unknown cause) in nature.

Therapeutic Management

Treatment may include close monitoring and frequent follow-up visits with the health care provider if the polyhydramnios is mild to moderate. In severe cases in which the woman is in pain and experiencing shortness of breath, an amniocentesis or artificial rupture of the membranes is done to reduce the fluid and the pressure. Removal of fluid by amniocentesis is only transiently effective. A noninvasive treatment may involve the use of a prostaglandin synthesis inhibitor (indomethacin) to decrease amniotic fluid volume by decreasing fetal urinary output, but this may cause premature closure of the fetal ductus arteriosus (King et al., 2015).

Nursing Assessment

Begin the assessment with a thorough history, being alert to risk factors such as maternal diabetes or multiple gestations. Review the maternal history for information about possible fetal anomalies including fetal esophageal or intestinal atresia, neural tube defects, chromosomal deviations, fetal hydrops, CNS or cardiovascular anomalies, and hydrocephaly.

Determine the gestational age of the fetus and measure the woman's fundal height. With polyhydramnios, there is a discrepancy between fundal height and gestational age, or a rapid growth of the uterus is noted. Assess the woman for complaints of discomfort in her abdomen, such as being severely stretched and tight. Also note any reports of uterine contractions, which may result from overstretching of the uterus. Assess for shortness of breath resulting from pressure on her diaphragm and inspect her lower extremities for edema, which results from increased pressure on the vena cava. Palpate the abdomen and obtain fetal heart rate. Often the fetal parts and heart rate are difficult to obtain because of the excess fluid present.

Prepare the woman for possible diagnostic testing to evaluate for the presence of possible fetal anomalies. An ultrasound usually is done to measure the pockets of amniotic fluid to estimate the total volume. In some cases, ultrasound also is helpful in finding the etiology of polyhydramnios, such as multiple pregnancy or a fetal structural anomaly.

Nursing Management

Nursing management of the woman with polyhydramnios focuses on ongoing assessment and monitoring for symptoms of abdominal pain, dyspnea, uterine contractions, and edema of the lower extremities. Explain to the woman and her family that this condition can cause her uterus to become overdistended and may lead to preterm labor and preterm rupture of membranes. Outline the signs and symptoms of both conditions and instruct the woman to contact her health care provider if they occur. If a therapeutic amniocentesis is performed, assist the health care provider and monitor maternal and fetal status throughout for any changes.

Oligohydramnios

Oligohydramnios is a decreased amount of amniotic fluid (less than 500 mL) between 32 and 36 weeks' gestation. It occurs in approximately 4% of all pregnancies. Oligohydramnios may result from any condition that prevents the fetus from making urine or blocks it from going into the amniotic sac. Oligohydramnios occurs in about four out of every 100 pregnancies. It is most common in the last trimester of pregnancy, but it can develop at any time in the pregnancy. About one out of eight women whose pregnancies last 2 weeks past the due date develops oligohydramnios. This happens as amniotic fluid levels naturally decline. This condition puts the fetus at an increased risk of perinatal morbidity and mortality (March of Dimes, 2015e). Reduction in amniotic fluid reduces the ability of the fetus to move freely without risk of cord compression, which increases the risk for fetal death and intrapartal hypoxia.

Therapeutic Management

The woman with oligohydramnios can be managed on an outpatient basis with serial ultrasounds and fetal surveillance through nonstress testing and biophysical profiles. As long as fetal well-being is demonstrated with frequent testing, no intervention is necessary. If fetal well-being is compromised, however, birth is planned along with amnioinfusion (the transvaginal infusion of crystalloid fluid to compensate for the lost amniotic fluid). The fluid is introduced into the uterus through an intrauterine pressure catheter. The infusion is administered in a controlled fashion to prevent overdistention of the uterus. Amnioinfusion is thought to improve abnormal fetal heart rate patterns, decrease cesarean births, and possibly minimize the risk of neonatal meconium aspiration syndrome, but more studies need to be done to validate this (Carter & Boyd, 2015).

Nursing Assessment

Review the maternal history for factors associated with oligohydramnios, including:
' Uteroplacental insufficiency
' Premature rupture of membranes prior to labor onset
' Hypertension of pregnancy
' Maternal diabetes
' Intrauterine growth restriction
' Post-term pregnancy
' Fetal renal agenesis
' Polycystic kidneys
' Urinary tract obstructions

Assess the client for complaints of fluid leaking from the vagina. Leaking of amniotic fluid from the vagina occurs with rupture of the amniotic sac. Leaking in conjunction with a uterus that is small for expected dates of gestation also suggests oligohydramnios. Unfortunately, the woman may not present with any symptoms. Typically, the reduced volume of amniotic fluid is identified on ultrasound.

Nursing Management

Nursing management of the woman with oligohydramnios involves continuous monitoring of fetal well-being during nonstress testing or during labor and birth by identifying category II and III patterns on the fetal monitor. Variable decelerations indicating cord compression are common. Changing the woman's position might be therapeutic in altering this fetal heart rate pattern. After the birth, evaluate the newborn for signs of postmaturity, congenital anomalies, and respiratory difficulty.

Assist with amnioinfusion as indicated and continue to assess the woman's vital signs and contraction status and the fetal heart rate throughout the procedure. Provide comfort measures such as changing the bed linens and the woman's bed clothes frequently because of the constant leakage of fluid from the vagina. Also provide frequent perineal care during the infusion.

MULTIPLE GESTATION

Multiple gestation is defined as a pregnancy with two or more fetuses.. This includes twins, triplets, and higher-order multiples such as quadruplets. In the past two decades, the number of multiple gestations in the United States has jumped dramatically because of the widespread use of fertility drugs, older age of women having babies, and the development of assisted reproductive technologies to treat infertility. About one third of live births from assisted reproductive technology result in more than one infant, and twins represent 85% of those multiple-birth children (De Sutter, 2015).

In the United States, the overall prevalence of twins is approximately 12 per 1,000, and two thirds are dizygotic (derived from two separate ova [March of Dimes, 2015f]). The increasing number of multiple gestations is a concern because women who are expecting more than one infant are at high risk for preterm labor, polyhydramnios, hyperemesis gravidarum, anemia, preeclampsia, and antepartum hemorrhage. Fetal/newborn risks or complications include prematurity, respiratory distress syndrome, birth asphyxia/perinatal depression, congenital anomalies (CNS, cardiovascular, and gastrointestinal defects), twin-to-twin transfusion syndrome (transfusion of blood from one twin [i.e., donor] to the other twin [i.e., recipient]), intrauterine growth restriction, and becoming conjoined twins (Martin, Fanaroff, & Walsh, 2014).

The two types of twins are monozygotic and dizygotic (Fig. 19.6). Monozygotic twins develop when a single, fertilized ovum splits during the first 2 weeks after conception. Monozygotic twins also are called identical twins. Two sperm fertilizing two ova produce dizygotic twins, which are called fraternal twins. Separate amnions, chorions, and placentas are formed in dizygotic twins. Triplets can be monozygotic, dizygotic, or trizygotic.

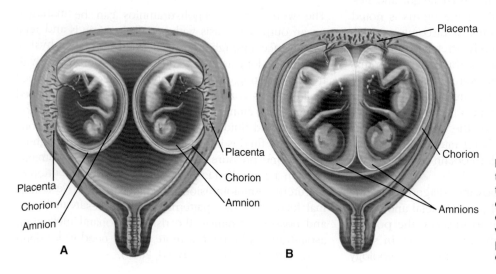

FIGURE 19.6 Multiple gestation with twins. **A.** Dizygotic twins, where each fetus has its own placenta, amnion, and chorion. **B.** Monozygotic twins, where the fetuses share one placenta, two amnions, and one chorion.

Therapeutic Management

When a multiple gestation is confirmed, the woman is followed with serial ultrasounds to assess fetal growth patterns and development. Biophysical profiles along with nonstress tests are ordered to determine fetal well-being. Many women are hospitalized in late pregnancy to prevent preterm labor and receive closer surveillance. During the intrapartum period the woman is closely monitored, with a perinatal team available to assist after birth. Operative delivery is frequently needed due to fetal malpresentation.

Nursing Assessment

Obtain a health history and perform a physical examination. Be alert for complaints of fatigue and severe nausea and vomiting. Assess the woman's abdomen and fundal height. Typically with a multiple gestation the uterus is larger than expected based on the estimated date of birth. Laboratory test results may reveal anemia. Prepare the woman for ultrasound, which typically confirms the diagnosis of a multiple gestation.

Nursing Management

During the prenatal period, provide education and support for the woman regarding nutrition, increased rest periods, and close observation for pregnancy complications such as anemia, excessive weight gain, proteinuria, edema, vaginal bleeding, and hypertension. Instruct the woman to be alert for and report immediately any signs and symptoms of preterm labor: contractions, uterine cramping, low back ache, increase in vaginal discharge, loss of mucus plug, pelvic pain, and pressure.

With the onset of labor, expect to monitor fetal heart rates continuously. Prepare the woman for an ultrasound to assess the presentation of each fetus to determine the best delivery approach. Ensure that extra nursing staff and the perinatal team are available for any birth or newborn complications.

After the babies are born, closely assess the woman for hemorrhage by frequently assessing uterine involution. Palpate the uterine fundus and monitor the amount and characteristics of lochia.

Throughout the entire pregnancy, birth, and hospital stay, inform and support the woman and her family. Encourage them to ask questions and verbalize any fears and concerns.

PREMATURE RUPTURE OF MEMBRANES

Premature rupture of membranes (PROMs) is the rupture of the bag of waters before the onset of true labor. There are a number of associated conditions and complications, such as infection, prolapsed cord, abruptio placentae, and preterm labor. High-risk factors associated with preterm PROM include low socioeconomic status, multiple gestation, low BMI, tobacco use, history of preterm labor, placenta previa, abruptio placentae, urinary tract infection, vaginal bleeding at any time in pregnancy, cerclage, and amniocentesis (Jazayeri, 2015).

If prolonged (greater than 24 hours), the woman's risk for infection (chorioamnionitis, endometritis, sepsis, and neonatal infections) increases and continues to increase the longer the time since the bag of waters ruptured. The time interval from rupture of membranes to the onset of regular contractions is termed the latent period.

Women with PROM present with leakage of fluid, vaginal discharge, vaginal bleeding, and pelvic pressure, but they are not having contractions. PROM is diagnosed by speculum vaginal examination of the cervix and vaginal cavity. Pooling of fluid in the vagina or leakage of fluid from the cervix, ferning of the dried fluid under microscopic examination, and alkalinity of the fluid as determined by nitrazine paper (ph indicator) confirm the diagnosis.

The terminology of PROM can be confusing. PROM is rupture of the membranes prior to the onset of labor and is used appropriately when referring to a woman who is beyond 37 weeks' gestation, has presented with spontaneous rupture of the membranes, and is not in labor. A related term is **preterm premature rupture of membranes (PPROM)**, which is defined as rupture of membranes prior to the onset of labor in a woman who is *less* than 37 weeks' gestation. Perinatal risks associated with PPROM may stem from immaturity, including respiratory distress syndrome, intraventricular hemorrhage, patent ductus arteriosus, and necrotizing enterocolitis. Eighty-five percent of neonatal morbidity and mortality is a result of prematurity. PPROM is associated with 30% to 40% of preterm deliveries and is the leading identifiable cause of preterm delivery. PPROM complicates 3% of all pregnancies and occurs in approximately 150,000 pregnancies yearly in the United States (Jazayeri, 2015).

The exact cause of PROM is not known, but may be associated with vaginal bleeding, placental abruption, microbial invasion of the amniotic cavity, and defective placentation. In many cases, PROM occurs spontaneously. Increasing evidence associates abnormalities in vaginal flora during pregnancy with preterm labor and birth with potential neonatal sequelae due to prematurity and poor perinatal outcome (Gilbert, 2014). A recent study found that women with previous PPROM are at increased risk for recurrence, and a short interval between pregnancies is associated with increased risk (Gibbins et al., 2014).

Therapeutic Management

Treatment of PROM typically depends on the gestational age. Under no circumstances is an unsterile digital cervical examination done until the woman enters active labor, to minimize infection exposure. If the fetal lungs are mature, induction of labor is initiated. PROM is not a lone indicator for surgical birth. If the fetal lungs are immature, expectant management is carried out with adequate hydration, reduced physical activity, pelvic rest, and close observation for possible infection, such as with frequent monitoring of vital signs and laboratory test results (e.g., the white blood cell count). Corticosteroids may be given to enhance fetal lung maturity if lungs are immature, although this remains controversial. Recent studies have shown clear benefits of antibiotics to decrease neonatal morbidity associated with PPROM (Mattson & Smith, 2016).

Nursing Assessment

Nursing assessment focuses on obtaining a complete health history and performing a physical examination to determine maternal and fetal status. An accurate assessment of the gestational age and knowledge of the maternal, fetal, and neonatal risks are essential to appropriate evaluation, counseling, and management of women with PROM and PPROM. Nurses need to be aware that the risk of infection increases with the duration of PPROM.

Health History and Physical Examination

Review the maternal history for risk factors such as infection, increased uterine size (polyhydramnios, macrosomia, multiple gestation), uterine and fetal anomalies, lower socioeconomic status, STIs, cervical insufficiency, vaginal bleeding, and cigarette smoking during pregnancy. Ask about any history or current symptoms of urinary tract infection (frequency, urgency, dysuria, or flank pain) or pelvic or vaginal infection (pain or vaginal discharge).

Assess for signs and symptoms of labor, such as cramping, pelvic pressure, or back pain. Also assess her vital signs, noting any signs indicative of infection such as fever and elevated white blood cell count (more than 18,000 cells/mm^3) (Nagtalon-Ramos, 2014).

Institute continuous electronic fetal heart rate monitoring to evaluate fetal well-being. Conduct a vaginal examination to ascertain the cervical status in PROM. If PPROM exists, a sterile speculum examination (where the examiner inspects the cervix but does not palpate it) is done rather than a digital cervical examination because it may diminish latency (period of time from rupture of membranes to birth) and increase newborn morbidity (Cunningham et al., 2014).

Observe the characteristics of the amniotic fluid. Note any evidence of meconium, or a foul odor. When meconium is present in the amniotic fluid, it typically indicates fetal distress related to hypoxia. Meconium stains the fluid yellow to greenish brown, depending on the amount present. A foul odor of amniotic fluid indicates infection. Also observe the amount of fluid. A decreased amount of amniotic fluid reduces the cushioning effect, thereby making cord compression a possibility. Some research shows that restoring the volume of lost amniotic fluid will help to reduce the risk of infection and reduce cord compression. See Evidence-Based Practice 19.1. Key assessments are summarized in Box 19.3.

EVIDENCE-BASED PRACTICE 19.1   A LOW-DOSE ASPIRIN FOR PREVENTING PREECLAMPSIA AND ITS COMPLICATIONS: A META-ANALYSIS

STUDY

Preeclampsia is a major cause of perinatal mortality and morbidity worldwide. The etiology of it remains unclear, but it is thought that the condition arises because of abnormal trophoblastic invasion of uterine vessels or endothelial cell activation and dysfunction. Low-dose aspirin is thought to prevent preeclampsia in high-risk pregnancy, but it is not universally used because of safety concerns. The World Health Organization (WHO) and the US Preventive Services Task Force (USPSTF) both recommend using low-dose aspirin in women at high risk for preeclampsia. A systematic review and meta-analysis were analyzed using 29 studies involving 21,403 women.

Findings

The meta-analysis showed that low-dose aspirin significantly reduced the incidence of preeclampsia. Risk of preeclampsia was reduced when initiated before 16 weeks gestation. Prophylactic low-dose aspirin, especially initiated before 16 weeks' gestation, is effective at preventing preeclampsia, preterm birth, and fetal growth restriction in high-risk pregnancies.

Nursing Implications

Based on the study's results, nurses can be involved in prenatal assessments of the high-risk mother to identify them early so that prophylactic low-dose aspirin can be prescribed if deemed appropriate by the health care provider. The nurse can provide instruction and rationales for the use and timing of this therapy to the clients. Two major professional health organizations have recommended this therapy to prevent preeclampsia, so nurses can view this therapy as an evidence-based intervention to promote better outcomes for mothers and their infants.

Adapted from Xu, T. T., Zhou, F., Deng, C. Y., Huang, G. Q., Li, J. K., & Wang, X. D. (2015). Low-dose aspirin for preventing preeclampsia and its complications: A meta-analysis. *The Journal of Clinical Hypertension. 17*(7), 567–573.

BOX 19.3

KEY ASSESSMENTS WITH PREMATURE RUPTURE OF MEMBRANES

For the woman with PROM, the following assessments are essential:
- Determining the date, time, and duration of membrane rupture by client interview.
- Ascertaining gestational age of the fetus based on date of mother's last menstrual period, fundal height, and ultrasound dating.
- Questioning the woman about possible history of or recent UTI or vaginal infection that might have contributed to PROM.
- Assessing for any associated labor symptoms, such as back pain or pelvic pressure.
- Assisting with or performing diagnostic tests to validate leakage of fluid, such as Nitrazine test, "ferning" on slide, and ultrasound. Contamination of Nitrazine tape with lubricant or insufficient fluid will render the assessment unreliable.
- Continually assessing for signs of infection including:
  - Elevation of maternal temperature and pulse rate
  - Abdominal/uterine tenderness
  - Fetal tachycardia more than 160 bpm
  - Elevated white blood cell count and C-reactive protein
  - Cloudy, foul-smelling amniotic fluid

Adapted from Nagtalon-Ramos, J. (2014). *Maternal-newborn nursing care: Best evidence-based practices*. Philadelphia, PA: F. A. Davis Company; Cunningham, F. G., Leveno, K. J., Bloom, S. L., Spong, C. Y., Dashe, J. S., Hoffman, B. L., et al. (2014). *Williams' obstetrics* (24th ed.). New York, NY: McGraw-Hill Education; and Magowan, B. A., Owen, P., & Thomson, A. (2014). *Clinical obstetrics & gynecology* (3rd ed.). St. Louis, MO: Saunders Elsevier.

Laboratory and Diagnostic Testing

To diagnose PROM or PPROM, several procedures may be used: the nitrazine test, fern test, or ultrasound. After the insertion of a sterile speculum, a sample of the fluid in the vaginal area is obtained. With a nitrazine test, the pH of the fluid is tested; amniotic fluid is more basic (7.0) than normal vaginal secretions (4.5). Nitrazine paper turns blue in the presence of amniotic fluid. However, false-positive results can occur if blood, urine, semen, or antiseptic chemicals are also present; all will increase the pH.

For the fern test, a sample of vaginal fluid is place on a slide to be viewed directly under a microscope. Amniotic fluid will develop a fern-like pattern when it dries because of sodium chloride crystallization. If both of these tests are inconclusive, a transvaginal ultrasound can also be used to determine whether membranes have ruptured by demonstrating a decreased amount of amniotic fluid (oligohydramnios) in the uterus (Jazayeri, 2015).

Other laboratory and diagnostic tests that may be used include:
- Urinalysis and urine culture for UTI or asymptomatic bacteriuria
- Cervical test or culture for chlamydia or gonorrhea
- Vaginal culture for bacterial vaginosis and trichomoniasis
- Vaginal introital/rectal culture for group B streptococcus

Nursing Management

Nursing management for the woman with PROM or PPROM focuses on preventing infection and identifying uterine contractions. The risk for infection is great because of the break in the amniotic fluid membrane and its proximity to vaginal bacteria. Therefore, monitor maternal vital signs closely. Be alert for a temperature elevation or an increase in pulse, which could indicate infection. Also monitor the fetal heart rate continuously, reporting any fetal tachycardia (which could indicate a maternal infection) or variable decelerations (suggesting cord compression). If variable decelerations are present, anticipate amnioinfusion based on agency policy. Evaluate the results of laboratory tests such as a CBC. An elevation in white blood cells would suggest infection. Administer antibiotics if ordered.

Encourage the woman and her partner to verbalize their feelings and concerns. Educate them about the purpose of the protective membranes and the implications of early rupture. Keep them informed about planned interventions, including potential complications and required therapy. As appropriate, prepare the woman for induction or augmentation of labor as appropriate if she is near term.

If labor does not start within 48 hours, the woman with PPROM may be discharged home on expectant management, which may include:
- Antibiotics if cervicovaginal cultures are positive
- Activity restrictions
- Education about signs and symptoms of infection and when to call with problems or concerns (Teaching Guidelines 19.3)
- Frequent fetal testing for well-being
- Ultrasound every 3 to 4 weeks to assess amniotic fluid levels
- Possible corticosteroid treatment depending on gestational age
- Daily kick counts to assess fetal well-being

Teaching Guidelines 19.3

TEACHING FOR THE WOMAN WITH PPROM

- Monitor your baby's activity by performing fetal kick counts daily.
- Check your temperature daily and report any temperature increases to your health care provider.
- Watch for signs related to the beginning of labor. Report any tightening of the abdomen or contractions.
- Avoid any touching or manipulating of your breasts, which could stimulate labor.
- Do not insert anything into your vagina or vaginal area—no tampons, avoid vaginal intercourse
- Do not swim in pools or in the ocean or sit in a hot tub or Jacuzzi.
- Take showers for daily hygiene needs; avoid sitting in a tub bath.
- Maintain any specific activity restrictions as recommended.
- Wash your hands thoroughly after using the bathroom and make sure to wipe from front to back each time.
- Keep your perineal area clean and dry.
- Take your antibiotics as directed if your health care provider has prescribed them.
- Call your health care provider with changes in your condition, including fever, uterine tenderness, feeling like your heart is racing, and foul-smelling vaginal discharge.

KEY CONCEPTS

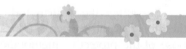

- Identifying risk factors early on and throughout the pregnancy is important to ensure the best outcome for every pregnancy. Risk assessment should start with the first prenatal visit and continue with subsequent visits.

- The three most common causes of hemorrhage early in pregnancy (first half of pregnancy) are spontaneous abortion, ectopic pregnancy, and GTD.

- Ectopic pregnancies occur in about 1 in 50 pregnancies and have increased dramatically during the past few decades.

- Having a molar pregnancy results in the loss of the pregnancy and the possibility of developing choriocarcinoma, a chronic malignancy from the trophoblastic tissue.

- The classic clinical picture presentation for placenta previa is painless, bright-red vaginal bleeding occurring during the third trimester.

- Treatment of abruptio placentae is designed to assess, control, and restore the amount of blood lost; to provide a positive outcome for both mother and infant; and to prevent coagulation disorders.

- DIC can be described in simplest terms as a loss of balance between the clot-forming activity of thrombin and the clot-lysing activity of plasmin.

- Hyperemesis gravidarum is a complication of pregnancy characterized by persistent, uncontrollable nausea and vomiting before the 20th week of gestation.

- Gestational hypertension is the leading cause of maternal death in the United States and the most common complication reported during pregnancy.

- HELLP is an acronym for hemolysis, elevated liver enzymes, and low platelets.

- Rh incompatibility is a condition that develops when a woman of Rh-negative blood type is exposed to Rh-positive fetal blood cells and subsequently develops circulating titers of Rh antibodies.

- Polyhydramnios occurs in approximately 3% to 4% of all pregnancies and is associated with fetal anomalies of development.

- Nursing care related to the woman with oligohydramnios involves continuous monitoring of fetal well-being during nonstress testing or during labor and birth by identifying category II and III patterns on the fetal monitor.

- The increasing number of multiple gestations is a concern because women who are expecting more than one infant are at high risk for preterm labor, hydramnios, hyperemesis gravidarum, anemia, preeclampsia, and antepartum hemorrhage.

- Nursing care related to PROM centers on infection prevention and identification of preterm labor contractions.

- Monitoring maternal vital signs for changes and the fetal hearth rate once PPROM occurs is essential to increasing the changes of a good outcome.

- It is essential that nurses educate all pregnant women how to detect the early signs of PROM and what action is needed if it happens.

References and Recommended Readings

Abu Hashim, H., Al-Inany, H., & Kilani, Z. (2014). A review of the contemporary evidence on rescue cervical cerclage. *International Journal of Gynecology & Obstetrics, 124*(3), 198–203.

Agarwal, N., & Odejinmi, F. (2014). Early abdominal ectopic pregnancy: Challenges, update and review of current management. *Obstetrician & Gynecologist, 16*(3), 193–198.

Agency for Healthcare Research and Quality [AHRQ] (2015). *Cerclage for the management of cervical insufficiency.* Retrieved from http://www.guideline.gov/content.aspx?id=47771

American Cancer Society [ACS] (2015). *Gestational trophoblastic disease.* Retrieved from http://www.cancer.org/cancer/gestation-altrophoblasticdisease/detailedguide/gestational-trophoblastic-disease-key-statistics

American College of Obstetricians and Gynecologists [ACOG] (2014a) Practice bulletin no. 142: Cerclage for the management of cervical insufficiency. *Obstetrics & Gynecology, 123*(2), 372–379.

American College of Obstetricians and Gynecologists [ACOG] (2014b). *Placenta accreta.* Retrieved from http://www.acog.org/Resources-And-Publications/Committee-Opinions/Committee-on-Obstetric-Practice/Placenta-Accreta

American College of Obstetricians and Gynecologists [ACOG] (2014c). ACOG task force on hypertension in pregnancy—A step forward in management. *Contemporary OB/GYN.* Retrieved from http://contemporaryobgyn.modernmedicine.com/contemporary-obgyn/news/acog-task-force-hypertension-pregnancy-step-forward-management?page=full

Amorim, M. M., Katz, L., Barros, A. S., Almeida, T. S., Souza, A. S. R., & Faúndes, A. (2015). Maternal outcomes according to mode of delivery in women with severe preeclampsia: a cohort study. *The Journal of Maternal-Fetal & Neonatal Medicine, 28*(6), 654–660.

Ananth, C. V., & Kinzler, W. L. (2015). Placental abruption: Clinical features and diagnosis. *UpToDate.* Retrieved from http://www.uptodate.com/contents/placental-abruption-clinical-features-and-diagnosis

Archibong, E. I., & Ahmed, E. S. (2015). Risk factors maternal and neonatal outcome in major placenta previa: A prospective study. *Annals of Saudi Medicine, 21*(3-4), 245–247.

Ardehali, A., & Casikar, I. (2015). Identification of risk factors of ectopic pregnancy. In T. Tulandi (Ed.), *Ectopic pregnancy A clinical casebook* (pp. 1–10). Switzerland: Springer International Publishing.

ARUP Laboratories (2016). *Disseminated intravascular coagulation.* Retrieved from https://arupconsult.com/content/disseminated-intravascular-coagulation

Atkinson, A. L., Santolaya-Forgas, J., Blitzer, D. N., Santolaya, J. L., Matta, P., Canterino, J., et al. (2015). Risk factors for perinatal mortality in patients admitted to the hospital with the diagnosis of placental abruption. *The Journal of Maternal-Fetal & Neonatal Medicine, 28*(5), 594–597.

Ayyavoo, A., Derraik, J. B., Hofman, P. L., & Cutfield, W. S. (2014). Hyperemesis gravidarum and long-term health of the offspring. *American Journal of Obstetrics & Gynecology, 210*(6), 521–525.

Berghella, V. (2014). Cervical insufficiency. *UpToDate.* Retrieved from http://www.uptodate.com/contents/cervical-insufficiency

Berkowitz, R. S., Goldstein, D. P., & Horowitz, N. S. (2014). Management options of gestational trophoblastic disease. *Current Obstetrics and Gynecology Reports, 3*(1), 76–83.

Boots, A. B., Sanchez-Ramos, L., Bowers, D. M., Kaunitz, A. M., Zamora, J., & Schlattmann, P. (2014). The short-term prediction of preterm birth: a systematic review and diagnostic metaanalysis. *American Journal of Obstetrics and Gynecology, 210*(1), 54.e1–54.e10.

Bourne, T. (2015). A missed opportunity for excellence: the NICE guideline on the diagnosis and initial management of ectopic pregnancy and miscarriage. *Journal of Family Planning and Reproductive Health Care, 41*(1), 13–19.

Bujold, E. (2015). Low-dose aspirin reduces morbidity and mortality in pregnant women at high-risk for preeclampsia. *Evidence Based Nursing, 18*(3), 71.

Carson, M. P., & Gibson, P. S. (2015). Hypertension and pregnancy. *eMedicine.* Retrieved from http://emedicine.medscape.com/article/261435-overview

Carter, B. S., & Boyd, R. L. (2015). Polyhydramnios and oligohydramnios. *eMedicine.* Retrieved from http://reference.medscape.com/article/975821-overview

Castillo, M. J., & Phillippi, J. C. (2015). Hyperemesis gravidarum: A holistic overview and approach to clinical assessment and management. *The Journal of Perinatal & Neonatal Nursing, 29*(1), 12–22.

Clausen, T. D., & Bergholt, T. (2014). Chronic hypertension during pregnancy. *BMJ: British Medical Journal. 348,* g2655.6.

Cohen, A., Zakar, L., Gil, Y., Amer-Alshiek, J., Bibi, G., Almog, B., & Levin, I. (2015). Methotrexate success rates in progressing ectopic pregnancies: A reappraisal. *Obstetrical & Gynecological Survey, 70*(2), 88–89.

Creasy, R. K., Resnik, R., Iams, J. D., Lockwood, C. J., Moore, T. R., & Greene, M. F. (2014). *Creasy and Resnik's maternal-fetal medicine: Principles and practice* (7th ed.). Philadelphia, PA: Elsevier.

Cunningham, F. G., Leveno, K. J., Bloom, S. L., Spong, C. Y., Dashe, J. S., Hoffman, B. L., et al. (2014). *Williams' obstetrics* (24th ed.). New York, NY: McGraw-Hill Education.

Dalia, S., Price, S., Forsyth, P., Sokol, L., & Jaglal, M. (2014). What is the optimal dose of high dose methotrexate in the initial treatment of primary Central Nervous System lymphoma?. *Leukemia & Lymphoma, 1*–7. doi:10.3109/10428194.2014.927458

Davidson, M. R. (2014). *Fast facts for the neonatal nurse: A nursing orientation & care guide in a nutshell.* New York, NY: Springer Publishing Company.

Davis, S. J., & Kessler, C. M. (2014). Disseminated intravascular coagulation: Diagnosis and management. In H. I. Saba & H. R. Roberts (Eds.), *Hemostasis and thrombosis: Practical Guidelines in Clinical Management* (pp. 151–168). Hoboken, NJ: Wiley Blackwell.

Deering, S. H. (2015). Abruptio placenta. *eMedicine.* Retrieved from http://emedicine.medscape.com/article/252810-overview

Dekker, G. A. (2014). Management of preeclampsia. *Pregnancy hypertension: An International Journal of Women's Cardiovascular Health, 4*(3), 246–247.

Desai, D., Lu, J., Wyness, S. P., Greene, D. N., Olson, K. N., Wiley, C. L., et al. (2014). Human chorionic gonadotropin discriminatory zone in ectopic pregnancy: does assay harmonization matter?. *Fertility and Sterility, 101*(6), 1671–1674.

De Sutter, P. (2015). The challenge of multiple pregnancies. In *Reducing risk in fertility treatment* (pp. 1–17). London, England: Springer Publishers.

Dickson, E. L., & Mullany, S. A. (2015). Gestational trophoblastic disease. In *Gynecologic oncology* (pp. 175–201). New York, NY: Springer.

Foley, M., Strong, T. M., & Garite, T. (2014). *Obstetric intensive care manual* (4th ed.), New York, NY: McGraw-Hill Publishers.

Foo, L., Tay, J., Lees, C. C., McEniery, C. M., & Wilkinson, I. B. (2015). Hypertension in pregnancy: Natural history and treatment options. *Current Hypertension Reports, 17*(5), 1–18.

Gibbins, K., Esplin, M. S., Varner, M., Eller, A., & Manuck, T. (2014). 835: Subsequent pregnancy outcomes among women with a history of preterm premature rupture of membranes (PPROM) <24.0 weeks gestation. *American Journal of Obstetrics & Gynecology, 210*(1), S405–S406.

Gilbert, R. (2014). Immediate delivery for group B streptococci-colonized women with preterm premature rupture of membranes. Don't forget the antibiotics. *BJOG: An International Journal of Obstetrics & Gynecology.* doi: 10.1111/1471-0528.12940

Hensley, J., & Shviraga, B. (2014). Metastatic choriocarcinoma in a term pregnancy: A case study. *MCN. The American Journal of Maternal Child Nursing, 39*(1), 8–15.

Herrera, K., & Lewis, D. (2014). Cervical insufficiency and cerclage. *Postgraduate Obstetrics & Gynecology, 34*(3), 1–5.

Holt, J. L. (2015). Multidisciplinary care of a woman experiencing obstetric hemorrhage. *Journal of Obstetric, Gynecologic, & Neonatal Nursing, 44*: S85–S86.

Hosein, H., Abdel-Kariem, R., & Shriki, J. E. (2014). Placental abruption imaging. *eMedicine.* Retrieved from http://emedicine.medscape.com/article/402314-overview

Humphrey, J. (2015). Primary cesarean delivery results in emergency hysterectomy due to placenta accreta: a case study. *AANA Journal, 83*(1), 28–34.

Infante, F., Menakaya, U., & Condous, G. (2014). Medical treatment of ectopic pregnancy. *Fertility and Sterility, 101*(3), e16–22. http://dx.doi.org/10.1016/j.fertnstert.2013.12.013

Jaju, K. G., Kulkarni, A. P., & Mundada, S. K. (2014). Study of perinatal outcome in relation to abruptio placentae. *International Journal of Recent Trends in Science and Technology, 11*(3), 355–358.

Jazayeri, A. (2015). Premature rupture of membranes. *eMedicine.* Retrieved from http://emedicine.medscape.com/article/261137-overview

Jena, S. K., Samal, S., Behera, B. K., & Allms, B. (2015). Cervical cerclage in modern obstetrics: A review. *Health, 3*(1), 9–14.

Jones, R. E., & Lopez, K. H. (2014). *Human reproductive biology* (4th ed.). Waltham, MA: Academic Press/Elsevier.

Joy, S., & Temming, L. (2015). Placenta previa. *eMedicine*. Retrieved from http://emedicine.medscape.com/article/262063-overview

Kao, L., Scheinfeld, M., Chernyak, V., Rozenblit, A., Oh, S., & Dym, R. (2014). Beyond ultrasound: CT and MRI of ectopic pregnancy. *American Journal of Roentgenology, 202*(4), 904–911.

Khan, H., & Meirowitz, N. B. (2015). HELLP syndrome. *eMedicine*. Retrieved from http://emedicine.medscape.com/article/1394126-overview

King, T. L., Brucker, M. C., Kriebs, J. M., Fahey, J. O., Grgor, C. L., & Varney, H. (2015). *Varney's midwifery* (5th ed.), Burlington, MA: Jones & Bartlett Learning.

Ko, J., & Cheung, V. (2014). Time to revisit the human chorionic gonadotropin discriminatory level in the management of pregnancy of unknown location. *Journal of Ultrasound in Medicine, 33*(3), 465–471.

Kobayashi, T. (2014). Obstetrical disseminated intravascular coagulation score. *Journal of Obstetrics and Gynecology Research, 40*(6), 1500–1506.

Knez, J., Day, A., & Jurkovic, D. (2014). Ultrasound imaging in the management of bleeding and pain in early pregnancy. *Best Practice & Research Clinical Obstetrics & Gynecology. 28*(5), 621–636.

Magee, L. A., Pels, A., Helewa, M., Rey, E., von Dadelszen, P., Audibert, F., et al. (2015). The hypertensive disorders of pregnancy (29.3). *Best Practice & Research Clinical Obstetrics & Gynecology, 29*(5):643–657.

Magowan, B. A., Owen, P., & Thomson, A. (2014). *Clinical obstetrics & gynecology* (3rd ed.). St. Louis, MO: Saunders Elsevier.

Maltepe, C., Popa, M. V., Bertucci, C., Farine, D., Koren, G., & Nulman, I. (2015). The effects of counseling and predictors of pregnancy outcomes in women with hyperemesis gravidarum [316]. *Obstetrics & Gynecology, 125*, 101S.

March of Dimes (2015a) *Pregnancy loss.* Retrieved from http://www.marchofdimes.com/loss/stillbirth.aspx

March of Dimes (2015b). *Ectopic pregnancy.* Retrieved from http://www.marchofdimes.com/loss/ectopic-pregnancy.aspx

March of Dimes (2015c). *Placenta accreta, increta, and percreta.* Retrieved from http://www.marchofdimes.com/pregnancy/placental-accreta-increta-and-percreta.aspx

March of Dimes (2015d). *Rh disease.* Retrieved from http://www.marchofdimes.com/baby/rh-disease.aspx

March of Dimes (2015e). *Oligohydramnios.* Retrieved from http://www.marchofdimes.com/pregnancy/oligohydramnios.aspx

March of Dimes (2015f). *Multiples: Twins, triplets and beyond.* Retrieved from http://www.marchofdimes.com/pregnancy/multiples-twins-triplets-and-beyond.aspx

Marik, P. E. (Ed.) (2015). Pregnancy related disorders. In *Evidence-based critical care* (pp. 759–772). Switzerland: Springer International Publishing.

Martin, R. J., Fanaroff, A. A., & Walsh, M. C. (2014). *Fanaroff & Martin's neonatal-perinatal medicine* (10th ed.), Philadelphia, PA: Elsevier Health Sciences.

Matthews, A., Haas, D. M., O'Mathúna, D. P., Dowswell, T., & Doyle, M. (2014). Interventions for nausea and vomiting in early pregnancy. *Cochrane Database of Systematic Reviews*, (3):CD007575.

Mattson, S., & Smith, J. E. (2016). *Core curriculum for maternal-newborn nursing* (5th ed.). St. Louis, MO: Saunders Elsevier.

Miller, M. A., & Carpenter, M. (2015). Hypertensive disorders of pregnancy. In *Medical management of the pregnant patient* (pp. 177–193). New York, NY: Springer Publishers.

Moore, T. R. (2015). Abnormal amniotic fluid. *Protocols for high-risk pregnancies: An evidence-based approach* (pp. 315–328). West Sussex, UK: John Wiley & Sons.

Moses, S. (2015a) Placental abruption. *Family Practice Notebook.* Retrieved from http://www.fpnotebook.com/ob/Bleed/PlcntlAbrptn.htm

Moses, S. (2015b) HELLP syndrome. *Family Practice Notebook.* Retrieved from http://www.fpnotebook.com/hemeonc/OB/HlpSyndrm.htm

Mukherjee, S., Bawa, A. K., Sharma, S., Nandanwar, Y. S., & Gadam, M. (2014). Retrospective study of risk factors and maternal and fetal outcome in patients with abruptio placentae. *Journal of Natural Science, Biology and Medicine, 5*(2), 425–428.

Nagtalon-Ramos, J. (2014). *Maternal-newborn nursing care: Best evidence-based practices.* Philadelphia, PA: F.A. Davis Company.

National High Blood Pressure Education Program Working Group on High Blood Pressure in Pregnancy. (2002). Working Group in High Blood Pressure in Pregnancy report. *American Journal of Obstetrics and Gynecology, 183*, S1–S22.

Nguyen, N., & Slim, R. (2014). Genetics and epigenetics of recurrent hydatidiform moles: Basic science and genetic counselling. *Current Obstetrics and Gynecology Reports, 3*, 55–64.

Norwitz, E. R. (2015). Eclampsia. *UpToDate*. Retrieved from http://www.uptodate.com/contents/eclampsia

Norwitz, E. R., & Conroy, K. E. (2015). Cervical insufficiency. *eMedicine*. Retrieved from http://emedicine.medscape.com/article/1979914-overview

Ogunyemi, D. A., Fong, A., & Herrero, T. C. (2015). Hyperemesis gravidarum. *eMedicine*. Retrieved from http://emedicine.medscape.com/article/254751-overview

Pauli, J. M., & Repke, J. T. (2015). Preeclampsia: Short-term and long-term implications. *Obstetrics and Gynecology Clinics of North America, 42*(2), 299–313.

Peled, Y., Melamed, N., Hiersch, L., Pardo, J., Wiznitzer, A., & Yogev, Y. (2014). The impact of total parenteral nutrition support on pregnancy outcome in women with hyperemesis gravidarum. *Journal of Maternal-Fetal & Neonatal Medicine, 27*(11), 1146–1150.

Randall, S., & LaMontagne, D. S. (2015). Screening for chlamydia: Seize the day. *Journal of Family Planning and Reproductive Health Care, 31*(2), 98–100.

Ross, M. G. (2015). Eclampsia. *eMedicine*. Retrieved from http://emedicine.medscape.com/article/253960-overview

Salem, L., & Singer, K. R. (2015). Rh incompatibility. *eMedicine*. Retrieved from http://emedicine.medscape.com/article/797150-overview

Schultz, W., & McConachie, I. (2015). Vital signs after hemorrhage–caution is appropriate. *Trends in Anesthesia and Critical Care.* doi: http://dx.doi.org/10.1016/j.tacc.2015.04.001

Sepilian, V., & Wood, E. (2015). Ectopic pregnancy. *eMedicine*. Retrieved from http://emedicine.medscape.com/article/2041923-overview

Sibai, B. M. (2015). HELLP syndrome. UpToDate. Retrieved from http://www.uptodate.com/contents/hellp-syndrome

Skidmore-Roth, L. (2015). *Mosby's 2015 nursing drug reference* (28th ed.). Philadelphia, PA: Elsevier Health Science.

Smith, J. A., Refuerzo, J. S., & Ramin, S. M. (2016). Nausea and vomiting of pregnancy: Beyond the basics. *UpToDate*, Retrieved from http://www.uptodate.com/contents/nausea-and-vomiting-of-pregnancy-beyond-the-basics

Staneva, A., Bogossian, F., Pritchard, M., & Wittkowski, A. (2015). The effects of maternal depression, anxiety, and perceived stress during pregnancy on preterm birth: A systematic review. *Women and Birth.* doi:10.1016/j.wombi.2015.02.003.

Strohl, A. E., & Lurain, J. R. (2014). Clinical epidemiology of gestational trophoblastic disease. *Current Obstetrics and Gynecology Reports, 3*(1), 40–43.

Szypulski, H. (2015). Practice guideline to prevent ectopic pregnancy rupture. *International Journal of Childbirth Education, 30*(1), 59–62.

Tan, P., Zaidi, S., Azmi, N., Omar, S., & Khong, S. (2014). Depression, anxiety, stress and hyperemesis gravidarum: Temporal and case controlled correlates. *Plos ONE, 9*(3), 1–7.

Taylor, T. (2014). Treatment of nausea and vomiting in pregnancy. *Australian Prescriber, 37*(2), 42–45.

Tulandi, T. (2015). Medical treatment of ectopic pregnancy. In Tulandi T. (Ed.), *Ectopic pregnancy: A clinical casebook* (pp. 49–53). Switzerland: Springer International Publishing.

Tulandi, T., & Al-Fozan, H. M. (2015). Spontaneous abortion: Risk factors, etiology, clinical manifestations, and diagnostic evaluation. *UpToDate*, Retrieved from http://www.uptodate.com/contents/spontaneous-abortion-risk-factors-etiology-clinical-manifestations-and-diagnostic-evaluation

Urquhart, C., Currell, R., Harlow, F., & Callow, L.. (2015) Home uterine monitoring for detecting preterm labor. *Cochrane Database of Systematic Reviews*, (1):CD006172.

U.S. Department of Health and Human Services. (2010). *Healthy People 2020.* Retrieved from http://www.healthypeople.gov/2020/topicsobjectives2020/

Verklan, T., & Walden, M. (2014). *Core curriculum for neonatal inten-sive care nursing* (4th ed.). St. Louis, MO: Saunders Elsevier.

Vigil-De Gracia, P. (2015). HELLP syndrome. *Ginecología Y Obstetricia De México, 83*(1), 48–57.

Wiedaseck, S., & Monchek, R. (2014). Placental and cord insertion pathologies: Screening, diagnosis, and management. *Journal of Midwifery & Women's Health, 59*(3), 328–335.

World Health Organization [WHO]. (2015). *Skilled birth attendants.* Retrieved from http://www.who.int/reproductivehealth/topics/mdgs/skilled_birth_attendant/en/

Xu, T. T., Zhou, F., Deng, C. Y., Huang, G. Q., Li, J. K., & Wang, X. D. (2015). Low-dose aspirin for preventing preeclampsia and its complications: A meta-analysis. *The Journal of Clinical Hyperten-sion. 17*(7), 567–573.

Zainul Rashid, M. R., Lim, J., Nawawi, N. M., Luqman, M., Zolkeplai, M., Rangkuty, H., et al. (2014). A pilot study to determine whether progestogen supplementation using dydrogesterone during the first trimester will reduce the incidence of gestational hyper-tension in primigravidae. *Gynecological Endocrinology, 30*(3), 217–220.

MULTIPLE CHOICE QUESTIONS

1. Which of the following women should receive Rho-GAM postpartum?
   a. Nonsensitized Rh-negative mother with an Rh-negative newborn
   b. Nonsensitized Rh-negative mother with an Rh-positive newborn
   c. Sensitized Rh-negative mother with an Rh-positive newborn
   d. Sensitized Rh-negative mother with an Rh-negative newborn

2. A woman is suspected of having abruptio placentae. Which of the following would the nurse expect to assess as a classic symptom?
   a. Painless, bright-red bleeding
   b. "Knife-like" abdominal pain
   c. Excessive nausea and vomiting
   d. Hypertension and headache

3. RhoGAM is given to Rh-negative women to prevent maternal sensitization. In addition to pregnancy, Rh-negative women would also receive this medication after which of the following?
   a. Therapeutic or spontaneous abortion
   b. Head injury from a car accident
   c. Blood transfusion after a hemorrhage
   d. Unsuccessful artificial insemination procedure

4. After teaching a woman about hyperemesis gravidarum and how it differs from the typical nausea and vomiting of pregnancy, which statement by the woman indicates that the teaching was successful?
   a. "I can expect the nausea to last through my second trimester."
   b. "I should drink fluids with my meals instead of in between them."
   c. "I need to avoid strong odors, perfumes, or flavors."
   d. "I should lie down after I eat for about 2 hours."

5. A pregnant woman, approximately 12 weeks' gestation, comes to the emergency department after calling her health care provider's office and reporting moderate vaginal bleeding. Assessment reveals cervical dilation and moderately strong abdominal cramps. She reports that she has passed some tissue with the bleeding. The nurse interprets these findings to suggest which of the following?
   a. Threatened abortion
   b. Inevitable abortion
   c. Incomplete abortion
   d. Missed abortion

6. When administering magnesium sulfate to a client with preeclampsia, the nurse explains to her that this drug is given to:
   a. Reduce blood pressure
   b. Increase the progress of labor
   c. Prevent seizures
   d. Lower blood glucose levels

7. A woman is being discharged after receiving treatment for a hydatidiform molar pregnancy. The nurse should include which of the following in her discharge teaching?
   a. Do not become pregnant for at least a year; use contraceptives to prevent it
   b. Have the client's blood pressure checked weekly in the clinic
   c. RhoGAM must be given within the next month to her at the clinic
   d. An amniocentesis can detect a recurrence of this disorder in the future

CRITICAL THINKING EXERCISE

1. A 16-year-old primigravida, presents to the maternity clinic complaining of continual nausea and vomiting for the past 3 days. She states that she is approximately 15 weeks pregnant and has been unable to hold anything down or take any fluids in without throwing up for the past 3 days. She reports she is dizzy and weak. On examination, Suzanne appears pale and anxious. Her mucous membranes are dry, skin turgor is poor, and her lips are dry and cracked.
   a. What is your impression of this condition?
   b. What risk factors does Suzanne have?
   c. What intervention is appropriate for this woman?

2. An obese 39-year-old primigravida of African–American descent who is diagnosed with gestational hypertension. Her history reveals that her sister developed preeclampsia during her pregnancy. When describing her diet to the nurse, this client mentions that she tends to eat a lot of fast food.
   a. What risk factors does this client have that increase her risk for gestational hypertension?
   b. When assessing this client, what assessment findings would lead the nurse to suspect that this client has developed severe preeclampsia?

STUDY ACTIVITIES

1. Ask a community health maternity nurse how the signs and symptoms of gestational hypertension (including preeclampsia and eclampsia) are taught, and how effective efforts have been to reduce the incidence in the area.

2. Find a website designed to help parents who have suffered a pregnancy loss secondary to a spontaneous abortion. What is its audience level? Is the information up to date?

3. A pregnancy in which the blastocyst implants outside the uterus is a/an _____ pregnancy.

4. The most serious complication of hydatidiform mole is the development of _____ afterward.

5. Discuss various activities a woman with a multiple gestation could engage in to help pass the time when ordered to be on bed rest at home for 2 months.

BRINGING IT ALL TOGETHER: CASE STUDY

A 21-year-old woman presented to the local Public Health maternity clinic with a chief complaint of intermittent vaginal bleeding, abdominal cramping, and nausea. She stated her last menstrual period was 8 weeks ago and she had done a home pregnancy test prior to coming here, which was positive. She was taking no medications and had no known drug allergies. She did admit that she was a half-pack a day smoker, but had been trying to quit.

ASSESSMENT

The nurse started to take her history which revealed that this client had been taking oral contraceptives until approximately 3 months ago when her copayment went up and she did not get her prescription filled because they did not have the money. She also reported that she had a dilation and curettage (D & C) for dysfunctional bleeding about a year ago because she did not respond to medications. Her sexual history revealed that she had five sexual partners in the past with inconsistent use of condoms with those partners. She had tested positive for gonorrhea and chlamydia and was treated for that about 6 months ago. Her retest was negative. Her vital signs were within normal range and the remainder of her physical examination was unremarkable.

Go to thePoint **to find questions to consider about this case.**

20

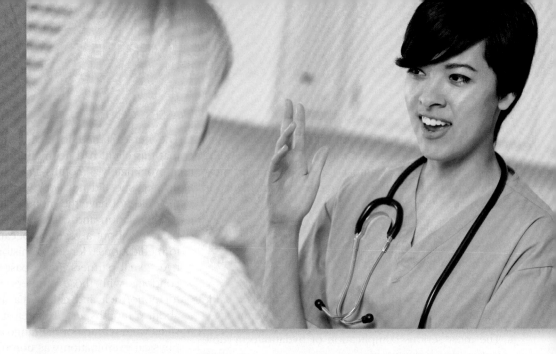

Nursing Management of the Pregnancy at Risk: Selected Health Conditions and Vulnerable Populations

Learning Objectives

Upon completion of the chapter, you will be able to:

1. Select at least two conditions present before pregnancy that can have a negative effect on a pregnancy.
2. Examine how a condition present before pregnancy can affect the woman physiologically and psychologically when she becomes pregnant.
3. Evaluate the nursing assessment and management for a pregnant woman with diabetes from that of a pregnant woman without diabetes.
4. Explore how congenital and acquired heart conditions can affect a woman's pregnancy.
5. Design the nursing assessment and management of a pregnant woman with cardiovascular disorders and respiratory conditions.
6. Differentiate among the types of anemia affecting pregnant women in terms of prevention and management.
7. Relate the nursing care needed for the pregnant woman with an autoimmune disorder.
8. Compare the most common infections that can jeopardize a pregnancy, and propose possible preventive strategies.
9. Develop a plan of care for the pregnant woman who is HIV positive.
10. Outline the nurse's role in the prevention and management of adolescent pregnancy.
11. Determine the impact of pregnancy on a woman over the age of 35.
12. Analyze the effects of substance abuse during pregnancy.

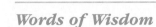

Rose, a thin 16-year-old appearing very pregnant, came into the clinic wheezing and having difficulty catching her breath. She had missed several previous prenatal visits but arrived at the clinic today in distress. Rose has a history of asthma since she was 5 years old. How might Rose's current condition affect her pregnancy? Is this picture typical of the pregnant woman with asthma?

Words of Wisdom
As the sun sets each day, nurses should make sure they have done something for others, and should try to be understanding even under the most difficult of conditions.

INTRODUCTION

Pregnancy and childbirth are exciting yet complex facets within the continuum of women's health. Pregnancy is a special time in most women's lives, but the 9-month waiting period can be very anxiety-producing if it is complicated by a medical condition which might complicate the pregnancy and jeopardize the fetal outcome. Ideally the pregnant woman is free of any conditions that can affect a pregnancy, but in reality many women enter pregnancy with a multitude of health-related or psychosocial issues that can have a negative impact on the outcome. Currently, because of the obesity epidemic in the nation and women postponing their pregnancies until later in their lives, nurses will increasingly see more women with medical conditions that affect their pregnancies.

Many pregnant women express the wish "I hope my baby is born healthy." Nurses can play a major role in helping this become a reality by educating women before they become pregnant. Conditions such as diabetes, cardiac and respiratory disorders, anemia, autoimmune disorders, and specific infections frequently can be controlled through close prenatal management so that their impact on pregnancy is minimized. Nurses can provide pregnancy prevention strategies when counseling teenagers. Meeting the developmental needs of pregnant adolescents is a challenge. Finally, lifestyle choices can place many women at risk during pregnancy, and nurses need to remain nonjudgmental when working with these special populations. Lifestyle choices such as use of alcohol, nicotine, and illicit substances during pregnancy are addressed in a *Healthy People 2020* goal.

Chapter 19 described pregnancy-related conditions that place the woman at risk. This chapter addresses common conditions that can have a negative impact on the pregnancy and special populations at risk, outlining appropriate nursing assessment and management for each condition or situation. The unique skills of nurses, in conjunction with the other members of the health care team, can increase the potential for a positive outcome in many high-risk pregnancies.

DIABETES MELLITUS

Diabetes mellitus is a chronic disease characterized by a relative lack of insulin or absence of the hormone that is necessary for glucose metabolism. The chronic hyperglycemia of diabetes is associated with long-term damage, dysfunction, and failure of the eyes, kidneys, nerves, heart, and blood vessels. The prevalence of diabetes in the United States is increasing at an alarming rate, already reaching epidemic proportions. Contributing factors to these increasing rates are more sedentary lifestyles, dietary changes, continued immigration by high-risk populations, and the growing epidemic of childhood and adolescent obesity. Currently, an estimated 20% of people over the age of 20 have undiagnosed prediabetes. This group of people is the pool from which childbearing women are drawn. Current estimates project that by 2025, one in three adults in the United States will have diabetes mellitus (Knox, Delaney, & Winterstein, 2014). The Institute for Alternative Futures estimates that the number of Americans living with diabetes (diagnosed and undiagnosed) will increase 64% by 2025. The resulting medical and societal cost of diabetes will be approximately $515 billion (Institute for Alternative Futures, 2015).

Diabetes commonly is classified based on disease etiology (American Diabetes Association [ADA], 2015a). These groups include:

- **Type 1 diabetes:** Absolute insulin deficiency (due to an autoimmune process); usually appears before the age of 30 years; approximately 5% % of those diagnosed have type 1 diabetes.
- **Type 2 diabetes:** Insulin resistance or deficiency (related to obesity, sedentary lifestyle); diagnosed primarily in adults older than 30 years of age but now being seen in children; the most common type of diabetes. It is more common in African Americans, Latinos, Native Americans, and Asian Americans/Pacific Islanders, as well as older adults.
- **Impaired fasting glucose *and* impaired glucose tolerance:** characterized by hyperglycemia at a level lower than what qualifies as a diagnosis of diabetes (fasting blood glucose level between 100 and 125 mg/dL; blood glucose level between 140 and 199 mg/dL after a 2-hour glucose tolerance test, respectively); symptoms of diabetes are absent; newborns are at risk for being large for gestational age (LGA).

HEALTHY PEOPLE 2020 • 20.1

Objective	Nursing Significance
Increase abstinence from alcohol, cigarettes, and illicit drugs among pregnant women	Will help to focus attention on measures for reducing substance exposure and use, thereby minimizing the effects of these substances on the fetus and newborn
Increase in reported abstinence in the past month from substances by pregnant women	
Alcohol from a baseline of 89.4% to 98.3%	
Binge drinking from a baseline of 95% to 100%	
Cigarette smoking from a baseline of 89.6% to 98.6%	
Illicit drugs from a baseline of 94.9% to 100%	

Healthy People objectives based on data from http://www.healthypeople.gov.

• **Gestational diabetes mellitus:** Glucose intolerance with its onset during pregnancy usually around the 24th week or first detected in pregnancy. The prevalence of gestational diabetes has been increasing in the United States and is as high as up to 10% in the United States.

During pregnancy, diabetes typically is categorized into two groups: **pregestational diabetes** (alteration in carbohydrate metabolism identified before conception), which includes women with type 1 or type 2 disease and gestational diabetes, which develops during pregnancy.

The International Association of Diabetes and Pregnancy Study Group has issued recommendations for diagnosing and classifying hyperglycemia in pregnancy (see Table 20.1).

Gestational diabetes is associated with either neonatal complications such as macrosomia, hypoglycemia, and birth trauma or maternal complications such as preeclampsia and cesarean birth. All women of childbearing age with diabetes should be counseled about the importance of strict glycemic control prior to conception. Observational studies show an increase risk of anencephaly, microcephaly, and congenital heart disease, which increases directly with elevations in their A1C (Lapolla & Dalfra, 2015).

Before the discovery of insulin in 1922, most women with diabetes were infertile or experienced spontaneous abortion (March of Dimes, 2015a). During the past several decades, great strides have been made in improving the outcomes of pregnancy in women with diabetes, but this chronic metabolic disorder remains a high-risk condition during pregnancy. A favorable outcome requires commitment on the woman's part to adhere to frequent prenatal visits, dietary restrictions, self-monitoring of blood glucose levels, frequent laboratory tests, intensive fetal surveillance, and perhaps hospitalization.

Pathophysiology

Diabetes is a complex and progressive disease that has major societal and economic impact. It is a multifactorial disease, the pathophysiology of which involves not only the pancreas but also the liver, skeletal muscle, adipose tissue, gastrointestinal tract, brain, and kidney. Reduced sensitivity to insulin in the liver, muscle, and adipose tissue, and a progressive decline in pancreatic beta cell function leads to impaired insulin secretion, eventually resulting in hyperglycemia, the hallmark of diabetes (Cornell, 2015). Current understanding of the pathophysiology of gestational diabetes includes two key components. These are the existence of pancreatic beta cell dysfunction prior to pregnancy and the unmasking of this problem by the development of insulin resistance during pregnancy, which requires enhanced insulin production to maintain normal blood glucose ranges.

Normal pregnancy is characterized by increasing peripheral resistance to insulin and a compensatory increase in insulin secretion. Therefore, pregnancy might be viewed as a stress test for the glucose homeostasis mechanisms. That is, women who have some degree of chronic insulin resistance and compensatory increased insulin production resulting in beta-cell dysfunction before pregnancy may be unable to mount a sufficiently robust beta-cell response to pregnancy-mediated insulin resistance. Pregnancy is accompanied by insulin resistance, mediated by placental secretion of diabetogenic hormones. These and other metabolic changes that occur during pregnancy ensure that the fetus has an ample supply of nutrients.

TABLE 20.1	RECOMMENDATIONS FOR DIAGNOSING AND CLASSIFYING HYPERGLYCEMIA IN PREGNANCY		
When	**Diagnosis**	**Test**	**Cutoff for Diagnosis**
First prenatal visit	Overt (pregestational) diabetes or high risk history—physical inactivity, first-degree relative with diabetes, hypertension, high risk race/ethnicity, obesity, polycystic ovarian syndrome, hypercholesterolemia, previous large infant >9 lb; and smoker.	Fasting HbA1C Random	126 mg/dL <7% 200 mg/dL
24–28 weeks	Gestational diabetes	Fasting 75 g OGTT–1 hr 75 g OGTT–2 hr	92 mg/dL 180 mg/dL 153 mg/dL

OGTT, oral glucose tolerance test.

Adapted from International Association of Diabetes and Pregnancy Study Group. (2012). Screening for gestational diabetes mellitus. *Diabetes Care, 35*(2). Retrieved from http://care.diabetesjournals.org/content/early/2012/01/23/dc11-1643; ACOG. (2014a). ACOG guidelines at a glance: Gestational Diabetes Mellitus. *Contemporary OB/GYN*. Retrieved from http://contemporaryobgyn. modernmedicine.com/contemporary-obgyn/news/acog-guidelines-glance-gestational-diabetes-mellitus?page=full; and Roglie, G., & Colagiuri, S. (2014). Gestational diabetes mellitus: Squaring the circle. *Diabetes Care, 37*(6), 143–144.

With diabetes, there is a deficiency of or resistance to insulin. This alteration interferes with the body's ability to obtain essential nutrients for fuel and storage. If a pregnant woman has pregestational diabetes or develops gestational diabetes, the profound metabolic alterations that occur during pregnancy and that are necessary to support the growth and development of the fetus are greatly affected.

Maternal metabolism is directed toward supplying adequate nutrition for the fetus. In pregnancy, placental hormones cause insulin resistance at a level that tends to parallel the growth of the fetoplacental unit. As the placenta grows, more placental hormones are secreted. Human placental lactogen (hPL) and growth hormone (somatotropin) increase in direct correlation with the growth of placental tissue, rising throughout the last 20 weeks of pregnancy and causing insulin resistance. Subsequently, insulin secretion increases to overcome the resistance of these two hormones. In the pregnant woman without diabetes, the pancreas can respond to the demands for increased insulin production to maintain normal glucose levels throughout the pregnancy (Toledano, Hadar, & Hod, 2015). However, the woman with glucose intolerance or diabetes during pregnancy cannot cope with changes in metabolism resulting from insufficient insulin to meet the needs during gestation.

Over the course of pregnancy, insulin resistance does change. It peaks in the last trimester to provide more nutrients to the fetus. The insulin resistance typically results in postprandial hyperglycemia, although some women also have an elevated fasting blood glucose level (Aktas et al., 2014). With this increased demand on the pancreas in late pregnancy, women with diabetes or glucose intolerance cannot accommodate the increased insulin demand; glucose levels rise as a result of insulin deficiency, leading to hyperglycemia. Subsequently, the mother and her fetus can experience major problems, as shown in Table 20.2.

Screening

Currently, there are inconsistent standards around the world for how women are tested for gestational diabetes, as well cut-off values to diagnose it. The American College of Obstetricians and Gynecologists (ACOG) and ADA currently recommend a risk analysis of all pregnant women at their first prenatal visit and additional screening of all high-risk pregnant women again at 24 to 28

TABLE 20.2	DIABETES AND PREGNANCY: EFFECTS ON THE MOTHER AND FETUS	
Effects on the Mother	**Effects on the Fetus/Neonate**
<ul><li>Hydramnios due to fetal diuresis caused by hyperglycemia</li><li>Gestational hypertension of unknown etiology</li><li>Ketoacidosis due to uncontrolled hyperglycemia</li><li>Preterm labor secondary to premature membrane rupture</li><li>Stillbirth in pregnancies complicated by ketoacidosis and poor glucose control</li><li>Hypoglycemia as glucose is diverted to the fetus (occurring in first trimester)</li><li>Urinary tract infections resulting from excess glucose in the urine (glucosuria), which promotes bacterial growth</li><li>Chronic monilial vaginitis due to glucosuria, which promotes growth of yeast</li><li>Difficult labor, cesarean birth, postpartum hemorrhage secondary to an overdistended uterus to accommodate a macrosomic infant</li></ul>	<ul><li>Cord prolapse secondary to polyhydramnios and abnormal fetal presentation</li><li>Congenital anomaly due to hyperglycemia in the first trimester (cardiac problems, neural tube defects, skeletal deformities, and genitourinary problems)</li><li>Macrosomia resulting from hyperinsulinemia stimulated by fetal hyperglycemia</li><li>Birth trauma due to increased size of fetus, which complicates the birthing process (shoulder dystocia)</li><li>Preterm birth secondary to polyhydramnios and an aging placenta, which places the fetus in jeopardy if the pregnancy continues</li><li>Fetal asphyxia secondary to fetal hyperglycemia and hyperinsulinemia</li><li>Intrauterine growth restriction secondary to maternal vascular impairment and decreased placental perfusion, which restricts growth</li><li>Perinatal death due to poor placental perfusion and hypoxia</li><li>Respiratory distress syndrome resulting from poor surfactant production secondary to hyperinsulinemia inhibiting the production of phospholipids, which make up surfactant</li><li>Polycythemia due to excessive red blood cell (RBC) production in response to hypoxia</li><li>Hyperbilirubinemia due to excessive RBC breakdown from hypoxia and an immature liver unable to break down bilirubin</li><li>Neonatal hypoglycemia resulting from ongoing hyperinsulinemia after the placenta is removed</li><li>Subsequent childhood obesity and carbohydrate intolerance</li></ul>

Adapted from Cunningham, F. G., Leveno, K. J., Bloom, S. L., Spong, C., & Dashe, J. (2014). *Williams' obstetrics* (24th ed.). New York, NY: McGraw-Hill Professional Publishing; Moore, T. R. (2015). Diabetes mellitus and pregnancy. *eMedicine*. Retrieved from http://emedicine.medscape.com/article/127547 and March of Dimes (2015a). *Gestational diabetes*. Retrieved from http://www.marchofdimes.com/pregnancy/gestational-diabetes.aspx

weeks, or earlier if risk factors are present. If the initial screening risk assessment is low, additional screening may not be necessary. Pregnant women who fulfill all of the following criteria need not be screened at their first prenatal visit:

• No history of glucose intolerance
• Less than 25 years old
• Normal body weight
• No family history (first-degree relative) of diabetes
• No history of poor obstetric outcome
• Not from an ethnic/racial group with a high prevalence of diabetes (ADA, 2015b)

If the initial risk assessment is high, rescreening should take place between 24 and 28 weeks. A woman with abnormal early results may have had diabetes before the pregnancy, and her fetus is at great risk for congenital anomalies. An elevated glycosylated hemoglobin supports the likelihood of gestational diabetes. Combining the use of HbA1c and plasma glucose measurements for the diagnosis of diabetes offers the benefits of each test and reduces the risk of systematic bias inherent in HbA1c testing alone (Petry, 2014).

There is little consensus regarding the appropriate screening method. Typically, screening is based on a 75-g 1-hour glucose challenge test, usually performed between 24 and 28 weeks of gestation (McIntyre, Dyer, & Metzger, 2015). A 75-g oral glucose load is given, without regard to the timing or content of the last meal. Blood glucose is measured 1 hour later; a level above 140 mg/dL is abnormal. If the result is abnormal, a 3-hour glucose tolerance test is done. Normal values are:

• Fasting blood glucose level: Less than 92 mg/dL
• At 1 hour: Less than 180 mg/dL
• At 2 hours: Less than 153 mg/dL
• At 3 hours: Less than 140 mg/dL

A diagnosis of gestational diabetes can be made only after an abnormal result is obtained on the glucose tolerance test. One or more abnormal values confirm a diagnosis of gestational diabetes (Farrar et al., 2015). A newer, more controlled screening (HbA1C) has been adopted by ADA and ACOG because of mounting evidence that diagnosing and treating even mild gestational diabetes reduces morbidity for both mother and infant (ADA, 2015c). If adopted universally, the new guidelines are expected to have immediate, widespread clinical implications.

Therapeutic Management

Care for the Woman with Pregestational Diabetes

Pregestational diabetes is a significant public health problem that increases the risk for structural birth defects affecting both maternal and neonatal pregnancy outcomes. Women who have pregestational diabetes (the alteration in carbohydrate metabolism is identified before conception) need comprehensive prenatal care. Achieving good metabolic control during the period prior to conception is essential to reducing congenital malformations that can occur in pregnancies complicated by diabetes. The primary goals of care are to maintain glycemic control and minimize the risks of the disease on the fetus. Key aspects of treatment include nutritional management, exercise, insulin regimens, and close maternal and fetal surveillance (Fig. 20.1).

Preconception counseling is essential for the woman with pregestational diabetes (the alteration in carbohydrate metabolism that is identified before conception) to ensure that her disease state is stable. The problem is that as many as half of all pregnancies in the United States

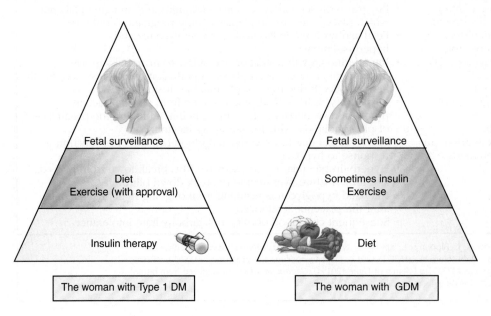

FIGURE 20.1 Treatment overview for diabetes in pregnancy. For women with pregestational type 1 DM, the foundation of glycemic management is insulin therapy along with dietary management, exercise, and fetal surveillance. For the woman who develops gestational diabetes, dietary modification is generally the foundation of treatment. Some women may require insulin along with dietary modifications, whereas others will not require insulin therapy, and others do not. Exercise and fetal surveillance are also important facets of care.

are unplanned. Thus women with chronic medical conditions such as diabetes might not have the opportunity to take steps to optimize management of their diabetes before becoming pregnant. When preconception care is possible, women with pregestational diabetes should be taught how to improve their metabolic control prior to conception to reduce the risk of birth defects. Nurses caring for women of reproductive age can contribute to preconception care by helping to counsel someone who is prediabetic to avoid progression to diabetes and its attendant risks during pregnancy. The goals of preconception care are to:

* integrate the woman into the management of her diabetes;
* achieve the lowest glycosylated hemoglobin A1C test results without excessive hypoglycemia;
* ensure effective contraception until stable glycemia is achieved;
* identify and evaluate long-term diabetic complications such as retinopathy, nephropathy, neuropathy, cardiovascular disease (CVD), and hypertension (Gabbay-Benziv et al., 2015).

Excellent control of blood glucose, as evidenced by normal fasting blood glucose levels and a **glycosylated hemoglobin (HbA1C) level** (a measurement of the average glucose levels during the past 100 to 120 days), is crucial to achieve the best pregnancy outcome. A glycosylated hemoglobin level of less than 7% indicates good control; a value of more than 8% indicates poor control and warrants intervention. A pregestational diabetic pregnant woman has up to a nine-fold increase in birth defects, compared with the rate seen in nondiabetic pregnancies if she does not have glycemic control (Mitanchez et al., 2015).

Preconception counseling is also important in helping to reduce the risk of congenital malformation. The most common malformations associated with diabetes occur in the renal, cardiac, skeletal, and central nervous systems. Since these defects occur by the eighth week of gestation, preconception counseling is critical. The rate of congenital anomalies in women with pregestational diabetes can be reduced if excellent glycemic control is achieved at the time of conception (Simeone et al., 2015). This information needs to be stressed with all women with diabetes who are contemplating a pregnancy. In addition, the woman with pregestational diabetes needs to be evaluated for complications of diabetes. This evaluation should be part of baseline screening and continuing assessment during pregnancy.

Care During Pregnancy for the Woman with Gestational Diabetes

Lifestyle modification, nutritional changes, and encouragement of physical activities forms the primary mode of

therapy for diabetes during pregnancy. Therapeutic management for the woman with gestational diabetes mellitus (defined as glucose intolerance with its onset during pregnancy or first detected during pregnancy) focuses on tight glucose control. The ADA (2015b) recommends maintaining a fasting blood glucose level below 92 mg/dL, with postprandial levels below 180 mg/dL at 1-hour and 2-hour postprandial levels below 153 mg/dL. In comparison, for pregnant women without diabetes, near-normal glucose values include a fasting value between 60 and 90 mg/dL, a 1-hour postprandial value of 100 to 120 mg/dL, and a 2-hour postprandial value of 60 to 120 mg/dL. Such tight control has been advocated because it is associated with a reduction in macrosomia. In addition, maternal prepregnancy weight and weight gain during pregnancy appear to be significant and independent risk factors for macrosomia in women with gestational diabetes also (Grandy et al. 2015).

Nutritional management focuses on maintaining balanced glucose levels and providing enough energy and nutrients for the pregnant woman, while avoiding ketosis, and minimizing the risk of hypoglycemia in women treated with insulin. Nutrition therapy is the cornerstone of therapy for women with gestational diabetes. Women should receive ethically appropriate nutritional advice on how to change their dietary habits from a dietitian. The diet counseling must be in keeping with their present cultural dietary patterns and not radically different to become adopted and followed. If rice is a staple of a Chinese client's diet, then it must be incorporated into the diet counseling plan and not eliminated (He et al., 2015). A low-glycemic index diet is considered safe and has positive effects on the glycemic control and pregnancy outcomes for both healthy women, those with type 2 diabetes and gestational diabetes. A moderately low carbohydrate diet with a carbohydrate content of 40% of the calories results in good glycemic control for most (Roskjaer et al., 2014). Eating for two during pregnancy for a woman who has diabetes means eating not volume for two, but rather quality and timing to support both mother and fetus. Women who receive dietary instruction and follow it have been shown to have a better pregnancy outcome than those who do not receive dietary advice (Ma et al., 2015).

PHARMACOLOGIC THERAPY FOR GESTATIONAL DIABETES

For the woman with gestational diabetes, nutritional management and exercise may be all that is necessary. Pharmacologic therapy is considered if nutrition and exercise fail to maintain target glucose levels. Blood glucose levels in the woman can be controlled by nutritional therapy and exercise, but in uncontrolled cases, where target glycemic levels cannot be reached, insulin is also required. Insulin, which does not cross the placenta, historically has been the medication of choice for treating hyperglycemia in pregnancy. Insulin is calculated based on the woman's weight. Combining intermediate and short-acting insulin yields the best result for most women. Two insulin doses are given daily with two thirds of the total insulin in the morning to cover energy needs of the active day and one third at night.

Oral Medications for Management of Gestational Diabetes. Women tend to manage oral medications better than insulin, so the standard of care may be moving toward the oral route (King et al., 2015). Recent studies have examined the use of oral hypoglycemic medications in pregnancy with much success. Several studies have used glyburide (DiaBeta) with promising results. Many health care providers are using glyburide and metformin as an alternative to insulin therapy because they do not cross the placenta and therefore do not cause fetal/neonatal hypoglycemia. Some oral hypoglycemic medications are considered safe and may be used if nutrition and exercise are not adequate alone. Maternal and newborn outcomes are similar to those seen in women who are treated with insulin. Oral hypoglycemic agents, however, must be further investigated to determine their safety with confidence and provide better treatment options for diabetes in pregnancy. Currently, there is a growing acceptance of glyburide (glibenclamide) use as a primary therapy for gestational diabetes Glyburide and metformin (Glucophage) have also been found to be safe, effective, and economical for the treatment of gestational diabetes, although neither drug has been approved by the FDA for use in pregnancy. Insulin, however, still has an important role to play in gestational diabetes (Buschur, Brown, & Wyckoff, 2015).) Gestational diabetes offers a window of opportunity, which needs to be seized, for prevention of diabetes in future life (Nagtalon-Ramos, 2014).

The ADA (2015c) recommends that women diagnosed with gestational diabetes by a 3-hour glucose tolerance test receive nutritional counseling from a registered dietitian. The ADA also recommends insulin therapy or oral diabetic medications if diet is unsuccessful in achieving a fasting glucose level below 92 mg/dL, a 1-hour postprandial level below 180 mg/dL, or 2-hour postprandial level below 153 mg/dL (ADA, 2015c).

The ACOG (2014a) recommends the use of diet or insulin or oral diabetic medications to achieve a 1-hour postprandial blood glucose level of 130 mg/dL. Randomized studies show that glyburide and insulin are equally effective in achieving glycemic control. Glycemic control—regardless of whether it involves diet, insulin, or oral agents—leads to fewer cases of shoulder dystocia, hyperbilirubinemia requiring phototherapy, nerve palsy, bone fracture, LGA status, and fetal macrosomia (ACOG, 2014a).

Exercise is another important component of comprehensive prenatal care for the pregnant woman with glucose intolerance. Regular exercise helps maintain glucose control by increasing the uptake of glucose into the cells and decreasing central obesity, hypertension, and dyslipidemia, which will ultimately decrease the woman's insulin requirements (Jordan et al., 2014). Regular physical activity has been proven to result in marked benefits for mother and fetus. Maternal benefits include improved cardiovascular function, limited pregnancy weight gain, decreased musculoskeletal discomfort, reduced incidence of muscle cramps and lower limb edema, mood stability, and reduction of gestational diabetes mellitus and gestational hypertension. Fetal benefits include decreased fat mass, improved stress tolerance, and advanced neurobehavioral maturation. Research also suggests the role of physical activity in prevention of gestational diabetes (Bain, Crane et al., 2015).

Insulin for Management of Gestational Diabetes. Insulin remains the medication of choice for glycemic control if oral medications, diet, or exercise fail to yield results in pregnant and lactating women with any type of diabetes (Moore, 2015). Generally, insulin doses are reduced in the first trimester to prevent hypoglycemia resulting from increased insulin sensitivity as well as from nausea and vomiting. Newer short-acting insulins such as lispro (Humalog) and aspart (NovoLog), which do not cross the placenta, may help reduce postprandial hyperglycemia, episodes of hypoglycemia between meals. Target fasting glucose values of 60 to 90 mg/dL and 1-hour postprandial values less than 120 mg/dL are necessary to provide good glycemic control and good pregnancy outcomes (Moore, 2015). Changes in diet and activity level add to the need for changes in insulin dosages throughout pregnancy.

Insulin regimens vary, and controversy remains over the best strategy for insulin delivery in pregnancy. Many health care providers use a split-dose therapy (two thirds of the daily dose in the morning and the remaining one third in the evening). Others advocate the use of an insulin pump to deliver a continuous subcutaneous insulin infusion. Regardless of which protocol is used, frequent blood glucose measurements are necessary, and the insulin dosage is adjusted on the basis of daily glucose levels. Insulin therapy or oral hypoglycemic agents, in addition to diet and exercise are main elements of achieving glycemic control. See Evidence-Based Practice 20.1.

Close maternal and fetal surveillance is also essential. Frequent laboratory tests are done during pregnancy to monitor the woman's status and glucose control. Fetal surveillance via diagnostic testing aids in evaluating fetal well-being and assisting in determining the best time for birth.

Care During and After Labor for the Woman with Gestational Diabetes

For the laboring woman with diabetes, intravenous saline or lactated Ringer's is given and blood glucose levels are

EVIDENCE-BASED PRACTICE 20.1   PREVENTION OF GESTATIONAL DIABETES IN PREGNANT WOMEN WITH RISK FACTORS FOR GESTATIONAL DIABETES: A SYSTEMATIC REVIEW AND META-ANALYSIS OF RANDOMIZED TRIALS

STUDY

Gestational diabetes mellitus (GDM) is defined as the diabetes diagnosed during pregnancy that is not clearly overt diabetes. According to this definition, glycemic levels meeting the thresholds of overt diabetes are considered to have pre-existing diabetes and the rest are given diagnosis of GDM. The objective of the systematic review was to identify any intervention that could be used for primary prevention of gestational diabetes in women with risk factors for it.

A systematic review and meta-analysis was conducted by including randomized controlled trials comparing any form of therapeutic intervention in comparison to usual antenatal care. A literature search was conducted using electronic databases together with a hand search of relevant journals and conference proceedings.

Findings

A total of 2,422 women from 14 randomized trials were included which compared diet, exercise, lifestyle changes, and metformin with standard care in women with risk factors for gestational diabetes. Dietary intervention was associated with statistically significant lower incidence of gestational diabetes and gestational hypertension compared to standard of care. There was no statistically significant difference in the incidence of gestational diabetes with exercise, lifestyle changes or metformin used compared to standard care.

Nursing Implications

Based on these findings, nurses can encourage healthy dietary changes as a primary prevention strategy to prevent gestational diabetes for high-risk women since this intervention was shown to be a statistically significant intervention over standard care. Instructing them on health dietary habits either preconceptually or at the first prenatal visit may help prevent gestational diabetes and turn the tide for better pregnancy outcomes for both the mother and the infant.

Adapted from Madhuvrata, P., Govinden, G., Bustani, R., Song, S., & Farrell, T. A. (2015). Prevention of gestational diabetes in pregnant women with risk factors for gestational diabetes: A systematic review and meta-analysis of randomized trials. *Obstetric Medicine: The Medicine of Pregnancy, 8*(2), 68–85.

monitored every 1 to 2 hours. Glucose levels are maintained below 110 mg/dL throughout labor to reduce the likelihood of neonatal hypoglycemia. If necessary, an infusion of regular insulin may be given to maintain this level (King et al., 2015). If the woman was receiving insulin during her pregnancy, adjustments in dosage may be necessary after birth since glucose diversion across the placenta to supply the growing fetus is no longer present and insulin resistance is now removed. Frequently, the woman with gestational diabetes can remain controlled through diet and weight management; the woman with type 1 diabetes usually returns to prepregnant levels of insulin administration (Kim, 2014).

After giving birth, the overt glycemic abnormalities of gestational diabetes usually resolve. This phenomenon suggests that the diabetes is transient and that the consequences of gestational diabetes end with the birth of the infant. However, for the woman, childbirth is not the end of the story. The diagnosis of gestational diabetes heralds future health risks. Knowledge of this "failed" stress test conveys new information about her future risk for type 2 diabetes, which warrants further screening and prevention efforts during the postpartum period and beyond.

Nursing Assessment

Nursing assessment begins at the first prenatal visit. A thorough history and physical examination in conjunction with specific laboratory and diagnostic testing aids in developing an individualized plan of care for the woman with diabetes.

Health History and Physical Examination

For the woman with pregestational diabetes, obtain a thorough history of the preexisting diabetic condition. Ask about her duration of disease, management of glucose levels (insulin injections, insulin pump, or oral hypoglycemic agents), dietary adjustments, presence of vascular complications and current vascular status, current insulin regimen, and technique used for glucose testing. Review any information that she may have received as part of her preconception counseling and measures that were implemented during this time.

Be knowledgeable about the woman's nutritional requirements and assess the adequacy and pattern of her dietary intake. Assess her blood glucose self-monitoring in terms of technique, frequency, and her ability to adjust the insulin dose based on the changing patterns. Ask about the frequency of episodes of hypoglycemia or hyperglycemia to ascertain the woman's ability to recognize and treat them. Continue to assess her for signs and symptoms of hypo- and hyperglycemia.

During antepartum visits, assess the client's knowledge about her disease, including the signs and symptoms of hypoglycemia, hyperglycemia, and diabetic

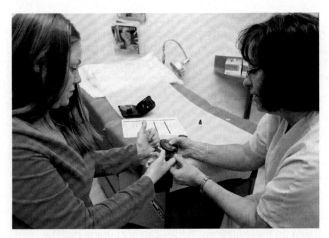

FIGURE 20.2 The nurse is demonstrating the technique for self-blood glucose monitoring with a pregnant client who has diabetes.

ketoacidosis, insulin administration techniques, and the impact of pregnancy on her chronic condition. If possible have the woman demonstrate her technique for blood glucose monitoring and insulin administration if appropriate. It is essential that the nurse keeps in mind that there is a huge learning curve for women with diabetes concerning the need for dietary changes, frequency of blood glucose monitoring, exercise, and insulin or oral medication administration. Suddenly, the woman is expected to make rapid changes in her life, which can be overwhelming. The nurse can help facilitate these changes by exercising patience and understanding and reinforcing all verbal instructions with written material. Frequent encouragement is also needed to assist the woman in her lifestyle changes. Although the client may have had diabetes for some time, do not assume that she has a firm knowledge base about her disease process or management of it (Fig. 20.2).

Assess the woman's risk for gestational diabetes at the first prenatal visit. The clinical presentation of diabetes mellitus in pregnancy may be quite varied, but the classical triad of the symptoms of polydipsia, polyphagia, and polyuria may not be reported by most women during pregnancy. Instead, the women may present with previous history of medical complications of diabetes (chronic hypertension/chronic renal disease) and obesity. All of these conditions can influence pregnancy outcome. The ADA (2015a) recommends assessing all women for risk factors and then determining the need for additional testing in the high-risk group only. Factors that place a woman at high risk include:

- Previous infant with congenital anomaly (skeletal, renal, central nervous system, cardiac)
- History of gestational diabetes or polyhydramnios in a previous pregnancy
- Family history of diabetes
- Medications: corticosteroids or antipsychotics

- Age 35 years or older
- Polycystic ovarian syndrome
- Multiple pregnancy (twins, triplets)
- Previous infant weighing more than 9 lb (4,000 g)
- Previous unexplained fetal demise or neonatal death
- Maternal obesity (body mass index [BMI] >30)
- Hypertension before pregnancy or in early pregnancy
- Hispanic, Native American, Pacific Islander, or African–American ethnicity
- Recurrent monilia infections that do not respond to treatment
- Signs and symptoms of glucose intolerance (polyuria, polyphagia, polydipsia, fatigue)
- Presence of glycosuria or proteinuria (Gupta, 2015).

Women with clinical characteristics consistent with a high risk for gestational diabetes should undergo glucose testing as soon as feasible.

Provide close ongoing assessment throughout the antepartal period. Women with gestational diabetes mellitus (GDM) are at increased risk for preeclampsia and glucose control–related complications such as hypoglycemia, hyperglycemia, and ketoacidosis. Gestational diabetes of any severity increases the risk of fetal macrosomia, as noted earlier. It is also associated with an increased frequency of maternal hypertensive disorders and operative births. This may be the result of fetal growth disorders (ADA, 2015a). Even though gestational diabetes is diagnosed during pregnancy, the woman may have had glucose intolerance before the pregnancy. Therefore, monitor the woman closely for signs and symptoms of possible complications.

Also assess the woman's psychosocial adaptation to her condition. This assessment is critical to gain her cooperation for a change in regimen or the addition of a new regimen throughout pregnancy. Identify her support systems and note any financial constraints, because she will need intense monitoring and frequent fetal surveillance.

Laboratory and Diagnostic Testing

The results of laboratory and diagnostic tests provide valuable information about maternal and fetal wellbeing. Women with pregestational diabetes and those discovered to have gestational diabetes require ongoing maternal and fetal surveillance to promote the best outcome.

SURVEILLANCE

Maternal surveillance may include the following:

- Urine check for protein (may indicate the need for further evaluation for preeclampsia) and for nitrates and leukocyte esterase (may indicate a urinary tract infection).
- Urine check for ketones (may indicate the need for evaluation of eating habits).

- Kidney function evaluation every trimester for creatinine clearance and protein levels.
- Eye examination in the first trimester to evaluate the retina for vascular changes.
- HbA1c every 4 to 6 weeks to monitor glucose trends (Jordan et al., 2014).

Fetal surveillance may include ultrasound to provide information about fetal growth, activity, and amniotic fluid volume and to validate gestational age. Alpha-fetoprotein levels may be obtained to detect congenital anomalies such as an open neural tube or ventral wall defects of omphalocele or gastroschisis, and a fetal echocardiogram may be necessary to rule out cardiac anomalies. A biophysical profile helps to monitor fetal well-being and uteroplacental profusion, and nonstress tests commonly are performed weekly after 28 weeks of gestation to evaluate fetal well-being. As the pregnancy progresses, an amniocentesis may be done to determine the lecithin/sphingomyelin (L/S) ratio and the presence of phosphatidyl glycerol (PG) to evaluate whether the fetal lung is mature enough for birth (Moore, 2015).

Nursing Management

The ideal outcome of every pregnancy is a healthy newborn and mother. Nurses can be pivotal in realizing this positive outcome for women with pregestational or gestational diabetes by implementing measures to minimize risks and complications. Since the woman with diabetes is considered to be at high risk, antepartal visits occur more frequently (every 2 weeks up to 28 weeks and then twice a week until birth), providing the nurse with numerous opportunities for ongoing assessment, education, and counseling (Nursing Care Plan 20.1).

Promoting Optimal Glucose Control

At each visit, review the mother's blood glucose levels, including any laboratory tests and self-monitoring results. Reinforce with the woman the need to perform blood glucose monitoring (usually four times a day: before meals and at bedtime) and to keep a record of the results. If appropriate, obtain a fingerstick blood glucose level to evaluate the accuracy of self-monitoring results. Also assess the woman's techniques for monitoring blood glucose levels and for administering insulin if ordered, and offer support and guidance. If the woman is receiving insulin therapy, assist with any changes needed if glucose levels are not controlled. Obtain a urine specimen and check for glucose, protein, and ketones. Ask the woman if she has had any episodes of hypoglycemia and what she did to alleviate them. Discuss dietary measures related to blood glucose control (Fig. 20.3). In addition, recommend the following:

- Avoid weight loss and dieting during pregnancy.
- Ensure that food intake is adequate to prevent ketone formation and promote weight gain.
- Eat three meals a day plus three snacks to promote glycemic control:
  - 40% of calories from good-quality complex carbohydrates
  - 35% of calories from protein sources
  - 25% of calories from unsaturated fats.
  - Small frequent feedings throughout the day are recommended.
  - Bedtime snacks are recommended for all women.
  - Include protein and fat at each meal (National Diabetes Information Clearing House, 2015).

Take Note!
Nutrient requirements and recommendations for weight gain for the pregnant woman with diabetes are the same as those for the pregnant nondiabetic woman.

If necessary, arrange for consultation with a dietitian or nutritionist to individualize the dietary plan. Also encourage the women to participate in an exercise program that includes at least three sessions which last at least 30 minutes daily. Exercise may lessen the need for insulin or dosage adjustments.

When caring for the laboring woman with pregestational or gestational diabetes, adjust the intravenous flow rate and the rate of supplemental regular insulin based on the blood glucose levels as ordered. Monitor blood glucose levels every 1 to 2 hours or more frequently if necessary. Keep a syringe with 50% dextrose solution Retrieved from the bedside to treat profound hypoglycemia. Monitor fetal heart rate patterns throughout labor to detect category II and III patterns. Assess maternal vital signs every hour, in addition to assessing the woman's urinary output with an indwelling catheter. If a cesarean birth is scheduled, monitor the woman's blood glucose levels hourly and administer short-acting insulin or glucose based on the blood glucose levels as ordered.

After birth, monitor blood glucose levels every 2 to 4 hours for the first 48 hours to determine the woman's insulin need and continue intravenous fluid administration as ordered. Encourage breast-feeding to assist in maintaining good glucose control. For the woman with pregestational diabetes and type 1 or 2 diabetes, expect insulin needs to decrease rapidly after birth: they may be reduced by half of the antepartum dose as meals are started (King et al., 2015). Some women may return to their prepregnancy insulin dosage. In addition, the nurse must monitor the infant of the diabetic mother for common problems see in them which includes macrosomia, respiratory distress syndrome, hypoglycemia, polycythemia, hypocalcemia, hyperbilirubinemia, and a variety of congenital anomalies (Green, 2016). Frequently,

Overview of the Pregnant Woman with Type 1 Diabetes

Donna, a 30-year-old woman with type 1 diabetes, presents to the maternity clinic for preconception care. She has had diabetes for 8 years and takes insulin twice daily by injection. She does blood glucose self-monitoring four times daily. She reports that her disease is fairly well controlled, but "I'm worried about how my diabetes will affect a pregnancy and my baby. Will I need to make changes in my routine? Will my baby be normal?" She reports that she recently had a foot infection and needed to go to the emergency department because it led to an episode of ketoacidosis. She states that her last glycosylated hemoglobin A1c test results were abnormal.

NURSING DIAGNOSIS: Ineffective health maintenance: Maternal related to deficient knowledge regarding care in diabetic condition in pregnancy as evidenced by questions about effect on pregnancy, possible changes in regimen, and pregnancy outcome

Outcome Identification and Evaluation

The client will demonstrate increased knowledge of type 1 diabetes and effects on pregnancy as evidenced by proper techniques for blood glucose monitoring and insulin administration, ability to modify insulin doses and dietary intake to achieve control, and verbalization of need for glycemic control prior to pregnancy, with blood glucose levels remaining within normal range.

Interventions: *Providing Client Teaching*

- Assess client's knowledge of diabetes and pregnancy to establish a baseline from which to develop an individualized teaching plan.
- Review the underlying problems associated with diabetes and how pregnancy affects glucose control to provide client with a firm knowledge base for decision making.
- Review signs and symptoms of hypoglycemia and hyperglycemia and prevention and management measures to ensure client can deal with them should they occur.
- Provide written materials describing diabetes and care needed for control to provide opportunity for client's review and promote retention of learning.
- Observe client administering insulin and self-glucose testing for technique and offer suggestions for improvement if needed to ensure adequate self-care ability.
- Discuss proper foot care to prevent future infections.
- Teach home treatment for symptomatic hypoglycemia to minimize risk to client and fetus.

- Outline acute and chronic diabetic complications to reinforce the importance of glucose control.
- Discuss use of contraceptives until blood glucose levels can be optimized before conception occurs to promote best possible health status before conception.
- Explain the rationale for good glucose control and the importance of achieving excellent glycemic control before pregnancy to promote a positive pregnancy outcome.
- Review self-care practices (blood glucose monitoring and frequency of testing; insulin administration; adjustment of insulin dosages based on blood glucose levels) to foster independence in self-care and feelings of control over the situation.
- Refer client for dietary counseling to ensure optimal diet for glycemic control.
- Outline obstetric management and fetal surveillance needed for pregnancy to provide client with information on what to expect.
- Discuss strategies for maintaining optimal glycemic control during pregnancy to minimize risks to client and fetus.

NURSING DIAGNOSIS: Anxiety related to threat to self and fetus as evidenced by questions about her condition's effect on the baby and baby being normal

NURSING CARE PLAN 20.1

Overview of the Pregnant Woman with Type 1 Diabetes (continued)

Outcome Identification and Evaluation

The client will openly express her feelings related to her diabetes and pregnancy as evidenced by statements of feeling better about her preexisting condition and pregnancy outlook, and statements of understanding related to future childbearing by linking good glucose control with positive outcomes for both her and offspring.

Interventions: *Minimizing Anxiety*

- Review the need for a physical examination to evaluate for any effects of diabetes on the client's health status.
- Explain the rationale for assessing client's blood pressure, vision, and peripheral pulses at each visit to provide information related to possible effects of diabetes on health status.
- Identify any alterations in present diabetic condition that need intervention to aid in minimizing risks that may increase client's anxiety level.
- Review potential effects of diabetes on pregnancy to promote client understanding of risks and ways to control or minimize them.
- Encourage active participation in decision making and planning pregnancy to promote feelings of control over the situation and foster self-confidence.
- Discuss feelings about future childbearing and managing pregnancy to help reduce anxiety related to uncertainties.
- Encourage client to ask questions or voice concerns to help decrease anxiety related to the unknown.
- Emphasize the use of frequent and continued surveillance of client and fetal status during pregnancy to reduce the risk of complications and aid in alleviating anxieties related to the unknown.
- Provide positive reinforcement for healthy behaviors and actions to foster continued use and enhancement of self-esteem.

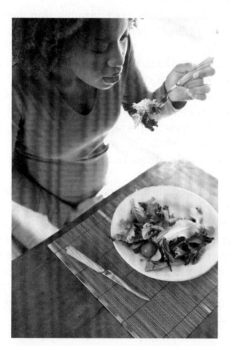

FIGURE 20.3 The pregnant client with diabetes eating a nutritious meal to ensure adequate glucose control.

admission to the neonatal intensive care unit (NICU) for close observational and glucose control is needed.

The therapy plan after childbirth is individualized. If recommended dietary modifications are carried out along with weight loss, the woman with gestational diabetes may return to her normal glucose levels. This is also true for the woman with pregestational diabetes, except that she will return to her prepregnancy insulin administration levels. This provides the nurse with a wonderful opportunity to reinforce healthy lifestyle interventions on the postpartum unit. Nurses can also become involved with community-based education to continue to offer their expertise.

Preventing Complications

Assess the woman closely for signs and symptoms of complications at each visit. Anticipate possible complications and plan appropriate interventions or referrals. Check the woman's blood pressure for changes and evaluate for proteinuria when obtaining a urine specimen. These might suggest the development of preeclampsia.

Measure fundal height and review gestational age. Note any discrepancies between fundal height and gestational age or a sudden increase in uterine growth. These may suggest polyhydramnios.

Encourage the woman to perform daily fetal movement counts to monitor fetal well-being. Tell her specifically when she should notify her health care provider. Also prepare the woman for the need for frequent laboratory and diagnostic testing to evaluate fetal status. Assist with serial ultrasounds to monitor fetal growth and with nonstress tests and biophysical profiles to assess fetal well-being.

Consider This

Scott and I had been busy all day setting up the new crib in our nursery, and we finally sat down to rest. I was due any day, and we had been putting this off until we had a long weekend to complete the task. I was excited to think about all the frilly pinks that decorated her room. I was sure that my new daughter would love it as much as I loved her already. A few days later I barely noticed any fetal movement, but I thought that she must be as tired as I was by this point.

That night I went into labor and kept looking at the worried faces of the nurses and the midwife in attendance. I had been diagnosed with gestational diabetes a few months ago and had tried to follow the instructions regarding diet and exercise, but old habits are hard to change when you are 38 years old. I was finally told after a short time in the labor unit that they couldn't pick up a fetal heartbeat and an ultrasound was to be done—still no heartbeat was detected. Scott and I were finally told that our daughter was a stillborn. All I could think about was that she would never get to see all the pink colors in the nursery.

Providing Client Education and Counseling

The pregnant woman with diabetes requires counseling and education about the need for strict glucose monitoring, diet and exercise, and signs and symptoms of complications. Encourage the client and her family to make any lifestyle changes needed to optimize the pregnancy outcome. Providing dietary education, weight control measures, and lifestyle advice that extends beyond pregnancy may lower the risk that the woman will have gestational diabetes in subsequent pregnancies as well as type 2 diabetes (Hashemi-Beni et al., 2015). At each visit stress the importance of performing blood glucose screening and documenting the results. With proper instruction, the client and her family will be able to cope with all the changes in her body during pregnancy (Teaching Guidelines 20.1).

Teaching Guidelines 20.1
TEACHING FOR THE PREGNANT WOMAN WITH DIABETES

- Be sure to keep your appointments for frequent prenatal visits and tests for fetal well-being.
- Perform blood glucose self-monitoring as directed, usually before each meal and at bedtime. Keep a record of your results and call your health care provider with any levels outside the established range. Bring your results to each prenatal visit.
- Perform daily "fetal kick counts." Document them and report any decrease in activity.
- Drink eight to ten 8-oz glasses of water each day to prevent bladder infections and maintain hydration.
- Wear proper, well-fitted footwear when walking to prevent injury.
- Engage in a regular exercise program such as walking to aid in glucose control, but avoid exercising in temperature extremes.
- Consider breast-feeding your infant to lower your blood glucose levels.
- If you are taking insulin:
  - Administer the correct dose of insulin at the correct time every day.
  - Eat breakfast within 30 minutes after injecting regular insulin to prevent a reaction.
  - Plan meals at a fixed time and snacks to prevent extremes in glucose levels.
- Avoid simple sugars (cake, candy, cookies), which raise blood glucose levels.
- Know the signs and symptoms of hypoglycemia and treatment needed:
  - Sweating, tremors, cold, clammy skin, headache
  - Feeling hungry, blurred vision, disorientation, irritability
  - Treatment: Drink 8 oz of milk and eat two crackers or take two glucose tablets
- Carry "glucose boosters" (such as Life Savers) to treat hypoglycemia.
- Know the signs and symptoms of hyperglycemia and treatment needed:
  - Dry mouth, frequent urination, excessive thirst, rapid breathing
  - Feeling tired, flushed, hot skin, headache, drowsiness
  - Treatment: Notify health care provider, because hospitalization may be needed
- Wear a diabetic identification bracelet at all times.
- Wash your hands frequently to prevent infections.
- Report any signs and symptoms of illness, infection, and dehydration to your health care provider, because these can affect blood glucose control.

Review discussions about the timing of birth and the rationale. Counsel the client about the possibility of cesarean birth for an LGA infant, or inform the woman who will be giving birth vaginally about the possible need for augmentation with oxytocin (Pitocin).

Take Note!

In the woman with well-controlled diabetes, birth is typically not induced before term unless complications arise, such as preeclampsia or fetal compromise. An early delivery date might be set for the woman with poorly controlled diabetes or a large size fetus who is having complications.

Instruct the client about the benefits of breast-feeding related to blood glucose control. Breast-feeding helps to normalize blood glucose levels. Therefore, encourage the woman to breast-feed her newborn. Also teach the woman receiving insulin for her diabetes that her insulin needs after birth will drastically decrease. Inform her that she will need a repeat glucose challenge test at a postpartum visit (ADA, 2015d).

For the woman with gestational diabetes, the focus is on lifestyle education. Women with gestational diabetes have a greater than 50% increased risk of developing type 2 diabetes (ADA, 2015d). Inform the woman that screening most likely will be done at the postpartum follow-up appointment in 6 weeks. Women with normal results at that visit typically are screened every 3 years thereafter (ADA, 2015d).). Teach her how to maintain an optimal weight to reduce her risk of developing diabetes. If necessary, refer the woman to a dietitian to help outline a balanced nutritious diet.

CARDIOVASCULAR DISORDERS

Despite an increase in awareness of a wide range of health concerns, the myth still exists that CVD is a man's disease and women do not need to be concerned about it. Every minute, an American woman dies of CVD and more than one in three women is living with a cardiovascular disorder, including nearly half of all African–American women and 34% of white women (American Heart Association [AHA], 2015). CVD is the leading cause of death for men and women in the United States and is more deadly than all forms of cancer. It kills nearly 500,000 women each year. Despite the prominent reduction in cardiovascular mortality among men, the rate has not declined for women. CVD has killed more women than men since 1984 (AHA, 2015). In addition to being the number-one killer of women, at the time of diagnosis women have both a poorer overall prognosis and a higher risk of death than men diagnosed with heart disease. Women represent 53% of deaths from CVD than the next three causes of death combined, including all forms of cancer (Worel & Hayman, 2015). In both men and women risk factors such as hypertension, high blood cholesterol level, smoking, lack of physical activity, and

obesity increase the probability of developing CVD. Menopause, gestational diabetes, oral contraceptive use, and bilateral oophorectomy in premenopausal women also affect the risk of CVD in women (Chomistek, Chiuve, & Eliassen, 2015).

More women die of heart disease, stroke, and other CVDs than men, yet many women do not realize they are at risk. These diseases kill more women each year than the next three causes of death combined, including all types of cancer (AHA, 2015). Approximately 3% of pregnant women have cardiac disease, which is responsible for 10% to 25% of maternal deaths (Cunningham et al., 2014). The prevalence of cardiac disease is increasing as a result of lifestyle patterns, including cigarette smoking, diabetes, and stress. As women are delaying childbearing, the incidence of cardiac disease in pregnancy will continue to increase. The cardiovascular adaptations during pregnancy are well tolerated by the normal heart, but may unveil undiagnosed underlying heart disease, or tip the hemodynamic balance and lead to decompensation in those with existing heart disease (Harvey, Coffman, & Miller, 2015).

Rheumatic heart disease used to represent the majority of cardiac conditions during pregnancy, but congenital heart disease now constitutes nearly half of all cases of heart disease encountered during pregnancy. Classic symptoms of heart disease mimic common symptoms of late pregnancy, such as palpitations, shortness of breath with exertion, and occasional chest pain. Few women with heart disease die during pregnancy, but they are at risk for other complications, such as heart failure, arrhythmias, and stroke. Their offspring are also at risk of complications, such as premature birth, low birth weight for gestational age, respiratory distress syndrome, intraventricular hemorrhage, and death (Gilstrap & Wood, 2014).

Congenital and Acquired Heart Disease

Congenital heart disease often involves structural defects that are present at birth but may not be discovered at that time (Table 20.3). Until recently, women with congenital heart disease did not live long enough to bear children. Today, due to new surgical techniques to correct these defects, many of these women can complete a successful pregnancy at relatively low risk when appropriate counseling and optimal care are provided. Increasing numbers of women with complex congenital heart disease are reaching childbearing age. Complications such as growth restriction, preterm and premature birth, and fetal and neonatal mortality are more common among children of women with congenital heart disease. The risk of complications is determined by the severity of the cardiac lesion, the presence of cyanosis, the maternal functional class, and the use of anticoagulation therapy (Choreño-Machain, Barrios, & Reta, 2015).

TABLE 20.3	SELECTED HEART CONDITIONS AFFECTING PREGNANCY	
Condition	**Description**	**Management**
Congenital		
Tetralogy of Fallot	Congenital defect involving four structural anomalies: obstruction to pulmonary flow; ventricular septal defect (abnormal opening between the right and left ventricles); dextroposition of the aorta (aortic opening overriding the septum and receiving blood from both ventricles); and right ventricular hypertrophy (increase in volume of the myocardium of the right ventricle).	Hospitalization and bed rest possible after the 20th week with hemodynamic monitoring via a pulmonary artery catheter to monitor volume status Oxygen therapy may be necessary during labor and birth.
Atrial septal defect (ASD)	Congenital heart defect involving a communication or opening between the atria with left-to-right shunting due to greater left-sided pressure. Arrhythmias present in some women.	Treatment with atrioventricular nodal blocking agents, and at times with electrical cardioversion.
Ventricular septal defect (VSD)	Congenital heart defect involving an opening in the ventricular septum, permitting blood flow from the left to the right ventricle. Complications include arrhythmias, heart failure, and pulmonary hypertension.	Rest with limited activity if symptomatic.
Patent ductus arteriosus	Abnormal persistence of an open lumen in the ductus arteriosus between the aorta and the pulmonary artery after birth; results in increased pulmonary blood flow and redistribution of flow to other organs.	Surgical ligation of the open ductus during infancy; subsequent problems minimal after surgical correction.
Acquired		
Mitral valve prolapse	Very common in the general population, occurring most often in younger women. Leaflets of the mitral valve prolapse into the left atrium during ventricular contraction. The most common cause of mitral valve regurgitation if present during pregnancy. Usually improvements in mitral valve function due to increased blood volume and decreased systemic vascular resistance of pregnancy; most women are able to tolerate pregnancy well.	Most women are asymptomatic; diagnosis is made incidentally. Occasional palpations, chest pain, or arrhythmias in some women, possibly requiring beta-blockers. Usually no special precautions are necessary during pregnancy.
Mitral valve stenosis	Most common chronic rheumatic valvular lesion in pregnancy. Causes obstruction of blood flow from the atria to the ventricle, thereby decreasing ventricular filling and causing a fixed cardiac output. Resultant pulmonary edema, pulmonary hypertension, and right ventricular failure. Most pregnant women with this condition can be managed medically.	General symptomatic improvement with medical management involving diuretics, beta blockers, and anticoagulant therapy. Activity restriction, reduction in sodium, and potentially bed rest if condition severe.
Aortic stenosis	Narrowing of the opening of the aortic valve, leading to an obstruction to left ventricular ejection Women with mild disease can tolerate hypervolemia of pregnancy; with progressive narrowing of the opening, cardiac output becomes fixed. Diagnosis can be confirmed with echocardiography. Most women can be managed with medical therapy, bed rest, and close monitoring.	Diagnosis confirmed with echocardiography Pharmacologic treatment with beta blockers and/or antiarrhythmic agents to reduce risk of heart failure and/or dysrhythmias. Bed rest/limited activity and close monitoring.

TABLE 20.3	SELECTED HEART CONDITIONS AFFECTING PREGNANCY (continued)	
Condition	**Description**	**Management**
Peripartum cardiomyopathy	Rare congestive cardiomyopathy that may arise during pregnancy. Multiparity, age, multiple fetuses, hypertension, an infectious agent, autoimmune disease, or cocaine use may contribute to its presence. Development of heart failure in the last month of pregnancy or within 5 months of giving birth without any preexisting heart disease or any identifiable cause.	Preload reduction with diuretic therapy Afterload reduction with vasodilators. Improvement in contractility with inotropic agents. Nonpharmacologic approaches include salt restriction and daily exercise such as walking or biking. The question of whether another pregnancy should be attempted is controversial due to the high risk of repeat complications.
Myocardial infarction (MI)	Rare during pregnancy but incidence is expected to increase as older women are becoming pregnant and the risk factors for coronary artery disease become more prevalent. Factors contributing to MI include family history, stress, smoking, age, obesity, multiple fetuses, hypercholesterolemia, and cocaine use. Increased plasma volume and cardiac output during pregnancy increase the cardiac workload as well as the myocardial oxygen demands; imbalance in supply and demand may contribute to myocardial ischemia.	Usual treatment modalities for any acute MI along with consideration for the fetus Anticoagulant therapy, rest, and lifestyle changes to preserve the health of both parties.

Adapted from Brickner, M. E. (2014). Cardiovascular management in pregnancy congenital heart disease. *Circulation, 130*(3), 273–282; Gilstrap, L. G., & Wood, M. J. (2014). Cardiovascular disease in women and pregnancy. In *MGH cardiology board review* (pp. 205–223). London, England: Springer Publishers; Jordan, R. G., Engstrom, J. L., Marfell, J. A., & Farley, C. L. (2014). *Prenatal and postnatal care: A woman-centered approach.* Ames, IO: John Wiley & Sons, Inc.; Mohamad, T. N., Fakhri, H. A., Bernal, J. M., Thatai, D., & Peterson, E. (2014). Cardiovascular disease and pregnancy. *eMedicine.* Retrieved from http://emedicine.medscape.com/article/162004-overview

Women with certain congenital conditions should avoid pregnancy. These include uncorrected tetralogy of Fallot or transposition of the great arteries, and Eisenmenger's syndrome, a defect with both cyanosis and pulmonary hypertension (Brickner, 2014).

Acquired heart diseases are conditions affecting the heart and its associated blood vessels that develop during a person's lifetime, in contrast with congenital heart diseases, which are present at birth. Acquired heart diseases include coronary artery disease, coronary heart disease, rheumatic heart disease, diseases of the pulmonary vessels and the aorta, diseases of the tissues of the heart, and diseases of the heart valves. The incidence of rheumatic heart disease has declined dramatically in the past several decades because of prompt identification of streptococcal throat infections and treatment with antibiotics. When the heart is involved, valvular lesions, such as mitral stenosis, prolapse, or aortic stenosis, are common (see Table 20.3).

Many women are postponing childbearing until their 30s and 40s. With advancing maternal age, underlying medical conditions such as hypertension, diabetes, and hypercholesterolemia contributing to ischemic heart disease become more common and increase the incidence of acquired heart disease complicating pregnancy. Coronary artery disease and myocardial infarction may result.

A woman's ability to function during the pregnancy is often more important than the actual diagnosis of the cardiac condition. The following is a functional classification system developed by the Criteria Committee of the New York Heart Association (1994) based on past and present disability and physical signs. It provides a simple way of classifying the extent of heart failure by placing people in one of four categories based on how much they are limited during physical activity, normal breathing, and varying degrees of shortness of breath and/or chest pain:

* *Class I:* Asymptomatic with no limitation of physical activity; no objective evidence of cardiac disease. Ordinary physical activity does not cause undue fatigue, palpitation, dyspnea, or chest pain.
* *Class II:* Symptomatic (dyspnea, chest pain) with increased activity resulting in slight limitation of physical activity. They are comfortable at rest. Ordinary physical activity results in fatigue, palpitation, dyspnea, or anginal pain. Minimal CVD present.

- *Class III:* Symptomatic (fatigue, palpitations) with normal activity resulting in marked limitation of physical activity. They are comfortable at rest. Less than ordinary activity causes fatigue, palpitation, dyspnea, or anginal pain. Moderately severe CVD present.
- *Class IV:* Symptomatic at rest or with any physical activity resulting in inability to carry on any physical activity without discomfort. Symptoms of heart failure or the anginal syndrome may be present even at rest. If any physical activity is undertaken, discomfort is increased. Severe CVD present.

The classification may change as the pregnancy progresses and the woman's body must cope with the increasing stress on the cardiovascular system resulting from the numerous physiologic changes taking place. Typically, a woman with class I or II cardiac disease can go through a pregnancy without major complications. A woman with class III disease usually has to maintain bed rest during pregnancy. A woman with class IV disease typically should be advised to avoid pregnancy (Grewal, Silversides, & Coleman, 2014). Women with cardiac disease may benefit from preconception counseling so that they know the risks before deciding to become pregnant.

Maternal mortality varies directly with the functional class at pregnancy onset. ACOG has adopted a three-tiered classification according to the risk of death during pregnancy (Box 20.1).

Pathophysiology

Numerous hemodynamic changes occur in all pregnant women. These normal physiologic changes can overstress the woman's cardiovascular system, increasing her risk for problems. Increased cardiac workload and greater myocardial oxygen demand during pregnancy place the woman's cardiovascular system at high risk for morbidity and mortality.

Pregnancy causes cardiac output to rise as early as the first trimester, reaching peak values at 20 to 24 weeks, and continues to increase until it plateaus between 28 and 34 weeks of gestation. This rise in cardiac output is due to a 30% to 50% increase in blood volume (stroke volume) and a 30% increase in heart rate. A normal resting heart rate for any pregnant woman can be on average 20 beats per minute above her normal values.

Take Note!

Uterine blood flow increases by at least 1 liter per minute, requiring the body to produce more blood during pregnancy. This results in a 25% increase in red blood cells, a 50% expansion of plasma volume during pregnancy, and an overall hemodilution. In addition, the increase in total red blood cellular volume includes an increase in clotting factors and platelets, defining the hypercoagulable state of pregnancy (Swan, 2014). These changes start as early as the second month of gestation.

BOX 20.1

CLASSIFICATION OF MATERNAL MORTALITY RISK

Group I (minimal risk) has a mortality rate of 1% and comprises women with:
- Patent ductus arteriosus
- Tetralogy of Fallot, corrected
- Atrial septal defect
- Ventricular septal defect
- Mitral stenosis, class I and II

Group II (moderate risk) has a mortality rate of 5% to 15% and comprises women with:
- Tetralogy of Fallot, uncorrected
- Mitral stenosis with atrial fibrillation
- Aortic stenosis, class III and IV
- Aortic coarctation without valvular involvement
- Artificial valve replacement

Group III (major risk) has a 25% to 50% mortality rate and comprises women with:
- Pulmonary hypertension
- Complicated aortic coarctation
- Previous myocardial infarction

Adapted from American Heart Association [AHA]. (2015). *Women and heart disease.* Retrieved from https://www.goredforwomen.org/about-heart-disease/facts_about_heart_disease_in_women-sub-category/statistics-at-a-glance/; Alonso-Gonzalez, R., & Swan, L. (2014). Treating cardiac disease in pregnancy. *Women's Health, 10*(1), 79–90; and Mohamad, T. N., Fakhri, H. A., Bernal, J. M., Thatai, D., & Peterson, E. (2014). Cardiovascular disease and pregnancy. *eMedicine.* Retrieved from http://emedicine.medscape.com/article/162004-overview

Similarly, cardiac output increases steadily during pregnancy by 30% to 50% over prepregnancy levels. Stroke volume increases 20% to 30% from prepregnant levels, and the maternal heart rate increases by 10 to 20 beats per minute (bpm). The increase is due to both the expansion in blood volume and the augmentation of stroke volume and heart rate. Other hemodynamic changes associated with pregnancy include a decrease in both the systemic vascular resistance and pulmonary vascular resistance, thereby lowering the systolic and diastolic blood pressure. In addition, the hypercoagulability associated with pregnancy might increase the risk of arterial thrombosis and embolization. These normal physiologic changes are important for a successful adaptation to pregnancy but create unique physiologic challenges for the woman with cardiac disease (Comparison Chart 20.1).

Therapeutic Management

Ideally, a woman with a history of congenital or acquired heart disease should consult her health care provider and undergo a risk assessment before becoming pregnant. This risk assessment must consider the woman's functional

COMPARISON CHART 20.1	CARDIOVASCULAR CHANGES: PREPREGNANCY VERSUS PREGNANCY	
Measurement	**Prepregnancy**	**Pregnancy**
Heart rate	72 (±10 bpm)	+10–20%
Cardiac output	4.3 (±0.9 L/min)	+30–50%
Blood volume	5 L	+20–50%
Stroke volume	73.3 (±9 mL)	+30%
Systemic vascular resistance	1,530 (±520 dyne/cm/sec)	−20%
Oxygen consumption	250 mL/min	+20–30%

Adapted from American Heart Association [AHA]. (2015). *Women and heart disease*. Retrieved from https://www.goredforwomen. org/about-heart-disease/facts_about_heart_disease_in_women-sub-category/statistics-at-a-glance/; Mohamad, T. N., Fakhri, H. A., Bernal, J. M., Thatai, D., & Peterson, E. (2014). Cardiovascular disease and pregnancy. *eMedicine*. Retrieved from http://emedicine. medscape.com/article/162004-overview; and King, T. L., Brucker, M. C., Kriebs, J. M., Fahey, J. O., Gegor, C. L., & Varney, H. (2015). *Varney's midwifery* (5th ed.), Burlington, MA: Jones & Bartlett Learning.

capacity, exercise tolerance, degree of cyanosis, medication needs, and history of arrhythmias. Data needed for risk assessment can be acquired from a thorough cardiovascular history and examination, a 12-lead electrocardiogram (ECG), and evaluation of oxygen saturation levels by pulse oximetry. The impact of heart disease on a woman's childbearing potential needs to be clearly explained, and providing information on how pregnancy may affect her and the fetus is important. This allows women to make an informed choice about whether they wish to accept the risks associated with pregnancy. When possible, any surgical procedures, such as valve replacement, should be done before pregnancy to improve fetal and maternal outcomes (Sliwa et al., 2015).

If the woman presents for care after she has become pregnant, prenatal counseling focuses on the impact of the hemodynamic changes of pregnancy, the signs and symptoms of cardiac compromise, and dietary and lifestyle changes needed. More frequent prenatal visits (every 2 weeks until the last month and then weekly) are usually needed to ensure the health and safety of the mother and fetus.

Nursing Assessment

Frequent and thorough assessments are crucial during the antepartum period to ensure early detection of and prompt intervention for problems. Assess the woman's vital signs, noting any changes. Auscultate the apical heart rate and heart sounds, being especially alert for abnormalities, including irregularities in rhythm or murmurs. Check the client's weight and compare with baseline and weights obtained on previous visits. Report any weight gain outside recommended parameters. Inspect the extremities for edema and note any pitting.

Question the woman about fetal activity, and ask if she has noticed any changes. Report any changes such as a decrease in fetal movements. Ask the woman about any symptoms of preterm labor, such as low back pain, uterine contractions, and increased pelvic pressure and vaginal discharge, and report them immediately. Assess the fetal heart rate and review serial ultrasound results to monitor fetal growth.

Assess the client's lifestyle and her ability to cope with the changes of pregnancy and its effect on her cardiac status and ability to function. Evaluate the client's understanding of her condition and what restrictions and lifestyle changes may be needed to provide the best outcome for her and her fetus. A healthy infant and mother at the end of pregnancy is the ultimate goal. As the client's pregnancy advances, expect her functional class to be revised based on her level of disability. Suggest realistic modifications.

The nurse plays a major role in recognizing the signs and symptoms of cardiac decompensation. Decompensation refers to the heart's inability to maintain adequate circulation. As a result, tissue perfusion in the mother and the fetus is impaired. Common complaints of normal pregnancy, such as dyspnea, fatigue, palpitations, orthpnea, and pedal edema, mimic symptoms of worsening cardiac disease and create challenges when trying to evaluate pregnant women with cardiac disease. The pregnant woman is most vulnerable for this complication from 28 to 32 weeks of gestation and in the first 48 hours postpartum (Gandhi & Martin, 2015). Assess the woman for the following signs and symptoms:

- Shortness of breath on exertion, dyspnea
- Cyanosis of lips and nail beds
- Swelling of face, hands, and feet
- Jugular vein engorgement
- Rapid respirations

- Abnormal heartbeats, reports of heart racing or palpitations
- Chest pain with effort or emotion
- Syncope with exertion
- Increasing fatigue
- Moist, frequent cough

Take Note!

Assessing the pregnant woman with heart disease for cardiac decompensation is vital because the mother's hemodynamic status determines the health of the fetus.

Nursing Management

Nursing management of the pregnant woman with heart disease focuses on assisting with measures to stabilize the mother's hemodynamic status, because a decrease in maternal blood pressure or volume will cause blood to be shunted away from the uterus, thus reducing placental perfusion. Pregnant women with cardiac disease also need assistance in reducing risks that would lead to complications or further cardiac compromise; therefore, education and counseling are critical. Collaboration between the cardiologist, obstetrician, perinatologist, and nurse is needed to promote the best possible outcome.

Drug therapy may be indicated for the pregnant woman with a cardiac disorder. Possible drugs include diuretics, such as Lasix, to prevent heart failure; digitalis to increase contractility and decrease heart rates; antiarrhythmic agents (lidocaine); beta blockers (labetalol); calcium channel blockers (nifedipine) to treat hypertension; and anticoagulants (low-molecular-weight heparin). Warfarin (Coumadin) is not recommended because it crosses the placenta and may have teratogenic effects. It has been associated with spontaneous abortion, multiple birth defects, fetal growth restriction, and stillbirth (Lichtin & Philipson, 2014).

The FDA has changed their drug risk categories as of 6/30/15. They are no longer using categories A, B, C, D, and X. The new rule requires removal of the previous letter pregnancy categories. The package inserts will now include three separate categories that provide information in a narrative format. The goal of the new labeling is to provide information about the drug to the consumer. They now use specific subheadings under each of the three categories: Pregnancy; Lactation; and Females and Males of Reproductive Potential. For specific changes under each category, please access the following FDA web site: http://www.fda.gov/Drugs/DevelopmentApprovalProcess/DevelopmentResources/Labeling/ucm425415.htm.

Encourage the woman to continue taking her cardiac medications as prescribed. Review the indications, actions, and potential side effects of the medications. Reinforce the importance of frequent antepartal visits and close medical supervision throughout the pregnancy.

Discuss the need to conserve energy. Help the client to prioritize household chores and child care to allow rest periods. Encourage the client to rest in the side-lying position, which enhances placental perfusion.

Encourage the client to eat nutritious foods and consume a high-fiber diet to prevent straining and constipation. Discuss limiting sodium intake if indicated to reduce fluid retention. Contact a dietitian to assist the woman in planning nutritionally appropriate meals.

Assist the woman in preparing for diagnostic tests to evaluate fetal well-being. Describe the tests that may be done, such as ECG and echocardiogram, and explain the need for serial nonstress testing, usually beginning at approximately 32 weeks of gestation. Instruct the woman in how to monitor fetal activity and movements. Urge her to do this daily and report any changes in activity immediately.

Although the morbidity and mortality rates of pregnant women with cardiac disease have decreased greatly, hemodynamic changes during pregnancy (increased heart rate, stroke volume, cardiac output, and blood volume) have a profound effect, which may increase cardiac work and might exceed the functional capacity of the diseased heart. These changes may result in pulmonary hypertension, pulmonary edema, heart failure, or maternal death (Alonso-Gonzalez, & Swan, 2014). Explain the signs and symptoms of these complications and review the sign and symptoms of cardiac decompensation, encouraging the woman to notify her health care provider if any occur.

Provide support and encouragement throughout the antepartal period. Assess the support systems available to the client and her family, and encourage her to use them. If necessary, assist with referrals to community services for additional support.

During labor, anticipate the need for invasive hemodynamic monitoring, and make sure the woman has been prepared for this beforehand. Monitor her fluid volume carefully to prevent overload. Anticipate the use of epidural anesthesia if a vaginal birth is planned. After birth, assess the client for fluid overload as peripheral fluids mobilize. This fluid shift from the periphery to the central circulation taxes the heart, and signs of heart failure such as cough, progressive dyspnea, edema, palpitations, and crackles in the lung bases may ensue before postpartum diuresis begins. Because hemodynamics do not return to baseline for several days after childbirth, women at intermediate or high risk require monitoring for at least 48 hours postpartum (Cunningham et al., 2014).

Pregnancy offers a unique window through which women at risk of future CVD may be identified. Nurses have the opportunity to implement health monitoring, lifestyle modifications, and other needed interventions to reduce the burden of future CVD in all of their pregnant clients. Dispelling the myths surrounding CVD in women verses men (it is a man's disease only) would be huge in promoting awareness.

Hypertension in Pregnancy

ACOG has recently published revised guidelines for management of hypertension in pregnancy. They have outlined four categories to describe hypertension in pregnancy: preeclampsia–eclampsia, chronic hypertension, chronic hypertension with superimposed preeclampsia, and gestational hypertension. "Mild" is no longer used to categorize the severity of preeclampsia. The woman has it or not, with or without severe features (thrombocytopenia, renal insufficiency, impaired liver function, pulmonary edema, visual, or cerebral changes). Proteinuria is no longer required to diagnose preeclampsia now. ACOG recommends women with preeclampsia without severe features should give birth at 37 0/7 weeks; women with preeclampsia with severe features give birth at 34 0/7 weeks (ACOG, 2013).

Chronic Hypertension

Entering pregnancy with chronic hypertension is increasingly common. It is an important risk factor for pregnancy complications, including for the fetus or newborn, poor fetal growth, preterm birth, low birth weight, admission to the NICU and death, and for the mother, superimposed preeclampsia/eclampsia, acute renal failure, pulmonary edema, surgical birth, placental abruption, stoke, postpartum cardiomyopathy, and mortality (Solomon & Greene, 2015). Chronic hypertension exists when the woman has high blood pressure before pregnancy or before the 20th week of gestation, or when hypertension persists for more than 12 weeks postpartum. The *Eighth Report of the Joint National Committee on Prevention, Detection, Evaluation, and Treatment of High Blood Pressure* (Joint National Committee [JNC 8], 2014) previously classified blood pressure that remained unchanged as follows:

- *Normal:* Systolic less than 120 mm Hg, diastolic less than 80 mm Hg.
- *Prehypertension:* Systolic 120 to 139 mm Hg, diastolic 80 to 89 mm Hg.
- *Mild hypertension:* Systolic 140 to 159 mm Hg, diastolic 90 to 99 mm Hg.
- *Severe hypertension:* Systolic 160 mm Hg or higher, diastolic 100 mm Hg or higher (James et al., 2014).

Chronic hypertension occurs in up to 22% of women of childbearing age, with the prevalence varying according to age, race, and BMI. It complicates at least 5% of pregnancies, with one in four women developing preeclampsia during pregnancy (Sibai, 2015). Chronic hypertension is typically seen in older, obese women with glucose intolerance. The most common complication is preeclampsia, which is seen in approximately 25% of women who enter the pregnancy with hypertension. Worldwide, about 60,000 women die from preeclampsia each year, corresponding to 12% of all maternal deaths (Raio, Bolla, & Baumann, 2015). (See Chapter 19 for more information about preeclampsia.)

Therapeutic Management

Preconception counseling is important in fostering positive outcomes. Typically, it involves lifestyle changes such as diet, exercise, weight loss, and smoking cessation. Treatment for women with chronic hypertension focuses on maintaining normal blood pressure, preventing superimposed preeclampsia/eclampsia, and ensuring normal fetal development.

Once the woman is pregnant, antihypertensive agents are typically reserved for severe hypertension >160 mm Hg systolic and >100 mm Hg diastolic. Methyldopa (Aldomet) is commonly prescribed because of its safety record during pregnancy. This slow-acting antihypertensive agent helps to improve uterine perfusion. Other antihypertensive agents that can be used include labetalol (Trandate), atenolol (Tenormin), and nifedipine (Procardia) (Foo et al., 2015).

The U.S. Preventive Services Task Force [USPTF] (2015) recommends daily low-dose aspirin (81 mg/day) after 12 weeks of pregnancy in women, with chronic hypertension and other risk factors, who are at high risk for preeclampsia to reduce its occurrence.

Lifestyle changes are needed and should continue throughout gestation. The woman with chronic hypertension will be seen more frequently (every 2 weeks until 28 weeks and then weekly until birth) to monitor her blood pressure and to assess for any signs of preeclampsia. At approximately 24 weeks of gestation, the woman will be instructed to document fetal movement. At this same time, serial ultrasounds will be ordered to monitor fetal growth and amniotic fluid volume. Additional tests will be included if the client's status changes.

Nursing Assessment

Nursing assessment of the woman with chronic hypertension involves a thorough history and physical examination. Review the woman's history closely for risk factors. The pathogenesis of hypertension is multifactorial and includes many modifiable risk factors such as smoking, obesity, caffeine intake, excessive alcohol intake, excessive salt intake, and use of nonsteroidal anti-inflammatory drugs (NSAIDs). Also be alert for nonmodifiable risk factors such as increasing age and African–American race (Miller & Carpenter, 2015). Ask if the woman has received any preconception counseling and what measures have been used to prevent or control hypertension.

Assess the woman's vital signs, in particular her blood pressure. Evaluate her blood pressure in all three positions (sitting, lying, and standing) and note any major differences in the readings. Assess her for orthostatic hypertension when she changes her position from sitting to standing. Document your findings.

Ask the woman if she monitors her blood pressure at home; if so, inquire about the typical readings. Ask the woman if she uses any medications for blood pressure control, including the drug, dosage, and frequency of administration, as well as any side effects. Ask the woman about lifestyle modifications that she has used to address any modifiable risk factors, and their effectiveness.

Hypertension during pregnancy decreases uteroplacental perfusion. Therefore, fetal well-being must be assessed and closely monitored. Anticipate serial ultrasounds to assess fetal growth and amniotic fluid volume. Question the woman about fetal movement and evaluate her report of daily "kick counts." Assess fetal heart rate at every visit.

Nursing Management

Preconception counseling is the ideal time to discuss lifestyle changes to prevent or control hypertension. One area to cover during this visit would be the Dietary Approaches to Stop Hypertension (DASH) diet, which contains an adequate intake of potassium, magnesium, and calcium. Sodium is usually limited to 2.4 g. Suggest aerobic exercise as tolerated. Encourage smoking cessation and avoidance of alcohol. If the woman is overweight, encourage her to lose weight before becoming pregnant, not during the pregnancy (Killion, 2015). Stressing the positive benefits of a healthy lifestyle might help motivate the woman to make the necessary modifications and change unhealthy habits.

Assist the woman in scheduling appointments for antepartum visits every 2 weeks until 28 weeks of gestation and then weekly. Prepare the woman for frequent fetal assessments. Explaining the rationale for the need to monitor fetal growth is important to gain the woman's cooperation. Carefully monitor the woman for signs and symptoms of abruptio placenta (abdominal pain, rigid abdomen, vaginal bleeding), as well as superimposed preeclampsia (elevation in blood pressure, weight gain, edema, proteinuria). Alerting the woman to these risks can mean early identification and prompt intervention.

Stress the importance of daily periods of rest (1 hour) in the left lateral recumbent position to maximize placental perfusion. Encourage women with chronic hypertension to use home blood pressure monitoring devices. Urge the woman to report any elevations. As necessary, instruct the woman and her family how to take and record a daily blood pressure, and reinforce the need for her to take her medications as prescribed to control her blood pressure and to ensure the well-being of her unborn child. Praising her for her efforts at each prenatal visit may motivate her to continue the regimen throughout her pregnancy.

The close monitoring of the woman with chronic hypertension continues during labor and birth and during the postpartum period to prevent or identify the onset of preeclampsia. Accurate and frequent blood pressure readings and careful administration of antihypertensive medications, if prescribed, are essential components of care. Stressing the need for continued medical supervision after childbirth is vital to motivate the woman to maintain or initiate lifestyle changes and dietary habits and stay compliant with her medication regimen.

RESPIRATORY CONDITIONS

During pregnancy, the respiratory system is affected by hormonal changes, mechanical changes, and prior respiratory conditions. These changes can cause a woman with a history of compromised respiration to decompensate during pregnancy. Although upper respiratory infections are typically self-limiting, chronic respiratory conditions, such as asthma or tuberculosis (TB), can have a negative effect on the growing fetus when alterations in oxygenation occur in the mother. The outcome of pregnancy in a woman with a respiratory condition depends on the severity of the oxygen alteration as well as the degree and duration of hypoxia on the fetus.

Asthma

Worldwide, the prevalence of asthma among pregnant women is on the rise; pregnancy leads to a worsening of asthma for many women (Nagtalon-Ramos, 2014). Asthma affects approximately up to 13% of pregnancies globally, ranging between 200,000 and 376,000 women annually in the United States. It affects over 20 million Americans and is one of the most common and potentially serious medical conditions to complicate pregnancy (Jordan et al., 2014). Maternal asthma is associated with an increased risk of infant death, preeclampsia, intrauterine growth restriction (IUGR), preterm birth, and low birth weight. These risks are linked to the severity of asthma: more severe asthma increases the risk (National Asthma Education and Prevention Program [NAEPP], 2015).

Remember Rose, the pregnant teenager with asthma in acute distress described at the beginning of the chapter? What therapies might be offered to control her symptoms? Should she be treated differently than someone who is not pregnant? Why or why not?

Pathophysiology

Asthma is an allergic-type inflammatory response of the respiratory tract to various stimuli such as allergens (pollen and animal dander), irritants (cigarette smoke and chemicals), stress, infections (colds or flu), and physical exertion. It is also known as reactive airway disease because the bronchioles constrict in response to these stimuli. Asthma is characterized by paroxysmal or persistent symptoms of bronchoconstriction including breathlessness, wheezing, chest tightness, cough, and sputum production. In addition to bronchoconstriction, inflammation of the airways produces thick mucus that further limits the movement of air and makes breathing difficult.

The normal physiologic changes of pregnancy affect the respiratory system. Although the respiratory rate does not change, hyperventilation increases at term by 48% due to high progesterone levels. Diaphragmatic elevation and a decrease in functional lung residual capacity occur late in pregnancy, which may reduce the woman's ability to inspire deeply to take in more oxygen. Oxygen consumption and the metabolic rate both increase, placing additional stress on the woman's respiratory system (American Academy of Allergy, Asthma, & Immunology [AAAAI], 2015).

Both the woman and her fetus are at risk if asthma is not well managed during pregnancy. When a pregnant woman has trouble breathing, her fetus also has trouble getting the oxygen it needs for adequate growth and development. Severe persistent asthma has been linked to the development of maternal hypertension, low birth weight, preterm birth, preeclampsia, placenta previa, uterine hemorrhage, and oligohydramnios. Women whose asthma is poorly controlled during pregnancy are at increased risk of preterm birth, low birth weight, and stillbirth (Vanders & Murphy, 2015).

The severity of the condition improves in one third of pregnant women, remains unchanged in one third, and worsens in one third (Cunningham et al., 2014). However, the effect of pregnancy on asthma is unpredictable. The greatest increase in asthma attacks usually occurs between 24 and 36 weeks of gestation; flare-ups are rare during the last 4 weeks of pregnancy and during labor (AAAAI, 2015).

Therapeutic Management

Asthma should be treated as aggressively in pregnant women as in nonpregnant women because the benefits of averting an asthma attack outweigh the risks of medications. The ultimate goal of asthma therapy is to prevent hypoxic episodes to preserve continuous fetal oxygenation; improved maternal and perinatal outcomes are achieved with optimal control of asthma. One third of women with asthma develop worsening of control during pregnancy; therefore, close monitoring and reevaluation are essential. Four important aspects of asthma treatment ensure optimal control: close monitoring, education of clients, avoidance of asthma triggers, and pharmacologic therapy.

Many women with asthma have positive skin tests to allergens, the most common being animal dander, dust mites, cockroach antigens, pollens, and molds. There are nonimmune triggers as well, including strong odors, tobacco smoke, air pollutants, and drugs such as aspirin and beta-blockers. For exercise-triggered asthma, the use of a bronchodilator 5 to 60 minutes before exercise may reduce symptoms. Avoidance of these allergens and triggers can significantly reduce the need for medication and the occurrence of exacerbations during and after pregnancy. All women should be strongly encouraged to stop smoking, but especially those with asthma because they are at increased risk for worsening chronic and acute asthma sequelae.

Allergy injections may benefit those with allergies and asthma, called allergic asthma. Also called immunotherapy, allergy shots do not "cure" asthma in the manner in which an injection of, say, antibiotics might cure an infection. Instead, allergy shots work a bit more like a vaccine. Allergy injections for asthma actually contain a very small amount of an allergen (substance causing allergy). Over time, the dosage is increased. Exposure to progressive amounts of the allergen is likely to help the body develop a tolerance to it. If the allergen buildup is effective, the allergic reaction will become much less severe. Allergy injections can reduce the symptoms of allergies and prevent the development of asthma.

Medical therapy includes a stepwise approach in an attempt to use the least amount of medication necessary to control a woman's asthma and keep her severity in the mild range. Goals of therapy include having normal or near-normal pulmonary function and minimal or no chronic symptoms, exacerbations, or limitations on activities. The final goal is to minimize the adverse effects of treatment. Inhaled corticosteroids are preferred for the management of all levels of persistent asthma in pregnancy. Corticosteroids are the most effective treatment for the airway inflammation of asthma and reduce the hyperresponsiveness of airways to allergens and triggers.

NAEPP (2015) recommends three specific drugs to be used during pregnancy to control asthma:
- Budesonide (inhaled corticosteroid)
- Albuterol (short-acting beta$_2$ agonist)
- Salmeterol (long-acting beta$_2$ agonist)

Oral corticosteroids are not recommended for the long-term treatment of asthma during pregnancy, but they can be used to treat severe asthma attacks during pregnancy (AAAAI, 2015). In addition, two prostaglandins (hemabate and misoprostol [Cytotec]) used for treating postpartum hemorrhage and cervical ripening are contraindicated for clients with asthma due to the risk of bronchial spasm and bronchoconstriction (King et al., 2015).

Nursing Assessment

Obtain a thorough history of the disease, including the woman's usual therapy and control measures. Question the woman about asthma triggers and strategies used to reduce exposure to them (Box 20.2). Review the client's medication therapy regimen.

Auscultate the lungs and assess respiratory and heart rates. Include the rate, rhythm, and depth of respirations; skin color; blood pressure and pulse rate; and signs of fatigue. Clients with an acute asthma attack often present with wheezing, chest tightness, tachypnea, nonproductive coughing, shortness of breath, and dyspnea. Lung auscultation findings might include diffuse wheezes and rhonchi, bronchovesicular sounds, and a more prominent expiratory phase of respiration compared to the inspiratory phase (Kelly, Massoumi, & Lazarus, 2015). If the

---

BOX 20.2

COMMON ASTHMA TRIGGERS

- Smoke and chemical irritants
- Air pollution
- Dust mites
- Animal dander
- Seasonal changes with pollen, molds, and spores
- Upper respiratory infections
- Esophageal reflux
- Medications, such as aspirin and nonsteroidal anti-inflammatory drugs (NSAIDs)
- Exercise
- Cold air
- Emotional stress

Adapted from American Academy of Allergy, Asthma & Immunology [AAAAI]. (2015). *Asthma and pregnancy*. Retrieved from http://www.aaaai.org/conditions-and-treatments/library/asthma-library/asthma-and-pregnancy.aspx; March of Dimes(2015l). *Asthma during pregnancy*. Retrieved from http://www.marchofdimes.org/pregnancy/asthma-during-pregnancy.aspx; and Cunningham, F. G., Leveno, K. J., Bloom, S. L., Spong, C., & Dashe, J. (2014). *Williams' obstetrics* (24th ed.). New York, NY: McGraw-Hill Professional Publishing.

---

pregnancy is far enough along, the fetal heart rate is measured and routine prenatal assessments (weight, blood pressure, fundal height, urine for protein) are completed.

Laboratory studies usually include a complete blood count with differential (to assess the degree of nonspecific inflammation and identify anemia) and pulmonary function tests (to assess the severity of an attack and to provide a baseline to evaluate the client's response to treatment).

Nursing Management

Nursing management focuses on client education about the condition and the skills necessary to manage it: self-monitoring, correct use of inhalers, identifying and limiting exposure to asthma triggers, and following a long-term plan for managing asthma and for promptly handling signs and symptoms of worsening asthma. Client education fosters adherence to the treatment regimen, thereby promoting an optimal environment for fetal growth and development.

Client education should begin at the first prenatal visit. The importance of optimal asthma control and the risks of poor control for the woman and her fetus should be discussed early in pregnancy. Clients should be taught signs and symptoms, and which should be of concern, as well as who to contact in emergent situations. Women should be observed using their inhalers and correct use reinforced. Frank discussion about the importance of continuing asthma medications and the possible severe consequences for the woman and her fetus with discontinuation is vital.

Ensure that the woman understands drug actions and interactions, the uses and potential abuses of asthma medications, and the signs and symptoms that require medical evaluation. Reviewing potential perinatal complications with the woman is helpful in motivating her to adhere to the prescribed regimen. At each antepartum visit, reassess the efficacy of the treatment plan to determine whether adjustments are needed.

Taking control of asthma in pregnancy is the responsibility of the client along with her health care team. Providing the client with the knowledge and tools to monitor her condition, control triggers and her environment (Teaching Guidelines 20.2), and use medications to prevent acute exacerbations assist the client in taking control. Facilitating a partnership with the woman will improve perinatal outcomes.

Teaching Guidelines 20.2
TEACHING TO CONTROL ASTHMA LINKED TO ENVIRONMENTAL TRIGGERS

- Remove any carpeting in the house, especially the bedroom, to reduce dust mites.
- Use allergen-proof encasing on the mattress, box spring, and pillows.
- Wash all bedding in hot water.
- Remove dust collectors in house, such as stuffed animals, books, knickknacks.
- Avoid pets in the house to reduce exposure to pet dander.
- Keep humidity <50% to reduce dust mites
- Use a high-efficiency particulate air-filtering system in the bedroom.
- Do not smoke, and avoid places where you can be exposed to passive cigarette smoke from others.
- Dust and vacuum frequently using vacuum with a high-efficiency HEPA air filter
- Avoid use of wood stove heaters within the house
- Stay indoors and use air conditioning when the pollen or mold count is high or air quality is poor.
- Wear a covering over your nose and mouth when going outside in the cold weather.
- Avoid exposure to persons with colds, flu, or viruses.

When teaching the pregnant woman with asthma, cover the following topics:
- Signs and symptoms of asthma progression and exacerbation
- Importance and safety of medication to the fetus and to herself
- Warning signs that indicate the need to contact the health care provider
- Potential harm to the fetus and to herself by under treatment or delay in seeking help
- Prevention and avoidance of known triggers
- Home use of metered-dose inhalers
- Adverse effects of medications

Nurses should instruct and strongly urge women to remain on asthma medications during pregnancy because one third of clients have worsening of their asthma, including those women with mild asthma. There are proven negative effects from exacerbations and poor control on pregnancy outcome, whereas there are clear benefits of good control. Client education about the importance of good asthma control is essential for improving pregnancy outcomes.

During labor, monitor the client's oxygenation saturation by pulse oximetry and provide pain management through epidural analgesia to reduce stress, which may trigger an acute attack. Continuously monitor the fetus for distress during labor and assess fetal heart rate patterns for hypoxia. Assess the newborn for signs and symptoms of hypoxia.

Rose, the pregnant teenager described earlier, is concerned about passing her asthma on to her baby. What should the nurse discuss with her? What questions should the nurse ask to help in identifying triggers in Rose's environment to prevent future asthma attacks?

Take Note!

Successful asthma management can reduce adverse perinatal outcomes: preeclampsia, preterm birth, and low birth weight.

Tuberculosis

TB is known as the great masquerader and manifestation of the disease can be vague and widespread. It is a disease that has been around for years but never seems to go away completely. TB is curable and preventable. Globally, TB is second only to HIV/AIDS as a cause of illness and death in adults, accounting for over 9 million cases of active disease and 2 million deaths each year. Someone in the world is newly infected with TB every second. Overall, one third of the world's population is currently infected with TB (World Health Organization [WHO], 2015b).

Although it is not prevalent in the United States, a resurgence was noted starting in the mid-1980s secondary to the AIDS epidemic and immigration. Left undiagnosed and untreated, each person with active TB will infect on average between 10 and 15 people each year (WHO, 2015b). The link between poverty and TB is strong. With the large numbers of immigrants coming to the United States, all nurses must be skilled in screening for and managing this condition.

In many cultures the social consequences associated with the diagnosis of TB fall most heavily on women. Difficulties finding a marriage partner and divorce or abandonment among those already married are significant consequences for women from Pakistan, Vietnam, and India. Fear of social consequences can translate into delayed or absent health-seeking behavior. In pregnancy, TB that is treated early and adequately has outcomes equivalent to those in nonpregnant women. By contrast, studies have reported an increase in obstetrical mortality with increased incidence of spontaneous abortion, preterm labor, and preeclampsia in cases where TB was diagnosed late (Bates et al., 2015).

A person becomes infected by inhaling the infectious organism *Mycobacterium tuberculosis,* which is carried on droplet nuclei and spread by airborne transmission. The lung is the major site of involvement, but the lymph glands, meninges, bones, joints, and kidneys can become infected. Women can remain asymptomatic for long periods of time as the organism lies dormant. Pregnant women with untreated TB are more likely to have an underweight infant, an infant with a low Apgar score, and perinatal death (Mehta et al., 2015). The newborn is at risk of postnatally acquired TB if the mother still has active TB at the time of birth. Therefore, prenatal diagnosis and effective treatment of the mother are essential.

Therapeutic Management

The WHO recommends that the treatment of TB in pregnant women should be the same as that in nonpregnant women and the rest of the general population. The only exception is that streptomycin should be avoided in pregnancy because it is ototoxic to the fetus.

Medications are the cornerstone of treatment to prevent infection from progressing. The FDA developed pregnancy categories that rank the risk of teratogenic effects of drugs to be used in drug labeling (see the list earlier in the chapter in the discussion of heart disease). The safety of the first-line drugs for the management of active TB in pregnancy has been established, and therapy improves both maternal and neonatal outcomes.

Pregnant women should start treatment as soon as TB is suspected. The preferred initial treatment regimen is INH, rifampin, and ethambutol daily for 2 months, followed by INH and rifampin daily, or twice weekly for 7 months. Women taking INH should also be taking pyridoxine (vitamin B6) supplementation (CDC, 2015b).

Nursing Assessment

Review the woman's history for risk factors such as immunocompromised status, recent immigration status, homelessness or overcrowded living conditions, and injectable drug use. Women emigrating from developing countries such as Latin America, Asia, the Indian subcontinent, Eastern Europe, Russia, China, Mexico, Haiti, and Africa with high rates of TB also are at risk.

At antepartum visits, be alert for clinical manifestations of TB, including fatigue, fever or night sweats, nonproductive cough, weakness, slow weight loss, anemia, hemoptysis, fatigue, and anorexia (Herchline & Amorosa, 2015). If TB is suspected or the woman is at risk for developing TB, anticipate screening with purified protein derivative (PPD) administered by intradermal injection. If the client has been exposed to TB, a reddened induration will appear within 72 hours. If the test is positive, anticipate a follow-up chest X-ray with lead shielding over the abdomen, as well as sputum cultures to confirm the diagnosis.

Nursing Management

Adherence to the multidrug therapy is critical to protect the woman and her fetus from progression of TB. Provide education about the disease process, the mode of transmission, prevention, potential complications, and the importance of adhering to the treatment regimen.

Stressing the importance of health promotion activities throughout the pregnancy is important. Some suggestions might include avoiding crowded living conditions, avoiding sick people, maintaining adequate hydration, eating a nutritious, well-balanced diet, keeping all prenatal appointments to evaluate fetal growth and well-being, and getting plenty of fresh air outside. Determining the woman's understanding of her condition and treatment plan is important for adherence. A language interpreter may be needed to validate and reinforce her understanding if she does not speak English.

Breast-feeding is not contraindicated during the time the mother is on the medication regimen and should in fact be encouraged. If the mother is untreated for TB at the time of childbirth they should not breastfeed or be in direct contact with their newborn until at least 2 weeks after starting antituberculin medications. Untreated mothers can be encouraged to pump their milk to feed their newborns until they can breastfeed directly (American Academy of Pediatrics [AAP, 2015]). Nurses should consult their hospital policies regarding mothers with tuberculosis for guidance. Management of the newborn of a mother with TB involves preventing transmission by teaching the parents not to cough, sneeze, or talk directly into the newborn's face. Nurses need to stay current about new therapies and screening techniques to treat this centuries-old disease.

HEMATOLOGIC CONDITIONS

Anemia, a reduction in red blood cell volume, is measured by hematocrit (Hct) or a decrease in the concentration of hemoglobin (Hgb) in the peripheral blood. This results in reduced capacity of the blood to carry oxygen to the vital organs of the mother and fetus. Anemia is a sign of an underlying problem but does not indicate its origin.

Iron-Deficiency Anemia

Iron deficiency is the most common pathologic cause of anemia in pregnancy. Increased risk during pregnancy is due to increased maternal iron needs and demands from the growing fetus, increased erythrocyte mas; and, in the third trimester, expanded maternal blood volume (Cantor et al., 2015). Anemia affects one fourth of the world's population, and iron deficiency is the predominate cause. Iron-deficiency anemia mainly reflects poor nutrition, principally attributed to poor economic status worldwide. A recent study supports that and found that iron-deficiency anemia is strongly associated with low socioeconomic status, which affects women's knowledge and health-seeking behaviors. The study concludes that empowering women in terms of education and economic status is the key factor in combating anemia in pregnancy to prevent the vicious cycle of associated problems (Friedman et al., 2015).

Iron-deficiency anemia accounts for 75% to 95% of the cases of anemia in pregnant women (affecting one in four pregnancies), and is usually related to an iron-deficient diet, gastrointestinal issues affecting absorption, or a short pregnancy interval (Jimenez et al., 2015). A woman who is pregnant often has insufficient iron stores to meet the demands of pregnancy.

The clinical consequences of iron-deficiency anemia include preterm delivery, perinatal mortality, and postpartum depression. Fetal and neonatal consequences include low birth weight and poor mental and psychomotor performance (Subramaniam & Girish, 2015). With significant maternal iron depletion, the fetus will attempt to store iron, but at a cost to the mother. Anemia at term increases the perinatal risk for both the mother and newborn. The risks of hemorrhage (impaired platelet function) and infection during and after birth also are increased. Clinical symptoms of iron-deficiency anemia include fatigue, diminished quality of life, impaired cognitive function, increased risk for thromboembolic events, headache, restless legs syndrome, and **pica** (consuming nonfood substances) eating behaviors (Camaschella, 2015).

Therapeutic Management

The goals of treatment for iron-deficiency anemia in pregnancy are to eliminate symptoms, correct the deficiency, and replenish iron stores. The Centers for Disease Control and Prevention (CDC), Health and Medicine Division (HMD), and ACOG recommend routine iron supplementation for all pregnant women starting at a low dose of 30 mg/day beginning at the first prenatal visit (Moses, 2015). Attempting to meet maternal iron requirements solely through diet in the face of diminished iron stores is difficult.

Nursing Assessment

Review the mother's history for factors that may contribute to the development of iron-deficiency anemia, including poor nutrition, hemolysis, pica (consuming nonfood substances), multiple gestation, limited intervals between pregnancies, and blood loss. Assess the woman's dietary intake as well as the quantity and timing of ingestion of substances that interfere with iron absorption, such as tea, coffee, chocolate, and high-fiber foods. Ask the woman if she has fatigue, weakness, malaise, anorexia, or increased susceptibility to infection, such as frequent colds. Inspect the skin and mucous membranes, noting any pallor. Obtain vital signs and report any tachycardia.

Prepare the woman for laboratory testing. Laboratory tests usually reveal low Hgb (<11 g/dL), low Hct (<35%), low serum iron (<30 mcg/dL), microcytic and hypochromic cells, and low serum ferritin (<100 mg/dL).

Take Note!

Hemoglobin and hematocrit decrease normally during pregnancy in response to an increase in blood plasma in comparison to red blood cells. This hemodilution can lead to physiologic anemia of pregnancy, which does not indicate a decrease in oxygen-carrying capacity or true anemia.

Nursing Management

Nursing management of the woman with iron-deficiency anemia focuses on encouraging adherence to drug therapy and providing dietary instruction about the intake of iron-rich foods. Although iron constitutes a minimal percentage of the body's total weight, it has several major roles: it assists in the transport of oxygen and carbon dioxide throughout the body, it aids in the production of red blood cells, and it plays a role in the body's immune response.

Stress the importance of taking the prenatal vitamin and iron supplement consistently. Encourage the woman to take the iron supplement with vitamin C–containing fluids such as orange juice, which will promote absorption, rather than milk, which can inhibit iron absorption. Taking iron on an empty stomach improves its absorption, but many women cannot tolerate the gastrointestinal discomfort it causes. In such cases, advise the woman to take it with meals. Instruct the woman about adverse effects, which are predominantly gastrointestinal and include gastric discomfort, nausea, vomiting, anorexia, diarrhea, metallic taste, and constipation. Suggest that the woman take the iron supplement with meals and increase her intake of fiber and fluids to help overcome the most common side effects.

Provide dietary counseling. Recommend foods high in iron, such as dried fruits, whole grains, green leafy vegetables, meats, peanut butter, and iron-fortified cereals (Dudek, 2014). Anticipate the need for a referral to a dietitian. Teaching Guidelines 20.3 highlights instructions for the pregnant woman with iron-deficiency anemia.

Teaching Guidelines 20.3
TEACHING FOR THE WOMAN WITH IRON-DEFICIENCY ANEMIA

- Take your prenatal vitamin daily; if you miss a dose, take it as soon as you remember.
- For best absorption, take iron supplements between meals.
- Awareness of the side effects of iron supplementation
- Avoid taking iron supplements with coffee, tea, chocolate, and high-fiber food.
- Eat foods rich in iron, such as:
  - Meats, green leafy vegetables, legumes, dried fruits, whole grains
  - Peanut butter, bean dip, whole-wheat fortified breads and cereals
- For best iron absorption from foods, consume the food along with a food high in vitamin C.
- Increase your exercise, fluids, and high-fiber foods to reduce constipation.
- Plan frequent rest periods during the day.

Thalassemia

Thalassemia is a group of hereditary anemias in which synthesis of one or both chains of the hemoglobin molecule (alpha and beta) is defective. Inheritance is autosomal recessive. A low Hgb and a microcytic, hypochromic anemia results. The prevalence and severity of thalassemia depend on the woman's racial background: persons of Mediterranean, Asian, Italian, or Greek heritage and African Americans are most frequently affected. Beta-thalassemia is the most common form found in the United States (March of Dimes, 2015b).

Thalassemia occurs in two forms: alpha-thalassemia and beta-thalassemia. Alpha-thalassemia (minor), the heterozygous form, results from the inheritance of one abnormal gene from either parent, placing the offspring in a carrier trait state. These women have little or no hematologic disease and are clinically asymptomatic (silent carrier state). Beta-thalassemia (major) is the form involving inheritance of the gene from both parents. Beta-thalassemia major can be very severe. Genetic counseling might be necessary when decisions about childbearing are being made.

Thalassemia minor has little effect on pregnancy, although the woman will have mild, persistent anemia. This anemia does not respond to iron therapy, and iron supplements should not be prescribed. Several recent studies suggest that pregnancy appears safe for a woman with well-treated beta thalassemia major who does not have heart disease (Rigby, 2015).

Management of thalassemia during pregnancy depends on the severity of the disease. Apart from the routine prenatal visit schedule, thalassemic pregnant women need additional care which includes regular and periodic evaluation of cardiac function by a cardiologist to prevent fluid overload; and frequent hemoglobin and ferritin levels should be monitored to avoid iron overload. Identification and screening are important to plan care. The woman's ethnic background, medical history, and blood studies are analyzed. If the woman is determined to be a carrier, screening of the father of the child is indicated. Knowledge of the carrier state of each parent provides the genetic counselor with knowledge about the risk that the fetus will be a carrier or will have the disease (Karimi, Cohan, & Parand, 2015). Mild anemia may be present, and instructions to rest and avoid infections are helpful. Nurses should provide supportive care and expectant management throughout the pregnancy.

Sickle Cell Anemia

Sickle cell anemia is an autosomal recessive inherited condition that results from a defective hemoglobin molecule (hemoglobin S). It is found most commonly in African Americans, Southeast Asians, and Middle Eastern populations. Sickle cell disease affects millions of people across the globe. In the United States, approximately 90,000, to 100,000 people have the disease, and 2 million have the sickle cell trait. Sickle cell disease occurs once in every 500 African–American births, and once in 36,000 Hispanic–American births. One in 12 African Americans has the sickle cell trait (CDC, 2015c).

Women with sickle cell disease can have more adverse maternal outcomes such as preeclampsia, eclampsia, preterm labor, placental abruption, intrauterine growth restriction, low birth weight, and maternal mortalities (Costa, Viana, & Aguiar, 2015). The gene offers protection against malaria, but can be a cause of chronic pain and early death. Life expectancy is shortened as a consequence of renal damage, cardiac damage, and infection (March of Dimes, 2015c). People with only one gene for the trait (heterozygous) will have sickle cell trait without obvious symptoms of the disease and with little effect on the pregnancy.

Pathophysiology

In the human body, the hemoglobin molecule serves as the oxygen-carrying component of the red blood cells. Most people have several types of circulating hemoglobin (HbA and HbA2) that make up the majority of their circulatory system. In sickle cell disease, the abnormal hemoglobin S (HbS) replaces HbA and HbA2. This abnormal hemoglobin (HbS) becomes "sickle" shaped as a result of any stress or trauma such as infection, fever, acidosis, dehydration, physical exertion, excessive cold

exposure, or hypoxia. The sickle shape of the hemoglobin causes clumping together, which blocks the microvasculature. Significant anemia usually results.

Sickle cell anemia during pregnancy is associated with more severe anemia and frequent vaso-occlusive crises, with increased maternal and perinatal morbidity and mortality. In pregnant women with sickle cell anemia, complications can occur at any time during gestation, labor and birth, or postpartum. This is believed to be secondary to hormonal modifications, hypercoagulable state, and increased susceptibility to infection. Microvascular sickling in the placental circulation is associated with miscarriages, placental abruption, preeclampsia, preterm labor, intrauterine growth restriction, fetal distress, and low birth weight (Vichinsky, 2015).

Therapeutic Management

Ideally, women with hemoglobinopathies are screened before conception and are made aware of the risks of sickle cell anemia to themselves and to the fetus. A blood hemoglobin electrophoresis (lab study used for both DNA and RNA analysis) is done for all women from high-risk ancestry at their first prenatal visit to determine the types and percentages of hemoglobin present. This information should help them in making reproductive decisions.

Treatment depends on the health status of the woman. The effect of sickle cell disease on pregnancy depends on which manifestations the woman is experiencing. For example, sickle cell anemia combined with the increased blood volume in pregnancy increases the risks for heart failure should fluid overload occur in therapy for the anemia (Cunningham et al., 2014).

Early and continuous prenatal care is needed to safeguard the fetus/infant from potential complications during the antepartum, intrapartum, and postpartum periods. Toward this end, prenatal visits for the first and second trimester should be scheduled more frequently. During pregnancy, only supportive therapy is used: blood transfusions for severe anemia, analgesics for pain, and antibiotics for infection.

Nursing Assessment

Assess the woman for signs and symptoms of sickle cell anemia. Ask the woman if she has anorexia, dyspnea, or malaise. Inspect the color of the skin and mucous membranes, noting any pallor. Be alert for indicators of sickle cell crisis, including severe abdominal pain, muscle spasms, leg pains, joint pain, fever, stiff neck, nausea and vomiting, and seizures (Jordan et al., 2014).

Nursing Management

Clients require emotional support, education, and follow-up care to deal with this chronic condition, which can have a great impact on the woman and her family. Monitor vital signs, fetal heart rate, weight gain, and fetal growth. Assess hydration status at each visit and urge the client to drink 8 to 10 glasses of fluid daily to prevent dehydration. Teach the client about the need to avoid infections (including meticulous hand hygiene), cigarette smoking, alcohol consumption, and temperature extremes.

Assist the woman in scheduling frequent fetal well-being assessments, such as biophysical profiles, nonstress tests, and contraction stress tests, and monitor laboratory test results for changes. Throughout the antepartal period, be alert for early signs and symptoms of crisis.

During labor, encourage rest and provide pain management. Oxygen supplementation is typically used throughout labor, along with intravenous fluids to maintain hydration. The fetal heart rate is monitored closely. After giving birth, the woman is fitted with antiembolism stockings to prevent blood clot formation. Before discharge from the facility after birth of the newborn, discuss family planning options.

The ability to predict the clinical course of sickle cell anemia during pregnancy is difficult. Outcomes have improved for pregnant women with the disease, and currently the majority can achieve a successful live birth. However, pregnancy is associated with an increased incidence of morbidity and mortality. Optimal management during pregnancy should be directed at preventing pain crises, chronic organ damage, and early mortality using a multidisciplinary team approach and prompt, effective, and safe relief of acute pain episodes. Although these measures do not remove the risk of maternal and fetal complications, they are thought to minimize them, promoting a successful pregnancy outcome. As part of the obstetric health care team, the nurse provides nursing interventions for the labor and postpartum client aimed at pain management, maternal/fetal safety, and client education. The overall objective is a healthy outcome for the childbearing family. The nurse has a vital role in making this happen.

AUTOIMMUNE DISORDERS

Autoimmune disorders are a group of more than 80 distinct diseases that emerge when the immune system launches an immune response against its own cells and tissues. Two distinct types of autoimmune disease occur:
1. Localized disorders target specific organs such as the thyroid gland in Hashimoto's thyroiditis and Graves' disease.
2. Systemic disorders affect multiple organs. For example, in systemic lupus erythematosus (SLE), the immune system can target the lungs, hearts, joints, kidneys, brain, and red blood cells.

Autoimmune disorders may cause mild insidious symptoms that come and go or debilitating conditions with high mortality.

Women suffer from autoimmune disease more than men. According to the CDC (2015d), autoimmune diseases affect approximately 8% of the population, 78% of whom are women. Autoimmune diseases are the third most common category of disease in the United States after cancer and heart disease; they affect approximately 5% to 8% of the population or 14 to 22 million people (CDC, 2015d). Previously, the general advice to women with autoimmune diseases, especially SLE, multiple sclerosis, or rheumatoid syndromes, was to avoid pregnancy because there was a high risk of maternal and fetal morbidity and mortality. However, it is now clear that these risks can be reduced in general by avoiding pregnancy when the diseases are active and continuing appropriate medication to reduce the chances of disease flare during pregnancy.

Systemic Lupus Erythematosus

Lupus disease, also known as **systemic lupus erythematosus (SLE)**, is diagnosed based on laboratory values, symptoms, and signs, SLE is a chronic, relapsing autoimmune disease of the connective tissues that can affect various organs, such as the skin, joints, kidneys, and serosal membranes. Lupus disease is of unknown etiology, but it is thought to be a failure of the regulatory mechanisms of the autoimmune system. It is usually managed with anti-inflammatory and antirheumatic medications. Several triggers that cause the disease to activate include estrogen; cigarette smoking; infections, especially Epstein–Barr virus; physical or psychologic stress; exposure to ultraviolet light; and pregnancy. Lupus symptoms may include swollen joints, extreme fatigue, oral ulcers, skin rashes, and sensitivity to sunlight (Mohindra & Marwah, 2015). Lupus is a complex disorder characterized by periods of relative inactivity and periods of disease exacerbation (flare-ups). To be diagnosed with SLE a woman must have at least four out of 11 positive American College of Rheumatology Criteria which include red rash on face, photosensitivity, oral ulcers, arthritis, serositis, renal disease, seizures, fatigue, weight changes, anemia, and a positive antinuclear antibody test (Wasserman & Clowse, 2014).

The overall incidence of lupus in the United States is 150 per 100,000 people. The peak onset occurs between ages 15 and 45 with over 80% of the cases being diagnosed in women who are in their childbearing years. SLE is more common among those of African American, Afro–Caribbean, Asian, Native American, and Hispanic descent (Schur & Hahn, 2015).

Pathophysiology

The autoimmune responses in SLE prevent the body from recognizing "self" from "nonself," thus allowing antibodies to be formed that attack the body's own cells and proteins. This activity causes suppression of the body's normal immunity and damage to the body tissue. The autoimmune response may initially involve one organ or several. The most common organs/organ systems involved are the cardiovascular, integumentary, musculoskeletal, nervous systems, kidneys, and lungs. In pregnancy, inflammation of the connective tissue of the deciduas can result in placental implantation problems and poor functioning (Bartels & Muller, 2015).

Women with SLE are at increased risk for adverse pregnancy outcomes and cardiovascular disease. A pregnancy with lupus is prone to complications, including flares of disease activity during pregnancy or in the postpartum period, preeclampsia, pregnancy loss, miscarriage, stillbirth, fetal growth restriction, and preterm birth. Active lupus nephritis poses the greatest risk. The recognition of a lupus flare during pregnancy may be difficult because the signs and symptoms may mimic those of normal pregnancy (Singh & Chowdhary, 2015).

Therapeutic Management

The focus of therapy is to control disease flare-ups, suppress symptoms, and prevent organ damage. Treatment decisions are based on severity of the condition and organ involvement. Treatment of SLE in pregnancy is generally limited to NSAIDs (e.g., ibuprofen [Advil]), prednisone (Deltasone), and an antimalarial agent, hydroxychloroquine (Plaquenil). During pregnancy in the woman with SLE, the goal is to keep drug therapy to a minimum (King et al., 2015).

Nursing Assessment

The time at which the nurse comes in contact with the woman in her childbearing life cycle will determine the focus of the assessment. If the woman is considering pregnancy, it is recommended that she postpone conception until the disease has been stable or in remission for 6 months. Active disease at time of conception and history of renal disease increase the likelihood of a poor pregnancy outcome (Cunningham et al., 2014). In particular, if pregnancy is planned during periods of inactive or stable disease, the result often is giving birth to healthy full-term babies without increased risks of pregnancy complications. Nonetheless, pregnancies in most autoimmune diseases are still classified as high risk because of the potential for major complications. Preconception counseling should include the medical and obstetric risks of spontaneous abortion, stillbirth, fetal death, fetal growth restriction, preeclampsia, preterm labor, and neonatal death and the need for more frequent visits for monitoring her condition (Hadar, Ashwal, & Hod, 2014).

If the woman is already pregnant when the nurse encounters her, the nurse needs to assess for the following:
- Duration and presence of SLE signs and symptoms (fatigue, fever, malaise, polyarthritis, skin rashes, and multiorgan involvement)

- Evidence of anemia, thrombocytopenia, and thrombophilias
- Underlying renal disease (check the urine for protein and specific gravity)
- Signs of flare-ups
- Abnormalities in laboratory tests
- Signs of infection (check at each prenatal visit especially urinary tract infections and upper respiratory infections since prednisone can mask signs of infection and lower resistance)
- Fetal well-being and growth (check using ultrasound, fundal height measurements, nonstress tests, and biophysical profiles)

Nursing Management

The nurse should discuss with the woman the importance of having good control over her SLE condition throughout the pregnancy. Discussions should focus on the effects of SLE during the pregnancy and possible risk for exacerbations. Emphasize the importance of frequent prenatal visits to detect early preeclampsia, preterm labor, or infections. Instruction should cover the implications and potential side effects of all drug therapies prescribed. Teach energy conservation techniques to prevent fatigue, signs and symptoms to report (extreme fatigue, edema, confusion, abdominal pain, weight loss, leg pain, anorexia), and the need for frequent and close monitoring for fetal well-being.

After childbirth, a discussion of birth control and the effects of the various methods on the disease is essential. Referral to self-help groups and local and national SLE organizations is important for further education of the woman and her family.

SLE can greatly complicate a pregnancy if close supervision is not maintained. The keys to a successful outcome for the mother and her infant include an accurate assessment of the disease and of the various systems involved, and vigilance during the pregnancy for disease progression, effects on the fetus, and development of complications. Nursing care should be directed at early detection of problematic signs and symptoms, education of the mother and family, careful evaluation of the fetal status, and providing support to assist the mother in strengthening her coping strategies.

Multiple Sclerosis

Multiple sclerosis (MS) is a chronic inflammatory, demyelinating autoimmune disorder of the central nervous system. The Multiple Sclerosis Association of America [MSAA] (2015) estimates that approximately 400,000 people in the United States have MS. It is more commonly seen in women than in men, and the mean age of onset is 30 years. Globally, approximately 2.5 million are affected. There is no cure for the disease, and the disease usually becomes a chronic condition (2015).

In the early, inflammatory course of MS, autoreactive T cells cross the blood–brain barrier, attacking myelin proteins and leading to inflammation and demyelination. As the inflammatory process continues, repeated injury results of the myelin membrane with progressive neurodegeneration. The pathologic hallmark of MS can be described as multicentric, multiphasic central nervous system inflammation with resultant demyelination (Armon et al. 2015).

Uncomplicated MS does not have adverse effects on fertility, labor, or birth. Rates of spontaneous abortion, congenital anomalies, and fetal mortality are no higher among women with MS when compared with women in the general population (Vukusic & Marignier, 2015). There is no indication that women with MS require different care or management during the labor and birth process. Pregnant women with MS tend to have fewer relapses during gestation with a subsequent increase in disease activity in the first 3 months postpartum. Breastfeeding does not seem to have an influence on severity or frequency of exacerbations or the health of mothers, and has been shown to decrease MS relapse rates during the first 6 months postpartum (Walker, 2014). Breastfeeding should be encouraged as long as the woman is not being treated with disease-modifying agents.

The clinical presentation of MS can be similar to common pregnancy-related symptoms, especially fatigue, weakness, constipation, urinary frequency, balance problems, back pain, and visual changes. The similarity of the symptoms makes it difficult to attribute any symptoms that may develop during an established pregnancy to the disease process. These symptoms should be assessed carefully to assess MS exacerbations (Novotna & Ehler, 2014).

The focus of therapy for MS is to prevent clinical relapse and postpone neurodegeneration and the subsequent disability. Current medications include anti-inflammatories, immunosuppressants, immunomodulators/biologic agents, and a variety of complementary and alternative therapies such as vitamin/mineral supplementation, homeopathy, botanical products, and antioxidants. The complementary or alternative therapies have not been proven to reduce relapse rates or disease progression, but many MS sufferers turn to them (King et al., 2015). Most medications used in MS treatment are not FDA-approved during pregnancy, but many have been used and have not shown to have adverse effects.

Nursing care is similar to that outlined previously under SLE. The need for support at this life-changing time is crucial. Continuity of care, access to information tailored to their needs, when requested by the woman or her family, and having a point of contact are all important aspects of nursing care.

Rheumatoid Arthritis

Rheumatoid arthritis (RA) is characterized by joint inflammation and progressive disability and is one of the most common chronic autoimmune disorders. It predominates in women, commonly affecting women of childbearing age and may complicate pregnancy. RA primarily affects synovial joints and tissues of the hands and feet, but any joint can be involved. Over time, bone and cartilage are damaged by the chronic inflammation process, resulting in joint deformity and loss of function. Progression of the disease and ensuing disability is unpredictable.

Rheumatoid arthritis affects approximately 1.3 million adults in the United States. It is present in nearly all geographic areas and affects all ethnic groups. The disease typically presents between 30 and 50 years of age and affects twice as many women as men (American College of Rheumatology, 2015). The course of RA during pregnancy is usually benign. In about three fourths of pregnancies, the symptoms of the disease lessen. In these cases, most women experience relief in the first trimester that continues throughout the pregnancy. For many women with RA, pregnancy can provide a reprieve from long-term joint pain and inflammation, but others will not experience remission and will continue to need medication. RA does not adversely affect pregnancy outcome. With occasional exceptions, RA returns after the third to fourth month postpartum (Strangfeld et al., 2015).

Individuals with RA typically present with pain, swelling, and tenderness in joints; decreased mobility; and stiffness after periods of inactivity. Treatment of RA focuses on reducing joint inflammation, managing pain, and preventing joint destruction. The categories of medications used to accomplish this are NSAIDs, glucocorticoids, hydroxychloroquine, methotrexate, immunomodulators/biologic agents, and complementary alternative therapies such as physical therapy, exercise, acupuncture, and joint splinting for pain relief. During pregnancy, medications are limited to hydroxychloroquine, glucocorticoids, and NSAIDs. Methotrexate is a, is contraindicated during pregnancy (King et al., 2015). Careful preconception counseling and risk assessment is important in women with rheumatoid arthritis. Antibody status and all medications need to be reviewed before pregnancy. Maintaining low disease activity before and during pregnancy is essential for optimal outcomes.

Nursing care should address the teratogenicity (the ability to cause birth defects) and adverse effects of some of the medications used to treat rheumatoid arthritis. Women with RA must be monitored closely following childbirth because most are likely to have arthritis flare-ups during the postpartum period. The general nursing care is similar to that outlined for the low-risk pregnant woman. Nurses caring for women with any disability (physical or cognitive) in general need to provide level-appropriate education on all reproductive health issues and improved access to health care. The woman's specific disability, her resources, and her approach to pregnancy and childbirth all help shape her experience. The nurse can play a role in making her experience a positive, memorable time in her life. Care for the woman with a disability should be well planned and coordinated by ensuring all documentation of the woman's needs and concerns is readily available to all personnel involved in her care. All members of the health care team should be involved in the plan of care and kept up to date of any changes. It is essential that the nurse facilitate care to ensure continuity of care throughout the woman's pregnancy and childbirth experience (Ostensen, 2014).

INFECTIONS

A wide variety of infections can affect the progression of pregnancy, possibly having a negative impact on the outcome. The effect of the infection depends on the timing and severity of the infection and the body systems involved. Common viral infections include cytomegalovirus, rubella, herpes simplex, hepatitis B, varicella, parvovirus B19, and several sexually transmitted infections (STIs; Table 20.4). Toxoplasmosis and group B streptococcus are common nonviral infections. Only the most common infections will be discussed here.

Cytomegalovirus

Human cytomegalovirus (CMV) infects greater than 50% of the human population. Humans are the only known hosts of CMV, which is transmitted via body fluids. Worldwide, the birth prevalence is estimated at seven per 1000 births with the highest rates seen in developing countries. It is typically asymptomatic in most individuals. CMV is the most common congenital and perinatal viral infection in the world (Fig. 20.4). CMV is the leading cause of congenital infection, with morbidity and mortality at birth and sequelae. Each year approximately 1% to 7% of pregnant women acquire a primary CMV infection (Kovacs & Briggs, 2015). Of these, about 30% to 40% transmit the infection to their fetuses. The risk of serious fetal injury is greatest when maternal infection develops in the first trimester or early in the second trimester. Between 10% and 15% of congenitally infected infants are acutely symptomatic at birth and most of the survivors have serious long-term complications (March of Dimes, 2015d). It is a leading cause of hearing loss and intellectual disability in the United States. As a result of its substantial disease burden, congenital CMV is associated with an estimated $1 billion to $2 billion in direct economic costs each year. However, there has been limited progress in developing interventions to prevent or treat CMV infection (Bialas, Swamy, & Permar, 2015). Pregnant women acquire active disease primarily from

sexual contact, blood transfusions, kissing, and contact with children in daycare centers. It can also be spread through vertical transmission from mother to child in utero (causing congenital CMV), during birth, or through breast-feeding. The virus can be found in virtually all body fluids. Prevalence rates in women in the United States range from 50% to 85% (CDC, 2015e). In the United States, approximately 1 in 60 people undergo seroconversion each year. Although prevalent in the United States population, CMV is not easily transmitted from host to recipient. The incidence of primary CMV infection in pregnant women in the United States ranges from 1% to 4% (CDC, 2015e).). CMV infection during pregnancy may result in abortion, stillbirth, low birth weight, IUGR, microcephaly, deafness, blindness, intellectual disability, jaundice, or congenital or neonatal infection. The first or primary infection, if it occurs during pregnancy, is the most dangerous to the fetus: the fetus has a 30% to 40% chance of being infected.

There are three time periods during which mother-to-child transmission can occur: in utero, during birth, and after birth. However, permanent disability only occurs in association with in utero infection. Such disability can result from maternal infection during any point in the pregnancy, but more severe disabilities are usually associated with maternal infection during the first trimester.

Most women are asymptomatic and do not know that they have been exposed to CMV. Symptoms of CMV in the fetus and newborn, known as CMV inclusion disease, include hepatomegaly, thrombocytopenia, IUGR, jaundice, microcephaly, hearing loss, chorioretinitis, and intellectual disability. Newborns that are asymptomatic at birth may go on to develop late neurodevelopmental sequelae, with sensorineural hearing loss being the most common condition (Silasi et al., 2015). Prenatal screening for CMV infection is not routinely performed. Unfortunately, a preventive vaccine remains elusive. Since there is no therapy to prevent or treat CMV infections, nurses are responsible for educating and supporting childbearing-age women at risk for CMV infection. Stressing the importance of good hand hygiene and the use of sound hygiene practices can help to reduce transmission of the virus. A few specific hygiene guidelines for pregnant women include the following:

- Wash hands frequently with soap and water and wear gloves, especially after diaper changes, feeding, wiping nose or drool, and handling children's toys.
- Do not share cups, plates, utensils, food, or toothbrushes.
- Do not share towels or washcloths.
- Do not put a child's pacifier in your mouth.
- Clean toys, countertops, and other surfaces that come in contact with children's urine or saliva.
- Practice safe sex, including limiting sexual partners and use condoms consistently.

TABLE 20.4	SEXUALLY TRANSMITTED INFECTIONS AFFECTING PREGNANCY	
Infection/Organism	Effect on Pregnancy and Fetus/Newborn	Implications
Syphilis (*Treponema pallidum*)	Maternal infection increases risk of premature labor and birth. Newborn may be born with congenital syphilis—jaundice, rhinitis, anemia, IUGR, and CNS involvement.	All pregnant women should be screened for this STI and treated with benzathine penicillin G 2.4 million units IM to prevent placental transmission.
Gonorrhea (*Neisseria gonorrhea*)	Majority of women are asymptomatic. It causes ophthalmia neonatorum in the newborn from birth through infected birth canal.	All pregnant women should be screened at first prenatal visit, with repeat screening in the third trimester. All newborns receive mandatory eye prophylaxis with tetracycline or erythromycin within the first hour of life. Mother is treated with ceftriaxone (Rocephin) 125 mg IM in single dose before going home.
Chlamydia (*Chlamydia trachomatis*)	Majority of women are asymptomatic. Infection is associated with infertility and ectopic pregnancy, spontaneous abortions, preterm labor, premature rupture of membranes, low birth weight, stillbirth, and neonatal mortality. Infection is transmitted to newborn through vaginal birth. Neonate may develop conjunctivitis or pneumonia.	All pregnant women should be screened at first prenatal visit and treated with erythromycin.
Human papillomavirus (HPV)	Infection causes warts in the anogenital area, known as condylomata acuminata. These warts may grow large enough to block a vaginal birth. Fetal exposure to HPV during birth is associated with laryngeal papillomas.	Warts are treated with trichloroacetic acid, liquid nitrogen, or laser therapy under colposcopy. Two HPV vaccines have been FDA approved (Gardasil and Cervarix) against the viral types most likely to cause cervical cancer (types 16 and 18) and genital warts (types 6 and 11) has been licensed in the United States for girls and women 9 to 26 years old. The vaccines are 95% to 100% effective. The vaccines are now recommended for young boys also.
Trichomonas (*Trichomonas vaginalis*)	Infection produces itching and burning, dysuria, strawberry patches on cervix, and vaginal discharge. Infection is associated with premature rupture of membranes and preterm birth.	Treatment is with a single 2-g dose of metronidazole (Flagyl).

Adapted from King, T. L., Brucker, M. C., Kriebs, J. M., Fahey, J. O., Gegor, C. L., & Varney, H. (2015). *Varney's midwifery* (5th ed.). Burlington, MA: Jones & Bartlett Learning; Kumar, B., & Gupta, S. (2014). *Sexually transmitted infections* (2nd ed.). Philadelphia, PA: Elsevier Health Sciences; and Centers for Disease Control and Prevention [CDC]. (2015r). *Sexually transmitted diseases*. Retrieved from http://www.cdc.gov/std/

Rubella

Rubella, commonly called German measles, is spread by droplets or through direct contact with a contaminated object. The risk of a pregnant woman transmitting this virus through the placenta to her fetus increases with earlier exposure to the virus. When infection occurs within the first month after conception, 50% of fetuses show signs of infection; in the second month following conception, 25% of fetuses will be infected; and in the third month, 10% of fetuses will be affected. Congenital rubella can manifest with a diverse range of symptoms in the newborn, including congenital cataracts, glaucoma, cardiac defects, microcephaly, as well as hearing and intellectual disabilities (Jyoti, Shirke, & Matalia, 2015).

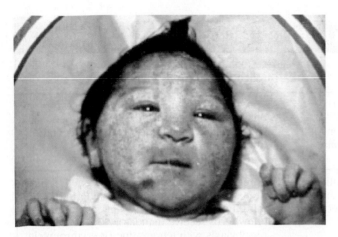

FIGURE 20.4 Clinical appearance of infant with congenital CMV with stigmata of disease, including petechial rash, microcephaly, jaundice, and abnormal posture of upper extremities secondary to CNS damage.

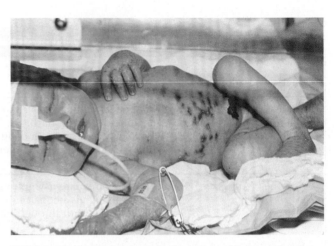

FIGURE 20.5 Newborn with disseminated herpes simplex virus infection. Note the healing ulcerations on the abdomen of the infant. From Sweet RL, Gibbs RS. (2009). *Infectious diseases of the female genital tract* (5th ed.). Philadelphia, PA: Lippincott Williams & Wilkins.

Preconception care has been defined as a set of interventions designed to identify and modify risks to a woman's health or pregnancy outcome through prevention and management. This care should be provided any time any health care provider sees a reproductive age woman. Personal and family history, physical exam, laboratory screening, reproductive plan, nutrition, supplements, weight, exercise, vaccinations, and injury prevention should be reviewed in all women. Folic acid 400 mcg per day, as well as proper diet and exercise, should be encouraged. Women should receive the influenza vaccine if planning pregnancy during flu season; the rubella and varicella vaccines if there is no evidence of immunity to these viruses; and tetanus/diphtheria/pertussis if lacking adult vaccination (Lambert et al., 2015).

Education for primary prevention is the key. Ideally, all women have been vaccinated and have adequate immunity against rubella. However, all women are still screened at their first prenatal visit to determine their status. A rubella antibody titer of 1:8 or greater proves evidence of immunity. Women who are not immune should be vaccinated during the immediate postpartum period so that they will be immune before becoming pregnant again (Agent, 2015). Nurses need to check the rubella immune status of all new mothers and should make sure all mothers with a titer of less than 1:8 are immunized prior to discharge after birth of the newborn.

Herpes Simplex Virus

Genital herpes is an STI caused by the herpes simplex virus (HSV) type 1 or type 2. Both types can cause genital infections, although in recent years HSV-1 has become the predominant cause of genital herpes. Approximately 45 million people are infected with genital herpes in the United States, and 1.5 million new cases are diagnosed annually, including 1,500 newborns. Untreated neonatal

HSV infection is associated with a mortality rate of 60%, and survivors experience considerable disability (Ural, 2015). Despite strategies designed to prevent perinatal transmission, the number of cases of newborn HSV infection continues to rise, mirroring the rising prevalence of genital herpes infection in women of childbearing age (Fig. 20.5) (James & Kimberlin, 2015).

HSV is a DNA virus with two subtypes: HSV-1 and HSV-2. HSV-1 infections were traditionally associated with oral lesions (fever blisters), whereas HSV-2 infections occurred in the genital region. Currently, either type can be found in either location, but HSV-1 is predominately causing genital herpes now (Ural, 2015).

Infection occurs by direct contact of the skin or mucous membranes with an active lesion through such activities as kissing, sexual (vaginal, oral, anal) contact, or routine skin-to-skin contact. HSV is associated with infections of the genital tract that when acquired during pregnancy can result in severe systemic symptoms in the mother and significant morbidity and mortality in the newborn. In addition, it may cause spontaneous abortion, birth anomalies, IUGR, or preterm labor. A 60% mortality rate may occur if the neonatal exposure is with an active primary infection (Silasi et al., 2015). Once the virus enters the body, it never leaves.

Infants born to mothers with a primary HSV infection have a 30% to 50% risk of acquiring the infection via perinatal transmission near or during birth. Recurrent genital HSV infections carry a 1% to 3% risk of neonatal infection if the recurrence occurs around the time of vaginal birth (March of Dimes, 2015e). About one in four pregnant women is infected with genital herpes, although most do not know it. Fortunately, only a small number pass the infection on to their newborns (March of Dimes, 2015e).

The greatest risk of transmission is when the mother develops a primary infection near term and it is not recognized. Most neonatal infections are acquired at or around the time of birth through either ascending infection after ruptured membranes or contact with the virus at the time of birth. The method and timing of birth in a woman with genital herpes are controversial. The CDC (2015f) recommends that in the absence of active lesions, a vaginal birth is acceptable, but if the woman has active herpetic lesions near or at term, a cesarean birth might be planned. All invasive procedures that might cause a break in the infant's skin should be avoided, such as artificial rupture of membranes, fetal scalp electrode, or forceps and vacuum extraction (Jordan et al., 2014).

Management for the woman with genital herpes during pregnancy involves caring for her as well as reducing the risk of newborn herpes. Some health care providers start the mother on prophylactic antiviral medications to prevent an active outbreak at the time of childbirth. No therapy can eradicate HSV, and this chronic infection is noted for its frequent asymptomatic viral shedding. Because the majority of newborn herpes cases result from perinatal transmission of the virus during vaginal birth, and because transmission can result in severe neurologic impairment or death, treatment of the mother with an antiviral agent such as acyclovir (Zovirax) must be started as soon as the culture comes back positive. Since the introduction of acyclovir, newer second-generation antivirals have been introduced (e.g., valacyclovir [Valtrex] and famciclovir [Famvir]) and are available (King et al., 2015). Use of condoms and antiviral mediations assist in preventing transmission. Evidence does not support routine HSV serologic screening among asymptomatic pregnant women currently (Workowski & Bolan, 2015), U, so nurses need to remain knowledgeable about current practice to provide accurate and sensitive care to all women. Despite the surge in vaccine research, there is unfortunately no readily available or preventative or therapeutic vaccine for HSV to date.

Hepatitis B Virus

Hepatitis B virus (HBV) is one of the most prevalent chronic diseases in the world. It is a serious global public health problem in Asia, Africa, Southern Europe, and Latin America especially. It has infected approximately 2 billion people worldwide, of whom more than 350 million are chronically infected. Life-threatening liver disease (cirrhosis, liver failure, and hepatocellular carcinoma) occurs in as many as 40% of people with hepatitis B. HBV infection causes about 5,000 deaths annually in the United States (Contag & Arrabal, 2015). HBV can be transmitted through contaminated blood, illicit drug use, and sexual contact. The virus is 100 times more infectious than HIV and, unlike HIV, it can live outside the body in dried blood for more than a week (Salman et al., 2015).

Sexual transmission accounts for most adult HBV infections in the United States. Acutely infected women develop hepatitis with anorexia, nausea, vomiting, fever, abdominal pain, and jaundice. In women with acute hepatitis B, vertical transmission occurs in approximately 10% of newborns when infection occurs in the first trimester and in 80% to 90% of newborns when acute infection occurs in the third trimester. Without intervention, 40% of infants born to women who are positive for hepatitis B will have chronic hepatitis B by 6 months of age (CDC, 2015g). In addition, hepatitis B infection during pregnancy is associated with an increased risk of preterm birth, fetal distress during labor, meconium peritonitis, low birth weight, and neonatal death. Newborns infected with HBV are likely to become chronic carriers of the virus, becoming reservoirs for continued infection in the population (CDC, 2015g). The fetus is at particular risk during birth because of the possible contact with contaminated blood at this time.

The CDC (2015g) recommends that all pregnant women should be tested for hepatitis B surface antigen (HBsAg) regardless of previous HBV vaccine or screening. Infants born to HBsAg-positive mothers should receive single-antigen HBV vaccine and hepatitis B immunoglobulin (HBIG) within 12 hours after birth. Completion of the vaccine schedule is recommended by HBV vaccination at 1 and 6 months (CDC, 2015g). There is a growing body of literature supporting the safety and efficacy of antiviral therapies administered in the third trimester of pregnancy to the reduce the vertical transmission of the HBV from the mother to the fetus, but to date there has not been any formal recommendations (Lamberth et al., 2015).

Nursing Assessment

Review the woman's history for factors placing her at high risk:
- History of STIs household contacts with HBV-infected persons
- Employment as a health care provider
- Abuse of intravenous drugs
- Prostitution
- Foreign born
- Multiple sexual partners
- Chinese, Southeast Asian, or African heritage
- Sexual partners who are HBV-infected (CDC, 2015g)

At the first prenatal visit, all pregnant women should be screened for HbsAg via blood studies, even if they were previously vaccinated or tested. Expect to repeat this screening later in pregnancy for women in high-risk groups (Park & Pan, 2014).

Nursing Management

If a woman tests positive for HBV, expect to administer HBV immune globulin (HBIG, Hep-B-Gammagee). The newborn will also receive HBV vaccine (Recombivax-HB, Engerix-B) within 12 hours of birth. The second and third doses of the vaccine are given at 1 and 6 months of age (CDC, 2015g). The CDC recommends routine vaccination of all newborns.

Women who are HbsAg negative may be vaccinated safely during pregnancy. No current research supports the use of surgical births to reduce vertical transmission of HBV. Breast-feeding by mothers with chronic HBV infection does not increase the risk of viral transmission to their newborns, nor is it a contraindication to breast-feeding, unless the woman is taking antiviral medication and has bleeding nipples. Women with bleeding nipples should abstain from breast-feeding until they are healed (Jhaveri, 2015).

Client education related to prevention of HBV is essential. Teach the woman about safer sex practices, good hand hygiene techniques, and the use of standard precautions (Teaching Guidelines 20.4). Protection can be afforded with the highly effective hepatitis B vaccine.

Teaching Guidelines 20.4
TEACHING TO PREVENT HEPATITIS B VIRUS PROGRESSION

- Abstain from alcohol and potentially hepatotoxic medications.
- Avoid intravenous drug exposure or sharing of needles.
- Encourage all household contacts and sexual partners to be vaccinated.
- Receive immediate treatment for any STI.
- Know that your newborn will receive the hepatitis B vaccine soon after birth.
- Use good hand hygiene techniques at all times.
- Avoid contact with blood or body fluids.
- Use barrier methods such as condoms during sexual intercourse.
- Avoid sharing any personal items, such as razors, toothbrushes, or eating utensils.
- Inform all health care providers of your HBV status.

Permanent remission of the disease even with treatment rarely occurs. Therefore, therapy is directed at long-term suppression of viral replication and prevention of end-stage liver disease. Urge the woman to consume a high-protein diet and avoid fatigue. A healthy lifestyle can help delay disease progression. Initiate an open discussion about the modes of transmission and use of condoms to prevent spread.

Varicella Zoster Virus

Varicella zoster virus (VZV), is one of the eight herpes family viruses. It is the virus that causes both varicella (chickenpox) and herpes zoster (shingles). Primary VZV leads to varicella (chicken pox) and establishes latency in dorsal root ganglia. Reactivation of VZV causes herpes zoster, commonly called shingles. Herpes zoster can occur once immune response against the virus wanes, usually with advancing age.

Pregnant women are at risk for developing varicella when they come in close contact with children who have active infection. Varicella occurs year round, but there is a higher incidence during winter and spring months. Maternal varicella can be transmitted to the fetus through the placenta, leading to congenital varicella syndrome, if the mother is infected during the first half of pregnancy, via an ascending infection during birth, or by direct contact with infectious lesions, leading to infection after birth. Varicella occurs in approximately 1/1,000 pregnancies (Charlier et al., 2014).

Congenital varicella syndrome can occur in newborns of mothers infected during early pregnancy. The vertical transmission rate is estimated to be between 2% and 10%. It is characterized by low birth weight, skin lesions in a dermatomal distribution, spontaneous abortion, chorioretinitis, cataracts, fetal growth restriction, delayed milestones, cutaneous scarring, limb hypoplasia, microcephaly, ocular abnormalities, intellectual disability, and early death (Swamy & Heine, 2015).

Preconception counseling is important for preventing this condition. A major component of counseling involves determining the woman's varicella immunity. Vaccination is the cornerstone of prevention. The vaccine is administered if needed. Varicella vaccine is a live attenuated viral vaccine. It should be administered to all adolescents and adults 13 years of age and older who do not have evidence of varicella immunity (King et al., 2015). Provide education to women who work in occupations that increase the risk of exposure to the virus, such as daycare workers, teachers of young children, and staff caring for children in institutional settings.

Varicella during pregnancy can be associated with severe illnesses for both the mother and her newborn. If contracted in the first half of pregnancy, some pregnant women are at risk for developing varicella pneumonia, which may put them at risk of life-threatening ventilatory compromise and death. Risk of varicella pneumonia appears to increase during pregnancy (Zhang, Patenaude, & Abenhaim, 2014). If the mother develops varicella rashes close to her due date, generalized neonatal varicella leading to death in about 20% of cases can be expected (Jordan et al. 2014).

Parvovirus B19

Parvovirus B19 infection, often referred to as Fifth disease, occurs worldwide and is extremely common. Most infected persons are asymptomatic. The incidence of acute B19 infection in pregnancy is about 3%.

Approximately 30% to 50% of pregnant women are not immune, and vertical transmission is common following maternal infection in pregnancy. Fetal infection may be associated with a normal outcome, but fetal death may also occur without ultrasound evidence of infectious sequelae (Desai & Brustman, 2014). Parvovirus B19 is a common, self-limiting, benign childhood virus that causes erythema infectiosum, also known as Fifth disease (referring to its fifth place in a list of common childhood infections). Approximately 65% of women of reproductive age have developed immunity to parvovirus B19. Infection with parvovirus B19 affects one in 400 pregnant women, but the majority has no adverse pregnancy outcome. Those that do may experience spontaneous abortion and severe fetal anemia. There is no treatment for the pregnant woman with parvovirus B19 infection (Malee, 2015).

Pathophysiology

The infection is spread transplacentally, by the oropharyngeal route in casual contact, and through infected blood. Infection of the fetus occurs through transplacental passage of the virus. Acute infection in pregnancy can cause B19 infection in the fetus, leading to nonimmune fetal hydrops (a serious abnormal accumulation of fluid in two or more fetal compartments, including ascites, pleural effusion, pericardial effusion, and skin edema), secondary to severe anemia or fetal loss, depending on the gestational age at the time of infection. The risk to the fetus is greatest when the woman is exposed and infected within the first 20 weeks of gestation. In addition to hydrops, other fetal effects of parvovirus include spontaneous abortion, congenital anomalies (central nervous system, craniofacial, and eye), and long-term effects such as hepatic insufficiency, myocarditis, and learning disabilities (Edwards, 2014). Fetal infection with B19V is also associated with intrauterine fetal death, nonimmune hydrops fetalis, thrombocytopenia, myocarditis, and neurologic manifestations. Fetal infection can also remain clinically unrecognized (Suliman & Seopela, 2015).

Therapeutic Management

Generally, a diagnosis of parvovirus is based on clinical symptoms and serologic antibody testing for parvovirus immunoglobulin G (IgG) and parvovirus immunoglobulin M (IgM). Parvovirus B19 infection is followed by lifelong immunity, which is shown by positive serum B19 IgG. Pregnant women who have been exposed to or who develop symptoms of parvovirus B19 require assessment to determine whether they are susceptible to infection (nonimmune). If the woman is immune, she can be reassured that she will not develop infection and that the virus will not adversely affect her pregnancy. If she is nonimmune, then referral to a perinatologist is recommended and counseling regarding the risks of

fetal transmission, fetal loss, and hydrops is necessary. Knowledge of how best to manage this infection during pregnancy lags behind our understanding of the potential adverse consequences.

Intrauterine B19 infection is a cause of fetal anemia, hydrops, and demise, and perhaps also of congenital anomalies. The best strategy for surveillance of the infected pregnant woman is serial ultrasounds for detection of hydropic changes and fetal anemia, and treatment for severe fetal anemia. Serial ultrasounds are advocated because the rates of fetal death and complications peak 4 to 6 weeks after exposure, but they can occur as late as 3 months following onset of symptoms. The infected newborn is assessed for any anomaly and followed for up to 6 years to identify any sequelae (Smith, 2015).

Nursing Assessment

Review the mother's history for any risk factors. Schoolteachers, daycare workers, and women living with school-aged children are at highest risk for being seropositive for parvovirus B19, especially if a recent outbreak has occurred in those settings. Also assess the woman for specific signs and symptoms. The characteristic rash starts on the face with a "slapped-cheeks" appearance and is followed by a generalized maculopapular rash. Fever, arthralgia, and generalized malaise are usually present in the mother. Prepare the mother for antibody testing.

Nursing Management

Prevention is the best strategy. Stress the need for hand hygiene after handling children; cleaning toys and surfaces that children have been in contact with; and avoiding the sharing of food and drinks. Screening for parvovirus B19 during early pregnancy may help in early diagnosis, but the cost effectiveness of a national screening program has not been accepted to date. The nurse can provide information regarding risk factors and potential complications if exposed and support the parent's decision.

Group B Streptococcus

Group B streptococcus (GBS) is a naturally occurring bacterium found in approximately 50% of healthy adults. Women who test positive for the GBS bacteria are considered carriers. Carrier status is transient and does not indicate illness. Approximately 25% of pregnant women carry GBS in the rectum or vagina, thus introducing the risk of colonization of the fetus during birth. GBS affects about 1 in every 2,000 newborns in the United States (March of Dimes, 2015f). Approximately 1 out of every 100 to 200 newborns born to mothers who carry GBS will develop signs and symptoms of GBS disease. Although

GBS is rarely serious in adults, it can be life threatening to newborns. GBS is the most common cause of sepsis and meningitis in newborns and is a frequent cause of newborn pneumonia (Puopolo, Madoff, & Baker, 2015). Newborns with early-onset (within a week after birth) GBS infections may have pneumonia or sepsis, whereas late-onset (after the first week) infections often manifest with meningitis (CDC, 2015i).

Genital tract colonization poses the most serious threat to the newborn because of exposure during birth and to the mother because of ascending infection after the membranes rupture. GBS colonization in the mother is thought to cause chorioamnionitis, endometritis, and postpartum wound infection.

Therapeutic Management

Antibiotic therapy usually is effective in treating women with GBS infections of the urinary tract or uterus, or chorioamnionitis without any sequelae. According to the CDC guidelines, all pregnant women should be screened for GBS at 35 to 37 weeks of gestation and treated (2015i). Vaginal and rectal specimens are cultured for the presence of the bacterium. Both pregnant women and women during labor who have positive cultures are treated with a penicillin-based anti-infective agent.

Penicillin G is the treatment of choice for GBS infection because of its narrow spectrum. Alternative antibiotics can be prescribed for clients with a penicillin allergy. The drug is usually administered intravenously at least 4 hours before birth so that it can reach adequate levels in the serum and amniotic fluid to reduce the risk of newborn colonization. Close monitoring is required during the administration of intravenous antibiotics because severe allergic reactions can occur rapidly.

Nursing Assessment

Review the woman's prenatal history, and ask about any previous infection. Determine if the woman's membranes have ruptured and the time of rupture. Rupture of amniotic membranes more than 18 hours increases the risk for infection. Monitor the mother's vital signs, reporting any maternal fever greater than 100.4° F (38° C). Assess the woman for other risk factors for perinatal transmission of GBS, including previous colonization with GBS, low socioeconomic status, African–American race, age less than 20 years, positive colonization at 35 to 37 weeks of gestation, GBS in urine sample, previous birth of GBS-positive newborn, preterm birth, and use of invasive obstetric procedures (March of Dimes, 2015f). Document this information to help prevent vertical transmission to the newborn.

Many women with GBS infection are asymptomatic, but they may have urinary tract infections, uterine infections, and chorioamnionitis.

Nursing Management

Nurses play major roles as educators and advocates for all women and newborns to reduce the incidence of GBS infections. Ensure that pregnant women between 35 and 37 weeks of gestation are screened for GBS infection during a prenatal visit. Record the results and notify the birth attendant if the woman has tested positive for GBS. During labor, be prepared to administer intravenous antibiotics to all women who are GBS positive.

Toxoplasmosis

Toxoplasmosis is a relatively widespread parasitic infection caused by a one-celled organism, *Toxoplasma gondii*. It is found all over the world, and can affect any warm-blooded animal, including humans, although the primary host is the cat. When a pregnant woman is exposed to this protozoan, the infection can pose serious risks to her fetus through transplacental transfer from the mother to the fetus. Between 1 in 1,000 and 8,000 newborns are born infected with toxoplasmosis in the United States (Hokelek, 2015). Cats are the definitive hosts of this parasite and shed it in their feces. It is transferred by hand to mouth after touching cat feces while changing the cat litter box or through gardening in contaminated soil. Consuming undercooked infected meat, such as pork, lamb, or venison drinking contaminated water, and eating unwashed fruits and vegetables can also transmit this organism.

A pregnant woman that contracts toxoplasmosis for the first time has an approximately 40% chance of passing the infection to her fetus. Toxoplasmosis acquired during pregnancy means high risk of damage for the fetus (March of Dimes, 2015g). Although the woman typically remains asymptomatic, transmission to her fetus can occur throughout pregnancy. A fetus that contracts congenital toxoplasmosis typically has a low birth weight, enlarged liver and spleen, chorioretinitis, jaundice, IUGR, hydrocephalus, microcephaly, neurologic damage, and anemia. Severity varies with gestational age; usually, the earlier the infection, the more severe the effects (Silasi et al., 2015).

Treatment of the woman during pregnancy to reduce the risk of congenital infection is a combination of pyrimethamine and sulfadiazine. Treatment with sulfonamides during pregnancy has been shown to reduce the risk of congenital infection.

Although there is much to learn about the best approach to the identification and treatment of toxoplasmosis, it is known that early treatment leads to the best neurodevelopmental outcomes in infants. Prevention is the key to managing this infection. Nurses play a key role in educating the woman about measures to prevent toxoplasmosis (Teaching Guidelines 20.5).

Teaching Guidelines 20.5

TEACHING TO PREVENT TOXOPLASMOSIS

- Avoid eating raw or undercooked meat, especially lamb or pork. Cook all meat to an internal temperature of 160° F (71° C) throughout.
- Clean cutting boards, work surfaces, and utensils with hot soapy water after contact with raw meat or unwashed fruits and vegetables.
- Peel or thoroughly wash all raw fruits and vegetables before eating them.
- Wash hands thoroughly with warm water and soap after handling raw meat.
- Avoid feeding the cat raw or undercooked meats.
- Avoid emptying or cleaning the cat's litter box. Have someone else do it daily.
- Keep outdoor sandboxes covered to prevent cat feces contamination
- Keep the cat indoors to prevent it from hunting and eating birds or rodents.
- Avoid uncooked eggs and unpasteurized milk.
- Wear gardening gloves when in contact with outdoor soil.
- Avoid contact with children's sandboxes, because cats can use them as litter boxes.

Women Who Are HIV Positive

The **human immunodeficiency virus (HIV)** infection is a chronic infection causes by the retrovirus HIV infection of T cells that express CD4 receptors causing immunodeficiency. Once the CD4-positive cell count falls below a certain level, HIV infection causes increased susceptibility to infections, cancers, and neurologic damage (Hardy, Esposti, & Nee, 2015). HIV is transmitted by blood and body fluids. The number of people contracting HIV infection annually is estimated at nearly 50 million, including approximately 20 million women of childbearing age and 2.5 million children, most of whom acquired HIV from mother-to-child transmission. According to the most recent incidence estimates, more than one million people in the United States are living with HIV infection, and almost one in six are unaware of their infection (CDC, 2015j).

Despite the revolutionary strides that have been made in treatment and detection and recent clinical advances and cautious optimism associated with combination therapies and vaccines, the number of individuals who are HIV-positive continues to climb worldwide. Intensive efforts notwithstanding, no real "cure" can be seen on the horizon. To achieve a durable end to the HIV pandemic, a vaccine remains essential in the fight against this virus (Fauci, Folkers, & Marston, 2014). Also, despite dramatic reductions in perinatal transmission of HIV in the United States, barriers to prevention still exist and perinatal HIV infections continue.

Historically, HIV/AIDS was associated with the male homosexual community and intravenous drug users, but currently the prevalence of HIV/AIDS is now increasing more rapidly among women than men. Women account for one in four people living with HIV in the United States, and are the fastest growing segment of persons becoming infected with HIV; transmission in women occurs most frequently from sexual contact (84%) and from intravenous drug use (15%) (CDC, 2015k). Most women, a large number of whom are mothers, have acquired the disease through heterosexual contact. The risk of acquiring HIV through heterosexual contact is greater for women due to exposure to the higher viral concentration in semen. In addition, sexual intercourse may cause breaks in the vaginal lining, increasing the chances that the virus will enter the woman's body. Fifty percent of all HIV/AIDS cases worldwide occur in women. AIDS is the third leading cause of death among all U.S. women aged 25 to 44 years and the leading cause of death among African–American women in this age group. At some point in their lifetimes, an estimated 1 in 32 African–American women will be diagnosed with HIV infection (CDC, 2015k).

Pathophysiology

The three recognized modes of HIV transmission are unprotected sexual intercourse with an infected partner, contact with infected blood or blood products, and perinatal transmission.

Take Note!

HIV is not transmitted by doorknobs, faucets, toilets, dirty dishes, mosquitoes, wet towels, coughing or sneezing, shaking hands, or being hugged or by any other indirect method.

The virus attacks the T4 cells, decreases the CD4 cell count, and disables the immune system. The HIV condition can progress to a severe immunosuppressed state termed **acquired immunodeficiency syndrome (AIDS)**. AIDS is a progressive, debilitating disease that suppresses cellular immunity, predisposing the infected person to opportunistic infections and malignancies. The CDC defines AIDS as an HIV-infected person with a specific opportunistic infection or a CD4 count of less than 200. Eventually, death occurs. The time from infection with HIV to development of AIDS is a median of 11 years but varies depending on whether the client is taking current antiretroviral therapy (ART) (Maartens, Celum, & Lewin, 2014). Research indicates that pregnancy does not accelerate the progression of HIV to AIDS or death (Calvert & Ronsmans, 2015).

TABLE 20.5	STAGES OF HIV INFECTION OUTLINED BY THE CDC	
Stages	Description	Clinical Picture
I	Acute infection	Early stage with pervasive viral production. Flu-like symptoms 2–4 weeks after exposure. Signs and symptoms: weight loss, low-grade fever, fatigue, sore throat, night sweats, and myalgia. Ability to spread HIV is highest during this stage because large amounts of HIV are being produced in the body and the CD4 count drops.
II	Asymptomatic infection or clinical latency	Viral replication continues within lymphatics, but slows down Usually free of symptoms; lymphadenopathy.
III	Persistent generalized lymphadenopathy	Possibly remaining in this stage for years; AIDS develops in most within 7–10 years. Opportunistic infections occur.
IV	End-stage disease (AIDS)	Severe immune deficiency; very vulnerable to infections. High viral load and low CD4 counts. Signs and symptoms: bacterial, viral, or fungal opportunistic infections, fever, wasting syndrome, fatigue, neoplasms, and cognitive changes.

Adapted from Centers of Disease Control and Prevention [CDC]. (2015s). *About HIV/AIDS*. Retrieved from http://www.cdc.gov/hiv/basics/whatishiv.html

Once infected with HIV, the woman develops antibodies that can be detected with the enzyme-linked immunosorbent assay (ELISA) and confirmed with the Western blot test. Antibodies develop within 6 to 12 weeks after exposure, although this latent period is much longer in some women. Table 20.5 highlights the four stages of HIV infection according to the CDC (2015l).

Impact of HIV on Pregnancy

When a woman who is infected with HIV becomes pregnant, the risks to herself, her fetus, and the newborn are great. The risks are compounded by problems such as drug abuse, lack of access to prenatal care, poverty, poor nutrition, and high-risk behaviors such as unsafe sex practices and multiple sex partners, which can predispose the woman to additional STIs such as herpes, syphilis, or human papillomavirus (HPV). Additional risk factors to assess for include women who exchange sex for money or drugs or have sex partners who do; a woman whose past or present sex partners were HIV infected; and women who had a blood transfusion between 1978 and 1985. Early identification of maternal HIV seropositivity allows early antiretroviral treatment to prevent mother-to-child transmission, allows a provider to avoid obstetric practices that may increase the risk for transmission, and allows an opportunity to counsel the mother against breast-feeding (also known to increase the risk for transmission) (U.S. Preventive Services Task Force [USPSTF], 2014). Subsequently, pregnant women who are HIV-positive are at risk for preterm delivery, fetal growth restriction, premature rupture of membranes, intrapartal or postpartum hemorrhage, postpartum infection, poor wound healing, and genitourinary tract infections (CDC, 2015m).

Perinatal transmission of HIV (from the mother to the fetus or child) also can occur. However, such cases have decreased in the past several years in the United States, primarily due to the use of antiretroviral therapy in pregnant women infected with HIV. This has not been the case in poor countries without similar resources. The Joint United Nations programs on HIV/AIDS (UNAIDS) estimate that over 2000 new infections due to mother-to-child transmission occur daily. This number is expected to increase rapidly as the prevalence rises in Southeast Asia (Rakhmanina & van den Anker, 2014). Perinatal transmission rates are as high as 35% when there is no intervention (ART) and below 1% when antiretroviral treatment and appropriate care are available African–American and Hispanic women make up 82% of HIV/AIDS cases among women and according to CDC data (2015j), the majority of prenatally infected children were African American or Hispanic. Lack of timely HIV testing during pregnancy is a major contributor to this outcome. Interventions are needed that will address knowledge barriers to HIV testing among African–American and Hispanic women. Research has found that women who have information about methods to prevent perinatal HIV transmission and the importance of testing for the baby's or mother's health are more likely to be HIV tested. Media campaigns addressing the benefits of HIV testing may be a significant intervention. Media campaigns are not only successful in promoting HIV testing but, in populations with high HIV prevalence, they also are cost effective (International AIDS Society, 2015).

With perinatal transmission, approximately half of children manifest AIDS within the first year of life, and about 80% have clinical symptoms of the disease within 3 to 5 years (Rivera & Frye, 2014). Breast-feeding is a major contributing factor for mother-to-child transmission, and the infected mother must be informed about this (March of Dimes, 2015i). The U.S. Public Health Service recommends that women who are HIV positive should avoid breast-feeding to prevent HIV transmission to the newborn. Given the devastating effects of HIV infection on children, preventing its transmission is critical (NIH, 2014).

In addition to perinatal transmission, the fetus and newborn also are at risk for prematurity, IUGR, low birth weight, and infection. Prompt treatment with antiretroviral medications for the infant with an HIV infection may slow the progression of the disease.

Therapeutic Management

Women who are seropositive for HIV require counseling about the risk of perinatal transmission and the potential for obstetric complications. The risk of perinatal transmission directly correlates with the viral load (Drake et al., 2014). A discussion of the options on continuing the pregnancy, medication therapy, risks, perinatal outcomes, and treatment is warranted. Women who elect to continue with the pregnancy should be treated with ART regardless of their CD4 count or viral load. Interventions to reduce HIV transmission include antiretroviral therapy to the mother and the newborn, consideration of elective cesarean section in women with elevated plasma viral load, and the avoidance of breastfeeding. With these interventions, the risk of HIV transmission is now less than 1% (Giles, 2015).

Drug therapy is the mainstay of treatment for pregnant women infected with HIV. The standard treatment is oral antiretroviral drugs given twice daily until giving birth, intravenous administration during labor, and oral zidovudine (AZT) for the newborn within 6 to 12 hours of birth (Vogler, 2014). The goal of therapy is to reduce the viral load as much as possible, which reduces the risk of transmission to the fetus.

Decisions about the birthing method to be used are made on an individual basis based on several factors involving the woman's health. Some reports suggest that cesarean birth may reduce the risk of HIV infection (King et al., 2015). Efforts to reduce instrumentation, such as avoiding the use of an episiotomy, fetal scalp electrodes, and fetal scalp sampling, will reduce the newborn's exposure to body fluids.

With appropriate therapies, the prognosis for pregnant women with HIV infection has improved significantly. In addition, the newborns of women with HIV infection who have received treatment usually do not become infected. Unfortunately, therapy is complicated and medications are expensive. Moreover, the medications are associated with numerous adverse effects and

possible toxic reactions. These therapies offer a dual purpose: reduce the likelihood of mother-to-infant transmission and provide optimal suppression of the viral load in the mother. The core goal of all medical therapy is to bring the client's viral load to an undetectable level, thus minimizing the risk of transmission to the fetus and newborn.

Nursing Assessment

Nursing assessment begins with a thorough history and physical examination. In addition, the woman is offered screening for HIV antibodies. Screening and effective intervention for women who are HIV positive are essential components of prenatal services, which also include education, counseling, testing, treatment, and continued care.

HEALTH HISTORY AND PHYSICAL EXAMINATION

Review the woman's history for risk factors, such as unsafe sex practices, multiple sex partners, and injectable drug use. Also have the woman complete a risk assessment survey. In addition, question the woman about any flu-like symptoms such as a low-grade fever, fatigue, sore throat, night sweats, diarrhea, cough, skin lesions, or muscle pain. Numerous factors influence perinatal transmission. Factors that increase risk of perinatal transmission include high maternal viral load; maternal immune depletion (low CD4 T cell counts); maternal genital tract infections; nutritional deficiencies; drug abuse; cigarette smoking; unprotected sexual intercourse; other opportunistic and coexisting infections (TB, malaria); prolonged ruptured membranes; and breast-feeding. Nurses need to take a thorough history to identify risk factors present.

Perform a complete physical examination. Obtain the woman's weight and determine if she has lost weight recently. Assess for signs and symptoms of STIs, such as vulvovaginal candidiasis, bacterial vaginosis, HSV, chancroid, CMV, or chlamydia because of the increased risk for STIs.

Take Note!

Women who request an HIV test despite reporting no individual risk factors should be considered at risk, since many are not likely to disclose their high-risk behaviors.

LABORATORY AND DIAGNOSTIC TESTING

The USPSTF (2014) recommends that all pregnant women be offered HIV antibody testing, regardless of their risk of infection, and that testing be done during the initial prenatal evaluation. Testing is essential because treatments are available that can reduce the likelihood of perinatal transmission and maintain the health of the woman.

Offer all women who are pregnant or planning a pregnancy HIV testing using ELISA. Prepare the woman with a reactive screening test for an additional test, such as the Western blot or an immunofluorescence assay. The Western blot is the confirmatory diagnostic test. A positive antibody test confirmed by a supplemental test indicates that the woman has been infected with HIV and can pass it on to others. HIV antibodies are detectable in at least 95% of women within 3 months after infection (Rayment, Asboe, & Sullivan, 2014).

In addition to the usual screening tests done in normal pregnancy, additional testing for STIs may be necessary. Women infected with HIV have high rates of STIs, especially HPV, vulvovaginal candidiasis, bacterial vaginosis, syphilis, HSV, chancroid, CMV, gonorrhea, chlamydia, and hepatitis B (March of Dimes, 2015i).

Nursing Management

Women infected with HIV should have comprehensive prenatal care, which starts with pretest and post-test counseling. In pretest counseling, the client completes a risk assessment survey and the nurse explains the meaning of positive versus negative test results, obtains informed consent for HIV testing, and educates the woman on how to prevent HIV infection by changing lifestyle behaviors if needed. Post-test counseling includes informing the client of the test results, reviewing the meaning of the results again, and reinforcing safer sex guidelines. All pretest and post-test counseling should be documented in the client's chart.

EDUCATING THE CLIENT

Pregnant clients are dealing with many issues at their first prenatal visit. The confirmation of pregnancy may be accompanied by feelings of joy, anxiety, depression, or other emotions. Simultaneously, the client is given many pamphlets and receives advice and counseling about many important health issues (e.g., nutrition, prenatal development, appointment schedules). This health teaching may be done while the woman feels excited, tired, and anxious. To expect women to understand detailed explanations of a complex disease entity (HIV/AIDS) too may be unrealistic. Determine the client's readiness for this discussion. Identify the client's individual needs for teaching, emotional support, and physical care. Nurses need to approach education and counseling

of HIV-positive pregnant women in a caring, sensitive manner. Address the following information:

- Infection control issues at home
- Safer sex precautions
- Stages of the HIV disease process and treatment for each stage
- Symptoms of opportunistic infections
- Preventive drug therapies for her unborn infant
- Avoidance of breast-feeding
- Referrals to community support, counseling, and financial aid
- Client's support system and potential caretaker
- Importance of continual prenatal care
- Need for a well-balanced diet
- Measures to reduce exposure to infections

Be knowledgeable about HIV infection and how HIV is transmitted and share this knowledge with all women. Nurses also can work to influence legislators, public health officials, and the entire health establishment toward policies to address the HIV epidemic. Research toward treatment and cure is tremendously important, but the major key to prevention of the spread of the virus is education. Nurses play a major role in this education.

SUPPORTING THE CLIENT

Be aware of the psychosocial sequelae of HIV/AIDS. A diagnosis of HIV can put a woman into an emotional tailspin, during which she is worried about her own health and that of her unborn infant. She may experience grief, fear, or anxiety about the future of her children. Along with the medications that are so important to her health maintenance, address the woman's mental health needs, family dynamics, capacity to work, and social concerns and provide appropriate support and guidance.

A stigma against both mothers and newborns who are HIV-exposed or infected persists as a challenge on many maternity care units. As nurses work to address this preventable disease, they should do so in a respectful conscientious manner. Beyond basic nursing care, nurses should strive to provide respectful care for all mothers and their newborns together. To accomplish this, be aware of your personal beliefs and attitudes toward women who are HIV positive or have AIDS. Incorporate this awareness in your actions as you help the woman face the reality of the diagnosis and treatment options. Empathy, understanding, caring, and assistance are key to helping the client and her family.

PREPARING FOR LABOR, BIRTH, AND AFTERWARD

Current evidence suggests that cesarean birth performed before the onset of labor and before the rupture of membranes significantly reduces the rate of perinatal transmission. ACOG recommends that HIV-positive women be offered elective cesarean birth to reduce the rate of transmission beyond that which may be achieved through

ART. They further suggest that operative births be performed at 38 weeks of gestation and that amniocentesis be avoided to prevent contamination of the amniotic fluid with maternal blood. Decisions concerning the method of delivery should be based on the woman's viral load, the duration of ruptured membranes, the progress of labor, and other pertinent clinical factors (USPSTF, 2014).

Prepare the woman physically and emotionally for the possibility of cesarean birth and assist as necessary. Ensure that she understands the rationale for the surgical birth.

After the birth of the newborn, the motivation for taking antiretroviral medications may be lower, thus affecting the woman's adherence to therapy. Encourage the woman to continue therapy for her own sake as well as that of the newborn. Nurses can make a difference in helping women to adhere to their complex drug regimens.

Reinforce family planning methods during this time, incorporating a realistic view of her disease status. It is clear that hormonal contraceptives are not protective against HIV infection and that dual protection with condoms should be the goal for women using hormonal contraception (U.S. Agency for International Development [USAID] 2014). Advise the woman that breast-feeding is not recommended. Instruct the woman who is HIV positive in self-care measures, including the proper method for disposing of perineal pads to reduce the risk of exposing others to infected body fluids. Finally, teach her the signs and symptoms of infection in newborns and infants, encouraging her to report any to the health care provider.

The evolution of HIV infection into a chronic disease has implications across all clinical care settings. Every nurse should be knowledgeable about the prevention, testing, treatment, and chronicity of the disease in order to provide high-quality care to people with or at risk for HIV. Breakthroughs in the prevention of HIV important to public health include male circumcision, antiretrovirals to prevent mother-to-child transmission, ART in HIV+ people to prevent transmission, and antiretrovirals for pre-exposure prophylaxis. Nurses, therefore, need to have an understanding of the changing epidemiology of the disease, the most recent testing recommendations, developments in screening technology, the implications of aging with HIV infection, and the nursing implications of this ongoing epidemic.

Take Note!

When providing direct care, **ALWAYS** follow standard precautions.

VULNERABLE POPULATIONS

Every year there are an estimated 208 million pregnancies worldwide, with about 6.6 million of them in the United States (Alan Guttmacher Institute, 2015b). Each pregnancy runs the risk of an adverse outcome for the mother and the baby, but risks are dramatically increased for certain vulnerable populations: adolescents, women over the age of 35, women who are obese, and women who abuse substances. Although risks cannot be totally eliminated once pregnancy has begun, they can be reduced through appropriate and timely interventions.

Every woman's experience with pregnancy is unique and personal. The circumstances each one faces and what pregnancy means to her involve emotions and experiences that belong solely to her. Many women in these special population groups go through this experience in confusion and isolation, feeling desperately in need of help but not knowing where to go. Although all pregnant women experience these emotions to a certain extent, they are heightened in women who have numerous psychosocial issues. Pregnancy is a stressful time. Pregnant women face wide-ranging changes in their lives, relationships, and bodies as they move toward parenthood. These changes can be challenging for a woman without any additional stresses but are even more so in the face of age extremes, illness, or substance abuse.

Skilled nursing interventions are essential to promote the best outcome for the client and her baby. Timely support and appropriate interventions during the perinatal period can have long-standing implications for the mother and her newborn, ultimately with the goal of stability and integration of the family as a unit.

Pregnant Adolescent

Adolescence lasts from the onset of puberty to the cessation of physical growth, roughly from 11 to 19 years of age. Adolescents vacillate between being children and being adults. They need to adjust to the physiologic changes their bodies are undergoing and establish a sexual identity during this time. They search for personal identity and desire freedom and independence of thought and action. However, they continue to have a strong dependence on their parents (Crockett & Crouter, 2014).

Adolescent pregnancy has emerged as one of the most significant social problems facing our society. The latest estimates show that approximately one million teens become pregnant each year in the United States (Alan Guttmacher Institute, 2015a; CDC, 2015a). Among these approximately half will give birth, slightly over one-third will opt for abortions, and the remaining 14% will have miscarriages or stillbirths. Despite being an advanced and relatively affluent nation, teens in the United States have higher rates of pregnancy and childbearing than any other industrialized country (Sedgh et al., 2015). It is estimated that 11% of births worldwide are to adolescents 15 to 19 years old (Ganchimeg et al., 2014). In addition, about half of all teen pregnancies occur within 6 months of first having sexual intercourse. About one in four teen mothers under age 18 have a second baby within 2 years after the birth of their first baby. Most of these girls are unmarried, and many are not ready for the emotional, psychological, and financial responsibilities of parenthood. Teens are least likely of all maternal age groups to get early and regular prenatal care (March of Dimes, 2015j). Adolescent pregnancy is further complicated by the adolescent's lack of financial resources: the income of teen mothers is half that of women who have given birth in their 20s (March of Dimes, 2015j).

Although the incidence of teenage pregnancy has steadily declined since the early 1990s, it continues to be higher in the United States than in any other industrialized country (Alan Guttmacher Institute, 2015a). Even this reduced incidence represents what is considered an unacceptably high level of pregnancy in an age group that is most likely to suffer the social consequences of early pregnancy. Although teen birth rates in the United States have declined, they remain high, especially among African–American and Hispanic teens and in southern states. The highest rate of unintended teenage pregnancies occurs in Hispanics and African Americans.

Currently, fewer high school students are having sexual intercourse, and more sexually active students are using some method of contraception. However, many teens who have had sexual intercourse have not spoken with their parents about sex, and use of contraceptives remains rare (Centers for Disease Control and Prevention [CDC] 2015a). Subsequently, adolescent pregnancy is considered a major health problem and is addressed in *Healthy People 2020* (see Healthy People 2020 20.1).

Impact of Pregnancy in Adolescence

The impact of adolescent pregnancy is evident in maternal and perinatal morbidity and mortality. Nonetheless, in addition to the age involved in precocious pregnancy, it also reflects previous conditions such as malnutrition, commu-

---

HEALTHY PEOPLE 2020 • 20.2

Objective	Nursing Significance
FP-8 Reduce pregnancy rates among adolescent females by 10% by 2020.	Will help to foster a continued decline in adolescent pregnancy rates by focusing on interventions related to pregnancy prevention, including safe sex practices and teaching about the complications associated with adolescent pregnancy.
FP-9 Increase the proportion of adolescents ages 17 years and under who have never had sexual intercourse by 10% by 2020.	
FP-10 Increase the proportion of sexually active persons ages 15 to 19 years who use condoms to both effectively prevent pregnancy and provide barrier protection against disease by 10% by 2020.	
FP-11 Increase the proportion of sexually active persons ages 15 to 19 years who use condoms and hormonal or intrauterine contraception to both effectively prevent pregnancy and provide barrier protection against disease by 10% by 2020.	
FP-12 Increase the proportion of adolescents who received formal instruction on reproductive health topics before they were 18 years old by 10% by 2020.	
FP-13 Increase the proportion of adolescents who talked to a parent or guardian about reproductive health topics before they were 18 years old by 10% by 2020.	
HIV-8 Reduce the number of perinatally acquired HIV and AIDS cases by 10% by 2020.	Education for the pregnant mothers about the need and rationale for antiretroviral drug therapy to prevent vertical transmission of HIV to their fetus will help reduce this incidence.
MICH-11 Increase abstinence from alcohol, cigarettes, and illicit drugs among pregnant women by 10% by 2020. **MICH-25** Reduce the occurrence of fetal alcohol syndrome (FAS) by 10% by 2020.	Education and support offered to pregnant women regarding the hazards of alcohol, cigarettes, and illicit drugs will reduce the abuse of these substances to enhance the perinatal outcomes.
NWS-22 Reduce iron deficiency among pregnant females.	Providing nutritional instruction on iron-rich foods will help reduce the incidence of iron deficiency anemia during pregnancy.

Healthy People objectives based on data from http://www.healthypeople.gov.

nicable diseases, and deficiencies in the health care given to pregnant adolescents. The most important impact lies in the psychosocial area: it contributes to a loss of self-esteem, societal discrimination, a destruction of life projects, and the maintenance of the circle of poverty (WHO, 2015a).

Adolescents are a unique group with special needs related to their stage of development. Adolescent pregnancy can be an emotionally charged situation, laden with ethical dilemmas and decisions. Topics such as abstinence, safer sex, abortion, and the decision to have a child are sensitive issues.

Adolescent pregnancy is an area when a nurse's moral convictions may influence the care that he or she provides to clients. Nurses need to examine their own beliefs about teen sexuality to identify personal assumptions. Putting aside one's moral convictions may be difficult, but it is necessary when working with pregnant adolescents. To be effective, health care providers must be able to communicate with adolescents in a manner they can understand and respect them as individuals.

The idea of it taking "a village to raise a child," as suggested by former First Lady Hillary Clinton in 1996, is perhaps even more valid than previously thought regarding teen pregnancy. The evidence suggests that it's not enough to teach teens to "just say no," nor is it enough to give them information about contraceptive methods; teens need to be connected to their parents, their peers, and their community (Whitworth & Cockerill, 2014). Nurses should feel that there is always hope and the chance of positive outcomes; nurses see that every day, often in the faces of their youngest clients. Nurses have to believe in that and work toward *'connecting'* with their teen clients. Nurses are on the front line of health care, and are often the first to interact and build rapport with teenagers. Teens that engage in risky sexual behavior may seek out nurses first. Nurse's scope of practice includes providing education and a source of comfort and support to all ages. It is therefore imperative for all nurses to be able to provide age appropriate information about sexual health. In providing this care, the quality of life and outcome of both mother and her infant can be improved.

Developmental Issues

An adolescent must accomplish certain developmental tasks to advance to the next stage of maturity. These developmental tasks include:

- Seeking economic and social stability
- Adjusting to sexually maturing bodies and feelings
- Developing a personal value system
- Building meaningful relationships with others (Fig. 20.6)
- Becoming comfortable with their changing bodies
- Working to become independent from their parents
- Learning to verbalize conceptually (CDC, 2015n)

Adolescents have special needs when working to accomplish their developmental tasks and making a

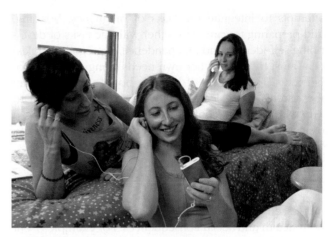

FIGURE 20.6 Adolescent girls sharing time together.

smooth transition to young adulthood. One of the biggest areas of need is sexual health. Adolescents commonly lack the information, skills, and services necessary to make informed choices related to their sexual and reproductive health. Developmentally, adolescents are trying to figure out who they are and how they fit into society. As adolescents mature, their parents become less influential and peers become more influential. Peer pressure can lead adolescents to participate in sexual activity, as can the typical adolescent's belief that "it won't happen to me" (Box 20.3). As a result, unplanned pregnancies occur. Work on the developmental tasks of adolescence, especially identity, can be interrupted as the adolescent

---

BOX 20.3

POSSIBLE FACTORS CONTRIBUTING TO ADOLESCENT PREGNANCY

- Early menarche
- Peer pressure to become sexually active
- Sexual or other abuse as a child
- Lack of accurate contraceptive information
- Fear of telling parents about sexual activity
- Feelings of invulnerability
- Poverty (85% of births occur in poor families)
- Culture or ethnicity (high incidence in Hispanic and African-American girls)
- Unprotected sex
- Low self-esteem and inability to negotiate
- Lack of appropriate role models
- Strong need for someone to love
- Drug use, truancy from school, or other behavioral problems
- Wish to escape a bad home situation
- Early dating without supervision

Adapted from Alan Guttmacher Institute. (2015a). *Facts on American teens' sexual and reproductive health*. Retrieved from http://www.guttmacher.org/pubs/FB-ATSRH.html; Ross, S., Baird, A.S., & Porter, C.C. (2014). Teenage pregnancy: Strategies for prevention. *Obstetrics, Gynecology, & Reproductive Medicine. 24*(9), 266–273.; and March of Dimes. (2015j). *Teenage pregnancy*. Retrieved from http://www.marchofdimes.com/professionals/14332_1159.asp

attempts to integrate the tasks of pregnancy, bonding, and preparing to care for another with the tasks of developing self-identity and independence. A pregnant adolescent must try to meet her own needs along with those of her fetus. The process of learning how to separate from the parents while learning how to bond and attach to a newborn brings conflict and stress. A pregnancy can exacerbate an adolescent's feeling of loss of control and helplessness (American Academy of Pediatrics, 2014).

Health and Social Issues

Adolescent pregnancy has a negative impact in terms of both health and social consequences. For example, 7 out of 10 adolescents will drop out of school. More than 75% will receive public assistance within 5 years of having their first child. In addition, children of adolescent mothers are at greater risk of preterm birth, low birth weight, child abuse, neglect, poverty, and death. The younger the adolescent is at the time of the first pregnancy, the more likely it is that she will have another pregnancy during her teens (March of Dimes, 2015j). Adolescent pregnancy also places them at high risk for obstetric complications such as preterm labor and births; low-birth-weight infants; STIs; poor maternal weight gain, preeclampsia, iron-deficiency anemia, poor eating habits, and inadequate nutrition and postpartum depression (Rajoriya & Kalra, 2015).

The psychosocial risks associated with early childbearing often have an even greater impact on mothers, families, and society than the obstetric or medical risks (Northridge & Coupey, 2015). Pregnant adolescents experience higher rates of domestic violence and substance abuse. Those experiencing abuse are more likely to abuse substances, receive inadequate prenatal care, and have lower pregnancy weight compared with those who are not (Jeha et al., 2015). Moreover, substance abuse (cigarettes, alcohol, or illicit drugs) can contribute to low birth weight, fetal growth restriction, preterm births, newborn addiction, and sepsis (March of Dimes, 2015j).

Although early childbearing (12 to 19 years of age) occurs in all socioeconomic groups, it is more prevalent among poor women and those from minority backgrounds, who face more obstetric and newborn risks than their more affluent counterparts (March of Dimes, 2015j). Poverty often contributes to delayed prenatal care and medical complications related to poor nutrition, such as anemia.

The financial burden of adolescent pregnancy is high and costs taxpayers an estimated $11 billion annually in the United States (Alan Guttmacher Institute, 2015b). Much of the expense stems from Medicaid, food stamps, state health department maternity clinics, the federal Aid to Families with Dependent Children program, and direct payments to health care providers. However, this amount does not address the costs to society in terms of the loss of human resources and the far-reaching intergenerational effects of adolescent parenting. For some adolescents, pregnancy may be seen as a hopeless situation: a grim story of poverty and lost dreams, of being trapped in a life that was never wanted. Health-related behaviors, such as smoking, diet, sexual behavior, and help-seeking behaviors, which are developed during adolescence often, endure into later life (Fedorowicz et al., 2014). The consequences associated with an adolescent's less-than-optimal health status at this age due to pregnancy can ultimately affect her long-term health and that of her children. However, some adolescents can create a happy, stable life for themselves and their children by facing their challenges and working hard to beat the odds.

Recall Rose, the pregnant teenager with asthma. What issues would be important for the nurse to discuss with her related to her pregnancy, her asthma, and her age?

Nursing Assessment

Assessment of the pregnant adolescent is the same as that for any pregnant woman. However, when dealing with pregnant teens, the nurse also needs to ask:
- How does the girl see herself in the future?
- Are realistic role models available to her?
- How much does she know about child development?
- What financial resources are available to her?
- Does she work? Does she go to school?
- What emotional support is available to her?
- Can she resolve conflicts and manage anger?
- What does she know about health and nutrition for herself and her child?
- Will she need help dealing with the challenges of the new parenting role?
- Does she need information about community resources?

Having an honest regard for adolescents requires getting to know them and being able to appreciate the important aspects of their life. Doing so forms a basis for the nurse's clinical judgment and promotes care that takes into account the concerns and practical circumstances of the teen and her family. Skillful practice includes knowing how and when to advise a teen and when to listen and refrain from giving advice. Giving advice can be misinterpreted as "preaching," and the adolescent will probably ignore the information. The nurse must be perceptive, flexible, and sensitive and must work to establish a therapeutic relationship.

Nursing Management

For adolescents, as for all women, pregnancy can be a physically, emotionally, and socially stressful time. The pregnancy is often both the result of and cause of social problems and stressors that can be overwhelming to them. Nurses must support adolescents during the transition from childhood into adulthood, which is complicated by their emergence into motherhood. Assist the adolescent in identifying family and friends who want to be involved and provide support throughout the pregnancy.

Help the adolescent identify the options for this pregnancy, such as abortion, self-parenting of the child, temporary foster care for the baby or herself, or placement of the child for adoption. Explore with the adolescent if the pregnancy was planned or unintended. Becoming aware of why she decided to have a child is necessary to help with the development of the adolescent and her ability to parent. Identify barriers to seeking prenatal care, such as lack of transportation, too many problems at home, financial concerns, the long wait for an appointment, and lack of sensitivity on the part of the health care system. Encourage the girl to set goals and work toward them. Assist her in returning to school and furthering her education. As appropriate, initiate a referral for career or job counseling.

Stress that the girl's physical well-being is important for both her and her developing fetus, which depends on her for its own health-related needs. Assist with arrangements for care, including stress management and self-care. Having a healthy newborn eases the transition to motherhood somewhat, rather than having to deal with the added stress of caring for an unhealthy baby (Rajoriya & Kalra, 2015). Monitor weight gain, sleep and rest patterns, and nutritional status to promote positive outcomes for both mother and child. Stress the importance of attending prenatal education classes. Provide appropriate teaching based on the adolescent's developmental level and emphasize the importance of continued prenatal and follow-up care. Monitor maternal and fetal well-being throughout pregnancy and labor (Fig. 20.7).

Nurses can also play a major role in preventing adolescent pregnancies, perhaps by volunteering to talk to teen groups. Teaching Guidelines 20.6 highlights the key areas for teaching adolescents about pregnancy prevention.

Teaching Guidelines 20.6
TOPICS FOR TEACHING ADOLESCENTS TO PREVENT PREGNANCY

- High-risk behaviors that lead to pregnancy.
- Involvement in programs such as Free Teens, Teen Advisors, or Postponing Sexual Involvement.
- Planning and goal setting to visualize their futures in terms of career, college, travel, and education.
- Choice of abstinence or taking a step back to become a "second-time virgin."
- Discussions about sexuality with a wiser adult—someone they respect can help put things in perspective.
- Protection against STIs and pregnancy if they choose to remain sexually active.
- Critical observation and review of peers and friends to make sure they are creating the right atmosphere for friendship.
- Empowerment to make choices that will shape their life for years to come, including getting control of their own lives now.
- Appropriate use of recreational time, such as sports, drama, volunteer work, music, jobs, church activities, and school clubs.

Adapted from Yoost, J. L., Hertweck, S. P., & Barnett, S. N. (2014). The effect of an educational approach to pregnancy prevention among high-risk early and late adolescents. *Journal of Adolescent Health, 55*(2), 222–227; Koh, H. (2014). The teen pregnancy prevention program: An evidence-based public health program model. *Journal of Adolescent Health, 54*(3), S1–S2; and March of Dimes. (2015j). *Teenage pregnancy.* Retrieved from http://www.marchofdimes.com/professionals/14332_1159.asp

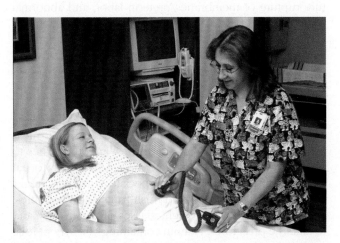

FIGURE 20.7 A pregnant adolescent receiving care during labor.

Tackling many issues surrounding adolescent pregnancy is difficult. Making connections with clients is crucial regardless of how complex their situation is. The future challenges nurses to find solutions to teenage pregnancies. Nurses must take proactive positions while working with adolescents, parents, schools, and communities to reduce the problems associated with early childbearing.

Nurses who provide care to adolescents have an opportunity to discuss future pregnancies and to use health care visits to teach about preconception health. Teaching adolescents who both express a desire for pregnancy and those who do not express such a desire is an important part of comprehensive nursing care. Teens require thorough teaching about health care risks such as smoking cessation, body weight control, interpersonal violence, and the need for folic acid. Adolescents should be the prime recipients of preconception education at every health care visit.

Teen childbearing is associated with adverse consequences for mothers and their children and imposes high public sector costs. Prevention of teen pregnancy requires evidence-based sex education, support for parents in talking with their children about pregnancy prevention and other aspects of sexual and reproductive health, and ready access to effective and affordable contraception for teens who are sexually active (CDC, 2015o).

The Advanced Maternal Age Woman

It is estimated that by the year 2025 about 25% of mothers will begin their childbearing period at an "advanced age." Advanced age is a risk factor for female infertility, pregnancy loss, fetal anomalies, stillbirth, and obstetric complications (Sauer, 2015). A few decades ago, a woman having a baby after the age of 35 probably was giving birth to the last of several children, but today she may be having her first. With advances in technology and the tendency of women to seek career advancement prior to childbearing, the dramatic increase in women having first pregnancies after the age of 35 will likely continue.

Impact of Pregnancy on the Advanced Maternal Age Woman

Whether childbearing is delayed by choice or by chance, women starting a family at age 35 or older are not doing so without risk. Women in this age group may already have chronic health conditions that can put the pregnancy at risk. In addition, numerous studies have shown that increasing maternal age is a risk factor for infertility and spontaneous abortions, gestational diabetes, chronic hypertension, postpartum hemorrhage, preeclampsia, preterm labor and birth, multiple pregnancy, genetic disorders and chromosomal abnormalities, placenta previa, fetal growth restriction, low Apgar scores, and surgical births (Schimmel et al., 2015). However, even though increased age implies increased complications, most women today, who become pregnant after age 34, have healthy pregnancies and healthy newborns. Today, one in five women in the United States has her first child after age 34 (March of Dimes, 2015m).

Nursing Assessment

Nursing assessment of the pregnant woman over age 34 is the same as that for any pregnant woman. For a woman of this age, a preconception visit is important to identify chronic health problems that might affect the pregnancy and also to address lifestyle issues that may take time to modify. Encourage the advanced maternal aged woman to plan for the pregnancy by seeing her health care provider before getting pregnant to discuss preexisting medical conditions, medications, and lifestyle choices. Assess the woman for risk factors such as cigarette smoking, poor nutrition, overweight or underweight, alcohol use, or illicit drug use.

A preconception visit also provides the opportunity to educate the woman about risk factors and provide information on how to modify her lifestyle habits to improve the pregnancy outcome. Assist the woman with lifestyle changes so that she can begin pregnancy in an optimal state of health. For example, if the woman is overweight, educate her about weight loss so that she can start the pregnancy at a healthy weight. If the woman smokes, encourage smoking cessation to reduce the effects of nicotine on herself and her fetus.

Prepare the woman for laboratory and diagnostic testing to establish a baseline for future comparisons. The risk of having a baby with Down syndrome increases with age, especially over age 34. Amniocentesis is routinely offered to all older women to allow the early detection of numerous chromosomal abnormalities, including Down syndrome. Additionally, a quadruple blood test screen (alpha fetoprotein [AFP], human chorionic gonadotropin [hCG], unconjugated estriol [UE], and inhibin A [placental hormone]) drawn between 15 and 20 weeks of pregnancy can be helpful in screening for Down syndrome and neural tube defects.

Nursing Management

During routine prenatal visits, the nurse can play a key role in promoting a healthy pregnancy. Consider social, genetic, and environmental factors that are unique to the advanced maternal aged pregnant women and prepare to address these factors when providing care. In a study by Mills& Lavender (2014), compared with the younger women, older women had statistically similar rates of gestational hypertension, gestational diabetes, preterm premature rupture of membranes/preterm labor, and abnormal placentation. Cesarean birth was higher in older women versus younger ones. Neonatal outcomes of gestational age and birth weight were excellent and similar between groups. Despite the increase risks, there are potential psychologic and social advantages to delaying childbirth and absolute numbers of complications are small.

Assess the woman's knowledge about risk factors and measures to reduce them. Educate her about measures to promote a positive outcome. Encourage her to get early and regular prenatal care. Advise her to eat a variety of nutritious foods, especially fortified cereals, enriched grain products, and fresh fruits and vegetables, and drink at least six to eight glasses of water daily and to take the prescribed vitamin containing 400 mcg of folic acid daily. Also stress the need for her to avoid alcohol intake during pregnancy, avoid exposure to second-hand smoke, and take no drugs unless they are prescribed. Provide continued surveillance of the mother and fetus throughout the pregnancy.

The Obese Pregnant Woman

Obese pregnant women are a particularly vulnerable group because their disability (obesity) is highly visible. In the United States, nearly 36% of adults are obese, including one out of three women (CDC, 2015p). Excess weight and obesity have gained attention as serious health care threats globally. Obesity during pregnancy is defined as a Body Mass Index (BMI) of 30 kg/m² or more calculated using the height and weight measured at the first prenatal visit. Compared to normal weight women, overweight and obese women tend to gain excessive weight in pregnancy and are high risk for maternal and birth outcomes. Excessive gestational weight gain is strongly associated with postpartum weight retention which increases the risk of additional weight gains in subsequent pregnancies (Chang et al., 2015). Obesity contributes to social, psychological, and economic problems throughout a woman's lifetime. Negative attitudes and discrimination by society can have negative consequences for the woman's quality of life. The number of women who are overweight or obese during pregnancy has also increased. During pregnancy, excess weight increases both obstetric and neonatal risks, including:

- Gestational diabetes
- Hypertension
- Thromboembolism
- Preeclampsia
- Preterm labor and birth
- Congenital anomalies
- Childhood and adolescent obesity
- Fetal macrosomia (birth weight. >4,000 g)
- Difficulty fighting postpartum infections
- Depression
- Tendency to remain overweight/obesity between pregnancies
- Prolongation of pregnancy/increased likelihood of post-term infant
- Increased risk of stillbirth
- Higher rate of cesarean births
- Increased risk of maternal mortality
- High risk for postpartum hemorrhage (ACOG, 2014b)

Negative or judgmental attitudes toward overweight or obese individuals can be encountered within the health care community and its providers, including nurses. Nurses can find it difficult to discuss weight issues during prenatal visits with obese women (Knight-Agarwal et al., 2014). Preconception assessment and counseling are needed for obese women and should include specific information about maternal and fetal risks of obesity in pregnancy, as well as encouragement to undertake a weight-reduction program including diet, exercise and behavior modification, enable achievement of a healthy weight prior to conception.

Obese pregnant women require individualized nursing care. Extra time may be needed to promote healthful practices, which should include dealing with issues of weight, diet, and exercise. Specialist dietary interventions and evidence-based guidelines for working with childbearing women must be seen as a public health priority by all nurses. This care must be done with honesty and respect for all of the woman's needs. There is an opportunity for health promotion aimed at disseminating information about the risks of obesity in pregnancy to overweight and obese women of childbearing age.

The Pregnant Woman and Substance Abuse

Substance abuse in pregnancy is a significant public health crisis causing increased morbidity in tow individuals, the mother, and the fetus. The epidemic of substance abuse continues to pose a significant challenge to all nations. Although there is a tendency to simply associate drug abuse with poverty, the problem affects every social stratum, gender, and race; and pregnant women are no exception. **Perinatal drug abuse** is the use of alcohol and other drugs by pregnant women. The incidence of substance abuse during pregnancy is highly variable because most pregnant women are reluctant to reveal the extent of their use. The National Institute on Drug Abuse (NIDA) (2015a) estimates that 7% or more of the women in the United States have used illicit drugs while pregnant. These include cocaine, marijuana, heroin, and psychotherapeutic drugs that were not prescribed by a health care provider. More than 20% used alcohol and 19% smoked cigarettes during their pregnancy (2015a).

Impact of Substance Abuse on Pregnancy

Substance use can be viewed along a continuum between social recreational drug use and addiction. Substance abuse is very prevalent remains and continues to remain undetected and underdiagnosed in many pregnant women. Substance abuse rarely starts during pregnancy. More often, women enter pregnancy already abusing or dependent on drugs.

Prenatal education and counseling is essential to successfully impacting this high-risk population. The positive overall impact of adequate prenatal care on birth outcomes is well documented. For pregnant substance users, the receipt of adequate prenatal care is especially critical. Several studies have reported that increasing the adequacy of prenatal care utilization in pregnant substance users reduces risks for prematurity, low birth weight, and perinatal mortality. However, many pregnant women who are substance users do not seek prenatal care for fear of being reported to Child Protective Services (SAMHSA, 2015).

The use of drugs, legal or not, increases the risk of medical complications in the mother and poor birth outcomes in the newborn. The placenta acts as an active transport mechanism, not as a barrier, and substances pass from a mother to her fetus through the placenta. Thus, along with the mother, the fetus experiences substance use, abuse, and addiction. Additionally, fetal vulnerability to drugs is much greater because the fetus has not developed the enzymatic system needed to metabolize drugs (Doulatram, Raj, & Govindaraj, 2015).

EFFECTS OF ADDICTION

Addiction is a multifaceted process that is affected by environmental, psychological, family, and physical factors. Women who use drugs, alcohol, or tobacco come from all socioeconomic backgrounds, cultures, and lifestyles. Factors associated with substance abuse during a pregnancy may include low self-esteem, inadequate support systems, low self-expectations, high levels of anxiety, socioeconomic barriers, involvement in abusive relationships, chaotic familial and social systems, and a history of psychiatric illness or depression. Women often become substance abusers to relieve their anxieties, previous physical, sexual, and emotional traumas in their life, depression, and feelings of worthlessness (Slater, 2015).

Societal attitudes regarding women and substance abuse may prohibit them from admitting the problem and seeking treatment. Society sanctions women for failing to live up to expectations of how a pregnant woman "should" behave, thereby possibly driving them further away from the treatment they so desperately need. For many reasons, pregnant women who abuse substances feel unwelcome in prenatal clinics or medical settings. Often they seek prenatal care late or not at all. They may fear being shamed or reported to legal or child protection authorities. A nonjudgmental atmosphere and unbiased teaching to all pregnant women regardless of their lifestyle is crucial. A caring, concerned manner is critical to help these women feel safe and respond honestly to assessment questions.

Pregnancy can be a motivator for some who want to try treatment. The goal of therapy is to help the client deal with pregnancy by developing a trusting relationship. Providing a full spectrum of medical, social, and emotional care is needed.

EFFECTS OF COMMONLY ABUSED SUBSTANCES

Substance abuse in pregnancy has increased during the past three decades in the United States, resulting in approximately 250,000 infants being born yearly with prenatal exposure to illicit substances (CDC, 2015q). Routine screening and education of women of childbearing age remain the most important ways to reduce addiction in pregnancy.

Substance abuse during pregnancy, particularly in the first trimester, has a negative effect on the health of the mother and the growth and development of the fetus. The fetus experiences the same systemic effects as the mother, but often more severely. The fetus cannot metabolize drugs as efficiently as the expectant mother and will experience the effects long after the drugs have left the women's system. Substance abuse during pregnancy is associated with preterm labor, abortion, IUGR, abruptio placenta, depressed Apgar scores, third trimester bleeding, meconium staining at birth, fetal demise, low birth weight, neurobehavioral abnormalities, and long-term childhood developmental consequences (WHO, 2015c). Table 20.6 summarizes the effects of selected drugs during pregnancy. *Healthy People 2020*

TABLE 20.6	EFFECTS OF SELECTED DRUGS ON PREGNANCY
Substance	Effect on Pregnancy
Alcohol	Spontaneous abortion, inadequate weight gain, IUGR, fetal alcohol spectrum disorder, the leading cause of intellectual disability
Caffeine	Vasoconstriction and mild diuresis in mother; fetal stimulation, but teratogenic effects not documented via research
Nicotine	Vasoconstriction, reduced uteroplacental blood flow, decreased birth weight, abortion, prematurity, abruptio placentae, fetal demise
Cocaine	Vasoconstriction, gestational hypertension, abruptio placentae, abortion, "snow baby syndrome," CNS defects, IUGR
Marijuana	Anemia, inadequate weight gain, "amotivational syndrome," hyperactive startle reflex, newborn tremors, prematurity, IUGR
Opiates and Narcotics	Maternal and fetal withdrawal, abruptio placentae, preterm labor, premature rupture of membranes, perinatal asphyxia, newborn sepsis and death, intellectual impairment, malnutrition
Sedatives	CNS depression, newborn withdrawal, maternal seizures in labor, newborn abstinence syndrome, delayed lung maturity

Adapted from Centers for Disease Control and Prevention [CDC]. (2015q). *Illegal drug use.* Retrieved from http://www.cdc.gov/nchs/fastats/drug-use-illegal.htm; March of Dimes. (2015k). *Smoking, alcohol, and drugs and pregnancy.* Retrieved from http://www.marchofdimes.org/pregnancy/illicit-drug-use-during-pregnancy.aspx; and McKeever, A. E., Spaeth-Brayton, S., & Sheerin, S. (2014). The role of nurses in comprehensive care management of pregnant women with drug addiction. *Nursing for Women's Health, 18*(4), 284–293.

(see Healthy People 2020 20.2) also addresses goals for perinatal substance abuse.

Alcohol. Alcohol abuse is a major public health issue in the United States. Alcohol is a teratogen, a substance known to be toxic to human development. The true rate of prenatal alcohol consumption is unknown. It is recognized that fetal alcohol spectrum disorder (FASD) is entirely preventable through alcohol abstinence, but worldwide approximately 30% of pregnant women consume alcohol during pregnancy (Vall et al., 2015). Theoretically, no mother would give a glass of wine, beer, or hard liquor to her newborn, but when she drinks, her embryo or fetus is exposed to the same blood alcohol concentration as she is.

The teratogenic effects of heavy maternal drinking have been recognized since 1973, when fetal alcohol syndrome was first described. Fetal alcohol syndrome is now a classification under the broader term of **fetal alcohol spectrum disorder (FASD)**; this disorder includes the full range of birth defects, such as structural anomalies and behavioral and neurocognitive disabilities caused by prenatal exposure to alcohol (Vaux & Chambers, 2015). FASD affects 1 in 100 infants each year, more than autism, Down syndrome, cerebral palsy, cystic fibrosis, spina bifida, and sudden infant death syndrome (SIDS) combined (National Organization on Fetal Alcohol Syndrome [NOFAS], 2015). Each year in the United States, up to 50,000 infants are born with FASD. It is the leading cause of nongenetic intellectual disability in the United States, possibly exceeding even Down syndrome, which is currently approaching 1 in 500 live births. Alcohol consumption during pregnancy results in brain, craniofacial, and heart defects, neurotoxicity, and immune systems dysfunction.

Characteristics of FASD include craniofacial dysmorphia (thin upper lip, small head circumference, and small eyes), IUGR, microcephaly, and congenital anomalies such as limb abnormalities and cardiac defects. Long-term sequelae include postnatal growth restriction, attention deficits, delayed reaction time, and poor scholastic performance (NOFAS, 2015).). The complex neurobehavioral problems typically manifest themselves insidiously. Children with prenatal alcohol exposure struggle with cognitive, academic, social, emotional, and behavioral challenges. These challenges reduce the child's ability to learn and function successfully in many structured environments (Mohammadzadeh & Farhat, 2014). Common cognitive and behavioral problems are listed in Box 20.4, and Figure 20.8 illustrates the characteristic facial features. See Chapter 24 for a more detailed discussion of the newborn with FASD.

The preferred action taken to prevent alcohol consumption during pregnancy is abstinence. However, the detection, diagnosis, and treatment of FASD remain major public health needs in this country and throughout the world. Not every woman who drinks during pregnancy

---

BOX 20.4

COMMON COGNITIVE AND BEHAVIORAL PROBLEMS ASSOCIATED WITH FASD AND ATTENTION DEFICIT/HYPERACTIVITY DISORDER

- Inability to foresee consequences
- Inability to learn from previous experience
- Lack of organization
- Intellectual disability or low IQ
- Difficulty in school, especially with math
- Learning difficulties
- Poor abstract thinking
- Poor reasoning and judgment skills
- Poor memory
- Poor impulse control
- Speech and language delays
- Poor judgment

Adapted from Centers for Disease Control and Prevention [CDC]. (2015h). *Fetal alcohol spectrum disorders.* Retrieved from http://www.cdc.gov/ncbddd/fasd/alcohol-use.html

---

will give birth to an affected child. Based on the best research available, the following is known about alcohol consumption during pregnancy:

- Intake increases the risk of alcohol-related birth defects, including growth deficiencies, facial abnormalities, central nervous system impairment, behavioral disorders, and intellectual development.
- No amount of alcohol consumption is considered safe during pregnancy.
- Damage to the fetus can occur at any stage of pregnancy, even before a woman knows she is pregnant.
- Cognitive defects and behavioral problems resulting from prenatal exposure are lifelong.
- Alcohol-related birth defects are completely preventable (ACOG, 2014c).

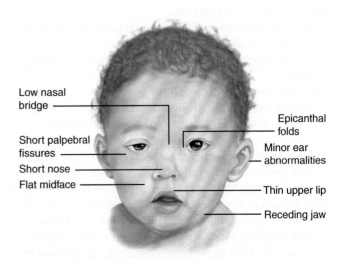

Low nasal bridge

Short palpebral fissures

Short nose

Flat midface

Epicanthal folds

Minor ear abnormalities

Thin upper lip

Receding jaw

FIGURE 20.8 Typical facial characteristics of a newborn with FASD.

Risk factors for giving birth to an alcohol-affected newborn include maternal age, socioeconomic status, ethnicity, genetic factors, poor nutrition, depression, family disorganization, unplanned pregnancy, and late prenatal care (ACOG, 2014d). Identification of risk factors strongly associated with alcohol-related birth outcomes could help identify high-risk pregnancies requiring intervention.

One of the biggest challenges in determining the true prevalence of FASD is how to recognize the syndrome, which depends in part on the age and physical features of the person being assessed. Difficulty identifying alcohol abuse results from the client's denial of alcohol use, unwillingness to report alcohol consumption, underreporting, and limited ability to recollect the frequency, quantity, and type of alcohol consumed. This makes it difficult to identify women who are drinking during pregnancy, institute preventive measures, or refer them for treatment.

Women who drink excessively while pregnant are at high risk for giving birth to children with birth defects. To prevent these defects, women should stop drinking during all phases of a pregnancy. Unfortunately, many women continue to drink during their pregnancy despite warnings from professionals.

Currently, it is not known whether there is a minimal amount of alcohol safe to drink during pregnancy; an occasional glass of wine might be harmless or might not be. Therefore, eliminating alcohol consumption during pregnancy is the ultimate goal to prevent FASD. Most women know they should not drink during pregnancy, but the window of vulnerability—i.e., the time lag between conception and the discovery of pregnancy—may put substantial numbers of children at risk. Additionally, traditional alcohol-screening questionnaires, such as the Michigan Alcoholism Screening Test (MAST) and the CAGE Questionnaire, are not sensitive enough to detect low levels of alcohol consumption among women.

Several challenges remain in preventing birth defects due to alcohol consumption:

- Ways to improve clinical recognition of high-risk women who drink alcohol.
- Ways to intervene more effectively to modify drinking behaviors.
- In utero approaches to prevent or minimize fetal injury.
- Strategies to address the neurodevelopmental problems of children affected by maternal alcohol ingestion.

Sedatives. Sedatives relax the central nervous system and are used medically for inducing relaxation and sleep, relieving tension, and treating seizures. Sedatives easily cross the placenta and can cause birth defects and behavioral problems. Infants born to mothers who abuse sedatives during pregnancy may be physically dependent on the drugs themselves and are more prone to respiratory problems, feeding difficulties, disturbed sleep, sweating, irritability, and fever (Alexander et al., 2014).

Nicotine. Cigarette smoking during pregnancy is the biggest preventable cause of death and illness in women and infants and is associated with numerous obstetric, fetal, and developmental complications, as well as an increased risk of adverse health consequences in the adult offspring. Nicotine replacement therapy has been developed as a pharmacotherapy for smoking cessation and is considered to be a safer alternative for women to smoking during pregnancy. The safety of nicotine replacement therapy (transdermal patches and bupropion) use during pregnancy has been evaluated in a limited number of short-term human trials, but there is currently no information on the long-term effects of developmental nicotine exposure in humans (Dhalwani, Szatkowski et al., 2015).

Nicotine is found in cigarettes, and is another substance that is harmful to the pregnant women and her fetus. Nicotine, which causes vasoconstriction, transfers across the placenta and reduces blood flow to the fetus, contributing to fetal hypoxia. When compared with alcohol, marijuana, and other illicit drug use, tobacco use is less likely to decline as the pregnancy progresses (Velez & Jansson, 2015). Smoking is associated with adverse pregnancy outcomes. However, these adverse outcomes can be avoided if the woman stops smoking before becoming pregnant.

Smoking increases the risk of spontaneous abortion, tubal ectopic pregnancy, preterm labor and birth, fetal growth restriction, stillbirth, premature rupture of membranes, low fetal iron stores, maternal hypertension, placenta previa, and abruptio placentae. The perinatal death rate among infants of smoking mothers is 20% to 35% higher than that of nonsmoking mothers (Varner et al., 2014). Perinatal and childhood risks associated with mothers smoking during their pregnancies include increased risk of cleft lip and palate, clubfoot, asthma, middle ear infections, SIDS, reduced head circumference, altered brainstem development, and cerebral palsy (Cunningham et al., 2014).

Smoking has also been considered an important risk factor for low birth weight, SIDS, and cognitive deficits, especially in language, reading, and vocabulary, as well as poorer performances on tests of reasoning and memory. Researchers have also reported behavior problems, such as increased activity, inattention, impulsivity, opposition, and aggression (Skoglund et al., 2014). Women who smoke during the pregnancy often continue to smoke after giving birth, and thus the infant will be exposed to nicotine after birth. This environmental or passive exposure affects the child's development and increases the risk of childhood respiratory disorders.

Caffeine. Caffeine is a widely used and accepted pharmacologically active substance. The socially sanctioned nature of caffeinated beverages promotes caffeine's popularity and at the same time obscures the fact that as a drug it can definitely be abused. The effect of caffeine intake during pregnancy on fetal growth and development is still unclear. A recent study found that caffeine intake of no more than 300 mg/day during pregnancy does not affect pregnancy duration and the condition of the newborn (Procter & Campbell, 2014). Caffeine, a stimulant of the central nervous system, is present in varying amounts in such common products as coffee, tea, colas, and chocolate. It is also in cold remedies and analgesics. Birth defects have not been linked to caffeine consumption, but maternal coffee consumption decreases iron absorption and may increase the risk of anemia during pregnancy.

Moderate caffeine consumption (less than 300 mg/day) does not appear to be a major contributing factor in miscarriage or preterm birth. The relationship of caffeine to growth restriction remains undetermined. A final conclusion cannot be made at this time as to whether there is a correlation between high caffeine intake and miscarriage due to lack of sufficient studies (Calhoun, & Lewis, 2016).

Energy drinks represent a new class of caffeinated beverages that are marketed to improve energy, athletic performance, concentration, endurance, and weight loss, although the claims have not been supported by rigorous scientific evidence (Higgins, Yarlagadda, & Yang, 2015). All energy drinks surpass the FDA official soft drink concentration of caffeine limit, typically two to four times the amount seen in one serving of soda or tea. Adverse effects of energy drinks can occur in healthy people, however pregnant women would be considered in an at risk group and should avoid excessive caffeine intake which has been linked to adverse reproductive outcomes, such as low birth weight. Consumption of energy drinks is associated with increased demand of the heart causing hypertension, tachycardia, dysrhythmias, coronary artery spasm, and sudden cardiac death (James, 2015). Given the rise in emergency room visits for complications of energy drink consumption, nurses should advise their pregnant clients to refrain from drinking them.

Marijuana. Marijuana is the most commonly used illicit drug in America, with over 90 million people having tried it at least once. Its estimated prevalence in pregnant women is about 10–15%. It is often called pot, reefer, herb, widow, hash, grass, weed, Mary Jane, or MJ (NIDA, 2015c). Marijuana is a preparation of the leaves and flowering tops of *Cannabis sativa,* the hemp plant, which contains a number of pharmacologically active agents. Tetrahydrocannabinol (THC) is the most active ingredient of marijuana. With heavy smoking, THC narrows the bronchi and bronchioles and produces inflammation of the mucous membranes. Smoking marijuana causes tachycardia and a reduction in blood pressure, resulting in orthostatic hypotension. Although the federal government considers marijuana a Schedule I substance (having

no medicinal uses and high risk for abuse), a few states have legalized it for adult recreational use, and many states have passed laws allowing its use as a treatment for medical conditions (pain, nausea and vomiting, HIV/AIDS, cancer).

The effects of marijuana smoking on pregnancy are not yet fully understood because there are very few studies on its long-term effects on child development. One can speculate that the effects of marijuana on the immature nervous system may be subtle and not detected until more complex functions are required, usually in a formal educational setting. There is some evidence that marijuana increases the risk of spontaneous abortion and preterm delivery (Desai, Mark, & Terplan, 2014). Although marijuana is not considered teratogenic, many newborns display altered responses to visual stimuli, increased tremulousness, and a high-pitched cry, which might indicate insults against the central nervous system (Volkow et al., 2014). A strong correlation exists between the use of marijuana and the use of alcohol and cigarettes.

Opiates and Narcotics. Opiates and narcotics include opium, heroin (known as horse, junk, smack, downtown), morphine, codeine, hydromorphone (Dilaudid; little D), oxycodone (Percodan, perkies), meperidine (Demerol, demise), and methadone (meth, dollies). Opiates can be inhaled, injected, snorted, ingested, or used subcutaneously. These drugs are central nervous system depressants that soothe and lull. They may be used medically for pain, but all have a high potential for abuse. Most cause an intense addiction in both mother and newborn.

Narcotic dependence is particularly problematic in pregnant women. It leads to medical, nutritional, and social neglect by the woman due to the long-term risks of physical dependence, malnutrition, compromised immunity, hepatitis, and fatal overdose (Alexander et al., 2014). Taking opiates or narcotics during pregnancy places the woman at increased risk for preterm labor, fetal growth restriction, abruptio placenta, perinatal mortality, preterm rupture of membranes, and preeclampsia (Prasad, 2014).

Heroin is the most common illicitly used opioid. It is derived from the seeds of the poppy plant and can be sniffed, smoked, or injected. It crosses the placenta via simple diffusion within 1 hour of maternal consumption (ACOG, 2014e). Use of heroin during pregnancy is believed to affect the developing brain of the fetus and may cause behavioral abnormalities in childhood. Risks of perinatal opiate exposure are not limited to the fetus. Maternal opiate overdose deaths have increased dramatically, which translates to 18 women dying per day, and for every woman who dies, 30 are being treated in emergency departments for abuse (Alexander et al., 2014).

The most common harmful effect of heroin and other narcotics on newborns is withdrawal, or **neonatal** abstinence syndrome (NAS) (see Chapter 24). This collection of symptoms may include irritability, hypertonicity, jitteriness, fever, excessive and often high-pitched cry, vomiting, diarrhea, feeding disturbances, respiratory distress, disturbed sleeping, excessive sneezing and yawning, nasal stuffiness, diaphoresis, fever, poor sucking, tremors, and seizures (Slater, 2015).

Withdrawal from opiates during pregnancy is extremely dangerous for the fetus, so a prescribed oral methadone maintenance program combined with psychotherapy is recommended for the pregnant woman. This closely supervised treatment program reduces withdrawal symptoms in the newborn, reduces drug cravings, and blocks the euphoric effects of narcotic drugs in order to reduce illicit drug use. Management of opioid addiction in pregnancy includes maintenance therapy with methadone or buprenorphine in addition to traditional prenatal care and psychosocial treatment of substance abuse, such as self-help, 12-step groups, individual and group substance abuse counseling, and psychotherapy. Maintenance therapy drugs provide a steady state of opiate levels, thus reducing the risk of withdrawal to the fetus and exposure to HIV and other STIs because the mother is no longer injecting drugs. However, maintenance therapy drugs have the same withdrawal consequences for women and newborns as heroin does (McKeever et al., 2014).

Methamphetamines. Methamphetamine use is now more common than cocaine use in pregnancy, and its use by women of childbearing age is increasing in the United States. This highly addictive stimulant is commonly known as speed, meth, or chalk. In its smoked form, it is often referred to as ice, crystal, crank, and glass. Smoking or injecting the drug quickly delivers it to the brain for an immediate, intense euphoria. Because the pleasure also fades quickly, users often take repeated doses, in a "binge and crash" pattern. It is a white, odorless, bitter-tasting powder that was developed from its parent drug, amphetamine, and was used originally in nasal decongestants and bronchial inhalers. The maternal effects include increased energy and alertness, an intense rush, decreased appetite, tachycardia, and tachypnea. Chronic use can lead to psychosis, including paranoia, hallucinations, memory loss, and aggressive or violent behavior. Signs of methamphetamine use include track marks from intravenous injection, malnutrition, severe dental decay (meth mouth), and skin abscesses from skin picking (ACOG, 2014f). Few studies have been done on the effects of methamphetamine abuse during pregnancy, but the few done indicate an increased risk for preterm births, low birth weight, placental abruption, fetal growth restriction, and congenital anomalies (NIDA, 2015d). These findings are hard to interpret, however, due to small sample size and polydrug use of the participants.

Cocaine. Cocaine use is second only to marijuana use in women who abuse drugs during pregnancy. The incidence of cocaine exposure in utero is approximately 1 to 10 per 1,000 live births (Brandt et al., 2014). There is evidence that cocaine affects infant development both directly, via in utero exposure, and indirectly via alterations in maternal care after birth.

Cocaine is a psychoactive drug derived from the leaves of the coca plant, which grows in the Andes Mountains of Peru, Ecuador, and Bolivia. The freebase form, called "crack" because of the cracking or popping noise made in its preparation, is less expensive, easily made, and smokable. Cocaine is a powerful vasoconstrictor. When sniffed into the mucous membranes of the nose, it produces an intense "rush" that some have compared to an orgasmic experience. Smoked crack is absorbed rapidly by the pulmonary vasculature and reaches the brain's circulation in 6 to 8 seconds (NIDA, 2015b).

Cocaine use produces vasoconstriction, dilates pupils, increases body temperature, tachycardia, and hypertension in both the mother and the fetus (Kahn, Mikhael, & Vadivelu, 2015). Uteroplacental insufficiency may result from reduced blood flow and placental perfusion. Chronic use can result in low birth weight, the most common effect of cocaine use in pregnancy (NIDA, 2015b).

Studies suggest that perinatal cocaine use increases the risk of preterm labor, abortion, abruptio placentae, fetal growth restriction, intrauterine fetal distress and demise, seizures, withdrawal, and cerebral infarcts. Cocaine may increase the risk of uterine rupture and congenital anomalies (NIDA, 2015b). Fetal anomalies associated with cocaine use in early pregnancy involve neurologic problems such as neural tube defects and microcephaly; cardiovascular anomalies such as congenital heart defects; genitourinary conditions such as prune belly syndrome, hydronephrosis, and ambiguous genitalia; and gastrointestinal system problems such as necrotizing enterocolitis (Connery, 2014). Some infants exposed to cocaine in utero show increased irritability and are difficult to calm and soothe to sleep.

Nonmedical Use of Prescription Drugs. In addition to alcohol and illicit drug use, a new worldwide trend has emerged and may soon exceed illicit drug use. That is, the nonmedical use of prescription drugs found in many home medicine cabinets. Prescription drug abuse has reached epidemic levels in the United States. Estimates of prescription drug abuse rates during pregnancy range from 5% to 20%. Common drugs of choice include analgesics, stimulants, sedatives, and tranquilizers. A frequent belief among abusers is that prescribed medications are less dangerous than street drugs and using a friend's medication is safe. Unfortunately, unintentional poisoning deaths occur frequently. In addition, the development of a counterfeit market has developed utilizing the Internet, thereby creating a global counterfeit drug market (McHugh, Nielsen, & Weiss, 2015).

Early detection through a comprehensive evaluation is essential to improve overall treatment outcomes. New research supports screening all pregnant women for substance abuse. A major role of the nurse is to focus on prevention by educating all women about the dangers associated with misuse of prescription medications. Community education is vital to manage risks to prevent problems from developing.

Nursing Assessment

Complete a thorough history and physical examination to evaluate a client for substance use and abuse. Substance abuse screening in pregnancy is done to detect the use of any substance known or suspected to exert a deleterious effect on the client or her fetus. Routinely ask about substance abuse with all women of childbearing age, inform them of the risks involved, and advise them against continuing. Screening questionnaires are helpful in identifying potential users, may reduce the stigma of asking clients about substance abuse, and may result in a more accurate and consistent evaluation. The questions in Box 20.5 may be helpful in assessing a client who is at risk for substance abuse during pregnancy. Using "accepting" terminology may encourage the woman to give honest answers without fear of reproach.

BOX 20.5

SAMPLE QUESTIONS FOR ASSESSING SUBSTANCE USE

- Have you ever used recreational drugs? If so, when and what?
- Have you ever taken a prescription drug other than as intended?
- What are your feelings about drug use during pregnancy?
- How often do you smoke cigarettes? How many per day?
- How often do you drink alcohol?
- Have you ever felt guilty about drinking or drug use?

If the assessment reveals substance use, obtain additional information by using the RAFFT questionnaire, which is a sensitive screening instrument for identifying substance abuse (Weekes & Lee, 2014):

R: Do you drink or take drugs to **R**elax, improve your self-image, or fit in?
A: Do you ever drink or take drugs while **A**lone?
F: Do you have any close **F**riends who drink or take drugs?
F: Does a close **F**amily member have a problem with alcohol or drugs?
T: Have you ever gotten in **T**rouble from drinking or taking drugs?

A woman who claims to have taken no drugs while pregnant may be unaware that substances such as hair dye, diet cola, paint, or over-the-counter medications for colds or headaches are still considered drugs. Thus, it is very difficult to get a true picture of the real use of drugs by pregnant women.

Many drugs are considered to have a teratogenic effect on growing fetuses. A **teratogen** is any environmental substance that can cause physical defects in the developing embryo and fetus. Pregnant women with substance abuse commonly present with polysubstance abuse, which is likely to be more damaging than the use of any single substance. Thus, it is inherently difficult to ascribe a specific perinatal effect to any one substance (McKeever, Spaeth-Brayton, & Sheerin, 2014).

A urine toxicology screen may also be helpful in determining drug use, although a urine screen identifies only recent or heavy use of drugs. The length of time a drug is present in urine is as follows:

- Cocaine: 24 to 48 hours in an adult, 72 to 96 hours in an infant.
- Heroin: 24 hours in an adult, 24 to 48 hours in an infant.
- Marijuana: 1 week to 1 month in an adult, up to a month or longer in an infant.
- Methadone: up to 10 days in an infant (Wang, 2015).

Nursing Management

If the woman's drug screen is positive, use this as an opportunity to discuss prenatal exposure to substances that may be harmful. The discussion may lead the nurse to refer the client for a diagnostic assessment or identify an intervention such as counseling that may be helpful. Being nonjudgmental is a key to success; a client is more apt to trust and reveal patterns of abuse if the nurse does not judge her and her lifestyle choices.

A positive drug screen in a newborn warrants an investigation by the state protection agency. In the interim, institute measures to reduce stress and stimuli to promote the newborn's comfort (see Chapter 24 for a more in-depth discussion).

Be proactive, supportive, and accepting when caring for the client. Assure women with substance abuse problems that sharing information of a confidential nature with health care providers will not render them liable to criminal prosecution. Provide counseling and education, emphasizing the following:

- Effects of substance exposure on the fetus
- Interventions to improve mother–child attachment and improve parenting
- Psychosocial support if treatment is needed to reduce substance abuse
- Referral to outreach programs to improve access to treatment facilities
- Hazardous legal substances to avoid during pregnancy

- Follow-up of children born to substance-dependent mothers
- Dietary counseling to improve the pregnancy outcome for both mother and child
- Drug screening to identify all drugs a client is using
- More frequent prenatal visits to monitor fetal well-being
- Maternal and fetal benefits of remaining drug free
- Cultural sensitivity
- Coping skills, support systems, and vocational assistance

There is nothing categorically different about addiction in pregnancy compared with addiction in general. Pregnant women who use drugs are women who use drugs, get pregnant, and cannot stop using drugs. The fact that they are condemned in society leads to their further marginalization, which does nothing to improve their lives or the lives of their children.

Substance abuse is a complex problem that requires sensitivity to each woman's unique situation and contributing factors. Be sure to address individual psychological and sociocultural factors to help the woman regain control of her life. Nurses must be aware of these women's unique needs and the related legal and ethical ramifications surrounding pregnancy. Treatment must combine different approaches and provide ongoing support for women learning to live drug free. Developing personal strengths, such as communication skills, assertiveness, and self-confidence, will help the woman to resist drug use. Encourage the use of appropriate coping skills. Enhancing self-esteem also helps provide a foundation to avoid drugs. Through therapeutic communication, nursing interventions, clinical assessment, and building trusting relationships, nurses can have a significant impact in managing clients with substance abuse.

KEY CONCEPTS

- Preconception counseling for the woman with diabetes is helpful in promoting blood glucose control to prevent congenital anomalies.

- The classification system for diabetes is based on disease etiology and not pharmacology management; the classification includes type 1 diabetes, type 2 diabetes, gestational diabetes, and impaired fasting glucose and impaired glucose tolerance.

- A functional classification for heart disease during pregnancy is based on past and present disability: class I, asymptomatic with no limitation of physical activity; class II, symptomatic (dyspnea, chest pain) with increased activity; class III, symptomatic (fatigue, palpitation) with normal activity; and class IV, symptomatic at rest or with any physical activity.

- Chronic hypertension exists when the woman has a blood pressure of 140/90 mm Hg or higher before pregnancy or before the 20th week of gestation or when hypertension persists for more than 12 weeks' postpartum.

- Successful management of asthma in pregnancy involves elimination of environmental triggers, drug therapy, and client education.

- Ideally, women with hematologic conditions are screened before conception and are made aware of the risks to themselves and to a pregnancy.

- A wide variety of infections, such as cytomegalovirus, rubella, herpes simplex, hepatitis B, varicella, parvovirus B19, and many sexually transmitted infections can affect a pregnancy, having a negative impact on its outcome.

- The prevalence of HIV/AIDS is increasing more rapidly among women than men: half of all the HIV/AIDS cases worldwide now occur in women. There are only three recognized modes of HIV transmission: unprotected sexual intercourse with an infected partner, contact with infected blood or blood products, and perinatal transmission. Breastfeeding is a major contributing factor in mother-to-child transmission of HIV.

- Cases of perinatal AIDS have decreased in the past several years in the United States, primarily because of the use of zidovudine (ZDV) therapy in pregnant women with HIV. The U.S. Preventive Services Task Force recommends that all pregnant women should be offered HIV antibody testing regardless of their risk of infection, and that testing should be done during the initial prenatal evaluation.

- The younger an adolescent is at the time of her first pregnancy, the more likely it is that she will have another pregnancy during her teens. About 1 million teenagers between the ages of 15 and 19 become pregnant each year; about half give birth and keep their infants.

- The nurse's role in caring for the pregnant adolescent is to assist her in identifying the options for this pregnancy, including abortion, self-parenting of the child, temporary foster care for the baby or herself, or placement for adoption.

- Pregnant women with substance abuse problems commonly abuse several substances, making it difficult to ascribe a specific perinatal effect to any one substance. Societal attitudes regarding pregnant women and substance abuse may prohibit them from admitting the problem and seeking treatment.

- Substance abuse during pregnancy is associated with preterm labor, abortion, low birth weight, central nervous system and fetal anomalies, and long-term childhood developmental consequences.

- Fetal alcohol spectrum disorder is a lifelong yet completely preventable set of physical, mental, and neurobehavioral birth defects; it is the leading cause of intellectual disability in the United States.

○ Nursing management for the woman with substance abuse focuses on screening and preventing substance abuse to reduce the high incidence of obstetric and medical complications as well as the morbidity and mortality among passively addicted newborns.

References and Recommended Readings

Aktas, G., Alcelik, A., Ozlu, T., Tosun, M., Tekce, B. K., Savli, H., et al. (2014). Association between omentin levels and insulin resistance in pregnancy. *Experimental and clinical endocrinology & diabetes, 122*(03), 163–166.

Alan Guttmacher Institute. (2015a). *Facts on American teens' sexual and reproductive health.* Retrieved from http://www.guttmacher.org/pubs/FB-ATSRH.html

Alan Guttmacher Institute. (2015b). *Pregnancy fact sheets.* Retrieved from http://www.guttmacher.org/in-the-know/pregnancy.html.

Alexander, L. L., LaRosa, J. H., Bader, H., & Garfield, S. (2014). *New dimensions in women's health* (6th ed.). Sudbury, MA: Jones & Bartlett.

Agent, O. E. (2015). 19 Classic viral exanthems. Clinical infectious disease. In *Clinical infectious diseases* (Chapter 19, 2nd ed.). Cambridge, MA: Cambridge University Press.

Alonso-Gonzalez, R., & Swan, L. (2014). Treating cardiac disease in pregnancy. *Women's Health, 10*(1), 79–90.

American Academy of Allergy, Asthma & Immunology [AAAAI]. (2015). *Asthma and pregnancy.* Retrieved from http://www.aaaai.org/conditions-and-treatments/library/asthma-library/asthma-and-pregnancy.aspx

American Academy of Pediatrics. (2014). Adolescent pregnancy: Current trends and issues. *AAP News, 35*(5), 19–25.

American Academy of Pediatrics [AAP]. (2015). *Serious illnesses and breastfeeding.* Retrieved from https://healthychildren.org/English/ages-stages/baby/breastfeeding/Pages/Serious-Illnesses-and-Breastfeeding.aspx

American College of Obstetricians & Gynecologists [ACOG]. (2013). Executive summary: Hypertension in pregnancy. *Obstetrics & Gynecology, 122151*, 1122–1131.

American College of Obstetricians & Gynecologists [ACOG], (2014a). ACOG guidelines at a glance: gestational diabetes mellitus. *Contemporary OB/GYN.* Retrieved from http://contemporaryobgyn.modernmedicine.com/contemporary-obgyn/news/acog-guidelines-glance-gestational-diabetes-mellitus?page=full

American College of Obstetricians & Gynecologists [ACOG]. (2014b). Obesity in pregnancy. *Obstetrics & Gynecology, 121.* 213–217.

American College of Obstetricians & Gynecologists [ACOG]. (2014c). *Fetal alcohol spectrum disorders prevention handbook.* Retrieved from http://www.acog.org/About-ACOG/ACOG-Districts/District-II/Fetal-Alcohol-Spectrum-Disorders-Prevention-Handbook

American College of Obstetricians & Gynecologists [ACOG]. (2014d). *Tobacco, alcohol, drugs, and pregnancy.* Retrieved from http://www.acog.org/Patients/FAQs/Tobacco-Alcohol-Drugs-and-Pregnancy

American College of Obstetricians & Gynecologists [ACOG]. (2014e). *Opioid abuse, dependence, and addiction in pregnancy.* Retrieved from http://www.acog.org/Resources-And-Publications/Committee-Opinions/Committee-on-Health-Care-for-Underserved-Women/Opioid-Abuse-Dependence-and-Addiction-in-Pregnancy

American College of Obstetricians & Gynecologists [ACOG]. (2014f). *Methamphetamine abuse in women of reproductive age.* Retrieved from http://www.acog.org/Resources-And-Publications/Committee-Opinions/Committee-on-Health-Care-for-Underserved-Women/Methamphetamine-Abuse-in-Women-of-Reproductive-Age

American College of Rheumatology. (2015). *Prevalence statistics.* Retrieved from http://www.rheumatology.org/Research/Prevalence_Statistics/

American Diabetes Association [ADA]. (2015a). *Diabetes basics.* Retrieved from http://www.diabetes.org/diabetes-basics/

American Diabetes Association [ADA]. (2015b). *What is gestational diabetes?* Retrieved from http://www.diabetes.org/diabetes-basics/gestational/what-is-gestational-diabetes.html

American Diabetes Association [ADA]. (2015c). *How to treat gestational diabetes.* Retrieved from http://www.diabetes.org/diabetes-basics/gestational/how-to-treat-gestational.html

American Diabetes Association [ADA]. (2015d). *Living with diabetes: After delivery.* Retrieved from http://www.diabetes.org/living-with-diabetes/

American Heart Association [AHA]. (2015). *Women and heart disease.* Retrieved from https://www.goredforwomen.org/about-heart-disease/facts_about_heart_disease_in_women-sub-category/statistics-at-a-glance/

Anderson, B., & Cu-Uvin, S. (2015). HIV and pregnancy (Beyond the basics). *UpToDate.* Retrieved from http://www.uptodate.com/contents/hiv-and-pregnancy-beyond-the-basics

Armon, C., Baquis, G. D., Howard, G. F., & Krupa, M. J. (2015). Neurologic disease and pregnancy. *eMedicine.* Retrieved from http://emedicine.medscape.com/article/1149405-overview#a7

Bain E, Crane M, Tieu J, Han S, Crowther CA, Middleton P. (2015). Diet and exercise interventions for preventing gestational diabetes mellitus. *Cochrane Database of Systematic Reviews,* (4): CD010443.

Bartels, C. M., & Muller, D. (2015). Systemic lupus erythematosus. *eMedicine.* Retrieved from http://emedicine.medscape.com/article/332244-overview

Bates, M., Ahmed, Y., Kapata, N., Maeurer, M., Mwaba, P., & Zumla, A. (2015). Perspectives on tuberculosis in pregnancy. *International Journal of Infectious Diseases, 32*, 124–127.

Bialas, K. M., Swamy, G. K., & Permar, S. R. (2015). Perinatal cytomegalovirus and varicella zoster virus infections: Epidemiology, prevention, and treatment. *Clinics in Perinatology, 42*(1), 61–75.

Brandt, L., Leifheit, A. K., Finnegan, L. P., & Fischer, G. (2014). Management of substance abuse in pregnancy: Maternal and neonatal aspects. In M. Galbally, M. Snellen, & A. Lewis (Eds.), *Psychopharmacology and pregnancy* (pp. 169–195). BerlinHeidelberg: Springer Publishers.

Brickner, M. E. (2014). Cardiovascular management in pregnancy congenital heart disease. *Circulation, 130*(3), 273–282.

Buschur, E., Brown, F., & Wyckoff, J. (2015). Using oral agents to manage gestational diabetes: What have we learned?. *Current Diabetes Reports, 15*(2), 1–8.

Calhoun, B.C., & Lewis, T. (2016) *Tobacco cessation and substance abuse treatment in women's healthcare: A clinical guide.* Switzerland: Springer International Publishing.

Calvert, C, Ronsmans, C. (2015). Pregnancy and HIV disease progression: A systematic review and meta-analysis. *Tropical Medicine & International Health, 20*, 122–145.

Camaschella, C. (2015). Iron-deficiency anemia. *New England Journal of Medicine, 372*(19), 1832–1843.

Cantor, A. G., Bougatsos, C., Dana, T., Blazina, I., & McDonagh, M. (2015). Routine iron supplementation and screening for iron deficiency anemia in pregnancy: A systematic review for the US Preventive Services Task Force. *Annals of Internal Medicine, 162*(8), 566–576.

Cennimo, D. J., & Dieudonne, A. (2015). Parvovirus B19 infection. *eMedicine.* Retrieved from http://emedicine.medscape.com/article/961063-overview

Chang, M. W., Brown, R., Nitzke, S., Smith, B., & Eghtedary, K. (2015). Stress, sleep, depression and dietary intakes among low-income overweight and obese pregnant women. *Maternal and Child Health Journal, 19*(5), 1047–1059.

Centers for Disease Control and Prevention [CDC]. (2015a). *Teen pregnancy in the United States.* Retrieved from http://www.cdc.gov/teenpregnancy/aboutteenpreg.htm

Centers for Disease Control and Prevention [CDC]. (2015b). *Tuberculosis and pregnancy.* Retrieved from http://www.cdc.gov/tb/publications/factsheets/specpop/pregnancy.htm

Centers for Disease Control and Prevention [CDC]. (2015c). *Fact sheet: Sickle cell disease.* Retrieved from http://www.cdc.gov/ncbddd/sicklecell/documents/scd-factsheet_what-is-scd.pdf

Centers for Disease Control and Prevention [CDC]. (2015d). *Women and autoimmune diseases.* Retrieved from http://wwwnc.cdc.gov/eid/article/10/11/14-0367_article

Centers for Disease Control and Prevention [CDC]. (2015e). *Cytomegalovirus and pregnant women*. Retrieved from http://www.cdc.gov/cmv/risk/preg-women.html

Centers for Disease Control and Prevention [CDC]. (2015f). *Genital herpes – CDC fact sheet*. Retrieved from http://www.cdc.gov/std/herpes/stdfact-herpes.htm

Centers for Disease Control and Prevention [CDC]. (2015g). *Hepatitis B information for health professionals: Perinatal transmission*. Retrieved from http://www.cdc.gov/hepatitis/HBV/PerinatalXmtn.htm

Centers for Disease Control and Prevention [CDC]. (2015h). *Fetal alcohol spectrum disorders*. Retrieved from http://www.cdc.gov/ncbddd/fasd/alcohol-use.html

Centers for Disease Control and Prevention [CDC]. (2015i). *Group B strep (GBS)*. Retrieved from http://www.cdc.gov/groupbstrep/about/fast-facts.html

Centers for Disease Control and prevention [CDC]. (2015j). *HIV in the United States: At a glance*. Retrieved from http://www.cdc.gov/hiv/statistics/basics/ataglance.html

Centers for Disease Control and Prevention [CDC]. (2015k). *HIV among women*. Retrieved from http://www.cdc.gov/hiv/risk/gender/women/facts/index.html

Centers for Disease Control and Prevention [CDC]. (2015l). *HIV transmission*. Retrieved from http://www.cdc.gov/hiv/basics/transmission.html

Centers for Disease Control and Prevention [CDC]. (2015m). *HIV among pregnant women, infants, and children*. Retrieved from http://www.cdc.gov/hiv/risk/gender/pregnantwomen/facts/

Centers for Disease Control and Prevention [CDC]. (2015n). *Child Development: Teenagers (15-17 years old)*. Retrieved from http://www.cdc.gov/ncbddd/childdevelopment/positiveparenting/adolescence2.html

Centers for Disease Control and Prevention [CDC]. (2015o). *Health care providers and teen pregnancy prevention*. Retrieved from http://www.cdc.gov/teenpregnancy/healthcareproviders.htm

Centers for Disease Control and Prevention [CDC]. (2015p). *Pregnancy complications: Obesity*. Retrieved from http://www.cdc.gov/reproductivehealth/maternalinfanthealth/pregcomplications.htm#n5

Centers for Disease Control and Prevention [CDC]. (2015q). *Illegal drug use*. Retrieved from http://www.cdc.gov/nchs/fastats/drug-use-illegal.htm

Centers for Disease Control and Prevention [CDC]. (2015r). *Sexually transmitted diseases*. Retrieved from http://www.cdc.gov/std/

Centers of Disease Control and Prevention [CDC]. (2015s). *About HIV/AIDS*. Retrieved from http://www.cdc.gov/hiv/basics/whatishiv.html

Charlier, C., Le Mercier, D., Salomon, L. J., Ville, Y., Kermorvant-Duchemin, E., Frange, P., et al. (2014). Varicella-zoster virus and pregnancy. *Presse Medicale*, *43*(6), 665–675.

Chomistek, A. K., Chiuve, S. E., & Eliassen, A. H. (2015). Healthy lifestyle in young women greatly reduces CHD and development of CVD risk factors. *Journal of American College of Cardiology*, *65*(1), 43–51.

Choreño-Machain, T. C., Barrios, J., & Reta, E. B. (2015). Congenital and acquired heart disease in pregnancy. *Journal of the American College of Cardiology*, *65*(10).

Connery, H. S. (2014). *Substance abuse during pregnancy. An issue of obstetrics and gynecology clinics*. *41*(2). Philadelphia, PA: Elsevier Health Sciences.

Contag, S. A., & Arrabal, P. P. (2015). Hepatitis in pregnancy. *eMedicine*. Retrieved from http://emedicine.medscape.com/article/1562368-overview#a1

Cornell, S. (2015). Continual evolution of type 2 diabetes: An update on pathophysiology and emerging treatment options. *Therapeutics and Clinical Risk Management*, *11*, 621–632.

Costa, V. M., Viana, M. B., & Aguiar, R. A. (2015). Pregnancy in patients with sickle cell disease: Maternal and perinatal outcomes. *The Journal of Maternal-Fetal & Neonatal Medicine*, *28*(6), 685–689.

Crockett, L. J., & Crouter, A. C. (Eds.). (2014). *Pathways through adolescence: Individual development in relation to social contexts*. New York, NY: Psychology Press.

Cunningham, F. G., Leveno, K. J., Bloom, S. L., Spong, C., & Dashe, J. (2014). *Williams' obstetrics* (24th ed.). New York, NY: McGraw-Hill Professional Publishing.

Desai, A., Mark, K., & Terplan, M. (2014). Marijuana use and pregnancy: prevalence, associated behaviors, and birth outcomes. *Obstetrics and Gynecology*, *123*, 46S--46S.

Desai, K. N., & Brustman, L. E. (2014). Parvovirus in pregnancy. *Postgraduate Obstetrics & Gynecology*, *34*(8), 1–5.

Dhalwani, N. N., Szatkowski, L., Coleman, T., Fiaschi, L., & Tata, L. J. (2015). Nicotine replacement therapy in pregnancy and major congenital anomalies in offspring. *Pediatrics*, *135*(5), 859–867.

Dillon, M. E. (2014). Adolescent pregnancy and mental health. In *International handbook of adolescent pregnancy* (pp. 79–102). New York, NY: Springer Publishers.

Doulatram, G., Raj, T. D., & Govindaraj, R. (2015). Pregnancy and substance abuse. In A. D. Kaye, N. Vadivelu, & R. D. Urman *Substance abuse* (pp. 453–494). New York, NY: Springer Publishers.

Drake, A. L., Wagner, A., Richardson, B., & John-Stewart, G. (2014). Incident HIV during pregnancy and postpartum and risk of mother-to-child HIV transmission: A systematic review and meta-analysis. *PLoS Medicine*, *11*(2), e1001608. doi: 10.1371/journal.pmed.1001608

Dudek, S. G. (2014). *Nutrition essentials for nursing practice* (7th ed.). Philadelphia, PA: Lippincott Williams & Wilkins.

Edwards, M. S. (2014). Adverse fetal outcomes: Expanding the role of infection. *JAMA*, *311*(11), 1115–1116.

Farrar D, Duley L, Medley N, Lawlor DA. (2015). Different strategies for diagnosing gestational diabetes to improve maternal and infant health. *Cochrane Database of Systematic Reviews*, (1), CD007122.

Fauci, A. S., Folkers, G. K., & Marston, H. D. (2014). Ending the global HIV/AIDS pandemic: The critical role of an HIV vaccine. *Clinical Infectious Diseases*, *59*(Suppl. 2), S80--S84.

Fedorowicz, A. R., Hellerstedt, W. L., Schreiner, P. J., & Bolland, J. M. (2014). Associations of adolescent hopelessness and self-worth with pregnancy attempts and pregnancy desire. *American Journal of Public Health*, *104*(8), e133--e140.

Foo, L., Tay, J., Lees, C. C., McEniery, C. M., & Wilkinson, I. B. (2015). Hypertension in pregnancy: Natural history and treatment options. *Current Hypertension Reports*, *17*(5), 1–18.

Friedman, A. J., Shander, A., Martin, S. R., Calabrese, R. K., Ashton, M. E., Lew, I., et al. (2015). Iron deficiency anemia in women: A practical guide to detection, diagnosis, and treatment. *Obstetrical & Gynecological Survey*, *70*(5), 342–353.

Gabbay-Benziv, R., Reece, E. A., Wang, F., & Yang, P. (2015). Birth defects in pregestational diabetes: Defect range, glycemic threshold and pathogenesis. *World Journal of Diabetes*, *6*(3), 481–488.

Ganchimeg, T., Ota, E., Morisaki, N., Laopaiboon, M., Lumbiganon, P., Zhang, J., et al. (2014). Pregnancy and childbirth outcomes among adolescent mothers: a World Health Organization multicountry study. *BJOG: An International Journal of Obstetrics & Gynecology*, *121*(s1), 40–48.

Gandhi, M., & Martin, S. R. (2015). Cardiac disease in pregnancy. *Obstetrics and Gynecology Clinics of North America*, *42*(2), 315–333.

Giles, M. L. (2015). HIV in pregnancy-Diagnosis, management and follow up of the neonate. *Pathology*, *47*, S49.

Gilstrap, L. G., & Wood, M. J. (2014). Cardiovascular disease in women and pregnancy. In H. K. Gaggin & J. L. Januzzi (Eds.), *MGH cardiology board review* (pp. 205–223). London, England: Springer Publishers.

Grandy, M., Purnell, J. Q., Thornburg, K. L., & Marshall, N. E. (2015). Gestational weight gain and maternal diet composition [272]. *Obstetrics & Gynecology*, *125*, 87S--88S.

Green, C. J. (2016). *Maternal newborn nursing care plans* (3rd ed). Burlington, MA: Jones & Bartlett Learning.

Grewal, J., Silversides, C. K., & Colman, J. M. (2014). Pregnancy in women with heart disease: Risk assessment and management of heart failure. *Heart Failure Clinics*, *10*(1), 117–129.

Gupta, Y. (2015). Updated guidelines on screening for gestational diabetes. *International Journal of Women's Health*, *7*, 539–550.

Hadar, E., Ashwal, E., & Hod, M. (2014). The preconceptional period as an opportunity for prediction and prevention of non-communicable disease. *Best Practice & Research Clinical Obstetrics & Gynecology*, *29*(1), 54–62.

Hamdan, A. H. (2015). Neonatal abstinence syndrome. *eMedicine*. Retrieved from http://emedicine.medscape.com/article/978763-overview

Hardy, E. J., Degli Esposti, S., & Nee, J. (2015). Viral infection in pregnancy: HIV and viral hepatitis. In K. Rosene-Montella (Ed.), *Medical management of the pregnant patient* (pp. 197–216). New York, NY: Springer Publishers.

Harvey, R. E., Coffman, K. E., & Miller, V. M. (2015). Women-specific factors to consider in risk, diagnosis and treatment of cardiovascular disease. *Women's Health, 11*(2), 239–257.

Hashemi-Beni, M., Rahimi-Madiseh, M., Khosravi, A., Malekpur-Thehrani, A., Alijani, Z., & Ayazi, Z. (2015). Educational needs assessment of gestational diabetes in pregnant women for safe delivery and healthy baby birth. *Journal of Clinical Nursing and Midwifery, 4*(1), 59–67.

He, J. R., Yuan, M. Y., Chen, N. N., Lu, J. H., Hu, C. Y., Mai, W. B., et al. (2015). Maternal dietary patterns and gestational diabetes mellitus: A large prospective cohort study in China. *British Journal of Nutrition, 113*(08), 1292–1300.

Herchline, T. E. & Amorosa, J. K. (2015). Tuberculosis. *eMedicine.* Retrived from http://emedicine.medscape.com/article/230802-overview

Higgins, J. P., Yarlagadda, S., & Yang, B. (2015). Cardiovascular complications of energy drinks. *Beverages, 1*(2), 104–126.

Hilfiker-Kleiner, D., & Arany, Z. (2014). Focus on pregnancy-mediated heart and vascular disease. *Cardiovascular Research, 101*(4), 543–544.

Hokelek, M., (2015). Toxoplasmosis. *eMedicine.* Retrieved from http://emedicine.medscape.com/article/229969-overview

Institute for Alternative Futures (2015). *Diabetes 2015 – U.S., state, and metropolitan trends.* Retrieved from http://altfutures.org/diabetes2025/

International AIDS Society. (2015). *Mass media campaigns effective for condom use and HIV knowledge.* Retrieved from http://www.iasociety.org/Default.aspx?pageId=5&elementId=15969

James, J. E. (2015). Review: higher caffeine intake during pregnancy increases risk of low birth weight. *Evidence Based Nursing, 18*(4), 111.

James, P. A., Oparil, S., Carter, B. L., Cushman, W. C., Dennison-Himmelfarb, C., Handler, J., et al. (2014). 2014 evidence-based guideline for the management of high blood pressure in adults: report from the panel members appointed to the Eighth Joint National Committee (JNC 8). *JAMA, 311*(5), 507–520.

James, S. H., & Kimberlin, D. W. (2015). Neonatal herpes simplex virus infection: Epidemiology and treatment. *Clinics in Perinatology, 42*(1), 47–59.

Jhaveri, R. (2015). Prevention of hepatitis B virus vertical transmission: Time for the next step. *Pediatrics, 135*(5), e1286–e1287.

Jimenez, K., Kulnigg-Dabsch, S., & Gasche, C. (2015). Management of iron deficiency anemia. *Gastroenterology & Hepatology, 11*(4), 241–250.

Joint National Committee. (2014). *Eighth report of the Joint National Committee on prevention, detection, evaluation, and treatment of high blood pressure* (NIH Publication No. 035233). Washington, DC: National Institutes of Health.

Jordan, R. G., Engstrom, J. L., Marfell, J. A., & Farley, C. L. (2014). *Prenatal and postnatal care: A woman-centered approach.* Ames, IO: John Wiley & Sons, Inc.

Jyoti, M., Shirke, S., & Matalia, H. (2015). Congenital rubella syndrome: Global issue. *Journal of Cataract & Refractive Surgery, 41*(5), 1127–1134.

Kahn, E., Mikhael, H., & Vadivelu, N. (2015). Cocaine abuse. In *Substance abuse* (pp. 143–154). New York, NY: Springer Publishers.

Karimi, M., Cohan, N., & Parand, S. (2015). Thalassemia and women's health. *Women's Health Bulletin, 2*(3), E29440.

Kelly, W., Massoumi, A., & Lazarus, A. (2015). Asthma in pregnancy: Physiology, diagnosis, and management. *Postgraduate Medicine, 127*(4), 349–358.

Killion, M. (2015). New hypertension in pregnancy guidelines. *MCN: The American Journal of Maternal/Child Nursing, 40*(2), 128.

Kim, C. (2014). Maternal outcomes and follow-up after gestational diabetes mellitus. *Diabetic Medicine, 31*(3), 292–301.

King, T. L., Brucker, M. C., Kriebs, J. M., Fahey, J. O., Gegor, C. L., & Varney, H. (2015). *Varney's midwifery* (5th ed.). Burlington, MA: Jones & Bartlett Learning

Knight-Agarwal, C. R., Kaur, M., Williams, L. T., Davey, R., & Davis, D. (2014). The views and attitudes of health professionals providing antenatal care to women with a high BMI: A qualitative research study. *Women and Birth, 27*(2), 138–144.

Knox, C. A., Delaney, J. A., & Winterstein, A. G. (2014). Anti-diabetic drug utilization of pregnant diabetic women in us managed care. *BMC Pregnancy and Childbirth, 14*(1), 28–34.

Koh, H. (2014). The teen pregnancy prevention program: An evidence-based public health program model. *Journal of Adolescent Health, 54*(3), S1–S2.

Kovacs, G., & Briggs, P. (2015). Infections during pregnancy–varicella, herpes, cytomegalovirus, toxoplasma, listeria, Group B streptococcus. In *Lectures in obstetrics, gynecology and women's health* (pp. 133–137). Springer International Publishing.

Kumar, B., & Gupta, S. (2014). *Sexually transmitted infections* (2nd ed.). Philadelphia, PA: Elsevier Health Sciences.

Lambert, N., Strebel, P., Orenstein, W., Icenogle, J., & Poland, G. A. (2015). Rubella. *Lancet, 385*(9984):2297–2307

Lamberth, J. R., Reddy, S. C., Pan, J. J., & Dasher, K. J. (2015). Chronic hepatitis B infection in pregnancy. *World Journal of Hepatology, 7*(9), 1233–1237.

Lapolla, A., & Dalfrà, M. G. (2015). Pregnancy and diabetes. In *Frontiers in diabetes Vol 24.* (pp. 11–22). Karger Medical & Scientific-Publishers.

Lichtin, A., & Philipson, E. H. (2014). Pregnancy. In *The coagulation consult* (pp. 249–269). New York, NY: Springer Publishers.

Ma, W. J., Huang, Z. H., Huang, B. X., Qi, B. H., Zhang, Y. J., Xiao, B. X., et al. (2015). Intensive low-glycemic-load dietary intervention for the management of glycemia and serum lipids among women with gestational diabetes: a randomized control trial. *Public Health Nutrition, 18*(08), 1506–1513.

Maartens, G., Celum, C., & Lewin, S. R. (2014). HIV infection: Epidemiology, pathogeneses, treatment, and prevention. *The Lancet, 384*(9939), 258–271.

Madhuvrata, P., Govinden, G., Bustani, R., Song, S., & Farrell, T. A. (2015). Prevention of gestational diabetes in pregnant women with risk factors for gestational diabetes: A systematic review and meta-analysis of randomized trials. *Obstetric Medicine: The Medicine of Pregnancy, 8*(2), 68–85.

Malee, M. P. (2015). Protocol 30: Parvovirus B19 infection. *Protocols for high-risk pregnancies: An evidence-based approach* (pp. 245–250). Chichester, UK: John Wiley & Sons.

March of Dimes. (2015a). *Gestational diabetes.* Retrieved from http://www.marchofdimes.com/pregnancy/gestational-diabetes.aspx

March of Dimes. (2015b). *Thalassemia.* Retrieved from http://www.marchofdimes.com/baby/thalassemia.aspx

March of Dimes. (2015c). *Sickle cell disease and pregnancy.* Retrieved from http://www.marchofdimes.com/pregnancy/sickle-cell-disease-and-pregnancy.aspx

March of Dimes. (2015d). *Cytomegalovirus and pregnancy.* Retrieved from http://www.marchofdimes.com/pregnancy/cytomegalovirus-and-pregnancy.aspx

March of Dimes. (2015e). *Genital herpes.* Retrieved from http://www.marchofdimes.com/pregnancy/genital-herpes.aspx

March of Dimes. (2015f). *Group B strep infection.* Retrieved from http://www.marchofdimes.com/pregnancy/group-b-strep-infection.aspx

March of Dimes. (2015g). *Toxoplasmosis.* Retrieved from http://www.marchofdimes.com/pregnancy/toxoplasmosis.aspx

March of Dimes. (2015h). *Keeping breastfeeding safe.* Retrieved from http://www.marchofdimes.org/baby/keeping-breastfeeding-safe.aspx

March of Dimes. (2015i). *Pregnancy complications: Sexually transmitted diseases.* Retrieved from http://www.marchofdimes.org/sexually-transmitted-diseases.aspx

March of Dimes. (2015j). *Teenage pregnancy.* Retrieved from http://www.marchofdimes.org/materials/teenage-pregnancy.pdf

March of Dimes. (2015k). *Smoking, alcohol, and drugs and pregnancy.* Retrieved from http://www.marchofdimes.org/pregnancy/illicit-drug-use-during-pregnancy.aspx

March of Dimes. (2015l). *Asthma during pregnancy.* Retrieved from http://www.marchofdimes.org/pregnancy/asthma-during-pregnancy.aspx

March of Dimes. (2015m). *A mommy after 35.* Retrieved from http://www.marchofdimes.org/pregnancy/a-mommy-after-35.aspx?gclid=CKqBr5zEwMACFWoR7AoddGQASQ

McHugh, R. K., Nielsen, S., & Weiss, R. D. (2015). Prescription drug abuse: from epidemiology to public policy. *Journal of Substance Abuse Treatment, 48*(1), 1–7.

McIntyre, H. D., Dyer, A. R., & Metzger, B. E. (2015). Odds, risks and appropriate diagnosis of gestational diabetes. *The Medical Journal of Australia, 202*(6), 309–311.

Mehta, N., Chen, K., Hardy, E., & Powrie, R. (2015). Respiratory disease in pregnancy. *Best Practice & Research Clinical Obstetrics & Gynecology, ;29*(5), 598–611.

Miller, M. A., & Carpenter, M. (2015). Hypertensive disorders of pregnancy. In *Medical management of the pregnant patient* (pp. 177–193). New York, NY: Springer Publishers.

Mills, T. A., & Lavender, T. (2014). Advanced maternal age. *Obstetrics, Gynecology & Reproductive Medicine, 24*(3), 85–90.

McKeever, A. E., Spaeth-Brayton, S., & Sheerin, S. (2014). The role of nurses in comprehensive care management of pregnant women with drug addiction. *Nursing for Women's Health, 18*(4), 284–293.

Mitanchez, D., Yzydorczyk, C., Siddeek, B., Boubred, F., Benahmed, M., & Simeoni, U. (2015). The offspring of the diabetic mother– short-and long-term implications. *Best Practice & Research Clinical Obstetrics & Gynecology, 29*(2), 256–269.

Mohamad, T. N., Fakhri, H. A., Bernal, J. M., Thatai, D., & Peterson, E. (2014). Cardiovascular disease and pregnancy. *eMedicine.* Retrieved from http://emedicine.medscape.com/article/162004-overview

Mohammadzadeh, A., & Farhat, A. (2014). Fetal alcohol syndrome. *Asia Pacific Journal of Medical Toxicology, 3,* 10–-10.

Mohindra, R., & Marwah, S. (2015). Systemic lupus erythematosus in pregnancy-intricate, but wieldy. *International Journal of Reproduction, Contraception, Obstetrics and Gynecology, 4*(2), 295–300.

Moore, T. R. (2015). Diabetes mellitus and pregnancy. *eMedicine.* Retrieved from http://emedicine.medscape.com/article/127547-overview

Moses, S. (2015). Anemia in pregnancy. *Family practice notebook.* Retrieved from http://www.fpnotebook.com/hemeonc/OB/AnmIn-Prgncy.htm

Multiple Sclerosis Association of America [MSAA]. (2015). *MS overview.* Retrieved from http://mymsaa.org/about-ms/overview/

Nagtalon-Ramos, J. (2014). *Best evidence-based practices: Maternal-newborn nursing care.* Philadelphia, PA: F.A. Davis Company.

National Asthma Education and Prevention Program [NAEPP]. (2015). *Guidelines for the diagnosis and management of asthma.* Retrieved from http://www.nhlbi.nih.gov/health-pro/guidelines/current/asthma-guidelines/index.htm

National Diabetes Information Clearing House. (2015). *What is gestational diabetes?* Retrieved from http://www.diabetes.niddk.nih.gov/dm/pubs/pregnancy

National Institute on Drug Abuse [NIDA]. (2015a). *What are the unique needs pf pregnant women with substance abuse disorders?* Retrieved from http://www.drugabuse.gov/publications/principles-drug-addiction-treatment-research-based-guide-second-edition/frequently-asked-questions/what-are-unique-needs-pregnant-women

National Institute on Drug Abuse [NIDA]. (2015b). *Drug facts: Cocaine.* Retrieved from http://www.drugabuse.gov/publications/drugfacts/cocaine

National Institute on Drug Abuse [NIDA]. (2015c). *Drug facts: Marijuana.* Retrieved from http://www.drugabuse.gov/publications/drugfacts/marijuana

National Institute on Drug Abuse [NIDA]. (2015d). *Drug facts: Methamphetamine.* Retrieved from http://www.drugabuse.gov/publications/drugfacts/methamphetamine

National Institutes of Health [NIH]. (2014). Recommendations for use of antiretroviral drugs in pregnant HIV-infected women for maternal health and interventions to reduce perinatal transmission in the United States. United Public Health Service. Retrieved from http://aidsinfo.nih.gov/contentfiles/lvguidelines/PerinatalGL.pdf

National Organization on Fetal Alcohol Syndrome [NOFAS]. (2015). *What is fetal alcohol syndrome?* Retrieved from http://www.nofas.org/main/what_is_FAS.htm.

New York Heart Association, Criteria Committee. (1994). *Nomenclature and criteria for diagnosis of diseases of the heart and great vessels* (9th ed., pp. 253–256). Boston, MA: Little, Brown.

Northridge, J. L., & Coupey, S. M. (2015). Realizing reproductive health equity for adolescents and young adults. *American Journal of Public Health, 105*(7), 1284–-1284.

Novotna, A., & Ehler, E. (2014). Multiple sclerosis and pregnancy. *Clinical Neurophysiology, 125*(5), e27.

Østensen, M. (2014). Contraception and pregnancy counseling in rheumatoid arthritis. *Current Opinion in Rheumatology, 26*(3), 302–307.

Park, J. S., & Pan, C. (2014). Current recommendations of managing HBV infection in preconception or pregnancy. *Frontiers of Medicine, 8*(2), 158–165.

Petry, C. J. (2014). *Gestational diabetes: Origins, complications, and treatment.* Boca Raton, FL: CRC Press Taylor & Francis Group

Prasad, M. (2014). When opiate abuse complicates pregnancy. *Contemporary OB/GYN* (Online, February 1, 2014).

Procter, S. B., & Campbell, C. G. (2014). Position of the academy of nutrition and dietetics: Nutrition and lifestyle for a healthy pregnancy outcome. *Journal of the Academy of Nutrition and Dietetics, 114*(7), 1099–1103.

Puopolo, K. M., Madoff, L. C., & Baker, C. J. (2015). Group B streptococcal infection in pregnant women. *UpToDate.* Retrieved from http://www.uptodate.com/contents/group-b-streptococcal-infection-in-pregnant-women

Raio, L., Bolla, D., & Baumann, M. (2015). Hypertension in pregnancy. *Current Opinion in Cardiology, 30*(4), 411–415.

Rajoriya, M., & Kalra, R. (2015). Challenges of motherhood in adolescent girls. *International Journal of Reproduction, Contraception, Obstetrics and Gynecology, 4*(3), 696–700.

Rakhmanina, N. Y., & van den Anker, J. N. (2014). Pharmacologic prevention of perinatal HIV infection. *Early Human Development, 90*(1), S13–-S15.

Rayment, M., Asboe, D., & Sullivan, A. K. (2014). HIV testing and management of newly diagnosed HIV. *British Medical Journal, 349,* g4275.

Rigby, F.B. (2015). Anemias in pregnancy. *eMedicine.* Retrieved from http://emedicine.medscape.com/article/261586-overview

Rivera, D. M., & Frye, R. E. (2014). Pediatric HIV infection. *eMedicine.* Retrieved from http://emedicine.medscape.com/article/965086-overview

Roglie, G., & Colagiuri, S. (2014). Gestational diabetes mellitus: Squaring the circle. *Diabetes Care, 37*(6), 143–144.

Roskjær, A. B., Andersen, J. R., Ronneby, H., Damm, P., & Mathiesen, E. R. (2014). Dietary advices on carbohydrate intake for pregnant women with type 1 diabetes. *The Journal of Maternal-Fetal & Neonatal Medicine, 28*(2), 229–2331–15.

Ross, S., Baird, A. S., & Porter, C. C. (2014). Teenage pregnancy: Strategies for prevention. *Obstetrics, Gynecology and Reproductive Medicine, 24*(9), 266–273.

Salman, K., Priti, S., Molly, M., Kumar, V. S., & Zeenat, S. (2015). Hepatitis B virus infection in pregnant women and transmission to newborns. *Asian Pacific Journal of Tropical Disease, 5*(6), 421–429.

Sauer, M. V. (2015). Reproduction at an advanced maternal age and maternal health. *Fertility and Sterility, 103*(5), 1136–1143.

Schimmel, M. S., Bromiker, R., Hammerman, C., Chertman, L., Ioscovich, A., Granovsky-Grisaru, S., et al. (2015). The effects of maternal age and parity on maternal and neonatal outcome. *Archives of Gynecology and Obstetrics, 291*(4), 793–798.

Schur, P. H., & Hahn, B. H. (2015). Epidemiology and pathogenesis of systemic lupus erythematosus. *UpToDate.* Retrieved from http://www.uptodate.com/contents/epidemiology-and-pathogenesis-of-systemic-lupus-erythematosus

Sedgh, G., Finer, L. B., Bankole, A., Eilers, M. A., & Singh, S. (2015). Adolescent pregnancy, birth, and abortion rates across countries: Levels and recent trends. *Journal of Adolescent Health, 56*(2), 223–230.

Seely, E. W., & Ecker, J. (2014). Chronic hypertension in pregnancy. *Circulation, 129*(11), 1254–1261.

Sibai, B. M. (2015). In J. T. Queenan, C. Y. Spong & C. J. Lockwood (Eds.), *Protocols for high risk pregnancies: An evidence-based approach.* (6th edition, pp. 203–212). Chichester, UK: John Wiley & Sons, Ltd.

Silasi, M., Cardenas, I., Kwon, J. Y., Racicot, K., Aldo, P., et al. (2015). Viral infections during pregnancy. *American Journal of Reproductive Immunology, 73*(3), 199–213.

Simeone, R. M., Devine, O. J., Marcinkevage, J. A., Gilboa, S. M., Razzaghi, H., Bardenheier, B. H., et al. (2015). Diabetes and congenital heart defects: A systematic review, meta-analysis, and modeling project. *American Journal of Preventive Medicine, 48*(2), 195–204.

Singh, A. G., & Chowdhary, V. R. (2015). Pregnancy-related issues in women with systemic lupus erythematosus. *International Journal of Rheumatic Diseases, 18*, 172–181.

Skoglund, C., Chen, Q., D'Onofrio, B. M., Lichtenstein, P., & Larsson, H. (2014). Familial confounding of the association between maternal smoking during pregnancy and ADHD in offspring. *Journal of Child Psychology and Psychiatry, 55*, 61–68.

Slater, L. (2015). Substance use in pregnancy. *The Practicing Midwife, 18*(1), 10–13.

Sliwa, K., Johnson, M. R., Zilla, P., & Roos-Hesselink, J. W. (2015). Management of valvular disease in pregnancy: A global perspective. *European Heart Journal, 36*(13), 1078–1089.

Smith, B. (2015). *Neonatal-perinatal infections: An update, in issue of clinics in perinatology* (Vol.42(1), pp. 77–104). Philadelphia, PA: Elsevier Health Sciences.

Solomon, C. G., & Greene, M. F. (2015). Control of hypertension in pregnancy—If some is good, Is more worse? *New England Journal of Medicine, 372*(5), 475–476.

Strangfeld, A., Pattloch, D., Spilka, M., Manger, B., Krummel-Lorenz, B., Gräßler, A., et al. (2015). Pregnancies in patients with rheumatoid arthritis: Treatment decisions, course of the disease, and pregnancy outcomes. *Annals of the Rheumatic Diseases, 74*(Suppl 2), 70–71.

Subramaniam, G., & Girish, M. (2015). Iron deficiency anemia in children. *The Indian Journal of Pediatrics, 82*(6), 558–564.

Substance Abuse and Mental Health Services Administration [SAMHSA]. (2015). *Pregnant women, new mothers, and substance abuse.* Retrieved from http://www.samhsa.gov/samhsaNewsLetter/Volume_17_Number_3/PregnancySubstanceAbuse.aspx

Suliman, S., & Seopela, L. (2015). Congenital and neonatal infections: Review. In *Obstetrics and gynecology forum, 25*(2), 27–32.

Swamy, G. K., & Heine, R. (2015). Vaccinations for pregnant women. *Obstetrics & Gynecology, 125*(1), 212–226.

Swan, L. (2014). Congenital heart disease in pregnancy. *Best Practice & Research Clinical Obstetrics & Gynecology, 28*(4), 495–506.

Toledano, Y., Hadar, E., & Hod, M. (2015). Diabetes in pregnancy. In R. A. DeFronzo, E. Ferrannini, P. Zimmet , et al. (Eds.), *International textbook of diabetes mellitus* (4th ed.). Chichester, UK: John Wiley & Sons.

Ural, S. H. (2015). Genital herpes in pregnancy. *eMedicine.* Retrieved from http://emedicine.medscape.com/article/274874-overview

U.S. Agency for International Development [USAID]. (2014). *Contraceptives for clients with STIs, HIV, and AIDS.* Retrieved from https://www.fphandbook.org/contraceptives-clients-stis-hiv-and-aids

U.S. Department of Health and Human Services. (2010). *Healthy people 2020.* Retrieved from http://www.healthypeople.gov/2020/topicsobjectives2020

U.S. Preventive Services Task Force [USPSTF]. (2014). *Screening for HIV.* Retrieved from http://www.uspreventiveservicestaskforce.org/uspstf13/hiv/hivfinalrs.htm#summary

U.S. Preventive Services Task Force [USPTF]. (2015). *Low-dose aspirin use for the prevention of morbidity and mortality from preeclampsia: Preventive medication.* Retrieved from http://www.uspreventiveservicestaskforce.org/Page/Topic/recommendation-summary/low-dose-aspirin-use-for-the-prevention-of-morbidity-and-mortality-from-preeclampsia-preventive-medication

Vall, O., Salat-Batlle, J., & Garcia-Algar, O. (2015). Alcohol consumption during pregnancy and adverse neurodevelopmental outcomes. *Journal of Epidemiology and Community Health, 69*(10), 927–929.

Vanders, R. L., & Murphy, V. E. (2015). Maternal complications and the management of asthma in pregnancy. *Women's Health, 11*(2), 183–191.

Varner, M. W., Silver, R. M., Hogue, C. J., Willinger, M., Parker, C. B., Thorsten, V. R., et al. (2014). Association between stillbirth and illicit drug use and smoking during pregnancy. *Obstetrics & Gynecology, 123*(1), 113–125.

Vaux, K. K., & Chambers, C. (2015). Fetal alcohol syndrome. *eMedicine.* Retrieved from http://emedicine.medscape.com/article/974016-overview

Velez, M. L., & Jansson, L. M. (2015). Perinatal addictions: intrauterine exposures. In *Textbook of addiction treatment: International perspectives* (pp. 2333–2363). Springer Publishers.

Vinchinski, E. P. (2015). Pregnancy in women with sickle cell disease. *UpToDate.* Retrieved from http://www.uptodate.com/contents/pregnancy-in-women-with-sickle-cell-disease

Vogler, M. A. (2014). HIV and pregnancy. *Current Treatment Options in Infectious Diseases, 6*(2), 183–195.

Volkow, N. D., Baler, R. D., Compton, W. M., & Weiss, S. R. (2014). Adverse health effects of marijuana use. *New England Journal of Medicine, 370*(23), 2219–2227.

Vukusic, S., & Marignier, R. (2015). Multiple sclerosis and pregnancy in the 'treatment era'. *Nature Reviews Neurology, 11*, 280–289.

Wang, M. (2015). Perinatal drug abuse and neonatal withdrawal. *eMedicine.* Retrieved from http://emedicine.medscape.com/article/978492-overview

Walker, M. (2014). *Breastfeeding management for the clinician: Using the evidence* (3rd ed.). Burlington, MA: Jones & Bartlett Learning.

Wasserman, S., & Clowse, M. E. (2014). Systemic lupus erthematosus. In L. R. Sammaritano & B. L. Bermas (Eds.), *Contraception and pregnancy in patients with rheumatic disease* (pp. 79–97). New York, NY: Springer Publishers.

Weber, J. R., & Kelley, J. H. (2014). *Health assessment in nursing* (5th ed.), Philadelphia, PA: Lippincott Williams & Wilkins.

Weekes, A. J., & Lee, D. S. (2014). Pediatric cocaine abuse clinical presentation. *eMedicine.* Retrieved from http://emedicine.medscape.com/article/917385-clinical

Whitworth, M., & Cockerill, R. (2014). Antenatal management of teenage pregnancy. *Obstetrics, Gynecology & Reproductive Medicine, 24*(1), 23–28.

Worel, J. N., & Hayman, L. L. (2015). Cardiovascular disease prevention in women: Reducing the major threat to women's health. *Journal of Cardiovascular Nursing, 30*(1), 5–7.

Workowski, K. A., & Bolan, G. A. (2015). Sexually transmitted diseases treatment guidelines, 2015. *MMWR. Recommendations and reports: Morbidity and Mortality Weekly Report. Recommendations and reports/Centers for Disease Control, 64*(RR-03), 1–137.

World Health Organization [WHO]. (2015a). *Health for the World's Adolescents: A second chance in the second decade.* Department of Maternal, Newborn, Child and Adolescent Health. Geneva, Switzerland: WHO

World Health Organization [WHO]. (2015b). *Tuberculosis: Key facts.* Retrieved from http://www.who.int/mediacentre/factsheets/fs104/en/

World Health Organization [WHO]. (2015c). *Guidelines for the identification and management of substance abuse use disorders in pregnancy.* Retrieved from http://www.cdc.gov/nchs/fastats/drug-use-illegal.htm

Worley, J. (2014). Identification and management of prescription drug abuse in pregnancy. *The Journal of Perinatal & Neonatal Nursing, 28*(3), 196–203.

Yoost, J. L., Hertweck, S. P., & Barnett, S. N. (2014). The effect of an educational approach to pregnancy prevention among high-risk early and late adolescents. *Journal of Adolescent Health, 55*(2), 222–227.

Zhang, H. J., Patenaude, V., & Abenhaim, H. (2014). Maternal outcomes in pregnancies affected by varicella zoster virus infections. *Obstetrics & Gynecology, 123*, 86S–87S.

MULTIPLE CHOICE QUESTIONS

1. Which of the following would the nurse include when teaching a pregnant woman about the pathophysiologic mechanisms associated with gestational diabetes?
   a. Pregnancy fosters the development of carbohydrate cravings.
   b. There is progressive resistance to the effects of insulin.
   c. Hypoinsulinemia develops early in the first trimester.
   d. Glucose levels decrease to accommodate fetal growth.

2. When providing prenatal education to a pregnant woman with asthma, which of the following would be important for the nurse to do?
   a. Explain that she should avoid steroids during her pregnancy.
   b. Demonstrate how to assess her blood glucose levels.
   c. Teach correct administration of subcutaneous bronchodilators.
   d. Ensure she seeks treatment for any acute exacerbation.

3. Which of the following conditions would most likely cause a pregnant woman with type 1 diabetes the greatest difficulty during her pregnancy?
   a. Placenta previa
   b. Hyperemesis gravidarum
   c. Abruptio placentae
   d. Rh incompatibility

4. Women who drink alcohol during pregnancy:
   a. Often produce more alcohol dehydrogenase.
   b. Usually become intoxicated faster than before.
   c. Can give birth to an infant with fetal alcohol spectrum disorder.
   d. Gain fewer pounds throughout the gestation.

5. When explaining to a pregnant woman about HIV infection and transmission, which of the following would the nurse include?
   a. It primarily occurs when there is a large viral load in the blood.
   b. HIV is most commonly transmitted via sexual contact.
   c. It affects the majority of infants of mothers with HIV infection.
   d. Nurses are most frequently affected due to needle sticks.

6. Women who are obese have a greater risk of developing which of the following during pregnancy?
   a. Type 1 diabetes
   b. Hypotension
   c. Low birth weight infant
   d. Gestational hypertension

7. Maintenance on methadone or buprenorphine is the most common medical treatment for which of the following drug addictions?
   a. Alcohol
   b. Nicotine
   c. Opiates
   d. Marijuana

CRITICAL THINKING EXERCISE

1. A client at 26 weeks of gestation came to the clinic to follow up on her previous 1-hour glucose screening. Her results had come back outside the accepted screening range, and a 3-hour glucose tolerance test (GTT) had been ordered. It resulted in three abnormal values, confirming a diagnosis of gestational diabetes. As the nurse in the prenatal clinic you are seeing her for the first time.
   a. What additional information will you need to provide care for her?
   b. What education will she need to address this new diagnosis?
   c. How will you evaluate the effectiveness of your interventions?

2. A 14-year-old girl comes to the public health clinic with her mother. The mother tells you that her daughter has been "out messing around and has gotten herself pregnant." The girl is crying quietly in the corner and avoids eye contact with you. The mother reports that her daughter "must be following in my footsteps" because she became pregnant when she was only 15 years old. The client's mother goes back out into the waiting room and leaves the client with you.
   a. What is your first approach with the client to gain her trust?
   b. List the client's educational needs during this pregnancy.
   c. What prevention strategies are needed to prevent a second pregnancy?

3. A 27-year-old G3P2, is admitted to the labor and birth suite because of preterm rupture of membranes at an estimated 35 weeks of gestation. She has received no prenatal care and reports this was an unplanned

pregnancy. Linda appears distracted and very thin. She reports that her two previous children have been in foster care since birth because the child welfare authorities "didn't think I was an adequate mother." She denies any recent use of alcohol or drugs, but you smell alcohol on her breath. She has a spontaneous vaginal birth a few hours later, producing a 4-lb baby boy with Apgar scores of 8 at 1 minute and 9 at 5 minutes.

a. What aspects of this woman's history may lead the nurse to suspect that this infant may be at risk for fetal alcohol spectrum disorder?

b. What additional screening or laboratory tests might validate your suspicion?

c. What physical and neurodevelopmental deficits might present later in life if the infant has fetal alcohol spectrum disorder?

STUDY ACTIVITIES

1. In the maternity clinic or hospital setting, interview a pregnant woman with a preexisting medical condition (e.g., diabetes, asthma, sickle cell anemia) and find out how this condition affects her life and this pregnancy, especially her lifestyle choices.

2. You have a close friend who has a problem with alcohol but denies it. She now admits to you that she thinks she is pregnant because she missed her period. What specific information and advice should you give her concerning alcohol use during pregnancy?

3. Should marijuana be legalized in the United States? What impact might your view (pro or con) have on pregnant women and their offspring?

4. Outline a discussion you might have with an HIV-positive pregnant woman who doesn't see the need to take antiretroviral agents to prevent perinatal transmission.

5. The nurse is preparing a teaching session about breast-feeding for a group of pregnant women who have various infections listed below. The nurse would

include women with which of the following conditions? Select all that apply.
a. Hepatitis B
b. Parvovirus B19
c. Herpesvirus type 2
d. HIV-positive status
e. Cytomegalovirus
f. Varicella-zoster virus

BRINGING IT ALL TOGETHER: CASE STUDY

Linda is an 18 year old, very thin client who has been abusing alcohol since the age of 12. She lived in foster care for much of her life and is recently on her own with a part-time job. She reports she had experienced both emotional and sexual abuse during her childhood. At 16, she was introduced to crack cocaine. So many of her friends and relatives were using, that it was impossible for her to see any other lifestyle or want to seek help for her addiction. She states she wanted to start a new life and get clean when she found out she was pregnant, but admitted she ended up partying and using drugs for the past 4 months of this pregnancy. She presents today for her first prenatal visit. She claims that she is ready to commit to a positive change.

ASSESSMENT

Based on Linda's history, she is very vulnerable because of her young age, underweight, abusive history, substance abuse, and lack of a supportive network to assist her in making a "positive change" in her life. Although she states she is ready to "get clean" and get off drugs, she has been unable to move toward that goal on her own previously. At this stage of her pregnancy, her vital signs and fetal heart rates were within normal limits, her weight is below standard limits for her height and lab tests were normal except for low hemoglobin indicating iron deficient anemia.

Go to thePoint to find questions to consider about this case.

21

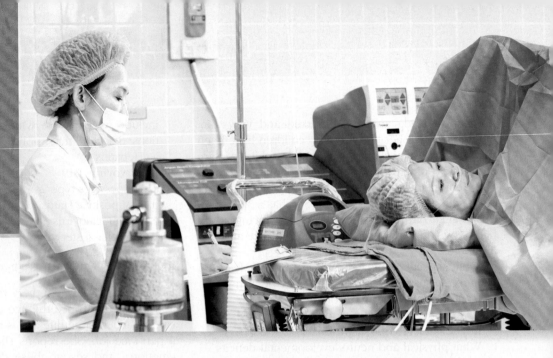

Nursing Management of Labor and Birth at Risk

Learning Objectives

Upon completion of the chapter, you will be able to:

1. Propose at least five risk factors associated with dystocia.

2. Differentiate the four major abnormalities or problems associated with dysfunctional labor patterns, giving examples of each problem.

3. Examine the nursing management for the woman with dysfunctional labor experiencing a problem with the powers, passenger, passageway, or psyche.

4. Devise a plan of care for the woman experiencing preterm labor.

5. Relate the nursing assessment and management of the woman experiencing a prolonged pregnancy.

6. Assess four obstetric emergencies that can complicate labor and birth, including appropriate management for each.

7. Compare and contrast the nursing management for the woman undergoing labor induction or augmentation, forceps- and vacuum-assisted birth.

8. Summarize the plan of care for a woman who is to undergo a cesarean birth.

9. Evaluate the key areas to be addressed when caring for a woman that undergoes a vaginal birth after cesarean (VBAC).

Jennifer, a 29-year-old G1P0, is at 41 weeks of gestation. Her health care provider has recommended that she come in for induction. She is very anxious about doing this since she has heard "horror stories" about the "hard painful contractions" that can result. What can the nurse do to calm her fears?

Words of Wisdom
In the face of a crisis or a potentially bad outcome, add a mixture of warmth and serenity to your technical abilities.

INTRODUCTION

Most women describe pregnancy as an exciting time in their lives, but the development of an unexpected problem can suddenly change this description dramatically. Consider the woman who has had a problem-free pregnancy and then suddenly develops a condition during labor, changing a routine situation into a possible crisis. Many complications occur with little or no warning and present challenges for the perinatal health care team as well as the family. The nurse plays a major role in identifying the problem quickly and coordinating immediate intervention, ultimately achieving a positive outcome.

National health goals address maternal and newborn outcomes involving complications of labor and birth and cesarean birth (U.S. Department of Health and Human Services, 2010). These goals are highlighted in *Healthy People 2020.*

This chapter will address several conditions occurring during labor and birth that may increase the risk of an adverse outcome for the mother and fetus. It also describes birth-related procedures that may be necessary for the woman who develops a condition that increases her risk or that may be needed to reduce the woman's risk for developing a condition, thus promoting optimal maternal and fetal outcomes. Nursing management of the woman and her family focuses on professional support and compassionate care.

DYSTOCIA

Dystocia, defined as abnormal or difficult labor, can be influenced by a vast number of maternal and fetal factors. Dystocia is said to exist when the progress of labor deviates from normal; it is characterized by a slow and abnormal progression of labor. It occurs in approximately 8% to 11% of all labors and is the leading indicator for primary cesarean birth in the United States (Joy, Lyon, & Scott, 2015). It is of concern because of its fatiguing factor for both mother and fetus and frequently requires medical or surgical interventions, which increases risk.

To characterize a labor as abnormal, a basic understanding of normal labor is essential. Normal labor starts with regular uterine contractions that are strong enough to result in cervical effacement and dilation. Early in labor, uterine contractions are irregular and cervical effacement and dilation occurs gradually. When cervical dilation reaches 5 to 6 cm and uterine contractions become more powerful, the active phase of labor begins. It is usually during the active phase that dystocia becomes apparent. Because dystocia cannot be predicted or diagnosed with certainty, the term "failure to progress" is often used. This term includes lack of progressive cervical dilation, lack of descent of the fetal head, or both. An adequate trial of labor is needed to declare with confidence that dystocia or "failure to progress" exists.

Early identification of and prompt interventions for dystocia are essential to minimize risk to the woman and fetus. According to the American College of Obstetricians and Gynecologists [ACOG] (2014a) factors associated with an increased risk for dystocia include epidural analgesia, excessive analgesia, multiple pregnancy, hydramnios, maternal exhaustion, ineffective maternal pushing technique, occiput posterior position, longer first stage of labor, nulliparity, short maternal stature (less than 5 ft tall), fetal birth weight (more than 8.8 lb), shoulder dystocia, abnormal fetal presentation or position (breech), fetal anomalies (hydrocephalus), maternal age older than 34 years, high caffeine intake, overweight, gestational age more than 41 weeks, chorioamnionitis, ineffective uterine contractions, and high fetal station at complete cervical dilation.

One in three women who gives birth in the United States today does so by a cesarean birth. The most common indications for primary cesarean births include, in order of frequency, labor dystocia, abnormal fetal heart rate tracing, fetal malpresentation, multiple gestations, and suspected macrosomia. It is time to revisit the definition of labor dystocia because recent studies show that contemporary labor progresses at a rate substantially slower than what was historically taught. Labors today are often longer which may in part be due to higher body mass index (BMI), higher rates of labor induction, and the significant increase in the use of epidural anesthesia (ACOG, 2014a).

Admitting women too early to the hospital while still in the early latent phase of labor may increase the diagnosis of dystocia and increase the risk of augmentation of labor and epidural analgesia. These two interventions may cascade into a surgical birth. Adequate hydration, rest, emotional and physical support, and, if needed, pharmacologic sedation can be encouraged as alternatives to early hospital admission. Patience should be the critical factor here.

HEALTHY PEOPLE 2020 • 21.1

Objective	Nursing Significance
MICH-9 Reduce preterm births	• Will help to focus attention on the need for close antepartum surveillance and identification of risks factors for preterm labor/births and provide appropriate interventions to reduce it.
MICH-7 Reduce cesarean births among low-risk (full-term, singleton, vertex presentation) women	• Will help to reduce the number of surgical births with accompanying risk factors and costs by appropriate labor management, continual labor support, and practice patterns, while helping to ensure positive maternal and newborn outcomes.

Healthy People objectives based on data from http://www.healthypeople.gov.

Dystocia can result from problems or abnormalities involving the expulsive forces (known as the "powers"); presentation, position, and fetal development (the "passenger"); the maternal bony pelvis or birth canal (the "passageway"); and maternal stress (the "psyche"). Table 21.1 summarizes the diagnosis, therapeutic management, and nursing management of the common problems associated with dystocia.

Problems with the Powers

When the expulsive forces of the uterus become dysfunctional, the uterus may either never fully relax (hypertonic contractions), placing the fetus in jeopardy, or relax too much (hypotonic contractions), causing ineffective contractions. Still another dysfunction can occur when the uterus contracts so frequently and with such intensity that a very rapid birth will take place (precipitate labor).

Hypertonic uterine dysfunction occurs when the uterus never fully relaxes between contractions. Subsequently, contractions are ineffectual, erratic, and poorly coordinated because they involve only a portion of the uterus and because more than one uterine pacemaker is sending signals for contraction. Women in this situation experience a prolonged latent phase, stay at 2 to 3 cm, and do not dilate as they should. Placental perfusion becomes compromised, thereby reducing oxygen to the fetus. These hypertonic contractions exhaust the mother, who is experiencing frequent, intense, and painful contractions with little progression. This dysfunctional pattern occurs in early labor and affects nulliparous women more than multiparous women (Hinshaw & Kenyon, 2015).

Hypotonic uterine dysfunction occurs during active labor (dilation more than 5 to 6 cm) when contractions become poor in quality and lack sufficient intensity to dilate and efface the cervix. Factors associated with this abnormal labor pattern include overstretching of the uterus, a large fetus, multiple fetuses, hydramnios, multiple parity, bowel or bladder distention preventing descent, and excessive use of analgesia. Clinical manifestations of hypotonic uterine dysfunction include weak contractions that become milder, a uterine fundus that can be easily indented with fingertip pressure at the peak of each contraction, and contractions that become more infrequent and briefer (King et al., 2015). The major risk with this complication is hemorrhage after giving birth because the uterus cannot contract effectively to compress blood vessels.

Labor refers to uterine contractions resulting in progressive dilation and effacement of the cervix, and accompanied by descent and expulsion of the fetus. *Abnormal labor*, *dystocia*, and *failure to progress* are imprecise terms that have been used to describe a difficult labor pattern that deviates from that observed in the majority of women who have spontaneous vaginal deliveries. A better classification is to characterize labor abnormalities as protraction disorders (i.e., slower than

normal progress) or arrest disorders (i.e., complete cessation of progress).

The term **protracted disorders** refers to a series of events including protracted active phase dilation (slower than normal rate of cervical dilation) and protracted descent (delayed descent of the fetal head in the active phase). A laboring woman with a slower than normal rate of cervical dilation is said to have a protraction labor pattern disorder. A slow progress may be the result of cephalopelvic disproportion. Most women, however, benefit greatly from adequate hydration and some nutrition, emotional reassurance, and position changes—these women may go on and give birth vaginally.

Arrest disorders include secondary arrest of dilation (no progress in cervical dilation in >2 hours), arrest of descent (fetal head does not descend for more than 1 hour in primip and more that 0.5 hour in multip), and failure of descent (no descent). About 20% of labors involve either protracted or arrest disorders (Ehsanipoor & Satin, 2016).

Precipitate labor is a labor that is completed in less than 3 hours from the start of contractions to birth. Not only can labor be too slow, but it can be abnormally rapid. The prevailing opinion has been that too rapid a labor can result in maternal injury and place the fetus at risk for traumatic or asphyxia insults (Suzuki, 2015). Women experiencing precipitate labor typically have soft perineal tissues that stretch readily, permitting the fetus to pass through the pelvis quickly, or abnormally strong uterine contractions. Maternal complications are rare if the maternal pelvis is adequate and the soft tissues yield to a fast fetal descent. However, if the fetus delivers too fast, it does not allow the cervix to dilate and efface, which leads to cervical lacerations and the potential for uterine rupture. Potential fetal complications may include head trauma, such as intracranial hemorrhage or nerve damage, and hypoxia due to the rapid progression of labor (Cunningham et al., 2014).

Precipitate labor is an anxiety-producing situation and frequently very painful with little rest between contractions. Continuous monitoring, frequent updates on her labor progress, pain management, and reassurance about her condition can assist in reducing the mother's anxious state of mind. Management includes readiness of the health care team for this rapid birth.

Problems with the Passenger

Any presentation other than occiput anterior (head down and anterior facing) or a slight variation of the fetal position or size increases the probability of dystocia. These variations can affect the contractions or fetal descent through the maternal pelvis. Common problems involving the fetus include occiput posterior position, breech presentation, multifetal pregnancy, excessive size (macrosomia) as it relates to cephalopelvic disproportion, and structural anomalies.

(text continues on page 765)

	Description	Diagnosis	Therapeutic Management	Nursing Management
Problems with the Powers				
Hypertonic uterine dysfunction	Occurring in the latent phase of the first stage of labor (cervical dilation of <4 cm); uncoordinated. Force of contraction typically in the midsection of uterus at the junction of the active upper and passive lower segments of the uterus rather than in the fundus. Loss of downward pressure to push the presenting part against the cervix. Woman commonly becomes discouraged due to lack of progress; also has increased pain secondary to uterine anoxia.	Characteristic hypertonicity of contractions and the lack of labor progress	Therapeutic rest with the use of sedatives to promote relaxation and stop the abnormal activity of the uterus. Identification and intervention of any contributing factors. Ruling out abruptio placentae (also associated with high resting tone and persistent pain). Onset of a normal labor pattern occurs in many women after a 4- to 6-h rest period.	Institute bed rest and sedation to promote relaxation and reduce pain. Assist with measures to rule out fetopelvic disproportion and fetal malpresentation. Evaluate fetal tolerance to labor pattern, such as monitoring of FHR patterns. Assess for signs of maternal infection. Promote adequate hydration through IV therapy. Provide pain management via epidural or IV analgesics. Assist with amniotomy to augment labor. Explain to woman and family about dysfunctional pattern. Plan for operative birth if normal labor pattern is not achieved.
Hypotonic uterine dysfunction	Often termed secondary uterine inertia because the labor begins normally and then the frequency and intensity of contractions decrease. Possible contributing factors: overdistended uterus with multifetal pregnancy or large single fetus, too much pain medicine given too early in labor, fetal malposition, and regional anesthesia.	Evaluation of the woman's labor to confirm that she is having hypotonic active labor rather than a long latent phase. Evaluation of maternal pelvis and fetal presentation and position to ensure that they are not contributing to the prolonged labor without noticeable progress.	Identification of possible cause of inefficient uterine action (a malpositioned fetus, a too small maternal pelvis, overdistention of the uterus with fluid or a macrosomic fetus). Rupture of amniotic sac (amniotomy) if all causes ruled out. Possible augmentation with oxytocin (Pitocin) to stimulate effective uterine contractions. Cesarean birth if amniotomy and augmentation ineffective.	Administer oxytocin as ordered once fetopelvic disproportion is ruled out. Assist with amniotomy if membranes are intact. Provide continuous electronic fetal monitoring. Monitor vital signs, contractions, and cervix continually. Assess for signs of maternal and fetal infection. Explain to woman and family about dysfunctional pattern. Plan for surgical birth if normal labor pattern is not achieved or fetal distress occurs.
Precipitate labor	Abrupt onset of higher-intensity contractions occurring in a shorter period of time instead of the more gradual increase in frequency, duration, and intensity that typifies most spontaneous labors.	Identification based on the rapidity of progress through the stages of labor	Vaginal delivery if maternal pelvis is adequate.	Closely monitor woman with previous history. Anticipate use of scheduled induction to control labor rate. Administer pharmacologic agents, such as tocolytics, to slow labor. Stay in constant attendance to monitor progress.

(continued)

TABLE 21.1 DIAGNOSIS AND MANAGEMENT OF COMMON PROBLEMS ASSOCIATED WITH DYSTOCIA (continued)

Description	Diagnosis	Therapeutic Management	Nursing Management
Problems with the Passenger			
Persistent occiput posterior position Engagement of fetal head in the left or right occipito-transverse position with the occiput rotating posteriorly rather than into the more favorable occiput anterior position (fetus born facing upward instead of the normal downward position). Labor usually much longer and more uncomfortable (causing increased back pain during labor) if fetus remains in this position. Possible extensive caput succedaneum and molding from the sustained occiput posterior position.	Leopold maneuvers and vaginal examination to determine position of fetal head in conjunction with the mother's complaints of severe back pain (back of fetal head pressing on mother's sacrum and coccyx).	Labor to proceed, preparing the woman for a long labor (spontaneous resolution possible). Comfort measures and maternal positioning to help promote fetal head rotation.	Assess for complaints of intense back pain in first stage of labor. Anticipate possible use of forceps to rotate to anterior position at birth or manual rotation to anterior position at end of second stage. Assess for prolonged second stage of labor with arrest of descent (common with this malposition). Encourage maternal position changes to promote fetal head rotation: hands and knees and rocking pelvis back and forth; side-lying position; side lunges during contractions; sitting, kneeling, or standing while leaning forward; squatting position to give birth and enlarge pelvic outlet. Prepare for possible cesarean birth if rotation is not achieved. Administer agents as ordered for pain relief (effective pain relief crucial to help the woman to tolerate the back discomfort). Apply low back counter pressure during contractions to ease the discomfort. Use other helpful measures to attempt to rotate the fetal head, including lateral abdominal stroking in the direction that that the fetal head should rotate; assisting the client into a hands-and-knees position (all fours); and squatting, pelvic rocking, stair climbing, assuming a side-lying position toward the side that the fetus should rotate, and side lunges. Provide measures to reduce anxiety. Continuously reinforce the woman's progress. Teach woman about measures to facilitate fetal head rotation.

Face and brow presentation	Face presentation with complete extension of the fetal head. Brow presentation: fetal head between full extension and full flexion so that the largest fetal skull diameter presents to the pelvis.	Diagnosis only once labor is well established via vaginal examination; palpation of facial features as the presenting part rather than the fetal head.	Vaginal birth possible with face presentation with an adequate maternal pelvis and fetal head rotation; cesarean birth if head rotates backward. Cesarean birth for brow presentation unless head flexes.	Assist with evaluating for fetopelvic disproportion. Anticipate cesarean birth if vertex position is not achieved. Explain fetal malposition to the woman and her partner. Provide close observation for any signs of fetal hypoxia, as evidenced by late decelerations on the fetal monitor.
Breech presentation	Fetal buttocks, or breech, presenting first rather than the head. 1. Frank breech: buttock as the presenting part, with hips flexed and legs and knees extended upward 2. Complete breech (or full breech): buttock as presenting part, with hips flexed and knees flexed in a "cannonball" position 3. Footling or incomplete breech: One or two feet as the presenting part, with one or both hips extended	Vaginal examination to determine breech presentation. Ideally, ultrasound to confirm a clinically suspected presentation and to identify any fetal anomalies.	The optimal method of birth is controversial: cesarean birth by some providers unless the fetus is small and the mother has a large pelvis; vaginal birth by others with each occurrence treated individually and labor monitored very closely. Regardless of the birth method selected, the risk for trauma is high. Breech vaginal births are not recommended by ACOG and come with a higher risk to the mother and infant than a planned surgical birth. Vaginal delivery: fetus allowed to spontaneously deliver up to the umbilicus; then maneuvers to assist in the delivery of the remainder of the body, arms, and head; fetal membranes left intact as long as possible to act as a dilating wedge and to prevent cord prolapse; anesthesiologist and pediatrician present. Cesarean birth; use of external cephalic version to reduce the chance of breech presentation at birth; attempted after the 35th week of gestation but before the start of labor (some fetuses spontaneously turn to a cephalic presentation on their own toward term, and some will return to the breech presentation if external cephalic version is attempted too early; variable success rates, with risk for fractured bones, ruptured viscera, abruptio placentae, fetomaternal hemorrhage, and umbilical cord entanglement. Tocolytic drugs to relax the uterus, as well as other methods, to facilitate external cephalic version at term. Individual evaluation of each woman for all factors before any interventions is initiated.	Assess for associated conditions such as placenta previa, hydramnios, fetal anomalies, and multifetal pregnancy. Arrange for ultrasound to confirm fetal presentation. Assist with external cephalic version possible after 36 weeks and administer tocolytics to assist with external cephalic version. Anticipate trial labor for 4 to 6 hours to evaluate progress if version is unsuccessful. Plan for cesarean birth if no progress is seen or fetal distress occurs. After external cephalic version, administer RhoGAM to the Rh-negative woman to prevent a sensitization reaction if trauma has occurred and the potential for mixing of blood exists.

(continued)

TABLE 21.1	DIAGNOSIS AND MANAGEMENT OF COMMON PROBLEMS ASSOCIATED WITH DYSTOCIA (continued)		
	Description	Diagnosis	Therapeutic Management	Nursing Management
Shoulder dystocia	Delivery of fetal head with neck not appearing; retraction of chin against the perineum; shoulders remaining wedged behind the mother's pubic bone, causing a difficult birth with potential for injury to both mother and baby. If shoulders still above the brim at this stage, no advancement. Newborn's chest trapped within the vaginal vault; chest unable to expand with respiration (although nose and mouth are outside). Risk of umbilical cord compression between the fetal body and the maternal pelvis.	Emergency, often unexpected complication. Diagnosis made when newborn's head delivers without delivery of neck and remaining body structures. Primary risk factors, including suspected infant macrosomia (weight > 4500 g), maternal diabetes mellitus, excessive maternal weight gain, abnormal maternal pelvic anatomy, maternal obesity, postdated pregnancy, short stature, a history of previous shoulder dystocia, and use of epidural analgesia.	If anticipated, preparatory tasks instituted: alerting of key personnel; education of woman and family regarding steps to be taken in the event of a difficult birth; emptying of woman's bladder to allow additional room for possible maneuvers needed for the birth. McRobert's maneuver: Suprapubic pressure (not fundal) (see Fig. 21.1). Combination of maneuvers effective in more than 50% of cases of shoulder dystocia. Newborn resuscitation team readily available.	Intervene immediately due to cord compression. Perform McRobert's maneuver and application of suprapubic pressure. Assist with positioning the woman in squatting position, hands-and-knees position, or lateral recumbent position for birth to free shoulder. Anticipate cesarean birth if no success in dislodging shoulders. Clear room of unnecessary clutter to make room for additional personnel and equipment. After the birth, assess newborn for crepitus, deformity, Erb's palsy, or bruising, which might suggest neurologic damage or a fracture.
Multiple pregnancy	More than one fetus, leading to uterine overdistention and possibly resulting in hypotonic contractions and abnormal presentations of the fetuses. Fetal hypoxia during labor a significant threat due to placenta providing oxygen and nutrients to more than one fetus.	Nearly all multiples are now diagnosed early by ultrasound. Most women go into labor before 37 weeks.	Admission to facility with specialized care unit if a woman goes into labor. Spontaneous progression of labor if woman has no complicating factors and first fetus is in longitudinal lie. Separate monitoring of each FHR during labor and birth. After birth of first fetus, clamping of cord and lie of the second twin assessed. Possible external cephalic version necessary to assist in providing a longitudinal lie. Second and subsequent fetuses at greater risk for birth-related complications, such as umbilical cord prolapse, malpresentation, and abruptio placentae. Cesarean birth if risk factors high.	Assess for hypotonic labor pattern due to overdistention. Evaluate for fetal presentation, maternal pelvic size, and gestational age to determine mode of delivery. Ensure presence of neonatal team for birth of multiples. Anticipate need for cesarean birth, which is common in multifetal pregnancy.

(continued)

Excessive fetal size and abnormalities	Macrosomia leading to fetopelvic disproportion (fetus unable to fit through the maternal pelvis to be born vaginally). Reduced contraction strength due to overdistention by large fetus leading to a prolonged labor and the potential for birth injury and trauma. Fetal abnormalities possibly interfering with fetal descent, leading to prolonged labor and difficult birth.	A diagnosis of fetal macrosomia can be confirmed by measuring the birth weight after birth. Suspicion of macrosomia based on the findings of an ultrasound examination before onset of labor (if suspected due to conditions such as maternal diabetes or obesity, estimation of fetal weight via ultrasound). Leopold's maneuvers to estimate fetal weight and position on admission to labor and birth unit.	Scheduled cesarean birth if diagnosis is made before the onset of labor to reduce the risk of injury to both the newborn and the mother. If identified by Leopold's maneuvers, possible trial of labor to evaluate progress; however, providers usually opt to proceed with a cesarean birth in a primigravida with a macrosomic fetus.	Assess for inability of fetus to descend. Anticipate need for vacuum and forceps-assisted births (common). Plan for cesarean birth if maternal parameters are inadequate to give birth to large fetus.
Problems with the Passageway	Contraction of one or more of the three planes of the pelvis. Poorer prognosis for vaginal birth in women with android and platypelloid types of pelvis. Contracted pelvis involving reduction in one or more of the pelvic diameters interfering with progress of labor: inlet, midpelvis, and outlet contracture. Obstruction in the birth canal, such as placenta previa that partially or completely obstructs the internal os of the cervix, fibroids in the lower uterine segment, a full bladder or rectum, an edematous cervix caused by premature bearing-down efforts, and human papillomavirus (HPV) warts.	Shortest A-P diameter <10 cm or greatest transverse diameter <12 cm. (Approximation of A-P diameter via measurement of diagonal conjugate, which in the contracted pelvis is <11.5 cm.) X-ray pelvimetry to determine the smallest A-P diameter through which the fetal head must pass. Interischial tuberous diameter of <8 cm possibly compromising outlet contracture (outlet and midpelvic contractures frequently occur together).	Focus on allowing natural forces of labor contractions to push the largest diameter (biparietal) of the fetal head beyond the obstruction or narrow passage. Possible forceps and vacuum extraction to assist navigation through this passageway.	Assess for poor contractions, slow dilation, prolonged labor. Evaluate bowel and bladder status to reduce soft tissue obstruction and allow increased pelvic space. Anticipate trial of labor; if no labor progression after an adequate trial, plan for cesarean birth.

TABLE 21.1 DIAGNOSIS AND MANAGEMENT OF COMMON PROBLEMS ASSOCIATED WITH DYSTOCIA (continued)

	Description	Diagnosis	Therapeutic Management	Nursing Management
Problems with the Psyche	Release of stress-related hormones (catecholamines, cortisol, epinephrine, beta-endorphin), which act on smooth muscle (uterus) and reduce uterine contractility. Excessive release of catecholamines and other stress-related hormones not therapeutic. Release also results in decreased uteroplacental perfusion and increased risk for poor newborn adjustment.	Ruling out of other possible causes of dystocia	Treatment dependent on woman's responses such as anxiety, fear, anger, frustration, or denial (highly variable due to woman's understanding of the condition itself, past experiences, previous coping mechanisms, and the amount of family and nursing support received). Appropriate medical or surgical interventions depending on the underlying condition.	Provide comfortable environment—dim lighting, music. Encourage partner to participate. Provide pain management to reduce anxiety and stress. Ensure continuous presence of staff to allay anxiety. Provide frequent updates concerning fetal status and progress. Provide ongoing encouragement to minimize the woman's stress and help her to cope with labor and to promote a positive, timely outcome. Assist in relaxation and comfort measures to help her body work more effectively with the forces of labor. Engage the woman in conversation about her emotional well-being; offer anticipatory guidance and reassurance to increase her self-esteem and ability to cope, decrease frustration, and encourage cooperation.

Adapted from American Academy of Pediatrics. (2015). *Delivery by cesarean section.* Retrieved from https://www.healthychildren.org/English/ages-stages/prenatal/delivery-beyond/Pages/Delivery-by-Cesarean-Section.aspx; Caughey, A. B., & Butler, J. R. (2015). Postterm pregnancy. *eMedicine.* Retrieved from http://emedicine.medscape.com/article/261369-overview; Cunningham, F. G., Leveno, K. J., Bloom, S. L., Spong, C. Y., Dashe, J., Hoffman, B. L., et al. (2014). *Williams' obstetrics* (24th ed.). New York, NY: McGraw-Hill; Fischer, R. (2015). Breech presentation. *eMedicine.* Retrieved from http://emedicine.medscape.com/article/262159-overview; Joy, S., Lyon, D., & Scott, P. L. (2015). Abnormal labor. *eMedicine.* Retrieved from http://emedicine.medscape.com/article/273053-overview; and King, T. L., Brucker, M. C., Kriebs, J. M., Fahey, J. O., Gegor, C. L., & Varney, H. (2015). *Varney's midwifery* (5th ed.). Burlington, MA: Jones & Bartlett Learning.

Persistent occiput posterior is the most common malposition, occurring in about 15% of laboring women. The reasons for this malposition are often unclear. This position presents slightly larger diameters to the maternal pelvis, thus slowing fetal descent. A fetal head that is poorly flexed may be responsible. In addition, poor uterine contractions may not push the fetal head down into the pelvic floor to the extent that the fetal occiput sinks into it rather than being pushed to rotate in an anterior direction.

Face and brow presentations are rare and are associated with fetal abnormalities (anencephaly), pelvic contractures, high parity, placenta previa, hydramnios, low birth weight, or a large fetus (World Health Organization [WHO], 2014a).

By 35 to 36 weeks of gestation, the majority of fetuses will spontaneously settle into the vertex presentation (head down, toward the birth canal). In about 3% to 4% of cases, however, the fetus will remain in a breech presentation with the buttocks or feet presenting. There is less risk to the fetus and mother when the head is down at the time of birth. This presentation frequently is associated with multifetal or multiple pregnancies, grand multiparity (more than five births), pregnancy over age 35 (advanced maternal age), placenta previa, hydramnios, preterm births, uterine malformations or fibroids, a scarred uterus, a female infant, and fetal anomalies such as hydrocephaly (Sharshiner & Silver, 2015). In a persistent breech presentation, an increased frequency of prolapsed cord, placenta previa, low birth weight from preterm birth, fetal or uterine anomalies, and perinatal morbidity and mortality from a difficult birth may occur (Cunningham et al., 2014). A breech presentation may be an indicator for subtle fetal abnormalities, as apparently healthy breech infants have on average poorer long-term neurodevelopmental scores than cephalic infants (Hofmeyr, 2015). Perinatal mortality is increased two- to fourfold with a breech presentation, regardless of the mode of delivery.

External cephalic version refers to a procedure in which the fetus is rotated from the breech to the cephalic presentation by manipulation through the mother's abdominal wall at or near term. Several national organizations (ACOG, WHO, AFP), recommend that this maneuver be offered to women between 36 and 38 weeks of gestation. It is performed only in a hospital setting under direct ultrasound guidance and continuous fetal monitoring. External cephalic version is successful in approximately 50% of cases. Women with a breech presentation today are often advised to have a surgical birth with no attempt to rotate the fetal position (Hofmeyr, Kulier, & West, 2015).

Shoulder dystocia is defined as the obstruction of fetal descent and birth by the axis of the fetal shoulders after the fetal head has been delivered. The incidence of shoulder dystocia is increasing due to increasing birth weight, with reports of it in up to 2% of vaginal births. It is an obstetric emergency that requires a coordinated

team response, as there is no reliable way to predict it, and thus decrease the rate at which adverse outcomes occur (Gherman, 2015). It is one of the most anxiety-provoking emergencies encountered in labor. Failure of the shoulders to deliver spontaneously places both the woman and the fetus at risk for injury. Postpartum hemorrhage, secondary to uterine atony, vaginal lacerations, anal tears, and uterine rupture are major complications to the mother. Transient Erb's or Duchenne's brachial plexus palsies and clavicular or humeral fractures are the most common fetal injuries encountered with shoulder dystocia. The occurrence of neonatal brachial plexus palsy in the United States is 1.5 per 1,000 live births, with about one-third suffering permanent upper extremity functional insufficiencies (Mehlman, 2015). Newborns experiencing shoulder dystocia typically have greater shoulder-to-head and chest-to-head disproportions compared with those delivered without dystocia (Cunningham et al., 2014). Prompt recognition and appropriate management, such as with McRobert's maneuver or suprapubic pressure, can reduce the severity of injuries to the mother and newborn (Fig. 21.1).

Take Note!

Prompt recognition and appropriate management of shoulder dystocia can reduce the severity of injuries to the mother and infant. Immediately assess the infant for signs of trauma such as a fractured clavicle, Erb's palsy, or neonatal asphyxia. Assess the mother for excessive vaginal bleeding and blood in the urine from bladder trauma.

Multiple or multifetal gestation refers to twins, triplets, or more infants within a single pregnancy (Box 21.1). The incidence is increasing, primarily as a result of infertility treatment (both ovarian stimulation and in vitro fertilization) and an increased number of women giving birth at older ages. The incidence of twins, triples, and higher order multiple gestations have now reached approximately 3% of all pregnancies (March of Dimes, 2015a). The incidence of twins is approximately 1 in 30 conceptions, with about two thirds of them due to the fertilization of two ova (dizygotic or fraternal) and about one-third occurring from the splitting of one fertilized ovum (monozygotic or identical twins). One in approximately 8,100 pregnancies results in triplets (March of Dimes, 2015a). The most common maternal complication is postpartum hemorrhage resulting from uterine atony. Compared with singletons (one fetus), the risk of perinatal morbidity and mortality is markedly increased in multiple gestations. Based on recent level 1 evidence from a randomized-controlled study, it was found that there was no difference in newborn outcomes between a planned surgical birth versus a planned vaginal birth for twins between 32 to 39 weeks of gestation. As long as the presenting twin is vertex, a vaginal birth should be considered (Bibbo & Robinson, 2015).

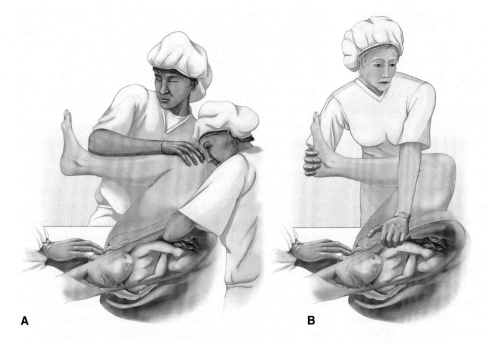

A   **B**

FIGURE 21.1 Maneuvers to relieve shoulder dystocia. **A.** McRobert's maneuver. The mother's thighs are flexed and abducted as much as possible to straighten the pelvic curve. **B.** Suprapubic pressure. Light pressure is applied just above the pubic bone, pushing the fetal anterior shoulder downward to displace it from above the mother's symphysis pubis. The newborn's head is depressed toward the mother's anus while light suprapubic pressure is applied.

Excessive fetal size and abnormalities can also contribute to labor and birth dysfunctions. **Macrosomia**, in which a newborn weighs 4,000 to 4,500 g (8.13 to 9.15 lb) or more at birth, complicates approximately 10% of all pregnancies. It is the result of a change in body composition in the neonate with an increase in both percentage of fat and fat mass. Macrosomia is associated with later life obesity, diabetes, and cardiovascular disease (Jazayeri, 2015). Fetal abnormalities may include hydrocephalus, ascites, or a large mass on the neck or head. Complications associated with dystocia related to excessive fetal size and anomalies include an increased risk for postpartum hemorrhage, shoulder dystocia, low Apgar scores, dysfunctional labor, fetopelvic disproportion, soft tissue laceration during vaginal birth, fetal injuries or fractures, and perinatal asphyxia (Hobbins, 2015a).

Problems with the Passageway

Problems with the passageway (pelvis and birth canal) are related to a contraction of one or more of the three planes of the maternal pelvis: inlet, midpelvis, and outlet.

BOX 21.1

MULTIPLE GESTATION

As the name implies, a multiple gestation or a multifetal pregnancy involves more than one fetus. These fetuses can result from fertilization of a single ovum or multiple ova. Monozygotic (identical) twins develop from one single ovum that divides into equal halves during early cleavage phase. Monozygotic twins are genetically identical; always the same gender, and look very similar in appearance. The number of amnions and chorions depends on the timing of division (cleavage). One fertilized ovum splitting into two separate individuals is termed *natural clones*. This type of twinning occurs in approximately 1 of 250 live births (March of Dimes, 2015a).

Twin pregnancies that are multiple-ova conceptions (dizygotic twins) result from two ova fertilized by two sperms. They are referred to as fraternal twins. Genetically, dizygotic twins are as alike (or unlike) as any other pair or siblings. There are separate amnions and chorions although the chorions and placentas may be fused. The incidence of dizygotic twinning is approximately 1 in 500 Asians, 1 in 125 Whites, and as high as 1 in 20 in African populations (March of Dimes, 2015a). Fraternal twins account for two-thirds of all twins and there is a tendency to repeat within families. Currently the incidence of fraternal twins is increasing secondary to advancing maternal age when pregnancy occurs and an increase in use of fertility drugs and procedures being done.

Multiple births other than twins can be of the identical type, the fraternal type, or combinations of the two. Triplets can occur from the division of one zygote into two, with one dividing again, producing identical triplets, or they can come from two zygotes, one dividing into a set of identical twins, and the second zygote developing as a single fraternal sibling, or from three separate zygotes. Triplets are said to occur once in 7,000 births and quadruplets once in 660,000 births (March of Dimes, 2015a). In recent years, fertility drugs used to induce ovulation have resulted in a greater frequency of quadruplets, quintuplets, sextuplets, and even octuplets.

The female pelvis can be classified into four types based on the shape of the pelvic inlet, which is bounded anteriorly by the posterior border of the symphysis pubis, posteriorly by the sacral promontory, and laterally by the linea terminalis. The four basic types are: gynecoid, anthropoid, android, and platypelloid (see Chapter 12 for additional information). Contraction of the midpelvis is more common than inlet contraction and typically causes an arrest of fetal descent. Obstructions in the maternal birth canal, such as swelling of the soft maternal tissue and cervix, termed soft tissue dystocia, also can hamper fetal descent and impede labor progression outside the maternal bony pelvis.

Problems with the Psyche

Many women experience an array of emotions during labor, which may include fear, anxiety, helplessness, isolation, and weariness. These emotions can lead to psychological stress, which indirectly can cause dystocia. Hormones released in response to anxiety can cause dystocia. Intense anxiety stimulates the sympathetic nervous system, which releases catecholamines that can lead to myometrial dysfunction. Norepinephrine and epinephrine then lead to uncoordinated or increased uterine activity (Cheng & Caughey, 2015).

Nursing Assessment

Begin the assessment by reviewing the client's history to look for risk factors for dystocia which may include maternal short stature, obesity, hydramnios, uterine abnormalities, fetal malpresentation, cephalopelvic disproportion, over stimulation with oxytocin, maternal exhaustion, ineffective pushing, excessive size fetus, poor maternal positioning in labor, and maternal anxiety and fear (Green, 2016). Include in the assessment the mother's frame of mind to identify fear, anxiety, stress, lack of support, and pain, which can interfere with uterine contractions and impede labor progress. Helping the woman to relax will promote normal labor progress.

Assess the woman's vital signs. Note any elevation in temperature (might suggest an infection) or changes in heart rate or blood pressure (might signal hypovolemia). Evaluate the uterine contractions for frequency and intensity. Question the woman about any changes in her contraction pattern, such as a decrease or increase in frequency or intensity, and report these. Assess fetal heart rate (FHR) and pattern, reporting any abnormal patterns immediately.

Assess fetal position via *Leopold's maneuvers* (see Chapter 14 for more information) to identify any deviations in presentation or position, and report any deviations. Assist with or perform a vaginal examination to determine cervical dilation, effacement, and engagement of the fetal presenting part. Evaluate for evidence of membrane rupture. Report any malodorous fluid.

Nursing Management

Nursing management of the woman with dystocia, regardless of the etiology, requires patience. The nurse should provide physical and emotional support to the client and her family. The final outcome of any labor depends on the size and shape of the maternal pelvis, the quality of the uterine contractions, and the size, presentation, and position of the fetus. Thus, dystocia is diagnosed after labor has progressed for a time, not at the beginning of labor.

PROMOTING THE PROGRESS OF LABOR

The nurse plays a major role in determining the progress of labor. Continue to assess the woman, frequently monitoring cervical dilation and effacement, uterine contractions, and fetal descent, and document that all assessed parameters are progressing. Evaluate progress in active labor by using the simple rule of 1 cm per hour for cervical dilation. When the woman's membranes rupture, if they have not already ruptured, observe for visible cord prolapse.

Take Note!

If a dysfunctional labor occurs, contractions will slow or fail to advance in frequency, duration, or intensity; the cervix will fail to respond to uterine contractions by dilating and effacing; and the fetus will fail to descend.

Throughout labor, assess the woman's fluid balance status. Check skin turgor and mucous membranes. Monitor intake and output. Also monitor the client's bladder for distention at least every 2 hours and encourage her to empty her bladder often. In addition, monitor her bowel status. A full bladder or rectum can impede descent.

Continue to monitor fetal well-being. If the fetus is in the breech position, be especially observant for visible cord prolapse and note any variable decelerations in heart rate. If either occurs, report it immediately.

Be prepared to administer a labor stimulant such as oxytocin (Pitocin) if ordered to treat hypotonic labor contractions. Anticipate the need to assist with manipulations if shoulder dystocia is diagnosed. Prepare the woman and her family for the possibility of a cesarean birth if labor does not progress.

PROVIDING PHYSICAL AND EMOTIONAL COMFORT

Employ physical comfort measures to promote relaxation and reduce stress. Offer blankets for warmth and a backrub, if the client wishes, to reduce muscle tension. Provide an environment conducive to rest so the woman can conserve her energy. Lower the lights and reduce external noise by closing the hallway door. Offer a warm shower to promote relaxation (if not contraindicated). Use pillows to support the woman in a comfortable

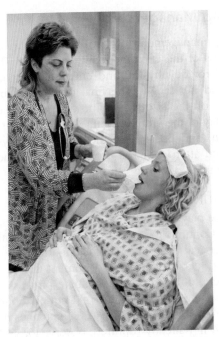

FIGURE 21.2 The nurse applies a cool, moist washcloth to the client's forehead and offers her ice chips to combat thirst and provide comfort to the woman experiencing dystocia.

position, changing her position every 30 minutes to reduce tension and to enhance uterine activity and efficiency. Offer her fluids/food as appropriate to moisten her mouth and replenish her energy (Fig. 21.2).

Assist with providing counter pressure along with backrubs if the fetus is in the occiput posterior position. Encourage the woman to assume different positions to promote fetal rotation. Upright positions are helpful in facilitating fetal rotation and descent. Also encourage the woman to visualize the descent and birth of the fetus.

Assess the woman's level of pain and degree of distress. Administer analgesics as ordered or according to the facility's protocol. Evaluate the mother's level of fatigue throughout labor, such as verbal expressions of feeling exhausted, inability to cope in early labor, or inability to rest or calm down between contractions. Praise the woman and her partner for their efforts. Provide empathetic listening to increase the client's coping ability, and remain with the client to demonstrate caring.

PROMOTING EMPOWERMENT

Educate the client and family about dysfunctional labor and its causes and therapies. Explain therapeutic interventions that may be needed to assist with the labor process. Encourage the client and her partner to participate in decision making about interventions.

Assist the woman and partner in expressing their fears and anxieties. Provide encouragement to help them to maintain control. Support the client and her partner in their coping efforts. Keep the woman and her partner informed of progress and advocate for them.

ALTERNATIVE/NONTRADITIONAL FAMILIES

There is a growing awareness of nontraditional families in the world. If one considers family forms cross-nationally, a variety of configurations exists. This awareness requires nurses to shift away from heterosexist thinking in caring for the childbearing family. Nurses must be adequately educated about lesbian-gay-bisexual-transgender-queer (LGBTQ) health issues to be empathetic and conscious of the needs of this population. With increasing numbers of LGBTQ couples getting married, and availability of alternative methods of conception, these couples are coming in contact with nurses through the birthing process. LGBTQ couples may face making complex childbearing decisions, navigating a health care system designed for heterosexual couples and confronting barriers such as insurance issues, non-accepting negative attitudes by health care workers, and uncertain legal rights (Holley & Pasch, 2015).

LGBTQ individuals are not a homogeneous group and they are shaped by a range of factors including race, sexual orientation, ethnicity, socioeconomic status, and age. This community has been previously marginalized in society. Nurses caring for LGBTQ clients need to allow them to have their own identity, values, and beliefs. Every client should be treated with the kindness, with an individualized approach, and be an advocate for their needs. Nurses need to consider the following when they are caring for the childbearing LGBTQ family by using appropriate language/identification and cultural representation by asking how they wish to be identified; and by personalizing their care that includes all intersecting aspects of their identity (Westwood et al., 2015).

PRETERM LABOR

Preterm labor is defined as the occurrence of regular uterine contractions accompanied by cervical effacement and dilation before the end of the 37th week of gestation. If not halted, it leads to preterm birth. Preterm births remain one of the biggest contributors to perinatal morbidity and mortality in the world. According to the March of Dimes (2015b), about 12% of births (one in eight infants) in the United States are premature.

Preterm birth is one of the most common obstetric complications, and its sequelae have a profound effect on the survival and health of the newborn. The rate of preterm births in the United States has increased 35% in the past 20 years. Preterm births account for 75% of neurodevelopmental disorders and other serious morbidities, as well as behavioral and social problems. They account for 85% of all perinatal morbidity and mortality. In addition, up to $30 billion is spent on maternal and infant care related to prematurity annually (March of Dimes, 2015b). Infants born prematurely also are at risk for serious sequelae such as respiratory distress syndrome, infections, congenital heart defects, thermoregulation problems that can lead to acidosis and weight loss, intraventricular hemorrhage, jaundice, hypoglycemia, feeding difficulties resulting from diminished stomach capacity and an underdeveloped suck reflex, and neurologic disorders related to hypoxia and trauma at birth. Many will face the prospect of numerous lifelong disabilities, such as cerebral palsy, intellectual impairment, vision defects, and hearing loss. A recent study's findings indicated that a single course of corticosteroids prenatally improved most neonate's neurodevelopmental outcomes if given before 34 weeks of gestation (Sotiriadis et al., 2015). Although great strides have been made in neonatal intensive care, prematurity remains the leading cause of death within the first month of life and is the second leading cause of all infant deaths (March of Dimes, 2015b). The exact cause of preterm labor is not known. Currently, prevention is the goal.

Therapeutic Management

Predicting the risk of preterm labor is valuable only if there is an available intervention that is likely to improve the situation. According to ACOG, many factors must be considered before selecting an intervention. Many factors influence the decision to intervene when women present with symptoms of preterm labor, including the probability of progressive labor, gestational age, and the risks of treatment. ACOG (2014b) recommends the following as guidelines:

- There are no clear first-line **tocolytic** drugs (drugs that promote uterine relaxation by interfering with uterine contractions) to manage preterm labor, and the results of research on their efficacy are mixed. Clinical circumstances and the health care provider's preference should dictate treatment.
- Antibiotics do not appear to prolong gestation and should be reserved for group B streptococcal prophylaxis in women in whom birth is imminent.
- Tocolytic drugs may prolong pregnancy for 2 to 7 days; during this time, steroids can be given to improve fetal lung maturity and the woman can be transported to a tertiary care center.
- A single course of corticosteroids is recommended for all pregnant women between 24 and 34 weeks of gestation who are at risk of preterm birth within 7 days. Prenatal corticosteroids significantly reduce the incidence and severity of neonatal respiratory distress syndrome.

With these recommendations, health care providers continue to prescribe pharmacologic treatment for preterm labor at home and in the hospital setting. This treatment often includes oral or intravenous tocolytics and

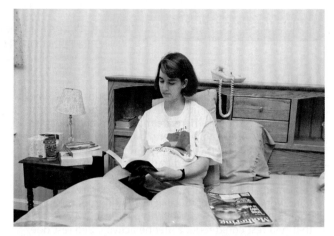

FIGURE 21.3 The mother with preterm labor resting in bed at home.

varying degrees of activity restriction (Fig. 21.3). Antibiotics may also be prescribed to treat presumed or confirmed infections. Steroids may be given to enhance fetal lung maturity between 24 and 34 weeks of gestation.

Tocolytic Therapy

The decision to stop preterm labor is individualized based on risk factors, extent of cervical dilation, membrane status, fetal gestational age, and presence or absence of infection. Tocolytic therapy is most likely ordered if preterm labor occurs before the 34th week of gestation in an attempt to delay birth and thereby to reduce the severity of respiratory distress syndrome and other complications associated with prematurity. Tocolytic therapy does not typically prevent preterm birth, but it may delay it. It is contraindicated for abruptio placentae, acute fetal distress or death, eclampsia or severe preeclampsia, active vaginal bleeding, dilation of more than 6 cm, chorioamnionitis, and maternal hemodynamic instability (Locatelli, Consonni, & Ghidini, 2015).

Medications commonly used for tocolysis include magnesium sulfate (which reduces the muscle's ability to contract), indomethacin (Indocin, a prostaglandin synthetase inhibitor), atosiban (Tractocile, Antocin, an oxytocin receptor antagonist), and nifedipine (Procardia, a calcium channel blocker) (see Evidence-Based Practice 21.1). These drugs are used "off label," which means that they are effective for this purpose but have not been officially tested and developed for this purpose by the U.S. Food and Drug administration (FDA) (Haas et al., 2014). In a recent Cochrane review study, calcium channel blockers were found to be better in preventing preterm labor when compared to betamimetics (Flenady et al., 2014). All of these medications have serious side effects, and the woman needs close supervision when they are being administered (Drug Guide 21.1).

EVIDENCE-BASED PRACTICE 21.1 · BED REST IN SINGLETON PREGNANCIES FOR PREVENTING PRETERM BIRTH

STUDY

Preterm birth, defined a birth occurring prior to 37 weeks of gestation occurs in up to 10% of all pregnancies worldwide. Although there are many different therapies available for preventing preterm birth, very few are proven to be effective and recommended for clinical use. One therapy, bed rest, has been traditionally been recommended for preventing preterm birth as a first step in treatment. This therapy is based on the observation that hard work and hard physical activity during pregnancy could be associated with preterm birth, and with the idea that bed rest could reduce uterine activity. Bed rest does have adverse effects such as increasing the incidence of venous thrombosis, muscle atrophy, and cardiovascular deconditioning. The purpose of this study was to evaluate the effect of bed rest in the hospital or at home for preventing preterm birth.

Findings

Randomized, cluster-randomized, and quasi-randomized control studies were sought. Two studies met the inclusion criteria with 1266 women participating. There was no evidence found to support or refute the use of bed rest at home or in the hospital to prevent preterm birth. Due to the potential adverse effects that bed rest can have on women, it is suggested that health care providers discuss this intervention thoroughly with their clients. Additional research is needed.

Nursing Implications

Although the study did not reveal results that were statistically significant, nurses need to be aware of the potential benefits and limitations associated with bed rest employed to delay a preterm birth so that they can provide women and their families with the most appropriate information about options to prolonged pregnancy. Potential benefits and harms should be discussed with women facing an increased risk of preterm birth. Nurses can integrate information from this study in their teaching about the risks associated with preterm labor and births. They can also use this information to help answer couple's questions about interventions currently used and their effectiveness as well as provide anticipatory guidance about the procedure. Doing so fosters empowerment of the woman and her family, promoting optimal informed decision making.

Adapted from Sosa, C. G., Althabe, F., Belizan, J. M., & Bergel, E. (2015). Bed rest in singleton pregnancies for preventing preterm birth. *Cochrane Database of Systematic Reviews*, (3), CD003581.

DRUG GUIDE 21.1 MEDICATIONS USED WITH PRETERM LABOR

Drug	Action/Indication	Nursing Implications
Magnesium sulfate	Relaxes uterine muscles to stop irritability and contractions, to arrest uterine contractions for preterm labor (off-label use). Has been used in seizure prophylaxis and treatment of seizures in preeclamptic and eclamptic clients for almost 100 years	Administer IV with a loading dose of 4–6 g over 15–30 min initially, and then maintain infusion at 1–4 g/hr. Assess vital signs and deep tendon reflexes (DTRs) hourly; report any hypotension or depressed or absent DTRs. Monitor level of consciousness; report any headache, blurred vision, dizziness, or altered level of consciousness. Perform continuous electronic fetal monitoring; report any decreased FHR variability, hypotonia, or respiratory depression. Monitor intake and output hourly; report any decrease in output (<30 mL/hr). Assess respiratory rate; report respiratory rate <12 breaths/min; auscultate lung sounds for evidence of pulmonary edema. Monitor for common maternal side effects, including flushing, nausea and vomiting, dry mouth, lethargy, blurred vision, and headache. Assess for nausea, vomiting, transient hypotension, lethargy. Assess for signs and symptoms of magnesium toxicity, such as decreased level of consciousness, depressed respirations and DTRs, slurred speech, weakness, and respiratory and/or cardiac arrest. Have calcium gluconate readily available at the bedside to reverse magnesium toxicity.

DRUG GUIDE 21.1   MEDICATIONS USED WITH PRETERM LABOR (continued)

Drug	Action/Indication	Nursing Implications
Indomethacin (Indocin)	Inhibits prostaglandins, which stimulate contractions; inhibits uterine activity to arrest preterm labor	Continuously assess vital signs, uterine activity, and FHR. Administer oral form with food to reduce GI irritation. Do not give to women with peptic ulcer disease. Schedule ultrasound to assess amniotic fluid volume and function of ductus arteriosus before initiating therapy; monitor for signs of maternal hemorrhage. Be alert for maternal adverse effects such as nausea and vomiting, heartburn, rash, prolonged bleeding time, oligohydramnios, and hypertension. Monitor for neonatal adverse effects, including constriction of ductus arteriosus, premature ductus closure, necrotizing enterocolitis, oligohydramnios, and pulmonary hypertension. Contraindicated in >32 weeks of gestations, fetal growth restriction, history of asthma, urticaria, or allergic type reactions to aspirin or NSAIDS.
Nifedipine (Procardia)	Blocks calcium movement into muscle cells, inhibits uterine activity to arrest preterm labor	Use caution if giving this drug with magnesium sulfate because of increased risk for hypotension. Monitor blood pressure hourly if giving with magnesium sulfate; report a pulse rate >110 bpm. Monitor for fetal effects such as decreased uteroplacental blood flow manifested by fetal bradycardia, which can lead to fetal hypoxia. Monitor for adverse effects, such as flushing of the skin, headache, transient tachycardia, palpitations, postural hypertension, peripheral edema, and transient fetal tachycardia. Contraindicated in women with cardiovascular disease or hemodynamic instability.
Betamethasone (Celestone)	Promotes fetal lung maturity by stimulating surfactant production; prevents or reduces risk of respiratory distress syndrome and intraventricular hemorrhage in the preterm neonate less than 34 weeks of gestation	Administer two doses intramuscularly 24 h apart. Monitor for maternal infection or pulmonary edema. Educate parents about potential benefits of drug to preterm infant. Assess maternal lung sounds and monitor for signs of infection.

Adapted from Chandrasekaran, S., & Srinivas, S. K. (2014). Antenatal corticosteroid administration: understanding its use as an obstetric quality metric. *American Journal of Obstetrics and Gynecology, 210*(2), 143–150; Jørgensen, J. S., Weile, L. K., & Lamont, R. F. (2014). Preterm labor: Current tocolytic options for the treatment of preterm labor. *Expert Opinion on Pharmacotherapy, 15*(5), 585–588; and King, T. L., Brucker, M. C., Kriebs, J. M., Fahey, J. O., Gegor, C. L., & Varney, H. (2015). *Varney's midwifery* (5th ed.). Burlington, MA: Jones & Bartlett Learning.

Corticosteroids

Corticosteroids given to the mother in preterm labor can help prevent or reduce the frequency and severity of respiratory distress syndrome in premature infants delivered between 24 and 34 weeks of gestation. The beneficial effects of corticosteroids on fetal lung maturation have been reported within 48 hours of initial administration. A recent Cochrane review found that corticosteroids repeatedly administered to the woman in preterm labor provided short-term benefits to the preterm infant of less respiratory distress and fewer serious health problems in the first few weeks after birth. They supported the use of repeat dose(s) of prenatal corticosteroids for women still at risk of preterm birth 7 days or more after an initial course. These benefits were associated with a small reduction in size at birth. The current available evidence reassuringly shows no significant harm in early childhood, although no benefit. Further research is needed on the long-term benefits and risks for the woman and baby. Individual client data meta-analysis may clarify how to maximize benefit and minimize harm (Cabbad et al., 2015). These drugs require at least 24 hours to become effective, so timely administration is crucial.

Nursing Assessment

The preterm birth rate cannot be reduced until there are ways to predict the risk for preterm birth. Because the etiology is often multifactorial, an individualized approach is needed.

Health History and Physical Examination

The signs of preterm labor are subtle and may be overlooked by the client as well as the health care provider. Obtain a thorough health history and be alert for risk factors associated with preterm labor and birth (Box 21.2).

BOX 21.2

RISK FACTORS ASSOCIATED WITH PRETERM LABOR AND BIRTH

- African-American race (double the risk)
- Maternal age extremes (<16 years and >40 years old)
- Low socioeconomic status
- Alcohol or other drug use, especially cocaine
- Poor maternal nutrition
- Maternal periodontal disease
- Cigarette smoking
- Low level of education
- History of prior preterm birth (triples the risk)
- Uterine abnormalities, such as fibroids
- Low pregnancy weight for height
- Preexisting diabetes or hypertension
- Multiple pregnancy
- Premature rupture of membranes
- Late or no prenatal care
- Short cervical length
- Sexually transmitted infections: gonorrhea, *Chlamydia,* trichomoniasis
- Bacterial vaginosis (50% increased risk)
- Chorioamnionitis
- Hydramnios
- Gestational hypertension
- Cervical insufficiency
- Short interpregnancy interval (<1 year between births)
- Placental problems, such as placenta previa and abruption placenta
- Maternal anemia
- Urinary tract infection
- Domestic violence
- Stress, acute and chronic

Adapted from March of Dimes. (2015b). *Preterm labor and birth: A serious pregnancy complication.* Retrieved from http://www.marchofdimes.com/pregnancy/preterm_indepth.html

Frequently, women are unaware that uterine contractions, effacement, and dilation are occurring, thus making early intervention ineffective in arresting preterm labor and preventing the birth of a premature newborn. Ask the woman about any complaints, being alert for the subtle symptoms of preterm labor, which may include:

- Change or increase in vaginal discharge with mucous, water, or blood in it
- Pelvic pressure (pushing-down sensation)
- Low, dull backache
- Menstrual-like cramps
- Urinary tract infection symptoms
- Feeling of pelvic pressure or fullness
- Gastrointestinal upset: nausea, vomiting, and diarrhea
- General sense of discomfort or unease
- Heaviness or aching in the thighs
- Uterine contractions, with or without pain
- More than six contractions per hour
- Intestinal cramping, with or without diarrhea (Jordan et al., 2014).

Assess the pattern of the contractions: the contractions must be persistent, such that four contractions occur every 20 minutes or 8 contractions occur in 1 hour. Evaluate cervical dilation and effacement: cervical effacement is 80% or greater and cervical dilation is greater than 1 cm (ACOG, 2014b). On examination, engagement of the fetal presenting part will be noted.

Laboratory and Diagnostic Testing

Commonly used diagnostic testing for preterm labor risk assessment includes a complete blood count to detect infection, which may be a contributing factor to preterm labor; urinalysis to detect bacteria and nitrites, which are indicative of a urinary tract infection; and an amniotic fluid analysis to determine fetal lung maturity and the presence of subclinical chorioamnionitis.

Other tests that may be used for preterm labor prediction include fetal fibronectin testing and cervical length evaluation by transvaginal ultrasound., Fetal fibronectin and cervical length examinations have a high negative predictive value and are thus better at predicting which pregnant women are unlikely to have a preterm birth as opposed to predicting those who will (van Baaren et al., 2015).

FETAL FIBRONECTIN

Fetal fibronectin, a glycoprotein produced by the chorion, is found at the junction of the chorion and decidua (fetal membranes and uterus). It acts as biologic glue, attaching the fetal sac to the uterine lining. It normally is present in cervicovaginal secretions up to 22 weeks of pregnancy and again at the end of the last trimester (1 to 3 weeks before labor). It usually cannot be detected between 24 and 34 weeks of pregnancy (5½ to 8½ months) unless there has been a disruption between the chorion and decidua. It is present in cervicovaginal fluid prior to delivery, regardless of gestational age.

The test is a useful marker for impending membrane rupture within 7 to 14 days if the level increases to >0.05 mcg/mL. The accuracy of fetal fibronectin is decreased in the presence of lubricants, blood, recent intercourse, or cervical manipulation within the previous 24 hours. Conversely, a negative fetal fibronectin test is a strong predictor that preterm labor in the next 2 weeks is unlikely (Abbott et al., 2015).

A sterile applicator is used to collect a cervicovaginal sample during an examination by speculum. The result is either positive (fetal fibronectin is present) or negative (fetal fibronectin is not present). Interpretation of fetal fibronectin results must always be viewed in conjunction with the clinical findings; it is not used as a lone indicator for predicting preterm labor. The primary importance of cervicovaginal fetal fibronectin lies in the high negative predictive values of the test for reducing preterm birth risk. Fibronectin testing can be a useful tool in the triaging of women symptomatic for preterm labor.

CERVICAL LENGTH MEASUREMENT

Transvaginal ultrasound of the cervix has been used as a tool to predict preterm labor in high-risk pregnancies and to differentiate between true and false preterm labor. Three parameters are evaluated during the transvaginal ultrasound: cervical length and width, funnel width and length, and percentage of funneling. Measurement of the closed portion of the cervix visualized during the transvaginal ultrasound is the single most reliable parameter for prediction of preterm delivery in high-risk women (van Baaren et al., 2014).

Cervical length varies during pregnancy and can be measured fairly reliably after 16 weeks of gestation using an ultrasound probe inserted in the vagina. A cervical length of 3 cm or more indicates that delivery within 14 days is unlikely. Women with a short cervical length of 2.5 cm during the mid-trimester have a substantially greater risk of preterm birth prior to 35 weeks of gestation. As with fetal fibronectin testing, negative results can be reassuring and prevent unnecessary interventions (Souka et al., 2015).

Nursing Management

Nurses play a key role in reducing preterm labor and births to improve pregnancy outcomes for both mothers and their infants. Early detection of preterm labor is currently the best strategy to improve outcomes. Because of the numerous factors associated with preterm labor, it is challenging to identify and address all of them, especially when women experiencing contractions are frequently falsely reassured and not assessed thoroughly to determine the cause. This delay impedes initiation of interventions to reduce infant death and morbidity.

Preterm birth prevention programs for women at high risk have used self-monitoring of symptoms and patterns, weekly cervical examinations, clinical markers, telephone monitoring, home visiting, alone or in combination, with disappointing results. Preterm labor is currently thought to be a chronic, long-term multifactorial process with a genetic component. A recent study found a multiple pregnancy, prior preterm birth, low socioeconomic status, maternal medical disorders, and maternal infections were statistically significant risk factors for predicting spontaneous preterm labor (Patel, Pitre, & Bhooker, 2015). Despite technologic and pharmacologic advances in the identification and treatment of preterm labor, the incidence remains high and is growing in the United States.

Supportive nursing care is needed for the woman in preterm labor whether the contractions are stopped with tocolytic therapy or not. Nursing tasks include monitoring vital signs, measuring intake and output, encouraging bed rest on the woman's left side to enhance placental perfusion, monitoring the fetal heart rate via an external monitor continuously, limiting vaginal examinations to prevent an ascending infection, and monitoring the mother and fetus closely for any adverse effects from the tocolytic agents. Offering the couple ongoing explanations will help prepare them for the birth.

Administering Tocolytic Therapy

Tocolysis is the use of drugs to inhibit uterine contractions. The primary goals of tocolytic therapy are to arrest labor and delay birth long enough to initiate prophylactic corticosteroid therapy when indicated for stimulation of fetal lung maturity and to arrange for maternal-fetal transport to a perinatal tertiary care hospital. A firm diagnosis of preterm labor is necessary before treatment is considered. Diagnosis requires the presence of both uterine contractions and cervical change (or an initial cervical examination of more than 2 cm and/or more than 80% effacement in a nulliparous client). A cause for preterm labor should always be sought.

Absolute contraindications to administering tocolytic agents to stop labor include intrauterine infection, active hemorrhage, fetal distress, fetus before viability, fetal abnormality incompatible with life, fetal growth restriction severe preeclampsia, heart disease, prolonged premature rupture of the membranes (PPROM), and intrauterine demise (Callahan, 2016). Bed rest and hydration are commonly recommended, but without proven efficacy.

Prevention of preterm labor remains an elusive goal. Presently, women at high risk for preterm labor are offered progesterone therapy at the start of their second trimester. Although progesterone therapy is recommended by ACOG, it has not been FDA approved for this purpose and has mixed results (Iams, 2015).

Magnesium sulfate may be ordered. This agent acts as a physiologic calcium antagonist and a general inhibitor of neurotransmission. Expect to administer it intravenously. Monitor the woman for nausea, vomiting, headache, weakness, hypotension, and cardiopulmonary arrest. Frequent monitoring of maternal respiratory effort and deep tendon reflexes is essential for early recognition of overdose. Because magnesium is exclusively excreted by the kidneys, adequate renal function is essential for safe administration. Assess the fetus for decreased FHR variability, drowsiness, and hypotonia. Magnesium has a wide margin of safety, but is not any more effective in delaying preterm birth as any other tocolytic agent. However, if administered prenatally, it is effective in helping women who develop preeclampsia and helping to protect fetal brains (Nakazawa et al., 2015).

Calcium channel blockers promote uterine relaxation by decreasing the influx of calcium ions into myometrium cells to inhibit contractions. Although calcium channel blockers may be prescribed to manage preterm labor, available literature provides little evidence that they have better efficacy in treating preterm labor than any other tocolytic agent. The perfect tocolytic drug that is 100% efficacious and 100% safe does not exist yet (van den Bosch, Ruys, & Roos-Hesselink, 2015). Administer calcium channel blockers (nifedipine) orally or sublingually every 4 to 8 hours as ordered. Monitor the woman for hypotension, reflex tachycardia, headache, nausea, and facial flushing.

Prostaglandin synthetase inhibitor (indomethacin [Indocin]) reduces prostaglandin synthesis from decidual macrophages. It readily crosses the placenta and can cause oligohydramnios due to a decrease in fetal renal blood flow if used for more than 48 hours. During treatment, urine output, maternal temperature, and amniotic fluid index (AFI) should be evaluated periodically. The initial recommended dose is 50 to 100 mg orally or per rectum followed by 25 to 50 mg every 6 hours for 8 doses. Indomethacin therapy is not recommended for gestations of 32 weeks or greater (Ross, 2015).

Educating the Client

Ensure that every pregnant woman receives basic education about preterm labor, including information about harmful lifestyles, the signs of genitourinary infections and preterm labor, and the appropriate response to these symptoms. Teach the client how to palpate for and time uterine contractions. Provide written materials to support this education at a level and in a language appropriate for the client. Also educate clients about the importance of prenatal care, risk reduction, and recognizing the signs and symptoms of preterm labor. Teaching Guidelines 21.1 highlights important instructions related to preventing preterm labor.

Teaching Guidelines 21.1
TEACHING TO PREVENT PRETERM LABOR

- Avoid traveling for long distances in cars, trains, planes, or buses.
- Avoid lifting heavy objects, such as laundry, groceries, or a young child.
- Avoid performing hard, physical work, such as yard work, moving of furniture, or construction.
- Mild to moderate levels of exercise are permitted such as walking daily.
- Achieve an appropriate prepregnancy weight.
- Achieve adequate iron stores through balanced nutrition.
- Wait at least 18 months between pregnancies.
- Visit a dentist in early pregnancy to evaluate and treat periodontal disease.
- Enroll in a smoking cessation program if you are unable to quit on your own.
- Curtail sexual activity until after 37 weeks if experiencing preterm labor symptoms.
- Consume a well-balanced nutritional diet to gain appropriate weight.
- Avoid the use of substances such as marijuana, cocaine, and heroin.
- Identify factors and areas of stress in your life, and use stress management techniques to reduce them.
- If you are experiencing intimate partner violence, seek resources to modify the situation.

Recognize the signs and symptoms of preterm labor and notify your birth attendant if any occur:
- Uterine contractions, cramping, or low back pain
- Feeling of pelvic pressure or fullness
- Increase in vaginal discharge
- Nausea, vomiting, and diarrhea
- Leaking of fluid from vagina

If you are experiencing any of these signs or symptoms, do the following:
- Stop what you are doing and rest for 1 hour.
- Empty your bladder.
- Lie down on your side.
- Drink two to three glasses of water.
- Feel your abdomen and make note of the hardness of the contraction. Call your health care provider and describe the contraction as
  - Mild if it feels like the tip of the nose
  - Moderate if it feels like the tip of the chin
  - Strong if it feels like your forehead

Adapted from Jordan, R. G., Engstrom, J. L., Marfell, J. A., & Farley, C. L. (2014). *Prenatal and postnatal care: A woman-centered approach.* Ames, Iowa: John Wiley & Sons, Inc.; and Ross, M. G. (2015). Preterm labor. *eMedicine.* Retrieved from http://emedicine.medscape.com/article/260998-overview#aw2aab6b7

Explaining to the couple what is happening in terms of labor progress, the treatment regimen, and the status of the fetus is important to reduce the anxiety associated with the risk of giving birth to a preterm infant. Educate them about the importance of promotion of fetal lung maturity with corticosteroids. Include supportive family members in all education. Allow time for the woman and her family to express their concerns about the possible outcome for the infant and the possible side effects of the tocolytic therapy. Encourage them to vent any feelings, fears, and anger they may experience. Provide the woman and her family with an honest appraisal of the situation and plan of treatment throughout her care.

Providing Psychological Support

Preterm labor and birth present multifactorial challenges for everyone involved. If the woman's activities are restricted, additional stresses may be placed on the family, contributing to the crisis. Assess the stress levels of the client and family, and make appropriate referrals. Emphasize the need for more frequent supervision and office visits, and encourage clients to talk to their health care provider for reassurance.

Every case of spontaneous preterm labor is unique. Care must take into account the clinical circumstances, and the full and informed consent of the woman and her partner is needed. Half of all women who ultimately give birth prematurely have no identifiable risk factors. Nurses should be sensitive to any complaint and should provide appropriate assessment, information, and follow-up. Sensitivity to the subtle differences between normal pregnancy sensations and the prodromal symptoms of preterm labor is a key factor in ensuring timely care. Offer validation and clarification of the woman's symptoms.

If tocolytic therapy is not successful in stopping uterine contractions, support the couple through this stressful period to prepare them for the birth. Keep them informed of all progress and changes; for example, continuously monitor maternal and fetal vital signs, especially the maternal temperature to detect signs of early infection. Offer one-on-one contact and be available throughout this difficult and anxiety-producing period.

POST-TERM PREGNANCY

A term pregnancy usually lasts 38 to 42 weeks. A post-term or prolonged pregnancy is one that continues past the end of the 42nd week of gestation, or 294 days from the first day of the last menstrual period. A **post-term or prolonged pregnancy** is defined as a pregnancy that extends to 42 0/7 weeks and beyond. Within the United States, about 7% of singleton pregnancies extend beyond 41 weeks (Walker & Gan, 2015). Incorrect dates account for the majority of these cases: many women have irregular menses and thus cannot identify the date of their last menstrual period accurately.

Recall Jennifer described at the beginning of the chapter, who was at 41 weeks of gestation. What information would be most important to determine on admission to the facility? What interventions might the nurse anticipate when she arrives?

The exact etiology of a post-term or prolonged pregnancy is unknown because the mechanism for the initiation of labor is not completely understood. Theories suggest there may be a deficiency of estrogen and continued secretion of progesterone that prohibits the uterus from contracting, but no evidence has validated this. A woman who has one prolonged pregnancy is at greater risk for another in subsequent pregnancies.

Post-term pregnancies may adversely affect both the mother and fetus or newborn. Maternal risk is related to the large size of the fetus at birth, which increases the chances that a cesarean birth will be needed. Other issues might include dystocia, birth trauma, postpartum hemorrhage, and infection. Mechanical or artificial interventions such as forceps or vacuum-assisted birth and labor induction with oxytocin may be necessary. In addition, maternal exhaustion and feelings of despair over this prolonged gestation can add to the woman's anxiety level and reduce her coping ability. Women often blame themselves for prolonging the pregnancy, and a woman's negative feelings about herself can bring about strained relationships with the people closest to her.

Fetal risks associated with a post-term pregnancy include macrosomia, shoulder dystocia, brachial plexus injuries, low Apgar scores, postmaturity syndrome (loss of subcutaneous fat and muscle and meconium staining), and cephalopelvic disproportion. All of these conditions predispose this fetus to birth trauma or a surgical birth. The perinatal mortality rate at more than 42 weeks of gestation is twice that at term and increases sixfold and higher at 43 weeks of gestation and beyond. Uteroplacental insufficiency, meconium aspiration, and intrauterine infection contribute to the increased rate of perinatal deaths (Callahan, 2016). As the placenta ages, its perfusion decreases and it becomes less efficient at delivering oxygen and nutrients to the fetus. Amniotic fluid volume also begins to decline after 38 weeks of gestation, possibly leading to oligohydramnios, subsequently resulting in fetal hypoxia and an increased risk of cord compression because the cushioning effect offered by adequate fluid is no longer present. Hypoxia and oligohydramnios predispose the fetus to aspiration of meconium, which is released by the fetus in response to a hypoxic insult (Caughey & Butler, 2015). All of these issues can compromise fetal well-being and lead to fetal distress.

Nursing Assessment

Obtain a thorough history to determine the estimated date of birth. Many women are unsure of the date of their last menstrual period, so the date given may be unreliable. Despite numerous methods used to date pregnancies, many are still misdated. Accurate gestational dating via ultrasound is essential.

When expectant management is chosen versus labor induction for the post-term pregnancy, the nurse should anticipate that assessments for a post-term pregnancy will typically include daily fetal movement counts done by the woman, nonstress tests with amniotic fluid assessments as part of the biophysical profile done twice weekly, and weekly cervical examinations to evaluate for ripening. Induction can be deferred until 42 weeks if the fetal surveillance is reassuring. In addition, assess the following:

- Client's understanding of the various fetal well-being tests
- Client's stress and anxiety concerning her lateness
- Client's coping ability and support network

Nursing Management

Once the dates have been established and post-term status is confirmed, monitoring fetal well-being becomes critical. When determining the plan of care for a woman with a prolonged pregnancy, the first decision is whether to deliver the baby or wait. If the decision is to wait, then fetal surveillance is the key. If the decision is to have the woman give birth, labor induction is initiated. Both decisions remain controversial, and there is no clear answer about which option is more appropriate. Therefore, the plan must be individualized.

Think back to Jennifer, who is scheduled for labor induction. What ongoing nursing assessments would be important when providing care for her?

Providing Support

The intense surveillance is time consuming and intrusive, adding to the anxiety and worry already being experienced by the woman about her overdue status. Be alert to the woman's anxiety and allow her to discuss her feelings. Provide reassurance about the expected time range for birth and the well-being of the fetus based on the assessment tests. Validating the woman's stressful state due to the post-term pregnancy provides an opportunity for her to verbalize her feelings openly.

Educating the Woman and Her Partner

Teach the woman and her partner about the testing required and the reasons for each test. Also describe the methods that may be used for cervical ripening if indicated. Explain about the possibility of induction if the woman's labor is not spontaneous or if a dysfunctional labor pattern occurs. Also prepare the woman for the possibility of a surgical delivery if fetal distress occurs.

Providing Care During the Intrapartum Period

During the intrapartum period, continuously assess and monitor FHR to identify potential fetal distress early (e.g., late or variable decelerations) so that interventions can be initiated. Also monitor the woman's hydration status to ensure maximal placental perfusion. When the membranes rupture, assess amniotic fluid characteristics (color, amount, and odor) to identify previous fetal hypoxia and prepare for prevention of meconium aspiration. Report meconium-stained amniotic fluid immediately when the woman's membranes rupture. Anticipate the need for amnioinfusion to minimize the risk of meconium aspiration by diluting the meconium in the amniotic fluid expelled by the hypoxic fetus. In addition, monitor the woman's labor pattern closely because dysfunctional patterns are common (Soni, Vaishnav, & Gohil, 2015). Encourage the woman to verbalize her feelings and concerns, and answer all her questions. Provide support, presence, information, and encouragement throughout this time.

WOMEN REQUIRING LABOR INDUCTION AND AUGMENTATION

Ideally, all pregnancies go to term, with labor beginning spontaneously. However, many women need help to initiate or sustain the labor process. **Labor induction** involves the stimulation of uterine contractions by medical or surgical means before the onset of spontaneous labor. The labor induction rate is at an all-time high in the United States. The widespread use of artificial induction of labor for convenience has contributed to the recent increase in the number of cesarean births. Evidence is compelling that elective induction of labor significantly increases the risk of cesarean birth, instrumented delivery, use of epidural analgesia, and neonatal intensive care unit admission, especially for nulliparous women (Caughey, 2014a).

Labor induction is not an isolated event: it brings about a cascade of other interventions that may or may not produce a favorable outcome. Labor induction also involves intravenous therapy, bed rest, continuous electronic fetal monitoring, significant discomfort from stimulating uterine contractions, epidural analgesia/anesthesia, and a prolonged stay on the labor and birth unit (Vogel et al., 2014). Labor augmentation (stimulating the uterus, typically with oxytocin) enhances ineffective contractions after labor has begun. Continuous electronic FHR monitoring is necessary.

The World Health Organization ([WHO], 2014b) has put forth recommendations regarding labor induction which includes:

- Labor induction should be performed only for a clear medical indication
- Women being induced should not be left unattended
- Labor induction should only be performed after CPD has been ruled out
- Labor induction should be applied to women with abnormal fetal presentations
- Close monitoring is needed of the fetal heart rate and uterine contraction pattern

There are multiple medical and obstetric reasons for inducing labor, the most common being prolonged gestation. Other indications for inductions include PPROM, gestational hypertension, cardiac disease, renal disease, chorioamnionitis, dystocia, intrauterine fetal demise, iso-immunization, and diabetes (Jordan et al., 2014). Contraindications to labor induction include complete placenta previa, abruptio placentae, transverse fetal lie, prolapsed umbilical cord, a prior classic uterine incision that entered the uterine cavity, pelvic structure abnormality, previous myomectomy, vaginal bleeding with unknown cause, invasive cervical cancer, active genital herpes infection, and abnormal FHR patterns (Cunningham et al., 2014). In general, labor induction is indicated when the benefits of birth outweigh the risks to the mother or fetus for continuing the pregnancy. However, the balance between risk and benefit remains controversial.

Take Note!

Before labor induction is started, fetal maturity (dating, ultrasound, amniotic fluid studies) and cervical readiness (vaginal examination, Bishop scoring; see Table 21.2) must be assessed. Both need to be favorable for a successful induction.

Therapeutic Management

The decision to induce labor is based on a thorough evaluation of maternal and fetal status. Typically, this includes an ultrasound to evaluate fetal size, position, and gestational age and to locate the placenta; engaged presenting fetal part; pelvimetry to rule out fetopelvic disproportion; a nonstress test to evaluate fetal well-being; a phosphatidylglycerol (PG) level to assess fetal lung maturity; confirmation of Category I fetal heart rate pattern; complete blood count and urinalysis to rule out infection; and a vaginal examination to evaluate the cervix for inducibility (Kriebs, 2015). Accurate dating of the pregnancy also is essential before cervical ripening and induction are initiated to prevent a preterm birth.

Cervical Ripening

Cervical ripening is a process by which the cervix softens via the breakdown of collagen fibrils. It is the first step in the process of cervical effacement and dilation so that, on average, the cervix is approximately 50% effaced and 2 cm dilated at the onset of labor, although wide differences do exist. There has been increasing awareness that if the cervix is unfavorable or unripe, a successful vaginal birth is unlikely. Cervical ripeness is an important variable when labor induction is being considered. A ripe cervix is shortened, centered (anterior), softened, and partially dilated. An unripe cervix is long, closed, posterior, and firm. Cervical ripening usually begins prior to the onset of labor contractions and is necessary for cervical dilation and the passage of the fetus.

Various scoring systems to assess cervical ripeness have been introduced, but the Bishop score is most commonly used today. The Bishop score helps identify women who would be most likely to achieve a successful induction (Table 21.2). The duration of labor is inversely correlated with the Bishop score: a score over 8 indicates a successful vaginal birth. Bishop scores of less than 6 usually indicate that a cervical ripening method should be used prior to induction (Goldberg, 2015). Medical induction of labor has two components: cervical ripening and induction of contractions. When induction of labor is indicated, cervical readiness for labor is evaluated by pelvic exam and determination of a Bishop score is documented.

Score	Dilation (cm)	Effacement (%)	Station	Cervical Consistency	Position of Cervix
0	Closed	0–30	−3	Firm	Posterior
1	1–2	40–50	−2	Medium	Midposition
2	3–4	60–70	−1 or 0	Soft	Anterior
3	5–6	80	+1 or +2	Very soft	Anterior

TABLE 21.2 BISHOP SCORING SYSTEM

Modified from International Childbirth Education Association [ICEA]. (2014). *ICEA position paper: Induction.* Retrieved from http://www.icea.org/sites/default/files/Induction%20PP-FINAL.pdf

COMPLEMENTARY AND ALTERNATIVE MEDICINE METHODS

Nonpharmacologic methods for cervical ripening are less frequently used today, but nurses need to be aware of them and question clients about their use. Methods may include herbal agents such as evening primrose oil, black haw, black and blue cohosh, and red raspberry leaves. In addition, castor oil, hot baths, and enemas are used for cervical ripening and labor induction. The risks and benefits of these agents are unknown. None have been evaluated scientifically, and thus, none can be recommended regarding their efficacy or safety.

Another nonpharmacologic method suggested for labor induction is sexual intercourse along with breast stimulation. This promotes the release of oxytocin, which stimulates uterine contractions. In addition, human semen is a biologic source of prostaglandins used for cervical ripening. According to a Cochrane review, sexual intercourse with breast stimulation would appear beneficial, but safety issues have not been fully evaluated, nor can this activity be standardized. It appears to shorten the latent phase of labor (King et al., 2015). Therefore, its use as a method for labor induction is not validated by research.

MECHANICAL METHODS

Mechanical methods are used to open the cervix and stimulate the progression of labor. All share a similar mechanism of action: application of local pressure stimulates the release of prostaglandins to ripen the cervix. Potential advantages of mechanical methods, compared with pharmacologic methods, may include simplicity or preservation of the cervical tissue or structure, lower cost, and fewer side effects. The risks associated with these methods include infection, bleeding, membrane rupture, and placental disruption (Sciscone, 2014). For example, an indwelling (Foley) catheter (e.g., 26 French) can be inserted into the endocervical canal to ripen and dilate the cervix. The catheter is placed in the uterus, and the balloon is filled. Direct pressure is then applied to the lower segment of the uterus and the cervix. This direct pressure causes stress in the lower uterine segment and probably the local production of prostaglandins. The risks, benefits, and expected side effects should be explained to the woman prior to the insertion of the balloon catheter (Fuks et al., 2015).

Hygroscopic dilators absorb endocervical and local tissue fluids; as they enlarge, they expand the endocervix and provide controlled mechanical pressure. The products available include natural osmotic dilators (laminaria, a type of dried seaweed) and synthetic dilators containing magnesium sulfate (Lamicel, Dilapan). Hygroscopic dilators are advantageous because they can be inserted on an outpatient basis and no fetal monitoring is needed. As many dilators are inserted in the cervix as will fit, and they expand over 12 to 24 hours as they absorb water.

Absorption of water leads to expansion of the dilators and opening of the cervix. They are a reliable alternative when prostaglandins are contraindicated or unavailable (Goldberg, 2015).

Recently there has been a reduction in the use of hygroscopic and osmotic dilators for the induction of labor in favor of pharmacologic agents. The increased risk of maternal and fetal infections with hygroscopic and osmotic dilators when compared with that associated with the use of other pharmacologic agents and the ease of pharmacologic administration may be reasons for the decline. Placement of dilators also requires additional training and may be associated with rupture of membranes, vaginal bleeding, and client discomfort or pain (Drunecky et al., 2015).

Recent systematic review of randomized trials that compared cervical ripening with mechanical methods versus alternative pharmacologic agents or placebo demonstrated that maternal infection was increased in clients who underwent cervical ripening with mechanical methods. Thus, mechanical methods for cervical ripening have fallen into disfavor and are used infrequently today when compared with pharmacologic or surgical methods for induction (McCarthy & Kenny, 2014).

SURGICAL METHODS

Surgical methods used to ripen the cervix and induce labor include stripping of the membranes and performing an amniotomy. Stripping of the membranes is accomplished by inserting a finger through the internal cervical os and moving it in a circular direction. This motion causes the membranes to detach. Manual separation of the amniotic membranes from the cervix is thought to induce cervical ripening and the onset of labor (Afzal, Asif, & Miraj, 2015). However, there is no strong evidence at this time that membrane stripping significantly shortens the duration of pregnancy.

An amniotomy involves inserting a cervical hook (Amniohook) through the cervical os to deliberately rupture the membranes. This promotes pressure of the presenting part on the cervix and stimulates an increase in the activity of prostaglandins locally. Risks associated with these procedures include umbilical cord prolapse or compression, maternal or neonatal infection, FHR deceleration, bleeding, and client discomfort (King et al., 2015).

When either of these techniques is used, amniotic fluid characteristics (such as whether it is clear or bloody, or meconium is present) and the FHR pattern must be monitored closely.

PHARMACOLOGIC METHODS

The use of pharmacologic agents has revolutionized cervical ripening. The use of prostaglandins to attain cervical ripening has been found to be highly effective in producing cervical changes independent of uterine contractions (Grobman, 2015). In some cases, women will go into labor and require no additional stimulants for induction. Induction of labor with prostaglandins offers the advantage of promoting both cervical ripening and uterine contractility. A drawback of prostaglandins is their ability to induce excessive uterine contractions, which can increase maternal and perinatal morbidity (Callahan, 2016). Prostaglandin analogs commonly used for cervical ripening include dinoprostone gel (Prepidil), dinoprostone inserts (Cervidil), and misoprostol (Cytotec). Misoprostol (Cytotec), a synthetic PGE1 analog, is a gastric cytoprotective agent used in the treatment and prevention of peptic ulcers. It can be administered intravaginally or orally to ripen the cervix or induce labor. It is available in 100-mcg or 200-mcg tablets, but doses of 25 to 50 mcg are typically used. It is important to note that only dinoprostone is approved by the FDA for use as a cervical ripening agent, although ACOG acknowledges the apparent safety and effectiveness of misoprostol for this purpose (King et al., 2015). A major adverse effect of the obstetric use of Cytotec is hyperstimulation of the uterus, which may progress to uterine tetany with marked impairment of uteroplacental blood flow, uterine rupture (requiring surgical repair, hysterectomy, and/or salpingo-oophorectomy), or amniotic fluid embolism (Ahmed et al., 2015; Drug Guide 21.2). Furthermore, it is contraindicated for women with prior uterine scars and therefore should not be used for cervical ripening in women attempting a vaginal birth after cesarean.

DRUG GUIDE 21.2   DRUGS USED FOR CERVICAL RIPENING AND LABOR INDUCTION

Drug	Action/Indication	Nursing Implications
Dinoprostone (Cervidil insert; Prepidil gel)	Directly softens and dilates the cervix/to ripen cervix and induce labor FDA approved for cervical ripening	Provide emotional support. Administer pain medications as needed. Frequently assess degree of effacement and dilation. Monitor uterine contractions for frequency, duration, and strength. Assess maternal vital signs and FHR pattern frequently. Monitor woman for possible adverse effects such as headache, nausea and vomiting, and diarrhea.
Misoprostol (Cytotec)	Ripens cervix/to induce labor	Instruct client about purpose and possible adverse effects of medication. Ensure informed consent is signed per hospital policy. Assess vital signs and FHR patterns frequently. Monitor client's reaction to drug. Initiate oxytocin for labor induction at least 4 hours after last dose was administered. Monitor for possible adverse effects such as nausea and vomiting, diarrhea, uterine hyperstimulation, and category II FHR patterns.
Oxytocin (Pitocin)	Acts on uterine myofibrils to contract/to initiate or reinforce labor	Administer as an IV infusion via pump, increasing dose based on protocol until adequate labor progress is achieved. Assess baseline vital signs and FHR and then frequently after initiating oxytocin infusion. Determine frequency, duration, and strength of contractions frequently. Notify health care provider of any uterine hypertonicity or abnormal FHR patterns. Maintain careful I&O, being alert for water intoxication. Keep client informed of labor progress. Monitor for possible adverse effects such as hyperstimulation of the uterus, impaired uterine blood flow leading to fetal hypoxia, rapid labor leading to cervical lacerations or uterine rupture, water intoxication (if oxytocin is given in electrolyte-free solution or at a rate exceeding 20 mU/min), and hypotension.

Adapted from Goldberg, A. E. (2015). Cervical ripening. *eMedicine.* Retrieved from http://emedicine.medscape.com/article/263311-overview#aw2aab6b7; King, T. L., Brucker, M. C., Kriebs, J. M., Fahey, J. O., Gegor, C. L., & Varney, H. (2015). *Varney's midwifery* (5th ed.). Burlington, MA: Jones & Bartlett Learning: and Goetzl, L. (2014). Methods of cervical ripening and labor induction: Pharmacologic. *Clinical Obstetrics and Gynecology, 57*(2), 377–390.

Oxytocin

Oxytocin is a potent endogenous uterotonic agent used for both artificial induction and augmentation of labor. It is produced naturally by the posterior pituitary gland and stimulates contractions of the uterus. For women with low Bishop scores, cervical ripening is typically initiated before oxytocin is used. Once the cervix is ripe, oxytocin is the most popular pharmacologic agent used for inducing or augmenting labor.

Frequently, a woman with an unfavorable cervix is admitted the evening before induction to ripen her cervix with one of the prostaglandin agents. Then induction begins with oxytocin the next morning if she has not already gone into labor. Doing so markedly enhances the success of induction.

Response to oxytocin varies widely: some women are very sensitive to even small amounts. The most common adverse effect of oxytocin is uterine hyperstimulation, leading to fetal compromise and impaired oxygenation (King, et al., 2015). The response of the uterus to the drug is closely monitored throughout labor so that the oxytocin infusion can be titrated appropriately. In addition, oxytocin has an antidiuretic effect, resulting in decreased urine flow that may lead to water intoxication. Symptoms to watch for include headache and vomiting.

Oxytocin is administered via an intravenous infusion pump piggybacked into the main intravenous line at the port most proximal to the insertion site. Typically, 10 units of oxytocin are added to 1 L of isotonic solution. The dose is titrated according to protocol to achieve stable contractions every 2 to 3 minutes lasting 40 to 60 seconds. Recent studies suggest that a more conservative oxytocin protocol with lower doses reduces the number of neonatal intensive care unit admissions and lower cesarean sections (Lewis et al., 2014; Manjula et al., 2015).

The uterus should relax between contractions. If the resting uterine tone remains above 20 mm Hg, uteroplacental insufficiency and fetal hypoxia can result. This underscores the importance of continuous FHR monitoring. Unfortunately, neither the optimal oxytocin administration regimen nor the maximum oxytocin dose has been established or agreed upon through research or expert opinion. Nurses assisting with labor inductions need to become familiar with their hospital protocols concerning dosage, infusion rates, and frequency of change.

Oxytocin has many advantages: it is potent and easy to titrate, it has a short half-life (1 to 5 minutes), and it is generally well tolerated. Induction using oxytocin has side effects (water intoxication, hypotension, and uterine hypertonicity), but because the drug does not cross the placental barrier, no direct fetal problems have been observed (Arrowsmith & Wray, 2014) (Fig. 21.4).

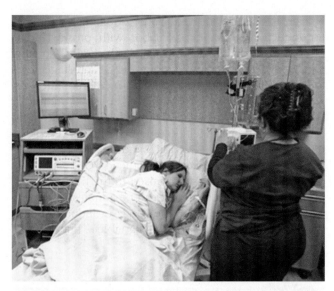

FIGURE 21.4 The nurse monitors an intravenous infusion of oxytocin being administered to a woman in labor who is being induced.

Remember Jennifer, the young woman described at the beginning of the chapter? After her cervix is ripened, an oxytocin infusion is started and her progress is slow. What encouragement can the nurse offer? After a few hours, her contractions begin to increase in intensity and frequency. What typical pain management measures can the nurse implement, and how would the nurse evaluate the effectiveness of these measures?

Nursing Assessment

Nursing assessment of the woman who is undergoing labor induction or augmentation involves a thorough history and physical examination. Review the woman's history for relative indications for induction or augmentation, such as diabetes, hypertension, post-term status, dysfunctional labor pattern, prolonged ruptured membranes, and maternal or fetal infection, and for contraindications such as placenta previa, over distended uterus, active genital herpes, fetopelvic disproportion, fetal malposition, or severe fetal distress.

Assist with determining the gestational age of the fetus to prevent a preterm birth. Assess fetal well-being to validate the client's and fetus's ability to withstand labor contractions. Evaluate the woman's cervical status, including cervical dilation and effacement, and station via vaginal examination as appropriate before cervical ripening or induction is started. Determine the Bishop score to determine the probable success of induction.

Take Note!

Nurses working with women in labor play an important role acting as the eyes and ears for the birth attendant because they remain at the client's bedside throughout the entire experience. Close, frequent assessment and follow-up interventions are essential to ensure the safety of the mother and her unborn child during cervical ripening and labor induction or augmentation.

Nursing Management

Explain to the woman and her partner about the induction or augmentation procedure clearly, using simple terms (Teaching Guidelines 21.2). Ensure that an informed consent has been signed after the client and her partner have received complete information about the procedure, including its advantages, disadvantages, and potential risks. Ensure that the Bishop score has been determined before proceeding. Nursing Care Plan 21.1 presents an overview of the nursing care for a woman undergoing labor induction.

Teaching Guidelines 21.2
TEACHING IN PREPARATION FOR LABOR INDUCTION

- Your health care provider may recommend that you have your labor induced. This may be necessary for a variety of reasons, such as elevated blood pressure, a medical condition, prolonged pregnancy over 41 weeks, or problems with fetal heart rate patterns or fetal growth.
- Your health care provider may use one or more methods to induce labor, such as stripping the membranes, breaking the amniotic sac to release the fluid, administering medication close to or in the cervix to soften it, or administering a medication called oxytocin (Pitocin) to stimulate contractions.
- Labor induction is associated with some risks and disadvantages, such as overactivity of the uterus; nausea, vomiting, or diarrhea; and changes in fetal heart rate.
- Prior to inducing your labor, your health care provider may perform a procedure to ripen your cervix to help ensure a successful induction.
- Medication may be placed around your cervix the day before you are scheduled to be induced.
- During the induction, your contractions may feel stronger than normal. However, the length of your labor may be reduced with induction.
- Medications for pain relief and comfort measures will be readily available.
- Health care staff will be present throughout labor.

Administering Oxytocin

If not already done, prepare the oxytocin infusion by diluting 10 units of oxytocin in 1,000 mL of lactated Ringer's solution or ordered isotonic solution. Use an infusion pump on a secondary line connected to the primary infusion. Start the oxytocin infusion in mU/min or milliliters per hour as ordered. Each hospital has its own standards/protocols for oxytocin infusion and dilution. The nurse needs to follow that procedure when administering this medication. Maintain the rate once the desired contraction frequency has been reached. To ensure adequate maternal and fetal surveillance during induction or augmentation, the nurse-to-client ratio should not exceed 1:2 (Mattson & Smith, 2016).

During induction or augmentation, monitoring of the maternal and fetal status is essential. Apply an external electronic fetal monitor or assist with placement of an internal device. Obtain the mother's vital signs and the FHR every 15 minutes during the first stage. Evaluate the contractions (frequency, duration, and intensity) and resting tone, and adjust the oxytocin infusion rate accordingly. Monitor the FHR, including baseline rate, baseline variability, and decelerations, to determine whether the oxytocin rate needs adjustment. Discontinue the oxytocin and notify the birth attendant if uterine hyperstimulation or a category II or III FHR pattern occurs. Perform or assist with periodic vaginal examinations to determine cervical dilation and fetal descent: cervical dilation of 1 cm per hour typically indicates satisfactory progress. Continue to monitor the FHR continuously and document it every 15 minutes during the active phase of labor and every 5 minutes during the second stage. Assist with pushing efforts during the second stage. Measure and record the intake and output to prevent excess fluid volume. Encourage the client to empty her bladder every 2 hours to prevent soft tissue obstruction.

Providing Pain Relief and Support

Assess the woman's level of pain. Ask her frequently to rate her pain and provide pain management as needed. Offer position changes and other nonpharmacologic measures. Note her reaction to any medication given, and document its effect. Monitor her need for comfort measures as contractions increase.

Throughout induction and augmentation, frequently reassure the woman and her partner about the fetal status and labor progress. Provide them with frequent updates on the condition of the woman and the fetus. Assess the woman's ability to cope with stronger contractions, and follow protocols of the hospital about how frequent pain assessments are performed for each phase and stage of labor (Nagtalon-Ramos, 2014). Provide support and encouragement as indicated.

After a very long day, Jennifer gives birth to a healthy baby boy with Apgar scores of 9 at 1 minute and 10 at 5 minutes. When transferring her to the postpartum unit, what information is essential to include for the accepting nurse? What specific

Overview of the Women Undergoing Labor Induction

Rose, a 29-year-old primipara, is admitted to the labor and birth suite at 40 weeks of gestation for induction of labor. Assessment reveals that her cervix is ripe and 80% effaced, and dilated to 2 cm. Rose says, "I'm a bit nervous about being induced. I've never been through labor before and I'm afraid that I'll have a lot of pain from the medicine used to start the contractions." She consents to being induced but wants reassurance that this procedure won't harm the baby. Upon examination, the fetus is engaged and in a cephalic presentation, with the vertex as the presenting part. Her partner is at her side. Induction is initiated with oxytocin. Rose reports that contractions have started and are beginning to get stronger.

NURSING DIAGNOSIS: Anxiety related to induction of labor and associated medical interventions needed as evidenced by statements about being nervous, not having gone through labor before, fear of pain, and potential harm to fetus.

Outcome Identification and Evaluation

The client will experience decrease in anxiety as evidenced by ability to verbalize understanding of procedures involved and use of positive coping skills to reduce anxious state.

Interventions: *Minimizing Anxiety*

- Provide a clear explanation of the labor induction process *to provide client and partner with a knowledge base.*
- Maintain continuous physical presence *to provide physical and emotional support and demonstrate concern for maternal and fetal well-being.*
- Explain each procedure before carrying it out and answer questions *to promote understanding of procedure and rationale for use and decrease fear of the unknown.*
- Review with client measures used in the past to deal with stressful situations *to determine*

effectiveness; encourage use of past effective coping strategies *to aid in controlling anxiety.*
- Instruct client's partner in helpful measures to assist client in coping and encourage their use *to foster joint participation in the process and feelings of being in control and to provide support to the client.*
- Offer frequent reassurance of fetal status and labor progress *to help alleviate client's concerns and foster continued participation in the labor process.*

NURSING DIAGNOSIS: Risk for injury (maternal or fetal) related to induction procedure risk factors: hypertonic uterine contractions, potential preterm birth as evidenced by client's concerns about fetal well-being and possible adverse effects of oxytocin administration.

Outcome Identification and Evaluation

The client will remain free of complications associated with induction as evidenced by progression of labor as expected, delivery of healthy newborn, and absence of signs and symptoms of maternal and fetal adverse effects.

Interventions: *Promoting Maternal and Fetal Safety*

- Follow agency's protocol for medication use and infusion rate *to ensure accurate, safe drug administration.*
- Set up oxytocin IV infusion to piggyback into the primary IV infusion line *to allow for prompt discontinuation should adverse effects occur.*
- Use an infusion pump *to deliver accurate dose as ordered.*
- Gradually increase oxytocin dose in increments based on assessment findings and protocol *to promote effective uterine contractions.*

NURSING CARE PLAN 21.1

Overview of the Women Undergoing Labor Induction (continued)

- Maintain oxytocin rate once desired frequency of contractions has been reached *to ensure continued progress in labor.*
- Accurately monitor contractions for frequency, duration, and intensity and resting tone *to prevent development of hypertonic contractions.*
- Maintain a nurse-to-client ratio of 1:2 *to ensure maternal and fetal safety.*
- Monitor FHR via electronic fetal monitoring during induction and continuously observe the FHR response to titrated medication rate *to ensure fetal well-being and identify adverse effects immediately.*
- Obtain maternal vital signs every 1 to 2 hours or as indicated by agency's protocol, reporting any deviations, *to promote maternal well-being and allow for prompt detection of problems.*
- Communicate with birth attendant frequently concerning progress *to ensure continuity of care.*
- Discontinue oxytocin infusion if tetanic contractions (>90 seconds), uterine hyperstimulation (<2 minutes apart), elevated uterine resting tone, or a distressed FHR pattern occurs *to minimize risk of drug's adverse effects.*
- Provide client with frequent reassurance of maternal and fetal status *to minimize anxiety.*

NURSING DIAGNOSIS: Pain related to uterine contractions as evidenced by client's statements about contractions increasing in intensity and expected effect of oxytocin administration

Outcome Identification and Evaluation

The client will report a decrease in pain as evidenced by statements of increased comfort and pain rating of 3 or less on numeric pain rating scale.

Interventions: *Promoting Maternal and Fetal Safety*

- Explain to the client that she will experience discomfort sooner than with naturally occurring labor *to promote client's awareness of events and prepare client for the experience.*
- Frequently assess client's pain using a pain rating scale *to quantify client's level of pain and evaluate effectiveness of pain relief measures.*
- Provide comfort measures, such as hygiene, backrubs, music, and distraction, and encourage the use of breathing and relaxation techniques *to help promote relaxation.*
- Provide support for her partner *to aid in alleviating stress and concerns.*
- Employ nonpharmacologic methods, such as position changes, birthing ball, hydrotherapy, visual imagery, and effleurage, *to help in managing pain and foster feelings of control over situation.*
- Administer pharmacologic agents such as analgesia or anesthesia as appropriate and as ordered *to control pain.*
- Continuously reassess client's pain level *to evaluate effectiveness of pain management techniques used.*

nursing information should be given to the nursery nurse regarding the laboring experience? With such a lengthy labor, what assessments might the postpartum nurse need to focus on for the first few hours after birth?

VAGINAL BIRTH AFTER CESAREAN

Vaginal birth after cesarean (VBAC) describes a woman who gives birth vaginally after having at least one previous cesarean birth. Despite evidence that some women who have had a cesarean birth are candidates for vaginal birth, most women who have had a cesarean birth once undergo another for subsequent pregnancies.

A multidisciplinary guideline group representing family medicine, epidemiology, obstetrics, and midwifery developed recommendations based on high-quality systematic evidence-based, peer-reviewed research, that individual assessment of risks and benefits be discussed with the pregnant woman with a history of one or more prior cesarean births who are deciding between a planned VBAC or a repeat cesarean birth. A planned VBAC is an appropriate option for most women with a history of prior cesarean birth (King et al., 2015).

Contraindications to VBAC include a prior classic uterine incision, prior transfundal uterine surgery (myomectomy), uterine scar other than low-transverse cesarean scar, contracted pelvis, and inadequate staff or facility if an emergency cesarean birth in the event of uterine rupture is required (Caughey, 2014b). Most women go through a trial of labor to see how they progress, but this must be performed in an environment capable of handling the emergency of uterine rupture. The use of cervical ripening agents increases the risk of uterine rupture and thus is contraindicated in VBAC clients. The woman considering induction of labor after a previous cesarean birth needs to be informed of the risks versus benefits with an induction than with spontaneous labor (Scott, 2015).

Women are the primary decision makers about the choice of birth method, but they need education about VBAC during their prenatal course. Management is similar for any women experiencing labor, but certain areas require special focus:

• *Consent:* Fully informed consent is essential for the woman who wants to have a trial of labor after cesarean birth. The client must be advised about the risks as well as the benefits. She must understand the ramifications of uterine rupture, even though the risk is small.
• *Documentation:* Record keeping is an important component of safe client care. If and when an emergency occurs, it is imperative to take care of the client, but also to keep track of the plan of care, interventions and their timing, and the client's response. Events and activities can be written right on the fetal monitoring tracing to correlate with the change in fetal status.
• *Surveillance:* A distressed fetal monitor tracing in a woman undergoing a trial of labor after a cesarean birth should alert the nurse to the possibility of uterine rupture. Terminal bradycardia must be considered an emergency situation, and the nurse should prepare the team for an emergency delivery.
• *Readiness for emergency:* According to ACOG (2010), criteria for a safe trial of labor for a woman who has had a previous cesarean birth, the physician, anesthesia provider, and operating room team must be immediately available. Anything less would place the women and fetus at risk.

Women and their health care providers are advised to consider VBAC in the context of potential risk, available resources, and the health care system. The ACOG (2010) guidelines state that VBACs are safe and appropriate for most women, but emphasize the need for thorough counseling, shared decision making, and client autonomy. Nurses must act as advocates, giving input on the appropriate selection of women who wish to undergo VBAC. Nurses also need to become experts at reading fetal monitoring tracings to identify fetal distress and set in motion an emergency birth. Including all of these nursing strategies will make VBAC safer for all.

INTRAUTERINE FETAL DEMISE

Pregnancy and childbirth are associated with hopes, expectations, joy, and happiness for the future. When an unborn life suddenly ends with fetal loss, the family members are profoundly affected. Intrauterine fetal demise (IUFD) is fetal death that occurs after 20 weeks of gestation but before birth. The cause of IUFD is often unknown. The sudden loss of an expected child is tragic and the family's grief can be very intense: it can last for years and can cause extreme psychological stress and emotional problems (Sousou & Smart, 2015). The family's anticipation of a joyous birth is supplanted by despair, confusion, and loss. To women and their families who have gone through this harrowing experience, culturally appropriate and sensitive care is crucial. Particularly for the mother, fetal death in the last trimester of pregnancy, when she feels very close to the fetus due to its frequent movement in the uterus, must be similar to losing a part of her body.

Fetal demise can be due to an extensive range of risk factors and possible causes, such as post-term pregnancy, renal disease, substance abuse, infection, hypertension, advanced maternal age, multiple gestation, Rh disease, uterine rupture, diabetes, congenital anomalies, obesity, smoking, cord accident, abruption, blunt trauma, premature rupture of membranes, or hemorrhage—or it may go unexplained (Hugin & Sultani, 2015). Trauma in pregnancy remains one of the major contributors to maternal and fetal morbidity and mortality. Potential complications include maternal injury or death, shock, internal hemorrhage, intrauterine fetal demise, direct fetal injury, abruptio placentae, and uterine rupture. The leading causes of obstetric trauma are motor vehicle accidents, falls, assaults, and gunshots, and ensuing injuries are classified as blunt abdominal trauma, pelvic fractures, or penetrating trauma. In view of the significant impact of trauma on the pregnant woman and her fetus, preventive strategies are paramount (Kilpatrick, 2014).

Early pregnancy loss may be through a spontaneous abortion (miscarriage), an induced abortion (therapeutic abortion), or a ruptured ectopic pregnancy. A wide spectrum of feelings may be expressed, from relief to sadness and despair. A fetal death can occur at any gestational age, and typically there is little or no warning other than reduced fetal movement. The effects of childbearing loss may affect women and their families for a lifetime. The need to reflect, share, and regain strength is universal for all families dealing with loss. Grief, the typical response to the loss of a valued object, is not an intellectual response. Rather, it is personally experienced as a deep emotion of sadness and sorrow. Feelings such as helplessness, disbelief, unreality, and powerlessness are common. Emotional recovery from the pain of perinatal loss occurs with time, but it varies with each couple.

The moment that fetal death is diagnosed can frequently be described very clearly and in detail by most women. In many cases, the death was sudden, and women have no chance to prepare for the impending grief. Once IUFD is confirmed, most women choose to immediately undergo induction of labor. Approximately 90% of women will go into spontaneous labor within two weeks of fetal death (Green, 2016). With the death of a fetus or neonate, a couple's dreams and hopes for their expected child suddenly dissolve. To women who have experienced a sudden fetal death, the following processes may take place: experiencing a quiet birth without the infant, eclipsed by emptiness, anger, anxiety, loneliness, and sorrow; living without their infant, making it very difficult to see others with young infants; and experiencing differences with their partner over the loss (Callister, 2014). The process of grieving a death is not completed within a specific time frame, and for some, it is never complete. In general, the grief accompanying the loss of a fetus proceeds in the following order:

1. Accepting the reality of the loss
2. Getting over suffering from the loss
3. Adapting to the new environment without the deceased
4. Emotionally relocating the deceased and getting on with life (Grunebaum & Chervenak, 2014)

The period following a fetal death is extremely difficult for the family. For many women, emotional healing takes much longer than physical healing. The feelings of loss can be intense. The grief response in some women may be so great that their relationships become strained, and healing can become hampered unless appropriate interventions and support are provided.

Fetal death also affects the health care staff. Despite the trauma that the loss of a fetus causes, some staff members avoid dealing with the bereaved family, never talking about or acknowledging their grief. This seems to imply that not discussing the problem will allow the grief to dissolve and vanish. As a result, the family's needs go unrecognized. Failing to keep the lines of communication open with a bereaved client and her family closes off some of the channels to recovery and healing that may be desperately needed. Subsequently, the bereaved family members may feel isolated.

Nursing Assessment

A woman experiencing an IUFD is likely to seek care when she notices that the fetus is not moving or when she experiences contractions, loss of fluid, or vaginal bleeding. History and physical examination frequently are of limited value in the diagnosis of fetal death, since many times the only history tends to be recent absence of fetal movement and no fetal heart beat heard. An inability to obtain fetal heart sounds on examination suggests fetal demise, but an ultrasound is necessary to confirm the absence of fetal cardiac activity. Once fetal demise is confirmed, induction of labor or expectant management is offered to the woman.

Nursing Management

IUFD is associated with posttraumatic stress disorder (PTSD) and anxiety in a subsequent pregnancy (Robinson, 2014). The nurse can play a major role in assisting the grieving family. Nurses who can deal honestly with their own feelings regarding loss will be better able to help others cope with theirs. By working with couples who have suffered a significant loss, the nurse can grow personally and professionally and gain a deeper perspective about life. With skillful intervention, the bereaved family may be better prepared to resolve their grief and move forward.

To assist families in the grieving process, include the following measures:

- Provide accurate, understandable information to the family.
- Acknowledge that the woman's feeling of loss is legitimate.
- Reassure mother that there was likely nothing that she could have done to prevent it.
- Be knowledgeable about the grief process and comfortable in sharing another's grief.
- Utilize active listening to provide needed encouragement to the family members to open up to their feelings.
- Create a warm, receptive, accepting, and caring environment conducive to dialogue.
- Dispel guilt by saying that nothing the woman did caused the fetal death.
- Acknowledge their grief by saying that their feeling sad is appropriate.
- Recognize that each family member may express their grief differently.
- Provide reassurance about successful future pregnancies.
- Encourage discussion of the loss and venting of feelings of grief and guilt.
- Provide the family with baby mementos and pictures to validate the reality of death.

- Allow unlimited time with the stillborn infant after birth to validate the death; provide time for the family members to be together and grieve; offer the family the opportunity to see, touch, and hold the infant.
- Use appropriate touch, such as holding a hand or touching a shoulder.
- Inform the chaplain or the religious leader of the family's denomination about the death and request his or her presence.
- Assist the parents with the funeral arrangements or disposition of the body.
- Provide the parents with brochures offering advice about how to talk to other siblings about the loss.
- Refer the family to the support group SHARE Pregnancy and Infant Loss Support, Inc., which is designed for those who have lost an infant through abortion, miscarriage, fetal death, stillbirth, or other tragic circumstances.
- Make community referrals to promote a continuum of care after discharge.

Openness to talking with couples about their loss and grief is the basis for support provided by nurses, which can have a positive influence on the long-term adjustment of couples and families coping with perinatal loss. A sensitive nurse who is comfortable talking about loss and is able to assist couples in navigating the process of grief provides a starting point for preparation for future pregnancy. Couples need to talk about their loss, its meaning, and the emotions that accompany it while the nurse listens. Nurses play a significant role in linking women and men to appropriate professional support. As couples move through their grief and begin to consider another pregnancy, sensitive nursing care may mediate the understandable anxiety and concern that accompany this process. Nurses are a vital part of the interdisciplinary health care team caring for families with IUFD, who continue to require timely and sensitive care throughout the grieving process.

WOMEN EXPERIENCING AN OBSTETRIC EMERGENCY

Obstetric emergencies are challenging to all labor and birth personnel because of the increased risk of adverse outcomes for the mother and fetus. Quick clinical judgment and good critical decision making will increase the odds of a positive outcome for both mother and fetus. This section discusses a few of these emergencies: umbilical cord prolapse, placenta previa, placental abruption, uterine rupture, and amniotic fluid embolism.

Umbilical Cord Prolapse

Umbilical cord prolapse is a rare obstetrical emergency that occurs when the cord precedes the fetus out. An **umbilical cord prolapse** is the protrusion of the umbilical cord alongside (occult) or ahead of the presenting part of the fetus (Fig. 21.5). This condition occurs in 1 out of every 300 births and requires prompt recognition and intervention for a positive outcome (March of Dimes, 2015c). Cord prolapse occurs in 3% of deliveries when the fetus is in the vertex position and in 3.7% of deliveries when the fetus is in the breech position. The risk is increased further when the presenting part does not fill the lower uterine segment, as is the case with incomplete breech presentations (5% to 10%), premature infants, and multiparous women (Bush, Eddleman, & Belogolovkin, 2015). With a 50% perinatal mortality rate, it is one of the most catastrophic events in the intrapartum period (Beall & Ross, 2014).

Pathophysiology

Prolapse usually leads to total or partial occlusion of the cord. Since this is the fetus's only lifeline, fetal perfusion deteriorates rapidly. Complete occlusion renders the

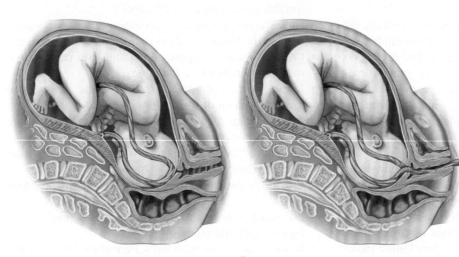

A **B**

FIGURE 21.5 Prolapsed cord. **A.** Prolapse within the uterus. **B.** Prolapse with the cord visible at the vulva.

fetus helpless and oxygen deprived. The fetus will die if the cord compression is not relieved.

Nursing Assessment

Prevention is the key to managing cord prolapse by identifying clients at risk for this condition. Carefully assess each client to help predict her risk status. Be aware that cord prolapse is more common in pregnancies involving malpresentation, growth restriction, prematurity, ruptured membranes with a fetus at a high station, hydramnios, grandmultiparity, and multiple gestation (Cunningham et al., 2014). Continuously assess the client and fetus to detect changes and to evaluate the effectiveness of any interventions performed.

Take Note!

When the presenting part does not fully occupy the pelvic inlet, prolapse is more likely to occur.

Nursing Management

Prompt recognition of a prolapsed cord is essential to reduce the risk of fetal hypoxia resulting from prolonged cord compression. Often the first sign of cord prolapse is a sudden fetal bradycardia or recurrent variable decelerations that become progressively more severe. Call for help immediately and do not leave the woman. Inform the woman of what is happening and what options may be discussed by her health care provider. When membranes are artificially ruptured, assist with verifying that the presenting part is well applied to the cervix and engaged into the pelvis. If pressure or compression of the cord occurs, assist with measures to relieve the compression. Typically, the examiner places a sterile gloved hand into the vagina and holds the presenting part off the umbilical cord until delivery. Changing the woman's position to a modified Sims, Trendelenburg, or knee–chest position also helps relieve cord pressure. Do not attempt to replace the cord in the uterus. Monitor fetal heart rate, maintain bed rest, and administer oxygen if ordered. Provide emotional support and explanations as to what is going on to allay the woman's fears and anxiety. If the mother's cervix is not fully dilated, prepare the woman for an emergency cesarean birth to save the fetus's life if that is the intervention planned for by her health care provider.

Placenta Previa

Placenta previa is placental implantation in the lower uterine segment over or near the internal os of the cervix, typically during the second or third trimester of pregnancy. With uterine segment formation and cervical dilation, placental implantation over or near the cervical os, instead of along the uterine wall, inevitably results in spontaneous placental separation—and subsequent hemorrhage. This position can create a barrier for the fetus from the uterus during the birthing process. As the cervix begins to thin and dilate (open up) in preparation for labor, blood vessels that connect the placenta to the uterus may tear and cause bleeding. It is the most common cause of bleeding in the second half of pregnancy and should be suspected in any woman beyond 24 weeks of gestation presenting with vaginal bleeding; ultrasonography (e.g., transvaginal) is used to diagnose it. During labor and birth, bleeding can be severe, which can place the mother and fetus at risk. Reported incidence is approximately 1 in 200 births (March of Dimes, 2015d).

There is a direct relationship between the number of previous cesarean births and the risk of placenta previa, probably due to uterine scarring. The degree of occlusion of the internal cervical os may depend on the degree of cervical dilation, so what may appear to be a low-lying or marginal placenta previa prior to the onset of labor can progress to become more serious as the cervix effaces and opens up (King et al., 2015).

The incidence of maternal mortality is less than 1%, but common morbidities include septicemia, renal failure, hemorrhage and hypovolemic shock, invasive placenta (accrete, increta, and percreta), and postpartum anemia. Risk factors for placenta previa include previous cesarean section, advanced maternal age > 34, multiparity, multiple gestation, prior placenta previa, and cigarette smoking. The risk for perinatal mortality is less than 10%, but common neonatal morbidities include stillbirth, prematurity, malpresentation, fetal growth restriction, and fetal anemia (Joy & Finneran, 2015).

Maternal signs and symptoms of placenta previa include sudden, painless bleeding (that may be heavy enough to be considered hemorrhaging), anemia, pallor, hypoxia, low blood pressure, tachycardia, soft and nontender uterus, and rapid, weak pulse. Bleeding may be episodic, with spontaneous initiation and cessation; in some cases, it is asymptomatic because there is intrauterine bleeding only without external signs.

Management of placenta previa varies by type and gestational age, and frequent medical surveillance may be sufficient in marginal cases; prompt treatment with bed rest, close monitoring, and control/replacement of blood loss greatly reduces risk for maternal and fetal complications and death. Vaginal delivery is possible when bleeding is minimal, placenta previa is marginal, or labor is rapid. Pregnancy termination, early birth by cesarean section, or a hysterectomy may be necessary in order to control severe bleeding, especially for clients with complete placenta previa. The overall maternal prognosis is good if hemorrhage is controlled and sepsis or other complications are prevented. Fetal prognosis is directly related to the amount of blood loss. The United States perinatal mortality rate associated with placental previa is 2% to 3%, and the maternal mortality rate is 0.03%. Risk for placenta previa recurrence in subsequent pregnancies is 4% to 8% (Lal & Hibbard, 2015).

Nursing management within the acute care setting includes the following: monitor maternal vital signs, intake and output, vaginal bleeding, and physiologic status for signs of hemorrhage, shock, or infection; closely monitor fetal heart tones for distress (e.g., bradycardia, tachycardia, baseline changes); and treat fetal distress, as ordered. Administer prescribed intravenous fluids, packed red blood cells platelets, and frozen plasma for transfusion, if ordered; Rho(D) immune globulin, if the client is Rh negative; intravenous-augmented oxytocin (Pitocin) to induce labor, if needed; and in cases of preterm labor, tocolytics (e.g., magnesium sulfate) to inhibit uterine contractions and corticosteroids (e.g., betamethasone) to enhance fetal lung maturity. Follow facility pre- and postsurgical protocols if woman becomes a surgical candidate (e.g., for cesarean section); reinforce pre- and postsurgical education and ensure completion of facility's informed consent documents; closely monitor postsurgically for bleeding, infection, and other complications; assess client's anxiety level and coping ability; and provide emotional support and reassurance.

Frequently there is expectant management for the woman after her first placenta previa bleed if it isn't severe and fetus well-being is validated. After she is assessed, she is released to go home. It is common for women to experience an initial bleeding episode, which then subsides. These women are monitored at home and instructed to report any additional bleeding episodes and come in to be evaluated (King et al., 2015).

Placental Abruption

Placental abruption refers to premature separation of a normally implanted placenta from the maternal myometrium. Placental abruption occurs in about 1% of all pregnancies throughout the world and is associated with significant perinatal mortality and morbidity (March of Dimes, 2015e). Risk factors include preeclampsia, gestational hypertension, seizure activity, advanced maternal age >34, uterine rupture, trauma, smoking, cocaine use, coagulation defects, chorioamnionitis, premature rupture of membranes, hydramnios, uterine trauma, external cephalic version for breech presentation, previous history of abruption, domestic violence, and placental pathology. These conditions may force blood into the underlayer of the placenta and cause it to detach (Deering, 2015).

Management of placental abruption depends on the gestational age, the extent of the hemorrhage, and maternal–fetal oxygenation perfusion/reserve status (see Chapter 19 for additional information on abruptio placentae). Treatment is based on the circumstances. Typically once the diagnosis is established, the focus is on maintaining the cardiovascular status of the mother and developing a plan to deliver the fetus quickly. A cesarean birth may take place quickly if the fetus is still alive with only a partial abruption. A vaginal birth may take place if there is fetal demise secondary to a complete abruption.

Uterine Rupture

Uterine rupture in pregnancy is a rare and often catastrophic complication with a high incidence of fetal and maternal morbidity. Uterine rupture is a catastrophic tearing of the uterus at the site of a previous scar into the abdominal cavity. Its onset is often marked only by sudden fetal bradycardia, and treatment requires rapid surgery for good outcomes. From the time of diagnosis to delivery, only 10 to 30 minutes are available before clinically significant fetal morbidity occurs. Fetal morbidity occurs secondary to catastrophic hemorrhage, fetal anoxia, or both.

Nursing Assessment

Review the mother's history for risk conditions such as uterine scars, prior cesarean births, prior rupture, trauma, prior invasive molar pregnancy, history of placenta percreta or increta, congenital uterine anomalies, multiparity, previous uterine myomectomy, malpresentation, labor induction with excessive uterine stimulation, and crack cocaine use (Nahum & Pham, 2015). Reviewing a client's history for risk factors might prove to be lifesaving for both mother and fetus.

Generally, the first and most reliable symptom of uterine rupture is sudden fetal distress. Other signs may include acute and continuous abdominal pain with or without an epidural, vaginal bleeding, hematuria, irregular abdominal wall contour, loss of station in the fetal presenting part, and hypovolemic shock in the woman, fetus, or both (Scott, 2015).

Timely management of uterine rupture depends on prompt detection. Because many women desire a trial of labor after a previous cesarean birth, the nurse must be familiar with the signs and symptoms of uterine rupture. It is difficult to prevent uterine rupture or to predict which women will experience rupture, so constant preparedness is necessary. Screening all women with previous uterine surgical scars is important, and continuous electronic fetal monitoring should be used during labor because this may provide the only indication of an impending rupture.

Nursing Management

Because the presenting signs may be nonspecific, the initial management will be the same as that for any other cause of acute fetal distress. Urgent delivery by cesarean birth is usually indicated. Monitor maternal vital signs and observe for hypotension and tachycardia, which might indicate hypovolemic shock. Assist in preparing for an emergency cesarean birth by alerting the operating room staff, anesthesia provider, and neonatal team. Insert an indwelling urinary (Foley) catheter if one is not in place already. Inform the woman of the seriousness of this event and remind her that the health care staff will be working quickly to ensure her health and that of her fetus. Remain calm and provide reassurance that everything is being done to ensure a safe outcome for both.

The life-threatening nature of uterine rupture is underscored by the fact that the maternal circulatory system delivers approximately 500 mL of blood to the term uterus every minute (Cunningham et al., 2014). Maternal death is a real possibility without rapid intervention. Newborn outcome after rupture depends largely on the speed with which surgical rescue is carried out. As in any case of acute obstetric emergency, preparation and timely mobilization of all necessary personnel is essential to optimizing outcome.

Take Note!

When excessive bleeding occurs during the childbirth process and it persists or signs such as bruising or petechiae appear, disseminated intravascular coagulation (DIC) should be suspected.

Amniotic Fluid Embolism

Amniotic fluid embolism (AFE) is an unforeseeable, life-threatening complication of childbirth. Amniotic fluid embolism remains an enigmatic, but devastating obstetric condition associated with significant maternal and newborn morbidity and mortality. It is a rare and often fatal event characterized by the sudden onset of hypotension, hypoxia, and coagulopathy. Amniotic fluid containing particles of debris (e.g., hair, skin, vernix, or meconium) enters the maternal circulation and obstructs the pulmonary vessels, causing respiratory distress and circulatory collapse (Sadera & Vasudevan, 2015). Prediction and diagnosis of the event are nearly impossible. However, timely recognition and response is critical in saving a woman's life. Although estimates vary, amniotic fluid embolism, also referred to as anaphylactoid syndrome of pregnancy, occurs in from 1 in 15,000 births, with a reported mortality rate reaching 60% despite technological advances in critical care life support (Moore, 2015).

Pathophysiology

The pathophysiology appears to involve an abnormal maternal response to fetal tissue exposure associated with breaches of the maternal-fetal physiologic barrier during the postpartum period. Normally, amniotic fluid does not enter the maternal circulation because it is contained within the uterus, sealed off by the amniotic

sac. An embolus occurs when the barrier between the maternal circulation and the amniotic fluid is broken and amniotic fluid enters the maternal venous system via the endocervical veins, the placental site (if the placenta is separated), or a site of uterine trauma. This condition has a high mortality rate: as many as 50% of women die within the first hour after the onset of symptoms, and about 85% of survivors have permanent hypoxia-induced neurologic damage (Sadera & Vasudevan, 2015).

Although medical science has supplied many answers to questions about this condition, health care providers remain largely unable to predict or prevent an amniotic fluid embolism or to decrease its mortality rate.

Nursing Assessment

Predisposing factors associated with amniotic fluid embolism include placental abruption, uterine over distention, fetal demise, uterine trauma, oxytocin-stimulated labor, amnioinfusion, multiparity, advanced maternal age, and ruptured membranes. However, many women present without any of the risk factors.

Nurses must stay a step ahead and be prepared at all times in this obstetric emergency. A team response is essential because every person will be needed. No test can diagnose an amniotic fluid embolism. Therefore, the nurse's assessment skills are critical. Immediate recognition and diagnosis of this condition are essential to improve maternal and fetal outcomes. Until recently, the diagnosis could be made only after an autopsy of the mother revealed squamous cells, lanugo hair, or other fetal and amniotic material in the pulmonary arterial vasculature (Baldisseri, 2014).

The clinical appearance is varied, but most women report difficulty breathing. Other symptoms include hypotension, cyanosis, hypoxemia, uterine atony, seizures, tachycardia, coagulation failure, disseminated intravascular coagulation (DIC), pulmonary edema, seizures, uterine atony with subsequent hemorrhage, adult respiratory distress syndrome, and cardiac arrest (Viswanathan, Venkateswaran, & Daniel, 2014).

Take Note!

Amniotic fluid embolism should be suspected in any pregnant women with an acute onset of dyspnea, hypotension, and DIC. By knowing how to intervene, the nurse can promote a better chance of survival for both the mother and her newborn. Most women are transferred to the intensive care unit.

Nursing Management

Upon recognizing the signs and symptoms of this life-threatening diagnosis, institute supportive measures: oxygenation (resuscitation and 100% oxygen), circulation (intravenous fluids, inotropic agents to maintain cardiac output and blood pressure), control of hemorrhage and coagulopathy (oxytocic agents to control uterine atony and bleeding), seizure precautions, and administration of steroids to control the inflammatory response. Monitor vital signs, pulse oximetry, skin color, and temperature and observe for clinical signs of coagulopathy (vaginal bleeding, bleeding from intravenous site, bleeding from gums) (Moses, 2015).

Care is largely supportive and aimed at maintaining oxygenation and hemodynamic function and correcting coagulopathy. There is no specific therapy that is lifesaving once this condition starts. Adequate oxygenation is necessary, with endotracheal intubation and mechanical ventilation for most women. Vasopressors are used to maintain hemodynamic stability. Management of DIC may involve replacement with packed red blood cells or fresh-frozen plasma as necessary. Oxytocin infusions and prostaglandin analogs can be used to address uterine atony.

Explain to the client and family what is happening and what therapies are being instituted. The woman is usually transferred to a critical care unit for intensive observation and care. Assist the family to express their feelings and provide support as needed. Inform and reassure the woman and family as much as possible during this crisis.

WOMEN REQUIRING BIRTH-RELATED PROCEDURES

Many women can give birth without the need for any operative obstetric interventions. Most do not anticipate the need for any medical intervention. However, in some situations interventions are necessary to safeguard the health of the mother and fetus. The most common birth-related procedures are amnioinfusion, forceps-assisted or vacuum-assisted birth, cesarean birth, episiotomy (see Chapter 14), and vaginal birth following a previous cesarean birth (see section earlier in this chapter). Nurses play a major role in helping couples to cope with any unanticipated procedures by offering thorough explanations of the procedure, its anticipated benefits and risks, and any other options available.

Amnioinfusion

Amnioinfusion is a technique in which a volume of warmed, sterile, normal saline or Ringer's lactate solution is introduced into the uterus transcervically through an intrauterine pressure catheter to increase the volume of fluid when oligohydramnios is present. It is a procedure used during labor. It is used to change the relationship of the uterus, placenta, cord, and fetus to improve placental and fetal oxygenation. Instilling an isotonic glucose-free solution into the uterus helps to cushion the umbilical cord to prevent compression or dilute thick meconium.

Studies support the use of this procedure a safe and effective in resolving FHR decelerations (Hofmeyr, Eke, & Lawrie, 2014).

This procedure is commonly indicated for severe variable decelerations due to cord compression, oligohydramnios due to placental insufficiency, postmaturity or rupture of membranes, preterm labor with premature rupture of membranes, and thick meconium fluid. However, it does not prevent meconium aspiration syndrome (Hofmeyr, Xu, & Eke, 2014). Contraindications to amnioinfusion include vaginal bleeding of unknown origin, umbilical cord prolapse, amnionitis, uterine hypertonicity, and severe fetal distress (Fong et al., 2014).

There is no standard protocol for amnioinfusion; nurses should follow their own institution protocols. After obtaining informed consent, a vaginal examination is performed to evaluate for cord prolapse, establish dilation, and confirm presentation. Next, 250 to 500 mL of warmed normal saline or lactated Ringer's solution is administered using an infusion pump over 20 to 30 minutes. Overdistention of the uterus is a risk, so the amount of fluid infused must be monitored closely. Amnioinfusion should reach therapeutic result or increase the amniotic fluid volume in approximately 30 minutes (Mattson & Smith, 2016).

When caring for the woman who is receiving an amnioinfusion, include the following:

- Explain the need for the procedure, what it involves, and how it may solve the problem.
- Inform the mother that she will need to remain on bed rest during the procedure.
- Assess the mother's vital signs and associated discomfort level.
- Maintain intake and output records.
- Assess the duration and intensity of uterine contractions frequently to identify overdistention or increased uterine tone.
- Assess for fluid leakage by evaluating the chuck or pad under the woman to determine that it is not being retained in the uterus, which could lead to increased uterine pressure.
- Monitor the FHR pattern to determine whether the amnioinfusion is improving the fetal status.
- Prepare the mother for a possible cesarean birth if the FHR does not improve after the amnioinfusion.

Forceps- or Vacuum-Assisted Birth

Forceps or a vacuum extractor may be used to apply traction to the fetal head or to provide a method of rotating the fetal head during birth. **Forceps** are stainless-steel instruments, similar to tongs, with rounded edges that fit around the fetus's head. Some forceps have open blades and some have solid blades. Outlet forceps are used when the fetal head is crowning and low forceps are used when the fetal head is at a +2 station or lower

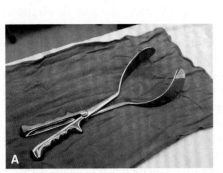
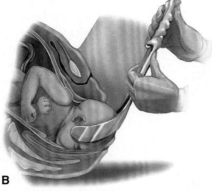
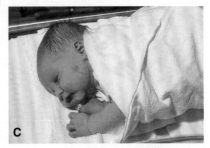

FIGURE 21.6 Forceps delivery (uncommon). **A.** Example of forceps. **B.** Forceps being applied to the fetus. **C.** Forceps marks are commonly found in newborns delivered by forceps. Such marks are transient and disappear in a day or two.

but not yet crowning. The forceps are applied to the sides of the fetal head. The type of forceps used is determined by the birth attendant. All forceps have a locking mechanism that prevents the blades from compressing the fetal skull. Use of forceps has declined in popularity recently because many obstetricians are not trained to use them in their residency since they are rarely used in obstetrical practice today (Fig. 21.6).

A **vacuum extractor** is a cup-shaped instrument attached to a suction pump used for extraction of the fetal head (Fig. 21.7). The suction cup is placed against the occiput of the fetal head. The pump is used to create negative pressure (suction) of approximately 50 to 60 mm Hg. The birth attendant then applies traction until the fetal head emerges from the vagina.

The indications for the use of either method are similar and include a prolonged second stage of labor, a distressed FHR pattern, failure of the presenting part to fully rotate and descend in the pelvis, limited sensation and inability to push effectively due to the effects of regional anesthesia, presumed fetal jeopardy or fetal

distress, maternal heart disease, acute pulmonary edema, intrapartum infection, maternal fatigue, or infection. There is a clear trend to choose vacuum extraction over forceps to assist delivery, but the evidence supporting that trend is unconvincing. Recent literature confirms some advantages for forceps (e.g., a lower failure rate) and some disadvantages for vacuum extraction (e.g., increased neonatal injury), depending on the clinical circumstances (O'Grady & St. Andre, 2015).

The use of forceps or a vacuum extractor poses the risk of tissue trauma to the mother and the newborn. Maternal trauma may include lacerations of the cervix, vagina, or perineum; hematoma; extension of the episiotomy incision into the anus; hemorrhage; and infection. Potential newborn trauma includes ecchymoses, facial and scalp lacerations, facial nerve injury, cephalhematoma, and caput succedaneum (Cunningham et al., 2014). For forceps or a vacuum extractor to be applied, the following criteria need to be met: membranes ruptured, cervix completely dilated, fetus vertex and engaged, and an adequate maternal pelvis size.

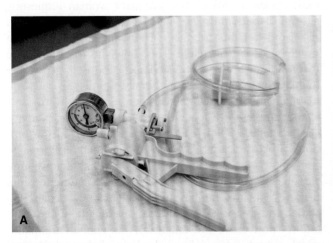
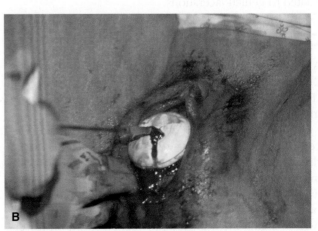

FIGURE 21.7 Vacuum extractor for delivery. **A.** Example of a vacuum extractor. **B.** Vacuum extractor applied to the fetal head to assist in delivery.

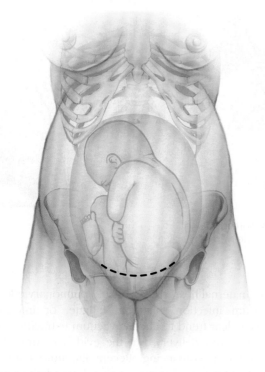

FIGURE 21.8 Low transverse incision for cesarean birth.

Prevention is the key to reducing the use of these techniques. Preventive measures include frequently changing the client's position, encouraging ambulation if permitted, frequently reminding the client to empty her bladder to allow maximum space for birth, and providing adequate hydration throughout labor. Additional measures include assessing maternal vital signs, the contraction pattern, the fetal status, and the maternal response to the procedure. Provide a thorough explanation of the procedure and the rationale for its use. Reassure the mother that any marks or swelling on the newborn's head or face will disappear without treatment within 2 to 3 days. Alert the postpartum nursing staff about the use of the technique so that they can observe for any bleeding or infection related to genital lacerations.

Cesarean Birth

A **cesarean birth** is the surgical birth of the fetus through an incision in the abdomen and uterine wall (Fig. 21.8) and is the most commonly performed surgery in the United States (Green, 2016).

High cesarean birth rates are an international concern. The cesarean birth rate in the United States is on the rise at an alarming rate. Today, approximately 33% or one in three births occurs this way. This is the 14th consecutive year the cesarean birth rate has risen, despite a number of medical organizations, including the WHO and ACOG, urging medical care providers to work on lowering the cesarean birth rate (Centers for Disease Control and Prevention, 2015). Cesarean births may result from

maternal, fetal, or placental factors that interfere with a vaginal birth. Several factors may explain this increased incidence of cesarean deliveries: the use of electronic fetal monitoring, which identifies fetal distress early; the reduced number of forceps-assisted births; older maternal age and reduced parity; increasing maternal obesity, with more nulliparous women having infants; convenience to the client and doctor; and an increase in malpractice suits. The leading indications for cesarean births are previous cesarean birth, breech presentation, dystocia, and fetal distress. Once a woman has experienced a primary cesarean birth, she has a 90% chance of having another one in a subsequent pregnancy (Joy & Contag, 2015).

Cesarean birth is a major surgical procedure with increased risks compared with a vaginal birth. The client is at risk for complications such as infection, hemorrhage, aspiration, pulmonary embolism, urinary tract trauma, thrombophlebitis, paralytic ileus, and atelectasis. Fetal injury and transient tachypnea of the newborn also may occur (Cunningham et al., 2014).

Spinal, epidural, or general anesthesia is used for cesarean births. Epidural anesthesia is most commonly used because it is associated with less risk and most women wish to be awake and aware of the birth experience.

Nursing Assessment

Review the woman's history for indications associated with cesarean birth and complete a physical examination. Any condition that prevents the safe passage of the fetus through the birth canal or that seriously compromises maternal or fetal well-being may be an indication for a cesarean birth. Controversy exists for the option of elective cesarean birth on maternal request. The Agency for Healthcare Research and Quality (AHRQ) has published a report on personal maternal request for a surgical birth, and although there is no high-quality medical evidence to support this, it is recognized that women have the right to be actively involved in choosing the route of her childbirth (Norwitz, 2015). The pregnant woman requesting a surgical birth must be made aware of the associated risks and benefits for the current and any subsequent pregnancies is reasonable. The clinician's role should be to provide the best evidence-based counseling possible to the woman and to respect her autonomy and decision-making capabilities when considering route of birth.

Examples of specific indications include active genital herpes, fetal macrosomia, fetopelvic disproportion, prolapsed umbilical cord, placental abnormality (placenta previa or abruptio placentae), previous classic uterine incision or scar, gestational hypertension, diabetes, positive human immunodeficiency virus (HIV) status, and dystocia. Fetal indications include malpresentation (nonvertex presentation), congenital anomalies (fetal neural tube defects, hydrocephalus, abdominal wall defects), and fetal distress (Joy & Contag, 2015).

Nursing Management

Once the decision has been made to proceed with a cesarean birth, assess the woman's knowledge of the procedure and necessary preparation. Assist with obtaining diagnostic tests as ordered. These tests are usually ordered to ensure the well-being of both parties and may include a complete blood count; urinalysis to rule out infection; blood type and cross-match so that blood is available for transfusion if needed; an ultrasound to determine fetal position and placental location; and an amniocentesis to determine fetal lung maturity if needed.

Although the nurse's role in a cesarean birth can be very technical and skill oriented at times, the focus must remain on the woman, not the equipment surrounding the bed. Care should be centered on the family, not the surgery. Provide education and minimize separation of the mother, father, and newborn. Remember that the client is anxious and concerned about her welfare as well as that of her child. Use touch, eye contact, therapeutic communication, and genuine caring to provide couples with a positive birth experience, regardless of the type of delivery.

PROVIDING PREOPERATIVE CARE

Client preparation varies depending on whether the cesarean birth is planned or unplanned. The major difference is the time allotted for preparation and teaching. In an unplanned cesarean birth, institute measures quickly to ensure the best outcomes for the mother and fetus. Ensure that the woman has signed an informed consent, and allow for discussion of fears and expectations. Provide essential teaching and explanations to reduce the woman's fears and anxieties.

Ascertain the client's and family's understandings of the surgical procedure. Reinforce the reasons for surgery given by the surgeon. Outline the procedure and expectations of the surgical experience. Ensure that all diagnostic tests ordered have been completed, and evaluate the results. Explain to the woman and her family about what to expect postoperatively. Reassure the woman that pain management will be provided throughout the procedure and afterward. Encourage the woman to report any pain. Ask the woman about the time she last had anything to eat or drink. Document the time and what was consumed. Throughout the preparations, assess maternal and fetal status frequently.

Provide preoperative teaching to reduce the risk of postoperative complications. Demonstrate the use of the incentive spirometer and deep-breathing and leg exercises. Instruct the woman on how to splint her incision.

Complete the preoperative procedures, which may include:

- Preparing the surgical site as ordered
- Starting an intravenous infusion for fluid replacement therapy as ordered
- Inserting an indwelling (Foley) catheter and informing the client about how long it will remain in place (usually 24 hours)
- Administering any preoperative medications as ordered; documenting the time administered and the client's reaction

Maintain a calm, confident manner in all interactions with the client and family. Help transport the client and her partner to the operative area.

PROVIDING POSTOPERATIVE CARE

Postoperative care for the mother who has had a cesarean delivery is similar to that for one who has had a vaginal birth, with a few additional measures. Assess vital signs and lochia flow every 15 minutes for the first hour, then every 30 minutes for the next hour, and then every 4 hours if stable. Assist with perineal care and instruct the client in the same. Inspect the abdominal dressing and document description, including any evidence of drainage. Assess uterine tone to determine fundal firmness. Check the patency of the intravenous line, making sure the infusion is flowing at the correct rate. Inspect the infusion site frequently for redness.

Assess the woman's level of consciousness if sedative drugs were administered. Institute safety precautions until the woman is fully alert and responsive. If a regional anesthetic was used, monitor for the return of sensation to the legs.

Assess for evidence of abdominal distention and auscultate bowel sounds. Assist with early ambulation to prevent respiratory and cardiovascular problems and to promote peristalsis. Monitor intake and output at least every 4 hours initially and then every 8 hours as indicated.

Encourage the woman to cough, perform deep-breathing exercises, and use the incentive spirometer every 2 hours. Enhance comfort and general well-being. Administer analgesics as ordered and provide comfort measures, such as splinting the incision and pillows for positioning. Assist the client to move in bed and turn side to side to improve circulation. Also encourage the woman to ambulate to promote venous return from the extremities. Prevent/minimize postoperative complications.

Encourage early touching and holding of the newborn to promote bonding. Promote family unity and bonding. Assist with breast-feeding initiation and offer continued support. Suggest alternate positioning techniques to reduce incisional discomfort while breast-feeding. (See Chapter 18 for breast-feeding positions.)

Review with the couple their perception of the surgical birth experience. Allow them to verbalize their feelings and assist them in positive coping measures. Promote a positive emotional response to the birth experience and parenting role. Prior to discharge, teach the woman about the need for adequate rest, activity restrictions such as lifting, and signs and symptoms of infection. Provide information about postpartum care at home upon discharge.

KEY CONCEPTS

○ Risk factors for dystocia include epidural analgesia, occiput posterior position, longer first stage of labor, nulliparity, short maternal stature (<5 ft tall), high birth weight, maternal age older than 35 years, gestational age more than 41 weeks, chorioamnionitis, pelvic contractions, macrosomia, and high station at complete cervical dilation.

○ Dystocia may result from problems in the powers, passenger, passageway, or psyche.

○ Problems involving the powers that lead to dystocia include hypertonic uterine dysfunction, hypotonic uterine dysfunction, and precipitate labor.

○ Management of hypertonic labor pattern involves therapeutic rest with the use of sedatives to promote relaxation and stop the abnormal activity of the uterus.

○ Any presentation other than occiput or a slight variation of the fetal position or size increases the probability of dystocia.

○ Multiple pregnancy may result in dysfunctional labor due to uterine overdistention, which may lead to hypotonic dystocia and abnormal presentations of the fetuses.

○ During labor, evaluation of fetal descent, cervical effacement and dilation, and characteristics of uterine contractions are paramount to determine progress or lack thereof.

○ Antepartum assessment for a post-term pregnancy typically includes daily fetal movement counts done by the woman, nonstress tests done twice weekly, amniotic fluid assessments as part of the biophysical profile, and weekly cervical examinations to check for ripening for induction.

○ Once the cervix is ripe, oxytocin is the most popular pharmacologic agent used for inducing or augmenting labor.

○ Generally, the first and most reliable symptom of uterine rupture is fetal distress.

○ Amniotic fluid embolism is a rare but often fatal event characterized by the sudden onset of hypotension, hypoxia, and coagulopathy.

○ Cesarean births have steadily risen in the United States; today, approximately one in three births occurs this way. Cesarean birth is a major surgical procedure and has increased risks over vaginal birth.

References and Recommended Readings

Abbott, D. S., Hezelgrave, N. L., Seed, P. T., Norman, J. E., David, A. L., Bennett, P. R., et al. (2015). Quantitative fetal fibronectin to predict preterm birth in asymptomatic women at high risk. *Obstetrics & Gynecology, 125*(5), 1168–1176.

Afzal, M., Asif, U., & Miraj, B. (2015). Induction of labor; Efficacy of sweeping of membranes at term in previous one C-section. *Professional Medical Journal, 22*(4), 385–389.

Ahmed, Z. D., Garba, I., Nafi'ah, T., & Yakasai, I. A. (2015). Misoprostol: An effective agent for cervical ripening and labor induction: A 2-year review in a tertiary center. *Open Journal of Obstetrics and Gynecology, 5*(05), 274–279.

American Academy of Pediatrics (2015) *Delivery by cesarean section.* Retrieved form http://www.healthychildren.org/English/ages-stages/prenatal/delivery-beyond/pages/Delivery-by-Cesarean-Section.aspx

American Academy of Pediatrics [AAP] and American College of Obstetricians and Gynecologists [ACOG]. (2010). *Guidelines for perinatal care* (6th ed.). Washington, DC: Author.

American College of Obstetricians and Gynecologists [ACOG]. (2010). ACOG practice bulletin no. 115: Vaginal birth after previous cesarean delivery. *Obstetrics and Gynecology, 116*, 450–463.

American College of Obstetricians & Gynecologists [ACOG]. (2014a). Safe prevention of primary cesarean delivery. *American Journal of Obstetrics & Gynecology. 123*(3), 693–711.

American College of Obstetricians & Gynecologists [ACOG]. (2014b). *Preterm labor practice guidelines.* Retrieved from http://www.acog.org/Womens-Health/Preterm-Premature-Labor-and-BirthAmerican

Arrowsmith, S., & Wray, S. (2014). Oxytocin: Its mechanism of action and receptor signaling in the myometrium. *Journal of Neuroendocrinology, 26*(6), 356–369.

Baldisseri, M. R. (2014). Amniotic fluid embolism syndrome. *UpToDate.* Retrieved from http://www.uptodate.com/contents/amniotic-fluid-embolism-syndrome

Beall, M. H., & Ross, M. G. (2014). Umbilical cord complications. *eMedicine.* Retrieved from http://emedicine.medscape.com/article/262470-overview

Bibbo, C., & Robinson, J. N. (2015). Management of twins: Vaginal or cesarean delivery?. *Clinical Obstetrics & Gynecology, 58*(2), 294–308.

Bush, M., Eddleman, K., & Belogovkin, V. (2015). Umbilical cord prolapse. *UpToDate.* Retrieved from http://www.uptodate.com/contents/umbilical-cord-prolapse

Cabbad, M. F., De Los Heros, D., Baltajian, K. Z., & Robertazzi, R. R. (2015). Corticosteroid use in the face of threatened preterm labor [165].*Obstetrics & Gynecology, 125*, 56S.

Callahan, T. L. (2016). *Tarascon Ob/Gyn Pocketbook.* Burlington, MA: Jones & Bartlett Publishers.

Callister, L. C. (2014). Global perspectives on perinatal loss. *MCN: The American Journal of Maternal/Child Nursing, 39*(3), 207.

Caughey A. B. (2014a). Induction of labor: does it increase the risk of cesarean delivery? *BJOG, 121*(6), 658–661.

Caughey, A. B. (2014b). Vaginal birth after cesarean delivery. *eMedicine.* Retrieved from http://emedicine.medscape.com/article/272187-overview

Caughey, A. B., & Butler, J. R. (2015). Postterm pregnancy. *eMedicine.* Retrieved from http://emedicine.medscape.com/article/261369-overview

Centers for Disease Control and Prevention [CDC] (2015). Primary cesarean delivery rates, by State. *National Vital Statistics Reports. 63*(1), Retrieved from http://www.cdc.gov/nchs/data/nvsr/nvsr63/nvsr63_01.pdf

Chandrasekaran, S., & Srinivas, S. K. (2014). Antenatal corticosteroid administration: understanding its use as an obstetric quality metric. *American Journal of Obstetrics and Gynecology, 210*(2), 143–150.

Cheng, Y., & Caughey, A. B. (2015). Normal labor and delivery. *eMedicine.* Retrieved from http://emedicine.medscape.com/article/260036-overview

Cunningham, F. G., Leveno, K. J., Bloom, S. L., Spong, C. Y., Dashe, J. S., Hoffman, B. L., et al. (2014). *Williams' obstetrics* (24th ed.). New York, NY: McGraw-Hill.

Deering, S. H. (2015). Abruptio placenta. *eMedicine.* Retrieved from http://emedicine.medscape.com/article/252810-overview

Drunecký, T., Reidingerová, M., Plisová, M., Dudič, M., Gdovinová, D., & Stoy, V. (2015). Experimental comparison of properties of natural and synthetic osmotic dilators. *Archives of Gynecology and Obstetrics, 292*(2), 349–354.

Ehsanipoor, R. M., & Satin, A. J. (2016) Overview of normal labor and protracted and arrest disorders. *UpToDate*. Retrieved from: http://www.uptodate.com/contents/overview-of-normal-labor-and-protraction-and-arrest-disorders

Fischer, R. (2015). Breech presentation. *eMedicine*. Retrieved from http://emedicine.medscape.com/article/262159-overview

Flenady, V., Wojcieszek, A. M., Papatsonis, D. N., Stock, O. M., Murray, L., Jardine, L. A., & Carbonne, B. (2014). Calcium channel blockers for inhibiting preterm labor and birth. *Cochrane Database of Systematic Reviews*, (6):CD002255.

Fong, A., Chau, C. T., Pan, D., & Ogunyemi, D. A. (2014). Amniotic fluid embolism: antepartum, intrapartum and demographic factors. *The Journal of Maternal-Fetal & Neonatal Medicine, 28*(7), 793–798.

Fuks, A. M., Robinson, J. V., Rothschild, T. J., Akinnawonu, K. F., & Salafia, C. (2015). Mechanical labor induction using the Foley catheter balloon compared with the cook cervical balloon [96]. *Obstetrics & Gynecology, 125*, 37S.

Gherman, R. (2015). Shoulder dystocia. In *Protocols for high-risk pregnancies: An evidence-based approach* (6th ed.). Hoboken, NJ: John Wiley & Sons.

Goetzl, L. (2014). Methods of cervical ripening and labor induction: Pharmacologic. *Clinical Obstetrics and Gynecology, 57*(2), 377–390.

Goldberg, A. E. (2015). Cervical ripening. *eMedicine*. Retrieved from http://emedicine.medscape.com/article/263311-overview

Green, C. J. (2016). *Maternal newborn nursing care plans* (3rd ed.). Burlington, MA: Jones & Bartlett Learning.

Grobman, W. A. (2015). Is it time for outpatient cervical ripening with prostaglandins? *BJOG: An International Journal of Obstetrics & Gynecology, 122*(1), 105.

Grunebaum, A., & Chervenak, F. A. (2014). Counseling parents after fetal demise and stillbirth. *UpToDate*. Retrieved from http://www.uptodate.com/contents/counseling-parents-after-fetal-demise-and-stillbirth

Haas, D. M., Benjamin, T., Sawyer, R., & Quinney, S. K. (2014). Short-term tocolytics for preterm delivery–current perspectives. *International Journal of Women's Health, 6*, 343–349.

Hinshaw, K., & Kenyon, S. (2015). Abnormal labor. In *Arias' practical guide to high-risk pregnancy & delivery* (4th ed.). New Delhi, India: Elsevier.

Hobbins, J. C. (2015a). Macrosomia. *OB/GYN Clinical Alert, 32*(2), 13–16.

Hofmeyr, G. J. (2015). Protocol 51: Breech delivery. In J. T. Queenan, C. Y. Spong., & C. J. Lockwood (Eds.), *Protocols for high-risk pregnancies: An evidence-based approach*. Chichester, UK: John Wiley & Sons. doi: 10.1002/9781119001256.ch51

Hofmeyr, G. J., Eke, A. C., & Lawrie, T. A. (2014). Amnioinfusion for third trimester preterm premature rupture of membranes. *Cochrane Database of Systematic Reviews*, (3), CD000942.

Hofmeyr G. J., Kulier, R., & West, H. M. (2015). External cephalic version for breech presentation at term. *Cochrane Database of Systematic Reviews*, (4), CD000083.

Hofmeyr, G. J., Xu, H., & Eke, A. C. (2014).Amnioinfusion for meconium-stained liquor in labor. *Cochrane Database of Systematic Reviews*, (1), CD000014.

Hobbins, J. C. (2015b). Macrosomia. *OB/GYN Clinical Alert, 32*(2), 13–16.

Holley, S. R., & Pasch, L. A. (2015). Counseling lesbian, gay, bisexual, and transgender patients. *Fertility counseling* (pp. 180–194). Cambridge, UK: Cambridge University Press.

Hugin, M. P. & Sultani, S. L. (2015). Evaluation of fetal death. *eMedicine*. Retrieved from http://emedicine.medscape.com/article/259165-overview

Iams, J. D. (2015). Clinical practice: Prevention of preterm parturition. *Obstetric Anesthesia Digest, 35*(1), 34–36.

International Childbirth Education Association [ICEA] (2014). *ICEA position paper: Induction*. Retrieved from http://www.icea.org/sites/default/files/Induction%20PP-FINAL.pdf

Jazayeri, A. (2015). Macrosomia. *eMedicine*. [Online] Available: http://emedicine.medscape.com/article/262679-overview

Jordan, R. G., Engstrom, J. L., Marfell, J. A., & Farley, C. L.(2014). *Prenatal and postnatal care: A woman-centered approach*. Ames, Iowa: John Wiley & Sons, Inc

Joy, S., & Contag, S. A. (2015). Cesarean delivery. *eMedicine*. Retrieved from http://emedicine.medscape.com/article/263424-overview

Jørgensen, J. S., Weile, L. K., & Lamont, R. F. (2014). Preterm labor: current tocolytic options for the treatment of preterm labor. *Expert Opinion on Pharmacotherapy, 15*(5), 585–588.

Joy, S., & Finneran, M. M. (2015). Placenta previa. *eMedicine*. Retrieved from http://emedicine.medscape.com/article/262063-overview

Joy, S., Lyon, D., & Scott, P. L. (2015). Abnormal labor. *eMedicine*. Retrieved from http://emedicine.medscape.com/article/273053-overview

Kilpatrick, S. J. (2014). Trauma in pregnancy. *UpToDate*. Retrieved from http://www.uptodate.com/contents/trauma-in-pregnancy

King, T. L., Brucker, M. C., Kriebs, J. M., Fahey, J. O., Gegor, C. L., & Varney, H. (2015). *Varney's midwifery* (5th ed.). Burlington, MA: Jones & Bartlett Learning.

King, V. J., Fontaine, P. L., Atwood, L. A., Powers, E., Leeman, L., Ecker, J. L., et al. (2015). Clinical practice guideline executive summary: Labor after cesarean/planned vaginal birth after cesarean. *The Annals of Family Medicine, 13*(1), 80–81.

Kriebs, J. M. (2015). Patient safety during induction of labor. *The Journal of Perinatal & Neonatal Nursing, 29*(2), 130–137.

Lal, A. K., & Hibbard, J. U. (2015). Placenta previa: an outcome-based cohort study in a contemporary obstetric population. *Archives of Gynecology and Obstetrics, 292*(2), 299–305.

Lewis, L., Pan, H., Heine, R., Brown, H., Brancazio, L., & Grotegut, C. (2014). Labor and pregnancy outcomes after adoption of a more conservative oxytocin labor protocol. *Obstetrics & Gynecology, 123* (Suppl 1), 66S.

Locatelli, A., Consonni, S., & Ghidini, A. (2015). Preterm labor: Approach to decreasing complications of prematurity. *Obstetrics and Gynecology Clinics of North America, 42*(2), 255–274.

Manjula, B. G., Bagga, R., Kalra, J., & Dutta, S. (2015). Labor induction with an intermediate-dose oxytocin regimen has advantages over a high-dose regimen. *Journal of Obstetrics & Gynecology, 35*(4), 362–367.

March of Dimes. (2015a). *Multiples: Twins, triplets and beyond*. Retrieved from http://www.marchofdimes.com/professionals/14332_4545.asp

March of Dimes. (2015b). Preterm labor and birth: A serious pregnancy complication. Retrieved from http://www.marchofdimes.com/pregnancy/preterm_indepth.html

March of Dimes. (2015c). *Umbilical cord abnormalities*. Retrieved from http://www.marchofdimes.com/professionals/681_4546.asp.

March of Dimes. (2015d). *Placenta previa*. Retrieved from http://www.marchofdimes.org/pregnancy/placenta-previa.aspx

March of Dimes. (2015e). *Placental abruption*. Retrieved from http://www.marchofdimes.org/pregnancy/placental-abruption.aspx

Mattson, S., & Smith, J. E. (2016). *Core curriculum for maternal-newborn nursing* (5th ed.). Philadelphia, PA: Elsevier Health Sciences.

McCarthy, F. P., & Kenny, L. C. (2014). Induction of labor. *Obstetrics, Gynecology & Reproductive Medicine, 24*(1), 9–15.

Mehlman, C. T. (2015). Neonatal brachial plexus palsy. *The pediatric upper extremity* (pp. 589–605). New York, NY: Springer Publishers.

Moore, L. E. (2015). Amniotic fluid embolism. *eMedicine*. Retrieved from http://emedicine.medscape.com/article/253068-overview#a5

Moses, S. (2015). Amniotic fluid embolism. *Family Practice Notebook*. Retrieved from http://www.fpnotebook.com/Lung/OB/AmntcFldEmblsm.htm

Nagtalon-Ramos, J. (2014). *Best evidence-based practices-Maternal-newborn nursing care*. Philadelphia, PA: F.A. Davis Company.

Nahum, G. G., & Pham, K. Q. (2015). Uterine rupture in pregnancy. *eMedicine*. Retrieved from http://emedicine.medscape.com/article/275854-overview

Nakazawa, H., Uchida, A., Minamitani, T., Makishi, A., Takamatsu, Y., Kiyoshi, K., et al. (2015). Factors affecting maternal serum magnesium levels during long-term magnesium sulfate tocolysis in singleton and twin pregnancy. *Journal of Obstetrics & Gynecology Research, 41*(8), 1178–1184.

Norwitz, E. R. (2015). Cesarean delivery on maternal request. *UpToDate*. Retrieved from http://www.uptodate.com/contents/cesarean-delivery-on-maternal-request

O'Grady, J. P. & St. Andre, C. (2015). Vacuum extraction. *eMedicine*. Retrieved from http://emedicine.medscape.com/article/271175-overview#aw2aab6b4

Patel, P. K., Pitre, D. S., & Bhooker, S. P. (2015). Predictive value of various risk factors for preterm labor. *Community Medicine, 6*(1), 121–125.

Robinson, G. E. (2014). Pregnancy loss. *Best Practice & Research Clinical Obstetrics & Gynecology, 28*(1), 169–178.

Ross, M. G. (2015). Preterm labor. *eMedicine*. Retrieved from http://emedicine.medscape.com/article/260998-overview#aw2aab6b7

Sadera, G., & Vasudevan, B. (2015). Amniotic fluid embolism. *Journal of Obstetric Anesthesia and Critical Care, 5*(1), 3–8.

Sciscione, A. C. (2014). Methods of cervical ripening and labor induction: Mechanical. *Clinical Obstetrics and Gynecology, 57*(2), 369–376.

Scott, J. R. (2015). Vaginal birth after cesarean. *Protocols for high-risk pregnancies: An evidence-based approach* (6th ed.). (pp. 428–432). Hoboken, NJ: John Wiley & Sons.

Sharshiner, R., & Silver, R. M. (2015). Management of fetal malpresentation. *Clinical Obstetrics and Gynecology, 58*(2), 246–255.

Soni, A., Vaishnav, G. D., & Gohil, J. (2015). Meconium and its significance and obstetric outcome. *Medicine Science| International Medical Journal, 4*(1), 1861–1868.

Sosa, C. G., Althabe, F., Belizan, J. M., & Bergel, E. (2015). Bed rest in singleton pregnancies for preventing preterm birth. *Cochrane Database of Systematic Reviews*, (3), CD003581.

Sotiriadis, A., Tsiami, A., Papatheodorou, S., Baschat, A. A., Sarafidis, K., & Makrydimas, G. (2015). Neurodevelopmental outcome after a single course of antenatal steroids in children born preterm: A systematic review and meta-analysis. *Obstetrics & Gynecology, 125*(6), 1385–1396.

Souka, A. P., Papastefanou, I., Papadopoulos, G., Chrelias, C., & Kassanos, D. (2015). Cervical length in late second and third trimester: a mixture model for predicting delivery. *Ultrasound in Obstetrics & Gynecology, 45*(3), 308–312.

Sousou, J., & Smart, C. (2015). Care of the childbearing family with intrauterine fetal demise. *Nursing for Women's Health, 19*(3), 236–246.

Suzuki, S. (2015). Clinical significance of precipitous labor. *Journal of Clinical Medicine Research, 7*(3), 150–153.

U.S. Department of Health and Human Services. (2010). *Healthy People 2020*. Retrieved from http://www.healthypeople.gov/2020/topicsobjectives2020/default.aspx

van Baaren, G. J., Bruijn, M. M., Vis, J. Y., Wilms, F. F., Oudijk, M. A., Kwee, A., et al. (2015). Risk factors for preterm delivery: Do they add to fetal fibronectin testing and cervical length measurement in the prediction of preterm delivery in symptomatic women? *European Journal of Obstetrics & Gynecology and Reproductive Biology, 192*, 150–153.

van Baaren, G. J., Vis, J. Y., Wilms, F. F., Oudijk, M. A., Kwee, A., Porath, M. M., et al. (2014). Predictive value of cervical length measurement and fibronectin testing in threatened preterm labor. *Obstetrics & Gynecology, 123*(6), 1185–1192.

van den Bosch, A. E., Ruys, T. P., & Roos-Hesselink, J. W. (2015). Use and impact of cardiac medication during pregnancy. *Future Cardiology, 11*(1), 89–100.

Viswanathan, M., Venkateswaran, V. K., & Daniel, S. (2014). Amniotic fluid embolism: a comprehensive review. *International Journal of Reproduction, Contraception, Obstetrics and Gynecology, 3*(2), 304–309.

Vogel, J. P., Gulmezoglu, A. M., Hofmeyr, G. J., & Temmerman, M. (2014). Global perspectives on elective induction of labor. *Clinical Obstetrics and Gynecology, 57*(2), 331–342.

Walker, N., & Gan, J. H. (2015). Prolonged pregnancy. *Obstetrics, Gynecology & Reproductive Medicine, 25*(3), 83–87.

Westwood, S., King, A., Almack, K., Suen, Y. T., & Bailey, L. (2015). Good practice in health and social care provision for LGBT older people in the UK. *Lesbian, gay, bisexual and trans health inequalities: International perspectives in social work* (pp. 145–158). Chicago, IL: Policy Press.

World Health Organization [WHO]. (2014a). *Managing complications in pregnancy and childbirth: A guide for midwives and doctors*. Retrieved from http://www.who.int/maternal_child_adolescent/documents/9241545879/en/

World Health Organization [WHO]. (2014b). *WHO recommendations for augmentation of labor*. Retrieved from http://apps.who.int/iris/bitstream/10665/112825/1/9789241507363_eng.pdf

MULTIPLE CHOICE QUESTIONS

1. When reviewing the medical record of a client, the nurse notes that the woman has a condition in which the fetus cannot physically pass through the maternal pelvis. The nurse interprets this as:
   a. Cervical insufficiency
   b. Contracted pelvis
   c. Maternal disproportion
   d. Fetopelvic disproportion

2. The nurse would anticipate a cesarean birth for a client who has which active infection present at the onset of labor?
   a. Hepatitis
   b. Herpes simplex virus
   c. Toxoplasmosis
   d. Human papillomavirus

3. After a vaginal examination, the nurse determines that the client's fetus is in an occiput posterior position. The nurse would anticipate that the client will have:
   a. Intense back pain
   b. Frequent leg cramps
   c. Nausea and vomiting
   d. A precipitous birth

4. When assessing the following women, which would the nurse identify as being at the greatest risk for preterm labor?
   a. Woman who had twins in a previous pregnancy
   b. Client living in a large city close to the subway
   c. Woman working full time as a computer programmer
   d. Client with a history of a previous preterm birth

5. The rationale for using a prostaglandin gel for a client prior to the induction of labor is to:
   a. Stimulate uterine contractions
   b. Numb cervical pain receptors
   c. Prevent cervical lacerations
   d. Soften and efface the cervix

6. A client who was in active labor and whose cervix had dilated to 4 cm experiences a weakening in the intensity and frequency of her contractions and exhibits no further progress in labor. The nurse interprets this as a sign of:
   a. Hypertonic labor
   b. Precipitate labor
   c. Hypotonic labor
   d. Dysfunctional labor

7. The nurse is developing a plan of care for a woman experiencing dystocia. Which of the following nursing interventions would be the nurse's high priority?
   a. Changing the woman's position frequently
   b. Providing comfort measures to the woman
   c. Monitoring the fetal heart rate patterns
   d. Keeping the couple informed of the labor progress

8. The nurse is caring for a woman experiencing hypertonic uterine dystocia. The woman's contractions are erratic in their frequency, duration, and of high intensity. The priority nursing intervention would be to:
   a. Encourage ambulation every 30 minutes
   b. Provide pain relief measures
   c. Monitor the Pitocin infusion rate closely
   d. Prepare the woman for an amniotomy

CRITICAL THINKING EXERCISE

1. A 26-year-old multipara, is admitted to the labor and birth suite in active labor. After a few hours, the nurse notices a change in her contraction pattern—poor contraction intensity and no progression of cervical dilatation beyond 5 cm. The client keeps asking about her labor progress and appears anxious about "how long this labor is taking."
   a. Based on the nurse's findings, what might you suspect is going on?
   b. How can the nurse address the client's anxiety?
   c. What are the appropriate interventions to change this labor pattern?

2. The woman activates her call light and states, "I feel increased wetness down below."
   a. What might be occurring?
   b. How will the nurse confirm the suspicions?
   c. What interventions are appropriate for this finding?

STUDY ACTIVITIES

1. Visit the SHARE Pregnancy and Infant Loss Support, Inc., website at the Point and assess its helpfulness to parents.

2. Outline the fetal and maternal risks associated with a prolonged pregnancy.

3. An abnormal or difficult labor describes _____.

BRINGING IT ALL TOGETHER: CASE STUDY

Tegan is a nulliparous woman who is now at 41 3/7 weeks of gestation with a male fetus. She presents for a routine prenatal visit. Fetal well-bring is reassuring at this point with FHR 144, active fetal movement, no complaints voiced except for fatigue and a mild backache when she stands for long periods of time. She expresses concern that she has not yet gone into labor.

ASSESSMENT

The mean duration of pregnancy is 40 weeks (280 days) dated from the first day of the last normal menstrual period. Post-term pregnancy is defined as a gestational age of >42 weeks (>292 days) dated from the last menstrual period. Approximately 10% of low risk pregnancies continue beyond the 42nd week gestation. Her fetal well-being assessment is within normal limits.

Go to thePoint **to find questions to consider about this case.**

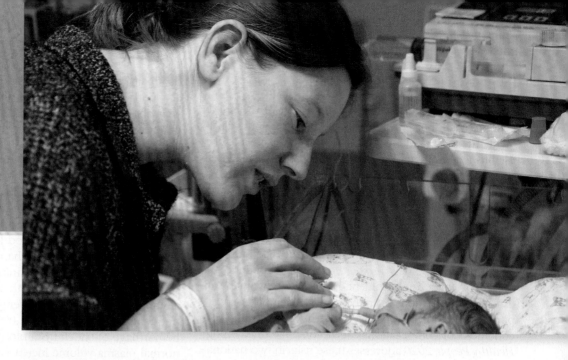

22

KEY TERMS
mastitis
metritis
postpartum
   depression (PPD)
postpartum
   hemorrhage (PPH)
subinvolution
uterine atony

Nursing Management of the Postpartum Woman at Risk

Learning Objectives

Upon completion of the chapter, you will be able to:

1. Examine the major conditions that place the postpartum woman at risk.

2. Analyze the risk factors, assessment, preventive measures, and nursing management of common postpartum complications.

3. Differentiate the causes of postpartum hemorrhage based on the underlying pathophysiologic mechanisms.

4. Outline the nurse's role in assessing and managing the care of a woman with a thromboembolic condition.

5. Characterize the nursing management of a woman who develops a postpartum infection.

6. Compare and contrast at least two affective disorders that can occur in women after birth, describing specific therapeutic management for each.

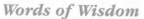

Joan gave birth about an hour ago to her fifth baby boy, who weighed 10 pounds, and she is resting in bed when the nurse comes in to assess her. She tells the nurse that she feels like there is "something really wet" between her legs. She also feels a bit light-headed. What would the nurse suspect is happening? What findings would support the nurse's suspicion? What should the nurse do first?

Words of Wisdom
Nurses should remain vigilant and observant throughout the childbirth experience all the way through discharge of the childbearing family.

INTRODUCTION

The postpartum period is the culmination of the child-bearing experience. Numerous adaptations and adjustments must be made to assimilate the newborn into the established family unit. It is a time designed for maternal recovery, family attachment, and new role development. Typically, recovery from childbirth progresses normally both physiologically and psychologically. Just like everything else in life, a woman's body faces significant changes in the weeks and months following childbirth. It is a time filled with many changes and wide-ranging emotions, and the new mother commonly experiences a great sense of accomplishment. However, the woman can experience deviations from the norm, developing a postpartum condition that places her at risk. These high-risk conditions or complications can become life threatening. *Healthy People 2020* addresses these risks in two national health goals that were retained from the 2010 document.

This chapter addresses the nursing management of the most common conditions that place the postpartum woman at risk: hemorrhage, thromboembolic disease, infections, and postpartum affective disorders.

POSTPARTUM HEMORRHAGE

Postpartum hemorrhage (PPH) is a potentially life-threatening complication that can occur after both vaginal and cesarean births. It is the leading cause of maternal

death in both developed and developing countries, accounting for about 35% of all maternal deaths. Every year about 14 million women globally suffer from PPH or approximately one in twenty births Agency for Healthcare Research and Quality [AHRQ], 2015). A hemorrhage occurs in 5% of all births and is responsible for a major part of maternal mortality. The majority of these deaths occur within 4 hours of childbirth, which indicates that they are a consequence of the third stage of labor management (Crowe & Faulkner, 2014; Ekin et al., 2015).

PPH is defined as a blood loss greater than 500 mL after vaginal birth or more than 1,000 mL after a cesarean birth. However, this definition is arbitrary, because estimates of blood loss at birth are subjective and generally inaccurate. Moreover, average blood loss from birth frequently exceeds 500 or 1,000 mL, and symptoms of hemorrhage or shock from blood loss may be hidden by normal plasma volume increases that occur during pregnancy. Morbidity from PPH can be severe, with sequelae including organ failure, shock, edema, thrombosis, acute respiratory distress, sepsis, anemia, intensive care admissions, and prolonged hospitalization (AHRQ, 2015). A major obstetric hemorrhage is defined as a blood loss of more than 1,500 to 2,500 mL or bleeding that required more than 5 units of transfused blood (Pavord & Maybury, 2015). Hemorrhage is the most common reason postpartum women are admitted to intensive care units and it is the most preventable cause of maternal death. Timely, accurate identification and initiation of appropriate interventions would improve outcomes (Clapp, 2015). Blood loss that occurs within 24 hours of birth is termed *primary (immediate or early) postpartum hemorrhage;* blood loss that occurs 24 hours to 12 weeks after birth is termed *delayed (late) postpartum hemorrhage.* A more objective definition of PPH would be any amount of bleeding that places the mother in hemodynamic jeopardy.

Pathophysiology

Excessive bleeding can occur at any time between the separation of the placenta and its expulsion or removal. The most common cause of PPH is **uterine atony**, failure of the uterus to contract and retract after birth. The uterus must remain contracted after birth to control bleeding from the placental site. Uterine atony is responsible for 80% of primary or immediate PPH, while obstetric lacerations, uterine inversion, and rupture compromise about 20% of all primary or early PPHs (Kamel & Mastrogiannis, 2015). Any factor that causes the uterus to relax after birth will cause bleeding—even a full bladder that displaces the uterus.

During the third stage of labor the muscles of the uterus contract downward, causing constriction of the blood vessels that pass through the uterine wall to the placental surface and stopping the flow of blood. This action

---

also causes the placenta to separate from the uterine wall. The absence of uterine contractions may result in excessive blood loss. Uterotonic medications promote uterine contractions to prevent atony and speed delivery of the placenta.

Over the course of pregnancy, maternal blood volume increases as much as 50% (from 4 to 6 L). The plasma volume increases twice as much in comparison to the total red blood cell volume. As a result, hemoglobin and hematocrit fall. The increase in blood volume meets the perfusion demands of the low-resistance uteroplacental unit and provides a reserve for the blood loss that occurs at delivery (Cunningham et al., 2014). Given this increase, the typical signs of hemorrhage (e.g., falling blood pressure, increasing pulse rate, and decreasing urinary output) do not appear until as much as 1,800 to 2,100 mL of blood has been lost. Current evidence on postpartum volume replacement suggests packed red blood cells, fresh frozen plasma, platelets, and recombinant factor VIIa be used for volume replacement (Nagtalon-Ramos, 2014). Clinical manifestations of shock resulting from blood loss are seen in Table 22.1.

In addition, accurate determination of actual blood loss is difficult because of blood pooling inside the uterus, on peripads, mattresses, and the floor. Because no universal clinical standard exists, nurses must remain vigilant, assessing for risk factors and checking clients carefully before the birth attendant leaves the birthing area.

Other causes of PPH include lacerations of the genital tract, episiotomy, retained placental fragments, uterine inversion, coagulation disorders, large for gestational age newborn, failure to progress during the second stage of labor, placenta accreta, induction or augmentation of labor with oxytocin, surgical birth, and hematomas of the vulva, vagina, or subperitoneal areas (Moses, 2015). A helpful way to remember the causes of postpartum hemorrhage is by using the 4 Ts:

1. **T**one: uterine atony, distended bladder
2. **T**issue: retained placenta and clots; uterine subinvolution
3. **T**rauma: lacerations, hematoma, inversion, rupture
4. **T**hrombin: coagulopathy (pre-existing or acquired)

Tone

Altered uterine muscle tone most commonly results from overdistention of the uterus. Overdistention can be caused by multiple gestation, fetal macrosomia, hydramnios, fetal abnormality, placenta previa, precipitous birth, or retained placental fragments. Other causes might include prolonged or rapid, forceful labor, especially if stimulated by oxytocin; bacterial toxins (e.g., chorioamnionitis, endomyometritis, septicemia); use of anesthesia, especially halothane; and magnesium sulfate used in the treatment of preeclampsia (Jordan et al., 2014). Overdistention of the uterus is a major risk factor for uterine atony, the most common cause of early postpartum hemorrhage, which can lead to hypovolemic shock. A distended bladder can also displace the uterus from the midline to either side, which impedes its ability to contract to reduce bleeding.

Tissue

Uterine contraction and retraction lead to detachment and expulsion of the placenta after birth. Classic signs of placental separation include a small gush of blood with lengthening of the umbilical cord and a slight rise of the uterus in the pelvis. Complete detachment and expulsion of the placenta permit continued contraction and optimal occlusion of blood vessels. Failure of complete placental separation and expulsion leads to retained fragments, which occupy space and prevent the uterus from contracting fully to clamp down on blood vessels; this can lead to hemorrhage. Clots can also occupy space, which inhibits uterine contractions.

After the placenta has been expelled, a thorough inspection is necessary to confirm its intactness; tears or fragments left inside may indicate an accessory lobe or placenta accreta (an uncommon condition in which the chorionic villi adhere to the myometrium, causing the placenta to adhere abnormally to the uterus and not separate and deliver spontaneously). Profuse hemorrhage results because the uterus cannot contract fully.

SUBINVOLUTION OF THE UTERUS

Subinvolution refers to incomplete involution of the uterus or failure to return to its normal size and condition after birth. Typically, subinvolution occurs when the myometrial fibers of the uterus do not contract effectively and

TABLE 22.1	CLINICAL MANIFESTATIONS OF SHOCK DUE TO BLOOD LOSS	
Degree of Shock	Blood Loss	Signs and Symptoms
Mild	20%	Diaphoresis, increased capillary refilling, cool extremities, maternal anxiety
Moderate	20–40%	Tachycardia, postural hypotension, oliguria
Severe	>40%	Hypotension, agitation/confusion, hemodynamic instability

Adapted from Kolecki, P., & Menckhoff, C. R. (2015). Hypovolemic shock. *eMedicine*. Retrieved from http://emedicine.medscape.com/article/760145-overview; Belfort, M. A. (2015). Overview of postpartum hemorrhage. *UpToDate*. Retrieved from http://www.uptodate.com/contents/overview-of-postpartum-hemorrhage; and Cunningham, F. G., Leveno, K. J., Bloom, S. L., Spong, C., Dashe, J. S., Hoffman, B. L., et al. (2014). *Williams' obstetrics* (24th ed.). New York, NY: McGraw-Hill.

causes relaxation. Complications of subinvolution include hemorrhage, pelvic peritonitis, salpingitis, and abscess formation (King et al., 2015). Causes of subinvolution include retained placental fragments, distended bladder, excessive maternal activity prohibiting proper recovery, uterine myoma, and infection. All of these conditions contribute to delayed postpartum bleeding. The clinical picture includes a postpartum fundal height that is higher than expected, with a boggy uterus; the lochia fails to change colors from red to serosa to alba within a few weeks. This condition is usually identified at the woman's postpartum examination 4 to 6 weeks after birth with a bimanual vaginal examination or ultrasound. Treatment is directed toward stimulating the uterus to expel fragments with a uterine stimulant, and antibiotics are given to prevent infection.

Trauma

Damage to the genital tract may occur spontaneously or through the manipulations used during birth. Lacerations and hematomas resulting from birth trauma can cause significant blood loss. Hematomas can present as pain or as a change in vital signs disproportionate to the amount of blood loss. Most often, hematoma formation is associated with episiotomy, instrumental birth, or nulliparity. Many hematomas can be prevented with gentle, controlled birth, and appropriate inspection and repair of lacerations or episiotomy (Jordan et al., 2014). Uterine inversion happens when the top of the uterus collapses into the inner cavity due to excessive fundal pressure or pulling on the umbilical cord when the placenta is still firmly attached to the fundus after the infant has been born. Treatment for uterine inversion includes giving uterine relaxants and immediate manual replacement by the health care provider. Additionally, uterine rupture can occur and cause damage to the genital tract and is more common in women with previous cesarean incisions or those who have undergone any procedure resulting in disruption of the uterine wall, including myomectomy, perforation of the uterus during a dilation and curettage, biopsy, or intrauterine system insertion. Classically, its signs and symptoms combine pain, fetal heart rate abnormalities, and vaginal bleeding. Uterine rupture is a catastrophic complication that requires a rapid diagnosis and intervention, but initial clinical manifestations may be nonspecific (Nahum & Pham, 2015).

Trauma can also occur after prolonged or vigorous labor, especially if the uterus has been stimulated with oxytocin or prostaglandins. Trauma can also occur after extrauterine or intrauterine manipulation of the fetus.

Cervical lacerations commonly occur during a forceps delivery or in mothers who have not been able to resist bearing down before the cervix is fully dilated. Vaginal sidewall lacerations are associated with operative vaginal births but may occur spontaneously, especially if the fetal hand presents with the head. Lacerations can arise during manipulations to resolve shoulder dystocia. Lacerations should always be suspected in the face of a contracted uterus with bright-red blood continuing to trickle out of the vagina.

Thrombin

Thrombosis (formation of a blood clot) helps to prevent PPH immediately after birth by providing hemostasis. Fibrin deposits and clots in supplying vessels play a significant role in the hours and days after birth. Disorders that interfere with the clot formation can lead to postpartum hemorrhage. Medication used to prevent hemorrhage by stimulating uterine contractions may delay the appearance of coagulation disorders. Coagulopathies should be suspected when postpartum bleeding persists without any identifiable cause (Agency for Healthcare Research and Quality [AHRQ], 2015).

Disorders of coagulation are relatively uncommon as a sole cause of PPH. Coagulation disturbances should be suspected in women with a family history of such abnormalities and women with a history of menorrhagia. Clinical circumstances may also suggest coagulation defect as a cause of PPH. Diagnosis of a coagulation disorder often requires a high index of suspicion and should not be overlooked in the evaluation of obstetric hemorrhage (Yiadom & Carusi, 2015).

Ideally, the client's coagulation status is determined during pregnancy. However, if she received no prenatal care, coagulation studies should be ordered immediately to determine her status. Abnormal results typically include decreased platelet and fibrinogen levels, increased prothrombin time, partial thromboplastin time, and fibrin degradation products, and a prolonged bleeding time (Cunningham et al., 2014). Selected conditions associated with coagulopathies in the postpartum client include idiopathic thrombocytopenic purpura, von Willebrand disease, and disseminated intravascular coagulation (DIC).

IDIOPATHIC THROMBO PURPURA

Idiopathic thrombocytopenia purpura (ITP) is an autoimmune disorder of increased platelet destruction caused by autoantibodies, which can increase a woman's risk of hemorrhaging. There is a decrease in the number of circulating platelets in the absence of toxic exposure or a disease associated with a low platelet count. It is most common in young women during childbearing age and may be associated with maternal and fetal complications. The incidence of ITP in adults is approximately 66 cases per 1,000,000 per year (Silverman, 2015). Glucocorticoids and immune globulin are the mainstays of medical therapy (Kessler & Sandler, 2015).

VON WILLEBRAND DISEASE

von Willebrand disease is a congenital bleeding disorder that is inherited as an autosomal dominant trait. It is characterized by a prolonged bleeding time, a deficiency of von Willebrand factor, and impairment of platelet adhesion Centers for Disease Control and Prevention [CDC], 2015a). It is the most common hereditary bleeding disorder, affecting approximately 1% of the general population (National Hemophilia Foundation, 2015). Although vWD is thought to affect men and women equally, it is diagnosed more frequently in women because of menorrhagia, and it is more common among white women than African-American women American College of Obstetrics and Gynecologists [ACOG], 2014a). Most cases remain undiagnosed due to lack of awareness, difficulty in diagnosis, a tendency to attribute bleeding to other causes, and variable symptoms.

The most common symptoms of vWD include bleeding gums, easy bruising, menorrhagia, blood in urine and stools, nosebleeds and hematomas. Prolonged bleeding from trivial wounds, oral cavity bleeding, and excessive menstrual bleeding are common. Gastrointestinal bleeding is rare. During pregnancy, the von Willebrand factor level increases in most women; thus, labor and birth usually proceed normally. However, all women should be monitored for excessive bleeding, particularly during the first week postpartum (Pollak, 2015).

DISSEMINATED INTRAVASCULAR COAGULATION

DIC is a life-threatening, acquired coagulopathy in which the clotting system is abnormally activated, resulting in widespread clot formation in the small vessels throughout the body, which leads to the depletion of platelets and coagulation factors. This is why DIC is also known as consumption coagulopathy.

DIC is not itself a specific illness; rather it is always a secondary diagnosis that occurs as a complication of abruptio placentae, amniotic fluid embolism, intrauterine fetal death with prolonged retention of the fetus, acute fatty liver of pregnancy, severe preeclampsia, HELLP syndrome (hemolysis, i.e., the breakdown of red blood cells, elevated liver enzymes, and low platelet count), septicemia, and postpartum hemorrhage. Clinical features include petechiae, ecchymoses, bleeding gums, fever, hypotension, acidosis, hematomas, tachycardia, proteinuria, uncontrolled bleeding during birth, and acute renal failure (Levi & Schmaier, 2015).Treatment goals are to maintain tissue perfusion through aggressive administration of fluid therapy, oxygen, heparin, and blood products. The most important treatment concept in DIC is that it is a secondary manifestation of an underlying disorder. The most important therapeutic maneuver is treating the initiating disorder, DIC will disappear, and the coagulation status will normalize Without this, supportive measures ultimately fail (Erez, Mastrolia, & Thachil, 2015).

Therapeutic Management

Prompt diagnosis and understanding of the underlying triggers of this complication is essential for a favorable outcome. Team work and prompt treatment are essential for the successful management of women with DIC. Therapeutic management focuses on the underlying cause of the hemorrhage. For example, uterine massage is used to treat uterine atony. If retained placental fragments are the cause, the fragments are usually manually separated and removed and a uterine stimulant is given to promote the uterus to expel fragments. Antibiotics are administered to prevent infection. Lacerations are sutured or repaired. Glucocorticoids and intravenous immunoglobulin, intravenous anti-RhoD, and platelet transfusions may be given for ITP. Perinatal management of ITP should also include maintenance of maternal platelet count and regular monitoring of fetal growth along with prediction and prevention of fetal passive immune thrombocytopenia (Silverman, 2015).

The mainstays of therapy for vWD are desmopressin and plasma concentrates that contain von Willebrand factor. Delayed postpartum hemorrhage may occur, despite adequate prophylaxis. Frequent monitoring and continued prophylaxis and/or treatment are recommended for at least 2 weeks after childbirth (Pollak, 2015).

Nursing Assessment

Most women will not have identifiable risk factors. Nonetheless, primary prevention of a PPH begins with an assessment of identifiable risk factors. Pregnancy and childbirth involve significant health risks, even for women with no pre-existing health problems. In the United States, where most births occur in hospitals and where resources are likely to be available as compared with developing countries, PPH still continues to be among the top causes of maternal deaths. Retrospective studies of these events suggest that some cases are preventable. As with many other sources of perinatal harm, delays in recognition, diagnosis, and treatment, problems with hierarchy and communication, and lack of knowledge, policies, and protocols were often cited as contributing factors (Shields et al., 2015).

The period after the birth and the first hours postpartum are crucial times for the prevention, assessment, and management of bleeding. Compared with other maternal risks such as infection, bleeding can rapidly become life threatening, and nurses, along with other health care providers, need to identify this condition quickly and intervene appropriately.

Begin by reviewing the mother's history, including labor and birth history, for risk factors associated with PPH (Table 22.2). The incidence of PPH has been rising, though the mortality has come down, suggesting improvement in the management of this condition. Although specific risk factors have been identified, PPH is often unanticipated and still occurs in approximately 5% of all births and increasing (Ekin et al., 2015).

TABLE 22.2	FACTORS PLACING A WOMAN AT RISK FOR POSTPARTUM HEMORRHAGE
Clinical Risk Factors	**Associated Clinical Conditions**
Tone (abnormalities of uterine contractions)	
Overdistention of uterus	Polyhydramnios Multifetal gestation Macrosomia
Uterine muscle exhaustion	Rapid labor Prolonged labor Oxytocin use
Uterine infection	Maternal fever Prolonged rupture of membranes
Tissue (retained in uterus)	
Products of conception	Incomplete placenta at birth
Retained blood clots	Atonic uterus
Trauma (of the genital tract)	
Lacerations anywhere	Precipitate birth or operative birth
Laceration extensions	Malposition of fetus Previous uterine surgery
Uterine inversion	Forceful pulling when placenta isn't separated yet; traction on the cord when uterus isn't contracted
Thrombin (coagulation abnormalities)	
Pre-existing conditions	Hereditary inheritance Hemophilia von Willebrand's disease History of previous PPH Acquired in pregnancy Idiopathic thrombocytopenia purpura Bruising, elevated blood pressure Disseminated intravascular coagulation

Adapted from Centers for Disease Control and Prevention [CDC]. (2015a). *Facts about von Willebrand Disease*. Retrieved from http://www.cdc.gov/ncbddd/vwd/facts.html; King, T. L., Brucker, M. C., Kriebs, J. M., Fahey, J. O., Gegor, C. L., & Varney, H. (2015). *Varney's midwifery* (5th ed.) Burlington, MA: Jones & Bartlett Learning; and Mattson, S., & Smith, J. E. (2015). *Core curriculum for maternal-newborn nursing* (5th ed.), St. Louis, MO: Saunders Elsevier.

Since the most common cause of immediate severe PPH is uterine atony (failure of the uterus to contract properly after birth), assess uterine tone after birth by palpating the fundus for firmness and location. A soft, boggy fundus indicates uterine atony.

Take Note!

A soft, boggy uterus that deviates from the midline suggests that a full bladder is interfering with uterine involution. If the uterus is not in correct position (midline), it will not be able to contract to control bleeding.

Assess the amount of bleeding. Visual estimation is the most frequently practiced method of determining blood loss during childbirth in the United States, and the results are usually included in the documentation of events pertaining to the birth. This method is used despite repeated studies showing its inaccuracy and underestimation. Weighing or counting peri pads or using a Signaling a Postpartum Hemorrhage Emergency mat would provide a more accurate estimate of blood loss. The mat was constructed so that each square on the mat would absorb up to 50 mL of blood. Blood loss is then calculated by multiplying the number of blood-saturated squares by 50 mL (Wilcox et al., 2015). In any method used, nurses should consult their hospital protocols and follow them. If bleeding continues even though there are no lacerations, suspect retained placental fragments.

The uterus remains large with painless, dark-red bleeding mixed with clots. This cause of hemorrhage can be prevented by carefully inspecting the placenta for intactness.

If trauma is suspected, attempt to identify the source and document it. Typically, the uterus will be firm with a steady stream or trickle of unclotted bright-red blood noted in the perineum. Most deaths from PPH are not due to gross bleeding, but rather to inadequate management of slow, steady blood loss (Clapp, 2015).

Assess for hematoma which may require surgical treatment. The uterus would be firm, with bright-red bleeding. Observe for a localized bluish bulging area just under the skin surface in the perineal area (Fig. 22.1). Often the woman will report severe perineal or pelvic pain and will have difficulty voiding. In addition, she may exhibit hypotension, tachycardia, and anemia. Frequently, the health care provider will incise the skin bulge to evacuate the hematoma of trapped blood. A pressure dressing is applied to this area to prevent further bleeding (Green, 2016).

Inspect the skin and mucous membranes for gingival bleeding or petechiae and ecchymoses. Check venipuncture sites for oozing or prolonged bleeding. These findings might suggest a coagulopathy as a cause of PPH. Also assess the amount of lochia, which would be much greater than usual. Urinary output would be diminished, with signs of acute renal failure. Vital signs would show an increased pulse rate and a decreased level of consciousness. However, signs of shock do not appear until hemorrhage is far advanced due to the increased fluid and blood volume of pregnancy.

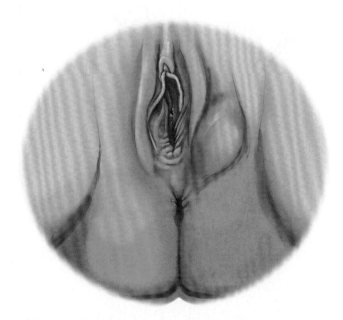

FIGURE 22.1 Perineal hematoma. Note the bulging swollen mass.

Nursing Management

When excessive bleeding is encountered, initial management steps are aimed at improving uterine tone with immediate fundal massage, intravenous fluid resuscitation, and administration of uterotonic medications. If these methods fail to control bleeding, additional resources are mobilized and more aggressive interventions such as bimanual compression, internal uterine packing, and/or balloon tamponade techniques are employed by the health care provider. Other potential causes of bleeding should be thoroughly explored, and laboratory tests such as a complete blood count, type and cross-match, and coagulations studies should be obtained immediately. Transfusion of blood products should be instituted without hesitation once estimates of bleeding reach 1,500 mL (Nagtalon-Ramos, 2014).

 Concept Mastery Alert

Priority Intervention for Uterine Atony

Before initiating fundal massage, the nurse must first place a hand over the symphysis pubis to anchor the uterus and prevent possible uterine inversion.

Clearly, in all cases of unexpected hemorrhage, the interventions discussed as follows must be performed without delay. Postpartum hemorrhage is best managed by using a stepwise progressive approach. Manual message and pharmacologic therapies are first-line treatments. If the bleeding continues, second-line interventions might include the use of intrauterine balloon (or gauze) tamponade and uterine compression sutures. If these second-line therapies still don't stop the bleeding, women may need to undergo radiologic embolization, pelvic devascularization, or hysterectomy. Peripartum hysterectomy remains the last-resort lifesaving measure and carries with it a higher mortality rate compared with nonobstetric hysterectomy. It is a most demanding obstetric surgery performed under very trying circumstances of life-threatening hemorrhage (Van de Velde, Diez, & Varon, 2015). Moreover, high-volume transfusions are often required, and there are significant postsurgical morbidity risks such as renal failure, hepatic failure, respiratory distress syndrome, coagulopathies, septicemia, tissue hypoxia, and pituitary necrosis (Sheehan syndrome) (Rong, Yuna, & Yan, 2014). Postpartum hemorrhage outcomes can be improved by thorough preparation, anticipating the risks of PPH, and coordinating consultants for interventional procedures if warranted.

PPH is a serious complication of pregnancy that is often unanticipated. Even with prompt aggressive management, postpartum bleeding can quickly evolve into a life-threatening event. Perinatal nurses are often the first to observe significant postpartum bleeding and their prompt initial response and continued assessments are pivotal in the anticipation and coordination of necessary interventions. Multidisciplinary team support is critical because obstetric caregivers need a full array of medical and surgical strategies to manage intractable bleeding. Because all postpartum women are at risk for hemorrhage, nurses need to possess the knowledge and skills to practice active management of the third stage of labor to prevent hemorrhage and to recognize, assess, and respond rapidly to excessive blood loss in their clients.

Massage the Uterus

Massage the uterus if uterine atony is noted. The uterine muscles are sensitive to touch; massage stimulates the muscle fibers to contract. Massage the boggy uterus to stimulate contractions and expression of any accumulated blood clots while supporting the lower uterine segment. As blood pools in the vagina, stasis of blood causes clots to form. These clots need to be expelled as pressure is placed on the fundus. Note, however, that overly forceful massage can tire the uterine muscles, resulting in further uterine atony and increased pain. See Nursing Procedure 22.1 for the steps in massaging the fundus.

Administer a Uterotonic Drug

Administer a uterotonic drug if repeated fundal massage and expression of clots fail; medication is probably needed to contract the uterus in order to control bleeding from the placental site. The injection of a uterotonic drug immediately after birth is an important intervention used to prevent PPH. Oxytocin (Pitocin); a synthetic analog of prostaglandin E1, misoprostol (Cytotec) or dinoprostone (Prostin E2); methylergonovine maleate (Methergine); and a derivative of prostaglandin (PGF2α), carboprost (Hemabate), are drugs used to manage postpartum hemorrhage (Drug Guide 22.1). However, misoprostol is not approved by the U.S. Food and Drug Administration (FDA) for this purpose. The choice of which uterotonic drug to use for management of bleeding depends on the judgment of the health care provider, the availability of drugs, and the risks and benefits of the drug.

All nurses need to be aware of the contraindications of administering each of the medications used to control postpartum hemorrhage as follows:
- *Pitocin*–never give undiluted as a bolus injection intravenously

NURSING PROCEDURE 22.1

Massaging the Fundus

Purpose: To Promote Uterine Contraction

1. After explaining the procedure to the woman, place one gloved hand on the area above the symphysis pubis (this helps to support the lower uterine segment).
2. Place the other gloved hand (usually the dominant hand) on the fundus.
3. With the hand on the fundus, gently massage the fundus in a circular manner. Be careful not to over massage the fundus, which could lead to muscle fatigue and uterine relaxation.
4. Assess for uterine firmness (uterine tissue responds quickly to touch).
5. If firm, apply gentle yet firm pressure in a downward motion toward the vagina to express any clots that may have accumulated.
6. Do not attempt to express clots until the fundus is firm because the application of firm pressure on an uncontracted uterus could cause uterine inversion, leading to massive hemorrhage.
7. Assist the woman with perineal care and applying a new perineal pad.
8. Remove gloves and wash hands.

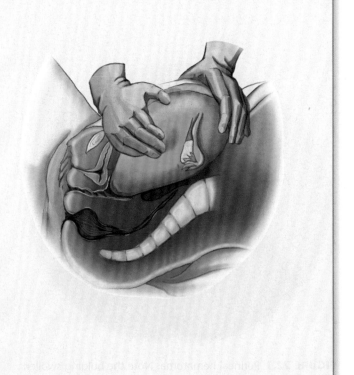

DRUG GUIDE 22.1   DRUGS USED TO CONTROL POSTPARTUM HEMORRHAGE

Drug	Action/Indication	Nursing Implications
Oxytocin (Pitocin) First-line therapy	Stimulates the uterus to contract/ to contract the uterus to control bleeding from the placental site 20–40 units in a liter IV or 10 units IM	Assess fundus for evidence of contraction and compare amount of bleeding every 15 min or according to orders. Monitor vital signs every 15 min. Monitor uterine tone to prevent hyperstimulation. Reassure client about the need for uterine contraction and administer analgesics for comfort. Offer explanation to client and family about what is happening and the purpose of the medication. Provide nonpharmacologic comfort measures to assist with pain management. Set up the IV infusion to be piggybacked into a primary IV line. This ensures that the medication can be discon- tinued readily if hyperstimulation or adverse effects occur while maintaining the IV site and primary infusion.
Misoprostol (Cytotec)	Stimulates the uterus to contract/ to reduce bleeding; a prosta- glandin analog 800 mcg per rectum, one dose (range, 400–1,000 mcg)	Contraindications: Never give undiluted as a bolus injec- tion IV. As above. Not FDA approved for this indication, but a very effective drug therapy for acute postpartum hemorrhage Contraindications: allergy, active CVD, pulmonary or hepatic disease; use with caution in women with asthma
Dinoprostone (Prostin E2)	20 mg vaginal or rectal suppository May be repeated every two hours	Monitor blood pressure frequently since hypotension is a frequent side effect along with vomiting and diarrhea, nausea, temperature elevation
Methylergonovine maleate (Methergine)	Stimulates the uterus/to prevent and treat postpartum hemor- rhage due to atony or subinvo- lution 0.2 mg IM injection May be repeated in 5 min Thereafter every 2–4 h	Assess baseline bleeding, uterine tone, and vital signs every 15 min or according to protocol. Offer explanation to client and family about what is hap- pening and the purpose of the medication. Monitor for possible adverse effects, such as hyperten- sion, seizures, uterine cramping, nausea, vomiting, and palpitations. Report any complaints of chest pain promptly. Contraindications: Hypertension
Prostaglandin (PGF2α), Carboprost, (Hemabate)	Stimulates uterine contractions/ to treat postpartum hemorrhage due to uterine atony when not controlled by other methods 0.25 mg IM injection May be repeated every 15–90 min up to 8 doses Stimulates uterine contractions to reduce bleeding when not controlled by the first-line therapy of oxytocin	Assess vital signs, uterine contractions, client's comfort level, and bleeding status as per protocol. Offer explanation to client and family about what is happening and the purpose of the medication. Monitor for possible adverse effects, such as fever, chills, headache, nausea, vomiting, diarrhea, flushing, and bronchospasm. Contraindications: asthma or active cardiovascular disease Same as above Contraindications: active cardiac, pulmonary, renal, or hepatic disease

Adapted from Callahan, T. L. (2016). *Tarascon's OB/GYN pocketbook*. Burlington, MA: Jones & Bartlett Learning.; Bohlmann, M.,
& Rath, W. (2014). Medical prevention and treatment of postpartum hemorrhage: a comparison of different guidelines. *Archives
of Gynecology & Obstetrics, 289*(3), 555–567.; and Skidmore-Roth, L. (2015). *Mosby's 2015 nursing drug reference* (28th ed.).
St. Louis, MO: Mosby Elsevier.

- *Cytotec*–allergy, active cardiovascular disease, pulmonary or hepatic disease
- *Prostin E2*–active cardiac, pulmonary, renal, or hepatic disease
- *Methergine*–if the woman is hypertensive, do not administer
- *Hemabate*–contraindicated with asthma due to risk of bronchial spasm

Remember Joan, the woman described at the beginning of the chapter? The nurse assesses her and finds that her uterus is boggy. What would the nurse do next? What additional nursing measures might be used if Joan's fundus remains boggy? When should the health care provider be notified?

Maintain the Primary Intravenous Infusion

Maintain the primary intravenous infusion and be prepared to start a second infusion at another site if blood transfusions are necessary. Draw blood for type and cross-match and send it to the laboratory. Administer oxytocics as ordered, correlating and titrating the infusion rate to assessment findings of uterine firmness and lochia. Assess for visible vaginal bleeding, and count or weigh perineal pads.

Take Note!

Postpartum hemorrhage outcomes can be improved by thorough preparation, anticipating the risks factors of PPH in every woman admitted, and coordinating consultants for interventional procedures if warranted.

Check Vital Signs

Check vital signs every 15 to 30 minutes, depending on the acuity of the mother's health status. Monitor her complete blood count to identify any deficit or assess the adequacy of replacement. Assess the woman's level of consciousness to determine changes that may result from inadequate cerebral perfusion.

A Foley catheter is typically in place to keep the bladder empty to avoid displacement of her uterus. A fundus above the umbilicus and deviated laterally indicates a full bladder and interferes with uterine contractions to slow the bleeding.

Prepare the Woman for Removal of Retained Placental Fragments

Prepare the woman for removal of retained placental fragments. These fragments usually are manually separated and removed by the health care provider. Be sure that the health care provider remains long enough after

birth to assess the bleeding status of the woman and determine the etiology. Assist the health care provider with suturing any lacerations immediately to control hemorrhage and repair the tissue.

Nurses should anticipate and prepare the woman for transfer to the operating room for surgical intervention if tamponade techniques fail to achieve hemostasis. The blood bank should be notified that additional transfusions may be required and the woman's condition closely monitored for signs of hypovolemic shock.

Continually Assess the Woman for Signs and Symptoms of Hemorrhagic Shock

Continually assess the woman for signs and symptoms of hemorrhagic shock, a condition in which inadequate perfusion of organs results in insufficient availability of oxygen to satisfy the metabolic needs of the tissues (Green, 2016). Hemorrhagic shock is the most common form of shock encountered in obstetric practice. Subsequently, a catabolic state develops, leading to inflammation, endothelial dysfunction, and disruption of normal metabolic processes in vital organs. Once these events become established, the process of shock is often irreversible, even if volume and red blood cell deficits are corrected. The main goals of treatment of hemorrhagic shock include fluid resuscitation, correction of the imbalance between oxygen delivery and consumption, and treating DIC (Tanczos, Nemeth, & Molnar, 2015).

A postpartum hemorrhage is a traumatic experience because medical complications are unexpected during what is anticipated as a joyful time. Assess the anxiety level of the woman; the woman going into hypovolemic shock is highly anxious and may lose consciousness. The woman's significant others experience a high level of anxiety as well and need a great deal of support.

Monitor the woman's blood pressure, pulse, capillary refill, mental status, and urinary output. These assessments allow estimation of the severity of blood loss and help direct treatment. If the woman develops hemorrhagic shock, interventions focus on controlling the source of blood loss; restoring adequate oxygen-carrying capacity; and maintaining adequate tissue perfusion. Successful treatment depends on efficient collaboration among all health care team members to meet the woman's specific needs.

For the woman with ITP, expect to administer glucocorticoids, intravenous immunoglobulin, intravenous anti-RhoD, and platelet transfusions. Prepare the woman for a splenectomy if the bleeding tissues do not respond to medical management. Be alert for women with abnormal bleeding tendencies, ensuring that they receive proper diagnosis and treatment. Teach them how to prevent severe hemorrhage by learning how to feel for and massage their fundus when boggy, assisting the nurse to keep track of the number of and amount of bleeding on perineal pads, and avoiding any medications with anti-platelet activity such as aspirin, antihistamines, or non-steroidal anti-inflammatory drugs (NSAIDs).

Institute Emergency Measures If DIC Develops

If the woman develops DIC, institute emergency measures to control bleeding and impending shock and prepare to transfer her to the intensive care unit. Identification of the underlying condition and elimination of the causative factor are essential to correct the coagulation problem. Be ready to replace fluid volume, administer blood component therapy, and optimize the mother's oxygenation and perfusion status to ensure adequate cardiac output and end-organ perfusion. Continually reassess the woman's coagulation status via laboratory studies.

Monitor vital signs closely, being alert for changes that signal an increase in bleeding or impending shock. Observe for early signs of ecchymosis, including spontaneous bleeding from gums or nose, petechiae, excessive bleeding from the cesarean incision site or intravenous site, hematuria, and blood in the stool. Late signs include progressive changes in vital signs, skin color, and reduction of urinary output. Collectively, these findings correlate with decreased blood volume, decreased organ and peripheral tissue perfusion, and clots in the microcirculation (Levi & Schmaier, 2015).

Take Note!

Always remember the five causes of postpartum hemorrhage and the appropriate intervention for each: (1) uterine atony—massage and oxytocics; (2) retained placental tissue—evacuation and oxytocics; (3) lacerations or hematoma—surgical repair; (4) thrombin (bleeding disorders)—blood products; and (5) uterine inversion caused by too much cord traction—gentle replacement of uterus and oxytocics.

Institute measures to avoid tissue trauma or injury, such as giving injections and drawing blood. Also provide emotional support to the client and her family throughout this critical time by being readily available and providing explanations and reassurance.

Preventing Postpartum Hemorrhage

Avoid an episiotomy unless an emergency birth is necessary and the perineum is a limiting factor. It is important to have the continuous intrapartum presence of an experienced labor and birth nurse. Provide active management of the third stage of labor, including administration of a uterotonic medication after birth of anterior shoulder, controlled and gentle cord traction to deliver the placenta, and uterine massage after the placenta is out. Authors of a Cochrane review concluded that active

management of the third stage of labor is associated with reduced blood loss, reduced risk of PPH, and a reduced prolonged third stage of labor (Mousa et al., 2014).

Frequent staff education and PPH drills will help keep skills up to date. Nurses must identify and correct anemia and screen for coagulopathies before labor and birth. After birth, it is important to inspect the placenta (once it is delivered) for completeness. Assess woman for lower genital tract lacerations immediately after birth and reevaluate the woman's vital signs and vaginal flow after childbirth. Finally, it is important to be aware of the mother's beliefs about blood transfusions. Recently a work-group representing all major women's health professional organizations developed an obstetric hemorrhage safety bundle for practice to improve PPH outcomes. Some of their selected readiness action domains include:

- Having a hemorrhage cart with supplies and instruction cards on every OB unit
- Having immediate access to medications used to treat a massive hemorrhage
- Establishing a response team within the hospital that can be called
- Developing emergency-release transfusion protocols in the blood bank
- Educating all staff on protocols and holding unit-based drills frequently (Main et al., 2015).

In summary, careful monitoring of the mother's vital signs, laboratory tests (in particular, coagulation testing) and immediate diagnosis of the cause of PPH are important key factors to reduce maternal morbidity and mortality. Nurses must always be prepared to identify signs and symptoms of PPH, recognize maternal compromise and deal with hemorrhage promptly. By identifying hemorrhage promptly and providing swift interventions, maternal mortality and morbidity can be reduced.

An intravenous oxytocin infusion is started for Joan. What assessments will need to be done frequently to make sure Joan is not losing too much blood? What discharge instructions need to be reinforced with Joan?

VENOUS THROMBOEMBOLIC CONDITIONS

Venous thromboembolism is one of the leading causes of maternal mortality and morbidity with an annual incidence of one per 1,000 pregnancies, a ten times higher risk than the nonpregnant population (Testa et al., 2015). A thrombosis (blood clot within a blood vessel) can cause an inflammation of the blood vessel lining (thrombophlebitis), which in turn can lead to a thromboembolism (obstruction of a blood vessel by a blood clot carried by the circulation from the site of origin).

Thrombi can involve the superficial or deep veins in the legs or pelvis. Superficial venous thrombosis usually involves the saphenous venous system and is confined to the lower leg. Superficial thrombophlebitis may be caused by the use of the lithotomy position during birth. Deep venous thrombosis (DVT) can involve deep veins from the foot to the calf, to the thighs, or pelvis. In both locations, thrombi can dislodge and migrate to the lungs, causing a pulmonary embolism (PE).

DVT is a common condition that can have serious complications. Deep venous thrombi have a high probability of propagating and leading to pulmonary emboli, which may cause chest pain, breathlessness, and sudden death. Thus, an accurate and timely diagnosis of DVT is imperative. Although DVT is often clinically silent, it may present with a number of signs, including calf pain, edema, and venous distention.

The three most common venous thromboembolic conditions occurring during the postpartum period are superficial venous thrombosis, DVT, and PE. Although venous thromboembolic disorders occur in less than 1% of all postpartum women, pulmonary embolus can be fatal if a clot obstructs the lung circulation; thus, early identification and treatment are paramount. Risk for postpartum venous thromboembolism is highest during the first three weeks after childbirth. Women with obstetric complications are at highest risk for this, and this risk remains elevated throughout the first twelve weeks postpartum (Tepper et al., 2014).

Pathophysiology

Thrombus (blood clot) formation typically results from venous stasis, injury to the innermost layer of the blood vessel, and hypercoagulation. Venous stasis and hypercoagulation are both common in the postpartum period.

If a clot dislodges and travels to the pulmonary circulation, PE can occur. PE is a potentially fatal condition that occurs when the pulmonary artery is blocked by a blood clot that has traveled from another vein into the lungs, causing an obstruction and infarction. When the clot is large enough to block one or more of the pulmonary vessels that supply the lungs, it can result in sudden death. Approximately 600,000 PEs occur yearly in the United States, resulting in 60,000 to 100,000 deaths (CDC, 2015b). Only 25% of all clients with PE are actually diagnosed, indicating that thousands of PEs go undetected. Many deaths due to PE are unrecognized and the diagnosis is often made at autopsy. PE is the leading cause of pregnancy-related death in the United States, occurring in 2 out of 100,000 live births. It most commonly occurs up to 3 weeks postpartum and following a surgical birth (Conti, et al., 2014). A national review of severe obstetric complications found a significant increase in the rate of PE associated with the increasing rate of cesarean births. Adequate treatment of thrombotic events in pregnancy is important to prevent progression of thrombosis to the development of pulmonary embolism (Sucker & Zotz, 2015).

Nursing Assessment

Assess the woman closely for risk factors and signs and symptoms of thrombophlebitis. Look for risk factors in the woman's history such as use of oral contraceptives before the pregnancy, smoking, employment that necessitates prolonged standing, history of thrombosis, thrombophlebitis, or endometritis, or evidence of current varicosities. Also look for other factors that can increase a woman's risk, such as prolonged bed rest, diabetes, obesity, cesarean birth, progesterone-induced distensibility of the veins of the lower legs during pregnancy, severe anemia, varicose veins, advanced maternal age (older than 34 years), and multiparity. The likelihood of thrombophlebitis is increased through most of pregnancy and for approximately 12 weeks after childbirth. This is partly due to increased platelet stickiness and partly due to reduced fibrinolytic activity (Guimicheva, Czuprynska, & Arya, 2015).

Ask the woman if she has pain or tenderness in the lower extremities. Suspect superficial venous thrombosis in a woman with varicose veins who reports tenderness and discomfort over the site of the thrombosis, most commonly in the calf area. The area appears reddened along the vein and is warm to the touch. The woman will report increased pain in the affected leg when she ambulates and bears weight.

Manifestations of DVT are often absent and diffuse. If present, they are caused by an inflammatory process and obstruction of venous return. Calf swelling, erythema, warmth, tenderness, and pedal edema may be noted. A positive Homans' sign (pain in the upper calf upon dorsiflexion) is not a definitive diagnostic sign as it is insensitive and nonspecific and is no longer recommended as an indicator of DVT. That is because calf pain can also be caused by a strained muscle, contusion, clients with herniated intervertebral discs, calf muscle spasm, neurogenic leg pain, ruptured Baker's cyst, and cellulitis (Heffline & Schmidt, 2014).

Be alert for signs and symptoms of pulmonary embolism, including unexplained sudden onset of shortness of breath and severe chest pain. The woman may be apprehensive and diaphoretic. Additional manifestations may include tachypnea, tachycardia, hypotension, syncope, distention of the jugular vein, decreased oxygen saturation (shown by pulse oximetry), cardiac arrhythmias, hemoptysis, and a sudden change in mental status as a result of hypoxemia (Quellette, Harrington, & Kamangar, 2015). Prepare the woman for a lung scan to confirm the diagnosis.

Nursing Management

Nursing management focuses on preventing thrombotic conditions, promoting adequate circulation if thrombosis occurs, and educating the client about preventive measures, anticoagulant therapy, and danger signs.

Preventing Thrombotic Conditions

Prevention of thrombotic conditions is an essential aspect of nursing management and can be achieved with the routine use of simple measures:

- Developing public awareness about risk factors, symptoms, and preventive measures
- Preventing venous stasis by encouraging activity that causes leg muscles to contract and promotes venous return (leg exercises and walking)
- Dorsi/plantar flexion of feet with prolonged sitting to promote venous return
- Using intermittent sequential compression devices to produce passive leg muscle contractions until the woman is ambulatory
- Elevating the woman's legs above her heart level to promote venous return
- Stopping smoking to reduce or prevent vascular vasoconstriction
- Applying compression stockings and removing them daily for inspection of legs
- Using postoperative deep-breathing exercises to improve venous return by relieving the negative thoracic pressure on leg veins
- Reducing hypercoagulability with the use of aspirin or anticoagulation therapy
- Preventing venous pooling by avoiding pillows under knees, not crossing legs for long periods, and not leaving legs up in stirrups for long periods
- Padding stirrups to reduce pressure against the popliteal angle
- Avoiding sitting or standing in one position for prolonged periods
- Avoiding trauma to legs to prevent injury to the vein wall
- Increasing fluid intake to prevent dehydration
- Avoiding the use of oral contraceptives

In women at risk, early ambulation is the easiest and most cost-effective method. Use of compression stockings decreases distal calf vein thrombosis by decreasing venous stasis and augmenting venous return (Wells, Forgie, & Rodger, 2014). Women who are at a high risk for thromboembolic disease based on risk factors or a previous history of DVT or PE may be placed on prophylactic anticoagulation therapy during pregnancy. A low-molecular-weight heparin such as enoxaparin (Lovenox) can be given or rivaroxaban (Xarelto), apixaban (Eliquis), or dabigatran etexilate (Pradaxa) can be given (Middeldorp, 2015). It is typically discontinued during labor and birth and then restarted during the postpartum period.

Promoting Adequate Circulation

The mainstay of venous thromboembolic conditions is anticoagulation, while interventions such as thrombolysis and inferior vena cava filters are reserved for limited circumstances. For the woman with superficial venous thrombosis, administer NSAIDs for analgesia, provide for rest and elevation of the affected leg, apply warm compresses to the affected area to promote healing, and use antiembolism stockings to promote circulation to the extremities.

Implement bed rest or limited ambulation if ordered and elevation of the affected extremity for the woman with DVT. These actions help to reduce interstitial swelling and promote venous return from that leg. Apply antiembolism stockings to both extremities as ordered. Fit the stockings correctly to avoid excess pressure and constriction and urge the woman to wear them at all times. Sequential compression devices can also be used for women with varicose veins, a history of thrombophlebitis, or a surgical birth.

Anticoagulant therapy using a continuous intravenous infusion of low molecular-weight heparin along with vitamin K antagonists usually is initiated to prolong the clotting time and prevent extension of the thrombosis. Monitor the woman's coagulation studies closely; these might include activated partial thromboplastin time (aPTT), whole-blood partial thromboplastin time, and platelet levels. A therapeutic aPTT value typically ranges from 35 to 45 seconds, depending on which standard values are used (Pagana, Pagana, & Pagana, 2014). Also apply warm moist compresses to the affected leg and administer analgesics as ordered to decrease the discomfort.

After several days of intravenous low molecular-weight heparin therapy, expect to begin oral anticoagulant therapy as ordered. In most cases, the woman will continue to take this medication for several months after discharge.

For the woman who develops a pulmonary embolism, institute emergency measures immediately. The objectives of treatment are to prevent growth or multiplication of thrombi in the lower extremities, prevent more thrombi from traveling to the pulmonary vascular system, and provide cardiopulmonary support if needed. Administer oxygen via mask or cannula as ordered and initiate intravenous low molecular-weight heparin therapy titrated according to the results of the coagulation studies. Maintain the client on bed rest, and administer analgesics as ordered for pain relief. Be prepared to assist with administering thrombolytic agents, such as alteplase (tPA), which might be used to dissolve pulmonary emboli and the source of the thrombus in the pelvis or deep leg veins, thus reducing the potential for a recurrence.

Educating the Client

Provide teaching about the use of anticoagulant therapy and danger signs that should be reported (Teaching Guidelines 22.1). Provide anticipatory guidance, support, and education about associated signs of complications and risks.

Teaching Guidelines 22.1

TEACHING TO PREVENT BLEEDING RELATED TO ANTICOAGULANT THERAPY

- Watch for possible signs of bleeding and notify your health care provider if any occur:
  - Nosebleeds
  - Bleeding from the gums or mouth
  - Black tarry stools
  - Brown "coffee grounds" vomitus
  - Red to brown speckled mucus from a cough
  - Oozing at incision, episiotomy site, cut, or scrape
  - Pink, red, or brown-tinged urine
  - Bruises, "black and blue marks"
  - Increased lochia discharge (from present level)
- Practice measures to reduce your risk of bleeding:
  - Brush your teeth gently using a soft toothbrush.
  - Use an electric razor for shaving.
  - Avoid activities that could lead to injury, scrapes, bruising, or cuts.
  - Do not use any over-the-counter products containing aspirin or aspirin-like derivatives.
  - Avoid consuming alcohol.
  - Inform other health care providers about the use of anticoagulants, especially dentists.
- Be sure to comply with follow-up laboratory testing as scheduled.
- If you accidentally cut or scrape yourself, apply firm direct pressure to the site for 5 to 10 minutes. Do the same after receiving any injections or having blood specimens drawn.
- Wear an identification bracelet or band that indicates that you are taking an anticoagulant.
- Elimination of modifiable risk factors for DVT (smoking, use of oral contraceptives, a sedentary lifestyle, and obesity).
- Importance of using compression stockings.
- Avoidance of constrictive clothing and prolonged standing or sitting in a motionless, leg-dependent position.
- Danger signs and symptoms (sudden onset of chest pain, dyspnea, and tachypnea) to report to the health care provider.

POSTPARTUM INFECTION

Infection during the postpartum period is a common cause of maternal morbidity and mortality. Overall, postpartum infection is estimated to occur in up to 8% of all births and accounts for 15% of global maternal mortality. There is a higher occurrence in cesarean births than in vaginal births (Mattson & Smith, 2016). Postpartum infection is defined as a fever of 100.4° F (38° C) or higher after the first 24 hours after childbirth, occurring on at least 2 of the first 10 days after birth, exclusive of the first 24 hours (Dalton & Castillo, 2014).

Risk factors include surgical birth, prolonged rupture of membranes, long labor with multiple vaginal examinations, inadequate hand hygiene, internal fetal monitoring, uterine manipulation, chorioamnionitis, instrumental birth, obesity, untreated infection prior to birth, retained placental fragments, obesity, gestational diabetes, extremes of client age, low socioeconomic status, and anemia during pregnancy (Jordan et al., 2014).

Infections can easily enter the female genital tract externally and ascend through the internal genital structures. Postpartum women possess an increased risk for infection due to tissue trauma during birth, vulnerability from placenta separation site, and the incision from cesarean section. In addition, the normal physiologic changes of childbirth increase the risk of infection by decreasing the vaginal acidity due to the presence of amniotic fluid, blood, and lochia, all of which are alkaline. An alkaline environment encourages the growth of bacteria.

Postpartum infections usually arise from organisms that constitute the normal vaginal flora, typically a mix of aerobic and anaerobic species. Generally, they are polymicrobial and involve the following microorganisms: *Staphylococcus aureus, Escherichia coli, Klebsiella, Gardnerella vaginalis,* gonococci, coliform bacteria, group A or B hemolytic streptococci, *Chlamydia trachomatis,* and the anaerobes that are common to bacterial vaginosis. Prevention can be achieved by screening and treating vaginal colonization during pregnancy (Callahan, 2016). Common postpartum infections include metritis, surgical site infections, urinary tract infections, and mastitis.

Metritis

Although usually referred to clinically as endometritis, postpartum uterine infections typically involve more than just the endometrial lining. **Metritis** is an infectious condition that involves the endometrium, decidua, and adjacent myometrium of the uterus. Extension of metritis can result in parametritis, which involves the broad ligament and possibly the ovaries and fallopian tubes, or septic pelvic thrombophlebitis, which results when the infection spreads along venous routes into the pelvis. It occurs within the first two days postpartum or as late as two to six weeks postpartum (King et al., 2015).

The uterine cavity is sterile until rupture of the amniotic sac. As a consequence of labor, birth, and associated manipulations, anaerobic and aerobic bacteria can contaminate the uterus. In most cases, the bacteria responsible for pelvic infections are those that normally reside in the bowel, vagina, perineum, and cervix, such as *E. coli, Klebsiella pneumoniae,* or *G. vaginalis.*

The risk of metritis increases dramatically after a cesarean birth; it complicates from 10% to 20% of cesarean births. This is typically an extension of chorioamnionitis that was present before birth (indeed, that may have been why the cesarean birth was performed). In addition, trauma to the tissues and a break in the skin (incision) provide entrances for bacteria to enter the body and multiply.

ACOG (2014b) recommends use of one dose of prophylactic antibiotic therapy administered one hour before any cesarean section and this has become standard practice in the United States today. Once rupture of the amniotic membranes occurs during labor and birth, the uterus becomes more susceptible to colonization and infection, especially if it is a prolonged labor. Any area traumatized during childbirth is susceptible to infection.

Surgical Site Infections

Any break in the skin or mucous membranes provides a portal for bacteria. In the postpartum woman, sites of wound infection include cesarean surgical incisions, the episiotomy site in the perineum, and genital tract lacerations (Fig. 22.2). Wound infections are usually not identified until the woman has been discharged from the hospital because symptoms may not show up until 24 to 48 hours after birth.

Urinary Tract Infections

Urinary tract infections are most commonly caused by bacteria often found in bowel flora, including *E. coli*, *Klebsiella*, *Proteus*, and *Enterobacter* species. Invasive manipulation of the urethra (e.g., urinary catheterization), frequent vaginal examinations, and genital trauma increase the likelihood of a urinary tract infection. It is the most common cause of a fever in the postpartum woman.

Mastitis

Mastitis is defined as inflammation of the mammary gland. A common problem that may occur within the

first 2 days to 2 weeks postpartum. An estimated 5% of breast-feeding women develop lactational mastitis (Spiliopoulos & Mastrogiannis, 2014). Risk factors associated with mastitis include stasis of milk due to infrequent, inconsistent breastfeeding, and nipple trauma. As well as causing significant discomfort, it is a frequent reason for women to stop breast-feeding. It can result from any event that creates milk stasis: insufficient drainage of the breast, rapid weaning, oversupply of milk, pressure on the breast from a poorly fitting bra, a blocked duct, missed feedings, and breakdown of the nipple via fissures, cracks, or blisters (Nagtalon-Ramos, 2014). The most common infecting organism is *S. aureus,* which comes from the breast-feeding infant's mouth or throat. *Staphylococcus albus*, *E. coli*, and streptococci are also causative agents, but found less frequently. Infection can be transmitted from the lactiferous ducts to a secreting lobule, from a nipple fissure to periductal lymphatics, or by circulation (Amir, 2014) (Fig. 22.3). A breast abscess may develop if mastitis is not treated adequately. Flu-like symptoms are often the first symptoms experienced by the mother. Breasts are red, tender, and hot to the touch. The upper, outer quadrant of the breast is the most common site for mastitis to occur because most of the breast tissue is located there with both the right and left breasts being equally affected. Effective milk removal, pain medication, and antibiotic therapy have been the mainstays of treatment.

Therapeutic Management

METRITIS

When metritis occurs, broad-spectrum antibiotics are used to treat the infection. Management also includes measures to restore and promote fluid and electrolyte balance, provide analgesia, and provide emotional support. In most treated women, fever drops and symptoms cease within 48 to 72 hours after the start of antibiotic therapy.

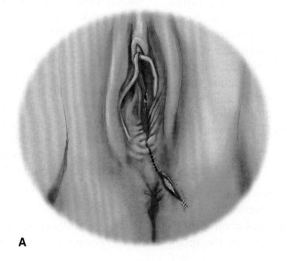
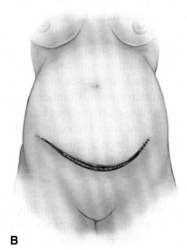

FIGURE 22.2 Postpartum wound infections. **A.** Infected episiotomy site. **B.** Infected cesarean birth incision.   **A**   **B**

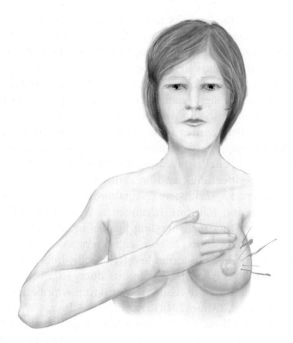

FIGURE 22.3 With mastitis, an area on one breast is tender, hot, red, and painful.

SURGICAL SITE INFECTIONS

Management for surgical site infections involves recognition of the infection, followed by opening of the wound to allow drainage. Aseptic wound management with sterile gloves and frequent dressing changes if applicable, good hand hygiene, frequent perineal pad changes, hydration, and ambulation to prevent venous stasis and improve circulation are initiated to prevent development of a more serious infection or spread of the infection to adjacent structures. Parenteral antibiotics are the mainstay of treatment. Analgesics are also important, because women often experience discomfort at the wound site.

URINARY TRACT INFECTIONS

Urinary tract infections are common during the postpartum period and could be prevented by timely removal of urinary catheters used during labor or surgical births. Risk factors include catheterization, epidural anesthesia, and vaginal procedures. If the woman develops a urinary tract infection, fluids are used to treat dehydration. General nutrition measures include acidifying the urine by taking large doses of vitamin C or a regular intake of cranberry juice. Cranberry juice contains a substance with biologic activity that inhibits the growth of *E. coli* in the urinary tract (Wong & Rosh, 2015). Antibiotics may also be ordered if appropriate.

MASTITIS

Treatment of mastitis focuses on two areas: emptying the breasts and controlling the infection. Frequent breast emptying helps both infectious and noninfectious mastitis. The breast can be emptied either by the infant sucking or by manual expression. Increasing the frequency of nursing is advised. Lactation need not be suppressed. Control of infection is achieved with antibiotics. In addition, ice or warm packs and analgesics may be needed. In addition to antibiotics, management of lactational breast infections includes symptomatic treatment, assessment of the infant's attachment to the breast, and reassurance, emotional support, education, and support for ongoing breast-feeding.

Take Note!

Regardless of the etiology of mastitis, the focus is on reversing milk stasis, maintaining milk supply, and continuing breast-feeding, along with providing maternal comfort and preventing recurrence.

Nursing Assessment

Perinatal nurses are the primary caregivers for postpartum women and have a unique opportunity to identify subtle changes that place women at risk for infection. Nurses play a key role in identifying signs and symptoms that suggest a postpartum infection. Today women are commonly discharged 24 to 48 hours after giving birth. Therefore, nurses must assess new mothers for risk factors and identify early, subtle signs and symptoms of an infectious process. Factors that place a woman at risk for a PPI are highlighted in Box 22.1.

Review the client's history and physical examination and labor and birth record for factors that might increase her risk for developing an infection. Then complete the assessment (using the "BUBBLE-EE" parameters discussed in Chapter 16), paying particular attention to areas such as the abdomen and fundus, breasts, urinary tract, episiotomy, lacerations, or incisions and being alert for signs and symptoms of infection (Table 22.3).

Take Note!

A PPI is commonly associated with an elevated temperature, as mentioned previously. Other generalized signs and symptoms may include chills, foul-smelling vaginal discharge, headache, malaise, restlessness, anxiety, and tachycardia. In addition, the woman may have specific signs and symptoms based on the type and location of the infection.

The acronym REEDA is frequently used for assessing a woman's perineum status. It is derived from five components that have been identified to be associated with the healing process of the perineum. These include:
1. Redness—area may also feel warm to touch
2. Edema—may indicate infection or a hematoma
3. Ecchymosis—may indicate vaginal trauma
4. Discharge—should follow the expected lochia pattern
5. Approximation of skin edges— should be well aligned without gaps

Each category is assessed and a number assigned (0 to 3 points) for a total REEDA score ranging from 0 to

BOX 22.1

FACTORS PLACING A WOMAN AT RISK FOR POSTPARTUM INFECTION

- Prolonged (>18 to 24 hours) premature rupture of membranes (removes the barrier of amniotic fluid so bacteria can ascend)
- Cesarean birth (allows bacterial entry due to break in protective skin barrier)
- Urinary catheterization (could allow entry of bacteria into bladder due to break in aseptic technique)
- Regional anesthesia that decreases perception of need to void (causes urinary stasis and increases risk of urinary tract infection)
- Staff attending to woman are ill (promotes droplet infection from personnel)
- Compromised health status, such as anemia, obesity, smoking, drug abuse (reduces the body's immune system and decreases ability to fight infection)
- Pre-existing colonization of lower genital tract with bacterial vaginosis, *Chlamydia trachomatis,* group B streptococci, *S. aureus,* and *E. coli* (allows microbes to ascend)
- Retained placental fragments (provides medium for bacterial growth)
- Manual removal of a retained placenta (causes trauma to the lining of the uterus and thus opens up sites for bacterial invasion)
- Insertion of fetal scalp electrode or intrauterine pressure catheters for internal fetal monitoring during labor (provides entry into uterine cavity)
- Instrument-assisted childbirth, such as forceps or vacuum extraction (increases risk of trauma to genital tract, which provides bacteria access to grow)
- Trauma to the genital tract, such as episiotomy or lacerations (provides a portal of entry for bacteria)
- Prolonged labor with frequent vaginal examinations to check progress (allows time for bacteria to multiply and increases potential exposure to microorganisms or trauma)
- Poor nutritional status (reduces body's ability to repair tissue)
- Gestational diabetes (decreases body's healing ability and provides higher glucose levels on skin and in urine, which encourages bacterial growth)
- Break in aseptic technique during surgery or birthing process (allows entry of bacteria)

Adapted from Salam, R. A., Mansoor, T., Mallick, D., Lassi, Z. S., Das, J. K., & Bhutta, Z. A. (2014). Essential childbirth and postnatal interventions for improved maternal and neonatal health. *Reproductive Health, 11*(Suppl 1), S3–20; Jordan, R. G., Engstrom, J. L., Marfell, J. A., & Farley, C. L. (2014). *Prenatal and postnatal care: A woman-centered approach.* Ames, Iowa: Wiley Blackwell; and Wong, A. W., & Rosh, A. J. (2015). Postpartum infections. *eMedicine.* Retrieved from http://emedicine.medscape.com/article/796892-overview

TABLE 22.3   SIGNS AND SYMPTOMS OF POSTPARTUM INFECTIONS

Postpartum Infection	Signs and Symptoms
Metritis	Lower abdominal tenderness or pain on one or both sides Temperature elevation (>38° C) Foul-smelling lochia Anorexia Nausea Fatigue and lethargy Leukocytosis and elevated sedimentation rate
Wound infection	Weeping serosanguineous or purulent drainage Separation of or unapproximated wound edges Edema Erythema Tenderness Discomfort at the site Maternal fever Elevated white blood cell count
Urinary tract infection	Urgency Frequency Dysuria Flank pain Low-grade fever Urinary retention Hematuria Urine positive for nitrates Cloudy urine with strong odor
Mastitis	Flu-like symptoms, including malaise, fever, and chills Tender, hot, red, painful area on one breast Inflammation of breast area Breast tenderness Cracking of skin around nipple or areola Breast distention with milk

Adapted from Dalton, E., & Castillo, E. (2014). Postpartum infections: A review for the non-OB/GYN. *Obstetric Medicine: The Medicine of Pregnancy,* (Online 2/27/14), 1753495X14522784. doi: 10.1177/1753495X14522784; Nagtalon-Ramos, J. (2014). *Maternal-newborn nursing care: Best evidence-based practices.* Philadelphia, PA: F.A. Davis Company; and Spiliopoulos, M., & Mastrogiannis, D. (2015). Normal and abnormal puerperium. *eMedicine.* Retrieved from http://emedicine.medscape.com/article/260187-overview#a1

Nursing Management

Nursing management focuses on preventing postpartum infections. Use the following guidelines to reduce the incidence of postpartum infections:

- Maintain aseptic technique when performing invasive procedures such as urinary catheterization, when changing dressings, and during all surgical procedures.

15. The higher scores indicate increased tissue trauma (Kaur et al., 2015). See Figure 22.4 for the REEDA method for assessing perineum healing.

Monitor the woman's vital signs, especially her temperature. Changes may also signal an infection.

REEDA Method for Assessing Perineum Healing

➤ **Redness**

   o   none = 0 points

   o   Redness within .25 cm of incision bilaterally = 1

   o   Redness within .50 cm of incision bilaterally = 2

   o   Redness reaching beyond .5 cm of incision bilaterally = 3

➤ **Edema** – the more swelling present, the high the score

   o   None = 0 points

   o   < 1 cm from incision = 1 point

   o   1 to 2 cm from incision = 2 points

   o   > 2 cm from incision = 3 points

➤ **Ecchymosis** – the more bruising observed, the higher the score

   o   None = 0 points

   o   1-2 cm from incision = 1 point

   o   .25 cm-1 cm bilaterally or .5-2 cm unilaterally = 2 points

   o   > 1 cm bilaterally or 2 cm unilaterally = 3 points

➤ **Discharge** – range would be from none present to profuse

   o   None = 0 points

   o   Serum discharge present = 1 point

   o   Serosanguineous discharge present = 2 points

   o   Bloody, purulent discharge present = 3 points

➤ **Approximation of skin edges**

   o   Closed, skin edges approximated well = 0 points

   o   Skin separated 3 cm or less = 1 point

   o   Skin and subcutaneous fat separated = 2 points

   o   Skin, subcutaneous fat and facial separation = 3 points

FIGURE 22.4 REEDA method for assessing perineum healing. Adapted from Davidson, N. (1974). REEDA: Evaluating postpartum healing. *Journal of Nurse Midwifery 19*(2), 6–8; and Nikpour, M., Shirvani, M. A., Azadbakht, M., Zanjani, R., & Mousavi, E. (2014). The effect of honey gel on abdominal wound healing in cesarean section: A triple blind randomized clinical trial. *Oman Medical Journal, 29*(4), 255–259.

- Use good hand hygiene technique before and after each client care activity.
- Reinforce measures for maintaining good perineal hygiene.
- Practice standard precautions whenever in contact with blood, body fluids, and excretions.
- Use adequate lighting and turn the client to the side to assess the episiotomy site.
- Use extreme caution when handling sharp instruments, specimens, and waste disposal.
- Screen all visitors for any signs of active infections to reduce the client's risk of exposure.
- Review the client's history for pre-existing infections or chronic conditions.
- Monitor vital signs and laboratory results for any abnormal values.
- Monitor the frequency of vaginal examinations and length of labor.
- Assess frequently for early signs of infection, especially fever and the appearance of lochia.
- Inspect wounds frequently for inflammation and drainage.
- Encourage rest, adequate hydration, and healthy eating habits.
- Reinforce preventive measures during any interaction with the client.

If the woman develops an infection, review treatment measures, such as antibiotic therapy if ordered, and any special care measures, such as dressing changes, that might be needed (Nursing Care Plan 22.1).

Postpartum women should be offered advice on the signs and symptoms of life-threatening conditions, including sepsis. Information should include the importance of good hand and perineal hygiene and of the need to seek immediate medical care if feeling unwell. Client teaching is a priority due to today's short lengths of stay after childbirth. Some infections may not manifest until after discharge. Review the signs and symptoms of infection, emphasizing the danger signs that need to be reported to the health care provider. Most importantly, stress proper hand hygiene, especially after perineal care and before and after breast-feeding. Also reinforce measures to promote breast-feeding, including proper breast care (see Chapter 16). Teaching Guidelines 22.2 highlights the major teaching points for a woman with a postpartum infection.

Teaching Guidelines 22.2
TEACHING FOR THE WOMAN WITH A POSTPARTUM INFECTION

- Continue your antibiotic therapy as prescribed.
- Take the medication exactly as ordered and continue with the medication until it is finished.
- Do not stop taking the medication even when you are feeling better.

- Check your temperature every day and call your health care provider if it is above 100.4° F (38° C).
- Watch for other signs and symptoms of infection, such as chills, increased abdominal pain, change in the color or odor of your lochia, or increased redness, warmth, swelling, or drainage from a wound site such as your cesarean incision or episiotomy. Report any of these to your health care provider immediately.
- Practice good infection prevention:
- Always wash your hands thoroughly before and after eating, using the bathroom, touching your perineal area, or providing care for your newborn.
- Wipe from front to back after using the bathroom.
- Remove your perineal pad using a front-to-back motion. Fold the pad in half so that the inner sides of the pad that were touching your body are against each other. Wrap in toilet tissue or place in a plastic bag and discard.
- Wash your hands before applying a new pad.
- Apply a new perineal pad using a front-to-back motion. Handle the pad by the edges (top and bottom or sides) and avoid touching the inner aspect of the pad that will be against your body.
- When performing perineal care with a peribottle, angle the spray of water to that it flows from front to back.
- Drink plenty of fluids each day and eat a variety of foods that are high in vitamins, iron, and protein.
- Be sure to get adequate rest at night and periodically throughout the day.

POSTPARTUM AFFECTIVE DISORDERS

The postpartum period involves extraordinary physiologic, psychological, and sociocultural changes in the life of a woman and her family. It is an exhilarating time for most women, but for others it may not be what they had expected. Women have varied reactions to their childbearing experiences, exhibiting a wide range of emotions. Typically, the delivery of a newborn is associated with positive feelings such as happiness, joy, and gratitude for the birth of a healthy infant. However, women may also feel weepy, overwhelmed, or unsure of what is happening to them. They may experience fear about loss of control; they may feel scared, alone, or guilty, or as if they have somehow failed. During the postpartum period, up to 85% of women experience some type of mood disorder (Joy, Mattingly, & Templeton, 2015).

Postpartum affective disorders have been documented for years, but only recently have they received medical attention. Plummeting levels of estrogen and progesterone immediately after birth can contribute to postpartum mood disorders. Reproductive hormones influence every biologic system and many women are particularly sensitive to the effects of perinatal changes in hormone

Overview of the Woman with a Postpartum Complication

Jennifer, a 16-year-old G1P1, gave birth to a boy 3 days ago. It was a cesarean birth due to cephalopelvic disproportion following 25 hours of labor with ruptured membranes. Her temperature is 102.6° F (39.2° C). She is complaining of chills and malaise and says, "My incision really hurts." Jennifer rates her pain as 7 to 8 out of 10. The incision site is red, swollen, and very warm to the touch. A 5-cm area of purulent drainage is noted on the dressing; a 3-cm area of the incision is slightly opened, with the wound edges separated. Jennifer's lochia is scant and dark red, with a strong odor. She asks the nurse to take her baby back to the nursery because she doesn't feel well enough to care for him.

NURSING DIAGNOSIS: Ineffective thermoregulation related to bacterial invasion as evidenced by fever, complaints of chills and malaise, and statement of not feeling well

Outcome Identification and Evaluation

The client will exhibit a return to normothermia as evidenced by a body temperature being maintained below 99° F (37.2° C), reports of a decrease in chills and malaise, and statements of feeling better.

Interventions: *Promoting Fever Reduction*

- Assess vital signs every 2 to 4 hours and record results *to monitor progress of infection.*
- Administer antipyretics as ordered *to reduce temperature and help combat infection.*
- Encourage fluid intake *to promote fluid balance.*
- Document intake and output *to assess hydration status.*

- Offer cool bed bath or shower *to reduce temperature.*
- Place cool cloth on forehead and/or back of neck *to provide comfort.*
- Change bed linen and gown when damp from diaphoresis *to provide comfort and hygiene.*

NURSING DIAGNOSIS: Impaired skin integrity related to wound infection as evidenced by purulent drainage, redness, swelling, and separation of wound edges

Outcome Identification and Evaluation

The client will experience a resolution of wound infection as evidenced by a reduction in redness, swelling, and drainage from wound; absence of purulent drainage; and beginning signs and symptoms of wound healing.

Interventions: *Promoting Wound Healing*

- Administer antibiotic therapy as ordered *to treat infection.*
- Perform frequent dressing changes and wound care as ordered *to promote wound healing;* monitor dressing for drainage, including amount, color, and characteristics, *to evaluate for resolution of infection.*
- Use aseptic technique *to prevent spread of infection.*
- Encourage fluid intake *to maintain fluid balance;* encourage adequate dietary intake, including protein, *to promote healing.*

NURSING DIAGNOSIS: Acute pain related to infectious process

Outcome Identification and Evaluation

The client will report a decrease in pain as evidenced by pain rating of 0 or 1 on pain scale, verbalization of relief with pain management, and statements of feeling better and ability to rest comfortably.

NURSING CARE PLAN 22.1

Overview of the Woman with a Postpartum Complication (continued)

Interventions: *Relieving Pain*

- Place client in semi-Fowler's position *to facilitate drainage and relieve pressure.*
- Assess pain level on pain scale of 0 to 10 to quantify pain level; reassess pain level after intervening *to determine effectiveness of intervention.*
- Assess fundus gently *to ensure appropriate involution.*
- Administer analgesics as needed and on time as ordered *to maintain pain relief.*
- Provide for rest periods *to allow for healing.*
- Assist with positioning in bed with pillows *to promote comfort.*
- Offer nonpharmacologic pain measures such as a backrub *to ease aches and discomfort if desired and enhance effectiveness of analgesics.*

NURSING DIAGNOSIS: Risk for impaired parent–infant attachment related to effects of postpartum infection as evidenced by mother's request to take baby back to the nursery

Outcome Identification and Evaluation

The client will begin to bond with newborn appropriately with each exposure as evidenced by desire to spend time with newborn, expression of positive feelings toward newborn when holding him, increasing participation in care of newborn as client's condition improves, and statements about help and support at home to care for self and newborn.

Interventions: *Promoting Mother–Newborn Interaction*

- Promote adequate rest and sleep *to ensure adequate energy for interaction and wound healing.*
- Bring newborn to mother after she is rested and has had an analgesic *to allow mother to focus her energies on the child.*
- Progressively allow the client to care for her infant or comfort him as her energy level and pain level improve *to promote self-confidence in caring for the newborn.*
- Offer praise and positive reinforcement for caretaking tasks; stress positive attributes of newborn to mother while caring for him *to facilitate bonding and attachment.*
- Contact family members to participate in care of the newborn *to allow mother to rest and recover from infection.*
- Encourage mother to care for herself first and then the newborn *to ensure adequate energy for newborn's care.*
- Arrange for assistance and support after discharge from hospital *to provide necessary backup.*
- Refer to community health nurse for follow-up care of mother and newborn at home *to foster continued development of maternal–infant relationship.*

levels after childbirth. It is believed that the greater the change in these hormone levels between pregnancy and postpartum, the greater the chance for developing a mood disorder (Schiller, Meltzer-Brody, & Rubinow, 2015).

Many types of affective disorders occur in the postpartum period. Although their description and classification may be controversial, the disorders are commonly classified on the basis of their severity as postpartum or baby blues, postpartum depression, and postpartum psychosis.

Postpartum Blues

Many postpartum women (approximately 80%) experience the "blues" (Callahan, 2016). The woman experiences rapid cycling mood symptoms during the first postpartum week typically. The woman exhibits mild depressive symptoms of anxiety, irritability, mood swings, tearfulness, increased sensitivity, despondency, feelings of being overwhelmed, difficulty thinking clearly, and fatigue (Pop et al., 2015). Emotional lability is the most prominent symptom of the maternity blues. The "blues" typically peak on postpartum days 4 and 5 and usually resolve by postpartum day 10. Biologic, psychological, and social factors have been hypothesized as relevant to blues causation, but no studies have validated this. Although the woman's symptoms may be distressing, they do not reflect psychopathology and usually do not affect the mother's ability to function and care for her infant.

Baby blues are usually self-limiting and require no formal treatment other than reassurance and validation of the woman's experience, as well as assistance in caring for herself and the newborn. However, follow-up of women with postpartum blues is important; because up to 20% go on to develop postpartum depression (Alexander et al., 2014).

Postpartum Depression

Depression is more prevalent in women than in men, which may be related to biologic, hormonal, and psychosocial factors. **Postpartum depression (PPD)** is a form of clinical depression that can affect women, and less frequently men, after childbirth. It affects as many as 20% of all mothers in the United States, and as many as 60% of adolescent mothers (ACOG, 2014c; CDC, 2015c; Joy et al., 2015). Unlike the postpartum blues, women with postpartum depression feel worse over time, and changes in mood and behavior do not go away on their own. Postpartum depression may persist for a minimum of six months if untreated. Different from the baby blues, the symptoms of PPD last longer, are more severe, and require treatment. Some signs and symptoms of PPD include feeling the following:

• Restless
• Worthless
• Guilty
• Hopeless
• Moody
• Sad
• Overwhelmed
• Loss of enjoyment
• Low energy level
• Loss of libido

The new mother may also:

• Cry a lot
• Exhibit a lack of energy and motivation
• Be unable to make decisions or focus
• Lose her memory
• Experience a lack of pleasure
• Have changes in, sleep, or weight
• Show a lack of concern for herself
• Withdraw from friends and family
• Have pains in her body that do not subside
• Feel negatively toward her baby
• Appetite disturbances

• Feelings of isolation from others
• Lack interest in her baby
• Worry about hurting the baby
• Act detached toward others and infant
• Have recurrent thoughts of suicide and death (Bobo & Yawn, 2014).

Postpartum depression affects not only the woman but also the entire family. Identifying depression early can substantially improve the client and family outcomes. PPD usually has a gradual onset and becomes evident within the first 6 weeks postpartum.

The cause of PPD is not known, but research suggests that it is multifactorial. According to ACOG (2014c), "postpartum depression is likely to result from body, mind, and lifestyle factors combined." The levels of estrogen, progesterone, serotonin, and thyroid hormone decrease sharply and return to normal during the immediate postpartum period, which can trigger depression and can change a woman's mood and behavior. Other aspects that can lead to PPD include:

• Unresolved feelings about the pregnancy
• Fatigue after delivery from lack of sleep or broken sleep
• Feelings of being less attractive
• Inadequate assistance from partner
• Lack of social support network
• History of sexual or physical abuse
• Unemployment or financial insecurity
• Doubts about the ability to be a good mother
• Stress from changes in work and home routines
• Loss of freedom and old identity (Finley & Brizendine, 2015).

PPD may lend itself to prophylactic intervention because its onset is predictable, the risk period for illness is well defined, and women at high risk potentially could be identified using a screening tool. This is not the case for all women, however (see Evidence-Based Practice 22.1). Prophylaxis starts with a prenatal risk assessment and education. Based on the woman's history of prior depression, prophylactic antidepressant therapy may be needed during the third trimester or immediately after giving birth. Management mirrors that of any major depression: a combination of antidepressant medication, antianxiety medication, adequate sleep and rest, and psychotherapy in an outpatient or inpatient setting (Callahan, 2016). Marital counseling may be necessary if marital problems are contributing to the woman's depressive symptoms.

The significant other's or partner's emotional health should not be overlooked during the woman's pregnancy and throughout the first postpartum year. PPD, once expected only in new mothers, occurs in new significant others or partners as well. Up to 50% of significant others or partners whose partners suffer from PPD also have depressive symptoms, and little is known

EVIDENCE-BASED PRACTICE 22.1   A SYSTEMATIC REVIEW OF THE RELATIONSHIP BETWEEN POSTPARTUM SLEEP DISTURBANCE AND POSTPARTUM DEPRESSION

STUDY

Sleep is closely associated with psychological well-being. Insufficient sleep leads to adverse medical and psychological consequences and a poorer quality of life. Despite commonly held beliefs of joy and happiness, women are vulnerable to mood disorders during the postpartum period. Nighttime feedings and frequent nocturnal awakenings contribute to sleep maternal disturbances. Poor and fragmented sleep patterns are associated with a poor quality of life, a decrease in attentiveness and general well-being. More importantly, it may be a risk factor for postpartum depression. Postpartum depression has been linked with a series of psychosocial sequelae for mothers and their newborns. The purpose of this review was to analyze the relationship between postpartum sleep disturbance and postpartum depression.

Findings

A systematic review was conducted on thirteen observational studies which included 3,793 women. The findings from all thirteen studies revealed a consistent strong relationship between sleep disturbance and postpartum depression. Short sleep duration and insomnia are related to a range of impaired functional outcomes that may negatively impact the daily life of postpartum women and their newborns.

Nursing Implications

Based on this evidence, nurses can counsel postpartum women about the importance of getting adequate sleep when they are discharged and the link between sleep disturbances to postpartum depression. Nurses can suggest several interventions to assist the new mother in obtaining adequate sleep such as bathing the newborn at night before bedtime, asking for help from family to assist in nighttime diaper changes, and taking naps throughout the day when the newborn sleeps. These simple helpful interventions may be a valuable prevention measure to assist in increasing the mother's wellness and reduce the risk of postpartum depression.

Adapted from Bhati, S., & Richards, K. (2015). A systematic review of the relationship between postpartum sleep disturbance and postpartum depression. *Journal of Obstetric, Gynecologic, & Neonatal Nursing, 44*(3), 350–357.

about the impact of maternal PPD on them. Depressive symptoms are likely to decrease their ability to provide maternal support. Significant other's or partner's PPD can be difficult to identify. New partners or significant others may seem more angry and anxious than sad, yet depression is present. When left untreated, partner's PPD limits the significant other's or partner's capacity to provide emotional support to their partners and children. The highest rates of depression among fathers have been reported between 3 and 6 months postpartum. Factors that increase the risk of paternal PPD include a personal history of depression and/or anxiety, a low level of marital satisfaction, excessive financial stressors, a lack of significant other or partner's parental leave, and the feeling that there is a great discrepancy between one's expectations of parenthood and its realities (Feeley et al., 2015).

Assessing partner's PPD is not easy. Nevertheless, it is important for all nurses who have contact with new partners to remain open to the notion that new partners are predisposed to PPD, particularly if their partner is afflicted. Delving deeper into understanding behaviors of withdrawing, indecisiveness, cynicism, avoiding, drinking, using drugs, fighting, partner violence, extramarital affairs, and feelings of heightened irritation will reveal important insights. Asking new partners candidly if they are feeling depressed, anxious, or angry can open the door to further exploration of these emotions (Weissman, 2014).

Although partner depression is only now beginning to be defined and measured, sufficient evidence exists to warrant nurses' attention and concern. Nurses may be most able to help a new partner devastated by PPD when they plant seeds of awareness that the disorder exists, that they are not alone, and that help is available.

Despite the negative outcomes associated with PPD, rates of diagnosis and treatment are low mainly because of lack of recognition by the health care provider. In addition, PPD is the most misinterpreted, frequently dismissed, and most undiagnosed postpartum complication. Early recognition of PPD can eliminate the length of time that women and men have to suffer with this debilitating condition and can decrease the potentially harmful effects on the infants involved.

Screening for symptoms of PPD in both men and women is an important preliminary step to diagnosis and treatment, but the effectiveness of depression screening is dependent on the reliability and validity of the screening instruments in the population. Both the Edinburgh Postnatal Depression Scale (EPDS) and the Postpartum Depression Predictor Scale (PDSS) have been used to screen mothers for PPD, but it is not clear which instrument best predicts a diagnosis of postpartum depression (Thombs et al., 2014).

The EPDS is a self-report, quick, and easy screening tool for PPD that consists of 10 questions with four possible responses. The couple fill out the tool according to their symptoms during the past 7 days, with each response given a score of 0 to 3 points, creating a maximum score of 30. Using a cutoff score of 9 or 10, the sensitivity is 86%; the specificity, 78%; and positive predictive value, 73% (Zhao et al., 2015).

The PDSS is a self-report, 35-item Likert-type response scale divided into seven conceptual domains:
1. Anxiety/insecurity
2. Sleep/eating disturbance
3. Emotional liability
4. Loss of self-esteem
5. Guilt/shame
6. Cognitive impairment
7. Suicidal thoughts

The scores range from 35 to 175. The scale has five symptoms for each domain, and the woman is asked to identify her degree of disagreement or agreement on the basis of her feelings over the past 2 weeks. The sensitivity of the PDSS is 91%; the specificity is 72% for detecting PPD. The PDSS takes 5 to 10 minutes to administer and is used during the postpartum period (King et al., 2015).

Early identification, screening, prevention, and treatment of PPD are crucial for improving overall outcomes for the mother and infant, as well as for decreasing mortality and morbidity. This is why it is crucial for nurses to understand and know about the risk factors, signs and symptoms, prevention, and use and interpretation of screening tools and to make appropriate referrals for treatment. Mass screening for PPD using a validated screening tool has been proven to improve the rates of detection and treatment of PPD and should be implemented in obstetricians' and pediatricians' offices and in primary care settings. The Edinburgh tool is shown in Figure 22.5.

Postpartum Psychosis

At the severe end of the continuum of postpartum emotional disorders is postpartum psychosis, which occurs in 1 in 1000 live births (Doyle, Carballedo, & O'Keane, 2015). Postpartum psychosis, an emergency psychiatric condition, can result in a significant increased risk for suicide and infanticide. Symptoms of postpartum psychosis, such as mood lability, delusional beliefs, hallucinations, and disorganized thinking, can be frightening for the women who are affected and for their families. It generally surfaces within 3 months of giving birth and is manifested by sleep disturbances, fatigue, depression, and hypomania. The mother will be tearful, confused, and preoccupied with feelings of guilt and worthlessness. Early symptoms resemble those of depression, but they may escalate to delirium, hallucinations, extreme disorganization of thought, anger toward herself and her infant, bizarre behavior, delusions, disorientation, depersonalization, delirium-like appearance, manifestations of mania, and thoughts of hurting herself and the infant. The mother frequently loses touch with reality and experiences a severe regressive breakdown, associated with a high risk of suicide or infanticide (del Corral Serrano, 2015). Women with

postpartum psychosis should not be left alone with their infants. Most women with postpartum psychosis are hospitalized for up to several months. Psychotropic drugs are almost always part of treatment, along with individual psychotherapy and support group therapy.

Take Note!

The greatest hazard of postpartum psychosis is suicide. Infanticide and child abuse are also risks if the woman is left alone with her infant. Early recognition and prompt treatment of this disorder are imperative.

Nursing Assessment

Postpartum affective disorders are often overlooked and go unrecognized despite the large percentage of women who experience them. The postpartum period is a time of increased vulnerability, but few women receive education about the possibility of depression after birth. In addition, many women may feel ashamed of having negative emotions at a time when they "should" be happy; thus, they do not seek professional help. Nurses can play a major role in providing guidance about postpartum affective disorders, detecting manifestations, and assisting women to obtain appropriate care.

Consider This

Even though I was an assertive practicing attorney in my thirties, my first pregnancy was filled with nagging feelings of doubt about this upcoming event in my life. Throughout my pregnancy I was so busy with trial work that I never had time to really evaluate my feelings. I was always reading about the bodily changes that were taking place, and on one level I was feeling excited, but on another level I was emotionally drained. Shortly after the birth of my daughter, those suppressed nagging feelings of doubt surfaced big time and practically immobilized me. I felt exhausted all the time and was only too glad to have someone else care for my daughter. I didn't breast-feed because I thought it would tie me down too much. Although at the time I thought this "low mood" was normal for all new mothers, I have since found out it was postpartum depression. How could any woman be depressed about this wondrous event?

Thoughts: Now that postpartum depression has been "taken out of the closet" and recognized as a real emotional disorder, it can be treated. This woman showed tendencies during her pregnancy but was able to suppress the feelings and go forward. Her description of her depression is very typical of many women who suffer in silence, hoping to get over these feelings in time. What can nurses do to promote awareness of this disorder? Can it be prevented?

Edinburgh Postnatal Depression Scale

Name: _____   Address: _____

Your Date of Birth: _____   _____

Baby's Date of Birth: _____   Phone: _____

As you are pregnant or have recently had a baby, we would like to know how you are feeling. Please check the answer that comes closest to how you have felt **IN THE PAST 7 DAYS**, not just how you feel today.

Here is an example, already completed.

I have felt happy:
- ☐ Yes, all the time
- ☒ Yes, most of the time   This would mean: "I have felt happy most of the time" during the past week.
- ☐ No, not very often   Please complete the other questions in the same way.
- ☐ No, not at all

In the past 7 days:

1. I have been able to laugh and see the funny side of things
   - ☐ As much as I always could
   - ☐ Not quite so much now
   - ☐ Definitely not so much now
   - ☐ Not at all

2. I have looked forward with enjoyment to things
   - ☐ As much as I ever did
   - ☐ Rather less than I used to
   - ☐ Definitely less than I used to
   - ☐ Hardly at all

*3. I have blamed myself unnecessarily when things went wrong
   - ☐ Yes, most of the time
   - ☐ Yes, some of the time
   - ☐ Not very often
   - ☐ No, never

4. I have been anxious or worried for no good reason
   - ☐ No, not at all
   - ☐ Hardly ever
   - ☐ Yes, sometimes
   - ☐ Yes, very often

*5 I have felt scared or panicky for no very good reason
   - ☐ Yes, quite a lot
   - ☐ Yes, sometimes
   - ☐ No, not much
   - ☐ No, not at all

*6. Things have been getting on top of me
   - ☐ Yes, most of the time I haven't been able to cope at all
   - ☐ Yes, sometimes I haven't been coping as well as usual
   - ☐ No, most of the time I have copied quite well
   - ☐ No, I have been coping as well as ever

*7 I have been so unhappy that I have had difficulty sleeping
   - ☐ Yes, most of the time
   - ☐ Yes, sometimes
   - ☐ Not very often
   - ☐ No, not at all

*8 I have felt sad or miserable
   - ☐ Yes, most of the time
   - ☐ Yes, quite often
   - ☐ Not very often
   - ☐ No, not at all

*9 I have been so unhappy that I have been crying
   - ☐ Yes, most of the time
   - ☐ Yes, quite often
   - ☐ Only occasionally
   - ☐ No, never

*10 The thought of harming myself has occurred to me
   - ☐ Yes, quite often
   - ☐ Sometimes
   - ☐ Hardly ever
   - ☐ Never

Administered/Reviewed by _____   Date _____

FIGURE 22.5 Adapted from Edinburgh Postnatal Depression Scale (EPDS). From Cox, J. L., Holden, J. M., & Sagovsky, R. (1987). Detection of postnatal depression: Development of the 10-item Edinburgh Postnatal Depression Scale. *British Journal of Psychiatry, 150,* 782–786.

Begin the assessment by reviewing the history to identify general risk factors that could predispose a woman to depression:

- Poor coping skills
- First pregnancy
- Low self-esteem
- Numerous life stressors
- History of abuse
- Mood swings and emotional stress
- Previous psychological problems or a family history of psychiatric disorders
- Substance abuse
- Limited or lack of social support network

Also review the history for specific pregnancy and birth factors that may increase the woman's risk for depression. These may include a history of PPD, evidence of depression during the pregnancy, prenatal anxiety, a difficult or complicated pregnancy, traumatic birth experience, or birth of a high-risk or special-needs infant (Callahan, 2016).

Be alert for physical findings. Assess the woman's activity level, including her level of fatigue. Ask about her sleeping habits, noting any problems with insomnia. When interacting with the woman, observe for verbal and nonverbal indicators of anxiety as well as her ability to concentrate during the interaction. Difficulty concentrating and anxious behaviors suggest a problem. Also assess her nutritional intake: weight loss due to poor food intake may be seen. Assessment can identify women with a high-risk profile for depression, and the nurse can educate them and make referrals for individual or family counseling if needed. Some common assessment findings associated with PPD are listed in Box 22.2.

Nursing Management

Nurses need to educate themselves about this disorder to facilitate early recognition of signs and symptoms of it, which, in turn, would make early treatment possible, thus supporting recovery. Furthermore, greater knowledge could contribute to providing more effective and compassionate care to these women. Nursing management focuses on assisting any postpartum woman to cope with the changes of this period. Encourage the client to verbalize what she is going through and emphasize the importance of keeping her expectations realistic. Assist the woman in structuring her day to regain a sense of control over the situation. Encourage her to seek help if necessary, using available support systems. Also reinforce the need for good nutrition and adequate exercise and sleep (Bobo & Yawn, 2014).

The nurse can play an important role in assisting women and their partners with postpartum adjustment. Providing facts about the enormous changes that occur during the postpartum period is critical. This

---

BOX 22.2

COMMON ASSESSMENT FINDINGS ASSOCIATED WITH POSTPARTUM DEPRESSION

- Loss of pleasure or interest in life
- Low mood, especially in the morning, sadness, tearfulness
- Exhaustion that is not relieved by sleep
- Feelings of guilt
- Weight loss
- Low energy
- Irritability
- Poor personal hygiene
- Constipated
- Preoccupied and unfocused
- Indecisiveness
- Diminished concentration
- Anxiety
- Despair
- Compulsive thoughts
- Loss of libido
- Loss of confidence
- Sleep difficulties (insomnia)
- Loss of appetite
- Bleak and pessimistic view of the future
- Not responding to infant's cries or cues for attention
- Social isolation, won't answer the door or the phone
- Feelings of failure as a mother

Adapted from American College of Obstetrics and Gynecology [ACOG]. (2014c). *Postpartum depression*. Retrieved from http://www.acog.org/Patients/FAQs/Postpartum-Depression#blues; Centers for Disease Control and Prevention [CDC]. (2015c). *Depression among women of reproductive age*. Retrieved from http://www.cdc.gov/reproductivehealth/depression/; and Joy, S., Mattingly, P. J., & Templeton, H. B. (2015). Postpartum depression: An overview of postpartum mood disorders. *eMedicine*. Retrieved from http://emedicine.medscape.com/article/271662-overview

---

information would include changes in the woman's body. Review the signs and symptoms of all three affective disorders. This information is typically included as part of prenatal visits and childbirth education classes. Know the risk factors associated with these disorders and review the history of clients and their families. Use specific, nonthreatening questions to aid in early detection, such as "Have you felt down, depressed, or hopeless lately?" and "Have you felt little interest or pleasure in doing things recently?"

Discuss factors that may increase a woman's vulnerability to stress during the postpartum period, such as sleep deprivation and unrealistic expectations, so couples can understand and respond to those problems if they occur. Stress that many women need help after childbirth and that help is available from many sources, including people they already know. Assisting women to learn how to ask for help is important so they can gain the support they need. Also provide educational materials about postpartum emotional disorders. Have available referral sources for psychotherapy and support groups appropriate for women experiencing postpartum adjustment difficulties. See Evidence-Based Practice 22.1.

KEY CONCEPTS

⦿ Postpartum hemorrhage is a potentially life-threatening complication of both vaginal and cesarean births. It is the leading cause of maternal mortality in the United States.

⦿ A good way to remember the causes of postpartum hemorrhage is the "5 Ts": tone, tissue, trauma, thrombin, and traction.

⦿ Uterine atony is the most common cause of early postpartum hemorrhage, which can lead to hypovolemic shock.

⦿ Oxytocin (Pitocin), misoprostol (Cytotec), dinoprostone (Prostin E2), methylergonovine maleate (Methergine), and prostaglandin PGF2α (carboprost [Hemabate]) are commonly used drugs used to manage postpartum hemorrhage.

⦿ Failure of the placenta to separate completely and be expelled interferes with the ability of the uterus to contract fully, thereby leading to hemorrhage.

⦿ Causes of subinvolution include retained placental fragments, distended bladder, uterine myoma, and infection.

⦿ Lacerations should always be suspected when the uterus is contracted and bright-red blood continues to trickle out of the vagina.

⦿ Conditions that cause coagulopathies may include idiopathic thrombocytopenic purpura, von Willebrand disease, and disseminated intravascular coagulation.

⦿ Pulmonary embolism is a potentially fatal condition that occurs when the pulmonary artery is obstructed by a blood clot that has traveled from another vein into the lungs, causing obstruction and infarction.

⦿ The major causes of a thrombus formation (blood clot) are venous stasis and hypercoagulation, both of which are common in the postpartum period.

⦿ Postpartum infection is defined as a fever of 100.4° F (38° C) or higher after the first 24 hours after childbirth, occurring on at least 2 of the first 10 days exclusive of the first 24 hours.

⦿ Common postpartum infections include metritis, wound infections, urinary tract infections, and mastitis.

⦿ Postpartum emotional disorders are commonly classified on the basis of their severity: "baby blues," postpartum depression, and postpartum psychosis.

⦿ Management of postpartum depression mirrors the treatment of any major depression: a combination of antidepressant medication, antianxiety medication, and psychotherapy in an outpatient or inpatient setting.

References and Recommended Readings

Agency for Healthcare Research and Quality [AHRQ]. (2015). *Evidence-based practice: Management of postpartum hemorrhage.* Retrieved from http://www.effectivehealthcare.ahrq.gov/ehc/products/552/2078/hemorrhage-postpartum-report-150427.pdf

Alexander, L. L., LaRosa, J. H., Bader, H., & Garfield, S. (2014). *New dimensions in women's health* (6th ed.). Sudbury, MA: Jones & Bartlett.

American College of Obstetrics and Gynecologists [ACOG]. (2014a). *Von Willebrand Disease in women.* Retrieved from http://www.acog.org/Resources-And-Publications/Committee-Opinions/Committee-on-Adolescent-Health-Care/Von-Willebrand-Disease-in-Women

American College of Obstetrics and Gynecologists [ACOG]. (2014b). *Use of prophylactic antibiotics in labor and delivery.* Retrieved from http://www.guideline.gov/content.aspx?id = 34024

American College of Obstetrics and Gynecology [ACOG]. (2014c). *Postpartum depression.* Retrieved from http://www.acog.org/Patients/FAQs/Postpartum-Depression#blues

Amir, L. H. (2014). The Academy of Breastfeeding Medicine Protocol Committee: Mastitis. *Breastfeeding Medicine, 9*(5), 239–243.

Anand, B., & Gujral, K. (2014). Monitoring of high-risk areas: Maternity wards. In *Hospital infection prevention* (pp. 133–136). New Delhi, India: Springer Publishers.

Belfort, M. A. (2015). Overview of postpartum hemorrhage. *UpToDate.* Retrieved from http://www.uptodate.com/contents/overview-of-postpartum-hemorrhage

Bhati, S., & Richards, K. (2015). A systematic review of the relationship between postpartum sleep disturbance and postpartum depression. *Journal of Obstetric, Gynecologic, & Neonatal Nursing, 44*(3), 350–357.

Bobo, W. V., & Yawn, B. P. (2014). Concise review for physicians and other clinicians: Postpartum depression. In *Mayo Clinic Proceedings, 89*(6), 835–844.

Bohlmann, M., & Rath, W. (2014). Medical prevention and treatment of postpartum hemorrhage: a comparison of different guidelines. *Archives of Gynecology & Obstetrics, 289*(3), 555–567.

Callahan, T. L. (2016). *Tarascon's OB/GYN pocketbook.* Burlington, MA: Jones & Bartlett Learning.

Centers for Disease Control and Prevention [CDC]. (2015a). *Facts about von Willebrand Disease.* Retrieved from http://www.cdc.gov/ncbddd/vwd/facts.html

Centers for Disease Control and Prevention [CDC]. (2015b). *Deep vein thrombosis (DVT)/Pulmonary embolism (PE) – Blood clot forming in a vein.* Retrieved from http://www.cdc.gov/ncbddd/dvt/data.html

Centers for Disease Control and Prevention [CDC]. (2015c). *Depression among women of reproductive age.* Retrieved from http://www.cdc.gov/reproductivehealth/depression/

Clapp, J. C. (2015). A multidisciplinary team approach to management of postpartum hemorrhage. *Journal of Obstetric, Gynecologic, & Neonatal Nursing, 44,* S22.

Conti, E., Zezza, L., Ralli, E., Comito, C., Sada, L., Passerini, J. et al., (2014). Pulmonary embolism in pregnancy. *Journal of Thrombosis and Thrombolysis, 37*(3), 251–270.

Cox, J., Holden, J., & Henshaw, C. (2014). *Perinatal mental health: The Edinburgh Postnatal Depression Scale (EPDS) Manual* (2nd ed). London, England: RCPsych Publications.

Cox, J. L., Holden, J. M., & Sagovsky, R. (1987). Detection of postnatal depression: Development of the 10-item Edinburgh Postnatal Depression Scale. *British Journal of Psychiatry, 150,* 782–786.

Crowe, S. D., & Faulkner, B. (2014). Lean management system application in creation of a postpartum hemorrhage prevention bundle on postpartum units. *Obstetrics and Gynecology, 123*, 45S–45S.

Cunningham, F. G., Leveno, K. J., Bloom, S. L., Spong, C., Dashe, J. S., Hoffman, B. L., et al. (2014). *Williams' obstetrics* (24th ed.). New York, NY: McGraw-Hill.

Dalton, E., & Castillo, E. (2014). Postpartum infections: A review for the non-OB/GYN. *Obstetric Medicine: The Medicine of Pregnancy*, (Online 2/27/14), 1753495X14522784. doi: 10.1177/1753495X14522784

del Corra l Serrano, J. (2015). Puerperal psychosis. In *Psychopathology in women* (pp. 497–510). Springer International Publishing.

Doyle, M., Carballedo, A., & O'Keane, V. (2015). Perinatal depression and psychosis: an update. *Advances in Psychiatric Treatment, 21*(1), 5–14.

Ekin, A., Gezer, C., Solmaz, U., Taner, C. E., Dogan, A., & Ozeren, M. (2015). Predictors of severity in primary postpartum hemorrhage. *Archives of Gynecology and Obstetrics, 292*(6):1247–1254.1–8.

Erez, O., Mastrolia, S. A., & Thachil, J. (2015). Disseminated intravascular coagulation in pregnancy: Insights in pathophysiology, diagnosis and management. *American Journal of Obstetrics and Gynecology, 213*(4):452–463. doi: http://dx.doi.org/10.1016/j.ajog.2015.03.054

Feeley, N., Bell, L., Hayton, B., Zelkowitz, P., & Carrier, M.E. (2015). Care for postpartum depression: What do women and their partners prefer? *Perspectives in Psychiatric Care*. doi: 10.1111/ppc.12107

Finley, P. R., & Brizendine, L. (2015). Enhancing our understanding of perinatal depression. *CNS Spectrums, 20*(1), 9–10.

Green, C. J. (2016). *Maternal newborn nursing care plans* (3rd ed.), Burlington, MA: Jones & Bartlett Learning.

Guimicheva, B., Czuprynska, J., and Arya, R. (2015). The prevention of pregnancy-related venous thromboembolism. *British Journal of Hematology, 168*, 163–174.

Heffline, M., & Schmidt, M. K. (2014). Superficial thrombophlebitis and deep vein thrombosis. *Core curriculum for vascular nursing.* Chapter 19, 370. Philadelphia, PA: Lippincott, Williams & Wilkins

Jordan, R. G., Engstrom, J. L., Marfell, J. A., & Farley, C. L. (2014). *Prenatal and postnatal care: A woman-centered approach.* Ames, Iowa: Wiley Blackwell.

Joy, S., Mattingly, P. J., & Templeton, H. B. (2015). Postpartum depression: An overview of postpartum mood disorders. *eMedicine.* Retrieved from http://emedicine.medscape.com/article/271662-overview

Kamel, I., & Mastrogiannis, D. S. (2015). The critically ill obstetric patient Part 1: Epidemiology and pathophysiology. *Postgraduate Obstetrics & Gynecology, 35*(11), 1–7.

Kaur, P., Sagar, N., Deol, R., & Kaur, J. (2015). Effectiveness of infrared therapy upon level of episiotomy pain and wound healing among postnatal mothers. *International Journal of Nursing Education, 7*(2), 184–187.

Kessler, C. M., & Sandler, S. G. (2015). Immune thrombocytopenic purpura. *eMedicine.* Retrieved from http://emedicine.medscape.com/article/202158-overview

King, T. L., Brucker, M. C., Kriebs, J. M., Fahey, J. O., Gegor, C. L., & Varney, H. (2015). *Varney's midwifery* (5th ed.). Burlington, MA: Jones & Bartlett Learning.

Kolecki, P., & Menckhoff, C. R. (2015). Hypovolemic shock. *eMedicine.* Retrieved from http://emedicine.medscape.com/article/760145-overview

Levi, M. M., & Schmaier, A. H. (2015). Disseminated intravascular coagulation. *eMedicine.* Retrieved from http://emedicine.medscape.com/article/199627-overview

Main, E. K., Goffman, D., Scavone, B. M., Low, L. K., Bingham, D., Fontaine, P. L., et al. (2015). National partnership for maternal safety: Consensus bundle on obstetric hemorrhage. *Journal of Obstetric, Gynecologic, & Neonatal Nursing, 44*(4):462–470.

Mattson, S., & Smith, J. E. (2015). *Core curriculum for maternal-newborn nursing* (5th ed.), St. Louis, MO: Saunders Elsevier

Middeldorp, S. (2015). New studies of low-molecular-weight heparin in pregnancy. *Thrombosis Research, 135*, S26–S29.

Moses, S. (2015). Postpartum hemorrhage. *Family Practice* Notebook. Retrieved from http://www.fpnotebook.com/ob/Bleed/PstprtmHmrhg.htm

Mousa H. A., Blum J., Abou El Senoun G., Shakur H., Alfirevic Z. (2014). Treatment for primary postpartum hemorrhage. *Cochrane Database of Systematic Reviews*, (2):CD003249..

Nagtalon-Ramos, J. (2014). *Maternal-newborn nursing care: Best evidence-based practices.* Philadelphia, PA: F.A. Davis Company.

Nahum, G. G., & Pham, K. Q. (2015). Uterine rupture in pregnancy. *eMedicine.* Retrieved from: http://reference.medscape.com/article/275854-overview

National Hemophilia Foundation. (2015). *Von Willebrand disease.* Retrieved from https://www.hemophilia.org/Bleeding-Disorders/Types-of-Bleeding-Disorders/Von-Willebrand-Disease

Nikpour, M., Shirvani, M. A., Azadbakht, M., Zanjani, R., & Mousavi, E. (2014). The effect of honey gel on abdominal wound healing in cesarean section: A triple blind randomized clinical trial. *Oman Medical Journal, 29*(4), 255–259.

Pagana, K. D., Pagana, T. J., & Pagana, T. N. (2014). *Mosby's diagnostic and laboratory test reference* (12th ed.). St. Louis, MO: Mosby Elsevier.

Pavord, S., & Maybury, H. (2015). How I treat postpartum hemorrhage. *Blood, 125*(18), 2759–2770.

Pollak, E. S. (2015). von Willebrand disease. *eMedicine.* Retrieved from http://emedicine.medscape.com/article/206996-overview

Pop, V. J., Truijens, S. E., Spek, V., Wijnen, H. A., van Son, M. J., & Bergink, V. (2015). A new concept of maternity blues: Is there a subgroup of women with rapid cycling mood symptoms?. *Journal of Affective Disorders, 177*, 74–79.

Quellette, D. R., Harrington, A., & Kamangar, N. (2015). Pulmonary embolism. *eMedicine.* Retrieved from http://emedicine.medscape.com/article/300901-overview

Rong, J., Yuna, G., & Yan, C. (2014). Risk factors associated with emergency peripartum hysterectomy. *Chinese Medical Journal, 127*(5), 900–904.

Salam, R. A., Mansoor, T., Mallick, D., Lassi, Z. S., Das, J. K., & Bhutta, Z. A. (2014). Essential childbirth and postnatal interventions for improved maternal and neonatal health. *Reproductive Health, 11*(Suppl 1), S3–S20.

Schiller, C. E., Meltzer-Brody, S., & Rubinow, D. R. (2015). The role of reproductive hormones in postpartum depression. *CNS Spectrums, 20*(1), 48–59.

Shields, L. E., Wiesner, S., Fulton, J., & Pelletreau, B. (2015). Comprehensive maternal hemorrhage protocols reduce the use of blood products and improve patient safety. *American Journal of Obstetrics and Gynecology, 212*(3), 272–280.

Silverman, M. A. (2015). Idiopathic thrombocytopenic purpura. *eMedicine.* Retrieved from http://emedicine.medscape.com/article/779545-overview

Skidmore-Roth, L. (2015). *Mosby's 2015 nursing drug reference* (28th ed.). St. Louis, MO: Mosby Elsevier.

Spiliopoulos, M., & Mastrogiannis, D. (2015). Normal and abnormal puerperium. *eMedicine.* Retrieved from http://emedicine.medscape.com/article/260187-overview#a1

Sucker, C., & Zotz, R. B. (2015). Prophylaxis and treatment of venous thrombosis and pulmonary embolism in pregnancy. *Reviews in vascular medicine.* doi:10.1016/j.rvm.2015.05.003

Tánczos, K., Németh, M., & Molnár, Z. (2015). What's new in hemorrhagic shock?. *Intensive Care Medicine, 41*(4), 712–714.

Tepper, N. K., Boulet, S. L., Whiteman, M. K., Monsour, M., Marchbanks, P. A., Hooper, W. C., et al. (2014). Postpartum venous thromboembolism: Incidence and risk factors. *Obstetrics & Gynecology, 123*(5), 987–996.

Testa, S., Passamonti, S. M., Paoletti, O., Bucciarelli, P., Ronca, E., Riccardi, A., et al. (2015). The "Pregnancy Health-care Program" for the prevention of venous thromboembolism in pregnancy. *Internal and Emergency Medicine, 10*(2), 129–134.

Thombs, B. D., Arthurs, E., Coronado-Montoya, S., Roseman, M., Delisle, V. C., Leavens, A., et al. (2014). Depression screening and patient outcomes in pregnancy or postpartum: a systematic review. *Journal of Psychosomatic Research, 76*(6), 433–446.

U.S. Department of Health and Human Services. (2010). *Healthy people 2020.* Retrieved from http://www.healthypeople.gov/2020/topicsobjectives2020

Van de Velde, M., Diez, C., & Varon, A. J. (2015). Obstetric hemorrhage. *Current Opinion in Anesthesiology, 28*(2), 186–190.

Weissman, M. M. (2014). Treatment of depression: men and women are different? *American Journal of Psychiatry, 171*(4), 384–387.

Wells, P. S., Forgie, M. A., & Rodger, M. A. (2014). Treatment of venous thromboembolism. *JAMA, 311*(7), 717–728.

Wilcox, L. L., Ramprasad, C., Gutierrez, A., Oden, M., Richards-Kortum, R., & Gandhi, M. (2015). Accuracy in estimation of blood loss using the SAPHE (Signaling a Postpartum Hemorrhage Emergency) Mat [51]. *Obstetrics & Gynecology, 125*, 25S.

Wong, A. W., & Rosh, A. J. (2015). Postpartum infections. *eMedicine.* Retrieved from http://emedicine.medscape.com/article/796892-overview

World Health Organization. (2010). WHO recommendations for the prevention of postpartum hemorrhage. Retrieved from http://www.who.int/making_pregnancy_safer/publications

World Health Organization [WHO]. (2014). *Postpartum hemorrhage.* Retrieved from http://www.who.int/medicines/areas/priority_medicines/Ch6_16PPH.pdf?ua = 1

Yiadom, M. Y., & Carusi, D. (2015). Postpartum hemorrhage in emergency medicine. *eMedicine.* Retrieved from http://emedicine.medscape.com/article/796785-overview

Zhao, Y., Kane, I., Wang, J., Shen, B., Luo, J., & Shi, S. (2015). Combined use of the postpartum depression screening scale (PDSS) and Edinburgh postnatal depression scale (EPDS) to identify antenatal depression among Chinese pregnant women with obstetric complications. *Psychiatry Research, 226*(1), 113–119.

MULTIPLE CHOICE QUESTIONS

1. A postpartum mother appears very pale and states she is bleeding heavily. The nurse should first:
   a. Call the client's health care provider immediately.
   b. Immediately set up an intravenous infusion of magnesium sulfate.
   c. Assess the fundus and ask her about her voiding status.
   d. Reassure the mother that this is a normal finding after childbirth.

2. A postpartum woman reports hearing voices and says, "The voices are telling me to do bad things to my baby." The clinic nurse interprets these findings as suggesting postpartum:
   a. Psychosis
   b. Anxiety disorder
   c. Depression
   d. Blues

3. When implementing the plan of care for a multigravida postpartum woman who gave birth just a few hours ago, the nurse vigilantly monitors the client for which complication?
   a. Deep venous thrombosis
   b. Postpartum psychosis
   c. Uterine infection
   d. Postpartum hemorrhage

4. Which of the following would the nurse expect to include in the plan of care for a woman with mastitis who is receiving antibiotic therapy?
   a. Stop breast-feeding and apply lanolin
   b. Administer analgesics and bind both breasts
   c. Apply warm or cold compresses and administer analgesics
   d. Remove the nursing bra and expose the breast to fresh air

5. While assessing a postpartum multiparous woman, the nurse detects a boggy uterus midline 2 cm above the umbilicus. Which intervention would be the priority?
   a. Assessing vital signs immediately
   b. Measuring her next urinary output
   c. Massaging her fundus
   d. Notifying the woman's obstetrician

6. Methergine has been ordered for a postpartum woman because of excessive bleeding. The nurse should question this order if which of the following is present?
   a. Mild abdominal cramping
   b. Tender inflamed breasts
   c. Pulse rate of 68 beats per minute
   d. Blood pressure of 158/96 mm Hg

7. Which of the following findings would lead the nurse to suspect that a woman is developing a postpartum complication?
   a. Moderate lochia rubra for the first 24 hours
   b. Clear lung sounds upon auscultation
   c. Temperature of 100° F
   d. Chest pain experienced when ambulating

8. Which of the following factors in a postpartum woman's history would lead the nurse to monitor the woman closely for an infection?
   a. Hemoglobin of 12 mg/dL
   b. Manually extracted placenta
   c. Labor of 10 hours length
   d. Multiparity of 5 pregnancies

CRITICAL THINKING EXERCISES

1. Mrs. Griffin had a 22-hour labor before a cesarean birth. Her membranes ruptured 20 hours before she came to the hospital. Her fetus showed signs of fetal distress, so internal electronic fetal monitoring was used. Her most recent test results indicate she is anemic.
   a. What postpartum complication is this new mother at highest risk for? Why?
   b. What assessments need to be done to detect this complication?
   c. What nursing measures will the nurse use to prevent this complication?

2. Tammy, a 32-year-old G9P9, had a spontaneous vaginal birth 2 hours ago. Tammy has been having a baby each year for the past 9 years. Her lochia has been heavy, with some clots. She hasn't been up to void since she had epidural anesthesia and has decreased sensation to her legs.
   a. What factors place Tammy at risk for postpartum hemorrhage?
   b. What assessments are needed before planning interventions?
   c. What nursing actions are needed to prevent a postpartum hemorrhage?

3. Lucy, a 25-year-old G2P2, gave birth 2 days ago and is expected to be discharged today. She had severe postpartum depression 2 years ago with her first child. Lucy has not been out of bed for the past 24 hours, is not eating, and provides no care for herself or her newborn. Lucy states she already has a boy at home and not having a girl this time is disappointing.
   a. What factors/behaviors place Lucy at risk for an affective disorder?
   b. Which interventions might be appropriate at this time?
   c. What education does the family need prior to discharge?

STUDY ACTIVITIES

1. Compare and contrast postpartum blues, postpartum depression, and postpartum psychosis in terms of their features and medical management.

2. Visit and select a website from the Student Resources for Chapter 22. Critique the website regarding its helpfulness to parents, the correctness of the information, and when it was last updated.

3. Interview a woman who has given birth and ask if she had any complications and what was most helpful to her during the experience.

4. The number one cause of postpartum hemorrhage is _____.

5. When giving report to the nurse who will be caring for a woman and her newborn in the postpartum period, what information should the labor nurse convey?

BRINGING IT ALL TOGETHER: CASE STUDY

Sheila is an 18-year-old G1P1 Hispanic who had her first child 2 days ago via primary cesarean section. Her pregnancy was uneventful, but she didn't attend prenatal clinic very often. She presented to the hospital in labor at 39 weeks of gestation with ruptured membranes. The client reported that her membranes had been ruptured for a "couple of days," but she wasn't really sure. Upon admission, she was dilated 2 cm/40% effacement. She labored for about 7 hours when the health care provider came in to check her. She was only 5 cm/completely effaced at that time. She was receiving IV antibiotics for her "prolonged rupture" status as per CDC guidelines. The health care provider inserted an internal fetal monitor with a scalp electrode and also an intrauterine pressure catheter because she was obese and the nurse was having difficulty in picking up the FHR tracing. She had no progress for the next four hours and the fetus was noted to develop tachycardia with a baseline heart rate increase to 170 bpm. A primary cesarean section was performed and she was given perioperative antibiotic prophylaxis at the time of surgery. Infant was LGA and Apgar scores were 9/9 at one minute and 5 minutes, respectively.

ASSESSMENT

On day 1, as the nurse caring for this client, you obtain a set of postpartum vital signs: T—101.6, P—102, BP—110/80, R—18. Sheila appears pale and is diaphoretic. Her lochia rubra is of moderate amount and foul smelling. She complains of uterine tenderness when you palpate her fundus. Her surgical site is intact without redness or drainage. She states she didn't have the breakfast that was served because she had no appetite. Her breasts are nontender and full upon palpation. She plans to bottle feed and has a supportive bra on. Sheila ambulates well and does her own peri-care.

Go to thePoint **to find questions to consider about this case.**

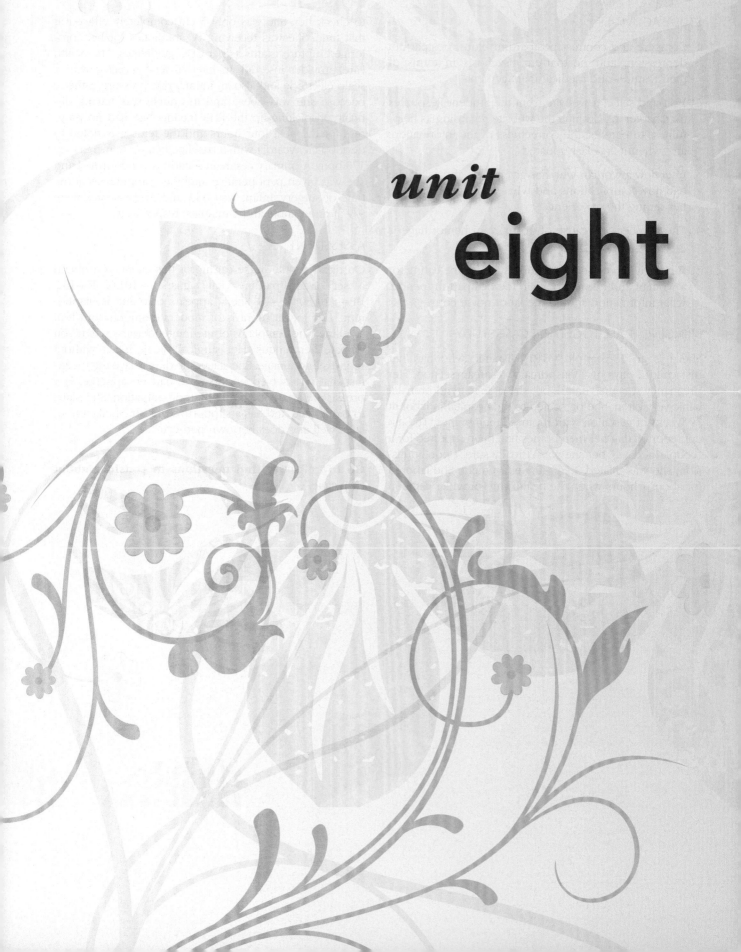

unit
eight

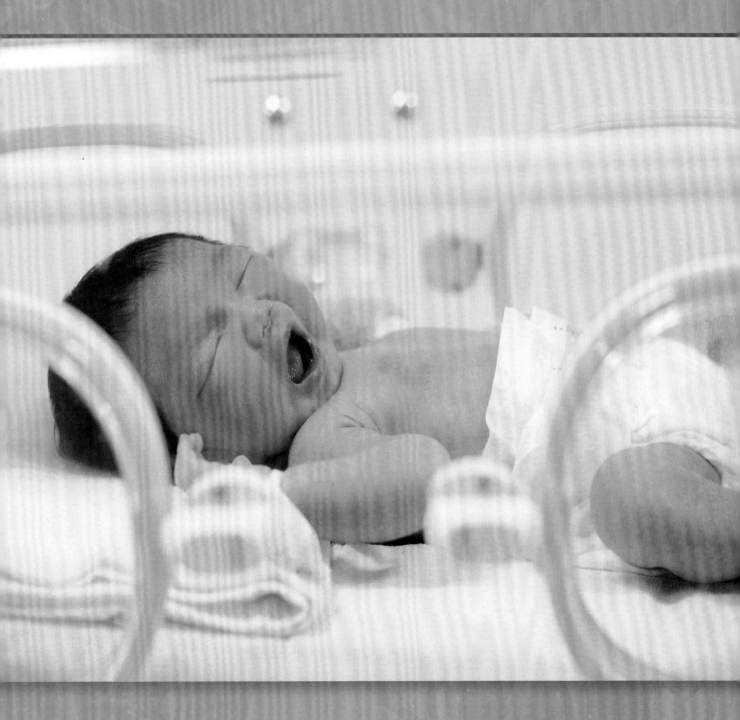

The Newborn at Risk

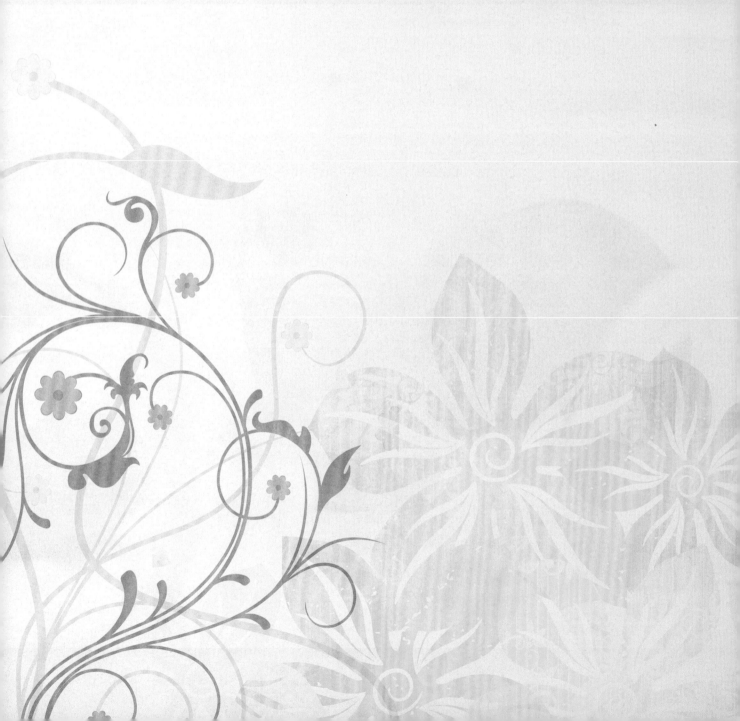

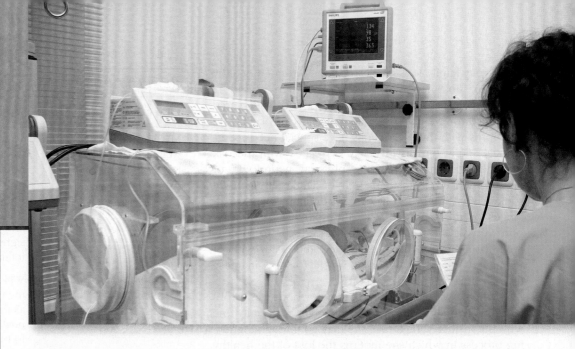

23

Nursing Care of the Newborn with Special Needs

KEY TERMS
appropriate for gestational age
asphyxia
extremely low birth weight
full term newborn
large for gestational age (LGA)
late preterm newborn
low birth weight (LBW)
post-term newborn
preterm newborn
retinopathy of prematurity (ROP)
small for gestational age (SGA)
very low birth weight

Learning Objectives

Upon completion of the chapter, you will be able to:

1. Examine factors that assist in identifying a newborn at risk due to variations in birth weight and gestational age.

2. Detect contributing factors and common complications associated with dysmature infants and their management.

3. Compare and contrast a small-for-gestational-age newborn and a large-for-gestational-age newborn; a post-term and preterm newborn.

4. Differentiate associated conditions that affect the newborn with variations in birth weight and gestational age, including appropriate management.

5. Outline the nurse's role in helping parents experiencing perinatal grief or loss.

6. Integrate knowledge of the risks associated with late preterm births into nursing interventions, discharge planning, and parent education.

Anna *and her husband were stunned when she went into labor at 7 months' gestation. They couldn't understand what would cause her to give birth early, but it happened. When they approached the neonatal intensive care unit (NICU), Anna took a deep breath and looked down at her tiny baby with tubes coming from everywhere. What feelings might they be experiencing at this moment?*

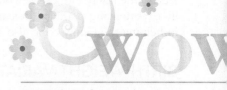

Words of Wisdom
Guiding a parent's hand to touch a frail or ill newborn demonstrates courage and compassion under very difficult circumstances and is a powerful tool in helping them to deal with the newborn's special needs.

Every family looks forward to the birth of a healthy newborn. Most newborns are born between 38 and 42 weeks' gestation and weigh 6 to 8 pounds, but variations in birth weight or gestational age can occur, and newborns with these variations have special needs. Gestational age at birth is inversely correlated with the risk that the infant will experience physical, neurologic, or developmental sequelae (March of Dimes, 2015a). In some cases, however, unexpected difficulties and challenges occur along the way and some newborns are born very ill and need special advanced care to survive. Some complications are unexpected and occur without warning. Other times, there are risk factors that increase the risk of problems in newborns.

When a woman gives birth to a newborn with problems involving immaturity or birth weight, especially one who is considered high risk, she may go through a grieving process in which she mourns the loss of the healthy full-term newborn she had expected. Through this process she learns to come to terms with the experience she now faces.

The development of new technologies and regionalized care centers for the care of newborns with special needs has resulted in significant improvements. Nurses need to have a sound knowledge base to identify the newborn with special needs and to provide coordinated care.

The key to identify a newborn with special needs related to birth weight or gestational age variation is an awareness of the factors that could place a newborn at risk. These factors are similar to those that would suggest a high-risk pregnancy. Being able to anticipate the birth of a newborn at risk allows the birth to take place at a health care facility equipped with the resources to meet the mother's and newborn's needs. This is important in reducing mortality and morbidity.

Healthy People 2020 identifies preterm births and low birth weight as important national health goals (U.S. Department of Health and Human Services, 2010). (See *Healthy People 2020* 23.1.)

This chapter discusses the nursing management of newborns with special needs related to variations in birth weight and gestational age. It also describes selected associated conditions affecting these newborns. Due to the frailty of these newborns, the care of the family experiencing perinatal loss and the role of the nurse in helping the family cope also are addressed.

BIRTH-WEIGHT VARIATIONS

Fetal growth is influenced by maternal nutrition, genetics, placental function, environment, and a multitude of other factors. Assigning size to a newborn is a way to measure and monitor the growth and development of the newborn at birth. Newborns can be classified according to their weight and weeks of gestation. Knowing the group into which a newborn fits is important.

HEALTHY PEOPLE *2020* • *23.1*	
Objective	**Nursing Significance**
MICH-8 Reduce low birth weight (LBW) and very low birth weight (VLBW) by 10% by 2020.	Will help to emphasize the issue of LBW as a risk factor associated with newborn death, helping to promote measures to reduce this risk factor and thus contributing to significant reductions in infant mortality.
MICH-9 Reduce preterm births by 10% by 2020.	Will help to emphasize the role of preterm birth as the leading cause of newborn deaths unrelated to birth defects.
MICH-33 Increase the proportion of VLBW infants born at level III hospitals or subspecialty perinatal centers by 10% by 2020.	Will aid in promoting an overall reduction in infant illness, disability, and death.

Healthy People objectives based on data from http://www.healthypeople.gov.

Appropriate for gestational age (AGA) characterizes approximately 80% of newborns and describes a newborn with a normal length, weight, head circumference, and body mass index (Panda, 2015). Being in the AGA group confers the lowest risk for any problems. These infants have lower morbidity and mortality than other groups.

Small for gestational age (SGA) describes newborns who typically weigh less than 2,500 grams (5 lb 8 oz) at term due to less growth in utero than expected. A newborn is also classified as SGA if his or her birth weight is at or below the 10th percentile as correlated with the number of weeks of gestation on a growth chart.

Large for gestational age (LGA) describes newborns whose birth weight is above the 90th percentile on a growth chart and who weigh more than 4,000 g (8 lb 13 oz) at term due to accelerated overgrowth for length of gestation (Sacks et al., 2015). The following terms describe other newborns with marginal weights at birth and of any gestational age:

- **Low birth weight:** less than 2,500 g (5.5 lb) (Fig. 23.1)
- **Very low birth weight:** less than 1,500 g (3 lb 5 oz)
- **Extremely low birth weight:** less than 1,000 g (2 lb 3 oz)

Small-for-Gestational-Age Newborns

Newborns are considered SGA when they weigh less than 2,500 g (5 lb 8 oz) or fall below the 10th percentile

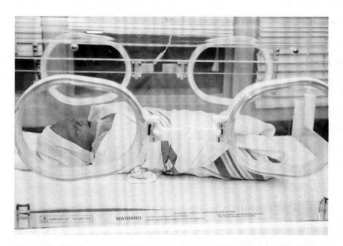

FIGURE 23.1 A low–birth-weight newborn in an isolette.

for length, weight, or head circumference on a growth chart for gestational age. These infants can be preterm, term, or post-term.

 Concept Mastery Alert

Planning Priority Care for the Small for Gestational Age Infant

Infants who are small for gestational age (SGA) are different from preterm infants who often have underdeveloped respiratory systems. SGA infants often have developed respiratory systems, but need frequent observations for hypoglycemia because of inadequate glycogen stores. This leads to the need for frequent and early feedings.

In some SGA newborns, the rate of growth does not meet the expected growth pattern. Termed fetal growth restriction, these newborns also are considered at risk, with the perinatal morbidity and mortality rate increased substantially compared with that of the AGA newborn (Cunningham et al., 2014). Fetal growth restriction is the pathologic counterpart of SGA. However, an important distinction to make between SGA and fetal growth restriction newborns is that not all who are SGA have growth restriction. The converse also is true: not all newborns who have fetal growth restriction are SGA. Some SGA newborns are constitutionally small; that is, they are statistically small but otherwise healthy.

Historically, fetal growth restriction has been categorized as symmetric or asymmetric. Symmetric fetal growth restriction (an insult that occurs early at less than 28 weeks in the gestation) refers to fetuses with equally poor growth rates of the head, the abdomen, and the long bones. All parameters of growth are affected. Typically these infants have the poorest long-term prognosis and are never able to catch up in size when compared with unaffected children (Nagtalon-Ramos, 2014). Asymmetric fetal growth restriction (insult occurs late—at more than 28 weeks' gestation) refers to infants whose head and long bones are

spared compared with their abdomen and internal organs. The brain and heart are spared and are larger, but overall weight and organ sizes are reduced. Generally, the asymmetrical fetal growth restriction infant has a better prognosis than one who is symmetrically fetal growth restriction. Once the infant is born, optimal nutrition usually restores normal growth potential. The current belief is that in most cases fetal growth restriction is a continuum from symmetrical (early stages) to asymmetrical (late stages). There is a strong association between stillbirth and fetal growth restriction. Early detection and management of fetal growth restriction can lead to reduced morbidity and mortality. A recent study found that combined screening of maternal factors and biophysical profiles conducted at 30 to 34 weeks' gestation can identify a large proportion of pregnancies that subsequently will have SGA newborns (Bakalis et al., 2015).

Fetal growth is dependent on genetic, placental, and maternal factors. Cognitive and motor development during infancy forms the basis for children's subsequent development. Newborns that experience nutritional deficiencies in utero and are born SGA are at risk for cognitive deficits that can undermine their academic performance throughout their lives. SGA infants are associated with increased neonatal morbidity and mortality as well as short stature, cardiovascular disease, insulin resistance, diabetes mellitus type 2, dyslipidemia, and end-stage renal disease in adulthood. In addition, SGA children have decreased levels of intelligence and cognition, although the effects are mostly subtle. The overall outcome of each child is the result of a complex interaction between intrauterine and extrauterine factors (Oros et al., 2014).

The fetus is thought to have an inherent growth potential that, under normal circumstances, yields a healthy newborn of appropriate size. The maternal–placental–fetal units act in harmony to meet the needs of the fetus during gestation. However, growth potential in the fetus can be limited, and this is analogous to failure to thrive in the infant. The causes of both can be intrinsic or environmental. Factors that can contribute to the birth of an SGA newborn are highlighted in Box 23.1.

Nursing Assessment

Assessment of the SGA infant begins by reviewing the maternal history to identify risk factors such as smoking, drug abuse, alcohol consumption, preeclampsia, anemia, uteroplacental insufficiency, intrauterine viral infection, cord prolapse, chronic maternal illness, hypertension, multiple gestation, or genetic disorders. This information allows the nurse to anticipate a possible problem and to be prepared to intervene quickly should one occur. At birth, perform a thorough physical examination, closely observing the newborn for typical characteristics, including:

- Head disproportionately large compared with rest of body
- Wasted appearance of extremities

POTENTIAL FACTORS CONTRIBUTING TO THE BIRTH OF SMALL-FOR-GESTATIONAL-AGE NEWBORNS

Maternal Causes
- Chronic hypertension
- Diabetes mellitus with vascular disease
- Autoimmune diseases
- Living at a high altitude (hypoxia)
- Smoking or exposure to passive smoke
- Periodontal disease of the mouth
- Maternal age of <20 or >34 years old
- Failure to seek any prenatal care
- Substandard living conditions
- Low socioeconomic status
- Abuse and violence
- Substance abuse (heroin, cocaine, methamphet-amines)
- Hemoglobinopathies (sickle cell anemia)
- Preeclampsia
- Exposure to occupational hazards
- Chronic renal disease
- Maternal nutrition (malnutrition or obesity)

- Extreme maternal stress
- TORCH group infections

Placental Factors
- Abnormal cord insertion
- Chronic abruption
- Decreased surface area, infarction
- Decreased placental weight
- Placenta previa
- Placental insufficiency

Fetal Factors
- Trisomy 13, 18, and 21
- Turner's syndrome
- Chronic fetal infection (cytomegalovirus, rubella, syphilis, toxoplasmosis)
- Congenital anomalies (heart, diaphragmatic hernia, tracheoesophageal fistula)
- Radiation exposure
- Multiple fetal gestation

Adapted from Kenner, C., & Lott, J. W. (2015). *Comprehensive neonatal care* (5th ed.). New York, NY: Springer Publishing Company; Fanaroff, A. A., & Fanaroff, J. M. (2014). *Klaus and Fanaroff's care of the high-risk neonate* (6th ed.) Philadelphia, PA: Elsevier; and Verklan, M. T., & Walden, M. (2014). *Core curriculum for neonatal intensive care nursing* (5th ed.). St. Louis, MO: Saunders Elsevier.

- Reduced subcutaneous fat stores
- Jittery secondary to hypoglycemia
- Temperature instability
- Decreased amount of breast tissue
- Scaphoid abdomen (sunken appearance)
- Wide skull sutures secondary to inadequate bone growth
- Poor muscle tone over buttocks and cheeks
- Loose and dry skin that appears oversized
- Thin umbilical cord

Also assess the SGA newborn for any congenital malformations, neurologic insults, or indications of infection. SGA newborns commonly face problems after birth because of the decrease in placental function during gestation. Table 23.1 highlights some of the common problems associated with SGA newborns and others experiencing a variation in birth weight or gestational age. Anticipate the need for and provide resuscitation as indicated by the newborn's condition.

Nursing Management

Interventions for the SGA infant may include obtaining weight, length, and head circumference, comparing them with standards, and documenting the findings. Perform frequent serial blood glucose measurements as ordered and monitor vital signs, being particularly alert for changes in respiratory status that might indicate respiratory distress. Institute measures to maintain a neutral thermal environment to prevent cold stress and acidosis.

Metabolic needs are increased for catch-up growth. Initiate early and frequent oral feedings unless contraindicated. At birth the newborn's glucose level is approximately 70% of the mother's serum glucose. Neonatal hypoglycemia is a major cause of brain injury since the brain needs glucose continuously as a primary source of energy (Chandran et al., 2015). Any newborn stressed at birth uses up available glucose stores with resulting hypoglycemia, a plasma glucose concentration at or below 40 mg/dL (Nagtalon-Ramos, 2014). With the loss of the placenta at birth, the newborn now must assume control of glucose homeostasis through intermittent oral feedings. If oral feedings are not accepted, an intravenous infusion with 10% dextrose in water may be needed to maintain the glucose level above 40 mg/dL. Weigh the newborn daily and ensure that he or she has adequate rest periods to decrease metabolic requirements. Monitor feeding tolerance, sucking, and swallowing ability.

POLYCYTHEMIA

Polycythemia is not uncommon and is a potentially serious disorder of newborns. It is defined as a venous hematocrit above 65% and hemoglobin of more than 20 g. The hematocrit in a newborn peaks between 6 to 12 hours of age and decreases gradually after that. Polycythemia occurs in up to 12% of neonates, and occurs commonly in SGA newborns 6 to 12 hours after birth (Lessaris, 2015). The relationship between hematocrit and viscosity is almost linear until 65% and exponential thereafter.

(text continues on page 840)

Problem	Occurrence	Etiology/Pathophysiology	Assessment Findings	Nursing Implications
Perinatal asphyxia	SGA newborns (common)	Poor tolerance to stress of labor, frequently leading to acidosis and hypoxia Living in hypoxic environment prior to birth due to placental insufficiency, leaving little to no oxygen reserves available to withstand stress of labor: – Uterine contractions increase hypoxic stress – Possible depletion of glycogen stores due to chronic hypoxic state, leading to fetal distress – Impaired uteroplacental circulation due to maternal and uterine conditions predisposing to perinatal depression Compromised newborn at birth experiencing difficulty adjusting to extrauterine environment	Fetal distress (bradycardia, decelerations) during labor Low Apgar scores Potential meconium passage into amniotic fluid	Anticipate possible problem; assess for maternal risk factors. Initiate resuscitation measures immediately at birth.
	Post-term newborns	Placental deprivation or oligohydramnios, leading to cord compression and subsequent reduction in perfusion to fetus		
	Preterm newborns (common)	Surfactant deficiency Unstable chest wall Immaturity of respiratory control centers in the CNS Small respiratory passages, increasing risk for obstruction Inability to clear mucus from airways		
Difficulty with thermoregulation	SGA newborns (common)	Less muscle mass, less brown fat, less heat-preserving subcutaneous fat, and limited ability to control skin capillaries	Temperature <36.4° C; temperature instability; skin cool to touch; cyanosis of hands and feet Bradypnea (<25 breaths/min) and tachypnea (>60 breaths/min) Tremors, irritability Wheezing, crackles, retractions Restlessness, lethargy Hypotonia Weak or high-pitched cry Seizures Poor feeding Grunting Acidosis	Maintain a neutral thermal environment to promote stabilization of newborn's temperature. Assess skin temperature and respiration characteristics. Monitor arterial blood gases and blood glucose levels. Eliminate sources of heat loss: – Dry newborn thoroughly. – Wrap in warmed blanket with stockinette cap on head –Use radiant heat source.
	Post-term newborns	Associated with depleted glycogen stores, poor subcutaneous fat stores, and disturbances in CNS thermoregulation due to hypoxia Increased risk for acidosis and hypoglycemia secondary to metabolic stress Loss of subcutaneous fat secondary to placental insufficiency Use of stored nutrients for nutrition due to lost ability of placenta to nourish fetus Subsequent wasting of subcutaneous fat, muscle, or both		

(continued)

TABLE 23.1 COMMON PROBLEMS ASSOCIATED WITH NEWBORNS EXPERIENCING A VARIATION IN BIRTH WEIGHT OR GESTATIONAL AGE (continued)

Problem	Occurrence	Etiology/Pathophysiology	Assessment Findings	Nursing Implications
	Preterm newborns (common)	Loss of natural insulation (subcutaneous fat) important in temperature regulation Immaturity of CNS (temperature-regulating center) interferes with ability to regulate body temperature Inadequate amounts of subcutaneous fat Lack of muscle tone and flexion to conserve heat		
	Late preterm infant (common)	Inadequate brown fat to generate heat Limited muscle mass activity, reducing ability to produce own heat Inability to shiver to generate heat		
Hypoglycemia	SGA newborns (common)	Increased metabolic rate and lack of adequate glycogen stores to meet newborn's metabolic needs	Often subtle Lethargy, tachycardia Respiratory distress Jitteriness Drowsiness Poor feeding, feeble sucking Hypothermia, temperature instability Diaphoresis Weak cry Seizures Hypotonia Blood glucose levels <40 mg/dL for term newborns, <20 mg/dL for preterm newborns	Monitor blood glucose levels, initially on arrival to nursery and hourly thereafter. Maintain fluid and electrolyte balance. Watch for subtle changes. Initiate early oral feedings if possible; if not, administer IV infusion with 10% dextrose in water.
	LGA newborns (common)	Commonly associated with infants of mothers with diabetes Abrupt cessation of high-glucose maternal blood supply with birth and continued insulin production by the newborn Limited ability to release glucagons and catecholamines, which normally stimulate glucagon breakdown and glucose release		
	Post-term newborns	Hypoxia secondary to depleted glycogen reserves Placental insufficiency secondary to placental aging contributing to chronic fetal nutritional deficiency further depleting glycogen stores		
	Preterm newborns	Immature sucking and swallowing leading to insufficient intake Perinatal hypoxia Increased energy expenditure		
	Late preterm infants	Decreased subcutaneous and brown fat with little to no glycogen stores		

Condition	Newborn type	Pathophysiology	Signs and symptoms	Nursing interventions
Polycythemia	SGA newborns	Chronic mild hypoxia secondary to placental insufficiency Stimulation of erythropoietin release, leading to increased RBC production	Venous hematocrit >65% Plethora (ruddy appearance) Weak sucking reflex Tachypnea Jaundice Lethargy Jitteriness Hypotonia Irritability Feeding Difficulties Difficulty in arousing Seizures	Ensure adequate hydration (orally or IV) Monitor hematocrit levels (goal is ~60%) Administer partial exchange transfusion, albumin, or normal saline IV to reduce RBC volume and increase fluid volume (controversial).
	LGA newborns	Secondary to fetal hypoxia, trauma with bleeding, increased erythropoietin production, or delayed cord clamping		
	Post-term newborns	Intrauterine hypoxia triggers increased RBC cell production to compensate for lower oxygen levels.		
Meconium aspiration	SGA newborns	Release of meconium into amniotic fluid prior to birth Inhalation of meconium-containing amniotic fluid by the newborn, leading to aspiration Commonly associated with chronic intrauterine hypoxia	Green amniotic fluid with rupture of membranes during labor Green staining of the umbilical cord or fingernails Difficulty initiating respirations	Initiate resuscitation measures as necessary. Suction airways and support ventilation (see Chapter 24 for more information).
	Post-term newborns	Struggling by fetus making respiratory efforts and bearing down with abdominal muscles, leading to expulsion of meconium into amniotic fluid Normal sucking and swallowing by fetus leads to meconium filling airways.		
Hyperbilirubinemia	LGA newborns (common)	Associated with polycythemia and RBC breakdown Inability to tolerate feedings in the first few days of life, leading to increased enterohepatic circulation of bilirubin	Elevated serum bilirubin levels Jaundice Tea-colored urine Clay-colored stools	Ensure adequate hydration. Institute early feedings if possible. Administer phototherapy (see Chapter 24 for more information).
	Preterm newborns	Excessive bruising secondary to birth trauma, leading to higher-than-normal bilirubin levels		
	Late preterm infants	Increased breakdown of RBCs and immature liver function to handle excess load		
Birth trauma	LGA newborns	Large size requiring use of operative birth procedure	Obvious deformities Bruising Edema Asymmetrical movement	Perform complete physical and neurologic assessment of the newborn. Note symmetry of structure and function. Assist parents in understanding situation (see Chapter 24 for more information).

Adapted from Fanaroff, A. A., & Fanaroff, J. M. (2014). *Klaus and Fanaroff's care of the high-risk neonate* (6th ed.). Philadelphia, PA: Elsevier; Creasy, R. K., Resnik, R., Iams, J. D., Lockwood, C. J., Moore, T., & Greene, M. F. (2014). *Creasy and Resnik's maternal-fetal medicine: Principles and practice* (7th ed.). St. Louis, MO: Saunders Elsevier; Nagtalon-Ramos, J. (2014). *Maternal-newborn nursing care: Best evidence-based practices*. Philadelphia, PA: F.A. Davis Company; and Verklan, M. T., & Walden, M. (2014). *Core curriculum for neonatal intensive care nursing*.(5th ed.). St. Louis, MO: Saunders Elsevier.

Increased viscosity of blood is associated with symptoms of hypoperfusion. Clinical features related to hyperviscosity may affect all organ systems. Hyperviscosity of blood results in increased resistance to blood flow and decreased oxygen delivery. In the newborn, hyperviscosity can cause abnormalities of central nervous system function, hypoglycemia, decreased renal function, cardiorespiratory distress, and coagulation disorders. Hyperviscosity has been reported to be associated with long-term motor and cognitive neurodevelopmental disorders (Fanaroff & Fanaroff, 2014). SGA newborns, infants of mothers with diabetes, newborns with jaundice, and multiple births are at risk for polycythemia. They should therefore undergo screening at 2, 12, and 24 hours of age (Alsafadi et al., 2014).

Observe for clinical signs of polycythemia (respiratory distress, cyanosis, jitteriness, jaundice, ruddy skin, lethargy) and monitor blood results. Asymptomatic newborns with a hematocrit between 65% and 70% may simply be supported with fluids, close observation, and a repeat hematocrit level in 12 hours (Mahajan, Une, & Bansal, 2015). If the newborn is symptomatic, a partial exchange transfusion with replacement of removed red blood cell volume with volume expanders may be used, but this treatment is considered controversial and not validated by current evidence-based practice research.

Provide anticipatory guidance to parents about any treatments and procedures that are being done. Emphasize the need for close follow-up and careful monitoring of the infant's growth in length, weight, and head circumference and feeding patterns throughout the first year of life to confirm any "catch-up" growth taking place.

Large-for-Gestational-Age Newborns

A newborn whose weight is above the 90th percentile on growth charts is defined as LGA. The range of weight is 4,000 to 5,000 g, or more than 9 lb. LGA infants may be preterm, term, or post-term. Based on these definitions, up to 10% of all births involve an LGA newborn. This large size can place the mother and fetus or newborn at risk for adverse outcomes (Creasy et al., 2014).

Because of the newborn's large size, vaginal birth may be difficult and occasionally results in birth injury. In addition, shoulder dystocia, clavicular fractures, and facial palsies are common. The incidence of cesarean births is very high with LGA newborns to avoid arrested labor and birth trauma.

Take Note!

Maternal diabetes is commonly associated with LGA newborns. However, due to poor placental perfusion, the newborn may experience fetal growth restriction and be SGA.

Nursing Assessment

Assessment of the LGA newborn begins with a review of the maternal history, which can provide clues as to whether the woman has an increased risk of giving birth to a LGA newborn. Maternal factors that increase the chance of bearing a LGA newborn include maternal diabetes mellitus or glucose intolerance, multiparity, prior history of a macrosomic infant, post-term gestation, maternal obesity, paternal height, gestational weight gain, male fetus, and genetics (Donnelley et al., 2014).

At birth, assess the newborn for common characteristics. The typical LGA newborn has a large body and appears plump and full faced. The increase in body size is proportional. However, the head circumference and body length are in the upper limits of intrauterine growth. These newborns have poor motor skills and have difficulty regulating behavioral states. LGA newborns are more difficult to arouse to a quiet alert state (Neonatal Handbook, 2015a).

Thoroughly assess the LGA newborn at birth to identify traumatic birth injuries such as fractured clavicles, brachial palsy, facial paralysis, phrenic nerve palsy, skull fractures, or hematomas. Perform a neurologic examination to identify any nerve palsies, looking for abnormalities such as immobility of the upper arm. Observe and document any injuries discovered to allow for early intervention and improved outcomes.

LGA infants are at risk for hypoglycemia related to early depletion of glycogen stores in the liver. Obtain frequent blood glucose levels as ordered to evaluate for hypoglycemia. The clinical signs are often subtle and include lethargy, apathy, drowsiness, irritability, tachypnea, weak crying, temperature instability, jitteriness, seizures, apnea, bradycardia, cyanosis or pallor, feeble sucking and poor feeding, hypotonia, and coma. Other disorders, including septicemia, severe respiratory distress, and congenital heart disease, may present with similar findings. In addition, be alert for other common problems, such as polycythemia and hyperbilirubinemia (see Table 23.1 earlier in this chapter).

Nursing Management

Hypoglycemia in a neonate is defined as blood glucose value below 40 mg/dL. It is commonly associated with a variety of neonatal conditions like prematurity, fetal growth restriction, fetal growth restriction, and maternal diabetes. It may be asymptomatic in some newborns. Screening for hypoglycemia in high-risk LGA infants is essential. Supervised breast-feeding or formula feeding may be initial treatment options in asymptomatic hypoglycemia. However, symptomatic hypoglycemia should always be treated with a continuous infusion of parenteral dextrose. LGA infants needing dextrose infusion rates above 12 mg/kg/min should be investigated for a definite cause of hypoglycemia. Hypoglycemia has been linked to poor neurodevelopmental outcome, and hence aggressive screening and treatment are recommended (Mitanchez et al., 2015).

Assist in stabilizing the LGA newborn. Monitor blood glucose levels within 30 minutes of birth and repeat the screening every hour. Recheck levels before feedings and also immediately in any infant suspected of having or showing clinical signs of hypoglycemia, regardless of age. To help prevent hypoglycemia, initiate feedings, which can be formula or breast milk, with intravenous glucose supplementation as needed. Monitor and record intake and output and obtain daily weights to aid in evaluating nutritional intake.

Observe for signs of polycythemia and hyperbilirubinemia and report any immediately to the health care provider so that early interventions can be taken to prevent poor long-term neurologic development outcomes. Polycythemia and hyperviscosity are associated with fine and gross motor delays, speech delays, and neurologic sequelae (Neonatal Handbook, 2015b). Increasing fluid volume aids in decreasing blood viscosity. Partial exchange transfusion with plasma or normal saline may be used to lower hematocrit and decrease blood viscosity, but this treatment remains controversial (Lessaris, 2015). Hydration, early feedings, and phototherapy are used to treat hyperbilirubinemia (see Chapter 24 for more information about hyperbilirubinemia). Provide parental guidance about the treatments and procedures being done and about the need for follow-up care for any abnormalities identified.

GESTATIONAL AGE VARIATIONS

The mean duration of pregnancy, calculated from the first day of the last normal menstrual period, is approximately 280 days, or 40 weeks. Gestational age is typically measured in weeks: a newborn born before completion of 37 weeks is classified as a preterm newborn and one born after completion of 42 weeks is classified as a post-term newborn. An infant born from the first day of the 38th week through 42 weeks is classified as a term newborn. An additional classification has been added, the late preterm newborn (near term)—one who is born between 34 weeks and 36 weeks, 6 days of gestation.

- **Preterm newborn:** before 37 completed weeks of gestation
- **Late preterm newborn** (near term): 34 to 36^6/$_7$ weeks
- **Full term newborn:** 38 through 41 completed weeks of gestation
- **Post-term newborn:** 42 weeks or more

Precise knowledge of a newborn's gestational age is imperative for effective postnatal management. Determination of gestational age by the nurse assists in planning appropriate care for the newborn and provides important information regarding potential problems that need interventions. See Chapter 18 for more information on assessing gestational age.

Take Note!

Although preterm and post-term newborns may appear to be at opposite ends of the gestational age spectrum and are very different in size and appearance, both are at high risk and need special care.

Preterm Newborn

A preterm newborn is one who is born before the completion of 37 weeks' gestation. There has been improved survival of preterm infants due to the advancing technology and improved evidence-based perinatal care. Although the national birth rate has been declining since the 1990s, the preterm birth rate has been climbing rapidly. Approximately one in nine infants, or nearly half a million infants, is born before the 37th week of gestation (March of Dimes, 2015b). Prematurity is now the leading cause of death worldwide, and can cause long-term health problems for these infants throughout their lives and affect their education and ability to work. Prematurity costs society more than $26 billion annually and takes a high toll on families.

The etiology of about 40% of all preterm births is unknown (March of Dimes, 2015c). Research suggests that four main etiologies may lead to spontaneous premature labor and birth:

- *Infections/inflammation.* Studies suggest that premature labor is often triggered by the body's natural immune response to certain bacterial infections, such as those involving the genital and urinary tracts and fetal membranes. Even infections far away from the reproductive organs, such as periodontal disease, may contribute to premature births.
- *Maternal or fetal stress.* Chronic psychosocial stress in the mother or physical stress (such as insufficient blood flow from the placenta) in the fetus appears to result in production of a stress-related hormone called corticotropin-releasing hormone (CRH). CRH may stimulate production of a cascade of other hormones that trigger uterine contractions and premature birth.
- *Bleeding.* The uterus may bleed because of problems such as placental abruption. Bleeding triggers the release of various proteins involved in blood clotting that also appear to stimulate uterine contractions.
- *Stretching.* The uterus may become overstretched by the presence of two or more fetuses, excessive amounts of amniotic fluid, or uterine or placental abnormalities, leading to the release of chemicals that stimulate uterine contractions (March of Dimes, 2015d).

Preterm births take an enormous financial toll, estimated to be in the billions of dollars. They also take an emotional toll on those involved.

Changes in perinatal care practices, including regional care, have reduced newborn mortality rates. Transporting high-risk pregnant women to a tertiary center for birth rather than transferring the neonate after birth is associated with a reduction in neonatal mortality and morbidity (Kaneko et al., 2015). Despite increasing survival rates, preterm infants continue to be at high risk for neurodevelopmental disorders such as cerebral palsy, intellectual disability, intraventricular hemorrhage, congenital anomalies, neurosensory impairment, behavioral problems, high frequency attention problems, psychiatric disorders, and chronic lung disease (Wilson-Costello & Payne, 2016). Making sure that all pregnant women receive quality prenatal care throughout pregnancy is a major method for preventing preterm births.

Effects of Prematurity on Body Systems

Since the preterm newborn did not remain in utero long enough, every body system may be immature, affecting the newborn's transition from intrauterine to extrauterine life and placing him or her at risk for complications. Without full development, organ systems are not capable of functioning at the level needed to maintain extrauterine homeostasis (Salam et al., 2014).

Recall Anna, who was described at the beginning of the chapter; she gave birth to a newborn at 7 months' gestation. What problems would you anticipate that her newborn might have?

RESPIRATORY SYSTEM

The respiratory system is one of the last body systems to mature. Therefore, the preterm newborn is at great risk for respiratory complications. A few of the problems that affect the preterm newborn's breathing ability and adjustment to extrauterine life include:

- Surfactant deficiency, leading to the development of respiratory distress syndrome
- Unstable chest wall, leading to atelectasis
- Immature respiratory control centers, leading to apnea
- Smaller respiratory passages, leading to an increased risk for obstruction
- Inability to clear fluid from passages, leading to transient tachypnea

CARDIOVASCULAR SYSTEM

The preterm newborn has great difficulty making the transition from intrauterine to extrauterine life in terms of changing from a fetal to a newborn circulation pattern. Higher oxygen levels in the circulation once air breathing begins spur this transition. If the oxygen levels remain low secondary to perinatal asphyxia, the fetal pattern of circulation may persist, causing blood flow to bypass the lungs. Another problem affecting the cardiovascular system is the increased incidence of congenital anomalies associated with continued fetal circulation—patent ductus arteriosus and an open foramen ovale. In addition, impaired regulation of blood pressure in preterm newborns may cause fluctuations throughout the circulatory system. Of special note is cerebral blood flow, which may predispose the fragile blood vessels in the brain to rupture, causing intracranial hemorrhage (Fanaroff & Fanaroff, 2014).

GASTROINTESTINAL SYSTEM

Preterm newborns usually lack the neuromuscular coordination required to maintain the sucking, swallowing, and breathing regimen necessary for sufficient calorie and fluid intake to support growth. Perinatal hypoxia causes shunting of blood from the gut to more important organs such as the heart and brain. Subsequently, ischemia and damage to the intestinal wall can occur. This combination of shunting, ischemia, damage to the intestinal wall, and poor sucking ability places the preterm infant at risk for malnutrition and weight loss.

In addition, preterm newborns have a small stomach capacity, weak abdominal muscles, compromised metabolic function, limited ability to digest proteins and absorb nutrients, and weak or absent suck and gag reflexes. All of these limitations place the preterm newborn at risk for nutritional deficiency and subsequent growth and development delays (Neonatal Handbook, 2015c).

The preterm infant's ability to coordinate sucking, swallowing, and breathing are challenged. As a result, preterm infants often require enteral or intravenous feeding. Enteral tube feeding will help to conserve energy even in an infant who is able to suck. The exact nutritional needs of preterm infants depend on their gestational age, postnatal age, weight, route of nutritional intake, growth rate, activity, and thermal environment. Preterm infants that are ill or experiencing stressful situations have higher energy requirements. Preterm infants take time to establish enteral intakes, and parenteral nutrition is now an integral component of care, but safe amounts of macronutrients, and the optimal amino acid and lipid composition remains an uncertainty (Embleton, Morgan, & King, 2015).

Currently, minimal enteral feeding is used to prepare the preterm newborn's gut to overcome the many feeding difficulties associated with gastrointestinal immaturity. It involves the introduction of small amounts, usually 0.5 to 1 mL/kg/hr, of enteral feeding to induce surges in gut hormones that enhance maturation of the intestine. This minute amount of breast milk or formula given via gavage (tube) feeding prepares the gut to absorb future introduction of nutrients. It builds mucosal bulk, stimulates development of enzymes, enhances pancreatic function, stimulates maturation of gastrointestinal hormones, reduces gastrointestinal distention and malabsorption, and enhances transition to oral feedings (Koletzko, Poindexter, & Uauy, 2014).

RENAL SYSTEM

The renal system of the preterm newborn is immature, reducing the baby's ability to concentrate urine and slowing the glomerular filtration rate. As a result, the risk for fluid retention, with subsequent fluid and electrolyte disturbances, increases. In addition, preterm newborns have limited ability to clear drugs from their systems, thereby increasing the risk of drug toxicity. Close monitoring of the preterm newborn's acid–base and electrolyte balance is critical to identify metabolic inconsistencies. Prescribed medications require strict evaluation to prevent overwhelming the preterm baby's immature renal system.

IMMUNE SYSTEM

The preterm newborn's immune system is very immature, increasing his or her susceptibility to infections. A deficiency of IgG may occur because transplacental transfer does not occur until after 34 weeks' gestation. This protection is lacking if the baby was born before this time. In addition, preterm newborns have an impaired ability to manufacture antibodies to fight infection if they were exposed to pathogens during the birth process. Moreover, the preterm newborn's thin skin and fragile blood vessels provide a limited protective barrier, adding to the increased risk for infection. Thus, anticipating and preventing infections is the goal; preventing infections has a better outcome than treating them.

CENTRAL NERVOUS SYSTEM

The preterm newborn is susceptible to injury and insult to the central nervous system, increasing the potential for long-term disability into adulthood. Like all newborns, preterm newborns have difficulty with temperature regulation and maintaining stability. However, their risk for heat loss is compounded by inadequate amounts of insulating subcutaneous fat; lack of muscle tone and flexion to conserve heat; inadequate brown fat to generate heat; limited muscle mass activity, reducing the possibility of producing their own heat; inability to shiver to generate heat; and an immature temperature-regulating center in the brain (Kenner & Lott, 2014). It is crucial to prevent cold stress, which would increase the newborn's metabolic and oxygen needs. The goal is to create a neutral thermal environment in which oxygen consumption is minimal but body temperature is maintained (Fanaroff & Fanaroff, 2014).

In addition, the preterm newborn is especially susceptible to hypoglycemia due to immature glucose control mechanisms, decreased glucose stores, and a reduced availability of alternative fuels such as ketone bodies.

Take Note!

Glucose is needed by the brain and central nervous system to maintain and support numerous body system functions.

Nursing Assessment

Preterm newborns are at high risk for numerous problems and require special care. When preterm labor develops and cannot be stopped by medical interventions, plans are necessary for appropriate management of the mother and the preterm newborn, such as transporting them to a regional center with facilities to care for preterm newborns or notifying the facility's NICU. Depending on the degree of prematurity, the preterm newborn may be kept in the NICU for months.

A thorough assessment of the preterm newborn upon admission to the nursery provides a baseline from which to identify changes in clinical status. Be aware of the common physical characteristics and be able to identify any deviation from the expected (Fig. 23.2). Common physical characteristics of preterm infants may include:

- Birth weight of less than 5.5 lb
- Scrawny appearance
- Head disproportionately larger than chest circumference
- Poor muscle tone
- Minimal subcutaneous fat
- Undescended testes in males
- Prominent clitoris and labia minora in females
- Plentiful lanugo (soft, downy hair), especially over the face and back
- Poorly formed ear pinna, with soft, pliable cartilage
- Fused eyelids
- Soft and spongy skull bones, especially along suture lines
- Matted scalp hair, woolly in appearance
- Absent-to-a-few creases in the soles and palms
- Minimal scrotal rugae in male infants;
- Thin, transparent skin with visible veins
- Breast and nipples not clearly delineated
- Abundant vernix caseosa (Verklan & Walden, 2014).

Be alert for evidence that might suggest that the preterm newborn is developing a complication (see Table 23.1).

Review the maternal history to identify risk factors for preterm birth and check antepartum and intrapartum records for maternal infections to anticipate the need for treatment. Maternal risk factors associated with preterm birth include a previous preterm delivery, low socioeconomic status, preeclampsia, hypertension, poor maternal nutrition, smoking, multiple gestation, infection, advanced maternal age, and substance abuse.

Assess the newborn's gestational age and assess for fetal growth restriction if appropriate. Inspect the

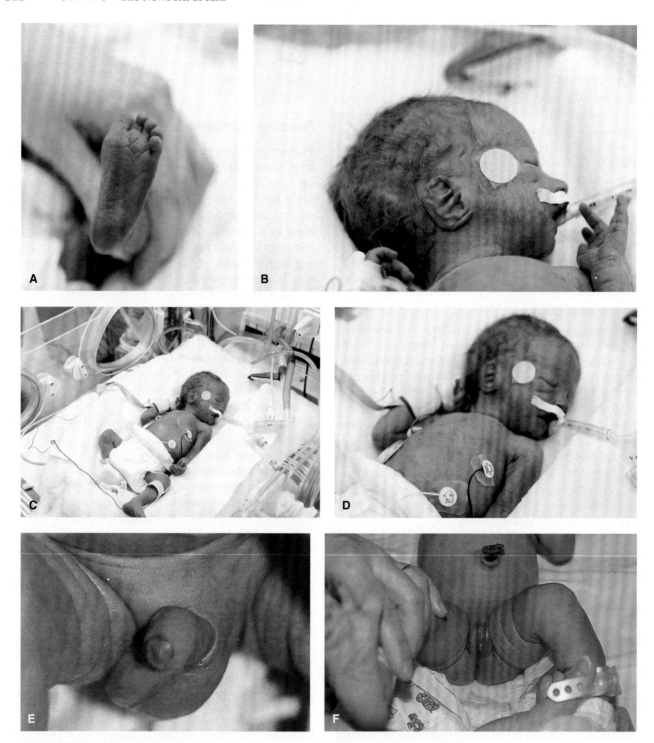

FIGURE 23.2 Characteristics of a preterm newborn. **A.** Few plantar creases. **B.** Soft, pliable ear cartilage, matted hair, and fused eyelids. **C.** Lax posture with poor muscle tone. **D.** Breast and nipple area barely visible. **E.** Male genitalia with minimal rugae on scrotum. **F.** Female genitalia with prominent labia and clitoris.

newborn's skin closely, especially skin color. Assess vital signs, including temperature via skin probe to identify hypothermia or fever, and heart rate for tachycardia or bradycardia. Evaluate the newborn's respiratory effort and respiratory rate. Observe for periods of apnea lasting longer than 20 seconds. Monitor oxygen saturation levels by pulse oximetry to validate perfusion status. Note and report any signs of respiratory distress. Auscultate lung and heart sounds, being especially alert for possible murmur, which would indicate the presence of patent ductus arteriosus in a preterm newborn. Assess neurologic status by observing the newborn's behavior.

Note any restlessness, hypotonia, or weak cry or sucking effort and report unusual findings.

Monitor laboratory studies such as hemoglobin and hematocrit for signs of polycythemia. Screen for hypoglycemia upon admission and then hourly, always observing for nonspecific signs of hypoglycemia such as lethargy, poor feeding, and seizures. Evaluate serum bilirubin concentrations.

Finally, assess the mother and family members. Identify family strengths and coping mechanisms to establish a basis for intervention.

Nursing Management

During the past 50 years in the United States, the rising preterm birth rate, a progressive decrease in preterm mortality, and a lowering of the limit of viability have made preterm birth a significant public health problem. It is estimated that, each day throughout the world, over 40,000 infants are born prematurely.

Preterm birth creates a crisis for the mother and family. Multiple studies have found that hospitalization for preterm newborns is often followed by negative mental health/behavioral outcomes, anxiety and depressive disorders, and long-term neurologic sequelae. Emerging evidence suggests that partners/significant others experience high rates of psychological stress in the first few months after a preterm birth (Treyvaud, 2014). Preterm newborns present with immaturity of all organ systems, abundant physiologic challenges, and significant morbidity and mortality globally (Salam et al., 2014). The nurse must be vigilant for complications when managing preterm newborns (Fig. 23.3 and Nursing Care Plan 23.1).

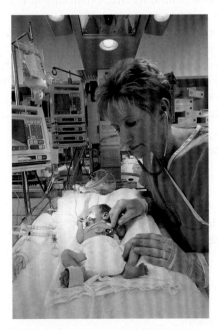

FIGURE 23.3 The physical condition of a preterm newborn demands skilled assessment and nursing care.

PROMOTING OXYGENATION

Newborns normally start to breathe without assistance and often cry after birth, being stimulated by a change in pressure gradients and environmental temperature. The work of taking that first breath is primarily due to overcoming the surface tension of the walls of the terminal lung units at the gas–tissue interface. Subsequent breaths require less inspiratory pressure since there is an increase in functional capacity and air retained. By 1 minute of age, most newborns are breathing well. A newborn who fails to establish adequate, sustained respiration after birth is said to have **asphyxia** (perinatal acidosis), which is the deprivation of oxygen during the birth process, resulting in fetal hypoxia that can lead to organ damage. Asphyxia is the most common clinical insult in the perinatal period that results in brain injury, which may lead to intellectual disability, cerebral palsy, or seizures (Herrera-Marschitz et al., 2015).

The preterm infant lacks surfactant. Surfactant lowers surface tension in the alveoli and stabilizes them to prevent their collapse. Even if preterm newborns can initiate respirations, they have a limited ability to retain air due to insufficient surfactant. Therefore, preterm newborns develop atelectasis quickly without alveoli stabilization. The inability to initiate and establish respirations leads to hypoxemia and ultimately hypoxia (decreased oxygen), acidosis (decreased pH), and hypercarbia (increased carbon dioxide). This change in the newborn's biochemical environment may inhibit the transition to extrauterine circulation, thus allowing fetal circulation patterns to persist.

Failure to initiate extrauterine breathing or failure to breathe well after birth leads to hypoxia (too little oxygen in the cells of the body). As a result, the heart rate falls, cyanosis develops, temperature decreases, blood pressure decreases, and respirations are altered (apnea, tachypnea, retractions, grunting, and nasal flaring) and the newborn becomes hypotonic and unresponsive. Although this can happen with any newborn, the risk is higher in preterm newborns.

Prevention and early identification of at risk newborns are essential. Prenatal risk factors that can help identify the newborn that may need resuscitation at birth secondary to asphyxia include:

- History of substance abuse
- Gestational hypertension
- Fetal distress due to hypoxia before birth
- Chronic maternal diseases such as diabetes or a heart or renal condition
- Maternal or perinatal infection
- Placental problems (placenta previa or abruptio placentae)
- Umbilical cord problems (nuchal or prolapsed)
- Difficult or traumatic birth
- Multiple births
- Congenital heart disease

(text continues on page 848)

NURSING CARE PLAN 23.1

Overview of the Care of a Preterm Newborn

Alice, an 18-year-old, felt that she had done everything right during her first pregnancy and certainly didn't anticipate giving birth to a preterm newborn at 32 weeks' gestation. When Mary Kaye was born, she had respiratory distress and hypoglycemia and couldn't stabilize her temperature. Assessment revealed the following: newborn described as scrawny in appearance; skin thin and transparent with prominent veins over abdomen; hypotonia with lax, extended positioning; weak sucking reflex when nipple offered; respiratory distress with tachypnea (70 breaths/min), nasal flaring, and sternal retractions; low blood glucose level suggested by lethargy, tachycardia, jitteriness; axillary temperature of 96.8° F (36° C) despite warmed blanket; weight 2,146 g (4.73 lb); length 45 cm (17.72 in).

NURSING DIAGNOSIS: Ineffective breathing pattern related to immature respiratory system and respiratory distress as evidenced by tachypnea, nasal flaring, and sternal retractions

Outcome Identification and Evaluation

The newborn's respiratory status will return to an adequate level of functioning as evidenced by rate remaining within 30 to 60 breaths/min, maintenance of acceptable oxygen saturation levels, and minimal to absent signs of respiratory distress.

Interventions: *Promoting Optimal Breathing Pattern*

- Assess gestational age and risk factors for respiratory distress *to allow early detection*.
- Anticipate need for bag and mask setup and wall suction *to allow for prompt intervention should respiratory status continue to worsen*.
- Assess respiratory effort (rate, character, effort) *to identify changes*.
- Assess heart rate for tachycardia and auscultate heart sounds *to determine worsening of condition*.
- Observe for cues (grunting, shallow respirations, tachypnea, apnea, tachycardia, central cyanosis, hypotonia, increased effort) *to identify need for additional oxygen*.
- Maintain slight head elevation *to prevent upper airway obstruction*.
- Assess skin color *to evaluate tissue perfusion*.

- Monitor oxygen saturation level via pulse oximetry *to provide objective indication of perfusion status*.
- Provide supplemental oxygen as indicated and ordered *to ensure adequate tissue oxygenation*.
- Assist with any ordered diagnostic tests, such as chest x-ray and arterial blood gases (ABGs), *to determine effectiveness of treatments*.
- Cluster nursing activities *to reduce oxygen consumption*.
- Maintain a neutral thermal environment *to reduce oxygen consumption*.
- Monitor hydration status *to prevent fluid volume deficit or overload*.
- Explain all events and procedures to the parents *to help alleviate anxiety and promote understanding of the newborn's condition*.

NURSING DIAGNOSIS: Ineffective thermoregulation related to lack of fat stores and hypotonia as evidenced by extended positioning, low axillary temperature despite warmed blanket, respiratory distress, and lethargy

Outcome Identification and Evaluation

The newborn will demonstrate ability to regulate temperature as evidenced by temperature remaining in normal range 97.7° to 99.5° F (36.5° to 37.5° C) and absent signs of cold stress.

Interventions: *Promoting Thermoregulation*

- Assess the axillary temperature every hour or use a thermistor probe *to monitor for changes*.
- Review maternal history *to identify risk factors contributing to problem*.

NURSING CARE PLAN 23.1

Overview of the Care of a Preterm Newborn (continued)

- Monitor vital signs, including heart rate and respiratory rate, every hour *to identify deviations*.
- Check radiant heat source or isolette *to ensure maintenance of appropriate temperature of the environment*.
- Assess environment for sources of heat loss or gain through evaporation, conduction, convection, or radiation *to minimize risk of heat loss*.
- Avoid bathing and exposing newborn *to prevent cold stress*.
- Warm all blankets and equipment that come in contact with newborn; place warmed cap on the newborn's head and keep it on *to minimize heat loss*.
- Encourage kangaroo care (mother or father holds preterm infant underneath clothing skin-to-skin and upright between breasts) *to provide warmth*.
- Educate parents on how to maintain a neutral thermal environment, including importance of keeping the newborn warm with a cap and double-wrapping with blankets and changing them frequently to keep dry *to promote newborn's adjustment*.
- Demonstrate ways *to safeguard warmth and prevent heat loss*.

NURSING DIAGNOSIS: Risk for imbalanced nutrition: less than body requirements related to poor sucking and lack of glycogen stores necessary to meet the newborn's increased metabolic demands as evidenced by weak sucking reflex, low birth weight, and signs and symptoms of hypoglycemia, including lethargy, tachycardia, and jitteriness

Outcome Identification and Evaluation

The newborn will demonstrate adequate nutritional intake, remaining free of signs of hypoglycemia as evidenced by blood glucose levels being maintained above 45 mg/dL, enhanced sucking ability, and appropriate weight gain.

Interventions: *Promoting Optimal Nutrition*

- Identify newborn at risk based on behavioral characteristics, body measurements, and gestational age *to establish a baseline and allow for early detection*.
- Assess blood glucose levels as ordered *to determine status and establish a baseline for interventions*.
- Obtain blood glucose measurements upon admission to nursery and every 1 to 2 hours as indicated *to evaluate for changes*.
- Observe behavior for signs of low blood glucose *to allow early identification*.
- Initiate early oral feedings or gavage feedings *to maintain blood glucose levels*.
- If oral or gavage feedings aren't tolerated, initiate an IV glucose infusion *to aid in stabilizing blood glucose levels*.
- Assess skin for pallor and sweating *to identify signs of hypoglycemia*.
- Assess neurologic status for tremors, seizures, jitteriness, and lethargy *to identify further drops in blood glucose levels*.
- Monitor weight daily for changes *to determine effectiveness of feedings*.
- Maintain temperature using warmed blankets, radiant warmer, or warmed isolette *to prevent heat loss and possible cold stress and reduce energy demands*.
- Monitor temperature *to prevent cold stress resulting in decreased blood glucose levels*.
- Offer opportunities for nonnutritive sucking on premature-size pacifier *to satisfy sucking needs*.
- Monitor for tolerance of oral feedings, including intake and output, *to determine effectiveness*.
- Administer IV dextrose if newborn is symptomatic *to raise blood glucose levels quickly*.
- Decrease energy requirements, including clustering care activities and providing rest periods, *to conserve glucose and glycogen stores*.
- Inform parents about procedures and treatments, including rationale for frequent blood glucose levels, *to help reduce their anxiety*.

- Maternal anesthesia or recent analgesia
- Preterm or post-term birth (Neonatal Handbook, 2015d).

Note the newborn's Apgar score at 1 and 5 minutes. If after 15 seconds of tactile stimulation without effective respirations or an increase in heart rate above 100 bpm, the infant should be resuscitated (Yousaf, Hayat, & Afzal, 2015). Several diagnostic studies may be done to identify underlying etiologies. For example, a chest x-ray helps to identify structural abnormalities that might interfere with respirations. Blood studies may be done, such as cultures to rule out an infectious process, a toxicology screen to detect any maternal drugs in the newborn, and a metabolic screen to identify any metabolic conditions (Fanaroff & Fanaroff, 2014). Monitor vital signs continually, check blood glucose levels for hypoglycemia secondary to stress, and maintain a neutral thermal environment to promote energy conservation and minimize oxygen consumption.

Resuscitating The Newborn. Any newborn can be born with asphyxia without warning. Approximately 10% of newborns require some assistance to begin breathing at birth. The aim of neonatal resuscitation is to prevent neonatal death and adverse long term neurodevelopmental sequelae associated with perinatal asphyxia. Anticipation, adequate preparation, accurate evaluation, and prompt initiation of support are critical for successful newborn resuscitation. Have all basic equipment immediately available and in working order. Ensure that the equipment is evaluated daily, and document its condition and any needed repairs. Box 23.2 lists the equipment needed for basic newborn resuscitation.

BOX 23.2

BASIC EQUIPMENT FOR NEWBORN RESUSCITATION

- A wall vacuum suction apparatus
- Infant size stethoscope
- Pulse oximeter
- Epinephrine
- Volume expander intravenous fluids
- A wall source or tank source of 100% oxygen with a flow meter
- A neonatal self-inflating ventilation bag with correctly sized face masks
- A selection of endotracheal tubes (2.5, 3.0, or 3.5 mm) with introducers
- A laryngoscope with a small, straight blade and spare batteries and bulbs
- Ampules of naloxone (Narcan) with syringes and needles
- A wall clock to document timing of activities and events
- A supply of disposable gloves in a variety of sizes for staff to use

---

Determine the need for resuscitation by performing a rapid assessment using the following three questions:
1. What is the newborn's heart rate?
2. What is the gestational age of this newborn?
3. Is the newborn breathing or crying now?
4. Does the newborn have good muscle tone?

If the answer to all questions is "yes," then routine care is initiated: provide warmth, clear the airway, dry the newborn, and assess color. If the answer to any of these questions is "no," the newborn should receive one or more of the following actions, according to this sequence:
1. Stabilization. Dry the newborn thoroughly with a warm towel; provide warmth by placing him or her under a radiant heater to prevent rapid heat loss through evaporation; position the head in a neutral position to open the airway; clear the airway with a bulb syringe or suction catheter; and stimulate breathing. At times, handling and rubbing the newborn with a dry towel may be all that is needed to stimulate respirations.
2. Assess for breathing – bag the newborn if not breathing
3. Place pulse oximeter on newborn's right hand to determine oxygen saturation
4. Ventilation if needed
5. Assess heart rate
6. Chest compressions if needed
7. Administration of epinephrine and/or volume expansion (Vali, Mathew, & Lakshminrusimha, 2015).

The decision to progress from one set of actions to the next and the need for further resuscitative efforts is determined by the assessment of respirations, heart rate, and color (American Academy of Pediatrics [AAP] & American Heart Association [AHA], 2014). Nurses need to remember that preterm infants have immature lungs that may be more difficult to ventilate and are also more vulnerable to injury by positive-pressure ventilation. They also have immature blood vessels in the brain that are prone to hemorrhage; thin skin and a large surface area, which contribute to rapid heat loss; increased susceptibility to infection; and increased risk of hypovolemic shock related to small blood volume. Anticipation, adequate preparation, accurate evaluation, and prompt initiation of support are critical for successful neonatal resuscitation.

When performing newborn resuscitation, use the mnemonic "ABCDs" (airway, breathing, circulation, and drugs) to remember the sequence of steps (Box 23.3).

Resuscitation measures are continued until the newborn has a pulse above 100 bpm, a good (healthy) cry, or good breathing efforts and a pink tongue. This last sign indicates a good oxygen supply to the brain. Effective ventilation is the key to successful neonatal resuscitation (AAP & AHA, 2014).

Throughout the resuscitation period, keep the parents informed of what is happening to their newborn and what is being done and why. Provide support through

BOX 23.3

ABCDS OF NEWBORN RESUSCITATION

- **A**irway
  - Place infant's head in "sniffing" position.
  - Suction mouth, then nose.
  - Suction trachea if meconium-stained and newborn is NOT vigorous (strong respiratory effort, good muscle tone, and heart rate >100 bpm).
- **B**reathing
  - Use positive-pressure ventilation (PPV) for apnea, gasping, or pulse <100 bpm.
  - Ventilate at rate of 40 to 60 breaths/min.
  - Listen for rising heart rate, audible breath sounds.
  - Look for slight chest movement with each breath.
  - Use carbon dioxide detector after intubation.
- **C**irculation
  - Start compressions if heart rate is <60 after 30 seconds of effective PPV.
  - Give three compressions: 1 breath every 2 seconds.
  - Compress one third of the anterior–posterior diameter of the chest.
- **D**rugs
  - Give epinephrine if heart rate is <60 after 30 seconds of compressions and ventilation.
  - *Caution:* Epinephrine dosage is different for endotracheal and IV routes!
  - Epinephrine: 1:10,000 concentration
  - 0.1 to 0.3 mL/kg IV
  - 0.3 to 1 mL/kg via endotracheal tube (AAP & AHA, 2014).

this initial crisis. Once the newborn has been stabilized, encourage bonding by having them stroke, touch, and, when appropriate, hold the newborn.

Administering Oxygen. Oxygen administration is a common therapy in newborn nurseries. Although it has been used in newborns for over 75 years, there is no universal agreement on the most appropriate range at which oxygen levels should be maintained for newborns experiencing hypoxia, nor is there a standard time frame for oxygen to be administered (Neonatal Handbook, 2015d). Although this uncertainty continues, nurses will experience a wide variation in practice in terms of modes of administration, monitoring, blood levels, and target ranges for both short- and long-term oxygen therapy.

A guiding principle, however, is that oxygen therapy should be targeted to levels appropriate to the condition, gestational age, oxygenation saturation level, and postnatal age of the newborn.

Oxygen therapy must be used judiciously to prevent **retinopathy of prematurity (ROP)**, a major cause of blindness in preterm newborns in the past. It is a disease that affects immature vasculature in the eyes of preterm

infants. It remains a significant threat to vision for preterm infants despite the availability of therapeutic modalities of treatment. ROP is a potentially blinding eye disorder that occurs when abnormal blood vessels grow and spread through the retina, eventually leading to retinal detachment. The incidence of ROP is inversely proportional to the preterm baby's birth weight. Despite current treatments, ROP remains a major cause of blindness in premature infants and the incidence is increasing with increased survival of infants born at very early gestational ages. ROP is a persistent and often devastating morbidity associated with premature and low–birth-weight infants. It continues to be a frequent diagnosis in the NICU, despite technological advances and increased knowledge.

The incidence of ROP varies with birth weight, but approximately 15,000 infants in the United States have ROP. About 90% of all infants with ROP have a mild form and do not need treatment. However, each year in the United States, about 400 to 600 infants do become legally blind or severely visually impaired from ROP (Hartnett, 2015).

The AAP has updated practice guideline recommendations for ROP screening and treatment that aid in creating a consistent and reliable ROP protocol (Sabri, 2016). Although the role of oxygen in the pathogenesis of ROP is unclear, current evidence suggests that it is linked to the duration of oxygen use rather than the concentration. Thus, the use of 100% oxygen to resuscitate a newborn should not pose a problem (National Eye Institute, 2015). However, an ophthalmology consult for follow-up after discharge is essential for preterm infants who have received extensive oxygen therapy.

Respiratory distress in preterm infants is commonly caused by a deficiency of surfactant, retained fluid in the lungs (wet lung syndrome), meconium aspiration, pneumonia, hypothermia, or anemia. The principles of care are the same regardless of the cause of respiratory distress:

- First, keep the newborn warm, preferably in a warmed isolette or with an overhead radiant warmer, to conserve the baby's energy and prevent cold stress.
- Handle the newborn as little as possible, because stimulation often increases the oxygen requirement.
- Provide energy through calories via intravenous dextrose or gavage or continuous tube feedings to prevent hypoglycemia.
- Treat cyanosis with an oxygen hood or blow-by oxygen placed near the newborn's face if respiratory distress is mild and short-term therapy is needed.
- Record the following important observations every hour or more frequently if indicated, and document any deterioration or changes in respiratory status:
  - Respiratory rate, quality of respirations, and respiratory effort
  - Airway patency, including removal of secretions per facility policy

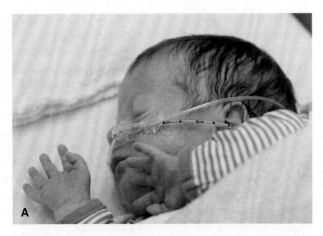
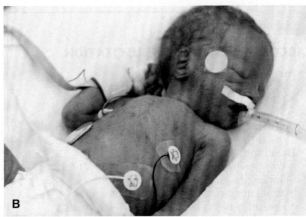

FIGURE 23.4 A. A preterm newborn receiving oxygen therapy via a nasal cannula. The newborn also has an enteral feeding tube inserted for nutrition. **B.** A preterm newborn receiving mechanical ventilation.

- Skin color, including any changes to duskiness, blueness, or pallor
- Lung sounds on auscultation to differentiate breath sounds in upper and lower fields
- Equipment required for oxygen delivery, such as:
  - Blow-by oxygen delivered via mask or tube for short-term therapy
  - Oxygen hood (oxygen is delivered via a plastic hood placed over the newborn's head)
  - Nasal cannula (oxygen is delivered directly through the nares) (Fig. 23.4A)
  - Continuous positive airway pressure, which prevents collapse of unstable alveoli and delivers high levels of inspired oxygen into the lungs
  - Mechanical ventilation, which delivers consistent assisted ventilation and oxygen therapy, reducing the work of breathing for the fatigued infant (see Fig. 23.4B)
- Correct placement of endotracheal tube (if present)
- Heart rate, including any changes
- Monitor the infant's respiratory status, clinically as well as by oxygen saturation, ABG, and chest x-ray
- Oxygen saturation levels via pulse oximetry to evaluate need for therapy modifications based on hemoglobin
- Suction as needed to remove secretions to maintain a patent airway and enhance oxygenation
- Maintenance of appropriate concentration of oxygen determined by ABG assay
- Nutritional intake, including calories provided, to prevent hypoglycemia and method of feeding, such as gavage, intravenous, or continuous enteral feedings
- Decrease stimulation; cluster all care to allow for rest
- Hydration status, including any signs and symptoms of fluid overload
- Maintain a neutral thermal environment
- Laboratory tests, including ABGs, to determine effectiveness of oxygen therapy

- Administration of medication, such as exogenous surfactant
- Offer emotional support and progress reports on infant's condition to the family

If the newborn shows worsening cyanosis or if oxygen saturation levels fall below 87%, prepare to give additional oxygen as ordered. Throughout, maintain trict asepsis, including hand hygiene, which is vital to reduce the risk of infection.

MAINTAINING THERMAL REGULATION

An optimal thermal environment is desirable for preterm infants. When an infant becomes chilled, it attempts to conserve body heat by vasoconstriction and thermogenesis by metabolizing brown adipose tissue and increasing oxygen consumption. This increase in energy expenditure reduces the newborn's ability to gain weight. Immediately after birth, dry the newborn with a warmed towel and then place him or her in a second warm, dry towel before performing the assessment. This drying prevents rapid heat loss secondary to evaporation. Newborns who are active, breathing well, and crying are stable and can be placed on their mother's chest ("kangaroo care") to promote warmth and prevent hypothermia. Preterm newborns who are not considered stable may be placed under a radiant warmer or in a warmed isolette after they have been dried with a warmed towel.

Typically newborns use nonshivering thermogenesis for heat production by metabolizing their own brown adipose tissue. However, the preterm newborn has an inadequate supply of brown fat because he or she left the uterus early, before the supply was adequate. The preterm newborn also has decreased muscle tone and thus cannot assume the flexed fetal position, which reduces the amount of skin exposed to a cooler environment. In addition, preterm newborns have large body surface areas compared with weight. This allows an increased transfer of heat from their bodies to the environment.

Usually, a preterm newborn who is having problems with thermal regulation is cool-to-cold to the touch. The hands, feet, and tongue may appear cyanotic. Respirations are shallow or slow, or signs of respiratory distress are present. The newborn is lethargic and hypotonic, feeds poorly, and has a feeble cry. Blood glucose levels are probably low, leading to hypoglycemia, due to the energy expended to keep warm.

When promoting thermal regulation for the preterm newborn:

- Remember the four mechanisms for heat transfer and ways to prevent loss:
  - *Convection*: heat loss through air currents (avoid drafts near the newborn)
  - *Conduction*: heat loss through direct contact (warm everything the newborn comes in contact with, such as blankets, mattress, stethoscope)
  - *Radiation*: heat loss without direct contact (keep isolettes away from cold sources and provide insulation to prevent heat transfer)
  - *Evaporation*: heat loss by conversion of liquid into vapor (keep the newborn dry and delay the first bath until the baby's temperature is stable)
- Frequently assess the temperature of the isolette or radiant warmer, adjusting the temperature as necessary to prevent hypo- or hyperthermia.
- Utilize plastic wraps and bags, skin-to-skin contact, or transwarmer mattresses if available to keep infants warmer and decrease the incidence of hypothermia
- Assess the newborn's temperature every hour until stable.
- Observe for clinical signs of cold stress, such as respiratory distress, central cyanosis, hypoglycemia, lethargy, weak cry, abdominal distention, apnea, bradycardia, and acidosis.
- Remember the complications of hypothermia and frequently assess the newborn for signs:
  - Metabolic acidosis secondary to anaerobic metabolism used for heat production, which results in the production of lactic acid
  - Hypoglycemia due to depleted glycogen stores
  - Pulmonary hypertension secondary to pulmonary vasoconstriction
- Monitor the newborn for signs of hyperthermia such as tachycardia, tachypnea, apnea, warm to touch, flushed skin, lethargy, weak or absent cry, and central nervous system depression; adjust the environmental temperature appropriately.
- Explain to the parents the need to maintain the newborn's temperature, including the measures used; demonstrate ways to safeguard warmth and prevent heat loss.

PROMOTING NUTRITION AND FLUID BALANCE

Providing nutrition is challenging for preterm newborns because their needs are great but their ability to take in

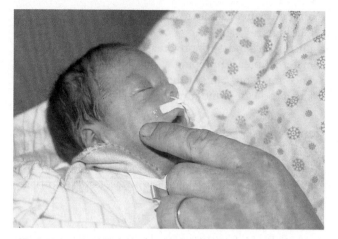

FIGURE 23.5 Infants who are ill at birth often need supplemental feedings by nasogastric or gastrostomy tubes. (Copyright Caroline Brown, RNC, MS, DEd.)

optimal amounts of energy/calories is reduced due to their compromised health status. Individual nutritional needs are highly variable.

Depending on their gestational age, preterm newborns receive nutrition orally, enterally, or parenterally via infusion. Several different methods can be used to provide nutrition: parenteral feedings administered through a percutaneous central venous catheter for long-term venous access with delivery of total parenteral nutrition, or enteral feedings, which can include oral feedings (formula or breast milk), continuous nasogastric tube feedings, or intermittent gavage tube feedings (Fig. 23.5). Gavage feedings are commonly used for compromised newborns to allow them to rest during the feeding process. Many have a weak suck and become fatigued and thus cannot consume enough calories to meet their needs.

Most newborns born after 34 weeks' gestation without significant complications can feed orally. Those born before 34 weeks' gestation typically start with parenteral nutrition within the first 24 hours of life. Then enteral nutrition is introduced and advanced based on the degree of maturity and clinical condition. Ultimately, enteral nutrition methods replace parenteral nutrition.

To promote nutrition and fluid balance in the preterm newborn:

- Measure daily weight and plot it on a growth curve.
- Monitor intake; calculate fluid and caloric intake daily.
- Assess fluid status by monitoring weight; urinary output; urine specific gravity; laboratory test results such as serum electrolyte levels, blood urea nitrogen, creatinine, and hematocrit; skin turgor; and fontanels (Koletzko, Poindexter, & Uauy, 2014). Be alert for signs of dehydration, such as a decrease in urinary output, sunken fontanels, temperature elevation, lethargy, and tachypnea.
- Continually assess for enteral feeding intolerance; measure abdominal girth, auscultate bowel sounds,

and measure gastric residuals before the next tube feeding.

• Encourage and support breast-feeding by facilitating maternal breast pumping.

• Encourage nuzzling at the breast in conjunction with kangaroo care if the newborn is stable.

Take Note!

When assessing the fluid status of a preterm newborn, palpate the fontanels. Sunken fontanels suggest dehydration; bulging fontanels suggest overhydration.

PREVENTING INFECTION

Prevention of infection is critical when caring for preterm newborns. Infections are the most common cause of morbidity and mortality in the NICU population (Ohlin et al., 2015). Nursing assessment and early identification of problems are imperative to improve outcomes.

Preterm newborns are at risk for infection because their early birth deprived them of maternal antibodies needed for passive protection. They are also susceptible to infection because of their limited ability to produce their own antibodies, asphyxia at birth, and thin, friable skin that is easily traumatized, providing a portal of entry for microorganisms.

Early detection is crucial. The clinical manifestations can be nonspecific and subtle: apnea, diminished activity, poor feeding, temperature instability, respiratory distress, seizures, tachycardia, hypotonia, irritability, pallor, jaundice, and hypoglycemia. Report any of these to the primary care provider immediately so that treatment can be instituted.

Include the following interventions when caring for a preterm or post-term newborn to prevent infection:

• Assess for risk factors in maternal history that place the newborn at increased risk.

• Monitor for changes in vital signs such as temperature instability, tachycardia, or tachypnea.

• Assess oxygen saturation levels and initiate oxygen therapy as ordered if oxygen saturation levels fall below acceptable parameters.

• Assess feeding tolerance, typically an early sign of infection.

• Monitor laboratory test results for changes.

• Avoid using tape on the newborn's skin to prevent tearing.

• Use equipment that can be thrown away after use.

• Adhere to standard precautions; use clean gloves to handle dirty diapers and dispose of them properly.

• Use sterile gloves when assisting with any invasive procedure; attempt to minimize the use of invasive procedures.

• Remove all jewelry on your hands prior to washing hands; wash hands upon entering the nursery and in between caring for newborns.

• Administer antibiotics as ordered and monitor for therapeutic and adverse effects

• Avoid coming to work when ill, and screen all visitors for contagious infections.

PREVENTING COMPLICATIONS

Preterm newborns face a myriad of possible complications as a result of their fragile health status or the procedures and treatments used. Some of the more common complications in preterm newborns include respiratory distress syndrome, apnea, periventricular–intraventricular hemorrhage, bronchopulmonary dysplasia, ROP, hyperbilirubinemia, anemia, necrotizing enterocolitis, hypoglycemia, infection or septicemia, delayed growth and development, and mental or motor delays (March of Dimes, 2015c). Several of these complications are described in Chapter 24.

Remember Anna, who was in a state of shock when she entered the NICU to see her preterm baby for the first time? How could the nurse have prepared her for this event? What information needs to be given at the isolette to reduce her anxiety and fear now?

PROVIDING APPROPRIATE STIMULATION

Newborn stimulation involves a series of activities to encourage normal development. Research on developmental interventions shows that when preterm newborns, in particular, receive sensorimotor interventions such as rocking, kangaroo (skin-to-skin) contact with parents, containment (swaddling and surrounded by blanket rolls), soft singing or music, nonnutritive sucking (Fig. 23.6), breast-feeding, cuddling, gentle stroking of the infant's skin, colorful mobiles, gentle massage, passive exercise involving flexion and extension of limbs, holding, or sleeping on waterbeds, they gain weight faster, progress in feeding abilities more quickly, and show improved interactive behavior compared with preterm newborns who were not stimulated. In the hospital, tactile and kinesthetic stimulation has shown to have a positive effect, contributing toward adjustment and self-regulation of behavior in the preterm infant (Sayed et al., 2015). Conversely, overstimulation may have negative effects by reducing oxygenation and causing stress. The NICU environment lends itself to persistent and unpredictable sounds that are in stark contrast to the protective sounds inside the mother. A newborn reacts to stress by flaying the hands or bringing an arm up to cover the face. When overstimulated (e.g., by noise, lights, excessive handling, alarms, and procedures) and stressed, heart and respiratory rates decrease and periods of apnea or bradycardia may follow (Gardner et al., 2016).

The NICU environment can be altered to provide periods of calm and rest for the newborn by dimming the lights, lowering the volume and tone of conversations, closing doors gently, setting the telephone ringer

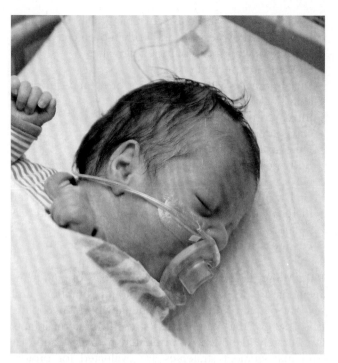

FIGURE 23.6 A preterm newborn receiving nonnutritive sucking with pacifier.

to the lowest volume possible, clustering nursing activities, and covering the isolette with a blanket to act as a light shield to promote rest at night.

Encourage parents to hold and interact with their newborn. Doing so helps to acquaint the parents with their newborn, promotes self-confidence, and fosters parent–newborn attachment (Fig. 23.7).

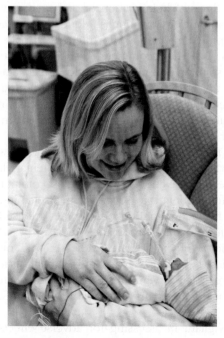

FIGURE 23.7 A mother bonding with her preterm newborn.

Think back to Anna, the woman who gave birth to a preterm newborn at 7 months' gestation. Anna will be discharged but her newborn will be staying in the NICU for a while. What interventions would be appropriate to facilitate bonding despite their separation? What support can be provided specifically to her family?

MANAGING PAIN

Pain control and prevention is imperative for ethical and clinical reasons and is required by the AAP and the Joint Commission as a standard of excellence. Pain is an unpleasant sensory and emotional experience felt by all humans. Unlike adults, infants are incapable of rating their pain on a scale of 0 to 10, and yet from the moment they take their first breath, newborns are exposed to heel sticks, circumcisions, injections, and immunizations, all which cause pain. Newborns feel pain and require the same level of pain assessment and management as adults. Awareness of the importance of pain in newborn babies has increased during recent years, but it remains a challenging area of clinical practice. Preterm infants show cortical, biochemical, physiologic, and behavioral responses to painful procedures. Common indicators of pain in the newborn who is unable to vocalize include facial expressions, body movements, and physiologic changes such as oxygen saturation (Hatfield & Ely, 2014). Untreated pain in newborns may result in increased morbidity and length of stay in the NICU, exaggerated responses to pain in later life, and altered psychosocial development (Valeri, Holsti, & Linhares, 2015). Parents commonly expect that health care providers will use appropriate measures to prevent pain in their newborns, but there are gaps in knowledge about the most effective way to accomplish this.

Assessing Pain in Newborns. Assessment of pain in the newborn remains a contentious and vexing problem. Newborns in the NICU are subjected to repeated procedures that cause them pain. Newborns, whether preterm, full term, or post-term, do experience pain, but the pain is difficult to validate with consistent behaviors. Considering that ill newborns undergo multiple noxious stimuli from invasive procedures, such as lumbar punctures, heel sticks, venipuncture, line insertions, chest tube placement, specimen collections, endotracheal intubation and suctioning, and mechanical ventilation. Common sense would suggest that newborns experience pain from these many activities and interventions. However, pain management in infants was not addressed formally until various professional and accrediting organizations issued position statements and clinical recommendations in an effort to promote effective pain management (Lee et al., 2014). An international consortium established principles

NEWBORN PAIN PREVENTION AND MANAGEMENT GUIDELINES

- Newborn pain frequently goes unrecognized and undertreated.
- Pain assessment is an essential activity prior to pain management.
- Newborns experience pain, and analgesics should be given.
- A procedure considered painful for an adult should also be considered painful for a newborn.
- Developmental maturity and health status must be considered when assessing for pain in newborns.
- Newborns may be more sensitive to pain than adults.
- Pain behavior is frequently mistaken for irritability and agitation.
- Newborns are more susceptible to the long-term effects of pain.
- Adequate pain management may reduce complications and mortality.
- Nonpharmacologic measures can prevent, reduce, or eliminate newborn pain.
- Sedation does not provide pain relief and may mask pain responses.
- A newborn's response to both pharmacologic and nonpharmacologic pain therapy should be assessed within 30 minutes of administration or intervention.
- Health care professionals are responsible for pain assessment and treatment.
- Written guidelines are needed on each newborn unit.

Adapted from Kenner, C., & Lott, J. W. (2014). *Comprehensive neonatal care* (5th ed.). New York, NY: Springer Publishing Company; and Sabic, D., Blattner, C., & Metts, M. (2015). Newborn and infant pain control. *Clinical Pediatrics, 54*(7), 613–614.

of newborn pain prevention and management that all nurses must be familiar with and apply (Box 23.4).

Several psychometric tools are available to assess pain in the newborn, but, unfortunately they are only rarely used in clinical practice examples include the Pain Assessment Tool (PAT), which evaluates respirations, heart rate, oxygen saturation, and blood pressure; the Premature Infant Pain Profile Revised, which assesses heart rate and oxygen saturation; the CRIES tool (cry, requires oxygen, increased vital signs, expression and sleeplessness); the Neonatal Infant Acute Pain Assessment Tool which assesses five behavioral and three physiologic indicators for pain; and the Neonatal Infant Pain Scale, which evaluates respiratory patterns. Most are based on facial expressions, crying patterns, changes in vital signs, and body movements (Reavey et al., 2014).

Nurses play a key role in assessing a newborn's pain level. Assess the newborn frequently. Pain is considered the "fifth vital sign" and should be assessed as frequently as the other four vital signs. Differentiate pain

from agitation by observing for changes in vital signs, behavior, facial expression, and body movement. Suspect pain if the newborn exhibits the following:

- Sudden high-pitched cry
- Facial grimace with furrowing of brow and quivering chin
- Increased muscle tone
- Oxygen desaturation
- Increase in heart rate
- Body posturing, such as squirming, kicking, and arching
- Limb withdrawal and thrashing movements
- Increase in heart rate, blood pressure, pulse, and respirations
- Fussiness and irritability (Verklan & Walden, 2014).

Pain Management Strategies. The goals of pain management are to minimize the amount, duration, and severity of pain and to assist the newborn in coping. It is essential that pain-related stress in preterm infants is accurately identified, appropriately managed, and that pain management strategies are evaluated for protective or adverse effects in the long term. Effective pain management strategies for newborns include preventing, limiting, or avoiding noxious stimuli; using nonpharmacologic techniques to reduce pain; and administering pharmacologic agents when appropriate. Box 23.5 lists some of the more commonly used nonpharmacologic pain management techniques for the preterm newborn.

Nonpharmacologic pain management strategies include nonnutritive sucking, breast-feeding, skin-to-skin contact, radiant heat source, and sweetened solutions. Recent research findings suggested that infants be given an appropriate-sized pacifier for comfort during painful procedures. Administration of oral sucrose with and without nonnutritive sucking is frequently used as a nonpharmacologic intervention for procedural pain relief in neonates also. The recommended sucrose concentration is a 24% solution and radiant heat for effective analgesia (Gray et al., 2015). Nurses need to be informed about the effectiveness of nonpharmacologic pain management strategies and how to use them and incorporate it into their practice.

The number of analgesics available for use with preterm newborns is limited. Morphine and fentanyl, usually administered intravenously, are the most commonly used opioids for moderate to severe pain. Acetaminophen is effective for mild pain. Benzodiazepines are used as sedatives during painful procedures and can be combined with opioids for more effectiveness. Local or topical anesthetics (e.g., EMLA cream) also may be used before procedures such as venipuncture, lumbar puncture, and intravenous catheter insertion (Sabic, Blattner, & Metts, 2014).

Be vigilant in assessing for adverse effects (respiratory depression or hypotension) when administering

NONPHARMACOLOGIC TECHNIQUES TO REDUCE PAIN IN THE PRETERM NEWBORN

- Gentle handling, rocking, caressing, cuddling, and massaging
- Rest periods before and after painful procedures
- Kangaroo care (skin-to-skin contact) during procedure
- Breast-feeding, if able, to reduce pain from minor procedures
- Use of a facilitated tuck (holding arms and legs in a flexed position)
- Application of topical anesthetics prior to venipuncture or lumbar puncture
- Swaddling and positioning to establish physical boundaries
- Non-nutritive sucking (pacifier dipped in sucrose) prior to procedure
- Minimal use of tape, with gentle removal to avoid skin tears
- Warm blankets for wrapping to facilitate relaxation
- Reduction of environmental stimuli by removing or turning down noxious stimuli such as noise from alarms, beepers, loud conversations, and bright lights
- Distraction, such as with colored objects or mobiles

Adapted from Hatfield, L. A., & Ely, E. A. (2014). Measurement of acute pain in infants: A review of behavioral and physiological variables. *Biological Research for Nursing*, (Online May 1, 2014). doi: 1099800414531448; Lee, G. Y., Yamada, J., Shorkey, A., & Stevens, B. (2014). Pediatric clinical practice guidelines for acute procedural pain: A systematic review. *Pediatrics, 133*(3), 500–515; and Sabic, D., Blattner, C., & Metts, M. (2015). Newborn and infant pain control. *Clinical Pediatrics*, (Online June 24, 2014), doi: 0009922814540043.

pharmacologic agents for pain management, especially in preterm newborns with neurologic impairment. These negative effects are usually dose and route related, so be knowledgeable about the pharmacokinetics and therapeutic dosing of any drug administered.

PROMOTING GROWTH AND DEVELOPMENT

In the late 1990s, researchers evaluated the NICU environment in terms of light and sound levels, caregiving activities, and handling of newborns. As a result of this research, many environmental modifications were made to reduce the stress and overstimulation of the NICU, and the concept of developmentally supportive care was introduced. Developmentally supportive care is defined as care of a newborn or infant to support positive growth and development. Developmental care focuses on what newborns or infants can do at that stage of development; it uses therapeutic interventions only to the point that they are beneficial; and it provides for the development of the newborn–family unit (White-Traut, 2015).

Developmental care is a philosophy of care that requires rethinking the relationships between newborns,

families, and health care providers. Family presence and participation in the care in the NICU is fundamental to the recovery and well-being of the sick neonate and family. The basis of family-centered, developmentally supportive care is the recognition that the newborn infant is a human being, in which caregivers need to be guided by the current needs of the infant and family, not their own. It includes a variety of activities designed to manage the environment and individualize the care of the preterm or high-risk ill newborn based on behavioral observations. Promoting kangaroo care in the NICU for preterm infants holds many benefits for the mother-infant dyad (see Evidence-Based Practice 23.1). Neonatal developmental care has evolved as a method of care that acknowledges that infant health depends on neonatal reactions to the environment and that each infant reacts to the environment favorably or unfavorably in an individual manner that depends on gestational and neurodevelopmental maturity. Key aspects of this care approach include attention to environmental infant stressors such as ambient light and sound levels, as well as individual infant and family needs including privacy and respect for diversity of cultural or other beliefs. Developmental care and family centered care notably not only improve parental satisfaction but influence the infant's health and well-being long after the NICU stay (Kiechl-Kohlendarfer et al., 2015).

Parents of NICU infants experience stress related to feelings of helplessness, exclusion and isolation, and lack sufficient knowledge regarding parenting and interacting with their newborn. There are several developmental interventions that nurses can do to help parents and newborns while in the NICU. Developmental care includes these strategies:

- Clustering care to promote rest and conserve the infant's energy
- Flexed positioning to simulate in utero positioning
- Environmental management to reduce noise and visual stimulation
- Kangaroo care to promote skin-to-skin sensation
- Placement of twins in the same isolette or open crib to reduce stress
- Activities to promote self-regulation and state regulation:
  - Surrounding the newborn with nesting rolls/devices
  - Swaddling with a blanket to maintain the flexed position
  - Providing sheepskin or a waterbed to simulate the uterine environment
    - Providing nonnutritive sucking (calms the infant)
    - Providing objects to grasp (comforts the newborn)
- Promotion of parent–infant bonding by making parents feel welcome in the NICU
- Open, honest communication with parents and staff
- Collaboration with the parents in planning the infant's care (Gardner et al., 2016).

EVIDENCE-BASED PRACTICE 23.1   UNDERSTANDING KANGAROO CARE AND ITS BENEFITS

STUDY

Holding an infant with ventral skin-to-skin contact in an upright position on the chest of the parent is referred to as kangaroo care. The purpose of kangaroo care is to facilitate infant transition to extrauterine life, promote early bonding, relieve pain, and establish exclusive breast-feeding. Numerous benefits of its use have been reported which include physiologic (thermoregulation, cardiorespiratory stability), behavioral (better sleep, breastfeeding duration, and degree of exclusivity), relieves procedural pain, and improves neurodevelopment. This review analyses current literature about the benefits of kangaroo care for preterm infants.

Findings

After the review of the literature and meta-analysis and two Cochrane reviews, there is current evidence that

supports kangaroo care improves sleep, neurodevelopment, and growth, length of breastfeeding, homeostasis, maternal-infant bonding, and relieves pain from procedures. Evidence supports the influence of kangaroo care increases maternal milk volume and increases breastfeeding duration in preterm infants. Yet, despite beneficial findings of kangaroo care, the adoption of it as routine clinical practice remains variable in many NICU settings.

Nursing Implications

The evidence is strong regarding the ability of kangaroo care to offer benefits to both mothers and their preterm infants. Nurses can be encouraging families to exercise this cost-effective, feasible, natural intervention that yields so many benefits for their preterm infant. It would be reasonable to recommend this intervention for all stable infants as soon as possible after birth and continued in the home setting.

Adapted from Campbell-Yeo, M. L., Disher, T. C., Benoit, B. L., & Johnston, C. C. (2015). Understanding kangaroo care and its benefits to preterm infants. *Pediatric Health, Medicine, and Therapeutics, 6,* 15–32.

Developmental care can be fostered by clustering the lights in one area so that no lights are shining directly on newborns, installing visual alarm systems and limiting overhead pages to minimize noise, and monitoring continuous and peak noise levels. Nurses can play an active role by serving on committees that address these issues. In addition, nurses can provide direct developmentally supportive care. Doing so involves careful planning of nursing activities to provide the ideal environment for the newborn's development. For example:

- Dim the lights and cover isolettes at night to simulate nighttime.
- Support early extubation from mechanical ventilation.
- Encourage early and consistent feedings with breast milk.
- Administer prescribed antibiotics judiciously.
- Position the newborn as if he or she was still in utero (a nesting fetal position).
- Promote kangaroo care by encouraging parents to hold the newborn against the chest for extended periods each day.
- Coordinate care to respect sleep and awake states.

Throughout the newborn's stay, work with the parents to develop a collaborative partnership so they feel comfortable caring for their newborn. Be prepared to make referrals to community support groups to enhance coping (Cano Gimenez & Sanchez-Luna, 2015).

PROMOTING PARENTAL COPING

Generally, pregnancy and the birth of a newborn are exciting times, but when the newborn has serious, perhaps life-threatening problems, the exciting experience

suddenly changes to one of anxiety, fear, guilt, loss, and grief. The birth of a preterm infant is an acutely stressful event for parents/partners, significant others.

Parents are typically unprepared for the birth of a preterm newborn and commonly experience an array of emotions, including disappointment, fear for the survival of the newborn, and anxiety due to the separation from their newborn immediately after birth. Gaining insight into the experience of parents of premature infants can help nurses ensure services more effectively meet the needs of these families (Vitale & Falco, 2014). Early interruptions in the bonding process and concern about the newborn's survival can create extreme anxiety and interfere with attachment (Yaman & Altay, 2015).

Nursing interventions aimed at reducing parental anxiety include:

- Reviewing with them the events that have occurred since birth
- Providing simple relaxation and calming techniques (visual imagery, breathing)
- Exploring their perception of the newborn's condition and offering explanations
- Validating their anxiety and behaviors as normal reactions to stress and trauma
- Providing a physical presence and support during emotional outbursts
- Exploring the coping strategies they used successfully in the past and encouraging their use now
- Encouraging frequent visits to the NICU
- Providing individualized support to parents while in NICU
- Encouraging parental involvement with their newborn in NICU

- Addressing their reactions to the NICU environment and explaining all equipment used
- Identifying family and community resources available to them (Stacey, Osborn, & Salkovskis, 2015).

PREPARING FOR DISCHARGE

Discharge planning typically begins with evidence that recovery of the newborn is certain. However, the exact date of discharge may not be predictable. The goal of the discharge plan is to make a successful transition to home care. Essential elements for discharge are a physiologically stable infant, a family who can provide the necessary care with appropriate support services in place in the community, and a pediatrician or family practice physician or nurse practitioner available for ongoing care.

The care of each high-risk newborn after discharge requires careful coordination to provide ongoing multidisciplinary support for the family. The discharge planning team typically includes the parents, primary care physician, neonatologists, neonatal nurses, and a social worker. Other health care providers, such as surgical specialists and pediatric subspecialists, occupational, physical, speech, and respiratory therapists, nutritionists, home health care nurses, and a case manager, may be included as needed. Critical components of discharge planning are summarized in Box 23.6.

Nurses involved in the discharge process are instrumental in bridging the gap between the hospital and home. Interventions typically include:

- Assessing the physical status of the mother and the newborn

- Discussing the early signs of complications and what to do if they occur
- Reinforcing instructions for infant care and safety
- Stressing the importance of proper car seat use
- Providing instructions for medication administration
- Reinforcing instructions for equipment operation, maintenance, and troubleshooting
- Teaching infant cardiopulmonary resuscitation and emergency care
- Demonstrating techniques for special care procedures such as dressings, ostomy care, artificial airway maintenance, chest physiotherapy, suctioning, and infant stimulation
- Providing breast-feeding support or instruction on gavage feedings
- Assisting with defining roles in the adjustment period at home
- Assessing the parents' emotional stability and coping status
- Providing support and reassurance to the family
- Reporting abnormal findings to the health care team for intervention
- Following up with parents to assure them that they have a "lifeline"

Late Preterm ("Near Term") Newborn

A late preterm newborn is an infant born between 34 0/7 and 36 6/7 weeks of gestation. In recent years, the subject of late preterm birth has received much attention, since this population of preterm newborns represents more than 72% of all preterm births in the United States and has increased by 30% in the past 20 years (CDC, 2015). The rise in elective induced births in the past decade is believed to have contributed to the rise in number of late preterm births. The largest increase in incidence of late preterm births is in the non-Hispanic White population. The underlying causes are poorly understood, although genetic, social, and environmental factors all likely play a role. Reasons for this might include an increased demand for assisted reproductive technology, older couples having babies, and higher rates of surgical births and inductions of labor (Horgan, 2015).

With birth weights typically ranging from 2,000 to 2,500 grams, late preterm infants may appear physically well developed when compared with their more premature counterparts. Consequently, it may be easy for nurses to overlook the fact that biologically and developmentally, these infants may be 4 to 6 weeks less mature than their full-term counterparts. Recent research has indicated that these infants are at heightened risk for a number of complications that are not normally seen in the healthy newborn population. They have more clinical problems, longer lengths of stay, and higher costs when compared with full-term infants (Kenner & Lott, 2015).

BOX 23.6

CRITICAL COMPONENTS OF DISCHARGE PLANNING

- Parental education—involvement and support in newborn care during NICU stay will ensure their readiness to care for the infant at home
- Evaluation of unresolved medical problems—review of the active problem list and determination of what home care and follow-up is needed
- Implementation of primary care—completion of newborn screening tests, immunizations, examinations such as funduscopic examination for ROP, and hematologic status evaluation
- Development of home care plan, including assessment of:
  - Equipment and supplies needed for care
  - In-home caregiver's preparation and ability to care for infant
  - Adequacy of the physical facilities in the home
  - An emergency care and transport plan if needed
  - Financial resources for home care costs
  - Family needs and coping skills
  - Community resources, including how they can be accessed

Late preterm babies are more likely than term babies to suffer complications at birth such as respiratory distress; require intensive and prolonged hospitalization; incur higher medical costs; die within the first year of life; and suffer brain injury that can result in long-term neurodevelopmental problems. Accordingly, increased high levels of late preterm births are an important public health issue (Baker, 2015). Perinatal nurses need to understand the risks of late preterm births and the unique needs of this population to facilitate timely assessment and intervention to improve outcomes.

Some additional challenges also facing the late preterm newborn include respiratory distress (secondary to cesarean births, maternal gestational diabetes, pulmonary hypertension, sepsis, chorioamnionitis, premature rupture of membranes, and fetal distress); thermoregulation issues related to limited ability to flex the trunk and extremities to decrease exposed surface area; hypoglycemia related to the first two challenges (respiratory distress and cold stress); jaundice and hyperbilirubinemia related to a gestational age of 36 weeks or less; sepsis; and feeding difficulties related to immature sucking and swallowing reflexes (Bird, 2014).

Recent research suggests that after the neonatal period, the risks continue with behavioral problems, 80% increased risk for attention-deficit/hyperactivity disorder (ADHD), and developmental and school-readiness delays (Ramenghi, 2015). These challenges are similar to those facing the preterm newborn and require similar management. Parents should be taught about these risks so that they will be aware of the unique risks and the need to remain vigilant. Health risks for the late preterm infant include:

- *Respiratory system dysfunction*—due to surfactant deficiency leading to distress
- *Glycemic instability*—due to increased energy demands needed for temperature regulation and increased respiratory effort, which cause the blood glucose to remain low for prolonged periods of time
- *Jaundice*—due to feeding difficulties and inability of liver to conjugate bilirubin
- *Inadequate oral intake*—due to a decreased ability to suck and swallow
- *Susceptibility to infection*—due to immaturity of the immune system
- *Neurologic immaturity*—due to reduced cortical development, which occurs during the 34th and 40th week of gestation (Baker, 2015; Kenner & Lott, 2015).

Nurses and parents must be aware of the risks associated with late preterm births to optimize care and outcomes for this group of newborns. Late preterm infants should not be discharged home before at least 48 hours of age; they should have demonstrated thermal stability when clothed in an open crib, normal vital signs, the ability to take feeds orally, a weight loss of less than 7% of birth weight, and the ability to pass stools spontaneously. Other assessments before discharge include metabolic and genetic screening together with hearing screening and a successful car seat challenge (Pappas & Robey, 2014).

Encourage and empower parents of a late preterm infant with appropriate teaching and ongoing support. Stress that although the infant may seem equivalent to the term infant in many ways, there are specific risks that should be addressed not only in the first year of life, but beyond. Close surveillance, follow-up, and referral to appropriate support services can optimize outcomes.

Post-Term Newborn

A pregnancy that extends beyond 42 weeks' gestation (294 days) produces a post-term newborn. Another term used to describe this late birth is *postmature infant*. Post-term newborns may be LGA, SGA, or dysmature (newborn weighs less than established normal parameters for estimated gestational age [fetal growth restriction]), depending on placental function. A postmature infant's appearance typically shows the effects of progressive placental insufficiency.

The reason why some pregnancies last longer than others is not completely understood. What is known is that women who experience one post-term pregnancy are at increased risk of doing so again in subsequent pregnancies. The incidence of prolonged pregnancy, beyond 42 weeks, is approximately 10% (Walker & Gan, 2015).

The ability of the placenta to provide adequate oxygen and nutrients to the fetus after 42 weeks' gestation is thought to be compromised, leading to perinatal mortality and morbidity. After 42 weeks, the placenta begins aging. Deposits of fibrin and calcium, along with hemorrhagic infarcts occur and the placental blood vessels begin to degenerate. All of these changes affect diffusion of oxygen to the fetus. As the placenta loses its ability to nourish the fetus, the fetus uses stored nutrients to stay alive, and wasting occurs. This wasted appearance at birth is secondary to the loss of muscle mass and subcutaneous fat. A recent study found that mortality risk in post-term infants was strongly related to fetal growth restriction, not gestational age (Morken, Klungsoyr, & Skjaerven, 2014).

Nursing Assessment

A thorough assessment of the post-term newborn upon admission to the nursery provides a baseline from which to identify changes in clinical status. Review the maternal history for any risk factors associated with post-term birth. Also be aware of the common physical characteristics and be able to identify any deviation from the expected. Post-term newborns typically exhibit the following characteristics:

- Dry, cracked, peeling, wrinkled skin
- Absence of vernix caseosa and lanugo

- Long, thin extremities
- Creases that cover the entire soles of the feet
- Wide-eyed, alert expression
- Abundant hair on scalp
- Thin umbilical cord
- Long fingernails
- Limited vernix and lanugo
- Meconium-stained skin and fingernails (Mattson & Smith, 2016)

Assess the newborn's gestational age and complete a physical examination to identify any abnormalities. Review the medical record to determine the color of the amniotic fluid when membranes ruptured and observe for a meconium-stained umbilical cord and fingernails to assess for possible meconium aspiration. Careful suctioning at the time of birth and afterward, if the condition dictates it, reduces the incidence of meconium aspiration. Also be alert for other typical complications associated with a post-term newborn, such as perinatal asphyxia (caused by placental aging or oligohydramnios [decreased amniotic fluid]), hypoglycemia (caused by acute episodes of hypoxia related to cord compression, which exhausts carbohydrate reserves), hypothermia (caused by loss of subcutaneous fat), and polycythemia (caused by an increased production of red blood cells to compensate for a reduced oxygen environment). Be prepared to initiate early interventions (see Table 23.1).

Nursing Management

The birth of a post-term newborn may create stress for the mother and her family. In most situations, birth of a newborn requiring special care was not anticipated. Post-term newborns are susceptible to several birth challenges secondary to placental dysfunction that place them at risk for asphyxia, hypoglycemia, and respiratory distress. The nurse must be vigilant for complications when managing these newborns.

The post-term newborn is at high risk for perinatal asphyxia, which is usually attributed to placental deprivation or oligohydramnios that leads to cord compression, thereby reducing perfusion to the fetus. Anticipating the need for newborn resuscitation is a priority. The newborn resuscitation team needs to be available in the birthing suite for immediate backup. The newborn may require transport to the NICU for continuous assessment, monitoring, and treatment, depending on his or her status after resuscitation.

Monitor and maintain the post-term newborn's blood glucose levels once stabilized. Intravenous dextrose 10% and/or early initiation of feedings will help stabilize the blood glucose levels to prevent central nervous system sequelae. Also monitor the post-term newborn's skin temperature, respiration characteristics, results of blood studies, such as ABGs and serum bilirubin levels,

and neurologic status. Institute measures to prevent or reduce the risk of hypothermia by eliminating sources of heat loss: thoroughly dry the newborn at birth, wrap him or her in a warmed blanket, and place a stockinette cap on the newborn's head. Providing environmental warmth via a radiant heat source will help stabilize the newborn's temperature.

Closely assess all post-term newborns for polycythemia, which contributes to hyperbilirubinemia due to red blood cell destruction. Providing adequate hydration helps to reduce the viscosity of the newborn's blood to prevent thrombosis. Be alert to the early, often subtle signs to promote early identification and prompt treatment to prevent any neurodevelopmental delays.

Consider This

I had been waiting for this baby since I can remember and now I was told to wait even longer. I was into my third week past my due date and was just told that if I didn't go into labor on my own, the doctor would induce me on Monday. As I walked out of his office into the hot summer sun, I thought about all the comments that would await me at the office: "You're not still pregnant, are you?" "Weren't you due last month?" "You look as big as a house." "Are you sure you aren't expecting triplets?" I started to get into my car when I felt warm fluid slide down my legs. Although I was embarrassed at my wetness, I was thrilled I wouldn't have to go back to the office and drove myself to the hospital. Within hours my wait was finally over with the birth of my son, a post-term infant with peeling skin and a thick head of hair. He was certainly worth the wait!

Thoughts: *Although most due dates are within plus or minus 2 weeks, we can't "go to the bank with it" because so many factors influence the start of labor. This woman was anxious about her overdue status, but nature prevailed. The old adage "when the fruit is ripe, it will fall" doesn't always bring a good outcome: many women need a little push to bring a healthy newborn forth. What happens when the fetus stays inside the uterus too long? What other features are typical of post-term infants?*

Dealing With Perinatal Loss

It is estimated that over 7 million perinatal losses occur globally each year. More than 1 million fetal deaths occur in the United States each year. Social determinants associated with perinatal loss include lack of education, poverty, overcrowded living conditions, poor sanitation, poor air quality, malnourishment, and war zones (Callister, 2014). Perinatal loss, defined as any pregnancy loss and/or neonatal death up to 1 month of age, continues to be a common occurrence although major advances have taken place in perinatal health care. The prevalence of perinatal death reflects a very real possibility that all nurses will meet and care for a woman who has experienced the death of a baby. Openness to expressions of grief, helping couples mobilize support, considering readiness for another pregnancy, and directing couples to useful Internet sites are essential nursing interventions (Callister, 2014).

Perinatal loss is a profound experience for the family. It engenders a unique kind of mourning since the infant is so much a part of the parents' identity. Instead of celebrating a new life as they expected, parents are mourning the loss of dreams and hopes and the loss of an extension of themselves. NICU nurses face a difficult situation when caring for newborns who may not survive. Newborn death is incomprehensible to most parents/partners/significant others. They are commonly offered time to see their infant, memory items, and support. This frequently makes the grieving process more difficult because what is happening "can't be real." Deciding whether to see, touch, or hold the dying newborn is extremely difficult for many parents/partners/ significant others. Nurses play a major role in assisting parents to make their dying newborn "real" to them by providing them with as many memories as possible and encouraging them to see, hold, touch, dress, and take care of the infant and take photographs. These actions help to validate the parents' sense of loss, relive the experience, and attach significance to the meaning of loss. A lock of hair, a name card, a photo, or an identification bracelet may serve as important mementoes that can ease the grieving process. The memories created by these interventions can be useful allies in the grieving process and in resolving grief (Jaffe, 2014).

A nurse's willingness to sit quietly and observe, to remain open and nonjudgmental, and to explore what might be helpful is a useful strategy to bridge cultural differences. Statements such as "Help me understand how your family cares for someone who is dying" or "What would be important for me to know about how best to care for your baby's body?" convey a nurse's willingness to learn what is most important to each family. Parents' answers may help guide nurses in providing culturally appropriate care for diverse populations. Nurses who are attentive to learning what is most important to parents, and subsequently work to incorporate such interventions into their care, foster relationships between parents and their infant (Robinson, 2014).

Parent–newborn interaction is vital to the normal processes of attachment and bonding. The detachment process involved in a newborn's death is equally important for parents. Nurses can aid in this process by helping parents to see their newborn through the maze of equipment, explaining the various procedures and equipment, encouraging them to express their feelings about the newborn's status, and providing time for them to be with their dying newborn (Randolph, Hruby, & Sharif, 2015).

A common reaction by many people when learning that a newborn is not going to survive is one of avoidance. Nurses are no exception. It is difficult to initiate a conversation about such a sensitive issue without knowing how the parents are going to react and cope with the impending loss. One way to begin a conversation with the parents is to convey concern and acknowledge their loss. Active listening can give parents a safe place to begin the healing process. The relationship that the nurse establishes with the parents is a unique one, providing an opportunity for both the nurse and the parents to share their feelings.

Be aware of personal feelings about loss and how these feelings are part of one's own life and personal belief system. Actively listen to the parents when they are talking about their experiences. Communicate empathy (understanding and feeling what another person is feeling), respect their feelings, and respond to them in helpful and supportive ways (Verklan & Walden, 2014). Table 23.2 highlights appropriate interventions for a family experiencing a perinatal loss before and after a newborn dies.

In a time of crisis or loss, individuals are often more sensitive to other people's reactions. For example, the parents may be extremely aware of the nurse's facial expressions, choice of words, and tone of voice. Talking quickly, in a businesslike fashion, or ignoring the loss may inhibit parents from discussing their pain or how they are coping with it. Parents may need to vent their frustrations and anger, and the nurse may become the target. Validate their feelings and attempt to reframe or refocus the anger toward the real issue of loss. An example would be to say, "I understand your frustration and anger about this situation. You have experienced a tremendous loss and it must be difficult not to have an explanation for it at this time." Doing so helps to defuse the anger while allowing them to express their feelings.

The death of an infant will more than likely be one of the toughest moments in a family's life. Giving families some sense of control in an otherwise hopeless situation can provide some comfort. Some ideas to provide them a sense of control include:

- Ask the family who they wish to have present as the infant dies.
- Give the family a choice of rooms in which they can say good-bye to their infant.
- Provide privacy for the family during this time period by placing a sign on the door.
- Provide ideas for making or selecting memorial items for a memory box.
- The family should never be left to handle their emotions alone unless they request it.
- Respect a family's wishes if they refuse to be with their infant during the dying process or afterward. Everyone grieves differently.

When assisting bereaved parents, start where the parents are in the grief process to avoid imposing your

TABLE 23.2	ASSISTING PARENTS TO COPE WITH PERINATAL LOSS
Before the newborn's death	Respect variations in the family's spiritual needs and readiness. Assess cultural beliefs and practices that may bring comfort; respect culturally appropriate requests for truth telling and informed refusal. Initiate spiritual comfort by calling the hospital clergy if appropriate; offer to pray with the family if appropriate. Encourage the parents to take photographs, make memory boxes, and record their thoughts in a journal. Explore with family members how they dealt with previous losses. Discuss techniques to reduce stress, such as meditation and relaxation. Recommend that family members maintain a healthy diet and get adequate rest and exercise to preserve their health. Participate in early and repeated care conferencing to reduce family stress. Allow family to be present at both medical rounds and resuscitation; provide explanations of all procedures, treatments, and findings; answer questions honestly and as completely as possible. Provide opportunities for the family to hold the newborn if they choose to. Assess the family's support network. Provide suggestions as to how friends can be helpful to the family.
After the newborn's death	Help the family to accept the reality of death by using the word "died." Acknowledge their grief and the fact that their newborn has died. Help the family to work through their grief by validating and listening. Provide the family with realistic information about the causes of death. Offer condolences to the family in a sincere manner. Encourage the father to cry and grieve with his partner. Provide opportunities for the family to hold the newborn if they desire.
At the time of the release of the newborn's body	Reassure the family that their feelings and grieving responses are normal. Encourage the parents to have a funeral or memorial service to bring closure. Suggest that the parents plant a tree or flowers to remember the infant. Address attachment issues concerning subsequent pregnancies. Provide information about local support groups. Provide anticipatory guidance regarding the grieving process. Present information about any impact on future childbearing, and refer the parents to appropriate specialists or genetic resources.

Adapted from Callister, L. C. (2014). Global perspectives on perinatal loss. *MCN: The American Journal of Maternal/Child Nursing*, *39*(3), 207; Chertok, I. R., McCrone, S., Parker, D., & Leslie, N. (2014). Review of interventions to reduce stress among mothers of infants in the NICU. *Advances in Neonatal Care*, *14*(1), 30–37; Jaffe, J. (2014). The reproductive story: Dealing with miscarriage, stillbirth, or other perinatal demise. In *Women's reproductive mental health across the lifespan* (pp. 159–176). Springer International Publishing; and Kissane, D. W., & Parnes, F. (Eds.). (2014). *Bereavement care for families*. New York, NY: Routledge.

own agenda on them. You may feel uncomfortable at not being able to change the situation or take the pain away. The nurse's role is to provide immediate emotional support and facilitate the grieving process. Supporting and strengthening the family bond in the face of perinatal loss is essential.

Comforting the family after the infant's death is vital to give them a sense of closure and start the healing process. Some things the nurse can do to help the family during this time include:

- Sending the family a card from the nursing staff, signed by all who worked with their infant within a week of leaving the hospital.
- Attending the funeral to allow for a public good-bye and to support others in their time of loss.
- Providing the family with a memory box, which might contain an outfit worn by their infant, a blanket used

to cover their infant, a lock of hair, and a card with hand and foot prints, a photo with someone holding their infant, etc.

- Remembering their infant at various anniversaries by sending a card or calling the family to see how they are doing.
- Donating to a charity such as March of Dimes in memory of the infant.
- Providing the family with resources that might help them. Information might include listings of local or online support groups as well as grief web sites such as Share.org.

Being present during this traumatic event for families is tough. Serving infants and their families by bearing witness to their pain and grief is a special privilege. Being present for the family with compassion, comfort, support, and resources during their time of loss is truly an honorable gesture. Nurses are remembered years later for their kindness and guidance of the family members through this adverse event with dignity (Green et al., 2015).

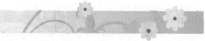

Take Note!

Infants born prematurely between 34 0/7 and 36 6/7 weeks are at higher risk for morbidity and mortality than those born before 28 weeks or after 37 weeks due to their physiologic and metabolic immunity (Boyle et al., 2015).

KEY CONCEPTS

- Variations in birth weight and gestational age can place a newborn at risk for problems that require special care.

- Variations in birth weight include the following categories: small for gestational age, appropriate for gestational age, and large for gestational age. Newborns who are small or large for gestational age have special needs.

- The SGA newborn faces problems related to a decrease in placental function in utero; these problems may include perinatal asphyxia, hypothermia, hypoglycemia, polycythemia, and meconium aspiration.

- Risk factors for the birth of a LGA infant include maternal diabetes mellitus or glucose intolerance, multiparity, prior history of a macrosomic infant, postdated gestation, maternal obesity, male fetus, and genetics. LGA newborns face problems such as birth trauma due to cephalopelvic disproportion, hypoglycemia, and jaundice secondary to hyperbilirubinemia.

- Variations in gestational age include post-term and preterm newborns. Post-term newborns may be large or small for gestational age or dysmature, depending on placental function.

- The post-term newborn may develop several complications after birth, including fetal hypoxia, hypoglycemia, hypothermia, polycythemia, and meconium aspiration.

- Preterm birth is the leading cause of death within the first month of life and the second leading cause of all infant deaths.

- The preterm newborn is at risk for complications because his or her organ systems are immature, thereby impeding the transition from intrauterine life to extrauterine life.

- Newborns can experience pain, but their pain is difficult to validate with consistent behaviors.

- Newborns with gestational age variations, primarily preterm newborns, benefit from developmental care, which includes a variety of activities designed to manage the environment and individualize the care based on behavioral observations.

- Nurses play a key role in assisting the parents and family of a newborn with special needs to cope with this crisis situation, including dealing with the possibility that the newborn may not survive. Nurses working with parents experiencing a perinatal loss can help by actively listening, understanding the parents' experiences, and communicating empathy.

- The goal of discharge planning is to make a successful transition to home care.

References and Recommended Readings

Alsafadi, T. R., Hashmi, S. M., Youssef, H. A., Suliman, A. K., Abbas, H. A. M. et al., (2014). Polycythemia in neonatal intensive care unit, risk factors, symptoms, pattern, and management controversy. *Journal of Clinical Neonatology, 3*(2), 93–100.

American Academy of Pediatrics [AAP] and American Heart Association [AHA]. (2014). Documentation of neonatal resuscitation. *23*(1), Retrieved from http://www2.aap.org/nrp/docs/IU/2014_SpringSummer_iu.pdf

Bakalis, S., Peeva, G., Gonzalez, R., Poon, L. C., & Nicolaides, K. H. (2015). Prediction of small-for-gestational-age neonates: Screening by biophysical and biochemical markers at 30–34 weeks. *Ultrasound in Obstetrics & Gynecology, 46*(4):446–451.

Baker, B. (2015). Evidence-based practice to improve outcomes for late preterm infants. *Journal of Obstetric, Gynecologic, & Neonatal Nursing, 44,* 127–134.

Bird, C. (2014). *Health concerns of the late preterm infant.* Retrieved from http://preemies.about.com/od/preemiehealthproblems/a/LatePretermBirth.htm

Boyle, E. M., Johnson, S., Manktelow, B., Seaton, S. E., Draper, E. S., Smith, L. K.,et al., (2015). Neonatal outcomes and delivery of care for infants born late preterm or moderately preterm: a prospective population-based study. *Archives of Disease in Childhood-Fetal and Neonatal Edition, 100*(6):F479–F485.

Callister, L. C. (2014). Global perspectives on perinatal loss. *MCN: The American Journal of Maternal/Child Nursing, 39*(3), 207.

Campbell-Yeo, M. L., Disher, T. C., Benoit, B. L., & Johnston, C. C. (2015) Understanding kangaroo care and its benefits to preterm infants. *Pediatric Health, Medicine, and Therapeutics, 6,* 15–32.

Cano Giménez, E., & Sánchez-Luna, M. (2015). Providing parents with individualised support in a neonatal intensive care unit reduced stress, anxiety and depression. *Acta Paediatrica, 104*(7), e300–e305.

Centers for Disease Control and Prevention [CDC]. (2015). *Birth weight and gestation – fast facts.* Retrieved from: http://www.cdc.gov/nchs/fastats/birthweight.htm

Chandran, S., Rajadurai, V. S., Haium, A., Alim, A., & Hussain, K. (2015). Current perspectives on neonatal hypoglycemia, its management, and cerebral injury risk. *Research & Reports in Neonatology, 5,* 17–30.

Chertok, I. R., McCrone, S., Parker, D., & Leslie, N. (2014). Review of interventions to reduce stress among mothers of infants in the NICU. *Advances in Neonatal Care, 14*(1), 30–37.

Creasy, R. K., Resnik, R., Iams, J. D., Lockwood, C. J., Moore, T., & Greene, M. F. (2014). *Creasy and Resnik's maternal-fetal medicine: Principles and practice* (7th ed.). St. Louis, MO: Saunders Elsevier.

Cunningham, F. G., Leveno, K. J., Bloom, S. L., Spong, C. Y., Dashe, J. S., Hoffman, B. L., et al. (2014). *Williams' obstetrics* (24th ed). New York, NY: McGraw-Hill.

Donnelley, E. L., Raynes-Greenow, C. H., Turner, R. M., Carberry, A. E., & Jeffery, H. E. (2014). Antenatal predictors and body composition of large-for-gestational-age newborns: perinatal health outcomes. *Journal of Perinatology, 34,* 698–704.

Embleton, N. D., Morgan, C., & King, C. (2015). Balancing the risks and benefits of parenteral nutrition for preterm infants: Can we define the optimal composition?. *Archives of Disease in Childhood-Fetal and Neonatal Edition, 100*(1), F72–F75.

Fanaroff, A. A., & Fanaroff, J. M. (2014). *Klaus and Fanaroff's care of the high-risk neonate* (6th ed.), Philadelphia, PA: Elsevier.

Gardner, S. L., Carter, B. S., Enzman-Hines, M., & Hernandez, J. A. (2016). *Merenstein & Gardner's handbook of neonatal intensive care* (8th ed.), St. Louis, MO: Elsevier.

Gray, L., Garza, E., Zageris, D., Heilman, K. J., & Porges, S. W. (2015). Sucrose and warmth for analgesia in healthy newborns: An RCT. *Pediatrics, 135*(3), e607–e614.

Green, J., Darbyshire, P., Adams, A., & Jackson, D. (2015). Desperately seeking parenthood: Neonatal nurses reflect on parental anguish. *Journal of Clinical Nursing, 24,* 1885–1894.

Hartnett, M. E. (2015). Pathophysiology and mechanisms of severe retinopathy of prematurity. *Ophthalmology, 122*(1), 200–210.

Hatfield, L. A., & Ely, E. A. (2014). Measurement of acute pain in infants: A review of behavioral and physiological variables. *Biological Research for Nursing,* 17(1):100-11.

Herrera-Marschitz, M., Neira-Peña, T., Leyton, L., Gebicke-Haerter, P., Rojas-Mancilla, E., Morales, P. et al., (2015). Short-and long-term consequences of perinatal asphyxia: Looking for neuroprotective strategies. In *Perinatal programming of neurodevelopment* (pp. 169–198). New York, NY: Springer Publishers.

Horgan, M. J. (2015). Management of the late preterm infant: Not quite ready for prime time. *Pediatric Clinics of North America, 62*(2), 439–451.

Jaffe, J. (2014). The reproductive story: Dealing with miscarriage, stillbirth, or other perinatal demise. In *Women's reproductive mental health across the lifespan* (pp. 159–176). Springer International Publishing.

Kaneko, M., Yamashita, R., Kai, K., Yamada, N., Sameshima, H., & Ikenoue, T. (2015). Perinatal morbidity and mortality for extremely low-birthweight infants: A population-based study of regionalized maternal and neonatal transport. *Journal of Obstetrics and Gynecology Research,* 41(7):1056–1066.

Kenner, C., & Lott, J. W. (2014). *Comprehensive neonatal care* (5th ed.). New York, NY: Springer Publishing Company.

Kenner, C., & Lott, J. W. (2015). *Comprehensive neonatal care* (5th ed.). New York, NY: Springer Publishing Company.

Kiechl-Kohlendorfer, U., Merkle, U., Deufert, D., Neubauer, V., Peglow, U. P., & Griesmaier, E. (2015). Effect of developmental care for very premature infants on neurodevelopmental outcome at 2 years of age. *Infant Behavior & Development, 39* 166–172.

Kissane, D. W., & Parnes, F. (Eds.). (2014). *Bereavement care for families.* New York, NY: Routledge.

Koletzko, B., Poindexter, B., & Uauy, R. (Eds.). (2014). *Nutritional care of preterm infants: Scientific basis and practical guidelines.* Basel, Switzerland: KargerMedical and Scientific Publishers.

Lee, G. Y., Yamada, J., Shorkey, A., & Stevens, B. (2014). Pediatric clinical practice guidelines for acute procedural pain: A systematic review. *Pediatrics, 133*(3), 500–515.

Lee, L. A., Carter, M., Stevenson, S. B., & Harrison, H. A. (2014). Improving family-centered care practices in the NICU. *Neonatal Network: The Journal of Neonatal Nursing, 33*(3), 125–132.

Lessaris, K. J., (2015). Polycythemia of the newborn. *eMedicine.* Retrieved from http://emedicine.medscape.com/article/976319-overview

Mahajan, R. C., Une, L., & Bansal, S. (2015). Study of clinical features and in newborn with polycythemi antenatal and natal factors. *MedPulse – International Medical Journal, 2*(2), 66–71.

March of Dimes. (2015a). *Preterm labor and birth.* Retrieved from http://www.marchofdimes.org/pregnancy/preterm-labor-and-birth.aspx

March of Dimes. (2015b). *The impact of premature birth on society.* Retrieved from http://www.marchofdimes.org/mission/the-economic-and-societal-costs.aspx

March of Dimes. (2015c). *Premature babies.* Retrieved from http://www.marchofdimes.org/baby/premature-babies.aspx

March of Dimes. (2015d). *Finding the causes of prematurity.* Retrieved from http://www.marchofdimes.org/research/finding-the-causes-of-prematurity.aspx

Mattson, S., & Smith, J. E. (2016). *Core curriculum for maternal-newborn nursing* (5th ed.). St. Louis, MO: Saunders Elsevier.

Mitanchez, D., Yzydorczyk, C., Siddeek, B., Boubred, F., Benahmed, M., & Simeoni, U. (2015). The offspring of the diabetic mother–short- and long-term implications. *Best Practice & Research Clinical Obstetrics & Gynecology, 29*(2), 256–269.

Morken, N. H., Klungsøyr, K., & Skjaerven, R. (2014). Perinatal mortality by gestational week and size at birth in singleton pregnancies at and beyond term: a nationwide population-based cohort study. *BMC Pregnancy and Childbirth, 14*(1), 172.

Nagtalon-Ramos, J. (2014) *Maternal-newborn nursing care: Best evidence-based practices.* Philadelphia, PA: F.A. Davis Company.

National Eye Institute. (2015). *Facts about retinopathy of prematurity (ROP).* Retrieved from http://www.nei.nih.gov/health/rop/rop.asp#2

Neonatal Handbook. (2015a). *Large for gestational age infants.* Retrieved from http://www.health.vic.gov.au/neonatalhandbook/

Neonatal Handbook. (2015b). *Polycythemia in neonates.* Retrieved from http://www.health.vic.gov.au/neonatalhandbook/conditions/polycythaemia.htm

Neonatal Handbook. (2015c). *Nutrition.* Retrieved from http://www.health.vic.gov.au/neonatalhandbook/nutrition/index.htm

Neonatal Handbook. (2015d). *Resuscitation of neonates.* Retrieved from http://www.health.vic.gov.au/neonatalhandbook/procedures/resuscitation.htm

Ohlin, A., Björkman, L., Serenius, F., Schollin, J., & Källén, K. (2015). Sepsis as a risk factor for neonatal morbidity in extremely preterm infants. *Acta Paediatrica.* doi: 10.1111/apa.13104

Oros, D., Altermir, I., Elia, N., Tuquet, H., Pablo, L. E., Fabre, E., et al., (2014). Pathways of neuronal and cognitive development in children born small-for-gestational age or late preterm. *Ultrasound in Obstetrics & Gynecology, 43*(1), 41–47.

Panda, U. (2015). *McGraw-Hill nurse's dictionary* (4th ed.). New Delhi, India: Jaypee.

Pappas, B. E., & Robey, D. L. (2014). 23 Care of the late preterm infant. *Core curriculum for neonatal intensive care nursing,* 439–446. St. Louis, MO: Saunders Elsevier.

Platt, M. J. (2014). Outcomes in preterm infants. *Public Health. 128*(5), 399–403.

Ramenghi, L. A. (2015). Late preterm babies and the risk of neurological damage. *Acta Bio Medica Atenei Parmensis, 86*(1S), 36–40.

Randolph, A. L., Hruby, B. T., and Sharif, S. (2015), Counseling women who have experienced pregnancy loss: A Review of the literature. *Adultspan Journal, 14,* 2–10.

Reavey, D. A., Haney, B. M., Atchison, L., Anderson, B., Sandritter, T., & Pallotto, E. K. (2014). Improving pain assessment in the NICU: A quality improvement project. *Advances in Neonatal Care, 14*(3), 144–153.

Robinson, G. E. (2014). Pregnancy loss. *Best Practice & Research Clinical Obstetrics & Gynecology, 28*(1), 169–178.

Rozance, P. J. (2014). Update on neonatal hypoglycemia. *Current Opinion in Endocrinology, Diabetes and Obesity, 21*(1), 45–50.

Sabic, D., Blattner, C., & Metts, M. (2014). Newborn and infant pain control. *Clinical Pediatrics* (Online June 24, 2014), doi: 0009922814540043.

Sabri, K. (2016). Global challenges in retinopathy of prematurity screening: Modern solutions for modern times. *Pediatrics.* 137(1). Retrieved from http://pediatrics.aappublications.org/content/early/2015/12/13/peds.2015-3914

Sacks, D. A., Black, M. H., Li, X., Montoro, M. N., & Lawrence, J. M. (2015). Adverse pregnancy outcomes using the International Association of the Diabetes and Pregnancy Study Group's criteria: Glycemic thresholds and associated risks. *Obstetrics & Gynecology, 126*(1), 67–73.

Salam, R. A., Mansoor, T., Mallick, D., Lassi, Z. S., Das, J. K., & Bhutta, Z. A. (2014). Essential childbirth and postnatal interventions for improved maternal and neonatal health. *Reproductive Health, 11* (Suppl 1), S3, 1–17.

Sayed, A. M., Youssef, M. M., Hassanein, F. E. S., & Mobarak, A. A. (2015). Impact of tactile stimulation on neurobehavioral development of premature infants in Assiut city. *Journal of Education and Practice, 6*(8), 93–101.

Stacey, S., Osborn, M., & Salkovskis, P. (2015). Life is a rollercoaster... What helps parents cope with the Neonatal Intensive Care Unit (NICU)?. *Journal of Neonatal Nursing, 21* (4), 136–141.

Treyvaud, K. (2014). Parent and family outcomes following very preterm or very low birth weight birth: A review. In *Seminars in fetal and neonatal medicine. 19*(2), 131–135): WB Saunders.

U.S. Department of Health and Human Services. (2010). *Healthy People2020*. Retrieved from http://www.healthypeople.gov/hp2020/Comments/default.asp

Valeri, B. O., Holsti, L., & Linhares, M. B. (2015). Neonatal pain and developmental outcomes in children born preterm: A systematic review. *The Clinical Journal of Pain, 31*(4), 355–362.

Vali, P., Mathew, B., & Lakshminrusimha, S. (2015). Neonatal resuscitation: Evolving strategies. *Maternal Health, Neonatology and Perinatology, 1*(1), 4–23.

Verklan, M. T., & Walden, M. (2014) *Core curriculum for neonatal intensive care nursing* (5th ed.). St. Louis, MO: Saunders Elsevier.

Vinall, J., & Grunau, R. E. (2014). Impact of repeated procedural pain-related stress in infants born very preterm. *Pediatric Research, 75*(5), 584–587.

Vitale, S. A., & Falco, C. (2014). Children born prematurely: Risk of parental chronic sorrow. *Journal of Pediatric Nursing, 29*(3), 248–251.

Walker, N., & Gan, J. H. (2015). Prolonged pregnancy. *Obstetrics, Gynecology & Reproductive Medicine, 25*(3), 83–87.

Westrup, B. (2014). Family-centered developmentally supportive care. *NeoReviews, 15*(8), e325–e335.

White-Traut, R. (2015), Nurse management of the NICU environment is critical to optimal infant development. *Journal of Obstetric, Gynecologic, & Neonatal Nursing, 44,* 169–170.

Wilson-Costello, D., & Payne, A. (2016). Long-term neurodevelopmental outcomes of preterm infants: Epidemiology and risk factors. *UpToDate.* Retrieved from: http://www.uptodate.com/contents/long-term-neurodevelopmental-outcome-of-preterm-infants-epidemiology-and-risk-factors

Yaman, S., & Altay, N. (2015). Posttraumatic stress and experiences of parents with a newborn in the neonatal intensive care unit. *Journal of Reproductive & Infant Psychology, 33*(2), 140–152.

Yousaf, U. F., Hayat, S., & Afzal, N. (2015). Resuscitation of newborns in high risk deliveries. *Journal of Ayub Medical College Abbottabad, 27*(2), 343–345.

MULTIPLE CHOICE QUESTIONS

1. The nurse documents that a newborn is post-term based on the understanding that he was born after:
   a. 38 weeks' gestation
   b. 40 weeks' gestation
   c. 42 weeks' gestation
   d. 44 weeks' gestation

2. SGA and LGA newborns have an excessive number of red blood cells because of:
   a. Hypoxia
   b. Hypoglycemia
   c. Hypocalcemia
   d. Hypothermia

3. Because subcutaneous and brown fat stores were used for survival in utero, the nurse would assess an SGA newborn for which of the following?
   a. Hyperbilirubinemia
   b. Hypothermia
   c. Polycythemia
   d. Hypoglycemia

4. In assessing a preterm newborn, which of the following findings would be of greatest concern?
   a. Milia over the bridge of the nose
   b. Thin transparent skin
   c. Poor muscle tone
   d. Heart murmur

5. In dealing with parents experiencing a perinatal loss, which of the following nursing interventions would be most appropriate?
   a. Sheltering the parents from the bad news
   b. Making all the decisions regarding care
   c. Encouraging them to participate in the newborn's care
   d. Leaving them by themselves to allow time to grieve

6. The nurse is providing care to several newborns with variations in gestational age and birth weight. When developing the plan of care for these newborns, the nurse focuses on energy conservation to promote growth and development. Which measures would the nurse include in the nursing plans of care? Select all that apply.
   a. Keeping the handling of the newborn to a minimum
   b. Maintaining a neutral thermal environment
   c. Decreasing environmental stimuli
   d. Initiating early oral feedings
   e. Using thermal warmers in all cribs
   f. Promoting kangaroo care by caretakers

7. Which of the following concepts would the nurse incorporate into the plan of care when assessing pain in a newborn with special needs?
   a. Newborns experience pain primarily with surgical procedures.
   b. Preterm newborns in the NICU are at the least risk for pain.
   c. Pain assessment needs to be comprehensive and frequent.
   d. A newborn's facial expression is the primary indicator of pain.

8. The term *evidence-based* refers to the use of which of the following to validate a nurse's practice interventions?
   a. Research findings
   b. Written guidelines
   c. Unit procedure manual
   d. Institutional policies

9. A preterm infant is placed under the radiant heat warmer after birth. The nurse evaluates the temperature frequently to prevent which of the following:
   a. Cold stress
   b. Respiratory depression
   c. Tachycardia
   d. Thermogenesis

10. Which of the following lab values need to be monitored by the nurse when providing care for a large for gestational age infant?
    a. White cell count
    b. Direct Coombs test
    c. Blood glucose
    d. Potassium level

CRITICAL THINKING EXERCISE

1. After fetal distress was noted on the monitor, a post-term newborn was delivered via a difficult vacuum extraction. The newborn had low Apgar scores and had to be resuscitated before being transferred to the nursery. Once admitted, the nurse observed the following behaviors: jitteriness, tremors, hypotonia, lethargy, and rapid respirations.
   a. What might these behaviors indicate?
   b. For what other conditions might this newborn be at high risk?
   c. What intervention is needed to address this newborn's condition?

2. A preterm newborn was born at 35 weeks following an abruptio placentae due to a car accident. He was transported to the NICU at a nearby regional medical center. After being stabilized, he was placed in an isolette close to the door and placed on a cardiac monitor. A short time later, the nurse notices that he is cool to the touch and lethargic, has a weak cry, and has an axillary temperature of 36° C.
   a. What might have contributed to this newborn's hypothermic condition?
   b. What transfer mechanism may have been a factor?
   c. What intervention would be appropriate for the nurse to initiate?

3. A term SGA newborn weighing 4 lb was brought to the nursery for admission a short time after birth. The labor and birth nurse reports the mother was a heavy smoker, a cocaine addict, and experienced physical abuse throughout her pregnancy. After stabilizing the newborn and correcting the hypoglycemia with oral feedings, the nurse observes the following: acrocyanosis, ruddy color, poor circulation to the extremities, tachypnea, and irritability
   a. What complication might this SGA newborn be manifesting?
   b. What factors may have contributed to this complication?
   c. What would be an appropriate intervention for managing this condition?

STUDY ACTIVITIES

1. At a community health department maternity clinic, secure permission to interview the parents of a special needs child. Ask about their feelings throughout the experience. How are they managing and coping now?

2. Visit the March of Dimes web site and review this group's national campaign to reduce the incidence of prematurity. Are their strategies workable or not? Explain your reasoning.

3. A common metabolic disorder present in both SGA and LGA newborns after birth is _____.

4. A 10-lb LGA newborn is brought to the nursery after a difficult vaginal birth. The nursery nurse should focus on detecting birth injuries such as _____.

BRINGING IT ALL TOGETHER: CASE STUDY

A pregnant woman drops in to the local hospital emergency room in labor. She has been inconsistent in attending her prenatal clinic appointments and is not sure of the date of her last menstrual period. She admits to smoking a pack of cigarettes per day, but states she has cut back from a two-pack a day habit prior to this pregnancy. Her membranes rupture for meconium stained fluid and she gives birth to a female infant weighing 2,200 g with low Apgar scores, who is taken to the nursery for observation.

ASSESSMENT

Upon admission to the nursery, the nurse observes the following: loose, wrinkled, peeling dry skin, long, thin extremities, small amounts of vernix caseosa and lanugo, and long green finger nails. When plotted on a weight for gestational age chart, the infant falls below the 10th percentile. A physical examination was done to identify any abnormalities.

Go to the Point **to find questions to consider about this case.**

24

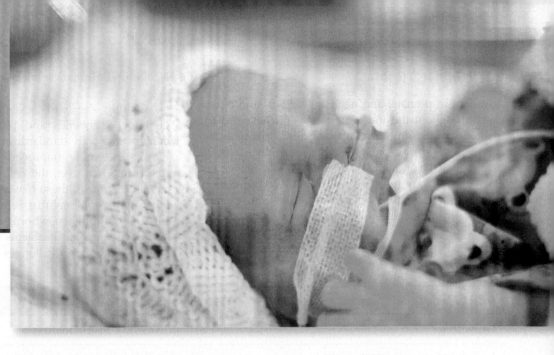

Nursing Management of the Newborn at Risk: Acquired and Congenital Newborn Conditions

Learning Objectives

Upon completion of the chapter, you will be able to:

1. Describe the most common acquired conditions affecting the newborn.
2. Construct the nursing management of a newborn experiencing respiratory distress syndrome.
3. Outline the birthing room preparation and procedures necessary to prevent meconium aspiration syndrome in the newborn at birth.
4. Devise parent education for the follow-up care needed by newborns with retinopathy of prematurity (ROP).
5. Select risk factors for the development of necrotizing enterocolitis.
6. Examine the impact of maternal diabetes on the newborn and the care needed.
7. Research the assessment and interventions for a newborn experiencing substance withdrawal after birth.
8. Outline the assessment and nursing management needed for newborns sustaining birth trauma.
9. Plan the assessment, interventions, prevention, and management of hyperbilirubinemia in newborns.
10. Summarize the interventions appropriate for a newborn with neonatal sepsis.
11. Compare and contrast the four classifications of congenital heart disease.
12. Evaluate the major acquired congenital anomalies affecting the central nervous system, respiratory system, gastrointestinal system, genitourinary system, and musculoskeletal system that can occur in a newborn.
13. Distinguish between three inborn errors of metabolism.
14. Formulate a plan of care for a newborn with an acquired or congenital condition.
15. Characterize the importance of parental participation in care of the newborn with an acquired or congenital condition, including the nurse's role in facilitating parental involvement.

WOW

Kelly, a 27-year-old G2P1, comes to the labor and birth area in active labor. She tells you she is overdue and relieved to finally be giving birth. Her membranes rupture on admission, revealing meconium-stained fluid. What additional nursing assessments need to be carried out now? What risk factors need to be considered when developing Kelly's plan of care?

Words of Wisdom
Courage and faith in oneself project onto others, giving them the strength to persevere.

INTRODUCTION

Advances in prenatal and neonatal medical and nursing care throughout the industrialized world have led to a marked increase in the number of newborns who have survived a high-risk pregnancy but experience acquired or congenital conditions. These newborns are considered one of our most vulnerable at-risk populations; that is, they are susceptible to morbidity and mortality because of the acquired or congenital disorder. Several national health goals address the issues of acquired and congenital conditions in newborns (U.S. Department of Health and Human Services, 2010). See *Healthy People 2020* 24.1.

During the past several decades, technological, genomic discoveries and pharmacologic advances, in conjunction with standardized policies and procedures have significantly improved survival rates for at-risk newborns. However, the risk of morbidity remains. For example, some of these newborns are at risk for continuing health problems that require long-term technological support. Other newborns remain at risk for physical and developmental problems into the school years and beyond. Although challenges remain in application of

---

HEALTHY PEOPLE *2020* • *24.1*

Objective	Nursing Significance
1. Reduce fetal and infant deaths: Decrease the number of all infant deaths (within 1 year) from a baseline of 6.2/1,000 live births to 5.6/1,000 live births (a 10% improvement). Decrease the number of neonatal deaths (within the first 28 days of life) from a baseline of 4.5 to 4.1 deaths/1,000 live births (a 10% improvement). Decrease the number of postneonatal deaths from a baseline of 2.2 to 2.0 deaths/1,000 live births (a 10% improvement). Reduce the number of deaths related to all birth defects from a baseline of 1.4 to 1.3 deaths/1,000 live births (a 10% improvement).	• Will foster early and consistent prenatal care, including education to place infants on their backs for naps and sleeping to prevent SIDS and avoidance of exposing the newborn to cigarette smoke.
2. Reduce the occurrence of developmental disabilities: Reduce the number of children with cerebral palsy who were born as low-weight infants (<2,500 g) from 50% to 45%. Reduce the number of children with autism spectrum disorder.	• Will promote measures for close antepartal and intrapartal monitoring of women at risk, subsequently reducing the incidence of disabilities, leading to a reduction in long-term effects and costs of care.
3. Reduce the occurrence of spina bifida and other neural tube defects: Reduce the number of new cases of spina bifida or other neural tube defects from a baseline of 34.2 to 30.8 new cases/100,000 live births.	• Will help to increase awareness of the need for all women of childbearing age to take a multivitamin containing at least 400 mg of folic acid and consume foods high in folic acid.
4. Reduce the occurrence of fetal alcohol syndrome. No target goal set for 2020.	• Will foster programs for at-risk groups, including adolescents, about the effects of substance abuse, especially alcohol, during pregnancy.
5. Ensure appropriate newborn blood spot screening, follow-up testing, and referral to services: Ensure all newborns are screened at birth for conditions as mandated by their state-sponsored newborn screening programs. Ensure that follow-up diagnostic testing for screening positives is performed within an appropriate time period. Ensure that infants with diagnosed disorders are enrolled in appropriate service interventions within an appropriate time period.	• Will help in the development of protocols and procedures to ensure appropriate screening and follow-up for all newborns.

Healthy People objectives based on data from http://www.healthypeople.gov.

these advances to improve the newborn's health, the high-risk newborn will increasingly benefit from them in the future. Providing the complex care needed to maintain the child's health and well-being will have a tremendous emotional and economic impact on the family. Nurses are challenged to provide support to mothers and their families when neonatal well-being is threatened.

Acquired disorders typically occur at or soon after birth. They may result from problems or conditions experienced by the woman during her pregnancy or at birth, such as diabetes, maternal infection, or substance abuse or conditions associated with labor and birth, such as prolonged rupture of membranes or fetal distress. However, there may be no identifiable cause for the disorder.

Congenital disorders can be defined as structural or functional or metabolic abnormalities which are present at birth. According to the World Health Organization (WHO), an estimated 1 in 33 infants or over 3 million fetuses and infants globally are born each year with major congenital disorders. They are found in approximately 3% of all newborns. The most common serious congenital disorders are congenital heart defects, neural tube defects (NTDs), and Down syndrome (WHO, 2015a). Congenital disorders, which typically involve a problem with inheritance, include structural anomalies (commonly referred to as birth defects), chromosomal disorders, and inborn errors of metabolism. Most congenital disorders have a complex etiology, involving many interacting genes, gene products, and social and environmental factors during organogenesis (the origin and development of organs). Some alterations can be prevented or compensated for with pharmacologic, nutritional, or other types of interventions, while others cannot be changed. The field of genomics and genetic medicine has witnessed an explosion of new knowledge, much of it learned from the Human Genome Project. Advances in understanding of the genetic basis of development and function, as well as the interaction of genes and the environment, continue to foster new insights into human health. Only through increased insight into the complex interplay of genetic, environmental, social, and cultural factors can these devastating and life-changing outcomes be prevented (Francine, Pascale, & Aline, 2014).

This chapter addresses selected acquired and congenital newborn conditions. In addition, it describes the nurse's role in assessment and management, emphasizing parental education and support. Nurses play a key role in helping the parents cope with the stress of having an ill newborn.

ACQUIRED DISORDERS

Congenital disorders are passed genetically from a parent to their offspring. These disorders are attained prior to birth. Acquired disorders are not passed genetically or caused by hereditary or developmental factors; they are obtained after birth, by a reaction to environmental influences outside of the body. A few examples might include respiratory distress syndrome (RDS), retinopathy of prematurity (ROP), birth trauma, hyperbilirubinemia, and newborn infections.

Perinatal Asphyxia

At birth, the lungs of newborns are filled with fluid. This fluid must be cleared and replaced with air after birth. As the newborn makes the transition to life outside the fluid-filled intrauterine environment, dramatic changes must occur to facilitate newborn respirations.

Perinatal asphyxia occurs when pulmonary oxygenation is delayed or interrupted. This insult can lead to death if not reestablished. Perinatal asphyxia interferes with newborn development, resulting in long-term deficits associated with mental and neurologic conditions with delayed onsets (Herrera-Marschitz et al., 2014).

Asphyxia is the most common clinical insult in the perinatal period. As many as 10% of newborns require some degree of active resuscitation to stimulate their breathing at birth (Cunningham et al., 2014). According to the World Health Organization (WHO, 2015b), up to 10 million cases of neonatal asphyxia occur annually worldwide, accounting for approximately 24% of all newborn deaths. More than a million newborns who survive asphyxia at birth develop long-term problems such as cerebral palsy, intellectual disability, and speaking, hearing, visual, and learning disabilities (WHO, 2015b).

Pathophysiology

Physiologically, asphyxia can be defined as impaired gas exchange resulting in a decrease in blood oxygen levels (hypoxemia) and an excess of carbon dioxide (hypercarbia) or hypercapnia that leads to metabolic acidosis. Any condition that reduces oxygen delivery to the fetus can result in asphyxia. These conditions may include maternal hypoxia, such as from cardiac or respiratory disease, anemia, or postural hypotension; maternal vascular disease that leads to placental insufficiency, such as diabetes or hypertension; cord problems such as compression or prolapse; and post-term pregnancies, which may trigger meconium release into the amniotic fluid.

Initially, the newborn uses compensatory mechanisms including tachycardia and vasoconstriction to help bring oxygen to the vital organs for a time. However, without intervention, these mechanisms fail, leading to hypotension, bradycardia, and eventually cardiopulmonary arrest.

With failure to breathe well after birth, the newborn will develop hypoxia (too little oxygen in the cells of the body). As a result, the heart rate falls, cyanosis develops, and the newborn becomes hypotonic and unresponsive. Newborn resuscitation is needed to help initiate breathing in newborns who fail to breathe spontaneously at birth.

Think back to Kelly, described at the beginning of the chapter. She gives birth to a son weighing approximately 2,500 g; he appears post-term and small for gestational age. His skin is stained yellow-green and he is limp, cyanotic, and apneic at birth. The initial assessment once the newborn is under the radiant warmer indicates that resuscitation and tracheal suctioning are needed. What is the nurse's role during resuscitation? What assessments will be needed during this procedure?

Nursing Assessment

The key to successful treatment of newborn asphyxia is early identification and recognition of newborns who may be at risk. Review the perinatal history for risk factors, including:

- *Trauma*: injury to the central or peripheral nervous system secondary to a long or difficult labor, a precipitous birth, multiple gestation, abnormal presentation, cephalopelvic disproportion, shoulder dystocia, or extraction by forceps or vacuum.
- *Intrauterine asphyxia*: for example, fetal hypoxia secondary to maternal hypoxia, diabetes, hypertension, anemia, cord compression, fetal bradycardia, or meconium aspiration.
- *Sepsis*: acquired bacterial or viral organisms from infected amniotic fluid, maternal infection, or direct contact while passing through the birth canal.
- *Malformation*: congenital anomalies including facial or upper airway deformities, renal anomalies, pulmonary hypoplasia, neuromuscular disorders, esophageal atresia, or NTDs.
- *Hypovolemic shock*: secondary to abruptio placentae, placenta previa, or cord rupture resulting in blood loss to the fetus.
- *Medication*: drugs given to mother during labor that can affect the fetus by causing placental hypoperfusion and hypotension; use of hypnotics, analgesics, anesthetics, narcotics administered to the mother within 4 hours of birth, oxytocin, and street drugs during pregnancy.

At birth, assess the newborn immediately. Observe the infant's color, noting any pallor or cyanosis. Assess the work of breathing. Be alert for apnea, tachypnea, gasping respirations, grunting, nasal flaring, or retractions. Evaluate heart rate and note bradycardia. Assess the newborn's temperature, noting hypothermia. Based on the initial assessment if poor, begin resuscitation measures until the Apgar score is above 7.

Anticipate diagnostic testing to identify etiologies for the newborn's asphyxia. For example, a chest x-ray may identify structural abnormalities that might interfere with respiration. A blood culture may identify an infectious process. A blood toxicology screen may detect any maternal drugs in the newborn. Severe fetal and neonatal asphyxia impair the physiologic transitions to extrauterine life (Verklan & Walden, 2014).

Nursing Management

Management of the newborn experiencing asphyxia includes immediate resuscitation. Ensure that the equipment needed for resuscitation is readily available and in working order. Essential equipment includes:

- wall suction apparatus
- oxygen source
- newborn ventilation bag
- infant warmer
- surgical blue towels
- endotracheal tubes (2 to 3 mm)
- laryngoscope
- ampules of naloxone (Narcan) with syringes and needles for administration.

Effective ventilation is the key to successful newborn resuscitation. Ventilation is frequently initiated with a manual resuscitation bag and face mask followed by endotracheal intubation if respiratory depression continues. (See Chapter 23 for a more detailed discussion of resuscitation.)

Dry the newborn quickly with a warm towel and then place him or her under a radiant heater to prevent rapid heat loss through evaporation. Handling and rubbing the newborn with a dry towel may be all that is needed to stimulate breathing. If the newborn fails to respond to stimulation, then active resuscitation is needed.

The procedure for newborn resuscitation is easily remembered by the ABCDs—**a**irway, **b**reathing, **c**irculation, and **d**rugs (see Chapter 23, Box 23.3). Continue resuscitation until the newborn has a pulse above 100 bpm, a good (healthy) cry, or good breathing efforts and a pink tongue. This last sign indicates a good oxygen supply to the brain (Jaques & Kennea, 2015).

Take Note!

According to the American Heart Association (AHA) and American Academy of Pediatrics (AAP) Guidelines for Neonatal Resuscitation, resuscitation efforts may be stopped if the newborn exhibits no heartbeat and no respiratory effort after 10 minutes of continuous and adequate resuscitation (AHA & AAP, 2014).

Provide continued observation and assessment of the newborn who has been successfully resuscitated. Monitor the newborn's vital signs and oxygen saturation levels closely for changes. Maintain a neutral thermal environment to prevent hypothermia, which would increase the newborn's metabolic and oxygen demands. Check the blood glucose level and observe for signs of hypoglycemia; if this develops, it can further stress the newborn.

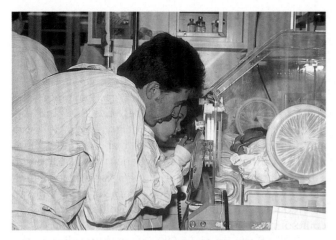

FIGURE 24.1 A father and sibling interacting with their newborn once the newborn's condition has stabilized.

The need for resuscitative measures can be extremely upsetting for the parents. Explain to them the initial resuscitation activities being performed and offer ongoing explanations about any procedures being done, equipment being used, or medications given. Provide physical and emotional support to the parents through the initial crisis and throughout the newborn's stay. When the newborn is stable, allow family to spend time with their newborn to promote bonding (Fig. 24.1). Point out the newborn's positive attributes (color, activity level, healthy cry) and give frequent updates on his or her status. Role-model techniques for holding, interacting with, and caring for the newborn to decrease the parents' anxiety post-resuscitation.

Remember Kelly, the young woman described at the beginning of the chapter? Her son is intubated and tracheal suctioning is performed. Positive-pressure ventilation is also started with a self-inflating bag and 50% oxygen. Ventilation is continued for 1 minute and then gradually discontinued. The heart rate is now 120 bpm, and spontaneous respirations are noted. When free-flow oxygen is administered, the newborn begins to cry and turn pink. What continued care is needed in the special care nursery? What explanation should be offered to Kelly regarding her son's treatment?

Transient Tachypnea of the Newborn

Transient tachypnea of the newborn (TTN) is a self-limiting condition involving a mild degree of respiratory distress. TTN is the result of a delay in clearance of fetal lung liquid. In the past, respiratory distress was thought to be a problem of relative surfactant deficiency, but is now characterized by an airspace-fluid burden secondary to the inability to absorb fetal lung liquid. It usually occurs within a few hours of birth and resolves over a 48- to 72-hour period. It occurs in approximately 1% of live births and incidence is higher in males than females (Subramanian et al., 2015). Although TTN is thought to be benign at birth, there is increasing data to link it to a newborn's risk to developing a wheezing syndrome early in life (Johnson, 2015).

Pathophysiology

Most newborns make the transition from fetal to newborn life without incident. During fetal life, the lungs are filled with a serous fluid because the placenta, not the lungs, is used for nutrient and gas exchange. During and after birth, this fluid must be removed and replaced with air. An infant born by cesarean birth is at risk of having excessive pulmonary fluid as a result of not having experienced all of the stages of labor. Passage through the birth canal during a vaginal birth compresses the thorax, which helps remove the majority of this fluid. Surgical births bypass the lessening of lung fluid for the newborn and place them at increased risk of TTN. Pulmonary circulation and the lymphatic drainage remove the remaining fluid shortly after birth. TTN occurs when the liquid in the lung is removed slowly or incompletely. The excess lung fluid results in decreased pulmonary compliance. Tachypnea develops to compensate for the increased workload of breathing associated with reduced compliance.

Nursing Assessment

Astutely observe the newborn with respiratory distress because TTN is a diagnosis of exclusion. Initially it might be difficult to distinguish this condition from RDS or group B streptococcal pneumonia, because the clinical picture is similar. However, the symptoms of transient tachypnea rarely last more than 72 hours. If symptoms progress beyond 72 hours, further investigation into another cause should be considered (Kim, Yang, & Kim, 2015).

HEALTH HISTORY AND PHYSICAL EXAMINATION

Review the perinatal history for contributing factors. TTN is commonly seen in newborns whose mothers have been heavily sedated in labor or have been born via cesarean birth. Also check the history for evidence of a prolonged labor, fetal macrosomia, inadequate initial resuscitation, breech births, when labor and birth are rapid, infants experiencing hypothermia, infants born before 38 weeks' gestation, infants born to a mother with diabetes, and maternal asthma and smoking. These factors are associated with a higher incidence of TTN.

Closely assess the newborn for signs of TTN. Within the first few hours of birth, observe for tachypnea, expiratory grunting, mild intercostal retractions, decreased breath sounds due to reduced air entry, labored breathing, nasal flaring, crackles on auscultation, and mild cyanosis. Mild to moderate respiratory distress is present by 6 hours of age, with respiratory rates as high as 100 to 140 breaths per minute (Lee, 2015). Also inspect the newborn's chest for hyperextension or a barrel shape. Auscultate breath sounds, which may be slightly diminished secondary to reduced air entry.

LABORATORY AND DIAGNOSTIC TESTING

To aid in the diagnosis, a chest x-ray may be done. It usually reveals mild symmetric lung hyperaeration and prominent perihilar interstitial markings and streaking. These findings correlate with lymphatic engorgement of retained fetal fluid. In addition, an arterial blood gas (ABG) assessment is important to ascertain the degree of gas exchange and acid–base balance. It typically demonstrates mild hypoxemia, mildly elevated CO_2 level, and a normal pH (Subramanian et al., 2015).

Nursing Management

Management of TTN is supportive. As the retained lung fluid is absorbed by the infant's lymphatic system, the pulmonary status improves. Nursing management focuses on providing adequate oxygenation and determining whether the newborn's respiratory manifestations appear to be resolving or persisting. Provide supportive care while the retained lung fluid is reabsorbed. Administer intravenous fluids and/or gavage feedings until the respiratory rate decreases enough to allow safe oral feeding. Withhold oral feedings until the respiratory status has improved. Provide supplemental oxygen via a nasal cannula or oxygen hood to maintain adequate oxygen saturation. Maintain a neutral thermal environment with minimal stimulation to minimize oxygen demand.

Provide ongoing assessment of the newborn's respiratory status. As TTN resolves, the newborn's respiratory rate declines to 60 breaths per minute or less, cyanosis resolves as do the nasal flaring and grunting sounds, the oxygen requirement decreases, the ABG values return to the normal range, bilateral breath sounds demonstrate good air entry, and the chest x-ray shows resolution of the perihilar streaking. Provide reassurance and progress reports to the parents to help them cope with this crisis.

Respiratory Distress Syndrome

Despite improved survival rates and advances in perinatal care, many high-risk newborns are at risk for respiratory problems, particularly **respiratory distress syndrome (RDS)**, a breathing disorder resulting from lung immaturity and lack of alveolar surfactant, which keeps the air sacs in the lungs from collapsing and allows them to inflate easily. Without surfactant, the alveoli collapse at the end of expiration. RDS is characterized by compromised lung expansion, poor gas exchange, and ventilator failure. Since the link between RDS and surfactant deficiency was discovered more than 30 years ago, tremendous strides have been made in understanding the pathophysiology and treatment of this disorder. The introduction of prenatal steroids to accelerate lung maturity and the development of synthetic surfactant can be credited with the dramatic improvements in the outcome of newborns with RDS.

RDS affects up to 25,000 infants born alive in the United States annually. The incidence declines with degree of maturity at birth. It occurs in 50% of preterm newborns of less than 28 weeks' gestation, 30% of those born at 28 to 34 weeks, and less than 5% of those born after 34 weeks. Intensive respiratory care, usually with mechanical ventilation, may be necessary.

Pathophysiology

Lung immaturity and surfactant deficiency contribute to the development of RDS. Surfactant is a complex mixture of phospholipids and proteins that adheres to the alveolar surface of the lungs. Anatomically, the immature lung cannot support oxygenation and ventilation because the alveolar sacs are insufficiently developed, causing a deficient surface area for gas exchange. Physiologically, the amount of surfactant is insufficient to prevent collapse of unstable alveoli. Surfactant forms a coating over the inner surface of the alveoli, reducing the surface tension and preventing alveolar collapse at the end of expiration. In the affected newborn, surfactant is deficient or lacking, and this deficit results in stiff lungs and alveoli that tend to collapse, leading to diffuse atelectasis (Fig. 24.2).

The work of breathing is increased because increased pressure similar to that required to initiate the first breath is needed to inflate the lungs with each successive breath. Hypoxemia and acidemia result, leading to vasoconstriction of the pulmonary vasculature. Right-to-left shunting occurs and alveolar capillary circulation is limited, further inhibiting surfactant production. As the disease progresses, fluid and fibrin leak from the pulmonary capillaries, causing hyaline membranes to form in the bronchioles, alveolar ducts, and alveoli. Hyaline membranes produce a glassy appearance in the lung membranes which is seen on x-rays. These membranes further decrease gas exchange. These factors decrease the total surface area of the gas exchange membrane. The end result is hypoxemia, academia, and worsening respiratory distress. A vicious circle is created, compounding the problem (Moses, 2015).

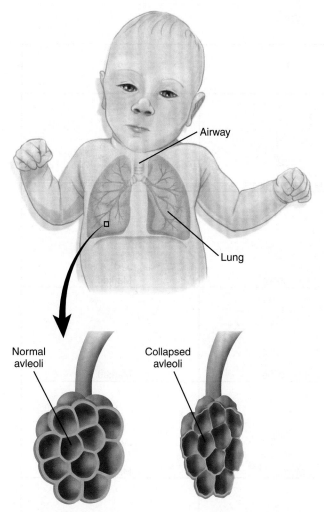

FIGURE 24.2 Pathophysiology of neonatal respiratory distress syndrome. Comparison of normal and collapsed alveoli.

Nursing Assessment

Nursing assessment focuses on keen observation to identify the signs and symptoms of respiratory distress. In addition, assessment aids in differentiating RDS from other respiratory conditions, such as TTN or group B streptococcal pneumonia.

HEALTH HISTORY AND PHYSICAL EXAMINATION

Review the history for risk factors associated with RDS. These include a preterm birth, perinatal asphyxia regardless of gestational age, neonatal sepsis, previous birth of an infant with RDS, cesarean birth in the absence of preceding labor (due to the lack of thoracic squeezing), male gender, perinatal asphyxia, cold stress, and maternal diabetes (produces high levels of insulin which inhibit surfactant production). It is believed that each of these conditions has an impact on surfactant production, thus resulting in RDS in the term infant (Saker & Martin, 2015).

> **Take Note!**
> Prolonged rupture of membranes, fetal growth restriction, gestational hypertension, maternal heroin addiction, and use of prenatal corticosteroids reduce the newborn's risk for RDS because of the physiologic stress imposed on the fetus. Chronic stress experienced by the fetus in utero accelerates the production of surfactant before the 35th week of gestation and, thus, reduces the incidence of RDS at birth.

The newborn with RDS usually demonstrates signs at birth or within a few hours of birth. Observe the infant for expiratory grunting, shallow breathing, nasal flaring, chest wall retractions (Fig. 24.3), see-saw respirations, and generalized cyanosis. Auscultate the heart and lungs, noting tachycardia (rates above 150 to 180), fine inspiratory crackles, and tachypnea (rates above 60 breaths per minute). Use the Silverman–Anderson index assessment tool to determine the degree of respiratory distress. The index involves observation of five features, each of which is scored as 0, 1, or 2 (Fig. 24.4). The higher the score, the greater the respiratory distress. A score over 7 suggests severe respiratory distress.

LABORATORY AND DIAGNOSTIC TESTING

The diagnosis of RDS is based on the clinical picture, a lung ultrasound or x-ray and ABGs which show hypoxemia and acidosis. A chest x-ray reveals hypoaeration, underexpansion, and a "ground-glass" pattern. Other lab tests are done to rule out infection and sepsis as a cause of the respiratory distress (Pramanik, Rangaswamy, & Gates, 2015).

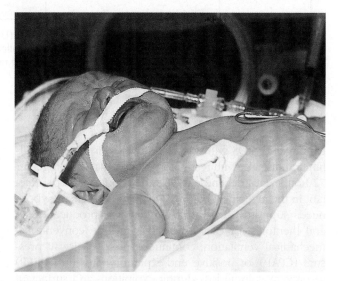

FIGURE 24.3 Sternal retractions are a sign of respiratory distress requiring immediate intervention, such as mechanical ventilation and other monitoring devices. (Copyright Caroline Brown, RNC, MS, DEd.)

Score

Feature observed	0	1	2
Chest movement	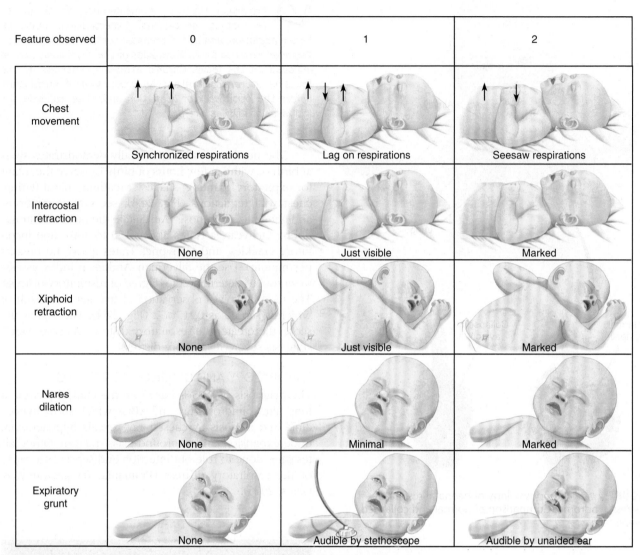Synchronized respirations	Lag on respirations	Seesaw respirations
Intercostal retraction	None	Just visible	Marked
Xiphoid retraction	None	Just visible	Marked
Nares dilation	None	Minimal	Marked
Expiratory grunt	None	Audible by stethoscope	Audible by unaided ear

FIGURE 24.4 Assessing the degree of respiratory distress. (Used with permission from Silverman, W. A., & Anderson, D. H. [1956]. A controlled clinical trial of effects of water mist on obstructive respiratory signs, death rate, and necroscopy findings among premature infants. *Pediatrics, 17*[4], 1–9.)

Nursing Management

If untreated, RDS will worsen. However, it can be a self-limiting disease, with respiratory symptoms declining after 72 hours. This decline parallels the production of surfactant in the alveoli (Rubarth & Quinn, 2015). The newborn needs supportive care until surfactant is produced. Several therapies for established RDS include conventional mechanical ventilation, continuous positive airway pressure (CPAP), or positive end-expiratory pressure (PEEP) to prevent volume loss during expiration, and surfactant therapy. The use of exogenous surfactant replacement therapy to stabilize the newborn's lungs until postnatal surfactant synthesis matures has become a standard of care, but is not necessarily evidence based. Knowledge of the surfactant proteins and lipids produced by the epithelial II cells was critical in the development of surfactant replacement preparations used to treat RDS, which enabled widespread use of these preparations used to prevent and treat RDS. This preparation has dramatically improved morbidity and mortality in preterm infants (Eibisberger, Resch, & Resch, 2015; Whitsett, Wert, & Weaver, 2015).

Despite recent advances in the perinatal management of neonatal RDS, controversies still exist. Strong evidence exists for the role of a single course of prenatal steroids in RDS prevention, but the potential benefit and long-term safety of repeated courses are unclear. A Cochrane review concluded that the incidence of RDS was reduced in infants born before 48 hours and between one and seven days of treatment of mothers with antenatal corticosteroids, but not those born <24 hours of administration (Gaur et al., 2015). Many practices involved in preterm neonatal stabilization at birth are not evidence based, including oxygen administration and positive-pressure lung inflation, and they may at times be harmful. Surfactant replacement therapy is crucial in the management of RDS, but the best preparation, optimal dose, and timing of administration at different gestations are not always clear. Respiratory support in the form of mechanical ventilation may also be lifesaving, but can cause lung injury, and protocols should be directed at avoiding mechanical ventilation where possible by using nasal CPAP or nasal ventilation. For newborns with RDS to experience the best outcomes, it is essential that they have optimal supportive care, including maintenance of a normal body temperature, proper fluid management, good nutritional support, and support of the circulation to maintain adequate tissue perfusion (Gardner et al., 2016).

As recommended, care of the newborn with RDS is primarily supportive and requires a multidisciplinary approach to obtain the best outcomes. Therapy focuses on improving oxygenation and maintaining optimal lung volumes. Expect to transfer the newborn to the neonatal intensive care unit (NICU) soon after birth. Apply the basic principles of newborn care, such as thermoregulation, cardiovascular and nutritional support, normal glucose level maintenance, and infection prevention, to achieve the therapeutic goals of reducing mortality and minimizing lung trauma.

Anticipate the administration of surfactant replacement therapy, prophylactically or as a rescue approach. With prophylactic administration, surfactant is given within minutes after birth, thus providing replacement surfactant before severe RDS develops. Rescue treatment is indicated for newborns with established RDS who require mechanical ventilation and supplemental oxygen. It is typically given within 2 hours after birth and repeated again at 4 hours. The earlier the surfactant is administered, the better the effect on gas exchange. Following surfactant administration, the newborn must be closely monitored, and preparation for reduced need for oxygenation and ventilation must be anticipated (Blennow & Bohlin, 2015).

Administer the prescribed oxygen concentration via nasal cannula. Anticipate the need for ventilator therapy, which has greatly improved in the past several years, with significant advances in conventional and high-frequency ventilation therapies (Fig. 24.5). Recent studies show no difference in outcomes for newborns who received early treatment with high-frequency oscillatory ventilation compared with those receiving conventional mechanical ventilation. They are both equally effective in prevention of bronchopulmonary dysplasia (BPD) without being associated with increased mortality or brain damage (Beam et al., 2014). Although mechanical ventilation has increased survival rates, it is also a contributing factor to BPD, pulmonary hypertension, and ROP (Cunningham et al., 2014).

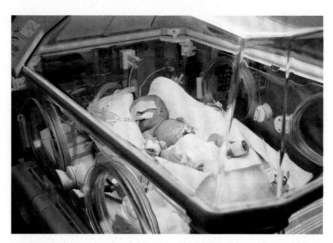

FIGURE 24.5 A newborn with RDS receiving mechanical ventilation.

In addition, support the newborn with RDS using the following interventions:
- Continuously monitor the infant's cardiopulmonary status via invasive or noninvasive means (e.g., arterial lines or auscultation, respectively).
- Monitor oxygen saturation levels continuously; assess pulse oximeter values to determine oxygen saturation levels.
- Closely monitor vital signs, acid–base status, and ABGs.
- Administer broad-spectrum antibiotics if blood cultures are positive.
- Administer sodium bicarbonate or acetate as ordered to correct metabolic acidosis.
- Provide fluids and vasopressor agents as needed to prevent or treat hypotension.
- Test blood glucose levels and administer dextrose as ordered for prevention or treatment of hypoglycemia.
- Cluster caretaking activities to avoid overtaxing and compromising the newborn.
- Place the newborn in the prone position to optimize respiratory status and reduce stress.
- Perform gentle suctioning to remove secretions and maintain a patent airway.
- Assess level of consciousness to identify intraventricular hemorrhage.
- Monitor x-ray studies to detect atelectasis or air leak.
- Provide a neutral thermal environment to reduce metabolic and oxygen demands.
- Provide sufficient calories via gavage and intravenous feedings.
- Maintain adequate hydration and assess for signs of fluid overload.
- Provide information to the parents about treatment modalities; give thorough but simple explanations about the rationales for interventions and provide support.
- Encourage the parents to participate in care (Mattson & Smith, 2015; Nagtalon-Ramos, 2014).

Provide ongoing assessment and be alert for complications. These may include air leak syndrome, BPD (chronic lung disease), patent ductus arteriosus, congestive heart failure, intraventricular hemorrhage, ROP, necrotizing enterocolitis (NEC), complications resulting from intravenous catheter use (infection, thrombus formation), and developmental delay or disability (Pramanik, Rangaswamy, & Gates, 2015).

Meconium Aspiration Syndrome

Meconium is a viscous green substance composed primarily of water and other gastrointestinal secretions that can be noted in the fetal gastrointestinal tract as early as 10 to 16 weeks' gestation. Meconium is sterile and does not contain bacteria, the primary factor that differentiates it from stool. Intrauterine distress can cause passage into the amniotic fluid. Factors that promote the passage in utero include placental insufficiency, maternal hypertension, preeclampsia, oligohydramnios, fetal hypoxia, transient umbilical cord compression, and maternal drug abuse, especially of tobacco and cocaine. Meconium can be aspirated before or during labor and after birth. Because meconium is rarely found in the amniotic fluid prior to 34 weeks' gestation, it mainly affects infants born at term and post-term (Haakonsen Lindenskov et al., 2015). It is usually expelled as the newborn's first stool after birth.

Meconium aspiration syndrome (MAS) occurs when the newborn inhales particulate meconium mixed with amniotic fluid into the lungs while still in utero or on taking the first breath after birth. It is a common cause of newborn respiratory distress and can lead to severe illness. Meconium staining of the amniotic fluid, with the possibility of aspiration, occurs in approximately 12% of pregnancies at term (Cunningham et al., 2014). Aspiration induces airway obstruction, surfactant dysfunction, hypoxia, and chemical pneumonitis with inflammation of pulmonary tissues. In severe cases, it progresses to persistent pulmonary hypertension and death (Cunningham et al., 2014). Of the up to 10% of infants born through meconium-stained amniotic fluid, only about 10% develop MAS and of that percentage, approximately 5% of infants with MAS die. The use of surfactant and inhaled nitric oxide has led to the decreased mortality and the need for extracorporeal membrane oxygenation use (Clark & Clark, 2015).

Pathophysiology

The pathophysiology of MAS is complex, and the timing of the insult resulting in it remains controversial. Meconium may be passed in utero secondary to hypoxic stress. Intrauterine fetal gasping, mechanical airway obstruction, pneumonitis, surfactant inactivation, persistent pulmonary hypertension, and damage of umbilical vessels all play roles in the pathophysiology of MAS.

Hypoxia induces the fetus to gasp or attempt to breathe. The fetus may bear down and pass meconium into the amniotic fluid or he or she may experience a vagal reflex that causes relaxation of the anal sphincter, allowing meconium to be passed into the amniotic fluid. The fetus then sucks or swallows this amniotic fluid in utero, or the infant may aspirate meconium with the first breath after birth as air rushes into the lungs.

Although the etiology is not well understood, the effects of meconium can be harmful to the fetus. Meconium alters the amniotic fluid by reducing antibacterial activity and subsequently increasing the risk of perinatal bacterial infection. Additionally, meconium is very irritating because it contains enzymes from the fetal pancreas.

When aspirated into the lungs, meconium blocks the bronchioles, causing an inflammatory reaction as well as a decrease in surfactant production. Gas exchange is impaired and atelectasis occurs. A ball-valve effect occurs when air is inspired into the alveoli but cannot be fully expired secondary to reduced airway diameter. Significant respiratory distress is followed by persistent pulmonary hypertension, right-to-left shunting of blood, and patent ductus arteriosus. Conventional mechanical ventilation, extracorporeal membrane oxygenation, nitric oxide, high-frequency ventilation, or liquid ventilation may be necessary.

Nursing Assessment

Review prenatal and birth records to identify newborns who may be at high risk for meconium aspiration. Predisposing factors for MAS include post-term pregnancy; breech, forceps, or vacuum extraction births; nulliparity; ethnicity (Pacific Islander, Indigenous Australian, African-American); intrapartum fever; low Apgar score; prolonged or difficult labor associated with fetal distress in a term or post-term newborn; birth weight of >4,500 g; Apgar score of <8 at 5 minutes of age; maternal infection; infants delivered by cesarean section; maternal hypertension or diabetes; oligohydramnios; fetal growth restriction; prolapsed cord; or acute or chronic placental insufficiency (Choi et al., 2015).

Assess the amniotic fluid for meconium staining when the maternal membranes rupture. Green-stained amniotic fluid suggests the presence of meconium in the amniotic fluid and should be reported immediately. After birth, note any yellowish-green staining of the umbilical cord, nails, and skin. This staining indicates that meconium has been present for some time.

Consider Kelly, the 27-year-old woman who gave birth to a son who required resuscitation. What findings would lead the nurse to suspect that her son had aspirated meconium? What risk factors in Kelly's history would support the diagnosis of meconium aspiration syndrome?

Take Note!

Standard prevention and treatment for MAS previously included suctioning the mouth and nares upon head delivery before body delivery. However, recent evidence suggests that aspiration occurs in utero, not at delivery; therefore, the infant's birth should not be impeded for suctioning. After full delivery, the infant should be handed to a neonatal team for evaluation and treatment. Although infants previously have been given intubation and airway suctioning, routine tracheal suction is recommended only for depressed infants (e.g., nonvigorous with depressed tone and respirations and/or heart rate <100 bpm) and those with respiratory symptoms. Use of orogastric suctioning to prevent MAS is not supported by evidence from current studies. Guidelines suggest not stimulating infants with vigorous sucking born with meconium staining at birth, to avoid aspiration (Hudson, 2015).

Observe the newborn for a barrel-shaped chest with an increased anterior–posterior chest diameter (similar to that found in a client with chronic obstructive pulmonary disease), prolonged tachypnea, progression from mild to severe respiratory distress, intercostal retractions, end-expiratory grunting, and cyanosis (Clark & Clark, 2015). Auscultate the lungs, noting coarse crackles and rhonchi.

Chest x-rays show patchy, fluffy infiltrates unevenly distributed throughout the lungs and marked hyperaeration mixed with areas of atelectasis. ABG analysis will indicate metabolic acidosis with a low blood pH, decreased PaO_2, and increased $PaCO_2$ (Karabayir, Demirel, & Bayramoglu, 2015). Direct visualization of the vocal cords for meconium staining using an appropriate size laryngoscope is needed. Expect to administer hyperoxygenation to dilate the pulmonary vasculature and close the ductus arteriosus or nitric oxide inhalation to decrease pulmonary vascular resistance, or to use high-frequency oscillatory ventilation to increase the chance of air trapping (Clark & Clark, 2015). In addition, administer vasopressors and pulmonary vasodilators as prescribed and administer surfactant as ordered to counteract inactivation by meconium. Monitor ABG results for changes and assist with measures to correct acid–base imbalances to facilitate perfusion of tissues and prevent pulmonary hypertension (Brooke-Vincent, 2015). If these measures are ineffective, be prepared to assist with the use of extracorporeal membrane oxygenation, a modified type of heart–lung machine. In addition, perform the following interventions:

- Cluster newborn care to minimize oxygen demand.
- Maintain an optimal thermal environment to minimize oxygen consumption.
- Prevent and treat any complications such as hypotension, metabolic acidosis, or anemia.
- Administer broad-spectrum antibiotics to treat bacterial pneumonia.
- Pay careful attention to systemic blood volume and blood pressure to decrease right-to-left shunting through the patent ductus.

- Administer sedation to reduce agitation and oxygen consumption.
- Continuously monitor the newborn's condition—cardiac and respiratory status, oximetry.
- Provide continuous reassurance and support to the parents throughout the experience (Gardner et al., 2016; Verklan & Walden, 2014).

Persistent Pulmonary Hypertension of the Newborn

Persistent pulmonary hypertension of the newborn (PPHN), previously referred to as persistent fetal circulation, is a cardiopulmonary disorder characterized by marked pulmonary hypertension that causes right-to-left extrapulmonary shunting of blood and hypoxemia. It occurs when the newborn's circulatory system does not have a normal transition after birth. PPHN can occur idiopathically or as a complication of perinatal asphyxia, MAS, maternal smoking, hypocalcemia, maternal obesity, maternal asthma, pneumonia, congenital heart defects, metabolic disorders such as hypoglycemia, hypothermia, hypovolemia, hyperviscosity, acute hypoxia with delayed resuscitation, sepsis, and RDS. It occurs in 1 per 1,000 live births of term, near-term, or post-term infants. Current research findings link increased risk of developing PPHN to exposure to selective serotonin reuptake inhibitors (SSRIs) (antidepressants) in late pregnancy (Gadot & Koren, 2015; Huybrechts et al., 2015). Treatment of depression with antidepressants is complicated by the mother's needs. Careful consideration must be given to the risks, benefits, and alternatives of in utero medication exposure and discussed with the woman.

Pathophysiology

Normally, pulmonary artery pressure decreases when the newborn takes the first breath. However, interference with this ability to breathe allows pulmonary pressures to remain increased. Hypoxemia and acidosis also occur, leading to vasoconstriction of the pulmonary artery. These events cause an elevation in pulmonary vascular resistance. Normally, the decrease in pulmonary artery pressure and pulmonary vascular resistance with breathing leads to the closure of the ductus arteriosus and foramen ovale. However, with PPHN, pulmonary vascular resistance is elevated to the point that venous blood is diverted to some degree through fetal shunts (i.e., the ductus arteriosus and foramen ovale) into the systemic circulation, bypasses the lungs, and results in systemic arterial hypoxemia.

Nursing Assessment

Assess the newborn's status closely. A newborn with persistent pulmonary hypertension demonstrates tachypnea within 12 hours after birth. Observe for marked cyanosis, grunting, respiratory distress with tachypnea, and retractions. Auscultate the heart, noting a systolic ejection harsh sound (tricuspid insufficiency murmur), and measure blood pressure for hypotension resulting from both heart failure and persistent hypoxemia (Kenner & Lott, 2014). Measure oxygen saturation via pulse oximetry and report low values. Prepare the newborn for an echocardiogram, which will reveal right-to-left shunting of blood that confirms the diagnosis.

Nursing Management

Nursing management focuses on ensuring adequate tissue perfusion and minimizing oxygen demand and energy expenditure. Caring for the newborn with PPHN includes identifying signs and symptoms associated with it which may include: murmur, respiratory distress, decreased pulmonary blood flow, hypoxia, hypercarbia, hypoglycemia, cyanosis, metabolic acidosis, and hypotension (late sign) (Kenner & Lott, 2014). Usually the newborn is transferred to the NICU for close monitoring.

Maintain a neutral thermal environment, including placing the newborn under a radiant warmer or in a warmed Isolette® to prevent hypothermia. In addition, minimize handling to reduce energy expenditure and oxygen consumption that could lead to further hypoxemia and acidosis.

Administer oxygen therapy as ordered via nasal cannula or with positive-pressure ventilation. Monitor oxygen saturation levels via pulse oximetry to evaluate the newborn's response to treatment and to detect changes. Increased pulmonary pressures associated with PPHN may cause blood to be shunted away from the lungs. The newborn may exhibit uneven pulmonary ventilation, with hyperinflation in some areas and atelectasis in others. This leads to poor perfusion and subsequent hypoxemia, which in turn may increase pulmonary vasoconstriction and a worsening of hypoxemia and acidosis. Blood is diverted to some degree through fetal structures such as the ductus arteriosus or foramen ovale, causing them to remain open, leading to a right-to-left shunting of blood into the systemic circulation. This diversion of blood bypasses the lungs, resulting in systemic arterial hypoxemia.

When caring for the newborn with persistent pulmonary hypertension, pay meticulous attention to detail, with continuous monitoring of the newborn's oxygenation and perfusion status and blood pressure. The goals of therapy include improving alveolar oxygenation, inducing metabolic alkalosis by administering sodium bicarbonate, correcting hypovolemia and hypotension with the administration of volume replacement and vasopressors, and anticipating use of extracorporeal membrane oxygenation when support has failed to maintain acceptable oxygenation (Davidson, 2014).

Provide immediate resuscitation after birth and administer oxygen therapy as ordered. Early and effective resuscitation and correction of acidosis and hypoxia are helpful in preventing persistent pulmonary hypertension. Monitor ABGs frequently to evaluate the effectiveness of oxygen therapy. Provide respiratory support, which frequently necessitates the use of mechanical ventilation. Administer prescribed medications, monitor cardiopulmonary status, cluster care to reduce stimulation, and provide ongoing support and education to the parents.

Take Note!

Almost any procedure, such as suctioning, weighing, changing diapers, or positioning, can precipitate severe hypoxemia due to the instability of the pulmonary vasculature. Therefore, minimize the newborn's exposure to stimulation as much as possible.

Bronchopulmonary Dysplasia/Chronic Lung Disease

BPD, a type of chronic lung disease, commonly occurs in infants who have experienced a lung injury resulting in the need for continued use of oxygen after the initial neonatal period (28 days of life). Approximately 5,000 to 10,000 new cases of BPD occur each year. White male infants seem to be at greatest risk for developing BPD (American Lung Association [ALA], 2015). The average length of intensive in-hospital care for infants with BPD is 120 days. The overall costs of treating BPD in the United States are estimated to be $2.5 billion annually (ALA, 2015). Newborns with BPD need intensive hospital care and home oxygen therapy after being discharged.

Pathophysiology

BPD results from an underlying lung injury. However, the etiology of the lung injury is multifactorial, complex, and remains incompletely understood. It is associated with surfactant deficiency, genetic predisposition, prematurity, oxygen toxicity, pulmonary edema, lung immaturity, lung injury from mechanical ventilation, inflammation, and fluid overload. Lung injury commonly occurs secondary to mechanical ventilation and oxygen toxicity, usually in infants who have had RDS. This lung damage results from the complex interplay between impairments in the premature lung such as surfactant deficiency, perinatal insults such as infection, and damage resulting from supportive care of the infant due to mechanical ventilation and oxygen toxicity from supplemental oxygen administration. These factors trigger an inflammatory cascade in the infant lung with recurring cycles of lung damage and repair that may impair alveolarization and vascularization in the developing lungs. High levels of inspired oxygen concentrations cause an inflammatory process in the lungs that leads to parenchymal damage. Various toxic factor exposure can injure small airways, which interferes with alveolarization (alveolar septation), leading to a reduction in the overall surface area for gas exchange (Zhang, Gien, & Dysart, 2015). This damage includes epithelial stretching, invasion by macrophages and polymorphonuclear leukocytes, airway edema interfering with the growth and development of lung structures, loss of cilia, and a decrease in the number of alveoli.

Therapeutic Management

BPD remains the most common severe adverse pulmonary outcome of preterm birth. It is associated with significant mortality, morbidity, and resource utilization. Low gestational age and birth weight are the strongest risk factors for the development of BPD, but the pathogenesis is complex. The strategy for respiratory support immediately after birth and during the initial neonatal period may have a critical impact on the development of BPD. The preterm lung is highly susceptible to injury. Excessive oxygen use in preterm infants increases the risk of BPD. The recently developed practices for oxygen saturation levels during the neonatal transition phase have become part of the newly revised resuscitation guidelines. For term neonates, starting resuscitation with air, rather than 100% oxygen, is now advised. Preterm infants may require a higher initial inspiratory oxygen concentration than term infants; however, the ideal level is not yet defined. Primary intubation is no longer a prerequisite for preterm survival. Recent studies have demonstrated that even very preterm infants can be safely stabilized after birth with CPAP and later be selectively treated with surfactant for RDS. This initially less invasive strategy has the advantage of reducing the need for mechanical ventilation and, thereby, the risk of lung injury (Iyengar & Davis, 2015).

BPD can be prevented by administering steroids to the mother in the antepartal period and exogenous surfactant to the newborn to help reduce the risk for RDS and its severity. In addition, the following better practices may help reduce the incidence of BPD:

- Use lower target oxygen saturation levels.
- Close the patent ductus arteriosus early, either medically or surgically.
- Monitor and minimize tidal volumes on ventilators.
- Use postnatal steroid therapy judiciously.
- Stem cell therapy.
- Inspired oxygen tensions should be kept as low as possible.
- Administer the antioxidant vitamin A.
- Maintain adequate nutritional status (Gardner et al., 2016).

Supplemental oxygen, antibiotics, and fluid restriction and diuretics to decrease fluid accumulation in the lungs are used. Bronchodilators are used to open the airways. Intravenous feedings are given to meet the infant's nutrition needs, and physical therapy is used to improve muscle performance and to help the lungs expel mucus.

Nursing Assessment

Although BPD is most common in preterm newborns, it can also occur in full-term ones who had respiratory problems during their first days of life. Thus, it is essential to assess the newborn's history for risk factors, including male gender, preterm birth (<32 weeks), nutritional deficiencies, White race, pulmonary hypertension, excessive fluid intake during the first few days of life, presence of patent ductus arteriosus, anemia, low Apgar score, severe RDS treated with mechanical ventilation for more than 1 week, and sepsis (Mattson & Smith, 2015). Also review the history for use of supplemental oxygen, the length of exposure to oxygen therapy, and the use of ventilatory support.

Assess the infant for signs and symptoms of BPD. These may include tachypnea, poor weight gain related to the increased metabolic workload, tachycardia, sternal retractions (see Fig. 24.2), episodes of cyanosis, nasal flaring, and bronchospasm with abnormal breath sounds (crackles, rhonchi, and wheezes). Hypoxia, as evidenced by abnormal blood gas results, and acidosis and hypercapnia also are noted. Chest x-rays will show hyperinflation, infiltrates, and cardiomegaly.

Nursing Management

The focus of management is to improve supportive care and minimize additional lung injury by decreasing the workload of breathing and normalizing gas exchange, thus promoting growth and development of the respiratory system. Nursing care includes providing continuous ventilatory and oxygen support and optimal nutrition to support growth, and administering bronchodilators, anti-inflammatory agents, and diuretics as ordered. Continuously monitor the newborn's respiratory status to determine the need for continued ventilatory assistance. When the newborn is clinically stable and ready, expect to wean him or her slowly so that he or she can compensate for the changes. Supplemental oxygen may be needed after discharge from the hospital. Provide a high caloric intake to promote growth and to compensate for the calories expended due to the increased work of breathing. Some infants may require high-calorie formulas to foster adequate growth.

Newborns with BPD may require continued care at home. When planning for discharge, educate the family caretaker about how to manage a chronically ill child who may be oxygen dependent for an extended time. Provide ongoing support to parents as they learn to meet their infant's needs. Also instruct the family about the safe use of oxygen in the home, including the need to notify emergency medical services and utility companies that a technology-dependent child is living in their district. In addition, initiate a social service referral to help the family access community resources and obtain necessary support (Bowen & Maxwell, 2014).

Despite decades of promising research, primary prevention of BPD has proven elusive. Future management of BPD will involve strategies that emphasize prevention. Because few accepted therapies currently prevent BPD, many therapeutic modalities are used to treat it, which may in fact exacerbate it.

Retinopathy of Prematurity

ROP is a potentially blinding retinal vascular eye disease that occurs in very low birth weight and preterm infants. Supplemental oxygen, birth weight, multiple births, White race, mechanical ventilation, and gestational age are the major risk factors for the development of ROP. The incidence of ROP in preterm newborns is inversely proportional to their birth weight. Of the approximately 4 million infants born in the United States annually, about 28,000 weigh 1,500 g (2.75 lb) or less. According to the National Eye Institute (NEI), each year an estimated 1,400 to 1,600 infants in the United States develop ROP severe enough to require medical treatment. Of these infants, 400 to 600 become legally blind from ROP annually (National Eye Institute [NEI] 2015). ROP can also lead to vitreous hemorrhage and retinal detachment, which is the major cause of visual impairment and blindness (Subramanian, Bahri, & Vicente, 2015).

Predisposing factors for the development of ROP include preterm birth, low birth weight, level of oxygen saturation, genetics, and the severity of underlying illnesses present at birth. Additionally, the level of oxygen saturation and genetics seem to play a role in the severity of ROP.

Pathophysiology

The eye begins to develop early in gestation, at approximately 16 weeks. Blood vessels begin to form and grow to supply the retina, which transmits visual information to the brain, with oxygen and nutrients. These vessels continue to grow gradually until about the last 12 weeks of pregnancy (between 28 and 40 weeks' gestation), at which time the eye undergoes rapid development. Thus, an infant born at term has retinal vessels that are almost completely developed. However, when the infant is born preterm, normal blood vessel development is interrupted. In terms of the developing retina, preterm birth interrupts the normal development of the vascular bed that will nourish the eye. The lack of blood vessels in the retina initiates anaerobic metabolism, further increasing the already existing hypoxia. Without blood flow

through the eye, the retina is deprived of oxygen and its metabolic needs go unmet.

ROP typically develops in both eyes secondary to an injury such as hyperoxemia due to prolonged assistive ventilation and high oxygen exposure, acidosis, and shock. Exposure to high oxygen concentrations leads to severe retinal vasoconstriction with endothelial damage and vessel obliteration. Abnormal blood vessels develop in an attempt to nourish the retina. These vessels, which proliferate in the retina, are highly fragile and bleed easily, leading to the formation of scar tissue. They also can enlarge and twist, pulling the retina away from the wall of the eye and resulting in retinal detachment.

Take Note!

Although the precise levels of hyperoxemia that can be sustained without causing retinopathy are not known, very immature newborns who develop respiratory distress often must be given high oxygen concentrations to maintain life (Cunningham et al., 2014).

ROP is classified in five stages, ranging from mild (stage I) to severe (stage V). The grades are based on three criteria: (1) severity, (2) location by zones in the retina, and (3) extent or proportion of the retinal circumference (Hartnett, 2015). The degree of abnormal blood vessel growth and evidence of retinal detachment are used to stage this disorder.

Therapeutic Management

With the increasing survival of premature infants and increased incidence of ROP, it is important to screen for ROP risk and treat at-risk clients in a timely manner to preserve their visual function and reduce complications. The key to treating ROP is prevention by minimizing the risk of preterm birth through providing quality prenatal care and health counseling to all pregnant women. When ROP does develop, treatment depends on the stage and degree of retinal findings. Typically, stages I and II resolve on their own and require only periodic evaluation by the ophthalmologist. For more advanced stages, surgical intervention such as laser photocoagulation therapy or cryotherapy can be done. Laser photocoagulation is the most common treatment modality. A laser is directed to a designated spot to destroy abnormal vessels and seal leaks. Vascular endothelial growth factor inhibitors such as bevacizumab are the newest treatment option, but more research into dosage, safety, and long-term outcomes must be performed (Jordan, 2014).

Nursing Assessment

The newborn who develops ROP exhibits no signs or symptoms, so assessment involves identifying the newborn at risk. Review the maternal prenatal history for risk factors such as substance abuse, hypertension, pre-eclampsia, heavy cigarette smoking, or evidence of placental insufficiency. Also assess the newborn's gestational age and weight. Be especially alert for newborns weighing 1,500 g or less or those born at 28 weeks' gestation or less. Evaluate the newborn's history for the duration of intubation and the use of oxygen therapy, intraventricular hemorrhage, and sepsis (Verklan & Walden, 2014). Prepare the infant for an ophthalmologic examination.

Nursing Management

By integrating the most recent evidence-based practice guidelines with clinical practice management, newborn outcomes can be improved. In light of the growing body of evidence regarding ROP prevention, many NICUs have adopted lower oxygen saturation ranges for preterm infants. Oxygen saturation target ranges in the mid-80s to lower mid-90s are usually safe and can reduce the severity of ROP in newborns <32 weeks' gestation. Recent research reported that using a low oxygen saturation approach reduced the severe ROP by 50% and BPD/lung problems by 25%, but further randomized trials are needed to provide definite conclusions and to assess whether reducing oxygen saturation has an impact on mortality among very and extremely low birth weight infants (Kaufman et al., 2014). Institute measures for prevention. Administer oxygen therapy cautiously and monitor oxygen saturation levels to ensure that the lowest oxygen concentration possible is used and for the shortest possible duration. Cover the Isolette® with a blanket and dim the surrounding lights to protect the newborn's eyes.

Clear evidence exists that lower oxygen saturation levels once considered insufficient are in fact safe, and have fewer harmful effects (Enomoto et al., 2015; Tataranno et al., 2015). It is essential that nurses understand the evidence base on which preventive strategies are founded, so they can help improve the visual outcomes for all preterm infants assigned to their care.

Take Note!

Any newborn with a birth weight of less than 1,500 g or born at less than 28 weeks' gestation should be examined by a pediatric ophthalmologist within 4 to 6 weeks after birth.

Assist with scheduling an ophthalmic examination for the newborn. Expect to administer a mydriatic eye agent to dilate the newborn's pupils approximately 1 hour prior to the examination as ordered. During this time, take extra care to protect the newborn's eyes from bright light. If necessary, provide assistance with the examination by holding the newborn's head. Assist with scheduling follow-up eye examinations, usually every 2 to 3 weeks depending on the severity of the clinical findings at the first examination (Mannan, Moni, & Shahidullah, 2015).

The AAP has issued practice guideline recommendations for ROP screening and treatment that aid in creating a consistent and reliable ROP protocol. Newborns with ROP are at risk of developing strabismus (abnormal alignment of the eyes), nystagmus (rapid involuntary movements of the eyes), high myopia (eyeball stretches and becomes too long which can lead to retinal detachment, and abnormal retinal structure and should therefore receive continued long-term follow-up. Challenges exist though in screening for and treating ROP, including delayed or omitted exams, lack of qualified examiners, and lack of parental adherence to instructions in following up after leaving the hospital (Subramanian, Bahri, & Vicente, 2015).

Provide support to the parents. This is an extremely difficult time for them; in addition to learning to meet the needs of their preterm newborn, they must also deal with the possibility that their baby may have a condition that could lead to blindness. Consider the family's needs and provide individualized support and guidance. Provide information about the newborn's condition and treatment options. Stress the need for follow-up vision screenings, because ROP is considered a lifelong disease. Post-discharge follow-up of infants who are still at risk for severe ROP is paramount for timely detection and treatment.

Periventricular–Intraventricular Hemorrhage

Periventricular–intraventricular hemorrhage (PVH–IVH) is defined as bleeding that usually originates in the subependymal germinal matrix region of the brain, with extension into the ventricular system. The germinal matrix is the embryonic structure that is unique to preterm infants, which provides vascular supply for 24 to 32 weeks of gestation. It is primitive, and made of smooth endothelial cells which are highly vascular and prone to bleeding (Ballabh, 2014). It is a common problem in preterm infants, especially in those born before 32 weeks. It remains a significant cause of both morbidity and mortality in infants who are born prematurely. Sequelae of PVH–IVH include lifelong neurologic deficits, such as cerebral palsy, developmental delay, and seizures (Annibale, 2015).

When a fetus is born prematurely, the infant is suddenly thrust from a well-controlled uterine environment into a highly stimulating, hostile one. The tremendous physiologic stress and shock experienced by a premature infant after birth may cause the periventricular capillaries to rupture. Bleeding occurs initially in the immediate periventricular areas causing a periventricular hemorrhage (PVH). If the bleeding persists, the expanding volume of blood dissects into the adjacent lateral ventricles leading to an intraventricular hemorrhage (IVH).

A significant number of these newborns will incur brain injury, leading to complications that may include hydrocephalus, seizure disorders, periventricular leukomalacia (an ischemic injury resulting from inadequate perfusion of the white matter adjacent to the ventricles), cerebral palsy, learning disabilities, vision or hearing deficits, language difficulties, behavioral and personality disorders, and intellectual disability. Unfortunately, the different areas of the cerebral cortex are not even used by an infant for months or even years after birth, so it may take this length of time before developmental problems resulting from damage to the cerebral cortex become evident. This emphasizes the need for long-term developmental follow-up for high-risk infants. Identifying preventive strategies to reduce the incidence of these brain insults is a national public health priority (Marcdante & Kliegman, 2015).

The incidence of ventricular hemorrhage depends on the gestational age at birth. Up to 50% of newborns weighing 1,500 g or less or born at 30 weeks' gestation or less will have evidence of hemorrhage, whereas only about 4% of term newborns show evidence of ventricular hemorrhage. Very low birth weight infants have the earliest onset of hemorrhage and the highest mortality rate (Annibale, 2015).

Pathophysiology

The pathogenesis of IVH is attributed to the intrinsic weakness of germinal vasculature and to the fluctuation in the cerebral blood flow. The fluctuation in the cerebral blood flow is attributed to the cardiorespiratory and hemodynamic instability associated with preterm infants, including hypotension, hypoxia, pneumothorax, and patent ductus arteriosus. Genetics appears to also play a role in this condition (Szpecht et al., 2015). The preterm newborn is at greatest risk for PVH–IVH because cerebrovascular development is immature, making it more vulnerable to injury. The more premature the newborn is, the greater the likelihood for brain damage. While all areas of the brain can be injured, the periventricular area is the most vulnerable.

Each ventricular area contains a rich network of capillaries that are very thin and fragile and can rupture easily. The causes of rupture vary and include fluctuations in systemic and cerebral blood flow, increases in cerebral blood flow from hypertension, intravenous infusions, seizure activity, increases in cerebral venous pressure due to vaginal delivery, hypoxia, and respiratory distress. With a preterm birth, the fetus is suddenly transported from a well-controlled uterine environment into a highly stimulating one. This tremendous physiologic stress and shock may contribute to the rupture of periventricular capillaries and subsequent hemorrhage. Most hemorrhages occur in the first 72 hours after birth (Cunningham et al., 2014).

The diagnosis of PVH–IVH is commonly done with a cranial ultrasound or a computed tomography (CT), or a magnetic resonance imaging (MRI) and then classified according to a grading system of I to V (least severe to most severe) (Wang et al., 2015). The prognosis is guarded, depending on the grade and severity of the hemorrhage. Generally, newborns with mild hemorrhage (grades I and II) have a much better developmental outcome than those with severe hemorrhage (grades III and IV).

Nursing Assessment

The signs of PVH–IVH vary significantly; no clinical signs may be evident. Approximately 50% of PVH–IVH occurs by 24 hours of age, and 90% occurs by 72 hours of age. Closely monitor newborns who are at an increased risk, such as those who are preterm or of low birth weight. Also assess for risk factors such as acidosis, asphyxia, unstable blood pressure, meningitis, seizures, acute blood loss, hypovolemia, respiratory distress with mechanical ventilation, intubation, apnea, hypoxia, suctioning, use of hyperosmolar solutions, rapid volume expansion, and activities that involve handling.

Evaluate the newborn for an unexplained drop in hematocrit, pallor, and poor perfusion as evidenced by respiratory distress and oxygen desaturation. Note seizures, lethargy or other changes in level of consciousness, bulging fontanel, weak sucking, metabolic acidosis, high-pitched cry, or hypotonia/flaccidity. Palpate the anterior fontanel for tenseness. Assess vital signs, noting bradycardia and hypotension. Evaluate laboratory data for changes indicating metabolic acidosis or glucose instability (Annibale, 2015). Frequently a bleed can progress rapidly and result in shock and death. Prepare the newborn for cranial ultrasonography, the diagnostic tool of choice to detect hemorrhage.

Nursing Management

Prevention of preterm birth is essential in preventing periventricular–intraventricular hemorrhage. Promote community awareness of factors that may contribute to PVH–IVH, such as a lack of prenatal care, maternal infection, alcohol consumption, and smoking (Kenner & Lott, 2014). Identify risk factors that can lead to hemorrhage and focus care on interventions to decrease the risk of hemorrhage. For example, institute measures to prevent perinatal asphyxia and birth trauma and provide developmental care in the NICU. If a preterm birth is expected, having the mother deliver at a tertiary care facility with a NICU would be preferable.

Care of the newborn with PVH–IVH is primarily supportive. Correct anemia, acidosis, and hypotension with fluids and medications. Administer fluids slowly to prevent fluctuations in blood pressure. Avoid rapid volume expansion to minimize changes in cerebral blood flow. Keep the newborn in a flexed, contained position with the head elevated to prevent or minimize fluctuations in intracranial pressure. Continuously monitor the newborn for signs of hemorrhage, such as changes in the level of consciousness, bulging fontanel, seizures, apnea, and reduced activity level. Also, measuring head circumference daily to assess for expansion in size is essential in identifying complications early.

Minimize handling of the newborn by clustering nursing care, and limit stimulation in the newborn's environment to reduce stress. Also reduce the newborn's exposure to noxious stimuli to avoid a fluctuation in blood pressure and energy expenditure. Provide adequate oxygenation to promote tissue perfusion but controlled ventilation to decrease the risk of pneumothorax. Developmental care principles include avoiding lifting the lower extremities above the midline with diaper changes, giving rapid fluid boluses, and high oxygen and ventilation, as these can all increase the chance of more cranial hemorrhage.

Support for the parents to cope with the diagnosis and potential long-term sequelae is essential. The long-term neurodevelopmental outcome is determined by the severity of the bleed. Provide education and emotional support for the parents throughout the newborn's stay. Discuss expectations for short-term and long-term care needs with the parents and assist them in obtaining the necessary support from appropriate community resources.

Necrotizing Enterocolitis

NEC is an inflammatory disease of the bowel which can cause ischemic and necrotic injury in the gastrointestinal tract. It is the most common and most serious acquired gastrointestinal disorder among hospitalized preterm neonates, and is associated with significant acute and chronic morbidity and mortality. This inflammatory bowel disease results in inflammation and bacterial invasion of the bowel wall. It represents a significant clinical problem and affects close to 10% of infants who weigh less than 1,500 g, with mortality rates of 50% or more depending on severity (Springer & Annibale, 2015). Population studies estimate the incidence of NEC at between 0.3 and 2.4 per 1,000 live births in the United States, with a predominance of cases among preterm neonates born at the earliest gestational ages. Also, more males than females are affected (about 3 to 1). The disease burden of NEC includes an overall disease-specific mortality rate of 15% to 20%, with yet higher rates among earliest gestations. The NEC burden also includes an increase in hospital costs approximating $100,000/case, as well as severe late sequelae including parenteral nutrition-associated liver disease and short bowel syndrome (Schanler, 2014).

Ways to improve gastrointestinal function and reduce the risk of NEC include enteral antibiotics, judicious administration of parenteral fluids, human breast milk feedings, antenatal corticosteroids, enteral probiotics (*Lactobacillus acidophilus*), and slow continuous-drip feedings. Meta-analysis of prospective randomized controlled trials evaluating probiotics as measures to prevent NEC have all provided encouraging results. Consequently, it has been argued that there is already evidence to warrant change in clinical practice and practice guidelines (Lau & Chamberlain, 2015) (see Evidence-Based Practice 24.1). Despite that, and despite major efforts

EVIDENCE-BASED PRACTICE 24.1

PROBIOTIC ADMINISTRATION CAN PREVENT NECROTIZING ENTEROCOLITIS IN PRETERM INFANTS: A META-ANALYSIS

STUDY

Necrotizing enterocolitis (NEC) is a serious disease that affects the bowel of premature infants in the first few weeks of life. Although the cause of NEC is not entirely known, milk feedings and bacterial growth play a role. Probiotics (dietary supplements containing potentially beneficial bacteria or yeast) have been used to prevent NEC. Early intervention and aggressive treatment have improved clinical outcomes, but considerable morbidity continues. This meta-analysis examines the impact of probiotics on the incidence of NEC and complications among very low birth weight infants.

Findings

A comprehensive review of the literature search was conducted for all published randomized controlled trials assessing the use of probiotics to prevent NEC. Twenty studies were found involving 5,982 preterm infants. The risk of NEC was reduced by 49% and overall mortality by

27% among infants receiving probiotics. An 8% reduction of sepsis was also observed in infants receiving probiotics. The meta-analysis found that the use of probiotic supplementation in preterm infants is associated with a significant reduction in the risk of NEC and overall mortality.

Nursing Implications

The study confirmed the effectiveness of probiotics in the prevention of neonatal NEC and the associated mortality. Enteral supplementation of probiotics prevents severe NEC and all-cause mortality in preterm infants. This updated review of available evidence strongly supports a change in practice. Nurses can integrate the findings of this study into their practice when caring for newborns who are at risk for developing NEC. Additional research studies are needed to assess the most effective preparations, timing, doses, and length of therapy to be used. Nurses can participate in collecting data for these future studies.

Adapted from Lau, C. S., & Chamberlain, R. S. (2015). Probiotic administration can prevent necrotizing enterocolitis in preterm infants: A meta-analysis. *Journal of Pediatric Surgery*. doi:10.1016/j.jpedsurg.2015.05.008

toward its eradication, NEC has persisted and appears to be increasing due to the increasing numbers of preterm births (Neu, 2014).

Pathophysiology

The pathophysiology of NEC is poorly understood and is thought to be multifactorial in nature. Current research points to five major pathologic mechanisms that lead to NEC: bowel hypoxic ischemia events, perinatal stressors, an immature intestinal barrier, abnormal bacterial colonization in the gut, and formula feeding. The intestine of a premature infant is characterized by underdeveloped immune defenses and compromised mucosal barrier function. As a result, the immature intestine is susceptible to bacterial colonization by opportunistic pathogens, which follows oral feeding, which in turn incites an inflammatory response culminating in the adverse sequelae of NEC (Lim, Golden, & Ford, 2015).

During perinatal or postnatal stress, oxygen is shunted away from the gut to more important organs such as the heart and brain. Ischemia and intestinal wall damage occur, allowing bacteria to invade. High-solute feedings allow bacteria to flourish. Mucosal or transmucosal necrosis of part of the intestine occurs (National Institutes of Health, 2015). Although any region of the bowel can be affected, the distal ileum and proximal colon are the regions most commonly involved. NEC usually occurs between 3 and 12 days of life, but it can occur weeks later in some newborns.

Nursing Assessment

NEC can be devastating, and astute assessment is crucial. Assessing the newborn for the development of NEC includes the health history and physical examination as well as laboratory and diagnostic testing. The onset of NEC is heralded by the development of feeding intolerance, abdominal distention, and bloody stools in a preterm infant receiving enteral feedings. As the disease worsens, the infant develops signs and symptoms of septic shock (respiratory distress, temperature instability, lethargy, hypotension, and oliguria). Nurses need to be suspicious of this condition in caring for this type of preterm infant.

HEALTH HISTORY AND PHYSICAL EXAMINATION

Assess the newborn's history for risk factors associated with NEC. In addition to preterm birth, prenatal and postnatal predisposing risk factors are highlighted in Box 24.1.

Also observe the newborn for common signs and symptoms, which may include:

- Cardiorespiratory baseline changes
- Feeding intolerance
- Abdominal distention and tenderness
- Bloody or hemoccult-positive stools
- Diarrhea

BOX 24.1

PREDISPOSING FACTORS FOR THE DEVELOPMENT OF NECROTIZING ENTEROCOLITIS

- Preterm labor
- Prolonged rupture of membranes
- Preeclampsia
- Maternal sepsis
- Amnionitis
- Uterine hypoxia

Postnatal Factors

- Respiratory distress syndrome
- Patent ductus arteriosus
- Congenital heart disease
- Exchange transfusion
- Low birth weight
- Polycythemia
- Acute hypoxic event
- Enteral feedings with formula
- Low Apgar scores
- Umbilical catheterization
- Hypothermia
- Gastrointestinal infection
- Hypoglycemia
- Perinatal stress and asphyxia

- Respiratory distress
- Metabolic acidosis
- Temperature instability
- Decreased or absent bowel sounds
- Signs of sepsis
- Lethargy
- Apnea
- Shock (Fox & Thacker, 2015).

Always keep the possibility of NEC in mind when dealing with preterm newborns, especially when enteral feedings are being administered. Note respiratory distress, cyanosis, lethargy, decreased activity level, temperature instability, feeding intolerance, diarrhea, bile-stained emesis, or grossly bloody stools. Assess blood pressure, noting hypotension. Evaluate the neonate's abdomen for distention, tenderness, and visible loops of bowel (Nagtalon-Ramos, 2014). Measure the abdominal circumference and if there is an increase or not. Determine residual gastric volume prior to feeding; when it is elevated, be suspicious for NEC.

LABORATORY AND DIAGNOSTIC TESTING

Tests used to diagnose NEC include ABGs (to assess for metabolic acidosis); complete blood count (to see counts of white blood cells and red blood cells, and platelets); blood culture (to identify the organism causing an infection); and an abdominal x-ray (to demonstrate dilated bowel loops, abnormal gas patterns, intramural air bubbles that occur from bacteria, and thickened bowel walls (Kenner & Lott, 2014; Springer & Annibale, 2015).

Nursing Management

Nursing management of the newborn with NEC focuses on maintaining fluid and nutritional status, providing supportive care, and teaching the family about the condition and prognosis. Therapeutic medical management initially consists of bowel rest and antibiotic therapy. Serial kidney, ureter, and bladder x-rays and C-reactive protein (CRP) levels are used to assess the resolution or progression of NEC. If medical treatment fails to stabilize the newborn or if free air is present on a left lateral decubitus film (where the infant is lying down on the left side), surgical intervention will be necessary to resect the portion of necrotic bowel while preserving as much of the intestinal length as possible. Surgery for NEC usually requires the placement of a proximal enterostomy until the anastomosis site is ready for reconnection. After surgery, postoperative supportive care includes fluids, total parenteral nutrition (TPN), antibiotics, and bowel rest for 10 to 14 days.

NEC is usually limited to a short period and resolves within 48 hours of stopping oral feedings, but surgically treated NEC can be a much lengthier process. The amount of bowel that has necrosed, as determined during the bowel resection, significantly increases the likelihood of long-term medical problems. Short bowel syndrome may result from a large resection of the bowel. Reassure the family that although some infants have more involved cases of NEC, today's improved parenteral nutrition formulations have improved the outcomes for these infants. Provide education about ostomy care if surgery is required. Promote interaction with the newborn. Nursing actions of active engagement with parents and the sick infant (providing NICU orientation and physical care), providing cautious guidance (offering information and instruction on infant care), and nurses' subtle presence (overseeing parents' interaction with their infant) all contribute to fostering a positive, trusting relationship with parents (Gardner et al., 2016).

MAINTAINING FLUID AND NUTRITIONAL STATUS

If NEC is suspected, immediately stop enteral feedings until a diagnosis is made. Administer intravenous fluids initially to restore proper fluid balance. If ordered, administer TPN to keep the newborn supported nutritionally. Give prescribed intravenous antibiotics to prevent sepsis from the necrotic bowel (if surgery is required, antibiotics may be needed for an extended period). Institute gastric decompression as ordered with an orogastric tube attached to low intermittent suction. Carefully monitor intake and output. Restart enteral feedings once the disease has resolved (normal abdominal examination and kidney, urinary, and bladder x-rays negative for pneumatosis) or as determined postoperatively by the surgeon.

PROVIDING SUPPORTIVE CARE

Manage pain by administering analgesics as ordered. Infection control is important, with an emphasis on careful hand hygiene. In addition, implement these interventions in an ongoing manner:

- Check stools for evidence of blood and report any positive findings.
- Measure the abdominal girth for an increase in size.
- Monitor blood pressure for hypotension.
- Palpate the abdomen for tenderness and rigidity.
- Monitor blood gases and oxygen saturation.
- Offer emotional support for parents.
- Auscultate for the presence or absence of bowel sounds in all four quadrants.
- Observe the abdomen for redness or shininess, which indicates peritonitis.

EDUCATING THE FAMILY

The diagnosis of NEC may cause significant family anxiety. Listen to the family's worries and fears. Answer their questions honestly. Inform the family that medically treated NEC places the infant at higher risk verses surgical treatment. Management of these risks is best achieved through comprehensive preconception care and making healthy choices, both prior to and during pregnancy.

Infant of a Diabetic Mother

An **infant of a diabetic mother (IDM)** is one born to a woman with pregestational or gestational diabetes (see Chapter 20 for additional information). The newborn of a woman who has diabetes is at high risk for numerous health-related complications, especially hypoglycemia. The prevalence of type 2 diabetes mellitus continues to rise worldwide. More women who are in the reproductive age group have diabetes, resulting in more pregnancies complicated by type 2 diabetes, thus placing both mother and fetus at risk for lifelong complications. In light of the increasing incidence of type 2 diabetes among women of childbearing age, it is important to educate women about the potential impact of poor glycemic control on their offspring.

Impact of Diabetes on the Newborn

For more than a century, it has been known that diabetes during pregnancy can have severe adverse effects on fetal and newborn outcomes. Infants of mothers with diabetes have increased morbidity and mortality in the perinatal period. The incidence of major congenital anomalies is much greater for these newborns than for other newborns. Poor glycemic control in the first trimester, during organogenesis, is thought to be a major reason for congenital malformations. The most common types of malformations in infants of mothers with diabetes involve the cardiovascular, skeletal, central nervous, gastrointestinal, and genitourinary systems. Cardiac anomalies are the most common (Nagtalon-Ramos, 2014).

Infants of mothers with diabetes can be large for gestational age (LGA) or small for gestational age (SGA), depending on the vascular impact of this chronic systemic disease on the mother prior to and during the pregnancy. Fetal macrosomia occurs in 25% to 42% of diabetic pregnancies because of hyperinsulinemia (Verklan, 2014). LGA infants (>90th percentile on growth chart) are longer and weigh more than 4,000 g with the majority of the excess weight composed of fat. They also have increased organ weights (organomegaly) and excessive fat deposits on their shoulders and trunk, contributing to the increased overall body weight and predisposing them to shoulder dystocia, brachial plexus injury, fracture, neonatal depression or cesarean birth (Korkmazer, Solak, & Tokgoz, 2015). These oversized newborns frequently require cesarean births for cephalopelvic disproportion and dysfunctional labor patterns. They are frequently hypoglycemic in the first few hours after birth.

SGA infants (<10th percentile on growth chart) of mothers with diabetes usually suffer from intrauterine malnutrition and have few glucose reserves to tolerate the rigors of labor and birth. Uteroplacental circulation is often impaired, leading to poor growth patterns and hypoxemia. Despite their increased or decreased size and weight, they may be remarkably frail, showing behaviors similar to those of a preterm newborn. Thus, birth weight may not be a reliable criterion of maturity. Newborns of women with diabetes but without vascular complications often tend to be LGA, whereas those of women with diabetes and vascular disease are usually SGA.

Pathophysiology

The large size of the IDM arises secondary to exposure to high levels of maternal glucose crossing the placenta into the fetal circulation. Maternal hyperglycemia acts as a fuel to stimulate increased production of fetal insulin, which in turn promotes somatic growth within the fetus. The fetus responds to these high levels by producing more insulin, which acts as a growth factor in the fetus (Potter & Kicklighter, 2016). How the fetus will be affected and the problems that the newborn will experience depend on the severity, duration, and control of the diabetes in the mother. Table 24.1 summarizes the common problems that may occur in infants of mothers with diabetes.

Nursing Assessment

Assessment begins in the prenatal period by identifying women with diabetes and taking measures to control maternal glucose levels. (See Chapter 20 for information on management of the pregnant woman with diabetes.)

PHYSICAL EXAMINATION

At birth, inspect the newborn for the following characteristic features (Fig. 24.6):

- Full rosy cheeks with a ruddy skin color
- Short neck (some describe "no-neck" appearance)
- Buffalo hump over the nape of the neck
- Massive shoulders with a full intrascapular area
- Distended upper abdomen due to organ overgrowth
- Excessive subcutaneous fat tissue, producing fat extremities

Be alert for hypoglycemia, which may occur immediately or within an hour after birth. Assess blood glucose levels, which should remain above 40 mg/dL. Closely assess the newborn for signs of hypoglycemia, including listlessness, hypotonia, apathy, poor feeding, apneic episodes with a drop in oxygen saturation, cyanosis, temperature instability, pallor and sweating, tremors, irritability, and seizures.

Pulmonary function may be affected in the IDM manifesting itself in TTN or RDS. Hyperinsulinemia has a negative impact on the maturity of the lung's surfactant system by reducing production and manufacturing an unstable surfactant. Polycythemia is another problem for the IDM because of the increased metabolic workload. Hyperinsulinemia and hyperglycemia increase fetal oxygen consumption and may lead to hypoxia, which stimulates the production of erythropoietin. Producing more red blood cells to compensate for the hypoxic environment may decrease the number of platelets produced. Frequency of congenital heart disease in IDM is typically over 50%. Careful evaluation and early diagnosis in this high risk group are needed along with an echocardiogram done on all IDMs as soon as possible (Muhammad et al., 2014).

Assess the newborn for signs of birth trauma involving the head (tense, bulging fontanels, cephalhematoma, skull fractures, and facial nerve paralysis), shoulders and extremities (posturing, paralysis), and skin (bruising). Inspect the newborn for compromised oxygenation by examining the skin for cyanosis, pallor, mottling, and sluggish capillary refill. Take the newborn's temperature frequently and provide a neutral thermal environment to prevent cold stress, which would increase the glucose utilization and contribute to the hypoglycemic state.

LABORATORY AND DIAGNOSTIC TESTING

Determine baseline serum calcium, magnesium, and bilirubin levels and monitor them frequently for changes (Table 24.2). Hypocalcemia is typically manifested in the first 2 to 3 days of life as a result of birth injury or a prolonged delay in parathyroid hormone production. Hypomagnesemia parallels calcium levels and is suspected only when hypocalcemia does not respond to calcium replacement therapy. Red blood cell breakdown leads to increased hematocrit and polycythemia. In addition, hyperbilirubinemia may be caused by slightly decreased extracellular fluid volume, hepatic immaturity, and birth trauma forming enclosed hemorrhages. It can appear

TABLE 24.1	COMMON PROBLEMS OF INFANTS OF MOTHERS WITH DIABETES	
Condition	**Description**	**Effects**
Macrosomia	Newborn with an excessive birth weight; arbitrarily defined as a birth weight >4,000 g (8 lb 13 oz) to 4,500 g (9 lb 15 oz) or >90th percentile for gestational age Complication in 10% of all pregnancies in the United States	Increased risk for shoulder dystocia, traumatic birth injury, birth asphyxia Risks for newborn hypoglycemia and hypomagnesemia, polycythemia, and electrolyte disturbances Increased maternal risk for surgical birth, postpartum hemorrhage and infection, and birth canal lacerations Increased risk of developing type 2 diabetes later in life for both Higher weight and accumulation of fat in childhood and a higher rate of obesity in adults
Respiratory distress syndrome (RDS)	Cortisol-induced stimulation of lecithin/sphingomyelin (phospholipids) necessary for lung maturation is antagonized due to the high-insulin environment within the fetus due to mother's hyperglycemia. Less mature lung development than expected for gestational age Decrease in the phospholipid phosphatidylglycerol (PG), which stabilizes surfactant, compounding risk	Most commonly, baby is breathing normally at birth but develops labored, grunting respiration with cough and a hoarse complaining cry within a few hours, with chest retractions and varying degrees of cyanosis. Infants of mothers with diabetes who also have vascular disease seldom develop RDS because the chronic stress of poor intrauterine perfusion leads to increased production of steroids, which accelerates lung maturation.
Hypoglycemia	Glucose is the major source of energy for organ function. Typical characteristics: • Poor feedings • Jitteriness • Lethargy • High-pitched or weak cry • Apnea • Cyanosis and seizures Some newborns are asymptomatic.	Low blood glucose levels are problematic during the early postbirth period due to abrupt cessation of high-glucose maternal blood supply and the continuation of insulin production by the newborn. Limited ability to release glucagon and catecholamines, which normally stimulate glucagon breakdown and glucose release Prolonged and untreated hypoglycemia leads to serious, long-term adverse neurologic sequelae such as learning disabilities and intellectual disability.
Hypocalcemia and hypomagnesemia	Hypocalcemia (drop in calcium levels) is manifested by tremors, hypotonia, apnea, high-pitched cry, and seizures due to abrupt cessation of maternal transfer of calcium to the fetus, which occurs primarily in the third trimester and if the infant experiences birth asphyxia Associated hypomagnesemia is directly related to the maternal level before birth. About half of infants of mothers with diabetes are affected.	Newborn is at risk for a prolonged delay in parathyroid hormone production and cardiac dysrhythmias.
Polycythemia	Venous hematocrit of >65% in the newborn Increased oxygen consumption by neonate secondary to fetal hyperglycemia and hyperinsulinemia Increased fetal erythropoiesis secondary to intrauterine hypoxia due to placental insufficiency from maternal diabetes Hypoxic stimulation of increased red blood cell (RBC) production as compensatory mechanism	Increased viscosity, resulting in poor blood flow that predisposes newborn to decreased tissue oxygenation and development of microthrombi

(continued)

TABLE 24.1	COMMON PROBLEMS OF INFANTS OF MOTHERS WITH DIABETES (continued)	
Condition	Description	Effects
Hyperbilirubinemia	Usually seen within the first few days after birth; manifested by a yellow appearance of the sclera and skin Excessive red cell hemolysis necessary to break down increased RBCs in circulation due to polycythemia Resultant elevated bilirubin levels Excessive bruising secondary to birth trauma of macrosomic infants, further adding to high bilirubin levels	If untreated, high levels of unconjugated bilirubin may lead to kernicterus (neurologic syndrome that results in irreversible damage) with long-term sequelae that include cerebral palsy, sensorineural hearing loss, and intellectual disability.
Congenital anomalies	Occur in up to 10% of infants of mothers with diabetes, accounting for 30% to 50% of perinatal deaths Incidence is greatest among SGA newborns. Overall, infants of mothers with diabetes have ~3 times the usual incidence of congenital anomalies compared to newborns from the nondiabetic general population.	Most common anomalies: • Coarctation of the aorta • Atrial and ventricular septal defects • Transposition of the great vessels • Sacral agenesis • Hip and joint malformations • Anencephaly • Spina bifida • Caudal dysplasia • Hydrocephalus

Adapted from Davidson, M. R. (2014). *Fast facts for the neonatal nurse: A nursing orientation and care guide in a nutshell.* New York, NY: Springer Publishers; Kenner, C., & Lott, J. W. (2014). *Comprehensive neonatal nursing care* (5th ed.). New York, NY: Springer Publishers; Marcdante, K., & Kliegman, R. M. (2015). *Nelson essentials of pediatrics* (7th ed.). St. Louis, MO: Saunders Elsevier; and Potter, C. F., & Kicklighter, S. D. (2016). Infant of a diabetic mother. *eMedicine.* Retrieved from http://emedicine.medscape.com/article/974230-overview

within the first 24 hours of life (pathologic) or after 24 hours of life (physiologic).

Nursing Management

The focus of care for these infants is early detection and initiation of therapy to address potential problems (Nursing Care Plan 24.1). Perform a head-to-toe physical assessment to identify congenital anomalies. Institute measures to correct hypoglycemia, hypocalcemia, hypomagnesemia,

dehydration, and jaundice. Provide oxygenation and ventilatory support as necessary. The focus of care includes correcting hypoglycemia, and hypocalcemia, providing phototherapy for jaundice, administering fluid therapy and maintaining oxygen and ventilation if required.

PREVENTING HYPOGLYCEMIA

Prevent hypoglycemia by providing early oral feedings with breast milk or formula at frequent intervals (every 2 to 3 hours). Feedings help to control glucose levels,

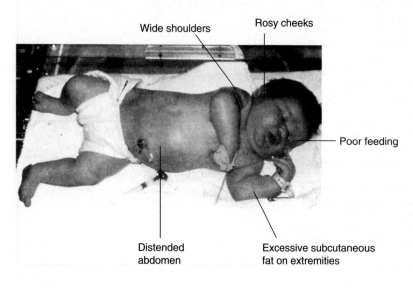

Wide shoulders
Rosy cheeks
Poor feeding
Distended abdomen
Excessive subcutaneous fat on extremities

FIGURE 24.6 Characteristics of an infant of a diabetic mother (IDM). A macrosomic IDM has head circumference and length that are at the 90th percentile; the IDM's body weight greatly exceeds the 90th percentile. The IDM has considerable fat deposition in the shoulder and intrascapular area. (MacDonald, M. G., Seshia, M. M. K., & Mullett, M. D. [2005]. *Avery's neonatology pathophysiology & management of the newborn* [6th ed.]. Philadelphia, PA: Lippincott Williams & Wilkins.)

TABLE 24.2	CRITICAL LABORATORY VALUES FOR INFANTS OF MOTHERS WITH DIABETES
Hypoglycemia	<50 mg/dL
Hypocalcemia	<7 mg/dL
Hypomagnesemia	<1.5 mg/dL
Hyperbilirubinemia	>12 mg/dL (term infant)
Polycythemia	>65% (venous hematocrit)

Adapted from Potter, C. F., & Kicklighter, S. D. (2016). Infant of a diabetic mother. *eMedicine*. Retrieved from http://emedicine.med-scape.com/article/974230-overview; Davidson, M. R. (2014). *Fast facts for the neonatal nurse: A nursing orientation and care guide in a nutshell*. New York, NY: Springer Publishers; Kenner, C., & Lott, J. W. (2014). *Comprehensive neonatal nursing care* (5th ed.). New York, NY: Springer Publishers; and King, T. L., Brucker, M. C., Kriebs, J. M., Fahey, J. O., Gegor, C. L., & Varney, H. (2015). *Varney's midwifery* (5th ed.). Burlington, MA: Jones & Bartlett Learning.

reduce hematocrit, and promote bilirubin excretion. Maintain a neutral thermal environment to avoid cold stress, which may stimulate the metabolic rate, thereby increasing the demand for glucose. Provide rest periods to decrease energy demand and expenditure.

Monitor blood glucose levels via heel stick every hour for the first 4 hours of life and then every 3 to 4 hours until stable. Document the results. Report unstable glucose values if oral feedings do not maintain and stabilize the newborn's blood glucose levels. If glucose levels are not stabilized, initiate intravenous glucose infusions as ordered and ensure that the infusions are flowing at the prescribed rate.

MAINTAINING FLUID AND ELECTROLYTE BALANCE

Monitor serum calcium levels for changes indicating the need for supplementation, such as with oral or intravenous calcium gluconate. Assess the newborn for signs of hypocalcemia, such as tremors, jitteriness, twitching, seizures, and high-pitched cry.

Also administer fluid therapy as ordered to maintain adequate hydration. Monitor serum bilirubin levels and institute phototherapy if the newborn is over 24 hours old.

PROVIDING PARENTAL SUPPORT

Good communication between the nurse and the family is essential. It should be supported by evidence-based, written information tailored to meet the woman's individual needs. Assist the parents and family in understanding the newborn's condition and need for frequent monitoring. Offer support and information to the parents and family about the benefits of breast-feeding for herself and the infant. They may erroneously interpret the newborn's large size as an indication that the newborn is free of problems.

Encourage open communication and listen with empathy to the family's fears and concerns. Provide frequent opportunities for the parents to interact with their newborn. Make appropriate referrals to social services and community resources as necessary to help the family cope.

Birth Trauma

Injuries to the newborn from the forces of labor and birth are categorized as birth trauma. In the past, numerous injuries were associated with difficult births requiring external or internal version or mid- or high forceps deliveries. Today, however, cesarean births have contributed to the decline in birth trauma. Damage occurs to the tissues and organs of the newborn caused by mechanical forces during childbirth often accompanied by impaired blood circulation and organ functioning. The most frequent and significant birth injuries are to the skull, brain, and spinal cord (Malcolm, 2015).

Significant birth trauma accounts for fewer than 3% of neonatal deaths and stillbirths in the United States. They estimate that birth trauma in the United States occurs in approximately 29 per 1,000 births with the three most frequently diagnosed birth trauma conditions being injuries to the scalp, injuries to the skeleton, and fracture of the clavicle (Laroia, 2015). Improved prenatal diagnosis and monitoring during labor have helped to reduce the incidence of birth injuries today.

Pathophysiology

The process of birth is a blend of compression, contractions, torques, and traction. When fetal size, presentation, or neurologic immunity complicates this process, the forces of labor and birth may lead to tissue damage, edema, hemorrhages, or fractures in the newborn. For example, birth trauma may result from the pressure of birth, especially in a prolonged or abrupt labor, abnormal or difficult presentation, cephalopelvic disproportion, or mechanical forces, such as forceps or vacuum used during delivery. Table 24.3 summarizes the most common types of birth trauma.

Nursing Assessment

Recognition of trauma and birth injuries is imperative so that early treatment can be initiated. Review the labor and birth history for risk factors, such as a prolonged or abrupt labor, abnormal or difficult presentation, cephalopelvic disproportion, or mechanical forces, such as forceps or vacuum used during delivery. Also review the history for multiple fetus deliveries, large-for-date infants, extreme prematurity, large fetal head, or newborns with congenital anomalies.

Complete a careful physical and neurologic assessment of every newborn admitted to the nursery to

NURSING CARE PLAN 24.1

Overview of the Infant of a Mother with Diabetes

Jamie, a 38-year-old Hispanic woman, gave birth to a term large-for-gestational-age newborn weighing 10 lb. She had a history of gestational diabetes but had not received any prenatal care. She arrived at the hospital in active labor. Despite macrosomia, the newborn's Apgar scores were 8 and 9 at 1 and 5 minutes, respectively. No resuscitative measures were needed.

One hour after birth, assessment revealed a pale, irritable newborn with sweating and several episodes of apnea. A glucose level obtained at this time via a heel stick was 35 mg/dL. Two hours later, the newborn begins exhibiting signs of respiratory distress—grunting, nasal flaring, retractions, tachypnea (respiratory rate 72 breaths/minute), and tachycardia (heart rate 176 bpm).

NURSING DIAGNOSIS: Risk for unstable glucose level related to hypoglycemia secondary to intrauterine hyperinsulinemic state resulting from maternal gestational diabetes as evidenced by low blood glucose level, irritability, pallor, sweating, and apnea.

Outcome Identification and Evaluation

The newborn will exhibit adequate glucose control as evidenced by maintaining blood glucose levels above 40 mg/dL and an absence of clinical signs of hypoglycemia.

Interventions: *Promoting Glucose Control*

- Monitor blood glucose levels hourly for the first 4 hours and then every 3 to 4 hours or as necessary *to detect hypoglycemia, which would be <40 mg/dL.*
- Continue to observe for manifestations of hypoglycemia, such as pallor, tremors, jitteriness, lethargy, and poor feeding, to allow for early *detection and prompt intervention, thereby minimizing the risk of complications associated with hypoglycemia.*
- Monitor temperature frequently and institute measures to maintain a neutral thermal environment *to prevent cold stress, which would increase metabolic demands and further deplete glycogen stores.*
- Initiate early feedings every 2 to 3 hours or as appropriate or administer glucose supplements

as ordered to prevent hypoglycemia caused by the newborn's *hyperinsulinemic state.* Administer IV glucose infusions as ordered *to correct hypoglycemia if glucose levels do not stabilize with feeding.*
- Cluster infant care activities and provide for rest periods *to conserve the newborn's energy and reduce use of glucose and glycogen stores.*
- Reduce environmental stimuli by dimming lights and speaking softly *to reduce energy demands and further utilization of glucose.*
- Explain all events and procedures to the mother *to help alleviate anxiety and promote understanding of the newborn's condition.*

NURSING DIAGNOSIS: Impaired gas exchange related to respiratory distress secondary to delayed lung maturity resulting from inhibition of pulmonary surfactant production due to fetal hyperinsulinemia as evidenced by grunting, nasal flaring, retractions, tachypnea, and tachycardia.

Outcome Identification and Evaluation

The newborn will demonstrate signs of adequate oxygenation without respiratory distress as evidenced by respiratory rate and vital signs within acceptable parameters, absence of nasal flaring, retractions, and grunting, and oxygen saturation and ABG levels within acceptable parameters.

Interventions: *Promoting Oxygenation*

- Monitor newborn's vital signs to establish a baseline and evaluate for changes.
- Assess airway patency and perform gentle suctioning as ordered to ensure patency and allow for adequate oxygen intake.
- Position the newborn prone to optimize respiratory status and reduce stress.

NURSING CARE PLAN 24.1

Overview of the Infant of a Mother with Diabetes (continued)

- Assess lung sounds for changes to allow early detection of change in status.
- Continuously monitor oxygen saturation levels via pulse oximetry to determine adequacy of tissue perfusion.
- Assess ABG results to detect changes indicating acidosis, hypoxemia, or hypercarbia, which would suggest hypoxia. Administer medications as ordered to correct acidosis.
- Administer oxygen as ordered to promote adequate tissue perfusion.
- Assess newborn's skin to identify cyanosis, pallor, and mottling to detect changes indicating compromised oxygenation.
- Administer surfactant replacement therapy as ordered to aid in stabilizing the newborn's lungs until postnatal surfactant synthesis improves.
- Institute measures to maintain normal blood glucose levels and a neutral thermal environment, cluster care activities, and reduce excessive stimuli to reduce oxygen demand and consumption.

---

establish whether injuries exist. Inspect the head for lumps, bumps, or bruises. Note if swelling or bruising crosses the suture line. Assess the eyes and face for facial paralysis, observing for asymmetry of the face with crying or appearance of the mouth being drawn to the unaffected side. Ensure that the newborn spontaneously moves all extremities. Note any absence of or decrease in deep tendon reflexes or abnormal positioning of extremities.

Assess and document symmetry of structure and function. Be prepared to assist with scheduling diagnostic studies to confirm trauma or injuries, which will be important in determining treatment modalities.

Nursing Management

Nursing management is primarily supportive and focuses on assessing for resolution of the trauma or any associated complications along with providing support and education to the parents. Provide the parents with explanations and reassurance that these injuries usually resolve with minimal or no treatment. Parents are alarmed when their newborn is unable to move an extremity or demonstrates asymmetric facial movements. Provide parents with a realistic picture of the situation to gain their understanding and trust. Be readily available to answer questions and teach them how to care for the newborn, including any modifications that might be necessary. Allow parents adequate time to understand the implications of the birth trauma or injury and what treatment modalities are needed, if any. Provide them with information about the length of time until the injury will resolve and when and if they need to seek further medical attention for the condition. Spending time with the parents and providing them with support, information, and teaching are important to allow them to make decisions and care for their newborn. Anticipate the need for community referral for ongoing follow-up and care, if necessary.

Newborns of Substance-Abusing Mothers

It is generally assumed that all pregnant women want to provide a healthy environment for their unborn child and know how to avoid harm. However, women who use tobacco, alcohol, or illicit substances during pregnancy place themselves and their newborns at risk for numerous complications before and after birth. Perinatal substance abuse is a persistent and significant public health issue particularly affecting children, with high rates of reported abuse, neglect, and foster care placement. The illicit drug abuse will only worsen as the use and misuse of prescription medications are significantly increasing in the United States.

Substance use during pregnancy also exposes the fetus to the possibility of IUGR, prematurity, neurobehavioral and neurophysiologic dysfunction, birth defects, infections, and long-term developmental sequelae. Infants of mothers who abuse substances are more likely to suffer substantiated harm, enter foster care, and have more negative child protection outcomes. The effects of fetal alcohol spectrum disorders (FASD) are well documented in the literature; studies attest to developmental delays, intellectual disabilities, attention disorders, and psychopathologies during the child's lifetime (AAP, 2015).

The full extent of the effects of prenatal drug exposure on a child is not known. However studies show that various drugs of abuse may result in premature birth, miscarriage, low birth weight, and a variety of behavioral

(text continues on page 894)

TABLE 24.3	COMMON TYPES OF BIRTH TRAUMA		
Type	**Description**	**Findings**	**Treatment**
Fractures	Most often occur during breech births or shoulder dystocia in newborns with macrosomia Midclavicular fractures are the most common type of fracture, secondary to shoulder dystocia. Long bone fractures of the humerus or femur, usually midshaft, also can occur.	Midclavicular fractures: the newborn is irritable and does not move the arm on the affected side either spontaneously or when the Moro reflex is elicited. Femoral or humeral long bone fractures: the newborn shows loss of spontaneous leg or arm motion, respectively; usually swelling and pain accompany the limited movement. X-rays confirm the fracture.	Midclavicular fractures typically heal rapidly and uneventfully; arm motion may be limited by pinning the newborn's sleeve to the shirt. Femoral and humeral shaft fractures are treated with splinting. Healing and complete recovery are expected within 2–4 weeks without incident. Explanation to the parents and reassurance are needed.
Brachial plexus injury	Primarily in large babies, babies with shoulder dystocia, or breech delivery Results from stretching, hemorrhage within a nerve, or tearing of the nerve or the roots associated with cervical cord injury Associated traumatic injuries include fracture of the clavicle or humerus or subluxations of the shoulder or cervical spine. Erb's palsy is an upper brachial plexus injury. Klumpke's palsy is an injury to the lower brachial plexus (lower brachial injuries are less common).	In Erb's palsy, the involved extremity usually presents adducted, prone, and internally rotated; shoulder movement is absent; Moro, bicep, and radial reflexes are absent, but the grasp reflex is usually present. Klumpke's palsy is manifested by weakness in the hand and wrist; grasp reflex is absent.	Erb's palsy usually involves immobilization of the upper arm across the upper abdomen/chest to protect the shoulder from excessive motion for the first week; then gentle passive range-of-motion exercises are performed daily to prevent contractures. There is usually no associated sensory loss, and this condition usually improves rapidly. Treatment for Klumpke's palsy involves placing the hand in a neutral position and using passive range-of-motion exercises. In some cases deficits may persist, requiring continuing observation.
Cranial nerve trauma	Most common is facial nerve palsy. Frequently attributed to pressure resulting from forceps May also result from pressure on the nerve in utero, related to fetal positioning such as the head lying against the shoulder	Physical findings include asymmetry of the face when crying; mouth may be drawn toward the unaffected side; wrinkles are deeper on the unaffected side. The paralyzed side may be smooth, with a swollen appearance. Eye is persistently open on the affected side.	Most infants begin to recover in the first week, but full resolution may take up to several months; parents need reassurance about this. In most cases, treatment is not necessary, only observation. If the eye is affected and unable to close, protection with patches and synthetic tears may be necessary. Parents need instruction about how to feed the newborn, since he or she cannot close the lips around the nipple without having milk seep out.

TABLE 24.3	COMMON TYPES OF BIRTH TRAUMA (continued)		
Type	**Description**	**Findings**	**Treatment**
Head trauma	Mild trauma can cause soft tissue injuries such as cephalhematoma and caput succedaneum; greater trauma can cause depressed skull fractures. **Cephalhematoma** (subperiosteal collection of blood secondary to the rupture of blood vessels between the skull and periosteum) occurs in 2.5% of all births and typically appears within hours after birth. **Caput succedaneum** (soft tissue swelling) is caused by edema of the head against the dilating cervix during the birth process. Subarachnoid hemorrhage (one of the most common types of intracranial trauma) may be due to hypoxia/ischemia, variations in blood pressure, and the pressure exerted on the head during labor. Bleeding is of venous origin, and underlying contusions also may occur. Subdural hemorrhage (hematomas) occurs less often today because of improved obstetric techniques. Typically, tears of the major veins or venous sinuses overlying the cerebral hemispheres or cerebellum (most common in newborns of primigravida and large newborns, or after an instrumented birth) are the cause. Increased pressure on the blood vessels inside the skull leads to tears. Depressed skull fractures (rare) may result from the pressure of a forceps delivery; can also occur during spontaneous or cesarean births and may be associated with other head trauma causing subdural bleeding, subarachnoid hemorrhage, or brain trauma.	In cephalhematoma, suture lines delineate its extent; usually located on one side, over the parietal bone. In caput succedaneum, swelling is not limited by suture lines: it extends across the midline and is associated with head molding. It does not usually cause complications other than a misshapen head. Swelling is maximal at birth and then rapidly decreases in size. In subarachnoid hemorrhage, some RBCs may appear in the cerebrospinal fluid (CSF) of full-term newborns. Newborns may present with apnea, seizures, lethargy, or abnormal findings on a neurologic examination. Subdural hemorrhage can be asymptomatic, or the neonate can exhibit seizures, enlarging head size, decreased level of consciousness, or abnormal findings on a neurologic examination, with hypotonia, a poor Moro reflex, or extensive retinal hemorrhages. Depressed skull fractures can be observed and palpated as depressions. Confirmation by x-ray is necessary.	Cephalhematoma resolves gradually over 2–3 weeks without treatment (see Chapter 18). Caput succedaneum usually resolves over the first few days without treatment (see Chapter 18). Subarachnoid hemorrhage requires minimal handling to reduce stress. Subdural hematoma requires aspiration; it can be life-threatening if it is in an inaccessible location and cannot be aspirated. Depressed skull fractures typically require a neurosurgical consultation.

Adapted from Cunningham, F. G., Leveno, K. J., Bloom, S. L., Spong, C. Y., Dashe, J. S., Hoffman, B. L., et al. (2014). *Williams' obstetrics* (24th ed.). New York, NY: McGraw-Hill; Davidson, M. R. (2014). *Fast facts for the neonatal nurse: A nursing orientation and care guide in a nutshell.* New York, NY: Springer Publishers; Laroia, N. (2015). Birth trauma. *eMedicine.* Retrieved from http://emedicine.medscape.com/article/980112-overview; and Verklan, M. T., & Walden, M. (2014). *Core curriculum for neonatal intensive care nursing* (5th ed.). St. Louis, MO: Saunders Elsevier.

and cognitive problems. It is difficult to establish the true prevalence of substance use in pregnant women; many women deny taking any nonprescribed substance because of the associated social stigma and legal implications. The National Institute on Drug Abuse (NIDA, 2015) suggests that approximately 6% of pregnant women 15 to 44 years old use illicit drugs. In the United States, approximately 225,000 infants yearly are exposed to illicit substances. Drug exposure may go unrecognized in these newborns, and they may be discharged from the newborn nursery at risk for medical and social problems, including abuse and neglect.

Tobacco, alcohol, and marijuana are the substances most commonly abused during pregnancy. The incidence of drug and alcohol abuse has increased dramatically during the past decade due to an increase in prenatal maternal opiate use. Other drugs may include opioids such as morphine, codeine, methadone, SSRIs, meperidine, and heroin; central nervous system stimulants such as methamphetamines and cocaine; central nervous system depressants such as barbiturates, diazepam (Valium), and sedative-hypnotics; and hallucinogens, such as lysergic acid diethylamide (LSD), inhalants, glue, paint thinner, nail polish remover, and nitrous oxide (NIDA, 2015). Table 24.4 highlights commonly used substances and their effects on the fetus and newborn.

Substance abuse during pregnancy is the subject of much controversy. The type of substance used, the timing of use during embryogenesis and fetal development, and the duration and amount used all contribute to the impact on a woman's pregnancy and to the fetal and newborn effects. Frequently, the woman uses more than one substance, which compounds the problem. Nurses must be knowledgeable about the issues of substance abuse and must be alert for opportunities to identify, prevent, manage, and educate women and families about this key public health issue.

Fetal Alcohol Spectrum Disorders

Alcohol abuse during pregnancy is currently among the fastest growing health care challenges in the United States. Years ago, alcohol was not commonly recognized as a teratogen, an agent that can disrupt the development of a fetus. Today, it is known that prenatal alcohol exposure induces a variety of adverse effects on physical, neurologic, and behavioral development. Alcohol now is recognized as the leading preventable cause of birth defects and developmental disorders in the United States (Glass, Ware, & Mattson, 2014). The adverse effects of alcohol consumption have been recognized for centuries, but the associated pattern of fetal anomalies was not labeled until the early 1970s. The distinctive pattern identified three specific findings: a distinct pattern of facial dysmorphology, pre- and postnatal growth deficiencies, and central nervous system dysfunction. These distinctive findings are called **fetal alcohol spectrum disorders (FASD)**, characterized by physical and mental disorders that appear at birth and remain problematic throughout the child's life. However, there are also circumstances in which the effects of prenatal alcohol exposure are apparent but the newborn does not meet all of the criteria. In an attempt to include those who do not meet the strict criteria, the terms *fetal alcohol effects*, *alcohol-related birth defects*, and *alcohol-related neurologic defects* are used to describe children with a variety of problems thought to be related to alcohol consumption during pregnancy. The Institutes of Medicine coined the term FASD as a way of describing the broader effects of prenatal alcohol exposure. Children with fetal alcohol syndrome (FAS) are at the severe end of the spectrum.

The disabilities associated with FASD can persist throughout life and place heavy emotional and financial burdens on individuals, families, and society (Artigas, 2015). Newborns with some but not all of the symptoms of FAS are described as having **alcohol-related birth defects** (ARBD). Fetal alcohol effects (FAE) may include such problems as low birth weight, developmental delays, and hyperactivity. The term FASD refers to a spectrum of conditions that includes FAS, FAE, alcohol-related neurodevelopmental disorder (ARND), and ARBD. Although disorders within the spectrum can be diagnosed, the term FASD itself is not intended for use as a clinical diagnosis (Substance Abuse and Mental Health Services Administration, 2015). Box 24.2 summarizes the manifestations of FAS.

Worldwide, the incidence of FAS is 1 to 3 cases per 1,000 live births, and that of FAE is 3 to 5 per 1,000 live births. About one in eight women drink alcohol during pregnancy (March of Dimes, 2015a). Current estimates indicate that approximately 19% of women of childbearing age are either problem drinkers or alcoholics; therefore, the number of fetuses exposed to alcohol in utero increases dramatically (March of Dimes, 2015a). Alcohol consumption during pregnancy results in brain, craniofacial, and heart defects, neurotoxicity, and immune dysfunction. The preferred action taken to prevent alcohol consumption during pregnancy is abstinence. However, the detection, diagnosis, and treatment of FASD remain major public health needs in this country and throughout the world. Despite the preventable nature of alcohol ingestion during pregnancy, the prevalence of alcohol consumption is increasing around the world. In addition, the majority of pregnancies are unintended, thus women are consuming alcohol while they are pregnant and are not even aware of the harm of it (Popova & Chambers, 2014).

Alcohol in the maternal circulation crosses the placenta, which results in direct fetal exposure. The mechanism of fetal exposure is likely related to three main factors: a teratogenic effect, hypoxia as a result of increased oxygen consumption, and a diminished ability

(text continues on page 898)

TABLE 24.4	SUBSTANCES AND THEIR EFFECTS ON THE FETUS AND NEWBORN		
Substance	**Description**	**Effects on Fetus and Newborn**	**Nursing Implications**
Alcohol	Consumption is pervasive and widely accepted, with use, abuse, and addiction affecting all levels of society. It is a common misconception that a substance sold to the public without restriction is safe.	Fetal alcohol syndrome (one of the most common known causes of intellectual disability) Fetal alcohol spectrum disorders Alcohol-related birth defects: Facial features—flattened philtrum (groove in upper lip up to nose), thin upper lip, short palpebral; growth deficit—in weight, height, and BMI; structural/functional CNS dysfunction—microcephaly, intellectual disability, psychiatric conditions, language, motor, and memory disorders. Symptoms of alcohol withdrawal: Hyperactivity, jitteriness, hyperreflexia, hypertonia, poor suck, tremors, seizures, poor sleep patterns, and diaphoresis	Provide education that decreasing or eliminating alcohol consumption during pregnancy is the only way to prevent fetal alcohol syndrome and fetal alcohol effects. Assist pregnant woman in finding a treatment program if possible. Inform all women who are pregnant or planning to become pregnant about the detrimental effects of alcohol during pregnancy. Educate women using a nonjudgmental, culturally connected approach. Warn women that there is no safe time to drink and that there is no safe amount of alcohol they can consume.
Tobacco/nicotine	Nicotine is an addictive substance. It causes epinephrine release from the adrenal cortex, leading to initial stimulation followed by depression and fatigue, causing the user to seek more nicotine. Increased numbers of women are smoking (at least 11% smoke during pregnancy). Over 2,500 chemicals are found in cigarette smoke, including nicotine, tar, carbon monoxide, and cyanide. It is unknown which are harmful, but nicotine and carbon monoxide are believed to play a role in causing adverse pregnancy outcomes.	Impaired oxygenation of mother and fetus due to nicotine crossing placenta and carbon monoxide combining with hemoglobin Increased risk for low birth weight (risk almost doubled), small for gestational age, and preterm birth Increased risk for sudden infant death syndrome (SIDS) and chronic respiratory illness	Provide teaching to women about healthy behaviors. Provide support for smoking cessation. Individualize counseling based on factors associated with the woman's smoking and challenges faced (why woman smokes, stressors in life, and social support network). Suggest options such as group smoking cessation programs, relaxation techniques, individual counseling, hypnosis, and partner-support counseling.
Marijuana	Most widely used illicit psychoactive substance in Western world and most commonly used illicit drug in the United States Derived from *Cannabis sativa* plant	Not shown to have teratogenic effects on fetus; no consistent types of malformations identified Fetal growth restriction is common due to delivery of carbon monoxide to fetus Increased risk for small for gestational age	Provide teaching to women about healthy behaviors. Provide support for cessation of marijuana use.

(continued)

TABLE 24.4	SUBSTANCES AND THEIR EFFECTS ON THE FETUS AND NEWBORN (continued)		
Substance	Description	Effects on Fetus and Newborn	Nursing Implications
		Altered responses to visual stimuli, sleep-pattern abnormalities, photophobia, lack of motor control, hyperirritability, increased tremulousness, and high-pitched cry noted in infants of mothers who smoked marijuana Research on long-term effects is continuing	
Methamphetamines	Addictive stimulant; use releases high levels of dopamine, which stimulates brain cells, enhancing mood and body movement High potential for abuse and addiction; can be inhaled, injected, smoked, or taken orally Many street names, such as speed, meth, ice, and chalk Primary effects include accelerated heart and respiratory rate, elevated blood pressure, papillary dilation; secondary effects include loss of appetite. Used medically as treatment for obesity and narcolepsy in adults and hyperactivity in children	Little research on use during pregnancy because its use is less common than cocaine or narcotics Fetal effects similar to cocaine (suggesting vasoconstriction as possible underlying mechanism) Possible maternal malnutrition, leading to problems with fetal growth and development Increased risk for preterm birth and low-birth-weight newborns Infants may have withdrawal symptoms, including dysphoria, agitation, jitteriness, poor weight gain, abnormal sleep patterns, poor feeding, frantic fist sucking, high-pitched cry, respiratory distress soon after birth, frequent infections, and significant lassitude. Long-term effects are not known.	Provide teaching to women about healthy behaviors. Provide support for cessation of methamphetamine use. Monitor the woman for weight changes; emphasize the need for adequate nutritional intake to support fetal growth and development.
Cocaine	Strong CNS stimulant that interferes with reabsorption of dopamine Physical effects: vasoconstriction; pupillary dilation; increased temperature, heart rate, and blood pressure Taken orally, sublingually, intranasally, intravenously, and via inhalation Estimated that 30%–40% of cocaine addicts are female Maternal cocaine use during pregnancy is a significant health problem Increased potential for use of multiple drugs if mother using cocaine	Preterm birth and lower birth weight Unclear impact on later development Speculation that cocaine interferes with infant's cognitive development, leading to learning and memory difficulties later in life Associated congenital anomalies: GU, cardiac, and CNS defects, and prune belly syndrome Other typical newborn characteristics: smaller head circumference, piercing cry (indicative of neurologic dysfunction), limb defects, ambiguous genitalia, poor feeding, poor visual and auditory responses, poor sleep patterns, decreased impulse control, stiff, hyperextended positioning, irritability and hypersensitivity (hard to console when crying), inability to respond to caretaker	Educate the woman about the effects of cocaine use on the fetus and newborn. Assess for use of other substances. Provide teaching to women about healthy behaviors. Provide support and guidance for cessation of cocaine and other substance use.

TABLE 24.4	SUBSTANCES AND THEIR EFFECTS ON THE FETUS AND NEWBORN (continued)		
Substance	**Description**	**Effects on Fetus and Newborn**	**Nursing Implications**
Heroin	Illegal, highly addictive opiate derived from morphine that can be sniffed, smoked, or injected Possible consequences include HIV infection, tuberculosis, crime, violence, and family disruption. Severe physical addiction; CNS depressant producing mental dullness and drowsiness	Newborns of heroin-addicted mothers are born dependent on heroin. Increased risk for transmission of hepatitis B and C and HIV to newborns when mothers share needles Significantly increased rates of stillbirth, IUGR, preterm birth, and newborn mortality (3–7 times greater) Small-for-gestational-age newborns, meconium aspiration, high incidence of SIDS, and delayed effects from subacute withdrawal (restlessness, continual crying, agitation, sneezing, vomiting, fever, diarrhea, seizures, irritability, and poor socialization [possibly persisting for 4–6 months]) Intrauterine death or preterm birth is possible with abrupt cessation of heroin use.	Educate the woman about the effects of heroin use on the fetus and newborn. Assess for use of other substances. Provide teaching to women about healthy behaviors. Warn the woman not to abruptly stop heroin use. Encourage her to enroll in a methadone maintenance program.
Methadone	Synthetic opiate narcotic used primarily as maintenance therapy for heroin addiction	Improvement in many of the detrimental fetal effects associated with heroin use Withdrawal symptoms are common in newborns. Possible low birth weight due to symmetric fetal growth restriction Increased severity and longer period of withdrawal (due to methadone's longer half-life) Seizures (commonly severe) do not usually occur until 2–3 weeks of age, when the newborn is at home. Increased rate of SIDS (3–4 times higher)	Methadone maintenance programs are the standard of care for women with narcotic addiction. Inform the woman about the benefits and risks of methadone use vs. heroin use. Advantages include improved fetal and newborn growth, reduced risk of fetal death, and reduced risk of HIV infections. Advise the woman that she will need to return consistently to receive the prescribed methadone dose. Reinforce the need for continued prenatal care. Inform the woman that she can breast-feed her newborn while receiving methadone. Teach mother and caregivers about signs and symptoms of methadone withdrawal.

Adapted from Centers for Disease Control and Prevention [CDC]. (2015b). *Fetal alcohol spectrum disorders.* Retrieved from http://www.cdc.gov/ncbddd/fasd/facts.html; Cunningham, F. G., Leveno, K. J., Bloom, S. L., Spong, C. Y., Dashe, J. S., Hoffman, B. L., et al. (2014). *Williams' obstetrics* (24th ed.). New York, NY: McGraw-Hill; Dörrie, N., Föcker, M., Freunscht, I., & Hebebrand, J. (2014). Fetal alcohol spectrum disorders. *European Child & Adolescent Psychiatry, 23*(10), 863–875; and Kocherlakota, P. (2014). Neonatal abstinence syndrome. *Pediatrics, 134*(2), e547–e561.

BOX 24.2

CLINICAL PICTURE OF FETAL ALCOHOL SYNDROME

- Microcephaly (head circumference <10th percentile)*
- Small palpebral (eyelid) fissures*
- Abnormally small eyes
- Intrauterine growth restriction
- Maxillary hypoplasia (flattened or absent)
- Epicanthal folds (folds of skin of the upper eyelid over the eye)
- Thin upper lip*
- Missing vertical groove in median portion of upper lip*
- Short upturned nose
- Short birth length and low birth weight
- Joint and limb defects
- Altered palmar crease pattern
- Prenatal or postnatal growth ≤10th percentile*
- Congenital cardiac defects (septal defects)
- Delayed fine and gross motor development
- Poor eye–hand coordination
- Clinically significant brain abnormalities*
- Intellectual disability
- Narrow forehead
- Performance substantially below expected level in cognitive or developmental functioning, executive or motor functioning, and attention or hyperactivity; social or language skills*
- Inadequate sucking reflex and poor appetite

*Diagnosis of fetal alcohol syndrome requires the presence of three findings:
1 Documentation of all three facial abnormalities
2 Documentation of growth deficits (height, weight, or both below 10th percentile)
3 Documentation of central nervous system abnormalities (structural, neurologic, or functional)

Adapted from Centers for Disease Control and Prevention [CDC]. (2015b). *Fetal alcohol spectrum disorders.* Retrieved from http://www.cdc.gov/ncbddd/fasd/facts.html; Hamdan, A. H. (2015). Neonatal abstinence syndrome. *eMedicine.* Retrieved from http://emedicine.medscape.com/article/978763-overview; and Substance Abuse and Mental Health Services Administration [SAMHSA]. (2015). *Fetal alcohol spectrum disorders.* Retrieved from http://fasdcenter.samhsa.gov/fasdfaqs.aspx

to use amino acids in protein synthesis. The expression of fetal alcohol exposure ranges from subtle to extreme and depends on the timing of exposure, the dose, length of exposure, and the genetic sensitivity of the fetus to the effects of alcohol (Centers for Disease Control and Prevention [CDC], 2015a).

FAS is one of the most common known causes of nongenetic intellectual disability, and it is the only cause that is entirely preventable. Recent studies suggest that deficits in attention, learning, impaired social cognition, and memory, emotional dysregulation, and executive functioning are core deficits present (Rangmar et al., 2015). The effects last a lifetime. Children with this syndrome have varying degrees of psychological and

behavioral problems and often find it difficult to hold a job and live independently. There is no cure for FASD, but research shows that early intervention treatment services can improve a child's development.

Decreasing or eliminating alcohol consumption during pregnancy is the only way to prevent fetal alcohol syndrome and fetal alcohol effects. No level of alcohol has been proven to be safe for the fetus, so alcohol should be completely avoided when planning for conception and during pregnancy and it is not recommended during breastfeeding. Nurses are in prime positions for primary prevention of FASD through work with women of childbearing age and secondary prevention through work with affected individuals whose lives can be greatly improved via tailored intervention. Women are frequently more receptive to making lifestyle changes during pregnancy than any other time during their lives. Offering nonjudgmental advice that can be easily understood is more effective than mass media in motivating women to choose to stop drinking. When more than a million infants are born each year with permanent brain damage from a known and preventable cause, a nurse's response should be immediate, determined, sustained, and educational for mothers who drink. Actions at every level of society are needed to encourage abstinence from alcohol during pregnancy to prevent its devastating impact.

Neonatal Abstinence Syndrome

Neonatal abstinence syndrome (NAS) comprises a constellation of drug-withdrawal symptoms that result from chronic intrauterine exposure to a variety of substances, including opioids, barbiturates, SSRIs, alcohol, benzodiazepines, caffeine, and nicotine. More than 6% of all live births occur in women who use illicit drugs during pregnancy. Maternal substance abuse is associated with adverse neonatal outcomes. Newborns of women who abuse tobacco, illicit substances (heroin, methamphetamines), prescription drugs (fentanyl, OxyContin, methadone, SSRIs, morphine, meperidine), caffeine, and alcohol can exhibit withdrawal behavior. These substances cross the placenta and may cause the fetus to develop a dependency; when fetal exposure to the substance(s) terminates at birth, the newborn is at risk for a spectrum of withdrawal symptoms (e.g., autonomic dysfunction, respiratory distress, gastrointestinal compromise) that may necessitate prolonged treatment, intensive monitoring, and extended hospitalization. Withdrawal symptoms usually result when an abrupt discontinuation of an addicting drug occurs, usually after prolonged drug exposure. Drug-exposed newborns begin a withdrawal process of varying degrees after birth.

Primary treatment for NAS consists of opioid replacement therapy with either morphine or methadone. Buprenorphine is emerging as a treatment option with promising results. Most nonopioid fetal drug exposures result in limited clinical manifestations, respond well to supportive care measures, and rarely require pharmacologic intervention. However, chronic opioid exposure does require pharmacotherapy to mitigate withdrawal signs in the newborn, especially when there has been maternal polysubstance consumption (Wiles et al., 2014).

NAS can be described as a generalized multisystem disorder of the drug-exposed newborn, which progresses to seizures. It manifests by central nervous system irritability, short, irregular sleep patterns, myoclonic jerks, gastrointestinal dysfunction—excessive sucking, poor feeding, vomiting, loose stools, poor weight gain, excessive, high-pitched crying, sleep and feeding disturbances, increased muscle tone and tremors, seizures, and excessive sneezing, yawning, and nasal stuffiness (Artigas, 2015). Although often treated as a single entity, NAS is not a single pathologic condition. The manifestations of withdrawal are a function of the drug's half-life, the specific drug or combination of drugs used, dosage, route of administration, timing of drug exposure, and length of drug exposure (Hamdan, 2015). NAS has both medical and developmental consequences for the newborn.

Nursing Assessment

A comprehensive prenatal medical and drug history, especially with respect to polydrug use, is vital. Fear of referral to child welfare agencies or the legal system has prompted women to conceal their drug abuse history. Frequently, the first inkling of drug use appears in the newborn when symptoms of withdrawal begin within 72 hours after birth. Typically the infant has been discharged by this time, unless the nurse has a high degree of suspicion that would prompt toxicology testing earlier. Several assessment tools can be used to assess a drug-exposed newborn. Figure 24.7 shows an example. Regardless of the tool used for assessment, address these key areas:

- Maternal history to identify risk behaviors for substance abuse:
  - Previous unexplained fetal demise
  - Lack of prenatal care
  - Incarceration
  - Prostitution
  - Cigarette smoking
  - Fetal growth restriction
  - Mental health disorders
  - History of intimate partner violence
  - History of missed prenatal appointments
  - Severe mood swings
  - Preterm birth
  - History of sexually transmitted infections (STIs) (hepatitis C and human immunodeficiency virus (HIV)
  - Precipitous labor
  - Poor nutritional status
  - Abruptio placentae

  - Hypertensive episodes
  - History of drug abuse
- Laboratory test results (toxicology) to identify substances in mother and newborn
- Signs of neonatal abstinence syndrome (use the "WITHDRAWAL" acronym; see Box 24.4)
- Evidence of seizure activity and need for protective environment

The newborn's behavior often prompts the health care provider or nurse to suspect intrauterine drug exposure (Box 24.3). The newborn physical examination may also reveal low birth weight for gestational age or drug- or alcohol-related birth defects and dysfunction. Assess the newborn for signs of NAS (see Box 24.4).

Take Note!

Cocaine-exposed newborns are typically fussy, irritable, and inconsolable at times. They demonstrate poor coordination of sucking and swallowing, making feeding time frustrating for the newborn and caregiver alike.

Assist with obtaining diagnostic studies to identify the severity of withdrawal. In general, a urine screen signifies only recent newborn exposure to maternal use of drugs. It can detect marijuana use up to a month earlier, cocaine use up to 96 hours earlier, heroin use 24 to 48 hours earlier, and methadone use up to 10 days earlier (Hamdan, 2015). Toxicology screening of the newborn's blood, urine, and meconium identifies the substances to which the newborn has been exposed.

Nursing Management

The needs of the substance-exposed newborn are multiple, complex, and costly, both to the health care system and to society. Substance abuse takes place among people of all colors, sizes, shapes, incomes, types, and conditions. Most pregnant women are unaware of the adverse impact their substance abuse can have on the newborn. Pregnant women dependent on opioids are maintained on methadone as the current standard of care, which provides multiple benefits including improved prenatal care, reduced fetal mortality, and improved fetal growth (Jansson, 2015).

Nurses are in a unique position to help because they interact with high-risk mothers and newborns in many settings, including the community, health care facilities, and family agencies. It is the responsibility of all nurses to identify, educate, counsel, and refer pregnant women with substance-abusing problems. For example, nurses can be instrumental in increasing the number of pregnant women who make a serious attempt to quit smoking by using the "5 A's" approach:

- *Ask*: ask all women if they smoke and would like to quit.
- *Advise*: encourage the use of clinically proven treatment plans.

CENTRAL NERVOUS SYSTEM DISTURBANCES

SIGNS AND SYMPTOMS	SCORE	AM							PM				
Excessive high-pitched cry	2												
Continuous high-pitched cry	3												
Sleeps <1 hour after feeding	3												
Sleeps <2 hours after feeding	2												
Sleeps <3 hours after feeding	1												
Hyperactive Moro reflex	2												
Markedly hyperactive Moro reflex	3												
Mild tremors disturbed	1												
Moderate–severe tremors disturbed	2												
Mild tremors undisturbed	1												
Moderate–severe tremors undisturbed	4												
Increased muscle tone	2												
Excoloration (specify area)	1												
Myoclonic jerks	3												
Generalized convulsions	5												

METABOLIC VASOMOTOR/RESPIRATORY DISTURBANCES

	SCORE												
Sweating													
Fever <101 (99–100.8°F/37.2–38.2°C)	1												
Fever >101 (38.2°C and higher)	2												
Frequent yawning (>3–4 times/interval)	1												
Mottling	1												
Nasal stuffiness	1												
Sneezing (>3–4 times/interval)	1												
Nasal flaring	2												
Respiratory rate >60 min	1												
Respiratory rate >60 min, with retractions	2												

GASTROINTESTINAL DISTURBANCES

	SCORE												
Excessive sucking	1												
Poor feeding	2												
Regurgitation	2												
Projectile vomiting	3												
Loose stools	2												
Watery stools	3												
TOTAL SCORE													

FIGURE 24.7 Neonatal abstinence scoring system. (From Cloherty, J. P., & Stark, A. P. [1998]. *Manual of neonatal care* [4th ed., pp. 26–27]. Boston: Little, Brown.)

BOX 24.3

MANIFESTATIONS OF NEONATAL ABSTINENCE SYNDROME

CNS Dysfunction
- Tremors
- Generalized seizures
- Hyperactive reflexes
- Restlessness
- Irritability
- Hypertonic muscle tone, constant movement
- Shrill, high-pitched cry
- Disturbed sleep patterns

Metabolic, Vasomotor, and Respiratory Disturbances
- Fever
- Frequent yawning
- Mottling of the skin
- Sweating
- Nasal stuffiness
- Temperature instability
- Frequent sneezing
- Nasal flaring
- Tachypnea >60 bpm
- Apnea

Gastrointestinal Dysfunction
- Poor feeding
- Frantic sucking or rooting
- Uncoordinated sucking
- Poor weight gain
- Loose or watery stools
- Regurgitation or projectile vomiting (Artigas, 2015)

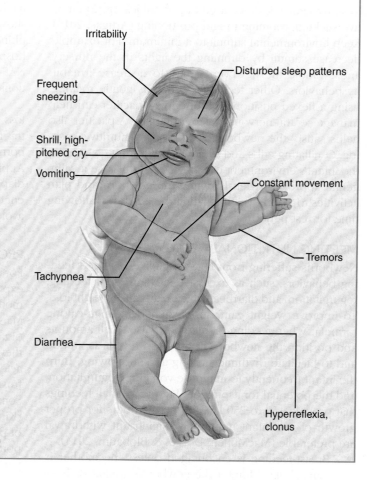

- *Assess*: provide motivation by discussing the "5 R's":
- *Relevance* of quitting to the woman
- *Risk* of continued smoking to the fetus
- *Rewards* of quitting for both
- *Roadblocks* to quitting
- *Repeat* at every visit

BOX 24.4

WITHDRAWAL ACRONYM

Assess the newborn for signs of NAS using the acronym WITHDRAWAL to focus the assessment:

W = **W**akefulness: sleep duration less than 3 hours after feeding
I = **I**rritability
T = **T**emperature variation, tachycardia, tremors
H = **H**yperactivity, high-pitched persistent cry, hyperreflexia, hypertonus
D = **D**iarrhea, diaphoresis, disorganized suck
R = **R**espiratory distress, rub marks, rhinorrhea
A = **A**pneic attacks, autonomic dysfunction
W = **W**eight loss or failure to gain weight
A = **A**lkalosis (respiratory)
L = **L**acrimation (Hamdan, 2015).

- *Assist*: help the woman to protect her fetus and newborn from the negative effects of smoking.
- *Arrange*: schedule follow-up visits to reinforce the woman's commitment to quit.

Although this approach is geared to smoking cessation, nurses can adapt it to focus on cessation for any substance use. Early, supportive, ongoing nursing care is critical to the well-being of the mother and her newborn. Nurses have an ethical responsibility to provide evidence-based and nonjudgmental care to this highly vulnerable aggregate.

Caring for a substance-exposed newborn remains a major challenge to health care providers. The major goals include providing comfort to the newborn by relieving symptoms, improving feeding and weight gain, preventing seizures, promoting parent–newborn interactions, and reducing the incidence of newborn mortality and abnormal development (Jordan et al., 2014).

PROMOTING COMFORT

Supportive interventions to promote comfort include swaddling, low lighting, gentle waking, quiet environment with little stimulation, use of soft voices, pacifiers to promote "self-soothing," frequent smaller feedings, vertical rocking during infant disorganization to decrease neurologic hyperactivity, increased opportunities for nonnutritive sucking, rooming-in and positioning (Artigas, 2015). Keep environmental stimuli to a minimum. For example, decrease stimuli by dimming the lights in the nursery, and swaddle the newborn tightly to decrease irritability behaviors. Other techniques such as gentle rocking, using a flexed position, and offering a pacifier can help manage central nervous system irritability. A pacifier also helps satisfy the newborn's need for nonnutritive sucking. Oscillating cribs and avoidance of abrupt changes in the infant's environment can also be helpful. Use a calm, gentle approach when handling the newborn and plan activities to avoid overstimulating the newborn, allowing time for rest periods.

MEETING NUTRITIONAL NEEDS

Newborns suffering from NAS may have impaired feeding behaviors, such as excessive sucking, poor feeding, regurgitation, and diarrhea, which may cause weight loss. To improve weight gain, supplement with high-calorie formula. When feeding the newborn, use small amounts and position the newborn upright to prevent aspiration and to facilitate rhythmic sucking and swallowing. Burp the infant frequently to minimize vomiting, regurgitation, and the potential for aspiration. Frequent, small feedings that provide 150 to 250 kcal/kg per 24 hours for proper growth of the infant undergoing significant withdrawal are preferable (MacMullen, Dulski, & Blobaum, 2014).

Breast-feeding is encouraged unless the mother is still using drugs. Monitor the newborn's weight daily to evaluate the success of food intake. Assess hydration; check skin turgor and fontanels. Assess the frequency and characteristics of bowel movements and monitor the newborn's fluid and electrolyte and acid–base status.

PREVENTING COMPLICATIONS

Pharmacologic treatment is warranted if conservative measures, such as swaddling and decreased environmental stimulation, are not adequate. The AAP recommends that, for newborns with confirmed drug exposure, drug therapy is indicated if the newborn has seizures, diarrhea, and vomiting, resulting in excessive weight loss and dehydration, poor feeding, inability to sleep, and fever unrelated to infection (Thigpen & Melton, 2014). The optimal treatment regimen for NAS has not been established. Based on the current literature, oral morphine and methadone are used as first-line therapies. Clonidine or phenobarbital is also recommended as an alternative therapy for those newborns who don't respond to a single pharmacologic agent (Artigas, 2015).

New research suggests that infants born to women addicted to opioids have fewer symptoms of NAS when their mothers receive buprenorphine, a partial mu-opioid agonist, during pregnancy compared with their counterparts whose mothers receive methadone. A multicenter randomized controlled trial comparing buprenorphine and methadone in pregnant women with opioid dependency showed that neonates whose mothers received buprenorphine required significantly less morphine, had shorter hospital stays, and had shorter duration of treatment for NAS (Maguire, 2014). Administer the prescribed medications and document the newborn's behavioral responses.

The newborn is at risk for skin breakdown. Weight loss, diarrhea, dehydration, and irritability can contribute to this risk. Provide meticulous skin care and protect the newborn's elbows and knees against friction and abrasions. Apply barrier ointments to avoid skin breakdown and diaper rash. If breakdown becomes severe, clear transparent dressings over reddened or excoriated areas may help avoid further progression of the skin breakdown.

PROMOTING PARENT–NEWBORN INTERACTION

For a mother who abuses substances, the birth of a drug-exposed newborn is both a crisis and an opportunity. The mother may feel guilty about the newborn's condition. Many of these newborns are unresponsive and have disorganized sleeping and feeding patterns. When awake, they can be easily overstimulated and irritated. Such characteristics make parent–newborn interactions difficult and frustrating, leading to possible detachment and avoidance. Some symptoms of withdrawal may last for up to 6 months (King et al., 2015). In addition, the mother may be a victim of physical and sexual abuse and may have a limited support system. Many of these mothers may have had poor parenting themselves, lack information about characteristic infant behaviors, and have unrealistic expectations about the newborn's abilities. Drug-exposed infants and their mothers experience a difficult early period together. Mothers need assistance in recognizing early cues from their infant signaling a need for caregiving. Communicate and provide referral to social services or other community agencies for follow-up post-discharge. Nursing support is essential if maternal–infant attachment is to occur and potential neglect and abuse are to be avoided (McKeever, Spaeth-Brayton, & Sheerin, 2014). Encourage the maternal–infant relationship through support for breast-feeding and rooming-in if there are no contraindications. Instruct the mother or caretaker on how to care for the newborn, including what to do after the newborn goes home (Teaching Guidelines 24.1).

Teaching Guidelines 24.1
CARING FOR YOUR NEWBORN AT HOME

- Position your newborn with the head elevated to prevent choking.
- To aid your newborn's sucking and swallowing during feeding, position the chin downward and support it with your hand. Do not overfeed.

- Place your newborn on his or her back to sleep or nap, never on the stomach.
- Keep a bulb syringe close by to suction your newborn's mouth in case of choking.
- Cluster newborn care (bathing, feeding, dressing) to prevent overstimulation.
- If your newborn is fussy or crying, try these measures to help calm him or her:
  - Wrap your newborn snugly in a blanket and gently rock in rocking chair.
  - Take the baby for a ride in the car (using a newborn car seat).
  - Play soothing music and "dance" with the newborn.
  - Use a wind-up swing with calming music.
- To help your newborn get to sleep, try these measures:
  - Schedule a bath with a gentle massage prior to bedtime.
  - Change diaper and clothes to make the baby comfortable.
  - Feed the baby just prior to bedtime.
  - If the newborn cries when put in crib and all needs are met, allow him or her to cry.
  - Use a rocking chair to feed and sing a soft lullaby.
- Call your primary care provider if you observe heightened withdrawal behaviors such as:
  - Slight tremors (shaking) of hands and legs
  - Stiff posture when held in your arms
  - Irritability and frequent fussiness
  - High-pitched cry, excessive sucking motions
  - Erratic sleep pattern
  - Frequent yawning, nasal stuffiness, sweating
  - Prolonged time needed to feed
  - Frequent vomiting after feeding

It is possible that the newborn may be a powerful motivator for the mother to undergo treatment and seek recovery. Refer the mother to community agencies to address her addiction and the infant's developmental needs (Nagtalon-Ramos, 2014). The nurse can play a pivotal role in assisting the mother to abstain from drug use and to promote effective parenting skills.

Hyperbilirubinemia

Jaundice is a yellow discoloration of the skin and sclera of the eyes caused by increased levels of unconjugated bilirubin in the newborn's circulation. Newborns produce large quantities of bilirubin, which is a by-product of the breakdown of red blood cells. It is processed in the liver and normally excreted out of the body in the urine and stools. In response to this increase, sometimes the skin and eyes turn yellow. It is usually harmless and clears up without treatment within 10 to 14 days. In some newborns, their bilirubin levels rise and further therapy

Consider This

I admit I had led a reckless life since I was a teen. I rebelled against my mother's authority and started smoking and doing drugs just to "check out" of my painful world. It was one big blast after another with a high and then a low. I never considered the consequences of my behavior then and never thought it would hurt anyone until I learned I was about 4 months pregnant. I convinced myself that if I cut back, everything would be fine.

Now, as I stand here in the NICU watching my tiny son struggle for air and tremble all over, I am not so convinced that I didn't hurt anyone except myself. As I witness my son fight against MY nicotine and drug addiction, my heart is heavy with guilt. I wonder how I could have thought that my troubles wouldn't become another's plight sooner or later. What must I have been thinking to isolate my addiction and not consider the impact that it would have on me as a mother and my son?

Thoughts: This woman honestly regrets what her addiction has done to her son as she stands watching him go through withdrawal. Her lifestyle choices do affect others, despite her previous denial. One problem with addiction is the difficulty in getting help after deciding to finally quit. There aren't enough rehab centers to deal with the large numbers of people needing their services and it can be difficult to get into one. What can be offered to pregnant women who abuse substances? How can nurses increase community awareness about the impact of this problem, especially during pregnancy?

is warranted because unconjugated bilirubin is neurotoxic and can cause mortality in newborns and lifelong neurologic issues in infants who survive.

Hyperbilirubinemia is a total serum bilirubin level above 5 mg/dL resulting from unconjugated bilirubin being deposited in the skin and mucous membranes (Hansen, 2015). The mean peak of total bilirubin plasma levels occur between 48 and 92 hours after birth and the average values are between 7 and 9 mg/dL (King et al., 2015). Hyperbilirubinemia is exhibited as jaundice (yellowing of the body tissues and fluids). Newborn jaundice is one of the most common reasons for hospital readmission. It occurs in up to 80% of term newborns in the first week of life and in virtually all preterm newborns (National Institute for Health and Care Excellence [NICE], 2015). African-American neonates have a lower overall risk for neonatal hyperbilirubinemia versus White, Greek, Native American, or Asian infants (Muchowski, 2014). Some infants are at higher risk for developing elevated bilirubin levels. Some of these risk factors include:
- Bruising at birth
- Prematurity

- Dehydration
- Congenital infection
- Maternal substance abuse
- History of a sibling with jaundice
- Inadequate breast-feeding
- Hemolytic disease
- Birth trauma
- Polycythemia
- Delayed cord clamping
- Biliary obstruction
- Prematurity
- Maternal diabetes
- Male infants
- Jaundice prior to 24 hours of age
- East Asian, American Indian, or Mediterranean descent
- Cephalhematoma (NICE, 2015; Wong & Bhutani, 2015).

Pathophysiology

Bilirubin has two forms—unconjugated or indirect, which is fat soluble and toxic to body tissues, and conjugated or direct, which is water soluble and nontoxic. Elevated serum bilirubin levels are manifested as jaundice in the newborn. Typically the total serum bilirubin level rises over the first 3 to 5 days and then declines.

Newborn jaundice results from an imbalance in the rate of bilirubin production and bilirubin elimination. This imbalance determines the pattern and degree of newborn hyperbilirubinemia (Mattson & Smith, 2015). During the newborn period, a rapid transition from the intrauterine to the extrauterine pattern of bilirubin physiology occurs. Fetal unconjugated bilirubin is normally cleared by the placenta and the mother's liver in utero, so total bilirubin at birth is low. After the umbilical cord is cut, the newborn must conjugate bilirubin (convert a lipid-soluble pigment into a water-soluble pigment) in the liver on his or her own. The rate and amount of bilirubin conjugation depend on the rate of red blood cell breakdown, the bilirubin load, the maturity of the liver, and the number of albumin-binding sites (Hansen, 2015). Bilirubin production increases after birth mainly because of a shortened red blood cell life span (70 days in the newborn vs. 90 days in the adult) combined with an increased red blood cell mass. Therefore, the amount of bilirubin the newborn must deal with is large compared with that of an adult.

PHYSIOLOGIC JAUNDICE

Physiologic jaundice is the manifestation of the normal hyperbilirubinemia seen in newborns, appearing during the third to fourth day of life, due to the limitations and abnormalities of bilirubin metabolism. By then, the newborn has been discharged home in the care of the parents. Serum bilirubin levels reach up to 10 mg/dL and then decline rapidly over the first week after birth (Cunningham et al., 2014). Most newborns have been discharged by the time this jaundice peaks (at about 72 hours).

Physiologic jaundice may result from an increased bilirubin load because of relative polycythemia, a shortened red blood cell life span, immature hepatic uptake and conjugation process, and increased enterohepatic circulation. Newborns with delayed passage of meconium are more likely to develop physiologic jaundice (El-Radhi, 2015).

Physiologic jaundice differs between breast-fed and bottle-fed newborns in relation to the onset of symptoms. Breast-fed newborns typically have peak bilirubin levels by the fourth day of life; levels for bottle-fed newborns usually peak on the third day of life. The rate of bilirubin decline is less rapid in breast-fed newborns compared with bottle-fed newborns because bottle-fed newborns tend to have more frequent bowel movements. Jaundice associated with breast-feeding presents in two distinct patterns: early-onset breast-feeding jaundice and late-onset breast-feeding jaundice.

Early-Onset Breast-Feeding Jaundice. Early-onset breast-feeding jaundice is probably associated with ineffective breast-feeding practices because of relative caloric deprivation in the first few days of life. Decreased volume and frequency of feedings may result in mild dehydration and the delayed passage of meconium. This delayed defecation allows enterohepatic circulation reuptake of bilirubin and an increase in the serum level of unconjugated bilirubin. To prevent this, strategies to promote early effective and frequent breast-feeding are important. The AAP guidelines that have recently been reaffirmed recommend early and frequent breast-feeding without supplemental water or dextrose-water because those supplements do not prevent hyperbilirubinemia and may lead to hyponatremia (Deshpande, 2015). Early frequent feedings can provide the newborn with adequate calories and fluid volume (via colostrum) to stimulate peristalsis and passage of meconium to eliminate bilirubin.

Late-Onset Breast-Feeding Jaundice. Late-onset breast-feeding jaundice occurs later in the newborn period, with the bilirubin level usually peaking in the 6th to 14th day of life. Total serum bilirubin levels may be 12 to 20 mg/dL, but the levels are not considered pathologic (Rosenthal, 2014). The specific cause of late-onset breast milk jaundice is not entirely understood, but it may be related to a change in the milk composition resulting in enhanced enterohepatic circulation. Additional research is needed to determine the cause. Interrupting breast-feeding is not recommended unless bilirubin levels reach dangerous levels; if this occurs, breast-feeding is stopped for only 1 or 2 days. Substituting formula during this short break usually results in a prompt decline of bilirubin levels, but interrupting breast-feeding is not necessary or advisable.

PATHOLOGIC JAUNDICE

Pathologic jaundice is manifested within the first 24 hours of life when total bilirubin levels increase by more than 5 mg/dL/day and the total serum bilirubin level is higher than 17 mg/dL in a full-term infant (Ives, 2015).

Conditions that alter the production, transport, uptake, metabolism, excretion, or reabsorption of bilirubin can cause pathologic jaundice in the newborn. A few conditions that contribute to red blood cell breakdown and thus higher bilirubin levels include polycythemia, blood incompatibilities, and systemic acidosis. These altered conditions can lead to high levels of unconjugated bilirubin, possibly reaching toxic levels and resulting in a severe condition called acute or chronic bilirubin encephalopathy.

The most common condition associated with pathologic jaundice is hemolytic disease of the newborn secondary to incompatibility of blood groups of the mother and the newborn. The most frequent conditions are Rh factor and ABO incompatibilities.

Bilirubin encephalopathy (yellow nucleus) is a preventable neurologic disorder characterized by encephalopathy, motor abnormalities, hearing and vision loss, and death (Cunningham et al., 2014). It can be acute or chronic in nature. Neurotoxicity develops because unconjugated bilirubin has a high affinity for brain tissue, and bilirubin not bound to albumin is free to cross the blood–brain barrier and damage cells of the central nervous system.

In the acute stage, acute bilirubin encephalopathy, the newborn becomes lethargic, sucks poorly, irritable, may have seizures, and can become hypotonic. If the hyperbilirubinemia is not treated, the newborn becomes hypertonic, with truncal arching and seizures. A high-pitched cry may be noted. These changes can occur rapidly, so all newborns must be assessed for jaundice and tested if indicated so that treatment can be initiated.

In the chronic stage, chronic bilirubin encephalopathy or kernicterus, the newborn may experience the following symptoms: severe cerebral palsy, dental enamel dysplasia, auditory dysfunction, and paralysis of their upward gaze. Cases of kernicterus should not be occurring today, but delays in diagnosing pathologic causes of prolonged jaundice are still being missed or overlooked (Ives, 2015).

Take Note!

Significant jaundice in a newborn less than 24 hours of age should be immediately reported to the physician, because it may indicate a pathologic process.

Nursing Assessment

Neonatal jaundice first becomes visible in the face and forehead. Identification is aided by pressure on the skin, since blanching reveals the underlying color. Jaundice then gradually becomes visible on the trunk and extremities. This cephalocaudal progression is well described. Jaundice disappears in the opposite direction. Nurses play an important role in early detection and identification of jaundice in the newborn. Keen observation skills are essential.

HEALTH HISTORY AND PHYSICAL EXAMINATION

Review the history for factors that might predispose the newborn to hyperbilirubinemia, such as:

- Polycythemia
- Significant bruising or cephalhematoma, which increases bilirubin production
- Infections such as TORCH (toxoplasmosis, hepatitis B, rubella, cytomegalovirus, herpes simplex virus)
- Use of drugs during labor and birth such as diazepam (Valium) or oxytocin (Pitocin)
- Prematurity
- Gestational age of 34 to 36 weeks
- Hemolysis due to ABO incompatibility or Rh isoimmunization
- Macrosomic infant of a mother with diabetes
- Delayed cord clamping, which increases the erythrocyte volume
- Decreased albumin binding sites to transport unconjugated bilirubin to the liver because of acidosis
- Delayed meconium passage, which increases the amount of bilirubin that returns to the unconjugated state and can be absorbed by the intestinal mucosa
- Siblings who had significant jaundice
- Inadequate breast-feeding leading to dehydration, decreased caloric intake, weight loss, and delayed passage of meconium
- Ethnicity, such as Asian American, Mediterranean, or Native American
- Male gender (Gardner et al., 2016; NICE, 2015).

Perform a complete physical examination. Assess the skin, mucous membranes, sclera, and body fluids (tears, urine) for a yellow color. Detect jaundice by observing the infant in a well-lit room and blanching the skin with digital pressure over a bony prominence. Typically, jaundice begins on the head and gradually progresses to the abdomen and extremities. Also inspect for pallor (anemia), excessive bruising (bleeding), and dehydration (sluggish circulation), which may contribute to the development of jaundice and the risk for kernicterus.

Assess the newborn for Rh incompatibility. Be alert for clinical manifestations such as ascites, anemia, congestive heart failure, edema, pallor, jaundice, hepatosplenomegaly, hydramnios, thick placenta, and dilation of the umbilical vein (Salem & Singer, 2015).

The hydropic newborn appears pale, edematous, and limp at birth and typically requires resuscitation. The newborn with immune hydrops exhibits severe generalized edema, organ hypertrophy and enlargement, and effusion of fluid into body cavities.

COMPARISON CHART 24.1   RH VERSUS ABO INCOMPATIBILITY

Clinical Picture	Rh Incompatibility	ABO Incompatibility
First-born	Rare	Common
Later pregnancies	More severe	No increase in severity
Jaundice	Moderate to severe	Mild
Hydrops fetalis	Frequent	Rare
Anemia	Frequently severe	Rare
Ascites	Frequent	Rare
Hepatosplenomegaly	Frequent	Common

LABORATORY AND DIAGNOSTIC TESTING

Determine maternal and fetal blood types, checking for incompatibilities (Comparison Chart 24.1). Assess laboratory values for bilirubin (both unconjugated and conjugated). Bilirubin levels establish the diagnosis of hyperbilirubinemia. The newborn with Rh incompatibility demonstrates a rapidly rising unconjugated bilirubin level at birth or in the first 24 hours. Also expect to obtain alkaline phosphatase, liver enzymes, and prothrombin time and partial thromboplastin time, as well as:

* *Direct Coombs test*—to identify hemolytic disease of the newborn; positive results indicate that the newborn's red blood cells have been coated with antibodies and thus are sensitized
* *Hemoglobin concentration*—for evidence of anemia
* *Blood type*—to determine Rh status and any incompatibility of the newborn
* *Total serum protein*—to detect reduced binding capacity of albumin
* *Reticulocyte count*—to identify an elevated level indicating increased hemolysis

Assist with obtaining blood specimens. Use cord blood for hemoglobin concentration measurements; use a heel stick for direct Coombs testing and bilirubin levels. Prepare the parents and newborn for radiologic evaluation if necessary to determine abnormalities that may be causing the jaundice.

Nursing Management

Nursing management of a newborn with hyperbilirubinemia requires a comprehensive approach. As members of the health care team, nurses share in the responsibility for early detection and identification, family education, management, and follow-up of the mother and newborn. Documentation of the timing of onset of jaundice is essential to differentiate between physiologic (>24 hours) and pathologic (<24 hours) jaundice. Nurses can improve care by offering their presence and support and by following the AAP guidelines for preventing hyperbilirubinemia:

* Promote and support successful breast-feeding.
* Establish nursery protocols for identifying jaundice, including when a serum bilirubin can be ordered by a nurse.
* Measure total serum bilirubin on jaundiced infants in the first 24 hours.
* Assess for risk factors that may increase bilirubin levels.
* Interpret all bilirubin levels according to the infant's age in hours.
* Do not use a visual estimation of jaundice, which is inaccurate; instead, use labs.
* Consider infants <38 weeks, particularly if breast-fed, at high risk for jaundice.
* Perform risk assessment on all newborns prior to discharge.
* Treat jaundiced newborns with phototherapy, if indicated.
* Provide parents with written and oral information about jaundice at discharge.
* Provide follow-up care and referrals based on time of discharge and risk.
* Empower parents to make appropriate decisions once home (Green, 2016;Griffin & Celenza, 2014).

REDUCING BILIRUBIN LEVELS

Encourage early initiation of feedings to prevent hypoglycemia and provide protein to maintain the albumin levels to transport bilirubin to the liver. Ensure newborn feedings (breast milk or formula) every 2 to 3 hours to promote prompt emptying of bilirubin from the bowel. Encourage the mother to breast-feed (8 to 12 feedings per day) to prevent inadequate intake and thus dehydration. Supplement breast milk with formula to supply protein if bilirubin levels continue to increase with breast-feeding only. Monitor serum bilirubin levels frequently to reduce the risk of severe hyperbilirubinemia.

Phototherapy. Phototherapy is the use of visible light for the treatment of hyperbilirubinemia in the newborn. This relatively common therapy lowers the serum bilirubin level by transforming bilirubin into water-soluble isomers that can be eliminated without conjugation in the liver. For the newborn with jaundice, regardless of its etiology, phototherapy is used to convert unconjugated bilirubin to the less toxic water-soluble form that can be excreted. Phototherapy, via special lights placed above the newborn or a fiber-optic blanket placed under the newborn and wrapped around him or her, uses blue wavelengths of light to alter unconjugated bilirubin in the skin.

For the newborn receiving phototherapy, place the newborn under the lights or on the fiber-optic blanket, exposing as much skin as possible. Cover the newborn's genitals and shield the eyes to protect them from becoming irritated or burned when using direct lights. Assess the intensity of the light source to prevent burns and excoriation (Fig. 24.8). Turn the newborn every 2 hours to maximize the area of exposure, removing the newborn from the lights only for feedings. Maintain a neutral thermal environment to decrease energy expenditure, and assess the newborn's neurologic status frequently. A recent study's findings indicated that intermittent phototherapy with 12 hours on and 12 hours off cycles was as efficacious as continuous phototherapy to lower bilirubin levels in term and late preterm infants (Sachdeva et al., 2014).

Assess the newborn's temperature every 3 to 4 hours as indicated. Monitor fluid intake and output closely and assess daily weights for gains or losses. Check skin turgor for evidence of dehydration.

With feedings, remove the newborn from the lights and remove the eye shields to allow interaction with the newborn. Encourage breast or bottle feedings every 2 to 3 hours. Follow agency policy about removing the eye shields periodically to assess the eyes for discharge or corneal irritation secondary to eye shield pressure. Typically, the eyes are assessed and eye shields are removed once a shift.

Monitor stool for consistency and frequency. Unconjugated bilirubin excreted in the feces will produce a greenish appearance, and typically stools are loose. Lack of frequent green stools is a cause for concern.

Provide meticulous skin care. Assess skin surfaces frequently for dryness and irritation secondary to the dehydrating effects of phototherapy and irritation from highly acidic stool to prevent excoriation and skin breakdown. Nursing responsibilities include ensuring effective irradiance delivery, maximizing skin exposure, providing eye protection and eye care, paying careful attention to thermoregulation, monitoring the newborn's skin turgor, maintaining adequate hydration, promoting elimination, and supporting parent–infant interactions (Nagtalon-Ramos, 2014). A summary of the nursing care for the newborn undergoing phototherapy is as follows:

- Support parents, encouraging them to interact with their infant.
- Support breast-feeding with one-on-one instruction and patience.
- Place infants on their back to expose as much naked skin as possible.
- Provide eye care/protection every time the infant is exposed to the phototherapy light.
- Check temperature and environment around infant to prevent overheating.
- Take daily weights to make sure the infant is not becoming dehydrated.

Exchange Transfusion. If the total serum bilirubin level remains elevated after intensive phototherapy, an exchange transfusion with albumin administered before the transfusion, the quickest method for lowering serum bilirubin levels, may be necessary (Hansen, 2015). In the presence of hemolytic disease, severe anemia, or a rapid rise in the total serum bilirubin level, an exchange transfusion is recommended. An exchange transfusion removes the newborn's blood and replaces it with nonhemolyzed red blood cells from a donor. During the transfusion, monitor the newborn's cardiovascular status continuously because serious complications can arise, such as acid–base imbalances, infection, hypovolemia, and fluid and electrolyte imbalances. Exchange transfusion is used only as a second-line therapy after phototherapy has failed to yield results. Intensive nursing care is needed.

Assist the physician with an exchange transfusion if necessary. Monitor the newborn's status closely for changes, especially in vital signs and heart rate and rhythm, before, during, and after the procedure.

PROVIDING PARENT TEACHING AND SUPPORT

Nurses can help the parents to understand the diagnostic tests and treatment modalities by offering individualized teaching. Nurses are the ones who give discharge instructions to the family. Explore with the family their

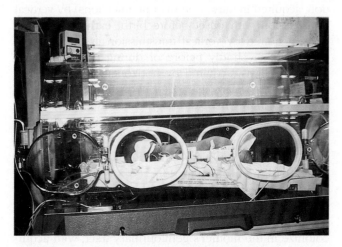

FIGURE 24.8 A newborn receiving phototherapy.

understanding of jaundice and treatment modalities to reduce anxiety and gain their cooperation in monitoring the infant. Teach the parents about jaundice and its potential risk using written and verbal material. Also show the parents how to identify newborn behaviors that might indicate rising bilirubin levels. Emphasize the need to seek treatment from their pediatrician should any of the following occur:

- Lethargy, sleepiness, poor muscle tone, floppiness
- Poor sucking, lack of interest in feeding
- High-pitched cry

Teach the parents how to assess their newborn for signs of jaundice because physiologic jaundice may not occur until after the newborn is discharged. Reinforce the need for appropriate follow-up with their pediatrician within 48 to 72 hours after discharge to assess jaundice status (Mattson & Smith, 2015). A general rule to follow is that any infant discharged at less than age 72 hours old should be seen within 2 days of discharge unless there is little risk of subsequent hyperbilirubinemia, in which case a later follow-up is appropriate. This follow-up can be provided in an office, clinic, or home and by a physician, physician's assistant, or nurse practitioner. Both written and oral information should be provided to all parents about newborn jaundice, for example the pamphlet titled *Jaundice and Your Newborn* published by the AAP (Maisels et al., 2014).

The need for phototherapy can be anxiety producing for the parents. Explain the rationale for the procedure and demonstrate techniques that the parents can use to interact with their newborn. Additional education about phototherapy may be necessary when home phototherapy is used (Teaching Guidelines 24.2).

Teaching Guidelines 24.2
CARING FOR YOUR NEWBORN RECEIVING HOME PHOTOTHERAPY

- Inspect your newborn's skin, eyes, and mucous membranes for a yellow color.
- Remember that a home health nurse will come to visit and help you set up the light system.
- Keep the lights about 12 to 30 inches above your newborn.
- Cover your newborn's eyes with patches or cotton balls and gauze to protect them.
- Keep the newborn undressed except for the diaper area; fold the diaper down below the newborn's navel in the front and as far as possible in the back to expose as much skin as possible.
- Turn your newborn every 2 hours so that all areas of the body are exposed.
- Remove the newborn from the lights only for feeding.
- Remove the eye patches during feedings so that you can interact with your newborn.

- Record your newborn's temperature, weight, and fluid intake daily.
- Document the frequency, color, and consistency of all stools; the stools should be loose and green as the bilirubin is broken down.
- Keep the skin clean and dry to prevent irritation.

Neonatal Sepsis

Neonatal sepsis is defined as a clinical syndrome of bacteremia with systemic signs and symptoms of infection in the first month of life (Molyneux & Gest, 2015). Newborns are susceptible to infections because their immune system is immature and slow to react, and they have a poorly developed skin barrier. The antibodies that newborns received from the mother during pregnancy and from breast milk help protect them from invading organisms. However, these need time to reach optimal levels.

Bacterial infections of the newborn remain a major cause of illness and death in the neonatal period. Making the diagnosis of sepsis in newborns is difficult due to its nonspecific symptoms. The mortality rate from newborn sepsis may be as high as 50% if untreated. Infection is a major cause of death during the first month of life, contributing to 13% to 15% of all neonatal deaths (Anderson-Berry, Bellig, & Ohning, 2015).

Pathophysiology

When a pathologic organism overcomes the newborn's defenses, infection and sepsis result. Neonatal sepsis is the presence of bacterial, fungal, or viral microorganisms or their toxins in blood or other tissues. Infections that have an onset within the first month of life are termed newborn infections. Exposure to a pathogenic organism, whether a virus, fungus, or bacteria, occurs, and it enters the newborn's body and begins to multiply.

Newborn infections are usually grouped into three classes according to their time of onset: congenital infection, acquired in utero (intrauterine infections) by vertical transmission with onset before birth; early-onset infections, acquired by vertical transmission in the perinatal period, either shortly before or during birth; and late-onset infections, acquired by horizontal transmission in the nursery. As many as 85% of neonatal infections have their onset in the first 2 days of life and usually are pneumonia and meningitis (Deleon, Shattuck, & Jain, 2015).

EARLY-ONSET NEONATAL INFECTIONS
Early-onset neonatal infections (<48 hours) are associated with acquisition of microorganisms from the mother. Transplacental infection or an ascending infection from the cervix may be caused by organisms that colonize in the mother's genitourinary tract, with acquisition of the microbe by passage through a colonized

birth canal at delivery. The microorganisms most commonly associated with early-onset infection include group B streptococci (GBS), *Escherichia coli*, coagulase-negative *Staphylococcus*, *Haemophilus influenzae*, and *Listeria monocytogenes*.

LATE-ONSET NEONATAL INFECTIONS

Late-onset infections (>48 hours), acquired in the postpartum period, are primarily through horizontal transmission from family members or caregivers or through environmental exposures. Infections can be acquired through breast-feeding (HIV and cytomegalovirus; discussed in more detail in Chapter 20) or by direct contact with family members or health care providers. These types of contacts and exposures are especially important in infants, primarily preterm, with prolonged hospital stays, where they are more likely to be exposed to multidrug-resistant hospital-associated organisms potentially from contact with caregivers or contaminated equipment. Organisms that cause late-onset sepsis include *Staphylococcus aureus*, *E. Coli*, *Klebsiella*, *Pseudomonas*, *Enterobacter*, *Candida*, and *Anaerobes*. Comparison Chart 24.2 compares the three classes of newborn infections.

Nursing Assessment

Diagnosis of neonatal infections is challenging. Most infants will have some risk factors and the presenting symptoms are many and nonspecific, including poor

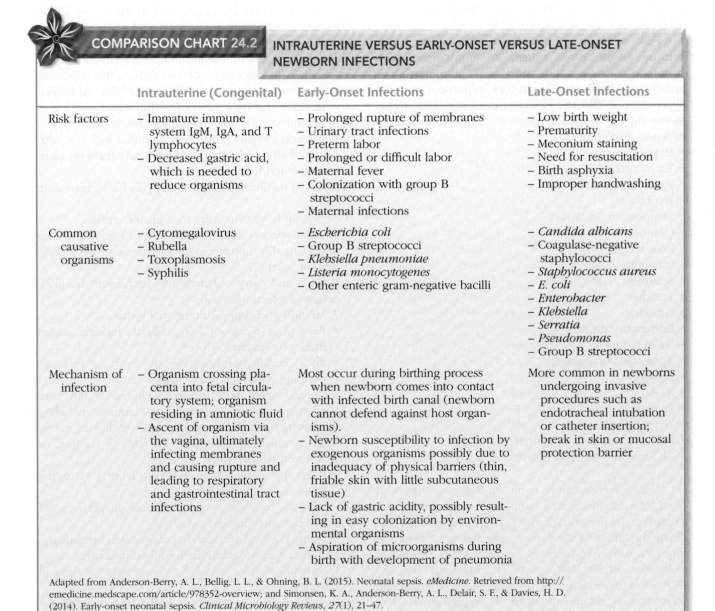

COMPARISON CHART 24.2   INTRAUTERINE VERSUS EARLY-ONSET VERSUS LATE-ONSET NEWBORN INFECTIONS

	Intrauterine (Congenital)	Early-Onset Infections	Late-Onset Infections
Risk factors	– Immature immune system IgM, IgA, and T lymphocytes – Decreased gastric acid, which is needed to reduce organisms	– Prolonged rupture of membranes – Urinary tract infections – Preterm labor – Prolonged or difficult labor – Maternal fever – Colonization with group B streptococci – Maternal infections	– Low birth weight – Prematurity – Meconium staining – Need for resuscitation – Birth asphyxia – Improper handwashing
Common causative organisms	– Cytomegalovirus – Rubella – Toxoplasmosis – Syphilis	– *Escherichia coli* – Group B streptococci – *Klebsiella pneumoniae* – *Listeria monocytogenes* – Other enteric gram-negative bacilli	– *Candida albicans* – Coagulase-negative staphylococci – *Staphylococcus aureus* – *E. coli* – *Enterobacter* – *Klebsiella* – *Serratia* – *Pseudomonas* – Group B streptococci
Mechanism of infection	– Organism crossing placenta into fetal circulatory system; organism residing in amniotic fluid – Ascent of organism via the vagina, ultimately infecting membranes and causing rupture and leading to respiratory and gastrointestinal tract infections	Most occur during birthing process when newborn comes into contact with infected birth canal (newborn cannot defend against host organisms). – Newborn susceptibility to infection by exogenous organisms possibly due to inadequacy of physical barriers (thin, friable skin with little subcutaneous tissue) – Lack of gastric acidity, possibly resulting in easy colonization by environmental organisms – Aspiration of microorganisms during birth with development of pneumonia	More common in newborns undergoing invasive procedures such as endotracheal intubation or catheter insertion; break in skin or mucosal protection barrier

Adapted from Anderson-Berry, A. L., Bellig, L. L., & Ohning, B. L. (2015). Neonatal sepsis. *eMedicine*. Retrieved from http://emedicine.medscape.com/article/978352-overview; and Simonsen, K. A., Anderson-Berry, A. L., Delair, S. F., & Davies, H. D. (2014). Early-onset neonatal sepsis. *Clinical Microbiology Reviews*, 27(1), 21–47.

feeding, breathing difficulty, apnea and bradycardia, gastrointestinal problems, increased oxygen requirement or ventilator support needs, lethargy or hypotension, decreased or elevated temperature, unusual skin rash or color change, persistent crying or irritability. Adding to the challenge of correctly identifying the infection, the list of conditions to consider in the differential diagnosis is extensive, including metabolic and congenital abnormalities (Randolph & McCulloh, 2014).

Nursing assessment focuses on early identification of a newborn at risk for infection to allow for prompt treatment, thus reducing mortality and morbidity. Be aware of the many risk factors associated with newborn sepsis. Among the factors that contribute to the newborn's overall vulnerability to infection are poor skin integrity, prematurity, poor maternal nutrition, low birth weight, birth trauma, invasive procedures, exposure to numerous caregivers, and an environment conducive to bacterial colonization (Green, 2016).

Few newborn infections are easy to recognize because manifestations usually are nonspecific. Early symptoms can be vague because of the newborn's inability to mount an inflammatory response. Often, the observation is that the newborn does not "look right." Assess the newborn for common nonspecific signs of infection, including:

- Hypotension
- Tachycardia
- Pallor or duskiness
- Hypotonia
- Temperature instability
- Cyanosis
- Poor weight gain
- Irritability
- Seizures
- Jaundice
- Grunting
- Respiratory distress
- Nasal flaring
- Apnea and bradycardia
- Lethargy
- Rash
- Petechiae
- Hypoglycemia
- Poor feeding (lack of interest in feeding)
- Abdominal distention (Gardner et al., 2016).

Since infection can be confused with other newborn conditions, laboratory and radiographic tests are needed to confirm the presence of infection. Be prepared to coordinate the timing of the various tests and assist as necessary. Evaluate the complete blood count with a differential to identify anemia, leukocytosis, or leukopenia. Elevated CRP levels may indicate inflammation. As ordered, obtain x-rays of the chest and abdomen, which may reveal infectious processes located there. Blood, cerebrospinal fluid (CSF), and urine cultures are indicated to identify the location and type of infection present. Positive cultures confirm that the newborn has an infection. Treatment is initially with ampicillin plus either gentamicin or cefotaxime, narrowed to organism-specific drugs as soon as the cultures identify the specific organism.

Nursing Management

To enhance the newborn's chance of survival, early recognition and diagnosis are key. Often the diagnosis of sepsis is based on a suspicious clinical picture. Antibiotic therapy is usually started before the laboratory results identify the infecting pathogen. Along with antibiotic therapy, circulatory, respiratory, nutritional, and developmental support is important. Antibiotic therapy is continued for 7 to 21 days if cultures are positive, or it is discontinued within 72 hours if cultures are negative. With the use of antibiotics along with early recognition and supportive care, mortality and morbidity rates have been reduced greatly.

Nurses possess the education and assessment tools to decrease the incidence of and reduce the impact of infections on women (see Chapter 20 for additional information) and their newborns. Implement measures for prevention and early recognition, including:

- Formulate a sepsis prevention plan that includes education of all members of the health care team on identification and treatment of sepsis.
- Maintain medical and surgical asepsis for all providing care.
- Screen all newborns daily for signs of sepsis.
- Monitor sepsis cases and outcomes to reinforce continued quality improvement measures or to modify current practices.
- Outline and carry out measures to prevent hospital-acquired infections, such as:
  - Monitor and support nutritional status.
  - Feed your newborn frequently to provide added fluid, protein, and calories.
  - Rock, cuddle, or hold the newborn to promote bonding when out of the lights.
  - Contact your pediatrician or home health care agency with any questions or changes, including refusing feedings, fewer than five wet diapers in one day, vomiting of complete amounts of feeding, or elevated temperature.
  - Keep appointments for follow-up laboratory testing to monitor bilirubin levels.
  - Provide frequent oral care and inspections of mucous membranes.
- Properly position and turn to prevent skin breakdown.
- Use strict aseptic technique for all wound care.
- Frequently monitor invasive catheter sites for signs of infection.
- Identify newborns at risk for sepsis by reviewing risk factors.

- Monitor vital sign changes and observe for subtle signs of infection.
- Monitor for signs of organ system dysfunction:
  - Cardiovascular compromise—tachycardia and hypotension
  - Respiratory compromise—respiratory distress and tachypnea
  - Renal compromise—oliguria or anuria
  - Systemic compromise—abnormal blood values
- Provide comprehensive sepsis treatment:
  - Circulatory support with fluids and vasopressors
  - Supplemental oxygen and mechanical ventilation
  - Obtaining culture samples as requested
  - Antibiotic administration as ordered, observing for side effects
  - Promoting newborn comfort
- Assess the family's educational needs and provide instructions as necessary.

Perinatal infections continue to be a public health problem, with severe consequences for those affected. By promoting a better understanding of newborn infections and appropriate use of therapies, nurses can lower the mortality rates associated with severe sepsis, especially with appropriate timing of interventions. The potential for nursing interventions to identify, prevent, and minimize the risk for sepsis is significant. Primary disease prevention must be a major focus for nurses. Family education plays a key role in the prevention of perinatal infections, in addition to following accepted practices in immunization.

CONGENITAL CONDITIONS

The human and economic toll of birth defects is significant and tragic—each year an estimated 8 million children—6% of the total births worldwide—are born with a serious birth defect. Approximately 120,000 infants are born with a birth defect in the United States annually (March of Dimes, 2015b).

Congenital conditions can arise from many etiologies, including single-gene disorders, chromosome aberrations, exposure to teratogens, and many sporadic conditions of unknown cause. Congenital conditions may be inherited or sporadic, isolated or multiple, apparent or hidden, gross or microscopic. They cause nearly half of all deaths in term newborns and cause long-term sequelae for many. The incidence varies according to the type of defect. When a serious anomaly is identified prenatally, the parents can decide whether or not to continue the pregnancy. When an anomaly is identified at or after birth, parents need to be informed promptly and given a realistic appraisal of the severity of the condition, the prognosis, and treatment options so that they can participate in all decisions pertaining to their child.

Congenital conditions can affect virtually any body system. This section describes common congenital conditions identified at or after birth. Some of these conditions warrant immediate treatment soon after birth. Other conditions, although identified in the newborn period, are long term with ongoing effects into childhood.

Ultimately, surveillance and research activities are translated into concrete strategies to prevent birth defects. In 1992, with solid evidence from epidemiologic research studies, the United States Public Health Service recommended that all women of childbearing age consume 400 mcg (0.4 mg) of folic acid daily to reduce the risk (up to 70%) of having a pregnancy affected by an NTD. This has spurred prevention activities at local and national levels to promote the folic acid message (CDC, 2015b).

Congenital Heart Disease

Congenital heart disease is a structural defect involving the heart, the great vessels, or both that is present at birth (AHA, 2015a). It is a broad term that can describe a number of abnormalities affecting the heart. At least 18 types of cardiovascular defects are recognized, with many additional anatomic variations. Approximately 8 newborns out of every 1,000 live births will have some form of congenital heart disease, or about 35,000 infants (1 out of every 125) are born with heart defects each year in the United States. Congenital heart disease causes more deaths during the first year of life than any other birth defect (AHA, 2015b). The defect may be very mild and the newborn appears healthy at birth, or it may be so severe that the newborn's life is in immediate jeopardy. Severe congenital cardiac defects usually present in the first few days or weeks of life, while the newborn's circulation is continuing to adapt to the demands of extrauterine life. Advances in diagnosis and medical and surgical interventions have led to dramatic increases in survival rates for newborns with serious heart defects.

Pathophysiology

In most cases, the exact cause of congenital heart disease is unknown. Most congenital heart defects develop during the first 8 weeks of gestation and are usually the result of genetic and environmental forces.

Typically, congenital heart disease is divided into four physiologic categories based on structural abnormalities and functional alterations (Table 24.5):
- *Septal wall defects*: defects causing increased pulmonary blood flow, such as atrial septal defect and ventricular septal defect
- *Obstruction defects*: defects causing obstructed blood flow out of the heart, such as pulmonary or aortic stenosis
- *Cyanotic heart lesions*: defects causing decreased pulmonary blood flow, such as tetralogy of Fallot

TABLE 24.5	CLASSIFICATIONS OF CONGENITAL HEART DISEASE		
Cardiac Defect	**Examples**	**Pathophysiology**	**Clinical Picture**
Increased pulmonary blood flow (left-to-right shunting)	Atrial septal defect (ASD) Ventricular septal defect (VSD) Patent ductus arteriosus (PDA)	Cardiac septum communication or abnormal connection between the great arteries permits blood to flow from higher pressure (left side of heart) to lower pressure (right side of heart).	Asymptomatic or murmur, fatigue with feedings, and symptoms of congestive heart failure (CHF): pallor, diminished peripheral blood flow, feeding difficulties, edema, diaphoresis, tachypnea, and tachycardia
Decreased pulmonary blood flow	Tetralogy of Fallot (TOF) Tricuspid atresia	Pulmonary blood flow obstruction accompanied by an anatomic defect such as ASD or VSD between the right and left sides of the heart, which allows desaturated blood to shunt right to left, causing desaturated blood to enter into the systemic circulation	Mild to severe oxygen desaturation, polycythemia, murmur, hypoxemia, dyspnea, increased cardiac workload, and marked exercise intolerance
Obstruction to blood flow out of the heart	Pulmonary stenosis Aortic stenosis Coarctation of the aorta	A narrowing or constriction of an opening causes pressure to rise in the area behind the obstruction and a decrease in blood available for systemic perfusion	CHF, decreased cardiac output, and pump failure
Mixed defects	Transposition of the great arteries Total anomalous pulmonary venous connection Truncus arteriosus Hypoplastic left heart syndrome	Fully saturated systemic blood flow mixes with desaturated pulmonary blood flow, causing desaturation of the systemic circulation. This leads to pulmonary congestion and a decrease in cardiac output. To support life, intervention must bring about a mixing of arterial and venous blood.	Decreased cardiac output, CHF, ruddiness, dusky or gray color, dyspnea

Adapted from Altman, C. A. (2015). Congenital heart disease in the newborn: Presentation and screening for critical CHD. *UpToDate*. Retrieved from http://www.uptodate.com/contents/congenital-heart-disease-chd-in-the-newborn-presentation-and-screening-for-critical-chd; American Academy of Pediatrics [AAP]. (2014). *Newborn screening for CCHD*. Retrieved from http://www.aap.org/en-us/advocacy-and-policy/aap-health-initiatives/PEHDIC/Pages/Newborn-Screening-for-CCHD.aspx; American Heart Association [AHA]. (2014a). *About congenital heart defects*. Retrieved from http://www.heart.org/HEARTORG/Conditions/CongenitalHeartDefects/AboutCongenitalHeartDefects/About-Congenital-Heart-Defects_UCM_001217_Article.jsp; and American Heart Association [AHA]. (2014b). *Common types of heart defects*. Retrieved from http://www.heart.org/HEARTORG/Conditions/CongenitalHeartDefects/AboutCongenitalHeartDefects/Common-Types-of-Heart-Defects_UCM_307017_Article.jsp

• *Defects of the great vessels*: defects involving mixing of saturated and desaturated blood, such as truncus arteriosus or transposition of the great arteries

These four categories are more descriptive than the system used previously, which classified the disorder only as cyanotic or acyanotic. This previous classification was imprecise because some newborns with "acyanotic" defects developed cyanosis and delayed symptoms that often became apparent during infancy and early childhood. With the hemodynamic classification, the clinical picture of each grouping is more uniform and predictable.

Critical congenital heart disease (CCHD) is a group of the seven most severe congenital heart diseases. They include coarctation of the aorta, transposition of the great arteries, hypoplastic left heart syndrome, total anomalous pulmonary venous return, tetralogy of Fallot, and truncus arteriosus. Treatment is needed very soon after birth or CCHD can be deadly (Altman, 2015).

Therapeutic Management

If the defect is mild, typically no treatment is necessary. However, for most congenital defects corrective surgery is necessary.

Nursing Assessment

Although most congenital heart defects cannot be prevented, several key areas need to be addressed to ensure the optimal health status for the woman and her fetus. A thorough health history of the woman and newborn and physical examination provide valuable information. Laboratory and diagnostic tests provide additional information about the defect and its severity.

HEALTH HISTORY AND PHYSICAL EXAMINATION

Ideally, nursing assessment begins prenatally by reviewing the maternal history for risk factors that might predispose the newborn to a congenital heart defect. Risk factors include:

- Maternal alcoholism
- Maternal diabetes mellitus
- Single-gene mutation or chromosomal disorders
- Maternal exposure to x-rays
- Maternal exposure to rubella infection
- Poor maternal nutrition during pregnancy
- Maternal age over 40
- Maternal use of amphetamines
- Genetic factors (family recurrence patterns)
- Maternal metabolic disorder of phenylketonuria
- Maternal use of anticonvulsants, estrogen, progesterone, lithium, warfarin (Coumadin), or isotretinoin (Accutane) (March of Dimes, 2015c).

After birth, carefully assess the newborn's cardiovascular and respiratory systems, looking for signs of respiratory distress, cyanosis, or congestive heart failure that might indicate a cardiac anomaly. Assess rate, rhythm, and heart sounds, reporting any abnormalities immediately. Note any signs of heart failure, including edema, diminished peripheral pulses, poor feeding, poor growth, cyanotic, depending on the lesion, hepatomegaly, tachycardia, diaphoresis, respiratory distress with tachypnea, peripheral pallor, and irritability. Pulse oximetry screening is now recommended by the Department of Health and Human Services (HHS) and AAP when the infant is at least 24 hours old to detect seven of the CCHDs, but is not mandated in many states (AAP, 2014; Wood, 2015).

LABORATORY AND DIAGNOSTIC TESTS

Assist with diagnostic testing, such as:

- ABGs to determine oxygenation levels and to differentiate lung disease from heart disease as the cause of cyanosis
- Chest x-rays to identify cardiac size, shape, and position
- Performing pulse oximetry and recording it when infant is at least 24 hours old
- Magnetic resonance imaging to evaluate for cardiac malformations
- Electrocardiogram to detect atrial or ventricular hypertrophy and dysrhythmias
- Echocardiogram to evaluate heart anatomy and flow defects
- Blood studies to assess anemia, blood glucose, and electrolyte levels
- Catheterization to obtain data for definitive diagnosis or in preparation for cardiac surgery

Nursing Management

Like nursing assessment, nursing management ideally focuses on prevention with measures during the prenatal period. For example, ensure that all women are tested prior to pregnancy for immunity to rubella so that they can be immunized if necessary. Any chronic health problems, such as diabetes, hypertension, seizures, and phenylketonuria (PKU), should be controlled and any medication or dietary adjustments should be made before attempting conception. Once pregnant, the woman should be encouraged to avoid alcohol, smoking, and the use of unprescribed drugs. Refer the woman and her partner for genetic counseling if cardiac defects are present in the family to provide the parents with a risk assessment for future offspring. Some defects can be discovered on routine prenatal ultrasound. Therefore, stress the importance of receiving prenatal care throughout pregnancy so that appropriate interventions can be initiated early if the need arises.

After birth of the newborn, nursing management focuses on ensuring adequate cardiac functioning. Provide continuous monitoring of the newborn's cardiac and respiratory status. Administer medications as ordered. Provide comfort measures to the newborn, who will be subjected to a variety of painful procedures. Be vigilant in ensuring the newborn's comfort, since he or she cannot report or describe pain. Assist in preventing pain as much as possible; interpret the newborn's cues suggesting pain and manage it appropriately.

Include the parents in the plan of care. Assess their ability to cope with the diagnosis, encouraging them to verbalize their feelings about the newborn's condition and treatment. Educate them about the specific cardiac defect; include written information and pictures to enhance understanding. Present an overview of the prognosis and possible interventions. Teach them about the medications prescribed, including side effects and doses, and how to observe for signs and symptoms indicating heart failure.

Assist them with making decisions about treatment, and support their decisions for the newborn's care. If surgical correction is planned, provide the parents with preoperative teaching and orient them to the NICU prior to surgery. Provide emotional support and guidance throughout the newborn's care.

The parents also need clear instructions about how to monitor the newborn at home, especially if the newborn will be discharged and then brought back later so the condition can be corrected. The parents also need instructions about caring for their newborn after the defect is corrected. Educate the parents about signs that need to be reported, such as weight loss, poor feeding, cyanosis, breathing difficulties, irritability, increased respiratory rate, and fever. Referrals to local support groups, national organizations, and websites also are helpful. Emphasize the importance of close supervision and follow-up care.

Neural Tube Defects

Neural tube defect (NTD) is the common name used to describe congenital central nervous system structural defects. NTDs are serious malformations involving the spine (spina bifida) and brain (anencephaly). NTDs affect approximately 3,000 newborns in the United States each year (Ellenbogen, 2015). NTD is the second most common major congenital anomaly worldwide, behind cardiac malformations, but NTD causes much more infant mortality and mortality. Worldwide there are more than 300,000 infants born annually with NTDs (CDC, 2015c). Significant ethnic differences in prevalence are recognized; people of Celtic origin have the highest rate of spina bifida. Hispanic women have higher rates of NTDs than non-Hispanic women in the United States. More females have NTDs, accounting for 60% to 70% of affected children (United States Preventive Services Task Force, 2014).

A worldwide decline in NTDs has occurred during the past few decades as a result of prevention (preconception folic acid supplementation and monitoring of maternal serum alpha-fetoprotein levels) and the use of ultrasonography and amniocentesis to identify affected fetuses. Based on this decline, the WHO recommends periconceptional folic acid supplementation to prevent NTD (Johnson & Prabhu, 2015). Despite this decline, still more infants could be born free of these birth defects if all women consumed the necessary amount (400 to 800 mg) of folic acid (CDC, 2015c).

Pathophysiology

NTDs occur when the neural tube that develops into the brain and spinal cord fails to close properly during early embryogenesis. The neural tube normally closes between the 17th and 30th day of gestation to form the brain and spinal cord of the embryo. NTDs develop during this first month, when most women are still unaware of their pregnancy and the embryo is estimated to be about the size of a grain of rice. In pregnancies in which the fetus has an NTD, the level of alpha-fetoprotein in the amniotic fluid and maternal serum is elevated. NTDs involve abnormalities in the region-specific neural tube closure junctions with the cranial and caudal levels of the neural tube. NTDs may be either closed (covered by skin or a membrane) or open (neural tissue exposed). These defects vary in their severity, depending on the type and level of the lesion. Common NTDs include anencephaly, spina bifida, meningocele, and myelomeningocele.

ANENCEPHALY

Anencephaly, the most severe NTD, is the congenital absence of the cranial vault, with the cerebral hemispheres completely missing or reduced to small masses. The brain has been replaced by an undifferentiated mass of connective tissue and vessels. It most commonly involves the forebrain and variable amounts of the upper brain stem, where there is no brain tissue above the brain stem. The incidence is approximately 1.2 per 10,000 births, and both genetic and environmental insults appear to be responsible (National Institute of Neurological Disorders and Stroke [NINDS], 2015a). Anencephaly is apparent on visual inspection after birth, with exposed neural tissue without a cranium surrounding it. Prenatally, alpha-fetoprotein levels are elevated late in the first trimester. Most newborns with anencephaly are stillborn, usually blind, deaf, and unconscious and most anencephalic infants born alive die within a few days.

SPINA BIFIDA

Spina bifida is a general term used to refer to caudal defects (below the level of T12) involving spinal cord tissue. It is a disorder involving incomplete development of the brain, spinal cord, and/or their protective coverings caused by the failure of the fetus's spine to close properly during the first month of pregnancy. Although the spinal opening can be surgically repaired shortly after birth, the nerve damage is permanent, resulting in varying degrees of paralysis of the lower limbs. Spina bifida is the leading cause of infantile paralysis in the world today, affecting up to 2,000 infants born annually in the United States (NINDS, 2015b).

Spina bifida may be classified by the degree of spinal cord involvement as spina bifida occulta or spinal bifida cystica (Fig. 24.9). Spina bifida occulta involves a defect in the vertebrae without any protrusion or herniation of the spinal cord or meninges. It is a closed defect and is not visible externally. A hairy patch, dermal sinus tract, dimple, hemangioma, or lipoma may be noted in the thoracic, lumbar, or sacral area. This form of spina bifida rarely causes disability or symptoms.

Spina bifida cystica is a more serious NTD. It includes meningocele and myelomeningocele. **Meningocele**, a less severe form of spina bifida cystica, is an opening in the spine through a bony defect (spina bifida) where a herniation of the meninges and spinal fluid has protruded. The spinal cord and nerve roots do not herniate into this dorsal dural sac. Some infants with meningocele may have few or no symptoms while others may experience such symptoms as complete paralysis with bladder and bowel dysfunction. Surgical treatment to close the defect is usually warranted.

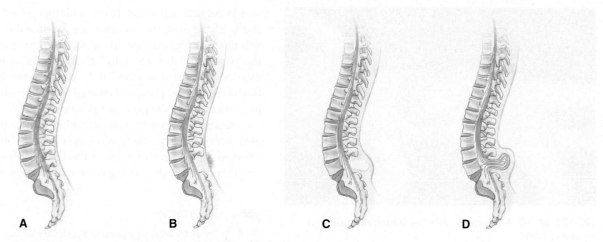

FIGURE 24.9 Neural tube defects. **A.** Normal spine. **B.** Spina bifida occulta. **C.** Meningocele. **D.** Myelomeningocele.

A **myelomeningocele** is the most severe form of spina bifida cystica in which the spinal cord and nerve roots herniate into the sac through an opening in the spine, compromising the meninges. It is the most common form, accounting for 94% of cases (Foster & Kolaski, 2016). The incidence is 1 in 1,000 births; it affects up to 1,500 newborns in the United States each year (International Society for Pediatric Neurosurgery [ISPN], 2015). This complex condition, resulting from a neurodevelopmental disruption early in gestation, affects not just the spine but also the central nervous system. Hydrocephalus (abnormal accumulation of CSF within the ventricles and subarachnoid spaces) frequently accompanies this anomaly (Avellino, 2015). This protrusion is typically covered partially or completely by skin but is very fragile and may leak CSF if traumatized.

Take Note!

Myelomeningoceles can arise at any point along the vertebral column, but they most commonly occur in the lower lumbar or sacral regions, causing neurologic deficits below the level of the defect. Paralysis, bladder and bowel incontinence, and hydrocephalus are the most common complications.

Therapeutic Management

No immediate treatment is needed for spina bifida occulta. However, surgical intervention may be necessary later in life to treat complications associated with degenerative changes or spinal or nerve root involvement. For meningocele, surgery is performed to close the defect. For myelomeningocele, surgical repair is completed as soon as possible, usually within 72 hours after birth, to prevent infection and preserve neurologic function. Due to the severity and life-threating nature of these defects, fetal surgery for the repair of myelomeningoceles in the

uterus is being advocated and done with encouraging results (Fuchs, 2015).

Nursing Assessment

Nursing assessment focuses on prevention. Assess all women of childbearing age for intake of folic acid and the use of folic acid supplementation. Review a pregnant woman's history for this supplementation throughout the pregnancy. In addition, monitor the pregnant woman's serum alpha-fetoprotein levels as indicated during pregnancy. Be alert for genetic and environmental risk factors associated with myelomeningocele, such as:

- Celtic or Hispanic ancestry (highest incidence)
- Female sex (accounting for 60% to 70% of affected newborns)
- Low socioeconomic status
- Maternal diabetes
- Use of anticonvulsants (valproic acid and carbamazepine)
- Previous newborn with an NTD
- Maternal obesity
- Maternal malnutrition
- Low folic acid intake (Cunningham et al., 2014).

Inspect the newborn for abnormalities of the spine and back. Look for dimpling or a tuft of hair, which would suggest spina bifida occulta. Observe for a protrusion along the back that may be partially or completely covered with skin. Note the head circumference: a newborn with myelomeningocele often exhibits hydrocephalus (Fig. 24.10).

Take Note!

Newborns with meningocele usually have normal examination findings and a covered (closed) dural sac. They typically do not have associated neurologic malformations.

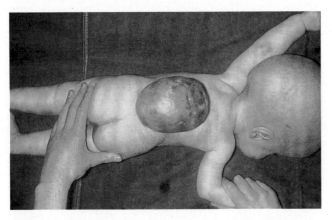

FIGURE 24.10 A newborn with myelomeningocele and hydrocephalus.

Nursing Management

Nursing management of the newborn with spina bifida occulta is primarily supportive. Be sure that the parents understand the term used and that they do not confuse their newborn's condition with a more serious form of NTD. Teach them about the possibility of surgery in the future should complications develop.

For the child with meningocele, closely monitor the skin covering the area for evidence of CSF leakage. Prepare the newborn and parents for surgery.

Nursing management for a newborn with myelomeningocele involves the following actions to reduce the risk of infection and injury to the defect site:

- Use strict aseptic technique when caring for the defect to prevent infection.
- Avoid trauma to the sac (to prevent leakage of CSF or damage to the nerve tissue) through prone or side-lying positioning.
- Avoid placing a diaper over the sac to prevent rupture or infection by fecal contamination.
- Apply a sterile dressing or protective covering over the sac to prevent rupture and drying, with frequent changes to prevent the dressing from adhering to the defect.
- Frequently monitor the sac for signs of oozing fluid or drainage.
- Preserve skin integrity on and around the spinal defect.
- Meticulously clean the genital area to avoid contamination of the sac.
- In addition, ensure a neutral thermal environment and avoid hypothermia. Heat can be lost through the defect opening, placing the newborn at increased risk for cold stress.

Corrective surgery (pre/postnatal) correction is the usual modality of treatment for these congenital malformations of the nervous system. Intrauterine fetal surgery to repair spina bifida early in the pregnancy has decreased the number of infants developing hydrocephalus that would require a postnatal ventricular shunt (Copp et al., 2015). If the surgery is performed postnatally, the nurse will need to prepare the infant preoperatively and inform the parents of the necessity of closing the spinal defect as soon after birth as possible to preserve the neurologic function present. Intravenous antibiotics are administered to prevent infection pre- and postoperatively.

Assess movement and sensation below the defect; also assess urinary and bowel elimination, which may be affected based on the level of the lesion. Measure head circumference daily to observe for hydrocephalus.

> **Take Note!**
>
> Infants with myelomeningocele are at increased risk for latex allergy due to their repeated and numerous exposures to products containing latex during surgery and other necessary treatments.

Provide support and information to help the parents cope. Allow them to verbalize their feelings and ask questions. Encourage open discussions regarding the baby's prognosis and long-term care. Provide education about the care of the newborn, including measures to reduce the risk of infection and trauma to the sac. Encourage the parents to participate in their newborn's care as much as possible. As necessary, refer the parents to a support group.

Microcephaly

Microcephaly is a condition in which a small brain is located within a normal-sized cranium. Infants born with microcephaly will have a smaller than normal head that will fail to grow as they progress through infancy. It can be caused by genetic abnormalities or by drugs, alcohol, Zika virus, and toxins that the fetus is exposed to during the pregnancy.

Microcephaly is rare, affecting more than 25,000 infants in the United States each year. It is generally defined as a head circumference that is more than 2 standard deviations below the mean for age and sex, and if not present at birth, it usually develops before 2 years of age. There is no treatment for microcephaly that can return an infant's head to a normal size and shape. Treatment focuses on ways to decrease the impact of the associated deformities and neurologic disabilities (Foundation for Children with Microcephaly [FCM], 2015).

This implies neurologic impairment. Diagnosis is confirmed by a CT scan or MRI. Care is supportive since there is no known treatment to reverse the disorder. This defect may be caused by a number of factors: genetic, chromosomal disorders, environment, and factors of unknown origin. Risk factors for this anomaly include maternal viral infections (toxoplasmosis, rubella, cytomegalovirus, herpes, and syphilis), radiation exposure, diabetes, PKU, street drug exposure, alcohol consumption during pregnancy, and malnutrition (NINDS, 2015c). Inform parents about the potential cognitive impairment of their newborn. Ensure that appropriate community referrals are made to assist the parents and the child, who will have developmental delays.

Hydrocephalus

Hydrocephalus is an increase in CSF in the ventricles of the brain due to overproduction or impaired circulation and absorption. It may be congenital or acquired. CSF is produced constantly inside each of the four spaces—ventricles—inside the brain. Approximately 400 and 600 mL of CSF is produced each day. The CSF normally flows from one ventricle to another, out of the brain and down the spinal cord. If this drainage is prevented at any point, fluid accumulates in the ventricles causing them to swell, resulting in compression of the surrounding tissue (Fig. 24.11A,B1). The term *hydrocephalus* stems from the Greek words *hydro* (water) and *kephale* (head). It occurs in about 3 per 1,000 live births (Gardner et al., 2016).

Pathophysiology

Congenital hydrocephalus usually arises as a result of a malformation in the brain or an intrauterine infection (toxoplasmosis or cytomegalovirus). Hydrocephalus rarely occurs as an isolated defect; it is usually associated with spina bifida or other neural tube anomalies. Normal growth of the brain is altered secondary to the increase in intracranial pressure from the CSF.

Therapeutic Management

No treatment is available that can counteract the accumulation of CSF in the brain, but a surgical placement of shunt system helps reduce the accumulation of CSF The management of congenital hydrocephalus consists primarily of early shunting as soon after birth as possible. Therefore, surgery with the insertion of a ventricular shunt is a frequent treatment to relieve pressure within the cranium.

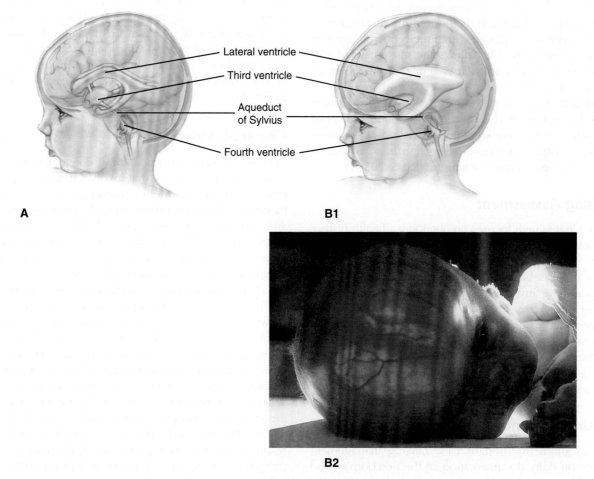

Lateral ventricle

Third ventricle

Aqueduct of Sylvius

Fourth ventricle

A

B1

B2

FIGURE 24.11 A. Infant *without* hydrocephalus. Note the ventricles of the brain and channels for the normal flow of cerebrospinal fluid. **B1, B2.** Infant *with* hydrocephalus. Note broadening of the forehead and large head size.

Concept Mastery Alert

Treatment of Hydrocephalus

An infant with hydrocephalus is unable to move cerebral spinal fluid out of the cranium. The increased fluid causes pressure on the brain and ultimately brain damage. The only treatment available is surgery in order to halt any further damage to the brain.

Shunts are designed to maintain normal intracranial pressure by draining off excess CSF. A ventriculoperitoneal shunt is inserted from the ventricle in the brain and threaded down into the peritoneal cavity to allow drainage of excess CSF. The long-term prognosis for this condition varies and depends on the patency of the shunt, the presence of other CNS anomalies and their impact on the newborn, and the quality of care the newborn receives. Historically, hydrocephalus treatment has almost exclusively consisted of ventricular-peritoneal (VP) shunting due to ease of insertion of the shunt by neurosurgeons and immediate clinical response. However, VP shunts do have high failure rates predominantly due to infection, and endoscopic third ventriculostomy (ETV) is fast becoming a frontline treatment despite its complexities. ETV creates an opening in the floor of the third ventricle using an endoscope placed within the ventricular system through a burr hole. This allows the movement of CSF out of the blocked ventricular system and into the interpeduncular cistern (a normal CSF space) thereby short-cutting any obstruction. ETV is an alternative treatment method, which keeps the CSF within the brain and spinal cord, and is now considered a safe method of choice in the treatment of obstructive hydrocephalus, particularly when following a failed VP shunt (NINDS, 2015d).

Nursing Assessment

Nursing assessment focuses on obtaining a health history and performing a physical examination. Be alert for risk factors in the maternal history such as intrauterine infection or preterm birth. Assess the infant's head circumference and note any increases. Also note any visible scalp veins (Fig. 24.11B2). Palpate the infant's head, noting any widened sutures and wide, opened fontanels. Typically the fontanels will feel tense and bulging. Also observe for other signs of hydrocephalus, including poor feeding, "setting sun" eyes, vomiting, lethargy, and irritability. A CT scan or MRI confirms the diagnosis.

Nursing Management

Prior to shunt insertion or ETV, nursing management focuses on daily documentation of the newborn's head circumference and associated neurologic behaviors that might indicate an increase in intracranial pressure: irritability, high-pitched cry, poor feeding and sucking, lethargy or sleepiness, vomiting, bulging anterior fontanel when newborn is quiet, seizures or posturing, or a decrease in consciousness. Gently palpate the fontanels for bulging and tenseness, and palpate the suture lines for increasing separation. Protect the enlarged head to prevent skin breakdown. Handle the head gently and use a sheepskin or a waterbed or egg-crate mattress. Change the newborn's position frequently to minimize pressure.

Postoperatively, strictly monitor the newborn's neurologic status and behavior and report any changes that might indicate increased intracranial pressure secondary to a blockage in the shunt. These findings may include pupillary dilation (increased intracranial pressure places pressure on the oculomotor nerve, producing dilation), increasing head size, bulging fontanels, and change in level of consciousness. Assess the abdomen for distention because drainage of CSF into the abdomen can cause peritonitis. Paralytic ileus is another possible postoperative complication due to distal catheter placement (Kenner & Lott, 2014).

After surgery, continue to provide protective and comfort measures for the enlarged head. Position the newborn's head so that he or she does not lie on the shunt area. Educate the parents about caring for the shunt and signs of infection or blockage. A referral for follow-up home care is appropriate. Stress the importance of close medical follow-up and prompt treatment of any health problems to prevent spread of infections to the shunt.

Choanal Atresia

Choanal atresia is an uncommon congenital malformation of the upper airway that involves a narrowing of the nasal airway due to membranous or bony tissue. It can be unilateral or bilateral and typically presents with other anomalies involving the heart and CNS. It occurs in 1 in approximately 8,000 live births, with a female preponderance. Half will have other congenital abnormalities in addition to choanal atresia (Kwong, 2015).

The cause of this congenital defect is unknown, but it is thought to result from persistence of the membrane between the nasal and oral spaces during fetal development. During attempted inspiration, the tongue is pulled to the palate and obstruction of the oral airway results. If the newborn cries and takes a breath through the mouth, the airway obstruction is momentarily relieved. When the crying stops, however, the mouth closes and the cycle of obstruction is repeated (Foster & Kolaski, 2016). This structural anomaly can result in significant respiratory distress in the newborn. If the nasal airway is completely obstructed, death from asphyxia may occur at birth.

Inability to pass a suction catheter through the nose into the pharynx is highly suggestive of choanal atresia.

Other signs include respiratory distress, noisy breathing, cyanosis unless newborn is crying, and inability to suck and breathe simultaneously. The diagnosis can be confirmed with a CT scan. Surgery to remove the obstruction and establish a patent airway is needed. Full recovery is the usual outcome.

Congenital Diaphragmatic Hernia

Congenital diaphragmatic hernia (CDH) is a severe anomaly of failure in the development of the diaphragm that results in an abnormal insertion onto the inner chest wall, allowing some or all of the abdominal organs/contents to protrude into the thoracic cavity, impeding fetal lung development. CDH is characterized by pulmonary hypoplasia and decreased pulmonary vasculature. Newborns with CDH often require prompt treatment of severe respiratory distress and pulmonary hypertension to prevent death. Incidence of CDH in the United States is 1 in 2,000 to 3,000 live births and accounts for 8% of all major congenital anomalies. It has a worldwide incidence of 1 in 2,500 to 3,000 live births. CDH accounts for 8% of all major congenital anomalies (Steinhorn & Porta, 2015).

CDH is associated with other anomalies, including congenital cardiac defects, genital or renal anomalies, NTDs, choanal atresia, or chromosomal anomalies, such as trisomy 13 and 18. The survival rate of newborns with a diaphragmatic hernia varies widely.

Pathophysiology

The pathogenesis of CDH is complex and remains poorly understood. Although there is strong evidence implicating genetic and environmental factors in pathogenesis, few causal genes have been identified. It is thought that the diaphragm fails to close properly during early embryonic development. The abdominal contents then herniate into the thoracic cavity through a defect in the diaphragm (Fig. 24.12). The timing of the herniation and the amount of abdominal contents in the thoracic cavity greatly influence the clinical picture at birth and the survival rate. The presence of the abdominal contents in the chest compresses the lung, leads to pulmonary hypoplasia, and promotes persistent pulmonary hypertension in the newborn. Signs and symptoms of CDH include acute respiratory distress, cyanosis, sterna retractions, grunting, nasal flaring, tachycardia, rapid breathing, barrel-shaped chest, and a concave-shaped abdomen (Gardner et al., 2016).

Nursing Assessment

Assess the newborn closely for evidence of respiratory distress, including cyanosis. Affected newborns present with profound respiratory distress because at least one of the lungs cannot expand or may not have fully developed, resulting in persistent pulmonary hypertension

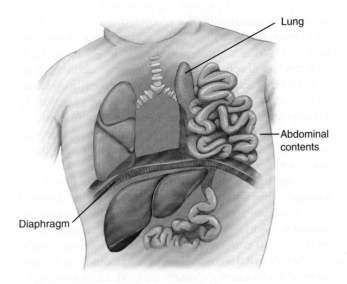

FIGURE 24.12 Congenital diaphragmatic hernia. Note how some of the abdominal contents have entered the thoracic cavity, compressing the lung.

shortly after birth. If present, institute resuscitation measures immediately.

Inspect the chest and abdomen, noting a barrel-shaped chest and scaphoid-shaped abdomen. During auscultation, note absent breath sounds on the affected side of the chest and heart sounds displaced to the right. Also listen for bowel sounds, which would be heard in the chest.

Prepare the newborn for a chest x-ray or ultrasound, which will reveal evidence of air-filled bowel in the chest.

 Take Note!

Prenatal diagnosis of CDH is possible through ultrasound. This diagnosis should be considered when polyhydramnios is present.

Nursing Management

Initial treatment involves respiratory support with the goal of maintaining oxygenation and cardiovascular stability. Surgery to correct the anatomic malformation is usually delayed until after the newborn's condition stabilizes. The surgical repair can also be delayed for months and done by minimally invasive surgery with the use of prosthetic material for closure of large defects. Extracorporeal membrane oxygenation, a process that mimics the gas exchange process of the lungs, may be ordered when the surgery is undertaken.

Nursing management focuses on maintaining optimal respiratory function until surgery is performed to correct the defect. Assist with endotracheal intubation and positive-pressure ventilation to aid in lung expansion and improvement of ventilation. Position the newborn on the affected side with the head and chest elevated to promote normal lung expansion. Monitor ventilatory pressures to prevent pneumothorax. If a pneumothorax occurs, assist with insertion of a chest tube and monitor chest tube drainage. Monitor oxygen saturation levels to evaluate systemic perfusion status. If the infant's condition does not stabilize, anticipate use of extracorporeal membrane oxygenation or high-frequency oscillatory ventilation. Be cognizant of potential complications postoperatively, which might include persistent pulmonary hypertension, gastric reflux, chronic lung disease, recurrent lung infections, and failure to thrive (McHoney, 2014).

Administer prescribed medications as ordered. For example, give inotropics (drugs that affect the force of muscle contractions) to support systemic blood pressure. Administer surfactant, steroids, and inhaled nitric oxide as ordered to correct hypoxia and acid–base imbalance.

Monitor vital signs, weight, urinary output, and serum electrolytes to identify changes early. Maintain nothing by mouth (NPO) status to prevent aspiration, and ensure a neutral thermal environment to prevent cold stress and reduce oxygen demands. Minimize environmental stimuli to reduce agitation and oxygen demand. Assist with placement of an orogastric tube for gastric decompression.

Counseling is an essential component in the management of CDH. Parents should be informed about the severity of this condition, the treatment plan, the risk of poor outcomes, and the potential for several long-term morbidities. Assess the parental anxiety level and coping ability; provide emotional support and educate about CDH pathophysiology, potential complications, treatment risks and benefits, long-term medical surveillance to reduce risk of complications, and individualized prognosis. Refer for counseling on coping strategies as appropriate; provide written information on CDH to reinforce verbal education. Provide the parents with continuing updates about the newborn's condition. Encourage the parents to see and touch the infant frequently to promote bonding. Assist parents with identifying newborn cues and responding to them.

Cleft Lip and Palate

Cleft lip with or without cleft palate is the most common congenital malformation of the head and neck. A cleft lip involves a congenital fissure or longitudinal opening in the lip; a cleft palate involves a congenital fissure or longitudinal opening in the roof of the mouth. The defect may be limited to the outer flesh of the upper lip or it may extend back through the midline of the upper jaw through the roof of the palate. It may occur as a single defect or as part of a syndrome of anomalies. It can be unilateral or bilateral. Unilateral cleft lip occurs more commonly on the left side. Bilateral cleft lip is usually accompanied by a cleft palate. Cleft palate can range from a cleft in the uvula to a complete cleft in the soft and hard palates that can be unilateral, bilateral, or in the midline (Fig. 24.13).

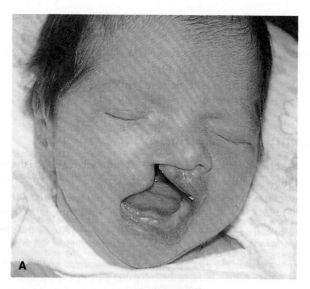

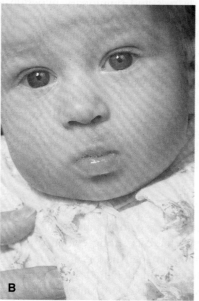

FIGURE 24.13 **A.** A newborn with a cleft lip. The defect may extend up through the roof of the palate. **B.** Infant with a surgical repair of a cleft lip. (Image **A** is from Moore, K. L., & Dalley, A. F. [2009]. *Clinical oriented anatomy* [6th ed.]. Baltimore, MD: Lippincott Williams & Wilkins.)

Cleft lip with cleft palate is a common craniofacial birth defect. It is more common in White and Asian males. It affects approximately 1 in 600 live births in the United States annually. In addition to immediate feeding difficulties, infants with cleft lip and palate may have problems with dentition, language acquisition, and hearing (Yadav et al., 2015).

Therapeutic Management

Repairing the facial anomaly as soon as possible is important to facilitate bonding between the newborn and the parents and to improve nutritional status. Treatment of cleft lip is surgical repair between the ages of 6 and 12 weeks. A rule of thumb for surgical readiness includes infant is 10 weeks old, weighs 10 pounds, and has hemoglobin of at least 10 g/dL. Successful surgery often leaves only a thin scar on the upper lip. The outcome of surgery depends on the severity of the defect: children with more severe cases will need additional surgery in stages (Crockett & Goudy, 2014).

The timing of the palate repair is more controversial, and there is not a universally correct recommendation. Surgical correction for cleft palate is typically done by 12 months of age to allow for developmental growth to occur. A plastic palate guard to form a synthetic palate may need to be used to allow for introduction of solid foods and to prevent aspiration in the interim.

Nursing Assessment

Obtain a thorough maternal history, noting the presence of any risk factors such as maternal use of phenytoin (Dilantin), alcohol, low folic acid intake, increased parental age, retinoic acid (Accutane), and cigarette smoking (Patel, 2014). Also assess for a family history of cleft lip or palate, which increases the risk. Keep in mind in the assessment that cleft lip and palate possess significant medical, psychological, social, and financial implications on the affected person and their family. In addition to the aesthetic disfigurement, the affected infant will suffer restricted maxillofacial growth, speech anomalies, swallowing and feeding difficulties, hearing loss and/or recurrent ear infections (Allam & Stone, 2014).

Inspect the lip for a visible deformity. Inspect and palpate the mouth for an opening, which may be small or involve the entire palate. Also observe for any feeding difficulties, which are common in newborns with cleft lip and palate.

Take Note!

Milk flow during feeding requires negative pressure and sucking pressure. Newborns with cleft lip and palate have feeding difficulties because they cannot generate a negative pressure in the mouth to facilitate sucking (Cleft Palate Foundation [CFF], 2015). Use special nipples, squeezable bottles, and feeders to help meet the nutritional needs of infants with this anomaly.

Nursing Management

Nursing management focuses on providing adequate nutrition, promoting parental bonding, and providing parental education. Prevention should be considered the ultimate objective through preconception education of couples.

PROVIDING ADEQUATE NUTRITION

Many infants born with cleft lip and palate cannot be breast-fed. Those with cleft palate cannot produce the negative pressure necessary for suction. Mothers of infants with a unilateral cleft lip may succeed with breast-feeding when the infant is positioned so that the cleft in the lip is obstructed by the mother's breast. No single right or correct method of feeding has been identified. Parents working together with the health care provider and nursing staff should choose the method that is best for their infant.

Nurses need to instruct the mother to feed the infant in an upright position to prevent aspiration, and assess for achievement of adequate suction during feeding. Use high-calorie formula to improve caloric intake. Burp the infant frequently to reduce the risk for vomiting and aspiration; burp him or her in the sitting position on your lap to prevent trauma to the mouth on your shoulder. Limit feeding sessions to avoid poor weight gain due to fatigue. After feeding, position the newborn on his or her side in an infant seat.

PROMOTING PARENTAL BONDING

Prenatal diagnosis of cleft lip and palate has been available for over 25 years. Three-dimensional ultrasound has significantly improved prenatal screening and perinatal care. Surface rendering of the fetal face is frequently asked by parents during exam and it has been shown to substantially improve parental–fetal bonding. Studies support that prenatal diagnosis of cleft lip and palate is known to improve parental well-being during the perinatal period. Furthermore, in addition to improved diagnosis, 3D ultrasound also provides a better understanding and acceptance of the malformation by parents. Nurses need to develop interventions to help parents deal with the impact of social stigmatization and physical concerns of the cleft lip and palate condition (Juneja & Juneja, 2014).

On first glance, parents may be upset with the appearance of their newborn. Encourage the parents to express their feelings about this highly visible anomaly. Emphasize the newborn's positive features and role-model nurturing behaviors when interacting with the infant. Encourage parents to interact with the newborn. Provide support to the parents, especially related to feeding difficulties. Allow them to vent their frustrations. Offer practical suggestions and continued encouragement for their efforts.

PROVIDING PARENTAL EDUCATION

The impact on quality of life for the infant and the family can be severe, particularly for unsuspecting families. Emotional and psychological needs must be recognized and addressed, in addition to surgical care, by all those caring for the infant. Outline treatment modalities and explain the staging of surgical interventions. Show the family photos taken before and after surgical repair in other babies. These photos can alleviate some of their anxiety. Start planning for discharge as soon as the parents feel comfortable with infant care. Provide anticipatory guidance and instructions for potential challenges they may face at home and into the future, which include feeding difficulties, frequent ear infections, speech difficulties, and dental problems. As part of the discharge plan, initiate appropriate referrals for community support and counseling as needed. Nurses can help parents/partners/significant others to trust in themselves and feel confident in their ability to nurture their newborns by listening, informing, and encouraging them (Tierney et al., 2015).

Esophageal Atresia and Tracheoesophageal Fistula

Esophageal atresia (EA) and tracheoesophageal fistula (TEF) are gastrointestinal anomalies in which the esophagus and trachea do not separate normally during early embryonic development (3 to 6 weeks). EA is a congenitally interrupted esophagus where the proximal and distal ends do not communicate; the upper esophageal segment ends in a blind pouch and the lower segment ends a variable distance above the diaphragm (Fig. 24.14). TEF is an abnormal communication between the trachea and esophagus. When associated with EA, the fistula most commonly occurs between the distal esophageal segment and the trachea. The lack of esophageal patency prevents swallowing. In addition to preventing normal feeding, this problem may cause infants to aspirate and literally drown in their own saliva, which quickly overflows the upper pouch of the obstructed esophagus. If a TEF is present, fluid (either saliva from above or gastric secretions from below) may flow directly into the lungs. The incidence of EA is 1 in 4,000 to 5,000 live births (Scorpio, 2014).

 Concept Mastery Alert

Priority Concern in Esophageal Atresia

The priority concern for the infant with esophageal atresia (EA) is the risk for respiratory distress. Many infants with EA also have a TEF, which is a connection between the esophagus and the trachea. This connection can put the infant at high risk for respiratory distress, especially if the child is fed any food by mouth.

Pathophysiology

Several types of EA exist, but the most common anomaly is a fistula between the distal esophagus and the trachea, which occurs in 90% of newborns with an esophageal defect. EA and TEF are thought to be the result of incomplete separation of the lung bed from the foregut during early fetal development. A large percentage (50% to 70%) of these newborns have other congenital anomalies involving the vertebrae, kidneys, heart, and musculoskeletal and gastrointestinal systems (Oermann, 2015). Most newborns have several anomalies.

Nursing Assessment

Review the maternal history for polyhydramnios. Often this is the first sign of EA because the fetus cannot swallow and absorb amniotic fluid in utero, leading to accumulation. Soon after birth, the newborn may exhibit copious, frothy bubbles of mucus in the mouth and nose, accompanied by drooling. Abdominal distention develops as air builds up in the stomach. In EA, an orogastric tube cannot be inserted beyond a certain point because the esophagus ends in a blind pouch. The newborn may have rattling respirations, excessive salivation and drooling, and "the three C's" (coughing, choking, and cyanosis) if feeding is attempted. The presence of a fistula increases the risk of respiratory complications such as pneumonitis and atelectasis due to aspiration of food and secretions (Davidson, 2014). Clinical manifestations of EA and TEF include:

*   Excessive secretions
*   Feeding intolerance
*   Inability to pass orogastric tube
*   Abdominal distention
*   Respiratory distress
*   Other anomalies involving the vertebrae, anus, cardiac system, and kidneys

 Take Note!

The "three C's" of choking, coughing, and cyanosis in conjunction with feeding are considered the classic signs of TEF and EA.

Prepare the newborn and parents for radiographic evaluation. Diagnosis is made by x-ray, an ultrasound, or MRI: if the gastric tube appears coiled in the upper esophageal pouch, with air in the gastrointestinal tract, this indicates the presence of a fistula (Mattson & Smith, 2015). Once a diagnosis of EA is established, begin preparations for surgery if the newborn is stable.

Nursing Management

Once the diagnosis is established, an orogastric tube is placed in the upper esophageal pouch and set to low continuous suction to prevent aspiration of oral secretions. Nursing management focuses on preparing the newborn and parents for surgery and providing meticulous postoperative care. The type of esophageal defect dictates the surgical approach needed.

PROVIDING PREOPERATIVE CARE

Preoperative nursing interventions include the following measures:

*   Initiate NPO status.

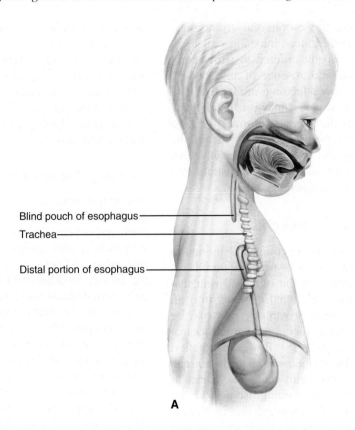

Blind pouch of esophagus
Trachea
Distal portion of esophagus

A

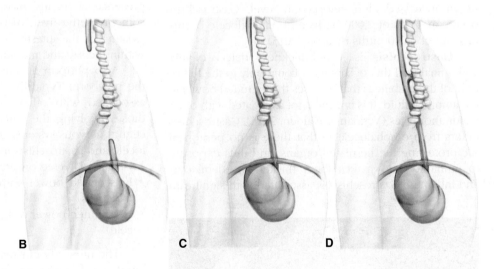

FIGURE 24.14 Esophageal atresia and tracheoesophageal fistula. **A.** The most common type of esophageal atresia, in which the esophagus ends in a blind pouch and a fistula connects the trachea with the distal portion of the esophagus. **B.** The upper and distal portions of the esophagus end in a blind pouch. **C.** The esophagus is one segment, but a portion of it is narrowed. **D.** The upper portion of the esophagus connects to the trachea via a fistula.

B   **C**   **D**

- Elevate the head of the bed 30 to 45 degrees to prevent reflux and aspiration.
- Monitor hydration status and fluid and electrolyte balance; administer and monitor parenteral intravenous fluid infusions.
- Assess and maintain the patency of the orogastric tube. Monitor the functioning of the tube, which is attached to low continuous suction. Avoid irrigation of the tube to prevent aspiration.
- Have oxygen and suctioning equipment readily available should the newborn experience respiratory distress.
- Assist with diagnostic studies to rule out other anomalies.

- Use comfort measures to minimize crying and prevent respiratory distress; provide nonnutritive sucking.
- Inform the parents about the rationales for the aspiration prevention measures.
- Document frequent observations of the newborn's condition (Kenner & Lott, 2014).

PROVIDING POSTOPERATIVE CARE

Surgery consists of closing the fistula and joining the two esophageal segments. Postoperative care involves closely observing all of the newborn's body systems to identify any complications. Expect to administer

TPN and antibiotics until the esophageal anastomosis is proven intact and patent. Before initiating oral feedings, an esophagram is usually ordered to verify complete anastomotic healing and absence of any leaks. If that validates healing, then oral feedings are started, usually within a week after surgery (Shawyer, Pemberton, & Flageole, 2014). Keep the parents informed of their newborn's condition and progress. Closely assess the newborn during feeding and report any difficulty with swallowing. Provide parent teaching. Demonstrate and reinforce all teaching prior to discharge.

Omphalocele and Gastroschisis

Omphalocele and gastroschisis are congenital anomalies of the anterior abdominal wall at or near the umbilicus. An **omphalocele** is a defect of the umbilical ring that allows evisceration of the abdominal contents into an external peritoneal sac. Defects vary in size; they may be limited to bowel loops or may include the entire gastrointestinal tract and liver (Fig. 24.15). Bowel malrotation is common, but the displaced organs are usually normal. Omphaloceles are associated with other anomalies in more than 50% of the cases, most often trisomies 12, 18, or 21. This anomaly is usually detected during routine prenatal ultrasound of the fetus or during investigation of an increased alpha-fetoprotein level. Gastroschisis occurs in 1 out of 2,000 births and omphalocele occurs in 1 out of 4,000 births (Glasser, 2015).

Gastroschisis is a full-thickness defect of the abdominal wall that occurs most commonly to the left or right of the umbilicus that exposes the extruded bowel to the amniotic fluid. It is typically not associated with other major anomalies (Verklan & Walden, 2014). Gastroschisis differs from omphalocele in that there is no peritoneal sac protecting the herniated organs, and thus exposure to amniotic fluid makes them thickened, edematous, and inflamed. Gastroschisis is associated with significant

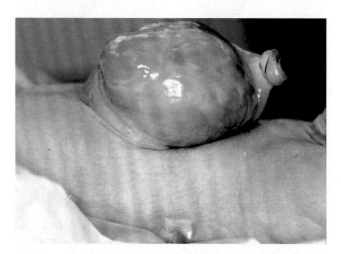

FIGURE 24.15 Omphalocele in a newborn. Note the large, protruding sac.

newborn mortality and morbidity rates. Despite surgical correction, feeding intolerance, short bowel syndrome, intestinal stricture, bowel obstruction, failure to thrive, and prolonged hospital stays occur in nearly all newborns with this anomaly (Markdante & Kliegman, 2014). Each of these diagnoses requires that a pediatric surgeon be available at birth to determine the extent of the defect and complications.

Nursing Assessment

Abdominal wall defects are readily diagnosed by prenatal ultrasound, which is helpful in planning for the birth and needed therapy. An early birth may be planned if the ultrasound reveals evidence of progressive bowel distention and thickening. Review the maternal history for factors associated with high-risk pregnancies, such as maternal illness and infection, drug use, smoking, and genetic abnormalities. These factors are also associated with omphalocele and gastroschisis. They contribute to placental insufficiency and the birth of an SGA or preterm newborn, the populations in which both of these abdominal defects most commonly occur.

Omphalocele and gastroschisis are readily observed. Note the appearance of the protrusion on the abdomen and evidence of a sac. Inspect the sac closely for the presence of organs, most commonly the intestines but sometimes the liver. Also inspect the contents for any twisting of the intestines. Note the color of the organs within the sac and measure the size of the omphalocele.

Also perform a complete physical examination of the newborn. Typically these congenital conditions are associated with other congenital anomalies, such as those involving the cardiovascular, genitourinary, and central nervous systems. Assessment findings of omphalocele and gastroschisis include:

- Usually detected on prenatal ultrasound exams
- Eviscerated bowel without peritoneal covering (gastroschisis)
- Eviscerated bowel with peritoneal covering (omphalocele)

The nurse should search for additional anomalies if omphalocele is diagnosed.

Nursing Management

Nursing management of newborns with omphalocele or gastroschisis focuses on preventing hypothermia, maintaining perfusion to the eviscerated abdominal contents by minimizing fluid loss, and protecting the exposed abdominal contents from trauma and infection. These objectives can be accomplished by placing the infant in a sterile drawstring bowel bag that maintains a sterile environment for the exposed contents, allows visualization, reduces heat and moisture loss, and allows heat from radiant warmers to reach the newborn. The newborn is placed feet-first into the bag and the drawstring is secured around the torso (Kallen, 2014a). Strict sterile technique is necessary to prevent contamination of the exposed abdominal contents.

An orogastric tube attached to low suction is used to prevent intestinal distention. Intravenous therapy is administered to maintain fluid and electrolyte balance and provide a route for antibiotic therapy. Monitor the newborn's fluid status frequently. Closely observe the exposed bowel for vascular compromise, such as changes in color or a decrease in temperature, and report these immediately.

PROVIDING POSTOPERATIVE CARE

Surgical repair of both defects occurs after initial stabilization and comprehensive evaluation for any other anomalies. It may have to occur in stages, depending on the defect (Box 24.5). Postoperative care involves providing pain management, monitoring respiratory and cardiac status, monitoring intake and output, assessing for vascular compromise, maintaining the orogastric tube to suction, documenting the amount and color of drainage, and administering ordered medications and treatments (Glasser, 2015). Also be alert for complications, such as short bowel syndrome.

PROMOTING PARENT–NEWBORN INTERACTION

The parents need continued support and progress reports on their newborn. They may be distraught at the sight of the anomaly, and they may be frightened to touch their newborn. Encourage the parents to touch the newborn and participate in care as much as possible. Because of the nature of this defect, bonding opportunities will be limited initially. However, strongly encourage frequent visiting. In addition, provide information to the parents about the defect, treatment modalities, and prognosis. After surgery, instruct the parents in care measures and give them care instructions. Anticipate the need for a referral to a home health care agency and community resources for support.

Imperforate Anus

An imperforate anus is a gastrointestinal system malformation of the anorectal area that may occur in several forms. The rectum may end in a blind pouch that does not connect to the colon, or it may have fistulas (openings) between the rectum and the perineum, the vagina in girls or the urethra in boys (Fig. 24.16). The malformations occur during early fetal development and are associated with anomalies in other body systems. The etiology of such malformations remains unclear and is likely multifactorial.

Imperforate anus occurs in about 1 of every 3,500 live births, and predominantly affects males more than females (Rosen, 2015). The defect can be further classified as a high or low type, depending on its level. A fistula connection to the perineum or the urogenital tract is frequently present. The level significantly influences fecal continence and management (Coppola, 2014).

Surgical intervention is needed for both high and low types of imperforate anus. Surgery for a high type of defect involves a colostomy in the newborn period, with corrective surgery performed in stages to allow for growth. Surgery for the low type of anomaly, which frequently includes a fistula, involves closure of the fistula, creation of an anal opening, and repositioning of the rectal pouch into the anal opening. A major challenge for either type of surgical repair is finding, using, or creating adequate nerve and muscle structures around the rectum to provide for normal evacuation.

Nursing Assessment

In the newborn, observe for an appropriate anal opening. If the anal opening exists, observe for passage of meconium stool within the first 24 hours of life. Assess urine output to identify genitourinary problems. For the newborn with an imperforate anus, inspection of the perineal area would reveal absence of the usual opening, and meconium generally is not passed or present within 24 hours of birth.

In the infant with suspected imperforate anus, assess for common signs of intestinal obstruction, which may occur as a result of the malformation. These include abdominal distention and bilious vomiting.

Prepare the newborn and family for a perineal ultrasound and an abdominal x-ray that will be ordered to identify the level of defect in the absence of a perineal fistula and also to assess for complications associated with imperforate anus.

BOX 24.5

SURGERY TO REPAIR OMPHALOCELE AND GASTROSCHISIS

Surgical repair of gastroschisis is an emergency due to the high risk of intestinal atresia, resulting in obstruction. Primary repair of gastroschisis is usually performed without incident unless the contents are unable to fit into the abdominal cavity. This occurs more often with a large omphalocele, requiring the surgeon to do a staged closure. This involves covering the defect with a synthetic material that is sequentially squeezed like toothpaste to reduce the defect into the abdominal cavity. After enough of the defect is in the abdominal cavity, a surgical repair is then performed (Glasser, 2015). If damage to the exposed organs occurs, such as necrosis, then the necrotic sections are removed during the repair. If a significant amount of small intestine is lost, then the complication of short bowel syndrome may occur.

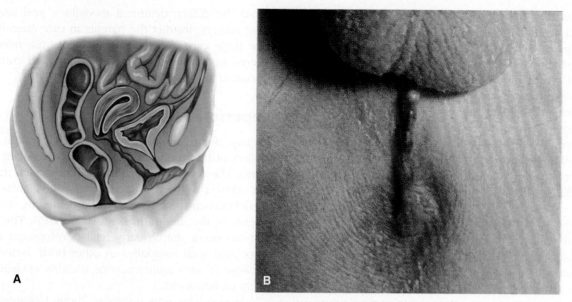

FIGURE 24.16 A. Imperforate anus, in which the rectum ends in a blind pouch. **B.** Imperforate anus without fistula. The visible meconium streak along the raphe is consistent with a low imperforate anus. (Courtesy of Kevin P. Lally, MD.)

Nursing Management

Nursing management focuses on preparing the newborn and parents for surgery and providing postoperative care. Preoperatively, maintain the newborn's NPO status and provide gastric decompression. Administer intravenous therapy and antibiotic therapy as ordered and monitor the newborn's hydration status. Provide a full explanation of the defect, surgical options, potential complications, typical postoperative course, and long-term care needed to the parents. Make sure they are aware of the available treatment modalities. Prepare them for the possibility that the newborn may require a colostomy. Provide support to the parents and family.

Postoperative care includes ensuring adequate pain relief, maintaining NPO status and gastric decompression until normal bowel function is restored, and providing colostomy care if applicable. Stoma care and teaching of the parents are paramount for home care of the infant.

Hypospadias

Hypospadias is a relatively common malformation of the male genital organ. It is an abnormal positioning of the urinary meatus on the underside of the penis (Fig. 24.17B). Scrotal and testicular anomalies are often associated, e.g., undescended testicle. Hypospadias is a relatively common

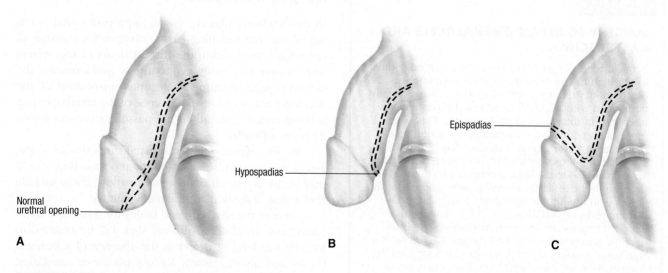

Normal urethral opening

Hypospadias

Epispadias

A   **B**   **C**

FIGURE 24.17 Genitourinary tract structural anomalies.

birth defect that occurs in approximately 1 of every 250 male births in the United States (Kallen, 2014b).

The malformation is the result of incomplete fusion of the urethral folds, which usually occurs between 8 and 20 weeks of gestation (Gatti, Snyder, & Kirsch, 2015). The cause is unknown, but it is thought to be of multifactorial inheritance because it occasionally occurs in more than one male in the same family.

The degree of hypospadias depends on the location of the opening. It is often accompanied by a downward bowing of the penis (chordee), which can lead to urination and erection problems and infertility in adulthood.

Hypospadias can be corrected surgically. Depending on the severity, the correction can be completed in one or more procedures with good results. The success of hypospadias repair can be measured according to functional results, such as urinary flow rate, straight urine stream and lack of urinary tract infection, as well as a normal appearance of the penis, with a slit-like meatus at the tip of the glans. Surgical intervention should be completed during the latter half of the first year of life to prevent any body image problems in the child.

Epispadias

Epispadias is a rare congenital genitourinary defect occurring in 1 in 10,000 to 50,000 male births. The male-to-female ratio is 2:1 (Kenner & Lott, 2014). The condition is usually diagnosed at birth or shortly thereafter. In boys with epispadias, the urethra generally opens on the top or side rather than the tip of the penis. In females, the urinary meatus is located between the clitoris and the labia. This anomaly often occurs in conjunction with exstrophy of the bladder (Foster & Kolaski, 2016). Surgical correction is necessary, and affected male newborns should not be circumcised. Surgery generally leads to the ability to control the flow of urine and a good cosmetic outcome (see Fig. 24.17C).

Bladder Exstrophy

In bladder exstrophy, the bladder protrudes onto the abdominal wall because the abdominal wall failed to close during embryonic development (Fig. 24.18). Wide separation of the rectus muscles and the symphysis pubis accompanies this defect. Virtually all affected male infants have associated epispadias. The upper urinary tract is usually normal. The incidence is approximately 1 in 30,000 live births, and happens in males slightly more than females (March of Dimes, 2015d).

Goals of therapy include restoring urinary continence, preserving renal function, and reconstructing functional and cosmetically acceptable genitalia. Initial bladder closure is completed within 48 hours after birth. Epispadias repair occurs at this time if possible. Further surgical reconstruction is performed in several stages at about 2 to 3 years of age (see Fig. 24.18B). Because of the potential long-term implications of exstrophy, family education is critical. Exstrophy support groups are established at several major medical centers.

Nursing management of the newborn with bladder exstrophy includes the following activities:

- Identify the genitourinary defect at birth so that immediate treatment can be provided.
- Cover the exposed bladder with a sterile clear nonadherent dressing to prevent hypothermia and infection.
- Irrigate the bladder surface with sterile saline after each diaper change to prevent infection.
- Assist with insertion and monitoring of a suprapubic catheter to drain the bladder and prevent obstruction.
- Administer antibiotic therapy as ordered to prevent infection.
- Schedule diagnostic tests to assess for additional anomalies.
- Assess the newborn frequently for any signs of infection.
- Inspect skin surfaces frequently to ensure skin integrity.

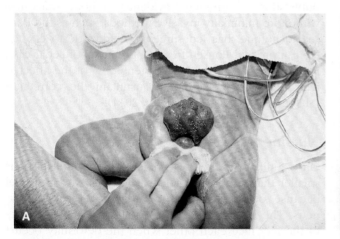
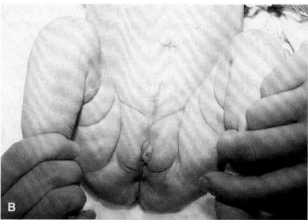

FIGURE 24.18 Bladder exstrophy. **A.** Before surgical repair. **B.** After surgery.

- Maintain modified Bryant traction for immobilization after surgery.
- Administer antispasmodics, analgesics, and sedatives as ordered to prevent bladder spasm and provide comfort.
- Educate the parents about the care of the urinary catheter at home if applicable.
- Support the parents throughout.
- Promote bonding by encouraging the parents to visit and touch the newborn.
- Refer the parents to a support group to enhance their coping ability.
- Be a therapeutic listener to the family (Davidson, 2014; Kenner & Lott, 2014).

Congenital Clubfoot

Clubfoot, or talipes equinovarus, is a common congenital deformity affecting approximately 1 to 2 per 1,000 live births. It is bilateral in about half of the cases and affects boys twice as often as girls. It is characterized by an excessive turned in foot. It typically has four components: inversion and adduction of the forefoot, inversion of the heel and hindfoot, limitation of extension of the ankle and subtalar joint, and internal rotation of the leg (Patel & Herzenberg, 2015) (Fig. 24.19). Reducing or eliminating all of the components of the deformity is the goal to ensure that the newborn has a functional, mobile, painless foot that does not require the use of special or modified shoes (Gray et al., 2014).

Pathophysiology

Clubfoot is a complex, multifactorial deformity with genetic and intrauterine factors. Heredity and race seem to factor into the incidence, but the means of transmission and the etiology are unknown. Most newborns with clubfoot have no identifiable genetic, syndromal, or extrinsic cause.

Clubfoot can be classified into extrinsic (supple) type, which is essentially a severe positional or soft tissue deformity, or intrinsic (rigid) type, where manual reduction is not possible.

Therapeutic Management

Its management must begin shortly after birth. The type of clubfoot deformity determines the treatment course. Treatment for the extrinsic (supple) type consists of serial casting, followed by maintenance splinting. Treatment for the intrinsic (rigid) type includes initial casting followed by surgery. It is generally agreed that the initial treatment should be nonsurgical and started soon after birth.

Treatment for either type starts with serial casting, which is needed due to the rapid growth of the newborn.

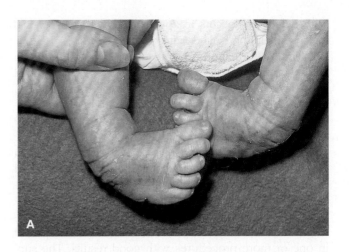

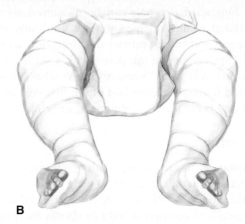

FIGURE 24.19 Clubfoot deformity. **A.** Initial appearance. **B.** Application of cast to correct clubfoot.

Casts initially are changed weekly and are applied until the deformity responds and is fully corrected. If serial casting is not successful in correcting the deformity, surgical intervention is necessary between 4 and 9 months of age. The standard treatment of clubfoot has changed greatly in the past 10 years. Previously, extensive surgery was common in children born with this condition. The publication of long-term evidence of good outcomes with more minimally invasive methods, such as the Ponseti technique, has led surgeons worldwide to change their approach. Ponseti treatment consists of serial casting and percutaneous Achilles tenotomy of the affected feet followed by bracing to maintain the correction (Shabtai, Specht, & Herzenberg, 2014).

Nursing Assessment

On examination, the foot appears "down and in." It is smaller than a normal foot, with a flexible, softer heel because of the hypoplastic (underdeveloped) calcaneus. The heel is internally rotated, making the soles of the feet face each other when the deformity occurs bilaterally.

Nursing Management

Nursing management focuses on education, anticipatory guidance, and pain management. Educate the parents about their newborn's condition and the treatment protocol to reduce their anxiety, and provide reassurance that the clubfoot is not painful and will not hinder the child's development. Discuss challenges associated with sleep, play, and dressing. Inform them that slight modifications will be necessary to accommodate the plaster casts. Review positioning, bathing, and skin care along with pain management when new casts are applied. Stress the need to provide a calm, quiet environment to promote relaxation and sleep for their newborn.

Developmental Dysplasia of the Hip

Developmental dysplasia of the hip (DDH) involves abnormal growth or development of the hip that results in instability. This includes hips that are unstable, subluxated, or dislocated (luxated) or have a malformed acetabulum. The instability allows the femoral head to become easily displaced from the acetabulum. The incidence of hip instability is about 1.5 to 25 per 1,000 live births and is more common in females and breech presentations (Schwend, 2014). The etiology of DDH is unclear.

Therapeutic Management

Treatment is started as soon as DDH is identified. If the newborn examination reveals DDH, the newborn is referred to an orthopedist. The goal of treatment is to relocate the femoral head in the acetabulum to facilitate normal growth and development. The Pavlik harness is the most widely used device; it prevents adduction while allowing flexion and abduction to accomplish the treatment goal (Fig. 24.20). The harness is worn continuously until the hip is stable, which may take several months. If harnessing is not successful, surgery is necessary.

Nursing Assessment

Assess the history for risk factors, including racial background (Native Americans), genetic transmission (runs in families), intrauterine positioning (breech), sex (female), oligohydramnios, birth order (first-born), and postnatal infant-carrying positions (swaddling, which forces the hips to be adducted). The risk increases in cultures that tightly swaddle infants with their hips forcefully maintained in extension and adduction.

Take Note!

DDH is frequently not identified during the newborn examination, so newborns require careful evaluation for hip dysplasia at subsequent visits throughout the first year.

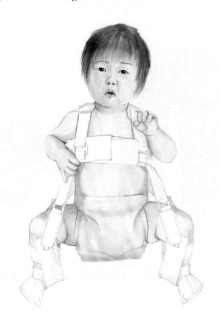

FIGURE 24.20 The Pavlik harness is used to treat developmental dysplasia of the hip.

Complete a physical examination. Typically, the newborn with DDH is otherwise healthy, usually without any other deformities. Pay particular attention to assessing hip instability. Perform Ortolani and Barlow maneuvers (see Chapter 18 for more information on these maneuvers). Ortolani's maneuver elicits the sensation of the dislocated hip reducing; Barlow's maneuver detects the unstable hip dislocating from the acetabulum. A hip "clunk" is felt when the infant's legs are abducted into a frog position. Although soft clicks are common, a sharp click indicates dislocation. Fractures may also be present and are characterized by limited movement and edematous, crepitant areas. Also observe for other physical signs of DDH, including an asymmetric number of skin folds on the thigh or buttock, an apparent or true short leg, and limited hip abduction (Rosenfeld, 2015) (Fig. 24.21).

Nursing Management

Nursing management related to DDH starts with recognition of the disorder and early reporting to the health care provider. Early diagnosis is the crucial aspect; education also is critical. Teach the parents how to care for their newborn while in the harness during treatment. Proper fit and adjustments for growth are essential for successful treatment. Frequent clinical assessment on an outpatient basis is needed to monitor progress. Through education, the nurse can be very effective in helping the parents to adhere to the treatment.

Inborn Errors of Metabolism

Inborn errors of metabolism are genetic disorders that disrupt normal metabolic function. Most are due to a

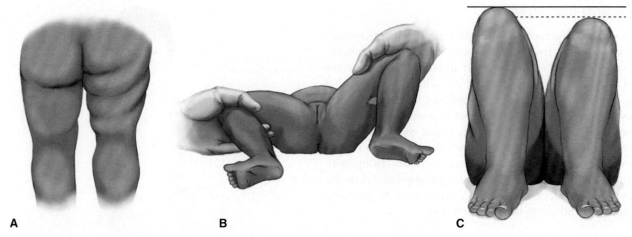

A   **B**   **C**

FIGURE 24.21 Characteristics of developmental dysplasia of the hip. **A.** Asymmetric number of skin folds on the thigh or buttock. **B.** Limited hip abduction. **C.** Unequal knee height.

defect in an enzyme or transport protein, resulting in a blocked metabolic pathway. Clinical symptoms are manifested secondary to toxic accumulations of substances before the block. When viewed individually, inborn errors of metabolism are rare, but collectively they are responsible for significant levels of infant mortality and morbidity. The incidence, collectively, is estimated to be approximately 1 in 4,000 live births (Weiner, 2015). Table 24.6 summarizes four common inborn errors.

A successful outcome depends on early diagnosis and prompt intervention. Most inborn errors present in the newborn period with nonspecific and subtle manifestations—lethargy, hypotonia, respiratory distress, poor feeding and weight gain, vomiting, and seizures (Sutton, 2015). Identification of an inborn error of metabolism in a newborn depends largely on the awareness of the nurse and clues from the maternal history, laboratory work, and clinical examination.

TABLE 24.6   INBORN ERRORS OF METABOLISM

Condition	Incidence and Etiology	Clinical Picture	Management
Phenylketonuria (PKU)	1:10,000–15,000 live births Autosomal recessive genetic disorder caused by a deficiency of the hepatic enzyme phenylalanine hydroxylase Enzyme deficiency with subsequent accumulation of amino acid phenylalanine	Newborns appear normal at birth, but by 6 months of age signs of slow mental development are evident. Vomiting, poor feedings, failure to thrive, overactivity, irritability, musty-smelling urine If not treated, possible intellectual disability	Screening of all newborns at about 48 h after birth to ensure adequate intake of protein Dietary restriction of phenylalanine, with regular monitoring of serum phenylalanine levels (effective when started before the first month of age) Lifelong dietary restriction of phenylalanine
Maple syrup urine disease (MSUR)	1:86,000–185,000 live births; most prevalent among the Mennonite population in Lancaster, Pennsylvania Autosomal recessive inherited disorder Enzyme metabolism of certain amino acids is affected, with the buildup of acids causing ketoacidosis.	Lethargy, poor feeding, vomiting, weight loss, seizures, shrill cry, shallow respirations, loss of reflexes, coma, sweet maple syrup odor to urine	Dialysis to remove accumulated acids Lifelong low-protein diet to prevent neurologic deficits of disease

TABLE 24.6	INBORN ERRORS OF METABOLISM (continued)		
Condition	**Incidence and Etiology**	**Clinical Picture**	**Management**
Galactosemia	1:60,000 live births Autosomal recessive inherited disorder in which an enzyme needed to convert galactose to glucose is missing and newborn cannot metabolize lactose	Vomiting, hypoglycemia, liver damage, hyperbilirubinemia, poor weight gain, cataracts, frequent infections	Routine newborn screening for galactosemia is performed in the majority of states. Lifelong lactose-restricted diet is needed to prevent intellectual disability, liver disease, and cataracts.
Congenital hypothyroidism	1:4,000 live births Multiple causes—absent or underdeveloped thyroid gland or biochemical defects in thyroid hormone	Large protruding tongue, slow reflexes, distended abdomen, large, open posterior fontanel, constipation, hypothermia, poor feeding, hoarse cry, dry skin, coarse hair, goiter, and jaundice If untreated, irreversible cognitive and motor impairment occurs. Decreased levels of thyroid hormone (T_4) and elevated levels of TSH	Newborn screening program in all states Lifelong thyroid replacement hormone therapy and continued monitoring of thyroid levels and clinical response to therapy

Adapted from Kenner, C., & Lott, J. W. (2014). *Comprehensive neonatal nursing care* (5th ed.). New York, NY: Springer Publishers; King, T. L., Brucker, M. C., Kriebs, J. M., Fahey, J. O., Gegor, C. L., & Varney, H. (2015). *Varney's midwifery* (5th ed.). Burlington, MA: Jones & Bartlett Learning; Marcdante, K., & Kliegman, R. M. (2014). *Nelson essentials textbook of pediatrics* (7th ed.). St. Louis, MO: Saunders Elsevier Health Science; and Malcolm, W. (2015). *Beyond the NICU: Comprehensive care of the high risk infant*. New York, NY: McGraw-Hill Education.

KEY CONCEPTS

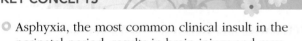

- Asphyxia, the most common clinical insult in the perinatal period, results in brain injury and may lead to intellectual disability, cerebral palsy, or seizures.

- Transient tachypnea of the newborn occurs when the liquid in the lung is removed slowly or incompletely.

- Common risk factors for respiratory distress syndrome (RDS) include young gestational age, perinatal asphyxia regardless of gestational age, cesarean birth in the absence of labor (related to the lack of thoracic squeeze), male gender, and maternal diabetes.

- Meconium aspiration has three major pulmonary effects: airway obstruction, surfactant dysfunction, and chemical pneumonitis.

- The management of persistent pulmonary hypertension of the newborn requires meticulous attention to detail, with continuous monitoring of oxygenation, blood pressure, and perfusion.

- Retinopathy of prematurity (ROP) is a developmental abnormality that affects the immature vasculature of the retina; abnormal growth of blood vessels (neovascularization) takes place within the retina and vitreous.

- Periventricular–intraventricular hemorrhage is bleeding that usually originates in the subependymal germinal matrix region of the brain with extension into the ventricular system.

- Necrotizing enterocolitis (NEC) is a serious gastrointestinal disease of unknown etiology in newborns that can result in necrosis of a segment of the bowel.

- Infants of mothers with diabetes are at risk for malformations most frequently involving the cardiovascular, skeletal, central nervous, gastrointestinal, and genitourinary systems; cardiac anomalies are the most common.

- Factors that place the newborn at risk for birth trauma include cephalopelvic disproportion, maternal pelvic anomalies, oligohydramnios, prolonged or rapid labor, abnormal presentation, fetal prematurity, fetal macrosomia, and fetal abnormalities.

- Women who use drugs during their pregnancy expose their unborn child to the possibility of intrauterine growth restriction, prematurity, neurobehavioral and neurophysiologic dysfunction, birth defects, infections, and long-term developmental sequelae.

- Newborns of women who use tobacco, illicit substances, caffeine, and alcohol can exhibit withdrawal behavior.

- Physiologic jaundice is a common, normal newborn phenomenon that appears during the second or third day of life and then declines over the first week after birth. Pathologic jaundice is manifested within the first 24 hours of life when total bilirubin levels increase by more than 5 mg/dL/day and the total serum bilirubin level is higher than 17 mg/dL in a full-term infant.

- Newborn infections are usually classified according to the time of onset and grouped into three categories: congenital infection, acquired in utero by vertical transmission with onset before birth; early-onset neonatal infections, acquired by vertical transmission in the perinatal period, either shortly before or during birth; and late-onset neonatal infections, acquired by horizontal transmission in the nursery.

- Congenital conditions can arise from many etiologies, including single-gene disorders, chromosomal aberrations, exposure to teratogens, and many sporadic conditions of unknown cause. Congenital structural anomalies may be inherited or sporadic, isolated or multiple, apparent or hidden, and gross or microscopic.

- Congenital heart disease is commonly classified physiologically as defects that result in increased pulmonary blood flow, defects that result in decreased pulmonary blood flow, defects that cause obstruction to blood flow out of the heart, and defects that are mixed.

- A worldwide decline in neural tube defects has occurred during the past few decades due to improved prevention secondary to preconception folic acid supplementation, maternal serum alphafetoprotein monitoring, and use of ultrasonography and amniocentesis.

- Congenital respiratory tract structural disorders include choanal atresia and congenital diaphragmatic hernia. Evidence of bowel sounds in the chest suggests congenital diaphragmatic hernia.

- Cleft lip with cleft palate is the most common craniofacial birth defect. The newborn has immediate feeding difficulties and may have problems with dentition, language acquisition, and hearing.

- Esophageal atresia refers to a congenitally interrupted esophagus where the proximal and distal ends do not communicate; the upper esophageal segment ends in a blind pouch and the lower segment ends a variable distance above the diaphragm. Tracheoesophageal fistula is an abnormal communication between the trachea and esophagus.

- Omphalocele and gastroschisis are congenital anomalies of the anterior abdominal wall. An omphalocele is a defect of the umbilical ring that allows evisceration of abdominal contents into an external peritoneal sac. Gastroschisis is a herniation of abdominal contents through an abdominal wall defect, usually to the left or right of the umbilicus.

- Hypospadias and epispadias are genitourinary system structural anomalies. Epispadias often occurs in conjunction with bladder exstrophy, where the bladder protrudes onto the abdominal wall.

- Congenital clubfoot usually involves inversion and adduction of the forefoot, inversion of the heel and hindfoot, limitation of extension of the ankle and subtalar joint, and internal rotation of the leg.

- Developmental dysplasia of the hip includes dislocation, subluxation, or malformation of the acetabulum. Early recognition and prompt treatment are crucial.

- Inborn errors of metabolism are genetic disorders that disrupt normal metabolic function. Most are due to a defect in an enzyme or transport protein, resulting in a blocked metabolic pathway.

References and Recommended Readings

Allam, E., & Stone, C. (2014). Cleft lip and palate: Etiology, epidemiology, preventive and intervention strategies. *Anatomy & Physiology*, *4*(150). doi: 10.4172/2161-0940.1000150

Altman, C. A. (2015). Congenital heart disease in the newborn: Presentation and screening for critical CHD. *UpToDate*. Retrieved from http://www.uptodate.com/contents/congenital-heart-disease-chd-in-the-newborn-presentation-and-screening-for-critical-chd

Ambalavanan, N. (2015). Bronchopulmonary dysplasia. *eMedicine*. Retrieved from http://emedicine.medscape.com/article/973717-overview

American Academy of Pediatrics [AAP]. (2014). *Newborn screening for CCHD*. Retrieved from http://www.aap.org/en-us/advocacy-and-policy/aap-health-initiatives/PEHDIC/Pages/Newborn-Screening-for-CCHD.aspx

American Academy of Pediatrics [AAP]. (2015). *Fetal alcohol spectrum disorders*. Retrieved from https://www.healthychildren.org/English/health-issues/conditions/chronic/Pages/Fetal-Alcohol-Spectrum-Disorders.aspx

American Heart Association [AHA]. (2015a). *About congenital heart defects*. Retrieved from http://www.heart.org/HEARTORG/Conditions/CongenitalHeartDefects/AboutCongenitalHeartDefects/About-Congenital-Heart-Defects_UCM_001217_Article.jsp

American Heart Association [AHA]. (2015b). *Common types of heart defects*. Retrieved from http://www.heart.org/HEARTORG/Conditions/CongenitalHeartDefects/AboutCongenitalHeartDefects/Common-Types-of-Heart-Defects_UCM_307017_Article.jsp

American Heart Association [AHA] & American Academy of Pediatrics [AAP]. (2014). *Neonatal resuscitation: Update and documentation.* Retrieved from http://www2.aap.org/nrp/docs/IU/2014_SpringSummer_iu.pdf

American Lung Association [ALA]. (2015). *Bronchopulmonary dysplasia.* Retrieved from http://www.lung.org/lung-disease/bronchopulmonary-dysplasia

Anderson-Berry, A. L., Bellig, L. L., & Ohning, B. L. (2015). Neonatal sepsis. *eMedicine.* Retrieved from http://emedicine.medscape.com/article/978352-overview

Annibale, D. J. (2015). Periventricular hemorrhage–intraventricular hemorrhage. *eMedicine.* Retrieved from http://emedicine.medscape.com/article/976654-overview

Artigas, V. (2015). Management of neonatal abstinence syndrome in the newborn nursery. *Nursing for Women's Health, 18*(6), 509–514.

Avellino, A. M. (2015). Hydrocephalus. In A. Agrawal & G. Britz (Eds.), *Emergency approaches to neurosurgical conditions* (pp. 71–78). Switzerland: Springer International Publishing.

Ballabh, P. (2014). Pathogenesis and prevention of intraventricular hemorrhage. *Clinics in Perinatology, 41*(1), 47–67.

Beam, K. S., Aliaga, S., Ahlfeld, S. K., Cohen-Wolkowiez, M., Smith, P. B., & Laughon, M. M. (2014). A systematic review of randomized controlled trials for the prevention of bronchopulmonary dysplasia in infants. *Journal of Perinatology, 34*(9), 705–710.

Blennow, M., & Bohlin, K. (2015). Surfactant and noninvasive ventilation. *Neonatology, 107*(4), 330–336.

Bowen, P., & Maxwell, N. C. (2014). Management of bronchopulmonary dysplasia. *Pediatrics and Child Health, 24*(1), 27–31.

Brooke-Vincent, F. (2015). Meconium aspiration syndrome and persistent pulmonary hypertension of the newborn. *Journal of Neonatal Nursing.* doi: 10.1016/j.jnn.2015.05.002

Centers for Disease Control and Prevention [CDC]. (2015a). *Fetal alcohol spectrum disorders.* Retrieved from http://www.cdc.gov/ncbddd/fasd/facts.html

Centers for Disease Control and Prevention [CDC]. (2015b). *Facts about birth defects.* Retrieved from http://www.cdc.gov/ncbddd/birthdefects/facts.html

Centers for Disease Control and Prevention [CDC]. (2015c). *Birth defects COUNT.* Retrieved from http://www.cdc.gov/ncbddd/folicacid/global.html

Choi, W., Jeong, H., Choi, S. J., Oh, S. Y., Kim, J. S., Roh, C. R., et al. (2015). Risk factors differentiating mild/moderate from severe meconium aspiration syndrome in meconium-stained neonates. *Obstetrics & Gynecology Science, 58*(1), 24–31.

Clark, D. A., & Clark, M. B. (2015). Meconium aspiration syndrome. *eMedicine.* Retrieved from http://emedicine.medscape.com/article/974110-overview

Cleft Palate Foundation [CFF]. (2015). *Feeding your baby.* Retrieved from http://www.cleftline.org/who-we-are/what-we-do/feeding-your-baby/

Copp, A. J., Adzick, N. S., Chitty, L. S., Fletcher, J. M., Holmbeck, G. N., & Shaw, G. M. (2015). Spina bifida. *Nature Reviews Disease Primers.* 15007.

Coppola, C. P. (2014). Imperforate anus and cloaca. In C. P. Coppola, A. P. Kennedy, & R. J. Scorpio (Eds.), *Pediatric surgery* (pp. 171–175). New York, NY: Springer International Publishing.

Crockett, D. J., & Goudy, S. L. (2014). Cleft lip and palate. *Facial Plastic Surgery Clinics of North America, 22*(4), 573–586.

Cunningham, F. G., Leveno, K. J., Bloom, S. L., Spong, C. Y., Dashe, J. S., Hoffman, B. L., et al. (2014). *Williams' obstetrics* (24th ed.). New York, NY: McGraw-Hill.

Davidson, M. R. (2014). *Fast facts for the neonatal nurse: A nursing orientation and care guide in a nutshell.* New York, NY: Springer Publishers.

Deleon, C., Shattuck, K., & Jain, S. K. (2015). Biomarkers of neonatal sepsis. *NeoReviews, 16*(5), e297–e308.

Deshpande, P. G., (2015). Breast milk jaundice treatment and management. *eMedicine.* Retrieved from http://emedicine.medscape.com/article/973629-treatment

Dörrie, N., Föcker, M., Freunscht, I., & Hebebrand, J. (2014). Fetal alcohol spectrum disorders. *European Child & Adolescent Psychiatry, 23*(10), 863–875.

Eibisberger, M., Resch, E., & Resch, B. (2015). Surfactant replacement therapy in extremely low gestational age newborns. *Indian Pediatrics, 52*(3), 227–230.

Ellenbogen, R. G. (2015). Neural tube defects in the neonatal period. *eMedicine.* Retrieved from http://emedicine.medscape.com/article/1825866-overview

El-Radhi, A. S. (2015). Management of common neonatal problems. *British Journal of Nursing, 24*(5), 258–265.

Enomoto, H., Miki, A., Matsumiya, W., & Honda, S. (2015). Evaluation of oxygen supplementation status as a risk factor associated with the development of severe retinopathy of prematurity. *Ophthalmologica, 234*(3):135–138.

Foster, M. R., & Kolaski, K. (2016). Spina bifida. *eMedicine.* Retrieved from: http://emedicine.medscape.com/article/311113-overview

Foundation for Children with Microcephaly [FCM]. (2015). *Microcephaly.* Retrieved from http://www.childrenwithmicro.org/

Fox, J. R., Thacker, L. R., & Hendricks-Muñoz, K. D. (2015). Early detection tool of intestinal dysfunction: Impact on necrotizing enterocolitis severity. *American Journal of Perinatology, 32*(10):927–932.

Francine, R., Pascale, S., & Aline, H. (2014). Congenital anomalies: Prevalence and risk factors. *Universal Journal of Public Health, 2*(2), 58–63.

Fuchs, H. E. (2015). Congenital neurosurgical problems. In A. Agrawal & G. Britz (Eds.), *Emergency approaches to neurosurgical conditions* (pp. 65–69). Switzerland: Springer International Publishing.

Gadot, Y., & Koren, G. (2015). Medications in pregnancy: Can we treat the mother while protecting the unborn? In S. Macleod, S. Hill, G. Koren, & A. Rane (Eds.), *Optimizing treatment for children in the developing world* (pp. 65–70). Switzerland: Springer International Publishing.

Gardner, S. L., Carter, B. S., Enzman-Hines, M., & Hernandez, J. A. (2016). *Merenstein & Gardner's handbook of neonatal intensive care* (8th ed.). St. Louis, MO: Elsevier.

Gatti, J. M., Snyder, H. M., & Kirsch, A. J. (2015). Hypospadias. *eMedicine.* Retrieved from http://emedicine.medscape.com/article/1015227-overview

Gaur, K. V., Nimbalkar, S. M., Desai, R., & Ganguly, B. P. (2015). Effect of single dose antenatal steroid for pregnant mothers with high risk of preterm delivery on the respiratory outcome of neonates. *Journal of Clinical Neonatology, 4*(3), 217.

Glass, L., Ware, A. L., & Mattson, S. N. (2014). Neurobehavioral, neurologic, and neuroimaging characteristics of fetal alcohol spectrum disorders. *Handbook of Clinical Neurology, 125*, 435–462.

Glasser, J. G. (2015). Omphalocele and gastroschisis. *eMedicine.* Retrieved from http://emedicine.medscape.com/article/975583-overview

Gray, K., Pacey, V., Gibbons, P, Little, D., & Burns, J. (2014). Interventions for congenital talipes equinovarus (clubfoot). *Cochrane Database Library, 2014*, CD008602.

Green, C. J. (2016). *Maternal newborn nursing care plans* (3rd ed.). Burlington, MA: Jones & Bartlett Learning.

Griffin, T., & Celenza, J. (2014). *Family-centered care for the newborn: The delivery room and beyond.* New York, NY: Springer Publishing Company.

Haakonsen Lindenskov, P. H., Castellheim, A., Saugstad, O. D., & Mollnes, T. E. (2015). Meconium aspiration syndrome: Possible pathophysiological mechanisms and future potential therapies. *Neonatology, 107*(3), 225–230.

Hamdan, A. H. (2015). Neonatal abstinence syndrome. *eMedicine.* Retrieved from http://emedicine.medscape.com/article/978763-overview

Hansen, W. R. (2015). Neonatal jaundice. *eMedicine.* Retrieved from http://emedicine.medscape.com/article/974786-overview

Hartnett, M. E. (2015). Pathophysiology and mechanisms of severe retinopathy of prematurity. *Ophthalmology, 122*(1), 200–210.

Herrera-Marschitz, M., Neira-Pena, T., Rojas-Mancilla, E., Espina-Marchant, P., Esmar, D., Perez, R., et al. (2014). Perinatal asphyxia: CNS development and deficits with delayed onset. *Frontiers in Neuroscience, 8*, 47–68.

Hudson, J. (2015). Facilitating normal physiology in the presence of meconium stained liquor. *The Practicing Midwife, 18*(6), 16–19.

Huybrechts, K. F., Bateman, B. T., Palmsten, K., Desai, R. J., Patorno, E., Gopalakrishnan, C., et al. (2015). Antidepressant use late in pregnancy and risk of persistent pulmonary hypertension of the newborn. *JAMA, 313*(21), 2142–2151.

International Society for Pediatric Neurosurgery [ISPN]. (2015). *Incidence and prevalence of myelomeningoceles.* Retrieved from http://ispn.guide/book/

Ives, N. K. (2015). Management of neonatal jaundice. *Pediatrics and Child Health, 25*(6), 276–281.

Iyengar, A., & Davis, J. M. (2015). Drug therapy for the prevention and treatment of bronchopulmonary dysplasia. *Frontiers in Pharmacology, 6*, 12.

Jallo, G. (2015). Neural tube defects. *eMedicine*. Retrieved from http://emedicine.medscape.com/article/1177162-overview

Jansson, L. M. (2015). Neonatal abstinence syndrome. *UpToDate*. Retrieved from http://www.uptodate.com/contents/neonatal-abstinence-syndrome

Jaques, S. C., & Kennea, N. (2015). Resuscitation of the newborn. *Obstetrics, Gynecology & Reproductive Medicine, 25*(3), 61–67.

Johnson, K. E. (2015). Transient tachypnea of the newborn. *UpToDate*. Retrieved from http://www.uptodate.com/contents/transient-tachypnea-of-the-newborn

Johnson, L. R., & Prabhu, S. (2015). Folic acid supplementation to prevent neural tube defects. *Academic Medical Journal of India, 3*(1), 47–48.

Jordan, C. O. (2014). Retinopathy of prematurity. *Pediatric Clinics of North America, 61*(3), 567–577.

Jordan, R. G., Engstrom, J. L., Marfell, J. A., & Farley, C. L. (2014). *Prenatal and postnatal care: A woman-centered approach*. Ames, IA: John Wiley & Sons.

Juneja, A., & Juneja, A. (2014). An exploratory study of socio-emotional experience and coping in mothers of cleft lip and palate children. *Journal of Behavioral Health, 3*(1), 65–70.

Källén, B. (2014a). Abdominal wall defects. In *Epidemiology of human congenital malformations* (pp. 137–141). New York, NY: Springer International Publishing.

Källén, B. (2014b). Hypospadias. In *Epidemiology of human congenital malformations* (pp. 95–98). New York, NY: Springer International Publishing.

Karabayir, N., Demirel, A., & Bayramoglu, E. (2015). Blood lactate level and meconium aspiration syndrome. *Archives of Gynecology and Obstetrics, 291*(4), 849–853.

Kaufman, D. A., Zanelli, S. A., Gurka, M. J., Davis, M., Richards, C. P., & Walsh, B. K. (2014). Time outside targeted oxygen saturation range and retinopathy of prematurity. *Early Human Development, 90*(2), S35–S40.

Kenner, C., & Lott, J. W. (2014). *Comprehensive neonatal nursing care* (5th ed.). New York, NY: Springer Publishers.

Kim, H. A., Yang, G. E., & Kim, M. J. (2015). Early neonatal respiratory morbidities in term neonates. *Neonatal Medicine, 22*(1), 8–13.

King, T. L., Brucker, M. C., Kriebs, J. M., Fahey, J. O., Gegor, C. L., & Varney, H. (2015). *Varney's midwifery* (5th ed.). Burlington, MA: Jones & Bartlett Learning.

Kocherlakota, P. (2014). Neonatal abstinence syndrome. *Pediatrics, 134*(2), e547–e561.

Korkmazer, E., Solak, N., & Tokgöz, V. Y. (2015). Gestational diabetes: Screening, management, timing of delivery. *Current Obstetrics and Gynecology Reports, 4*(2), 132–138.

Kwong, K. M. (2015). Current updates on choanal atresia. *Name: Frontiers in Pediatrics, 3*, 52–59.

Laroia, N. (2015). Birth trauma. *eMedicine*. Retrieved from http://emedicine.medscape.com/article/980112-overview

Lau, C. S., & Chamberlain, R. S. (2015). Probiotic administration can prevent necrotizing enterocolitis in preterm infants: A meta-analysis. *Journal of Pediatric Surgery, 50*(8):1405–1412.

Lee, K. G. (2015). Transient tachypnea – newborn. *MedlinePlus*. Retrieved from http://www.nlm.nih.gov/medlineplus/ency/article/007233.htm

Levitt, M. A., & Pena, A. (2015). Pediatric imperforate anus surgery. *eMedicine*. Retrieved from http://emedicine.medscape.com/article/933524-overview

Lim, J. C., Golden, J. M., & Ford, H. R. (2015). Pathogenesis of neonatal necrotizing enterocolitis. *Pediatric Surgery International, 31*(6), 509–518.

MacMullen, N. J., Dulski, L. A., & Blobaum, P. (2014). Evidence-based interventions for neonatal abstinence syndrome. *Pediatric Nursing, 40*(4), 165–174.

Maguire, D. (2014). Care of the infant with neonatal abstinence syndrome: Strength of the evidence. *The Journal of Perinatal & Neonatal Nursing, 28*(3), 204–211.

Maisels, M. J., Clune, S., Coleman, K., Gendelman, B., Kendall, A., McManus, S., et al. (2014). The natural history of jaundice in predominantly breastfed infants. *Pediatrics, 134*(2), e340–e345.

Malcolm, W. (2015). *Beyond the NICU: Comprehensive care of the high risk infant*. New York, NY: McGraw-Hill Education.

Mannan, M. A., Moni, S. C., & Shahidullah, M. (2015). Retinopathy of prematurity (ROP): Current understanding and management. *Bangladesh Journal of Child Health, 38*(3), 142–150.

Marcdante, K., & Kliegman, R. M. (2015). *Nelson essentials of pediatrics* (7th ed.). St. Louis, MO: Saunders Elsevier.

March of Dimes. (2015a). *Smoking, alcohol and drugs*. Retrieved from http://www.marchofdimes.org/pregnancy/alcohol-during-pregnancy.aspx

March of Dimes. (2015b). *Global report on birth defects*. Retrieved from http://www.marchofdimes.org/mission/march-of-dimes-global-report-on-birth-defects.aspx

March of Dimes. (2015c). *Congenital heart defects and CCHD*. Retrieved from http://www.marchofdimes.org/baby/congenital-heart-defects.aspx

March of Dimes. (2015d). *Genital and urinary tract defects*. Retrieved from http://www.marchofdimes.org/baby/genital-and-urinary-tract-defects.aspx

Mattson, S., & Smith, J. E. (2015). *Core curriculum for maternal-newborn nursing* (5th ed.). St. Louis, MO: Saunders Elsevier.

McHoney, M. (2014). Congenital diaphragmatic hernia. *Early Human Development, 90*(12):941–946.

McKeever, A. E., Spaeth-Brayton, S., & Sheerin, S. (2014). The role of nurses in comprehensive care management of pregnant women with drug addiction. *Nursing for Women's Health, 18*, 284–293.

Molyneux, E., & Gest, A. (2015). Neonatal sepsis: An old issue needing new answers. *The Lancet Infectious Diseases, 15*(5), 503–505.

Moses, S., (2015). Respiratory distress syndrome in the infant. *Family Practice Notebook*. Retrieved from http://www.fpnotebook.com/nicu/Lung/RsprtryDstrsSyndrmInThInfnt.htm

Muchowski, K. E. (2014). Evaluation and treatment of neonatal hyperbilirubinemia. *American Family Physician, 89*(11), 873–878.

Muhammad, A., Khan, M., Khan, I., & Anwar, T. (2014). Frequency of congenital heart diseases in infants of diabetic mothers referred to pediatrics departments. *Journal of Postgraduate Medical Institute, 28*(1). Retrieved from http://www.jpmi.org.pk/index.php/jpmi/article/view/1542

Nagtalon-Ramos, J. (2014). *Best evidence-based practices: Maternal-newborn nursing care*. Philadelphia, PA: F.A. Davis Company.

National Eye Institute [NEI]. (2015). *Facts about retinopathy of prematurity*. Retrieved from http://www.nei.nih.gov/health/rop/rop.asp#b

National Institute for Health and Care Excellence [NICE]. (2015). *Neonatal jaundice*. Retrieved from https://www.nice.org.uk/guidance/qs57/chapter/introduction

National Institute of Neurological Disorders and Stroke [NINDS]. (2015a). *What is anencephaly?* Retrieved from http://www.ninds.nih.gov/disorders/anencephaly/anencephaly.htm

National Institute of Neurological Disorders and Stroke [NINDS]. (2015b). *What is spina bifida?* Retrieved from http://www.ninds.nih.gov/disorders/spina_bifida/detail_spina_bifida.htm

National Institute of Neurological Disorders and Stroke [NINDS]. (2015c). *What is microcephaly?* Retrieved from http://www.ninds.nih.gov/disorders/microcephaly/microcephaly.htm

National Institute of Neurological Disorders and Stroke [NINDS]. (2015d). *What is hydrocephalus?* Retrieved from http://www.ninds.nih.gov/disorders/hydrocephalus/hydrocephalus.htm

National Institute on Drug Abuse [NIDA]. (2015). *Substance abuse while pregnant and breastfeeding*. Retrieved from http://www.drugabuse.gov/publications/substance-use-in-women/substance-use-while-pregnant-breastfeeding

National Institutes of Health. (2015). Necrotizing enterocolitis. *MedlinePlus*. Retrieved from http://www.nlm.nih.gov/medlineplus/ency/article/001148.htm

Neu, J. (2014). Necrotizing enterocolitis: The mystery goes on. *Neonatology, 106*(4), 289–295.

Oermann, C. M. (2015). Congenital anomalies of the intrathoracic airways and tracheoesophageal fistula. *UpToDate*. Retrieved from http://www.uptodate.com/contents/congenital-anomalies-of-the-intrathoracic-airways-and-tracheoesophageal-fistula

Patel, P. K. (2014). Unilateral cleft lip repair. *eMedicine*. Retrieved from http://emedicine.medscape.com/article/1279641-overview

Patel, M., & Herzenberg, J. (2015). Clubfoot. *eMedicine*. Retrieved from http://emedicine.medscape.com/article/1237077-overview

Popova, S., & Chambers, C. (2014). Fetal alcohol spectrum disorders must be recognized globally as a large public health problem. *The International Journal of Alcohol and Drug Research*, *3*(1), 1–3.

Potter, C. F., & Kicklighter, S. D. (2016). Infant of a diabetic mother. *eMedicine*. Retrieved from http://emedicine.medscape.com/article/974230-overview

Pramanik, A. K., Rangaswamy, N., & Gates, T. (2015). Neonatal respiratory distress: A practical approach to its diagnosis and management. *Pediatric Clinics of North America*, *62*(2), 453–469.

Randolph, A. G., & McCulloh, R. J. (2014). Pediatric sepsis: Important considerations for diagnosing and managing severe infections in infants, children, and adolescents. *Virulence*, *5*(1), 179–189.

Rangmar, J., Sandberg, A. D., Aronson, M., & Fahlke, C. (2015). Cognitive and executive functions, social cognition and sense of coherence in adults with fetal alcohol syndrome. *Nordic Journal of Psychiatry*, *69*(6), 472–478.

Rosen, N. G. (2015). Pediatric imperforate anus. *eMedicine*. Retrieved from http://emedicine.medscape.com/article/929904-overview

Rosenfeld, S. B. (2015). Developmental dysplasia of the hip: Clinical features and diagnosis. *UpToDate*. Retrieved from http://www.uptodate.com/contents/developmental-dysplasia-of-the-hip-clinical-features-and-diagnosis

Rosenthal, P. (2014). Another explanation for breast milk jaundice. *Journal of Pediatrics*, *165*(1), 10–11.

Rubarth, L. B., & Quinn, J. (2015). Respiratory development and respiratory distress syndrome. *Neonatal Network*, *34*(4), 231–238.

Sachdeva, M., Murki, S., Oleti, T. P., & Kandraju, H. (2014). Intermittent versus continuous phototherapy for the treatment of neonatal non-hemolytic moderate hyperbilirubinemia in infants more than 34 weeks of gestational age: A randomized controlled trial. *European Journal of Pediatrics*, 1–5.

Saker, F., & Martin, R. (2015). Prevention and treatment of respiratory distress syndrome in preterm infants. *UpToDate*. Retrieved from http://www.uptodate.com/contents/prevention-and-treatment-of-respiratory-distress-syndrome-in-preterm-infants

Salam, R. A., Mansoor, T., Mallick, D., Lassi, Z. S., Das, J. K., & Bhutta, Z. A. (2014). Essential childbirth and postnatal interventions for improved maternal and neonatal health. *Reproductive Health*, *11*(Suppl 1), 53–67.

Salem, L., & Singer, K. R. (2015). Rh incompatibility. *eMedicine*. Retrieved from http://emedicine.medscape.com/article/797150-overview#a0199

Saxena, A. K., Blair, G., & Konkin, D. E. (2015). Esophageal atresia with or without tracheoesophageal fistula. *eMedicine*. Retrieved from http://emedicine.medscape.com/article/935858-overview

Schanler, R. J. (2014). Clinical features and diagnosis of necrotizing enterocolitis in newborns. *UpToDate*. Retrieved from http://www.uptodate.com/contents/clinical-features-and-diagnosis-of-necrotizing-enterocolitis-in-newborns?source=see_link

Schwend, R. M. (2014). Developmental dysplasia of the hip. In R. A. Gosselin, D. A. Spiegel, & M. Foltz (Eds.), *Global orthopedics* (pp. 397–403). New York, NY: Springer Publishers.

Scorpio, R. J. (2014). Esophageal atresia and tracheoesophageal fistula. In B. J. Coventry (Ed.), *Pediatric surgery* (pp. 133–136). New York, NY: Springer International Publishing.

Shabtai, L., Specht, S. C., & Herzenberg, J. E. (2014). Worldwide spread of the Ponseti method for clubfoot. *World Journal of Orthopedics*, *5*(5), 585–590.

Shawyer, A. C., Pemberton, J., & Flageole, H. (2014). Post-operative management of esophageal atresia-tracheoesophageal fistula. *Journal of Pediatric Surgery*, *49*(5), 716–719.

Simonsen, K. A., Anderson-Berry, A. L., Delair, S. F., & Davies, H. D. (2014). Early-onset neonatal sepsis. *Clinical Microbiology Reviews*, *27*(1), 21–47.

Springer, S. C., & Annibale, D. J. (2015). Necrotizing enterocolitis. *eMedicine*. Retrieved from http://emedicine.medscape.com/article/977956-overview

Steinhorn, R. H., & Porta, N. (2015). Pediatric congenital diaphragmatic hernia. *eMedicine*. Retrieved from http://emedicine.medscape.com/article/978118-overview

Subramanian, K. N., Bahri, M., & Vicente, G. (2015). Retinopathy of prematurity. *eMedicine*. Retrieved from http://emedicine.medscape.com/article/976220-overview

Subramanian, K. N., Gupta, A. O., Bahri, M., & Kicklighter, S. D. (2015). Transient tachypnea of the newborn. *eMedicine*. Retrieved from http://emedicine.medscape.com/article/976914-overview

Substance Abuse and Mental Health Services Administration [SAMHSA]. (2015). *Fetal alcohol spectrum disorders*. Retrieved from http://fasdcenter.samhsa.gov/fasdfaqs.aspx

Sutton, V. R. (2015). Inborn errors of metabolism: Classification. *UpToDate*. Retrieved from http://www.uptodate.com/contents/inborn-errors-of-metabolism-classification

Szpecht, D., Szymankiewicz, M., Seremak-Mrozikiewicz, A., & Gadzinowski, J. (2015). Review paper: The role of genetic factors in the pathogenesis of neonatal intraventricular hemorrhage. *Folia Neuropathology*, *53*(1), 1–7.

Tamai, J., & McCarthy, J. J. (2015). Developmental dysplasia of the hip. *eMedicine*. Retrieved from http://emedicine.medscape.com/article/1248135-overview

Tataranno, M., Oei, J., Perrone, S., Wright, I., Smyth, J., Lui, K., et al. (2015). Resuscitating preterm infants with 100% oxygen is associated with higher oxidative stress than room air. *Acta Paediatrica*, *104*, 759–765.

Tewfik, T. L., Alrajhi, Y. A., & Hagr, A. A. (2015). Choanal atresia. *eMedicine*. Retrieved from http://emedicine.medscape.com/article/872409-overview

Thigpen, J., & Melton, S. T. (2014). Neonatal abstinence syndrome: A challenge for medical providers, mothers, and society. *The Journal of Pediatric Pharmacology and Therapeutics*, *19*(3), 144–146.

Tierney, S., Blackhurst, M., Scahill, R., & Callery, P. (2015). Loss and rebuilding: A qualitative study of late diagnosis of cleft palate. *Journal for Specialists in Pediatric Nursing*, *20*(4):280–289.

United States Preventive Services Task Force [USPSTF]. (2014). *Folic acid supplementation for the prevention of neural tube defects*. Retrieved from http://www.uspreventiveservicestaskforce.org/Page/Document/ResearchPlanDraft/folic-acid-supplementation-for-the-prevention-of-neural-tube-defects

U.S. Department of Health and Human Services. (2010). *Healthy People 2020*. Retrieved from http://www.healthypeople.gov/hp2020

Verklan, M. T. (2014). Infant of a diabetic mother: A preexisting disease? *The Journal of Perinatal & Neonatal Nursing*, *28*(1), 87–88.

Verklan, M. T., & Walden, M. (2014). *Core curriculum for neonatal intensive care nursing* (5th ed.). St. Louis, MO: Saunders Elsevier.

Wagle, S., & Deshpande, P. G. (2015). Hemolytic disease of the newborn. *eMedicine*. Retrieved from http://emedicine.medscape.com/article/974349-overview

Wang, S., Liao, C., Liang, S., Zhong, D., Liu, J., & Li, Z. (2015). Ultrasound findings of mild neonatal periventricular-intraventricular hemorrhage after different treatments. *International Journal of Clinical and Experimental Medicine*, *8*(4), 5085–5093.

Weiner, D. L. (2015). Inborn errors of metabolism. *eMedicine*. Retrieved from http://emedicine.medscape.com/article/804757-overview

Whitsett, J. A., Wert, S. E., & Weaver, T. E. (2015). Diseases of pulmonary surfactant homeostasis. *Annual Review of Pathology*, *10*, 371–393.

Wiles, J. R., Isemann, B., Ward, L. P., Vinks, A. A., & Akinbi, H. (2014). Current management of neonatal abstinence syndrome secondary to intrauterine opioid exposure. *The Journal of Pediatrics*, *165*(3):440–446.

Wong, R. J., & Bhutani, V. K. (2015). Patient information: Jaundice in newborn infants (beyond the basics). *UpToDate*. Retrieved from http://www.uptodate.com/contents/jaundice-in-newborn-infants-beyond-the-basics

Wood, J. (2015). Pulse oximetry screening for critical congenital heart defects. *Neonatal Network*, *34*(3), 156–164.

World Health Organization [WHO]. (2015a). *Congenital anomalies*. Retrieved from http://www.who.int/mediacentre/factsheets/fs370/en/

World Health Organization [WHO]. (2015b). *Newborn death and illness*. Retrieved from http://www.who.int/pmnch/media/press_materials/fs/fs_newborndealth_illness/en

Yadav, S. P., Sunil, K., Sajid, K., Manisha, U., Yash, R., & Gaurav, A. (2015). Cleft lip and palate. *British Journal of Material Sciences and Technology*, *1*(1), 11–14.

Zhang, H., Gien, J., & Dysart, K. (2015). Effects of prematurity, prolonged intubation, and chronic lung disease on the neonatal airway. In J. Lioy & S. E. Sobol (Eds.), *Disorders of the neonatal airway* (pp. 243–261). New York, NY: Springer Publishers.

CHAPTER WORKSHEET

MULTIPLE CHOICE QUESTIONS

1. Which finding would lead the nurse to suspect that a newborn is experiencing respiratory distress syndrome?
   a. Abdominal distention
   b. Acrocyanosis
   c. Depressed fontanels
   d. Nasal flaring

2. When assessing the substance-exposed newborn, which finding would the nurse expect?
   a. Calm facial appearance
   b. Daily weight gain
   c. Increasing irritability
   d. Feeding and sleeping well

3. A newborn with tracheoesophageal fistula is likely to present with which assessment finding?
   a. Subnormal temperature
   b. Absent Moro reflex
   c. Inability to swallow
   d. Drooling from mouth

4. The nurse would be most alert for the development of transient tachypnea in a newborn who:
   a. Was born by cesarean birth
   b. Received no sedation
   c. Has a mother with heart disease
   d. Is small for gestational age

5. Which of the following would the nurse include in the teaching plan for an infant with cleft lip and palate?
   a. Feed the infant in a semi-lying position.
   b. Continue feeding the infant for as long as it takes.
   c. Burp the infant frequently during feedings.
   d. Avoid use of high-calorie formulas.

6. Which finding would the nurse expect to assess in an infant with developmental dysplasia of the hip?
   a. Symmetrical thigh folds
   b. Even knee height
   c. Full abduction of the hip
   d. Audible clunk on hip abduction

7. A 30-week preterm male newborn is found to have tachypnea during the first few hours of life and oxygen administered via face mask at 100% doesn't improve his oxygen saturation level. Which of the following substances, if administered to the mother prenatally, could have prevented respiratory distress syndrome?
   a. Insulin
   b. Lecithin
   c. Folic acid
   d. Dexamethasone

8. A newborn suffering from respiratory distress syndrome is given supplemental oxygen. Which of the following is a possible consequence of oxygen therapy?
   a. Cardiac anomalies
   b. Blindness
   c. Anosmia
   d. Atelectasis

CRITICAL THINKING EXERCISES

1. As the nursery nurse, you receive a newborn from the labor and birth suite and place him under the radiant warmer. The nurse who reports states that the mother couldn't remember when her membranes broke before labor and that she ran a fever during labor for the past few hours. The Apgar scores were good, but the newborn seemed lethargic. As you begin your assessment, you note that he is pale and floppy and has a subnormal temperature; heart rate is 180 bpm and respiratory rate is 70 breaths per minute.
   a. What in the mother's history should raise a red flag to the nurse?
   b. What condition is this newborn at high risk for?
   c. What interventions are appropriate for this condition?

2. Terry, a day-old baby girl, is very fretful, and calming measures do not seem to work. As the nursery nurse you notice that she is losing weight and her formula intake is poor, even though she is manifesting hungry behavior. The mother received no prenatal care and denied drug use, but her drug screen was positive for heroin.
   a. What additional information do you need to obtain from the mother?
   b. What additional laboratory work might be needed for the infant?
   c. What specific measures need to be made for the infant's ongoing care?

3. A term newborn, was brought to the nursery. His mother received no prenatal care, but the newborn's Apgar scores were fine. As you carry out your newborn assessment, you note an imperforate anus and you palpate no testicles in the scrotal sac.
   a. What additional assessments should you complete?
   b. Are anorectal agenesis and genitourinary tract anomalies common?
   c. What diagnostic tests might be ordered? What might be included in the treatment plan for this newborn?

STUDY ACTIVITIES

1. Arrange for a tour of a regional NICU to see the nurse's role in caring for sick neonates. Ask the nurse to give a quick history of each newborn's condition. Was the nurse's role like you imagined? What was your impression of the NICU, and how would you describe it to expectant parents?

2. Visit and select a website from the list of resources that pertains to either an acquired or congenital newborn condition. What kind of information is given? How helpful would it be for parents with an infant diagnosed with a specific condition?

3. A herniation of a newborn's abdominal contents present at birth describes _____.

BRINGING IT ALL TOGETHER: CASE STUDY

A 4-day-old male infant born at 37 weeks to a 16-year-old G1P1 is brought to the well-baby clinic at the local health department. The young mother had an uneventful pregnancy and was induced with Pitocin for this birth. In the hospital, he was breast-fed every 3 hours, had adequate output, and had passed meconium. The newborn was discharged home on day 2 of life at which time his weight was down 4% from his birth weight, a cephalohematoma was present on his head and he had mild facial jaundice. The mother's chief concern was that her infant looked like a "yellow canary" to her; he wasn't interested in breast-feeding and was increasingly fussy.

ASSESSMENT

Upon examination, the nurse takes a transcutaneous bilirubin level, which is 14 mg%. Vital signs were taken: T-37.8; P-162, R-54 and found to be in normal range. The newborn was markedly jaundiced, scleras of both eyes were icteric and newborn was irritable during the exam. The anterior fontanel was slightly sunken, the oral mucosa was tacky, and a resolving cephalohematoma was noted. At today's visit, there had been a 7% weight loss from birth and a history of "fair" urine output since discharge. Muscle tone and movement are normal.

Go to thePoint **to find questions to consider about this case.**

Appendix A
Standard Laboratory Values

PREGNANT AND NONPREGNANT WOMEN		
Values	Nonpregnant	Pregnant
Hematologic		
Complete blood count (CBC)		
Hemoglobin, g/dL	12–16*	11.5–14*
Hematocrit, PCV, %	37–47	32–42
Red cell volume, mL	1,600	1,900
Plasma volume, mL	2,400	3,700
Red blood cell count, million/mm³	4–5.5	3.75–5.0
White blood cells, total per mm³	4,500–10,000	5,000–15,000
Polymorphonuclear cells, %	54–62	60–85
Lymphocytes, %	38–46	15–40
Erythrocyte sedimentation rate, mm/h	≤	30–90
MCHC, g/dL packed RBCs (mean corpuscular hemoglobin concentration)	30–36	No change
MCH (mean corpuscular hemoglobin per picogram)	29–32	No change
MCV/μm³ (mean corpuscular volume per cubic micrometer)	82–96	No change
Blood coagulation and fibrinolytic activity†		
Factors VII, VIII, IX, X		Increase in pregnancy, return to normal in early puerperium; factor VIII increases during and immediately after delivery
Factors XI, XIII		Decrease in pregnancy
Prothrombin time (protime), sec	12–14	Slight decrease in pregnancy
Partial thromboplastin time (PTT), sect	60–70	Slight decrease in pregnancy and again during second and third stages of labor (indicates clotting at placental site)
Bleeding time, min	1–3 (Duke) 2–4 (Ivy)	No appreciable change
Coagulation time, min	6–10 (Lee/White)	No appreciable change

PREGNANT AND NONPREGNANT WOMEN (continued)

Values	Nonpregnant	Pregnant
Platelets	150,000–350,000/mm³	No significant change until 3–5 days after delivery, then marked increase (may predispose woman to thrombosis) and gradual return to normal
Fibrinolytic activity		Decreases in pregnancy, then abrupt return to normal (protection against thromboembolism)
Fibrinogen, mg/dL	250	400
Mineral and vitamin Concentrations		
Serum iron, mcg	75–150	65–120
Total iron-binding capacity, mcg	250–450	300–500
Iron saturation, %	30–40	15–30
Vitamin B₁₂, folic acid, ascorbic acid	Normal	Moderate decrease
Serum protein		
Total, g/dL	6.7–8.3	5.5–7.5
Albumin, g/dL	3.5–5.5	3.0–5.0
Globulin, total, g/dL	2.3–3.5	3.0–4.0
Blood sugar		
Fasting, mg/dL	70–80	65
2-hour postprandial, mg/dL	60–110	Under 140 after a 100-g carbohydrate meal is considered normal
Cardiovascular		
Blood pressure, mm Hg	120/80‡	114/65
Peripheral resistance, dyne/s · cm⁻⁵	120	100
Venous pressure, cm H₂O		
Femoral	9	24
Antecubital	8	8
Pulse, rate/min	70	80
Stroke volume, mL	65	75
Cardiac output, L/min	4.5	6
Circulation time (arm-tongue), sec	15–16	12–14
Blood volume, mL		
Whole blood	4,000	5,600
Plasma	2,400	3,700
Red blood cells	1,600	1,900
Plasma renin, units/L	3–10	10–80

(continued)

PREGNANT AND NONPREGNANT WOMEN (continued)

Values	Nonpregnant	Pregnant
Chest x-ray studies		
Transverse diameter of heart	–	1–2-cm increase
Left border of heart	–	Straightened
Cardiac volume	–	70-mL increase
Electrocardiogram	–	15-degree left axis deviation
V_1 and V_2	–	Inverted T-wave
kV_4	–	Low T
III	–	Q + inverted T
aVr	–	Small Q
Hepatic		
Bilirubin total	Not more than 1 mg/dL	Unchanged
Cephalin flocculation	Up to 2+ in 48 hr	Positive in 10%
Serum cholesterol, mg/dL	110–300	↑ 60% from 16–32 wks of pregnancy; remains at this level until after delivery
Thymol turbidity	0–4 units	Positive in 15%
Serum alkaline phosphatase	2–4.5 units (Bodansky)	↑ from week 12 of pregnancy to 6 wks after childbirth
Serum lactate dehydrogenase		Unchanged
Serum glutamic-oxaloacetic transaminase		Unchanged
Serum globulin albumin, g/dL	1.5–3.0	↑ slight
	4.5–5.3	↓ 3.0 g by late pregnancy
A/G ratio		Decreased
α_2-globulin		Increased
β-globulin		Increased
Serum cholinesterase		Decreased
Leucine aminopeptidase		Increased
Sulfobromophthalein (5 mg/kg)	5% dye or less in 45 min	Somewhat decreased
Renal		
Bladder capacity, mL	1,300	1,500
Renal plasma flow (RPF), mL/min	490–700	Increase by 25%, to 612–875
Glomerular filtration rate (GFR), mL/min	105–132	Increase by 50%, to 160–198
Nonprotein nitrogen (NPN), mg/dL	25–40	Decreases
Blood urea nitrogen (BUN), mg/dL	20–25	Decreases

PREGNANT AND NONPREGNANT WOMEN (continued)

Values	Nonpregnant	Pregnant
Serum creatinine, mg/kg/24 hr	20–22	Decreases
Serum uric acid, mg/kg/24 hr	257–750	Decreases
Urine glucose	Negative	Present in 20% of gravidas
Intravenous pyelogram (IVP)	Normal	Slight to moderate hydroureter and hydronephrosis; right kidney larger than left kidney
Miscellaneous		
Total thyroxine concentration	5–12 mcg/dL thyroxine	↑ 9–16 mcg/dL thyroxine (however, unbound thyroxine not greatly increased)
Ionized calcium		Relatively unchanged
Aldosterone		↑ 1 mg/24 hr by third trimester
Dehydroisoandrosterone	Plasma clearance 6–8 L/24 hr	↑ plasma clearance 10-fold to 20-fold

Adapted from Cunningham, F. G. (2016). Normal reference ranges for laboratory values in pregnancy. *UpToDate*. Retrieved from http://www.uptodate.com/contents/normal-reference-ranges-for-laboratory-values-in-pregnancy; and Van Leeuwen, A. M., & Bladh, M. L. (2015). *Davis's comprehensive handbook of laboratory & diagnostic tests with nursing implications.* (6th ed.), Philadelphia, PA: F. A. Davis.

*At sea level. Permanent residents of higher levels (e.g., Denver) require higher levels of hemoglobin.
†Pregnancy represents a hypercoagulable state.
‡For the woman about 20 years of age.
10 years of age: 103/70.
30 years of age: 123/82.
40 years of age: 126/84.

Appendix B
Clinical Paths

	Active Phase	Expulsion/Pushing	Recovery First Hour Postpartum
CLIENT	Client coping with labor support Client utilizing appropriate labor options Client verbalizes satisfaction with plan Management interventions	Client demonstrates effective pushing technique Client coping effectively with pushing Support person coping effectively with labor	Bonding appropriately with baby
CLIENT'S STATUS	Cervix dilated 5 cm—complete Contraction regularly with progressive cervical change Maternal/fetal well-being maintained Hydration maintained If indicated: FSE and/or IUPC placed Pitocin IV started Epidural placed/WE encouraged Medicate with PRN pain meds	Vaginal birth	Placenta delivered Fundus firm Lochia small–moderate Without clots Perineum intact/repaired Hemodynamically stable EBL <500 mL
CONTINUUM OF CARE	Prenatal record available after 32 wks Prenatal labs WNL Preregistered to hospital Pediatrician identified Support after hospitalization identified Discharge plan discussed with client/family Communicates understanding of hospital and community resources		
ASSESSMENT/ TREATMENT	Assess: Continuous EFM or auscultation Q 15 of 30 min as indicated Vital signs hourly/temp Q4 hr if intact membranes/Q 2 hr if membranes ruptured Uterine by monitor or palpation Bladder for distention Hydration status Cervical dilation, effacement, station	Assess: Q 15 min monitoring of fetal well-being (low risk) and Q 5 min (high risk) Vital signs hourly/temp. Q 2–4 hr depending on membrane status Bladder for distention Hydration status Pushing effectiveness Descent of presenting part Caput	Assess: Uterus–fundus Vital signs Lochia Bladder Perineum Placenta
CLIENT EDUCATION	Reinforce comfort measures Encourage use of labor options Inform client/support person of plan of care	Teaching of upright pushing positions Discourage prolonged maternal breath holding Encourage to assume position of choice Inform client of progress	Baby status Breast-feeding

LABOR AND DELIVERY CLINICAL PATH—LABOR: EXPECTED OUTCOMES (continued)

	Interventions		
TESTS/ PROCEDURES	Hgb or Hct (if not done recently) T & S (if ordered) VE as indicated IV therapy AROM by MD or CNM: assess for color, amount, and odor, as appropriate FSE/IUPC placement if indicated	AROM: assess for color, amount, and odor, as appropriate	Cord blood or RhoGAM workup if appropriate Cord blood if O+ mother
THERAPIES	Comfort measures/birthing ball/ ambulate/telemetry/shower IV therapy Amnio infusion for variable decelerations If appropriate, pain management reviewed	Perineal massage Warm soaks to perineal area Allow to rest until feels the urge to push Frequent position changes Cool cloth/ice chips	Ice pack to perineum Warm blankets
MEDS	Antibiotics as indicated for + GBS Pitocin if indicated PRN pain medication (encourage WE if requesting this)	Pitocin if indicated	Pitocin IV
ACTIVITY/ SAFETY	Labor option usage Position changes	Provide wedge if supine Promote effective position for pushing: i.e., squatting, side lying, upright Breathing technique client/ support person most comfortable with	Assist with ambulate to bathroom Infant care Assist with positioning for breast-feeding Infant ID bands present
NUTRI- TION	Clear liquids Ice chips Others	Clear liquids Ice chips	Return to previous diet
UNIQUE CLIENT NEEDS			

INTEGRATED PLAN OF CARE FOR CESAREAN DELIVERY

Expected Client Outcomes

	Phase 1 Preadmission (Cesarean Delivery)	Phase 2 Surgery/ Immediate Postop/ Day of Surgery	Phase 3 Postop Day 1	
Usual time in phase assessment/ potential complications	**N/A Date Started:** VS WNL for client Hgb or Hct/values within normal SLH antepartum range	Up to 23 hr VS WNL for client Systems assessment: Skin warm, dry Clear ⇒ Alert & oriented ⇒ Neg. Homans sign ⇒ Breast soft/nipples intact ⇒ Lungs clear ⇒ Bowel sounds present ⇒ Fundus firm u/u or u 1–2 (–/+) Lochia sm—mod Dsg dry and intact No signs infiltration IV site Verbalizes comfort using pain rating scale 0–10	1 day VS WNL for client Afebrile Voiding without Foley ⇒ Passing flatus Incision without redness or drainage Lochia small amount Fundus firm u/1–2 Verbalizes comfort using pain scale 0–10 on oral pain meds	1–2 days Incision well approximated, without drainage or redness Passing flatus Lochia sm/mod amt Fundus firm u/1–2 Verbalizes comfort using pain medication as described
Client/family knowledge	**Date All Above Met** Verbalizes understanding of condition and need for surgery Verbalizes understanding of all preop teaching	**Date All Above Met** Verbalizes correct use of PCA/fentanyl pump and when to request pain medication Turn, cough, and deep breathe appropriately	**Date All Above Met** Can state criteria for when to call doctor for problems postdischarge ⇒ ↑ Bleeding ↑ Temperature ⇒ Incision redness, odor or drainage ⇒	**Date All Above Met** Verbalizes follow-up appointment date and time Verbalizes proper dosing of pain medication
ADLs/activity	**Date All Above Met** Verbalizes understanding of NPO status	**Date All Above Met** Able to ambulate with minimal assistance Tolerating clear/full liquid diet Bonding observed with newborn—taking-in phase ⇒	**Date All Above Met** Ambulating without assistance Tolerating soft to regular diet	**Date All Above Met** Ambulating in hall
	Date All Above Met	**Date All Above Met**	**Date All Above Met**	**Date All Above Met**
Unique client needs	**Date All Above Met Entire Phase Outcomes met; progress client to next phase**	**Date All Above Met Entire Phase Outcomes met; progress client to next phase**	**Date All Above Met Entire Phase Outcomes met; progress client to next phase**	**Date All Above Met Entire Phase Outcomes met; progress client to next phase**

INTEGRATED PLAN OF CARE FOR CESAREAN DELIVERY (continued)

		Plan of Care		
	#1 Preadmission	**#2 Surgery/ Immediate Postop/ Day of Surgery**	**#3 Postop Day 1**	**#4 Postop Day 2/ Discharge**
Assessments	Vital signs Fetal status immediately prior to surgery	VS per PACU then Q 4 hr Systems assessment: – Skin, LOC, FROM, Homans sign – Breasts, lungs, fundus, incision – Lochia, bladder, bowel sounds, IV, and site – I & O Q shift – Assess pain control 0–10 scale – Assess RhoGAM status – Assess Rubella titer status – ID band on mother	VS Q 6 hr Assess pain control 0–10 scale Incision Foley-volding Fundus/lochia Homans sign IV site Breasts ID band on mother Activity	Assess pain control 0–10 scale Incision Volding Fundus lochia Homans sign IV site as needed ID band on mother Activity
Consults	Anesthesia	Social work as needed, anesthesia, lactation, dietitian as needed	Social work, lactation, dietitian as needed	Social work, lactation, dietitian as needed
Client/family education discharge planning	Need for surgery Review cesarean delivery Review procedure, postop expectations Demonstrate/discuss equipment—PCA, fentanyl pump Tour of OR area and nursery	Review postop expectations Review equipment use PRN Instruct client on: Hospital/infant security systems Unity orientation Newborn orientation/ care/feeding (if breast-feeding problems, see decision trees)	Review dietary needs postsurgery Review bleeding/ lochia Precautions post– cesarean delivery Review follow-up care and doctor Appointments Review incision care, pericare Infant care Infant feeding	Verify follow-up appointment date and time Activity restrictions Follow-up for staple removal as needed Offer home follow-up care Discuss birth control
Tests and procedures	PAT; Hgb and Hct (if not done recently— within 1 mo) T & S (if ordered)			
Pharmacologic needs		IV fluids as ordered Pain control: PCA, fentanyl pump, IM to PO	IV lock PO pain meds Give RhoGAM if indicated Give rubella if indicated	DC IV lock as ordered

(continued)

INTEGRATED PLAN OF CARE FOR CESAREAN DELIVERY (continued)

Plan of Care

	#1 Preadmission	#2 Surgery/ Immediate Postop/ Day of Surgery	#3 Postop Day 1	#4 Postop Day 2/ Discharge
Activity/ rehabilitation	Client's usual	Change position Q 2 hr while in bed, OOB stand at bedside postop night/dangle and transfer to chair. Progress to client endurance. Observe bonding with infant. Observe family support system (if inadequate consult SW)	Progress endurance/ begin Ambulation in hall OOB in AM May shower	Ambulate in halls without assistance
Nutrition/ elimination		NPO then clear liquids to DAT Foley empty Q shift	DAT to regular or previous diet at home Foley discontinued	
Miscellaneous interventions		TCDB Q 2 hr while awake	Dressing removed by MD or RN with MD request	
Unique client needs				

Appendix C
Cervical Dilation Chart

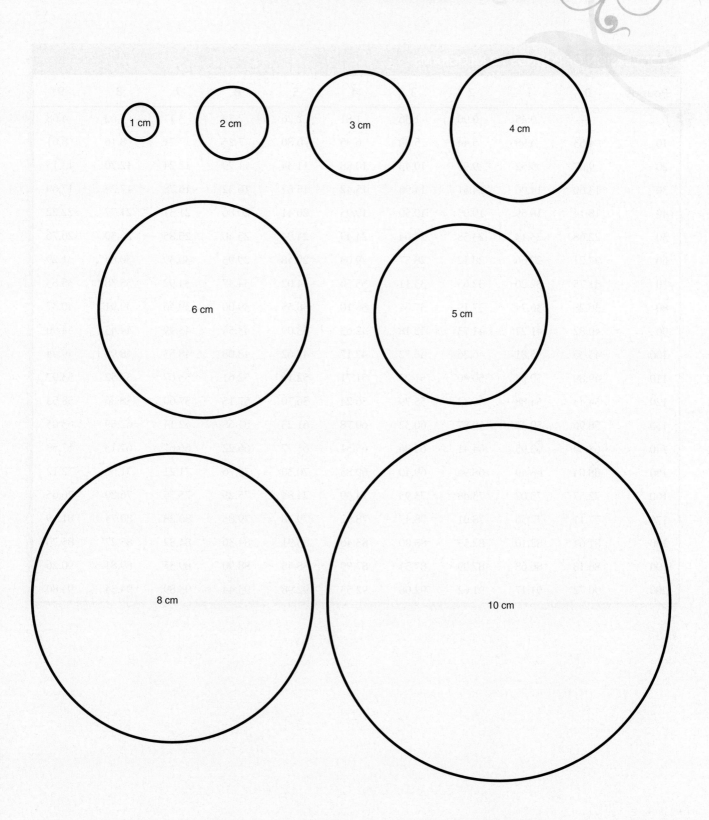

Appendix D
Weight Conversion Charts

Pounds	0	1	2	3	4	5	6	7	8	9
CONVERSION OF POUNDS TO KILOGRAMS										
0	—	0.45	0.90	1.36	1.81	2.26	2.72	3.17	3.62	4.08
10	4.53	4.98	5.44	5.89	6.35	6.80	7.25	7.71	8.16	8.61
20	9.07	9.52	9.97	10.43	10.88	11.34	11.79	12.24	12.70	13.15
30	13.60	14.06	14.51	14.96	15.42	15.87	16.32	16.78	17.23	17.69
40	18.14	18.59	19.05	19.50	19.95	20.41	20.86	21.31	21.77	22.22
50	22.68	23.13	23.58	24.04	24.49	24.94	25.40	25.85	26.30	26.76
60	27.21	27.66	28.12	28.57	29.03	29.48	29.93	30.39	30.84	31.29
70	31.75	32.20	32.65	33.11	33.56	34.02	34.47	34.92	35.38	35.83
80	36.28	36.74	37.19	37.64	38.10	38.55	39.00	39.46	39.91	40.37
90	40.82	41.27	41.73	42.18	42.63	43.09	43.54	43.99	44.45	44.90
100	45.36	45.81	46.26	46.72	47.17	47.62	48.08	48.53	48.98	49.44
110	49.89	50.34	50.80	51.25	51.71	52.16	52.61	53.07	53.52	53.97
120	54.43	54.88	55.33	55.79	56.24	56.70	57.15	57.60	58.06	58.51
130	58.96	59.42	59.87	60.32	60.78	61.23	61.68	62.14	62.59	63.05
140	63.50	63.95	64.41	64.86	65.31	65.77	66.22	66.67	67.13	67.58
150	68.04	68.49	68.94	69.40	69.85	70.30	70.76	71.21	71.66	72.12
160	72.57	73.02	73.48	73.93	74.39	74.84	75.29	75.75	76.20	76.65
170	77.11	77.56	78.01	78.47	78.92	79.38	79.83	80.28	80.74	81.19
180	81.64	82.10	82.55	83.00	83.46	83.91	84.36	84.82	85.27	85.73
190	86.18	86.68	87.09	87.54	87.99	88.45	88.90	89.35	89.81	90.26
200	90.72	91.17	91.62	92.08	92.53	92.98	93.44	93.89	94.34	94.80

CONVERSION OF POUNDS AND OUNCES TO GRAMS FOR NEWBORN WEIGHTS

Pounds	Ounces															
	0	1	2	3	4	5	6	7	8	9	10	11	12	13	14	15
0	—	28	57	85	113	142	170	198	227	255	283	312	340	369	397	425
1	454	482	510	539	567	595	624	652	680	709	737	765	794	822	850	879
2	907	936	964	992	1021	1049	1077	1106	1134	1162	1191	1219	1247	1276	1304	1332
3	1361	1389	1417	1446	1474	1503	1531	1559	1588	1616	1644	1673	1701	1729	1758	1786
4	1814	1843	1871	1899	1928	1956	1984	2013	2041	2070	2098	2126	2155	2183	2211	2240
5	2268	2296	2325	2353	2381	2410	2438	2466	2495	2523	2551	2580	2608	2637	2665	2693
6	2722	2750	2778	2807	2835	2863	2892	2920	2948	2977	3005	3033	3062	3090	3118	3147
7	3175	3203	3232	3260	3289	3317	3345	3374	3402	3430	3459	3487	3515	3544	3572	3600
8	3629	3657	3685	3714	3742	3770	3799	3827	3856	3884	3912	3941	3969	3997	4026	4054
9	4082	4111	4139	4167	4196	4224	4252	4281	4309	4337	4366	4394	4423	4451	4479	4508
10	4536	4564	4593	4621	4649	4678	4706	4734	4763	4791	4819	4848	4876	4904	4933	4961
11	4990	5018	5046	5075	5103	5131	5160	5188	5216	5245	5273	5301	5330	5358	5386	5415
12	5443	5471	5500	5528	5557	5585	5613	5642	5670	5698	5727	5755	5783	5812	5840	5868
13	5897	5925	5953	5982	6010	6038	6067	6095	6123	6152	6180	6209	6237	6265	6294	6322
14	6350	6379	6407	6435	6464	6492	6520	6549	6577	6605	6634	6662	6690	6719	6747	6776
15	6804	6832	6860	6889	6917	6945	6973	7002	7030	7059	7087	7115	7144	7172	7201	7228

Appendix E
Breast-Feeding and Medication Use

GENERAL CONSIDERATIONS
- Most medications are safe to use while breast-feeding; however, the woman should always check with the pediatrician, physician, or lactation specialist before taking any medications, including over-the-counter and herbal products.
- Inform the woman that she has the right to seek a second opinion if the physician does not perform a thoughtful risk-versus-benefit assessment before prescribing medications or advising against breast-feeding.
- Most medications pass from the woman's bloodstream into the breast milk. However, the amount is usually very small and unlikely to harm the baby.
- A preterm or other special needs neonate is more susceptible to the adverse effects of medications in breast milk. A woman who is taking medications and whose baby is in the neonatal intensive care unit or special care nursery should consult with the pediatrician or neonatologist before feeding her breast milk to the baby.
- If the woman is taking a prescribed medication, she should take the medication just after breast-feeding. This practice helps ensure that the lowest possible dose of medication reaches the baby through the breast milk.
- Some medications can cause changes in the amount of milk the woman produces. Teach the woman to report any changes in milk production.

Lactation Category	Risk	Rationale
L3	Probably compatible	There is possible risk to the infant; however, the risks are minimal or nonthreatening in nature. These medications should be given only when the potential benefit outweighs the risk to the infant.
L4	Possibly hazardous	There is positive evidence of risk to the infant; however, in life-threatening situations or for serious diseases, the benefit might outweigh the risk.
L5	No data: Hazardous	The risk of using the medication clearly outweighs any possible benefit from breast-feeding.

LACTATION RISK CATEGORIES (LRC)

Lactation Category	Risk	Rationale
L1	Compatible	Clinical research or long-term observation of use in many breast-feeding women has not demonstrated risk to the infant.
L2	Probably compatible	Limited clinical research has not demonstrated an increase in adverse effects in the infant.

POTENTIAL EFFECTS OF SELECTED MEDICATION CATEGORIES ON THE BREAST-FED INFANT

Narcotic Analgesics
- Codeine and hydrocodone appear to be safe in moderate doses. Rarely the neonate may experience sedation and/or apnea. (LRC: L3)
- Meperidine (Demerol) can lead to sedation of the neonate. (LRC: L3)
- Low to moderate doses of morphine appear to be safe. (LRC: L2)
- Trace-to-negligible amounts of fentanyl are found in human milk. (LRC: L2)

Nonnarcotic Analgesics and NSAIDs
- Acetaminophen and ibuprofen are approved for use. (LRC: L1)

- Naproxen may cause neonatal hemorrhage and anemia if used for prolonged periods. (LRC: L3 for short-term use and L4 for long-term use)
- The newer COX2 inhibitors, such as celecoxib (Celebrex), appear to be safe for use. (LRC: L2)

Antibiotics
- Levels in breast milk are usually very low.
- The penicillins and cephalosporins are generally considered safe to use. (LRC: L1 and L2)
- Tetracyclines can be safely used for short periods but are not suitable for long-term therapy (e.g., for treatment of acne). (LRC: L2)
- Sulfonamides should not be used during the neonatal stage (the first month of life). (LRC: L3)

Antihypertensives
- A high degree of caution is advised when antihypertensives are used during breast-feeding.
- Some beta blockers can be used.
- Hydralazine and methyldopa are considered to be safe. (LRC: L2)
- Angiotensin-converting enzyme (ACE) inhibitors are not recommended in the early postpartum period.

Sedatives and Hypnotics
- Neonatal withdrawal can occur when antianxiety medications, such as lorazepam, are taken. Fortunately withdrawal is generally mild.
- Phenothiazines, such as Phenergan and Thorazine, may lead to sleep apnea and increase the risk for sudden infant death syndrome.

Antidepressants
- The risk to the baby is often higher if the woman is depressed and remains untreated, rather than taking the medication.
- The older tricyclics are considered to be safe; however they cause many bothersome side effects, such as weight gain and dry mouth, which may lead to noncompliance on the part of the woman.

- The selective serotonin uptake inhibitors (SSRIs) are also considered to be safe and have a lower side effect profile, which makes them more palatable to the woman. (LRC: L2 and L3)

Mood Stabilizers (Antimanic Medication)
- Lithium is found in breast milk and is best not used in the breast-feeding woman. (LRC: L4)
- Valproic acid (Depakote) seems to be a more appropriate choice for the woman with bipolar disorder. The infant will need periodic lab studies to check platelets and liver function.

Corticosteroids
- Corticosteroids do not pass into the milk in large quantities.
- Inhaled steroids are safe to use because they do not accumulate in the bloodstream.

Thyroid Medication
- Thyroid medications, such as levothyroxine (Synthroid), can be taken while breast-feeding.
- Most are in LRC category L1.

MEDICATIONS THAT USUALLY ARE CONTRAINDICATED FOR THE BREAST-FEEDING WOMAN
- Amiodarone
- Antineoplastic agents
- Chloramphenicol
- Doxepin
- Ergotamine and other ergot derivatives
- Iodides
- Methotrexate and immunosuppressants
- Lithium
- Radiopharmaceuticals
- Ribavirin
- Tetracycline (prolonged use—more than 3 weeks)
- Pseudoephedrine (found in many over-the-counter medications)

Material in this appendix was adapted from information found in the following sources:
Wamback, K., & Riordan, J. (2015). *Breastfeeding and human lactation* (5th ed.), Burlington, MA: Jones & Bartlett Learning.
Lauwers, J., & Swisher, A. (2016). *Counseling the nursing mother: A lactation consultant's guide* (6th ed.), Burlington, MA: Jones & Bartlett Learning.
Brucker, M. C., & King, T. L. (2017). *Pharmacology for women's health* (2nd ed.), Burlington, MA: Jones & Bartlett Learning.

Index

Note: Page number followed by f, t, b, and d indicates figures, tables, box and display respectively.